Contents

ABOUT THE AUTHOR

H. Winter Griffith, M.D., authored 25 medical books, including the *Complete Guide to Symptoms, Illness & Surgery* and *Complete Guide to Sports Injuries*, each published by The Body Press/Perigee Books. Others include *Instructions for Patients; Drug Information for Patients; Instructions for Dental Patients; Information and Instructions for Pediatric Patients; Vitamins, Minerals and Supplements;* and *Complete Guide to Medical Tests*. Dr. Griffith received his medical degree from Emory University in Atlanta, Georgia. After 20 years in private practice, he established and was the first director of a basic medical science program at Florida State University. He then became an associate professor of Family and Community Medicine at the University of Arizona College of Medicine. Until his death in 1993, Dr. Griffith lived in Tucson, Arizona.

Editor

Stephen Moore, M.D.
  Family physician, Tucson, Arizona

Technical Consultants

Kevin Boesen, Pharm.D.
  Clinical Assistant Professor, College of Pharmacy, University of Arizona

Cindy Boesen, Pharm.D.
  Clinical Instructor, College of Pharmacy, University of Arizona

Drugs and You

A drug cannot "cure." It aids the body's natural defenses to promote recovery. Likewise, a manufacturer or doctor cannot guarantee a drug will be useful for everyone. The complexity of the human body, individual responses in different people and in the same person under different circumstances, past and present health, age and gender influence how well a drug works.

All effective drugs produce desirable changes in the body, but a drug can also cause undesirable adverse reactions or side effects in some people. Despite uncertainties, the drug discoveries of recent years have given us tools to save lives and reduce discomfort. Before you decide whether to take a drug, you or your doctor must ask, "Will the benefits outweigh the risks?"

The purpose of this book is to give you enough information about the most widely used drugs so you can make a wise decision. The information will alert you to potential or preventable problems. You can learn what to do if problems arise.

The information is derived from many authoritative sources and represents the consensus of many experts. Every effort has been made to ensure accuracy and completeness.

Each year, new drug charts are added and existing charts are updated when appropriate. However, because drug information is constantly changing, you should always talk to your doctor or pharmacist if you have any questions or concerns.

Information in this book applies to generic drugs in both the United States and Canada. Generic names do not vary in these countries, but brand names do.

In the United States, it is the responsibility of the Food and Drug Administration (FDA) to ensure that drugs are safe and effective. For more information, you may contact the FDA at 1-888-INFO-FDA or visit the website: www.fda.gov.

Be Safe! Tell Your Doctor

Some suggestions for wise drug use apply to all drugs. Always give your doctor, dentist, or health-care provider complete information about the drugs and supplements you take, including your medical history, your medical plans and your progress while under medication.

Medical History

Tell the important facts of your medical history including illness and previous experience with drugs. Include allergic or adverse reactions you have had to any medicine or other substance in the past. Describe the allergic symptoms you have, such as hay fever, asthma, eye watering and itching, throat irritation and reactions to food. People who have allergies to common substances are more likely to develop drug allergies.

List all drugs you take. Don't forget vitamin and mineral supplements; skin, rectal or vaginal medicines; eyedrops and eardrops; antacids; antihistamines; cold and cough remedies; inhalants and nasal sprays; aspirin, aspirin combinations or other pain relievers; motion sickness remedies; weight-loss aids; salt and sugar substitutes; caffeine; oral contraceptives; sleeping pills; laxatives; "tonics" or herbal preparations.

Future Medical Plans

Discuss plans for elective surgery (including dental surgery), pregnancy and breast-feeding. These conditions may require discontinuing or modifying the dosages of medicines you may be taking.

Questions

Don't hesitate to ask questions about a drug. Your doctor, nurse or pharmacist will be able to provide more information if they are familiar with you and your medical history.

Your Role

Learn the generic names and brand names of all your medicines. For example, acetaminophen is the generic name for the brand Tylenol. Write them down to help you remember. If a drug is a combination, learn the names of its generic ingredients.

Filling a Prescription

Once a prescription is written you may purchase the medication from various sources. Pharmacies are usually located in a drug or grocery store. You may need to consider your options: Does your health insurance limit where prescriptions can be filled? Is the location convenient? Does the pharmacy maintain patient records and are the employees helpful and willing to answer drug related questions?

Insurance companies or an HMO (Health Maintenance Organization) may specify certain pharmacies. Some insurance companies have chosen a mail-order pharmacy. Normally a prescription is sent to the mail-order pharmacy or phoned in by the physician. Mail order is best used for maintenance (long-term medications). Short-term medications such as antibiotics should be purchased at a local pharmacy.

Once a pharmacy has been chosen it is best to stay with that one so an accurate drug history can be maintained. The pharmacist can more easily check for drug interactions that may be potentially harmful to the patient or decrease the efficacy of one or more of the medications.

You can phone the pharmacy for a refill. Provide the prescription number, name of medication, and name of the patient.

Alcohol & Medications

Alcohol and drugs of abuse defeat the purpose of many medications. For example, alcohol causes depression; if you drink and are depressed, antidepressants will not relieve the depression. If you have a problem with drinking or drugs, discuss it with your doctor. There are many ways to help you conquer such a problem.

Taking A Drug

Never take medicine in the dark! Recheck the label before each use. You could be taking the wrong drug! Tell your doctor about any unexpected new symptoms you have while taking medicine. You may need to change medicines or have a dose adjustment.

Storage

Keep all medicines out of children's reach and in childproof containers. Store drugs in a cool, dry place, such as a kitchen cabinet or bedroom. Avoid medicine cabinets in bathrooms. They get too moist and warm at times.

Keep medicine in its original container, tightly closed. Don't remove the label! If directions call for refrigeration, keep the medicine cool, but don't freeze it.

Discarding

Don't save leftover medicine to use later. Discard it on or before the expiration date shown on the container. Dispose safely to protect children and pets. See page xiv.

Alertness

Many of the medicines used to treat disorders may alter your alertness. If you drive, work around machinery, or must avoid sedation, discuss the problem with your doctor; usually there are ways (e.g., the time of day you take the medicine) to manage the problem.

Learn About Drugs

Study the information in this book's charts regarding your medications. Read each chart completely. Because of space limitations, most information that fits more than one category appears only once. Any time you are prescribed a new medication, read the information on the chart for that drug, then take the time to review the charts on other medications you already take. Read any instruction sheets or printed warnings provided by your doctor or pharmacist.

Drug Advertising

Ads can cause confusion. Be sure and get sufficient information about any drug you think may help you. Ask your doctor or pharmacist.

Guide to Drug Charts

The drug information in this book is organized in condensed, easy-to-read charts. Each drug is described in a two-page format, as shown in the sample chart below and opposite. Charts are arranged alphabetically by drug generic names, such as ACETAMINOPHEN or by drug class name, such as *ANTIHISTAMINES*.

A generic name is the official chemical name for a drug. A brand name is a drug manufacturer's registered trademark for a generic drug. Brand names listed on the charts include those from the United States

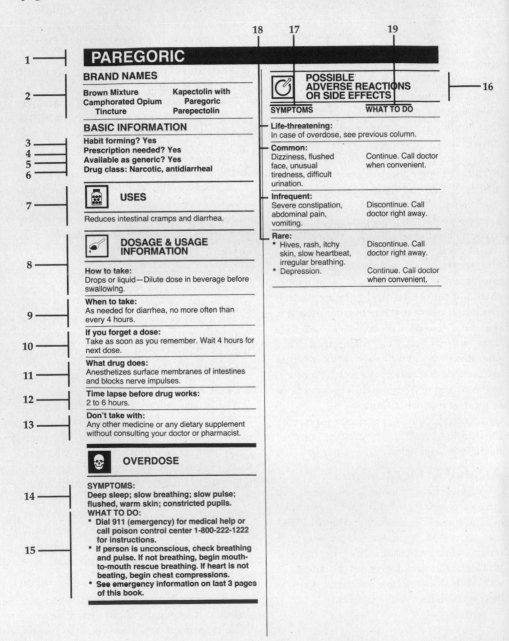

PAREGORIC

BRAND NAMES

Brown Mixture
Camphorated Opium
   Tincture
Kapectolin with
   Paregoric
Parepectolin

BASIC INFORMATION

Habit forming? Yes
Prescription needed? Yes
Available as generic? Yes
Drug class: Narcotic, antidiarrheal

USES

Reduces intestinal cramps and diarrhea.

DOSAGE & USAGE INFORMATION

How to take:
Drops or liquid—Dilute dose in beverage before swallowing.

When to take:
As needed for diarrhea, no more often than every 4 hours.

If you forget a dose:
Take as soon as you remember. Wait 4 hours for next dose.

What drug does:
Anesthetizes surface membranes of intestines and blocks nerve impulses.

Time lapse before drug works:
2 to 6 hours.

Don't take with:
Any other medicine or any dietary supplement without consulting your doctor or pharmacist.

OVERDOSE

SYMPTOMS:
Deep sleep; slow breathing; slow pulse; flushed, warm skin; constricted pupils.
WHAT TO DO:
• Dial 911 (emergency) for medical help or call poison control center 1-800-222-1222 for instructions.
• If person is unconscious, check breathing and pulse. If not breathing, begin mouth-to-mouth rescue breathing. If heart is not beating, begin chest compressions.
• See emergency information on last 3 pages of this book.

POSSIBLE ADVERSE REACTIONS OR SIDE EFFECTS

SYMPTOMS	WHAT TO DO
Life-threatening: In case of overdose, see previous column.	
Common: Dizziness, flushed face, unusual tiredness, difficult urination.	Continue. Call doctor when convenient.
Infrequent: Severe constipation, abdominal pain, vomiting.	Discontinue. Call doctor right away.
Rare: • Hives, rash, itchy skin, slow heartbeat, irregular breathing.	Discontinue. Call doctor right away.
• Depression.	Continue. Call doctor when convenient.

and Canada. A generic drug may have one or many brand names.

To find information about a generic drug, look it up in the index. To learn about a brand name, check the index, where each brand name is followed by the name(s) of its generic ingredients and their chart page number(s).

The chart design is the same for every drug. When you are familiar with the chart, you can quickly find information you want to know about a drug.

On the next few pages, each of the numbered chart sections below is explained. This information will guide you in reading and understanding the charts that begin on page 2.

PAREGORIC

20 — **WARNINGS & PRECAUTIONS**

21 — **Don't take if:**
You are allergic to any narcotic.*

22 — **Before you start, consult your doctor if:**
You have impaired liver or kidney function.

23 — **Over age 60:**
More likely to be drowsy, dizzy, unsteady or constipated.

24 — **Pregnancy:**
Risk factor varies with length of pregnancy. See category list on page xviii and consult doctor.

25 — **Breast-feeding:**
Drug filters into milk. May depress infant. Avoid.

26 — **Infants & children:**
Use only under medical supervision.

27 — **Prolonged use:**
Causes psychological and physical dependence.

28 — **Skin & sunlight:**
No problems expected.

29 — **Driving, piloting or hazardous work:**
Don't drive or pilot aircraft until you learn how medicine affects you. Don't work around dangerous machinery. Don't climb ladders or work in high places. Danger increases if you drink alcohol or take medicine affecting alertness and reflexes, such as antihistamines, tranquilizers, sedatives, pain medicine, narcotics and mind-altering drugs.

30 — **Discontinuing:**
May be unnecessary to finish medicine. Follow doctor's instructions.

31 — **Others:**
Great potential for abuse.

POSSIBLE INTERACTION WITH OTHER DRUGS

GENERIC NAME OR DRUG CLASS	COMBINED EFFECT
Analgesics*	Increased analgesic effect.
Anticholinergics*	Increased risk of constipation.
Antidepressants*	Increased sedation.
Antidiarrheal preparations*	Increased sedative effect. Avoid.
Antihistamines*	Increased sedation.
Central nervous system (CNS) depressants*	Increased central nerve system depression.
Naloxone	Decreased paregoric effect.
Naltrexone	Decreased paregoric effect.
Narcotics,* other	Increased narcotic effect.

— 32

POSSIBLE INTERACTION WITH OTHER SUBSTANCES

INTERACTS WITH	COMBINED EFFECT
Alcohol:	Increases alcohol's intoxicating effect. Avoid.
Beverages:	None expected.
Cocaine:	None expected.
Foods:	None expected.
Marijuana:	Impairs physical and mental performance.
Tobacco:	None expected.

— 33

1—Generic or Class Name

Each drug chart is titled by generic name or by the name of the drug class, such as DIGITALIS PREPARATIONS.

All drugs have a generic name. These generic names are the same worldwide. Sometimes a drug is known by more than one generic name. The chart is titled by the most common one. Less common generic names appear in parentheses. For example, vitamin C is also known as ascorbic acid. Its chart title is VITAMIN C (Ascorbic Acid). The index will include both names.

Your drug container may show a generic name, a brand name or both. If you have only a brand name, use the index to find the drug's generic name(s) and chart page number(s).

If your drug container shows no name, ask your doctor or pharmacist for the name and write it on the container.

2—Brand Names

A brand name is usually shorter and easier to remember than the generic name. The brand name is selected by the drug manufacturer

The brand names listed for each generic drug in this book do not include all brands available in the United States and Canada. The most common ones are listed. New brands appear on the market, and brands are sometimes removed from the market. No list can reflect every change. In the instances in which the drug chart is titled with a drug class name instead of a generic name, the generic and brand names all appear under the heading GENERIC AND BRAND NAMES. The GENERIC NAMES are in capital letters and the BRAND NAMES are in lower-case letters.

Inclusion of a brand name does not imply recommendation or endorsement. Exclusion does not imply that a missing brand name is less effective or less safe than the ones listed. Some drug charts have too many generic and brand names to list on the page. A complete list is on the page indicated on the chart.

Lists of brand names don't differentiate between prescription and nonprescription drugs. The active ingredients are the same.

If you buy a nonprescription drug, look for generic names of the active ingredients on the container. Common nonprescription drugs are described in this book under their generic components. Many are also listed in the index by brand name.

Most drugs contain inert, or inactive, ingredients that are fillers, dyes or solvents for active ingredients. Manufacturers choose inert ingredients that preserve the drug without interfering with the action of the active ingredients.

Inert substances are listed on labels of nonprescription drugs. They do not appear on prescription drugs. Your pharmacist can tell you all active and inert ingredients in a prescription drug.

Occasionally, a tablet, capsule or liquid may contain small amounts of sodium, sugar or potassium. If you are on a diet that severely restricts any of these, ask your pharmacist or doctor to suggest another form.

Some liquid medications contain alcohol. Avoid them if you are susceptible to the adverse effects of alcohol consumption.

BASIC INFORMATION

3—Habit Forming?

Yes—means the drug is capable of leading to physical and/or psychological dependence.

Physical dependence includes tolerance (requiring larger dosages or repeated use) and withdrawal symptoms (mental and physical) when it is stopped.

Psychological dependence involves repeated use of a drug to bring about effects that are pleasurable or satisfying, or it reduces undesirable feelings.

4—Prescription Needed?

Yes—means a doctor must prescribe the drug for you. "No" means you can buy the drug without prescription. Sometimes low strengths of a drug are available without prescription, while higher strengths require prescription.

The information about the drug applies whether it requires prescription or not. If the generic ingredients are the same, nonprescription drugs have the same dangers, warnings, precautions and interactions as prescription drugs. A nonprescription (over-the-counter) drug has dosing and other instructions printed on the container label. Always read them carefully before you take the drug. The information and warnings on containers for nonprescription drugs may not be as complete as the information in this book. Check both sources.

5—Available as Generic?

Some drugs have patent restrictions that protect the manufacturer or distributor of that drug. These drugs may be purchased only by a specific brand name.

Drugs purchased by generic name are usually less expensive than brand names. Once the patent expires, other drug companies can sell that particular drug. They will choose their own brand name.

Some states allow pharmacists to fill prescriptions by brand names or generic names (if one is available). This allows patients to buy the least expensive form of a drug.

A doctor may specify a brand name because he or she trusts a known source more than an unknown manufacturer of generic drugs. You and your doctor should decide together whether you should buy a medicine by generic name or brand name.

Generic drugs manufactured in other countries are not subject to regulation by the U.S. Food and Drug Administration. All drugs manufactured in the United States are subject to regulation.

6—Drug Class

Drugs that possess similar chemical structures or similar therapeutic effects are grouped into classes. Most drugs within a class produce similar benefits, side effects, adverse reactions and interactions with other drugs and substances. For example, all the generic drugs in the narcotic drug class will have similar effects on the body.

Some information on the charts applies to all drugs in a class. The index lists the classes (such as narcotics) and lists drugs in that class.

Names for classes of drugs are not standardized; classes listed in other references may vary from the classes in this book.

7— 🗓 Uses

This section lists the disease or disorder for which a drug is prescribed.

Most uses listed are approved by the U.S. Food and Drug Administration. Some uses are listed if experiments and clinical trials indicate effectiveness and safety. Still, other uses are included that may not be officially sanctioned, but for which doctors commonly prescribe the drug.

The use for which your doctor prescribes the drug may not appear. You and your doctor should discuss the reason for any prescription medicine you take. You alone will probably decide whether to take a nonprescription drug. This section may help you make a wise decision.

🥄 DOSAGE & USAGE INFORMATION

8—How To Take

Drugs are available in forms of tablets, capsules, chewables, liquids, suppositories, injections, transdermal patches (used on the skin), aerosol inhalants and topical forms such as drops, sprays, creams, gels, ointments and lotions. This section gives brief instructions for taking or using each form.

The information here supplements the drug label information. If your doctor's instructions differ from these suggestions, follow your doctor's instructions.

Instructions are left out for how much to take. Dose amounts can't be generalized. Dosages of prescription drugs must be individualized for you by your doctor. Be sure the dosage instructions are on the label. Advice to "take as directed" is not helpful if you forget the doctor's instructions or didn't understand them. Nonprescription drugs have instructions on the labels regarding how much to take.

9—When To Take

Dose schedules vary for medicines and for patients.

Drugs prescribed on a schedule should usually be taken at approximately the same times each day. Some must be taken at regular intervals to maintain a steady level of the drug in the body. If the schedule interferes with your sleep, consult your doctor.

Instructions to take on an empty stomach mean the drug is absorbed best in your body this way. Other drugs must be taken with liquid or food because they irritate the stomach.

Instructions for other dose schedules are usually on the label. Variations in standard dose schedules may apply because some medicines interact with others if you take them at the same time.

10—If You Forget a Dose

Suggestions in this section vary from drug to drug. Most tell you when to resume taking the medicine if you forget a scheduled dose.

Establish good habits so you won't forget doses. Forgotten doses decrease a drug's therapeutic effect.

11—What Drug Does

This is a simple description of the drug's action in the body. The wording is generalized and may not be a complete explanation of the complex chemical process that takes place. For some drugs, the method of action is unknown.

12—Time Lapse Before Drug Works

The times given are approximations. Times vary a great deal from person to person, and from time to time in the same person. The figures give you some idea of when to expect improvement or side effects.

13—Don't Take With

Some drugs create problems when taken in combination with other substances. Most problems are detailed in the Interaction section of each chart.

Occasionally, an interaction is singled out if the combination is particularly harmful.

☠ OVERDOSE

14—Symptoms

The symptoms listed are most likely to develop with accidental or purposeful overdose. Overdosage may not cause all symptoms listed. Sometimes symptoms are identical to ones listed as side effects. The difference is intensity and severity. You will have to judge. Consult a doctor or poison control center if you have any doubt.

15—What To Do

If you suspect an overdose, whether symptoms are apparent or not, get medical help or advice, and if needed, follow instructions in this section. Additional instructions for emergency treatment for overdose are at the end of the book.

16—🕐 Possible Adverse Reactions or Side Effects

Adverse reactions or side effects are symptoms that may occur when you take a drug. They are effects on the body other than the desired therapeutic effect.

The term side effects implies expected and usually unavoidable effects of a drug. Side effects have nothing to do with the drug's intended use.

For example, the generic drug paregoric reduces intestinal cramps and vomiting. It also often causes a flushed face. The flushing is a side effect that is harmless and does not affect the drug's therapeutic potential. Many side effects disappear in a short time without treatment.

The term adverse reaction is more significant. For example, paregoric can cause a serious adverse allergic reaction in some people. This reaction can include hives, rash and severe itch.

Some adverse reactions can be prevented, which is one reason this information is included in the book. Most adverse reactions are minor and last only a short time. With many drugs, adverse reactions that might occur will frequently diminish in intensity as your body adjusts to the medicine.

The majority of drugs, used properly for valid reasons, offer benefits that outweigh potential hazards.

17—Symptoms

Symptoms of commonly known side effects and adverse reactions are listed. Other drug responses may be listed under "Prolonged Use," "Skin & Sunlight" or "Others." You may experience a symptom that is not listed. It may be a side effect or adverse reaction to the drug, or it may be an additional symptom of the illness. If you are unsure, call your doctor.

18—Frequency

This is an estimation of how often symptoms occur in persons who take the drug. The four most common categories of frequency can be found under the SYMPTOMS heading and are as follows: Life-threatening means exactly what it says; seek emergency treatment immediately. Common means these symptoms are expected and sometimes inevitable. Infrequent means the symptoms occur in approximately 1% to 10% of patients. Rare means symptoms occur in fewer than 1%.

19—What To Do

Follow the guidelines provided opposite the symptoms that apply to you. These are general instructions. If you are concerned or confused, always call your doctor.

20—☞ Warnings & Precautions

Read these entries to determine special information that applies to you.

21—Don't Take If

This section lists circumstances when drug use is not safe. On some drug labels and in formal medical literature, these circumstances are called contraindications.

22—Before You Start, Consult Your Doctor If

This section lists conditions, especially disease conditions, under which a drug should be used only with caution and medical supervision.

23—Over Age 60

As a person ages, physical changes occur that require special considerations. Liver and kidney functions decrease, metabolism slows and the prostate gland enlarges in men.

Most drugs are metabolized or excreted at a rate dependent on kidney and liver functions. Smaller doses or longer intervals between doses may be necessary to prevent unhealthy concentration of a drug. Toxic effects and adverse reactions occur more frequently and cause more serious problems in older people.

24—Pregnancy

The best rule to follow during pregnancy is to avoid all drugs, including tobacco and alcohol. Any medicine—prescription or nonprescription—requires medical advice and supervision.

This section will alert you if there is evidence that a drug harms the unborn child. Lack of evidence does not guarantee a drug's safety.

The definitions of the pregnancy risk categories of drugs used by the Food and Drug Administration (FDA) are listed on page xviii.

25—Breast-feeding

Many drugs filter into a mother's milk. Some drugs have dangerous or unwanted effects on the nursing infant. This section suggests ways to minimize harm to the child.

26—Infants & Children

Many drugs carry special warnings and precautions for children because of a child's size and immaturity. In medical terminology, newborns are babies up to 2 weeks old, infants are 2 weeks to 1 year, and children are 1 to 12 years.

27—Prolonged Use

With the exception of immediate allergic reactions, most drugs produce no ill effects during short periods of treatment. However, relatively safe drugs taken for long periods may produce unwanted effects. These are listed. Drugs should be taken in the smallest doses and for the shortest time possible. Nevertheless, some diseases and conditions require a prolonged or even lifelong period of treatment. Therefore, follow-up medical examinations and laboratory tests recommended when a drug is used for long periods are listed. Your doctor may want to change drugs occasionally or alter your treatment regimen to minimize problems.

The words "functional dependence" sometimes appear in this section. This does not mean physical or psychological addiction. Sometimes a body function ceases to work naturally because it has been replaced or interfered with by the drug. The body then becomes dependent on the drug to continue the function.

28—Skin & Sunlight

Many drugs cause photosensitivity, which means increased skin sensitivity to ultraviolet rays from sunlight or artificial rays from a sunlamp. This section will alert you to this potential problem.

29—Driving, Piloting or Hazardous Work

Any drug that alters moods or that decreases alertness, muscular coordination or reflexes may make these activities particularly hazardous. The effects may not appear in all people, or they may disappear after a short exposure to the drug. If this section contains a warning, use caution until you determine how a new drug affects you.

30—Discontinuing

Some patients stop taking a drug when symptoms begin to go away, although complete recovery may require longer treatment.

Other patients continue taking a drug when it is no longer needed. This section gives warnings about prematurely discontinuing. Some drugs cause symptoms days or weeks after they have been discontinued.

31—Others

Warnings and precautions appear here if they don't fit into the other categories. This section includes special instructions, reminders, storage instructions, warnings to persons with chronic illness and other information.

32—Possible Interaction With Other Drugs

People often must take two or more drugs at the same time. Many of these drug combinations have the potential to interact adversely. Fortunately, this adverse reaction occurs in only a small proportion of people who take the interacting combinations. Drugs interact in your body with other drugs, whether prescription or non-prescription. Interactions affect absorption, metabolism, elimination or distribution of either drug. Other factors that can influence drug interactions are the patient's age, state of health and the way the drugs are administered: time taken, how taken, dosage, dosage forms and duration of treatment. The chart lists interactions by generic name, drug class or drug-induced effect. An asterisk (*) in this column reminds you to "See Glossary" in the back of the book, where that entry is further explained.

If a drug class appears, the drug you are looking up may interact with any drug in that class. Drugs in each class that are included in the book are listed in the index. Occasionally drugs that are not included in this book appear in the Interaction column.

Interactions are sometimes beneficial. You may not be able to determine from the chart which interactions are good and which are bad. Don't guess. Consult your doctor or pharmacist if you take drugs that interact. Some combinations can be fatal.

Some drugs have too many interactions to list on one chart. The additional inter-actions appear on the continuation page indicated at the bottom of the list.

Testing has not been done on all possible drug combinations. It is important to let your doctor or pharmacist know about any drugs you take, both prescription and nonprescription.

33— 🏃 Possible Interaction With Other Substances

The substances listed here are repeated on every drug chart. All people eat food and drink beverages. Many adults consume alcohol. Some people use cocaine and/or smoke tobacco or marijuana. This section shows possible interactions between these substances and each drug.

Checklist for Safer Drug Use

- Tell your doctor about any drug you take (even aspirin, allergy pills, cough and cold preparations, antacids, laxatives, vitamins, etc.) before you take any new drug.

- Learn all you can about drugs you may take *before* you take them. Information sources are your doctor, your nurse, your pharmacist, this book, other books in your public library and the Internet.

- Keep an up-to-date list of all the medicines you take in a wallet or purse. Include name, dose and frequency.

- Don't take drugs prescribed for someone else—even if your symptoms are the same.

- Keep your prescription drugs to yourself. Your drugs may be harmful to someone else.

- Tell your doctor about any symptoms you believe are caused by a drug—prescription or nonprescription—that you take.

- Take only medicines that are *necessary*. Avoid taking nonprescription drugs while taking prescription drugs for a medical problem.

- Before your doctor prescribes for you, tell him about your previous experiences with any drug—beneficial results, side effects, adverse reactions or allergies.

- Take medicine in good light after you have identified it. If you wear glasses to read, put them on to check drug labels. It is easy to take the wrong drug or take a drug at the wrong time.

- Don't keep any drugs that change mood, alertness or judgment—such as sedatives, narcotics or tranquilizers—by your bedside. These can cause accidental deaths. You may unknowingly repeat a dose when you are half asleep or confused.

- Know the names of your medicines. These include the generic name, the brand name and the generic names of all ingredients in a combination drug. Your doctor, nurse or pharmacist can give you this information.

- Study the labels on all nonprescription drugs. If the information is incomplete or if you have questions, ask the pharmacist for more details.

- If you must deviate from your prescribed dose schedule, tell your doctor.

- Shake liquid medicines before taking (if directed).

- Store all medicines away from moisture and heat. Bathroom medicine cabinets are usually unsuitable.

- If a drug needs refrigeration, don't freeze.

- Obtain a standard measuring spoon from your pharmacy for liquid medicines. Kitchen teaspoons and tablespoons are not accurate enough.

- Follow diet instructions when you take medicines. Some work better on a full stomach, others on an empty stomach. Some drugs are more useful with special diets. For example, medicine for high blood pressure may be more effective if accompanied by a sodium-restricted diet.

- Tell your doctor about any allergies you have to any substance (e.g., food) or adverse reactions to medicines you've had in the past. A previous allergy to a drug may make it dangerous to prescribe again. People with other allergies, such as eczema, hay fever, asthma, bronchitis and food allergies, are more likely to be allergic to drugs.

- Prior to surgery, tell your doctor, anesthesiologist or dentist about any drug you have taken in the past few weeks. Advise them of any cortisone drugs you have taken within two years.

- If you become pregnant while taking any medicine, including birth control pills, tell your doctor immediately.

- Avoid *all* drugs while you are pregnant, if possible. If you must take drugs during pregnancy, record names, amounts, dates and reasons.

- If you see more than one doctor, tell each one about drugs others have prescribed.

- When you use nonprescription drugs, report it so the information is on your medical record.

- Store all drugs away from the reach of children.

- Note the expiration date on each drug label. Discard outdated ones safely. If no expiration date appears and it has been at least one year since taking the medication, it may be best to discard it. Follow any specific disposal instructions on the drug label or patient information that came with the medication. Do not flush prescription drugs down the toilet unless this information specifically instructs you to do so. If no instructions are given, throw the drugs in the household trash, but first: Take them out of their original containers and mix them with an undesirable substance, such as used coffee grounds or kitty litter. Alternatively, check if local household hazardous-waste collection programs—where you're supposed to take motor oil and batteries—accept expired medicines.

- Pay attention to the information in the drug charts about safety while driving, piloting or working in dangerous places.

- Alcohol, cocaine, marijuana or other mood-altering drugs, as well as tobacco—mixed with some drugs—can cause a life-threatening interaction, prevent your medicine from being effective or delay your return to health. Be sure that you avoid them during illness.

- Some medications are subject to theft. For example, a repair person in your home who is abusing drugs may ask to use your bathroom, and while there "check out" your medicine cabinet. Sedatives, stimulants and analgesics are especially likely to be stolen, but almost any medication is subject to theft.

- If possible, use the same pharmacy for all your medications. Every pharmacy keeps a "drug profile," and if it is complete, the pharmacist may stop medications that are likely to cause serious interactions. Also, having a record of all your medications in one place helps your doctor or an emergency room doctor get a complete picture in case of an emergency.

- If you have a complicated medical history or a condition that might render you unable to communicate (e.g., diabetes or epilepsy), wear some type of medical identification (small tag, bracelet, neck chain or other) to identify your condition. (The MedicAlert Corporation provides this type of product. Call 888-633-4298 or go online www.medicalert.org for information.) Some people carry a wallet card with the information. A newer type of medical alert ID is the USB tag. It is basically a USB flash drive that contains a person's medical emergency information and can store much more information if desired. Emergency medical people can access the information using any available computer.

- If you are giving medicine to children, read all instructions carefully. Use the specific dosing device (dropper, cup, etc.) that comes with the product. Don't exceed recommended dose. It does not help and can cause health risks.

- Ask your pharmacist if they will provide an extra, prescription-labeled small bottle or container to use for one or two doses of your medication. It can be used when going out for a meal, during short trips or for a student in school. This avoids carrying all your medications with you.

Compliance with Doctors' Instructions

For medical purposes, compliance is defined as the extent to which a patient follows the instructions of a doctor and includes taking medications on schedule, keeping appointments and following directions for changes in lifestyle, such as changing one's diet or exercise.

Although the cost of obtaining medical advice and medication is one of the largest items in a family budget, many people defeat the health-care process by departing from the doctor's recommendations. This failure to carry out the doctor's instructions is the single most common cause of treatment failure. Perhaps the instructions were not presented clearly, or you may not have understood them or realized their importance and benefits.

Factors That Can Cause Problems With Compliance:
- Treatment recommendations that combine two or more actions (such as instructions to take medication, see a therapist and join a support group).
- Recommendations that require lifestyle changes (such as dieting).
- Recommendations that involve long-term treatment (such as taking a medication for life).
- Recommendations for very young patients or for the elderly (when another person has to be responsible for following the instructions).
- Other factors include traveling and time changes, busy work schedules and lack of organization.

Examples of Noncompliance:
- Medications are forgotten or discontinued too soon. Forgetting to take a medication is the most common of all shortcomings, especially if a medication must be taken more than once a day. If you need to take

a medication several times a day, set out a week's supply in an inexpensive pill box that you can carry with you.

- Side effects of medications are a common problem. Almost all medications have some unpleasant side effects. Often these disappear after a few days, but if they don't, let your doctor know right away. Side effects can often be controlled by changing dosage, switching to a similar medication or by adding medications that control the side effects.
- Not taking a drug because it is unpleasant (e.g., bad tasting). Ask your doctor about options.
- Cost is another reason why there are treatment failures; because of a tight budget, a person may take a medication less frequently than prescribed or just not purchase it. If you can't afford a medication, perhaps a less costly one can be prescribed or your doctor can find other ways to provide it.
- Laboratory tests, x-rays or other recommended medical studies are not obtained, perhaps due to concerns about costs or fear of the tests themselves.
- Recommendations about behavioral changes such as diet or exercise are ignored (old habits are difficult for anyone to change).
- Suggested immunizations are not obtained, sometimes due to fear of needles.
- Follow-up visits to the doctor are not made, or appointments are canceled, perhaps due to problems finding transportation or long waiting times in the doctor's office.

Communicating With Your Doctor:

- If you don't understand something, ask.
- If there are reasons why you cannot follow a recommendation, speak up.
- If you have reservations or fears about treatment, discuss them.

Remember, it is your health and your money that are at issue. You and your doctor are—or should be—working together to make you well and keep you healthy.

Cough and Cold Medicines

There are hundreds of nonprescription (over-the-counter or OTC) drugs available to treat symptoms of the common cold and other minor respiratory illnesses.

Some of these drugs contain a single active ingredient that relieves one specific symptom (such as a cough). Other drugs contain combinations of two or more ingredients intended to relieve a number of different symptoms (such as a cough, stuffy nose and pain).

Each of the active ingredients in a drug has a generic (or chemical) name. Generics are names such as acetaminophen, ibuprofen, aspirin, pseudoephedrine, guaifenesin, diphenhydramine and others.

Cough and cold drugs can be sorted into five categories (or classes). They include:

Antihistamines dry up secretions of the respiratory tract and help control allergy symptoms. Antihistamines may cause drowsiness, slow reflexes and decrease ability to concentrate. Therefore, don't drive vehicles or pilot aircraft until you learn how this medicine affects you. Don't work around dangerous machinery. Don't climb ladders or work in high places. The danger increases if you drink alcohol or take other medicines that affect alertness and reflexes. Antihistamines can cause other side effects or adverse reactions.

Decongestants relieve symptoms of nasal or bronchial congestion. Decongestants may cause nervousness, irregular heartbeats in some people, dizziness, confusion and other side effects. Conduct your daily activities with these effects in mind.

Antitussives (Cough suppressants) reduce the frequency and severity of a cough. These may be either narcotic (e.g., codeine and hydrocodone) or non-narcotic (e.g., dextromethorphan or carbetapentane). Narcotic cough suppressants are habit-forming and may cause some of the same mental changes that can take place with antihistamines. The most common non-narcotic antitussive medicine, dextromethorphan, is not habit-forming but has other side effects. Carbetapentane is similar (but not covered in this book).

Expectorants loosen secretions to make them easier to cough up. The most common expectorant is guaifenesin, which has very few side effects but doesn't loosen secretions very efficiently.

Analgesics relieve aches, pains and fever. Common analgesics in cough and cold medicines are aspirin, acetaminophen and ibuprofen.

These nonprescription drugs are generally recognized as safe, but they do have side effects, possible interactions with other drugs, and need to be used with caution in certain individuals.

There is no drug that will cure a cold (including antibiotics). If you decide to take a drug for specific symptoms, a single ingredient one is usually a better choice, unless each of the drug's ingredients is necessary to relieve your particular symptoms. Before taking a drug, read the label and follow all the directions. Also, read the information in this book about the drug's generic ingredients. To find information about a drug:

• Look on the label for the generic ingredients that are in the drug product.

• Consult the index for each generic name and find the page number for its drug chart. Then look up each drug chart. Read all the information, especially regarding the adverse reactions and side effects, precautions, and interactions with other drugs you may be taking.

Always consult a doctor if any cold symptoms cause you concern.

Practice prevention—wash your hands often and keep your hands away from your face.

Nonprescription cough and cold drugs in children

• Read the label to be sure it is approved for your child's age. Labels advise you not to use these medicines in children under age 4. Do not give children medications labeled only for adults.

• Choose nonprescription cough and cold medicines with child-resistant safety caps, when available. After using, make sure to close the cap tightly and store the medicine out of the sight and reach of children.

• Check the "active ingredients" section of the DRUG FACTS label of the medicines that you choose. This will help you know what symptoms the "active ingredients" in the medicine are intended to treat.

• Be careful about giving more than one medicine to a child. If you do, make sure they do not have the same type of "active ingredients." If you use two medicines that have the same or similar active ingredients, a child could get too much of an ingredient and that may hurt your child.

• Carefully follow the directions for how to use the medicine in the DRUG FACTS part of the label. The directions tell you how much medicine to give and how often you can give it. If you have a question about how to use the medicine, ask your pharmacist or doctor. Overuse or misuse of these products can lead to serious and potentially life threatening side effects.

• Only use measuring devices that come with the medicine or those specially made for measuring drugs. Do not use common household spoons to measure medicines for children because household spoons come in different sizes and are not meant for measuring medicines.

• Understand that using nonprescription cough and cold medicines does not cure the cold or cough. These medicines only treat the symptom(s) such as runny nose, congestion, fever and aches. They do not shorten the length of time your child is sick.

Pregnancy Risk Category Information

The pregnancy risk category assigned to a medication identifies the potential risk for that particular drug to cause birth defects or death to an unborn child (fetus). These categories are assigned by applying the definitions of the Food and Drug Administration (FDA) to the available clinical information about the drug. Most drugs are tested only on animals and not on humans for safety during pregnancy, because such testing would subject unborn children to unnecessary risks.

It is best to avoid all drugs during pregnancy, but this rating system can help you and your doctor to assess the risk-to-benefit ratio should drug treatment become necessary. You and your doctor should discuss these benefits and risks carefully before any drug treatment is initiated. You should not take any medications (including nonprescription drugs such as laxatives or cold remedies) without your doctor's approval.

A brief explanation and the definitions of the drug categories, labeled A, B, C, D, and X, are listed below:

- A: *No evidence of risk exists.* Adequate and well-controlled studies in pregnant women have not shown an increased risk of fetal abnormalities.

- B: *The risk of fetal harm is possible but remote.* Animal studies have revealed no evidence of harm to the fetus; however, there are no adequate and well-controlled studies in pregnant women, or animal studies have shown an adverse effect, but adequate and well-controlled studies in pregnant women have failed to demonstrate a risk to the fetus.

- C: *Fetal risk can't be ruled out.* Animal studies have shown an adverse effect, and there are no adequate and well-controlled studies in pregnant women, or no animal studies have been conducted, and there are no adequate and well-controlled studies in pregnant women.

- D: *Positive evidence of fetal risk exists, but, potential benefits from the drug may outweigh the risk. For example, the drug may be acceptable in a life-threatening situation or serious disease if safer drugs can't be used or are ineffective.* Adequate well-controlled or observational studies in pregnant women have demonstrated a risk to the fetus.

- X: *Contraindicated during pregnancy.* Adequate well-controlled or observational studies in animals or pregnant women have demonstrated positive evidence of fetal abnormalities. The use of the product is contraindicated in women who are or who may become pregnant.

- NR: Not rated.

Buying Prescription Drugs Online

The Food and Drug Administration (FDA) offers these suggestions. When it comes to buying medicine online, it is important to be very careful. Some websites sell medicine that may not be safe to use and could put your health at risk.

• Some websites that sell medicine:
1. Aren't U.S. state-licensed pharmacies or aren't pharmacies at all.
2. May give a diagnosis that is not correct and sell medicine that is not right for you or your condition.
3. Won't protect your personal information.

• Some medicines sold online:
1. Are fake (counterfeit or "copycat" medicines).
2. Are too strong or too weak.
3. Have dangerous ingredients.
4. Have expired (are out-of-date).
5. Aren't FDA-approved (haven't been checked for safety and effectiveness).
6. Aren't made using safe standards.
7. Aren't safe to use with other medicine or products you use.
8. Aren't labeled, stored, or shipped correctly.

What you should do:
1. Talk with your doctor and have a physical exam before you get any new medicine for the first time.
2. Use only medicine that has been prescribed by your doctor or another trusted professional who is licensed in the U.S. to write prescriptions for medicine.
3. Ask your doctor if there are any special steps you need to take to fill your prescription.

These tips will help protect you if you buy medicines online:

• Know your source to make sure it's safe.

• Make sure a website is a state-licensed pharmacy that is located in the United States. Pharmacies and pharmacists in the United States are licensed by a state's board of pharmacy. Your state board of pharmacy can tell you if a website is a state-licensed pharmacy, is in good standing, and is located in the United States. Find a list of state boards of pharmacy on the National Association of Boards of Pharmacy (NABP) website at www.nabp.info.

• The NABP has a program to help you find some of the pharmacies that are licensed to sell medicine online. Internet websites that display the seal of this program have been checked to make sure they meet state and federal rules. For more on this program and a list of pharmacies that display the Verified Internet Pharmacy Practice Sites™ Seal, (VIPPS® Seal), go to www.vipps.info.

• Look for websites with practices that protect you. A safe website should:
1. Be located in the United States and licensed by the state board of pharmacy where the website is operating.
2. Have a licensed pharmacist to answer your questions.
3. Require a prescription from your doctor or other health care professional who is licensed in the United States to write prescriptions for medicine.
4. Have a way for you to talk to a person if you have problems.

• Be sure your privacy is protected.
1. Look for privacy and security policies that are easy-to-find and easy-to-understand.
2. Don't give any personal information (such as social security number, credit card, or medical or health history), unless you are sure the website will keep your information safe and private.
3. Make sure that the site will not sell your information, unless you agree.

Report websites you are not sure of, or if you have complaints about a site.
Go to www.fda.gov/buyonline and click on "Notify FDA about problem websites."

Information about Substances of Abuse

Each of the drug charts list the interactions of alcohol, marijuana and cocaine. These three drugs are singled out because of their wide use and abuse.

Drugs of abuse include those that are addictive and harmful.

Common drugs of abuse:

Tobacco (nicotine)

What it does: Tobacco smoke contains noxious, addictive and cancer-producing ingredients. They include nicotine, carbon monoxide, ammonia and tars. Carcinogens probably come from the tars. Tars are present in chewing tobacco, snuff, cigarettes, cigars and pipes.

Short-term effects of average amount: Relaxation of mood if you are a steady smoker. Constriction of blood vessels.

Short-term effects of large amount inhaled: Headache, appetite loss, nausea.

Long-term effects: Risk of lung cancer and other cancers. Breathing problems and chronic lung disease, heart and blood vessel disease, risk of abortion and reduced birth weight of baby born to women who smoke during pregnancy.

Alcohol

What it does:

• *Central Nervous System*

It depresses normal mental activity and normal muscle function. Alcoholism is associated with accidents of all types. Marital, family, work, legal and social problems also occur. Abuse of alcohol may result in nerve damage and cause various types of brain disorders.

• *Gastrointestinal System*

Increases stomach acid, poisons liver function. Chronic alcoholism frequently leads to permanent damage to the liver.

• *Heart and Blood Vessels*

Decreased normal function, leading to heart diseases such as cardiomyopathy and disorders of the blood vessels and kidney, such as high blood pressure. Bleeding from the esophagus and stomach frequently accompany liver disease.

• *Unborn Fetus (teratogenicity)*

Alcohol abuse in the mother carrying a fetus causes *fetal alcohol spectrum disorder (FASD). It* includes mental deficiency, facial abnormalities, slow growth and other major and minor problems in a newborn.

Signs of Use:
Early signs: Smell of alcohol on the breath, behavior changes (aggressive; passive; lack of sexual inhibition; poor judgment; uncontrolled emotion, such as rage).
Intoxication signs: Unsteady gait, slurred speech, poor performance of any brain or muscle function, stupor or coma in *severe* alcoholic intoxication.

Long-term Effects:
Addiction: Compulsive alcohol use. Persons addicted to alcohol have severe withdrawal symptoms if alcohol is unavailable.
Liver disease: Usually cirrhosis.
Loss of sexual function: Impotence, erectile dysfunction, loss of libido.
Increased incidence of cancer: Lung and other types. Interferes with medications.

Marijuana (cannabis, hashish)

What it does: Heightens perception, causes mood swings, relaxes mind and body.
Signs of use: Red eyes, lethargy, uncoordinated body movements.
Long-term effects: Decreased motivation. Possible brain, heart, lung and reproductive system damage, schizophrenia.

Amphetamines (including ecstasy)

What they do: Speed up physical and mental processes to cause a false sense of energy and excitement. The moods are temporary and unreal.
Signs of use: Dilated pupils, insomnia, trembling.
Long-term effects or overdose: Violent

behavior, paranoia, inflammation of blood vessels, renal failure, possible death from overdose.

Anabolic Steroids

What they do: Enhance strength, increase muscle mass.

Signs of use: Significant mood swings, aggressiveness.

Long-term effects or overdose: Possible heart problems, paranoia and mania, liver damage, male infertility and impotence, male characteristics in females.

Barbiturates

What they do: Produce drowsiness and lethargy.

Signs of use: Confused speech, lack of coordination and balance.

Long-term effects or overdose: Disrupt normal sleep pattern. Possible death from overdose, especially with alcohol abuse.

Sedative-hypnotics (benzodiazepines, "party drugs" that include gammahydroxybutyrate and rohypnol)

What they do: Produce drowsiness and lethargy.

Signs of use: Slow breathing, low blood pressure, vomiting, delirium, amnesia, possible coma.

Long-term effects or overdose: Disrupt normal sleep pattern. Possible death from overdose, especially in combination with alcohol.

Cocaine

What it does: Stimulates the nervous system, heightens sensations and may produce hallucinations.

Signs of use: Trembling, intoxication, dilated pupils, constant sniffling.

Long-term effects or overdose: Soreness of nasal passages. Itching all over body, some with open sores. Possible brain damage or heart rhythm disturbance. Possible death from overdose.

Crystal Methamphetamine

What it does: Stimulates the nervous system, heightens sensations and has long-lasting euphoric effects.

Signs of use: Obsessively picking at the face or body, hallucinations, teeth grinding, extreme energy and no sleep for 2-3 days, major loss of weight.

Long-term effects or overdose: Rapid heart rate, high blood pressure, damaged blood vessels in the brain, fever, convulsions and death.

Opiates (codeine, heroin, morphine, methadone, opium)

What they do: Relieve pain, create temporary and false sense of well-being.

Signs of use: Small pupils, mood swings, slurred speech, sore eyes, lethargy, weight loss, sweating.

Long-term effects or overdose: Loss of appetite, infections, need to increase drug amount to produce same effects, death.

Phencyclidine (PCP, angeldust)

What they do: Produce euphoria along with a feeling of numbness.

Signs of use: Violent behavior, dizziness, loss of motor skills, disorientation.

Long-term effects or overdose: Seizures, high or low blood pressure, rigid muscles. Possible death from overdose.

Psychedelic Drugs (LSD, mescaline)

What they do: Produce hallucinations, either pleasant or frightening.

Signs of use: Dilated pupils, sweating, trembling, fever, chills.

Long-term effects or overdose: Lack of motivation, unpredictable behavior, hallucinations, death from overdose.

Volatile Substances (glue, solvents, nitrous oxide, other volatile compounds)

What they do: Produce hallucinations, false sense of well-being, unconsciousness.

Signs of use: Dilated pupils, flushed face, confusion, respiratory failure, coma.

Long-term effects or overdose: Permanent brain, liver, kidney damage; death.

Medical Conditions and Their Commonly Used Drugs

This list contains the names of many medical problems and the names of drugs that may be used for their treatment. The drugs are listed either as a generic name (e.g., Acetaminophen) or class name (e.g., Antihistamines). Specific brand or trade names of drugs are not shown. This list of drugs is intended only as a guide and is not meant to be 100% complete. Use it for a general reference.

The inclusion of a drug name does not mean it is necessarily an appropriate treatment for you. Also, your doctor may prescribe a drug for you that is not listed, but is quite appropriate for treatment. Your doctor knows your medical history and can prescribe the drug that should work best for you.

You can find information about the drugs listed by looking up the name in the General Index and referring to the page listed. Do not be concerned if the drug chart does not list your specific illness in the USES section. For example, that section may state that a drug is used for bacterial infections and not list specific bacterial disorders (such as a vaginal infection or urinary tract infection).

Acid Indigestion & Upset Stomach
Antacids
Bismuth Salts
Histamine H$_2$ Receptor
  Antagonists
Hyoscyamine
Proton Pump Inhibitors
Simethicone
Sodium Bicarbonate

Acne
Antiacne Cleansing (Topical)
Antibacterials for Acne
  (Topical)
Azelaic Acid
Benzoyl Peroxide
Erythromycins
Isotretinoin
Keratolytics
Nitroimidazoles
Retinoids (Topical)
Tetracyclines

Actinic Keratoses
Fluorouracil (Topical)
Masoprocol

Acute Myocardial Infarction
Angiotensin-Converting
  Enzyme (ACE) Inhibitors

Addison's Disease
Adrenocorticoids (Systemic)

Aging
Dehydroepiandrosterone
  (DHEA)

AIDS – See HIV Infection

Alcohol Withdrawal
Acamprosate
Benzodiazepines
Beta-Adrenergic Blocking
  Agents
Carbamazepine
Disulfiram
Hydroxyzine
Lithium
Naltrexone
Thiamine

Allergies & Allergic Reactions
Adrenocorticoids (Nasal
  Inhalation)
Adrenocorticoids (Oral
  Inhalation)
Adrenocorticoids (Systemic)
Antihistamines
Antihistamines (Nasal)
Antihistamines, Nonsedating
Antihistamines,
  Phenothiazine-Derivative
Cromolyn
Decongestants (Ophthalmic)
Ephedrine
Hydroxyzine
Leukotriene Modifiers

Alopecia
5-Alpha Reductase Inhibitors
Minoxidil

Altitude Illness
Carbonic Anhydrase
  Inhibitors

Alzheimer's Disease
Cholinesterase Inhibitors
Memantine

Amebiasis
Chloroquine
Iodoquinol
Nitroimidazoles

Amenorrhea
Bromocriptine
Progestins

Amyotrophic Lateral Sclerosis (ALS)
Riluzole

Anemia
Adrenocorticoids (Systemic)
Androgens
Cyclosporine
Folic Acid
Iron Supplements
Leucovorin
Vitamin B-12

Angina
Antithyroid Drugs
Beta-Adrenergic Blocking
  Agents
Calcium Channel Blockers
Dipyridamole
Nitrates
Ranolazine

Ankylosing Spondylitis
Adrenocorticoids (Systemic)
Anti-inflammatory Drugs,
  Nonsteroidal (NSAIDs)
Anti-inflammatory Drugs,
  Nonsteroidal (NSAIDs)
  COX-2 inhibitors
Aspirin
Methotrexate
Sulfasalazine

Tumor Necrosis Factor
Blockers

Anorexia
Antidepressants, Tricyclic
Progestins
Selective Serotonin
Reuptake Inhibitors
(SSRIs)

Anxiety
Antidepressants, Tricyclic
Barbiturates
Benzodiazepines
Beta-Adrenergic Blocking
Agents
Buspirone
Haloperidol
Hydroxyzine
Loxapine
Meprobamate
Phenothiazines
Selective Serotonin
Reuptake Inhibitors
(SSRIs)
Serotonin & Norepinephrine
Reuptake Inhibitors
(SNRIs)
Thiothixene

Appetite Stimulant
Antihistamines
Dronabinol

Appetite Suppressant
Appetite Suppressants
Sibutramine

Arthritis
Acetaminophen
Adrenocorticoids (Oral
Inhalation)
Adrenocorticoids (Systemic)
Anakinra
Antihistamines, Nonsedating
Anti-Inflammatory Drugs,
Nonsteroidal (NSAIDs)
Anti-Inflammatory Drugs,
Nonsteroidal (NSAIDs)
COX-2 Inhibitors
Aspirin
Azathioprine
Bronchodilators, Adrenergic
Bronchodilators, Xanthine
Capsaicin
Chloroquine
Cyclosporine
Diclofenac (Topical)
Gold Compounds
Hydroxychloroquine
Leflunomide
Leukotriene Modifiers
Meloxicam
Methotrexate
Salicylates
Tumor Necrosis Factor
Blockers

Asthma
Adrenocorticoids (Nasal
Inhalation)
Adrenocorticoids (Oral
Inhalation)
Adrenocorticoids (Systemic)
Bronchodilators, Adrenergic
Bronchodilators, Xanthine
Cromolyn
Ephedrine
Ipratropium
Leukotriene Modifiers

Athlete's Foot
Antibacterials, Antifungals
(Topical)
Antifungals (Topical)

**Attention Deficit
Hyperactivity Disorder
(ADHD)**
Amphetamines
Atomoxetine
Stimulant Medications
Stimulants, Amphetamine-
Related

Autism
Haloperidol
Olanzapine
Quetiapine
Selective Serotonin
Reuptake Inhibitors
(SSRIs)
Serotonin-Dopamine
Antagonists
Stimulant Medications

Bacterial Infections
Acetohydroxamic Acid (AHA)
Cephalosporins
Chloramphenicol
Clindamycin
Erythromycins
Fluoroquinolones
Kanamycin
Lincomycin
Linezolid
Macrolide Antibiotics
Neomycin (Oral)
Nitrofurantoin
Nitroimidazoles
Penicillins
Penicillins & Beta-Lactamase
Inhibitors
Rifamycins
Sulfonamides
Telithromycin
Tetracyclines
Trimethoprim
Vancomycin

Baldness – See Hair Loss

Bedwetting (Enuresis)
Antidepressants, Tricyclic
Desmopressin

Bipolar Disorder
Aripiprazole
Carbamazepine
Lithium
Divalproex
Quetiapine
Serotonin-Dopamine
Antagonists
Valproic Acid
Ziprasidone

**Birth Control – See
Contraception**

Bites & Stings
Adrenocorticoids (Topical)
Anesthetics (Topical)

**Bladder Infection – See
Cystitis**

Bladder Spasms
Clidinium
Propantheline

Bleeding
Antifibrinolytic Agents
Vitamin K

Blood Circulation
Cyclandelate
Intermittent Claudication
Agents
Isoxsuprine
Vitamin E

Blood Clots
Anticoagulants (Oral)
Dipyridamole
Platelet Inhibitors

Bronchial Spasms
Anticholinergics
Bronchodilators, Adrenergic

Bronchitis
Bronchodilators, Xanthine
Cephalosporins
Dextromethorphan
Fluoroquinolones
Ipratropium
Macrolide Antibiotics
Sulfonamides
Tetracyclines

Bulimia
Antidepressants, Tricyclic
Lithium
Selective Serotonin
Reuptake Inhibitors
(SSRIs)

Burns
Anesthetics (Topical)
Zinc Supplements

Bursitis
Adrenocorticoids (Systemic)
Anti-Inflammatory Drugs,
Nonsteroidal (NSAIDs)
Aspirin
Salicylates

Cancer
Adrenocorticoids (Systemic)
Aminoglutethimide
Androgens
Antiandrogens, Nonsteroidal
Antifungals, Azoles
Busulfan
Capecitabine
Chlorambucil
Cyclophosphamide
Estramustine
Estrogens
Etoposide
Hydroxyurea
Imatinib
Levamisole
Lomustine
Melphalan
Mercaptopurine
Methotrexate
Mitotane
Paclitaxel
Procarbazine
Progestins
Raloxifene
Tamoxifen
Thioguanine
Thyroid Hormones
Toremifene

Cancer Of The Skin
Fluorouracil (Topical)
Masoprocol
Mechlorethamine (Topical)

Canker Sores
Amlexanox
Anesthetics (Mucosal-Local)

Chickenpox
Acetaminophen
Antihistamines
Antivirals for Herpes Virus

Cholesterol, High
Cholestyramine
Colestipol
Ezetimibe
Gemfibrozil
HMG-CoA Reductase
Inhibitors
Neomycin (Oral)
Niacin
Raloxifene

**Chronic Obstructive
Pulmonary Disease (COPD)**
Adrenocorticoids (Systemic)
Bronchodilators, Adrenergic
Bronchodilators, Xanthine

Ipratropium
Tiotropium

Cirrhosis
Colchicine
Cyclosporine
Thiamine (Vitamin B-1)

Colds & Cough
Acetaminophen
Anticholinergics
Antihistamines
Antihistamines, Nonsedating
Anti-Inflammatory Drugs,
Nonsteroidal (NSAIDs)
Aspirin
Dextromethorphan
Ephedrine
Guaifenesin
Oxymetazoline
Phenylephrine
Phenylephrine (Ophthalmic)
Pseudoephedrine

Colic
Hyoscyamine
Simethicone

**Colitis – See Inflammatory
Bowel Disease**

Congestion, Chest
Bronchodilators, Adrenergic
Ephedrine
Oxymetazoline
Phenylephrine
Pseudoephedrine
Xylometazoline

Congestive Heart Failure
Angiotensin-Converting
Enzyme (ACE) Inhibitors
Digitalis Preparations
Beta-Adrenergic Blocking
Agents
Beta-Adrenergic Blocking
Agents & Thiazide
Diuretics
Diuretics, Loop
Diuretics, Potassium-Sparing
Diuretics, Potassium-Sparing
& Hydrochlorothiazide
Diuretics, Thiazide
Nitrates

Conjunctivitis (Pink Eye)
Antibacterials (Ophthalmic)
Antivirals (Ophthalmic)

**Conjunctivitis, Seasonal
Allergic**
Anti-Inflammatory Drugs,
Nonsteroidal (Ophthalmic)
Antiallergic Agents
(Ophthalmic)

Constipation
Laxatives, Bulk-Forming
Laxatives, Osmotic
Laxatives, Softener/Lubricant
Laxatives, Stimulant
Lubiprostone
Tegaserod

Contraception
Contraceptives, Oral & Skin
Contraceptives, Vaginal

**Convulsions (Epilepsy;
Seizures)**
Anticonvulsants, Hydantoin
Anticonvulsants, Succinimide
Barbiturates
Benzodiazepines
Carbamazepine
Divalproex
Felbamate
Gabapentin
Lacosamide
Lamotrigine
Levetiracetam
Oxcarbazepine
Primidone
Tiagabine
Topiramate
Valproic Acid
Zonisamide

Corneal Ulcers
Antibacterials (Ophthalmic)

**Crohn's Disease – See
Inflammatory Bowel Disease**

Cushing's Disease
Adrenocorticoids (Systemic)
Aminoglutethimide
Antifungals, Azoles
Metyrapone
Mitotane
Trilostane

Cystitis
Phenazopyridine
Sulfonamides &
Phenazopyridine
See also – Bacterial
Infections

Dandruff
Antifungals (Topical)
Antiseborrheics (Topical)
Coal Tar

Dementia
Buspirone
Cholinesterase Inhibitors
Ergoloid Mesylates
Haloperidol

Depression
Antidepressants, Tricyclic
Aripiprazole
Bupropion

Ergoloid Mesylates
Loxapine
Maprotiline
Mirtazapine
Monoamine Oxidase (MAO)
 Inhibitors
Monoamine Oxidase Type B
 (MAO-B) Inhibitors
Nefazodone
Selective Serotonin
 Reuptake Inhibitors
 (SSRIs)
Serotonin & Norepinephrine
 Reuptake Inhibitors
 (SNRIs)
Stimulant Medications
Trazodone

Dermatitis
Adrenocorticoids (Systemic)
Adrenocorticoids (Topical)
Anesthetics (Topical)
Antiseborrheics (Topical)
Coal Tar
Colchicine
Dapsone
Keratolytics

Dermatomyositis
Adrenocorticoids (Systemic)
Methotrexate

Diabetes
Acarbose
Colesevelam
DPP-4 Inhibitors
Exenatide
Insulin
Insulin Analogs
Meglitinides
Metformin
Miglitol
Pramlintide
Sulfonylureas
Thiazolidinediones

Diarrhea
Attapulgite
Bismuth Salts
Charcoal, Activated
Difenoxin & Atropine
Diphenoxylate & Atropine
Kaolin & Pectin
Kaolin, Pectin, Belladonna &
 Opium
Loperamide
Nitazoxanide
Paregoric
Rifaximin

Dietary Supplement
Calcium Supplements
Iron Supplements
Niacin
Vitamin A
Vitamin B-12
 (Cyanocobalamin)

Vitamin C (Ascorbic Acid)
Vitamin D
Vitamin E
Vitamin K
Zinc Supplements

Digestive Spasms
Clidinium
Dicyclomine
Difenoxin & Atropine
Hyoscyamine
Propantheline

Diverticulitis
Cephalosporins
Clindamycin
Fluoroquinolones
Nitroimidazoles
Penicillins

Drowsiness
Caffeine
Orphenadrine, Aspirin &
 Caffeine

Dry Eyes
Protectant (Ophthalmic)

Dry Mouth
Pilocarpine (Oral)

**Dysmenorrhea – See
Menstrual Cramps**

Ear Infections or Problems
Antibacterials (Otic)
Anti-Inflammatory Drugs,
 Steroidal (Otic)
Antipyrine & Benzocaine
 (Otic)
Phenylephrine
See also – Bacterial
 Infections

Ear Wax
Antipyrine & Benzocaine
 (Otic)

Eczema
Adrenocorticoids (Topical)
Antibacterials, Antifungals
 (Topical)
Coal Tar
Doxepin (Topical)
Keratolytics

Edema – See Fluid Retention

Emphysema
Adrenocorticoids (Systemic)
Bronchodilators, Adrenergic
Bronchodilators, Xanthine
Ipratropium
Tiotropium

Endometriosis
Danazol
Nafarelin

Epilepsy – See Convulsions

Erectile Dysfunction
Alprostadil
Erectile Dysfunction Agents
Papaverine

Esophagitis
Histamine H_2 Receptor
 Antagonists
Metoclopramide
Proton Pump Inhibitors

Estrogen Deficiency
Estrogens

Eye Allergies
Antiallergic Agents
 (Ophthalmic)

Eye Conditions
Antibacterials (Ophthalmic)
Cromolyn
Cycloplegic, Mydriatic
 (Ophthalmic)
Cyclopentolate (Ophthalmic)
Decongestants (Ophthalmic)
Natamycin (Ophthalmic)
Phenylephrine (Ophthalmic)

Fatigue
Caffeine

Fever
Acetaminophen
Anti-Inflammatory Drugs,
 Nonsteroidal (NSAIDs)
Aspirin
Barbiturates, Aspirin &
 Codeine
Narcotic Analgesics &
 Aspirin
Salicylates

Fibrocystic Breast Disease
Danazol
Vitamin E

Fibromyalgia
Pregabalin

Flu – See Influenza

Fluid Retention
Angiotensin-Converting
 Enzyme (ACE) Inhibitors &
 Hydrochlorothiazide
Carbonic Anhydrase
 Inhibitors
Clonidine & Chlorthalidone
Diuretics, Loop
Diuretics, Potassium-Sparing
Diuretics, Thiazide
Guanethidine &
 Hydrochlorothiazide
Hydralazine &
 Hydrochlorothiazide
Indapamide
Reserpine, Hydralazine &
 Hydrochlorothiazide

Eplerenone
Guanadrel
Guanethidine
Guanethidine &
  Hydrochlorothiazide
Hydralazine
Hydralazine &
  Hydrochlorothiazide
Indapamide
Mecamylamine
Minoxidil
Rauwolfia Alkaloids
Reserpine, Hydralazine &
  Hydrochlorothiazide

Hyperthyroidism
Antithyroid Drugs

Hypertriglyceridemia
Fibrates
Gemfibrozil
HMG-CoA Reductase
  Inhibitors
Omega-3-acid Ethyl Esters

Hypoglycemia
Glucagon

Hypothyroidism
Thyroid Hormones

**Impotence - See Erectile
Dysfunction**

Incontinence
Antidepressants, Tricyclic
Estrogens
Flavoxate
Muscarinic Receptor
  Antagonists

Indigestion – See Heartburn

Infertility
Bromocriptine
Clomiphene
Danazol
Progestins

Inflammation
Anti-Inflammatory Drugs,
  Nonsteroidal (NSAIDs)
Anti-Inflammatory Drugs,
  Nonsteroidal (NSAIDs)
  COX-2 Inhibitors
Aspirin
Mesalamine
Narcotic Analgesics &
  Aspirin
Salicylates

Inflammatory Bowel Disease
Adrenocorticoids (Systemic)
Cyclosporine
Infliximab
Mesalamine
Nitroimidazoles
Olsalazine

Influenza
Antivirals for Influenza
Antivirals for Influenza,
  Neuraminidase Inhibitors
Ribavirin

Insomnia
Barbiturates
Belladonna Alkaloids &
  Barbiturates
Benzodiazepines
Chloral Hydrate
Eszopiclone
Melatonin
Meprobamate
Ramelteon
Trazodone
Triazolam
Zaleplon
Zolpidem

Intermittent Claudication
Intermittent Claudication
  Agents
Pentoxifylline

**Irregular Heartbeat – See
Heart Rhythm Disorders**

Irritable Bowel Syndrome
Tegaserod

Itching
Adrenocorticoids (Topical)
Doxepin (Topical)

Jet Lag
Melatonin

Jock Itch
Antifungals (Topical)

Joint Pain
Anti-Inflammatory Drugs,
  Nonsteroidal (NSAIDs)
Anti-Inflammatory Drugs,
  Nonsteroidal (NSAIDs)
  COX-2 Inhibitors
Aspirin
Probenecid & Colchicine

Kidney Stones
Antigout Drugs
Cellulose Sodium Phosphate
Citrates
Diuretics, Thiazide
Penicillamine
Sodium Bicarbonate
Tiopronin

Labyrinthitis
Antihistamines,
  Phenothiazine-Derivative
Antihistamines, Piperazine
Benzodiazepines

Leg Pain or Cramps
Cyclandelate
Intermittent Claudication
  Agents
Orphenadrine
Pentoxifylline
Quinine

Leukemia
Imatinib
Thioguanine

Lice
Pediculicides

Lupus (Skin & Systemic)
Adrenocorticoids (Systemic)
Adrenocorticoids (Topical)
Anti-Inflammatory Drugs,
  Nonsteroidal (NSAIDs)
Anti-Inflammatory Drugs,
  Nonsteroidal (NSAIDs)
  COX-2 Inhibitors
Hydroxychloroquine
Methotrexate
Quinacrine

Lyme Disease
Cephalosporins
Erythromycins
Macrolide Antibiotics
Penicillins
Tetracyclines

Malabsorption
Quinacrine
Vitamin K

Malaria
Antimalarial
Atovaquone
Chloroquine
Hydroxychloroquine
Primaquine
Proguanil
Quinidine
Quinine
Sulfadoxine &
  Pyrimethamine
Tetracyclines

Male Hormone Deficiency
Androgens

Melanoma
Hydroxyurea
Levamisole
Melphalan

Meniere's Disease
Antihistamines
Antihistamines, Piperazine
Benzodiazepines
Scopolamine (Hyoscine)

Menopause
Estrogens
Progestins

Menstrual Cramps
Anti-Inflammatory Drugs,
Nonsteroidal (NSAIDs)
Anti-Inflammatory Drugs,
Nonsteroidal (NSAIDs)
COX-2 Inhibitors
Contraceptives, Oral & Skin

**Menstruation, Excessive
(Menorrhagia)**
Contraceptives, Oral & Skin
Danazol
Estrogens
Progestins

**Mental & Emotional
Disturbances**
Loxapine
Molindone
Rauwolfia Alkaloids
Serotonin-Dopamine
Antagonists

Motion Sickness
Antihistamines
Antihistamines, Nonsedating
Antihistamines,
Phenothiazine-Derivative
Antihistamines, Piperazine
Clotrimazole
Diphenidol
Scopolamine

Multiple Sclerosis
Adrenocorticoids (Systemic)
Baclofen
Tizanidine

**Muscle Cramp, Spasm,
Strain**
Baclofen
Cyclobenzaprine
Dantrolene
Muscle Relaxants, Skeletal
Orphenadrine
Orphenadrine, Aspirin &
Caffeine
Quinine
Tizanidine

Myasthenia Gravis
Adrenocorticoids (Systemic)
Antimyasthenics
Azathioprine
Cyclosporine

Narcolepsy
Amphetamines
Pemoline
Stimulant Medications
Stimulants, Amphetamine-
Related

Narcotic Withdrawal
Buprenorphine & Naloxone
Central Alpha Agonists
Naltrexone

Nasal Allergy
Adrenocorticoids (Nasal
Inhalation)
Antihistamines (Nasal)

Nausea & Vomiting
Antihistamines,
Phenothiazine-Derivative
Bismuth Salts
Diphenidol
Dronabinol
Hydroxyzine
Metoclopramide
Nabilone
Phenothiazines
Scopolamine
Trimethobenzamide

Nerve Disorders
Pregabalin

**Neural Tube Defects
(prevention)**
Folic Acid

Obesity
Appetite Suppressants
Orlistat
Selective Serotonin
Reuptake Inhibitors
(SSRIs)
Sibutramine

**Obsessive Compulsive
Disorder**
Antidepressants, Tricyclic
Selective Serotonin
Reuptake Inhibitors
(SSRIs)

Ocular Hypertension
Beta-Adrenergic Blocking
Agents (Ophthalmic)
Antiglaucoma, Carbonic
Anhydrase Inhibitors

Osteoarthritis – See Arthritis

Osteoporosis
Bisphosphonates
Bone Formation Agents
Calcitonin
Calcium Supplements
Estrogens
Raloxifene
Sodium Fluoride
Vitamin D

**Otitis Media – See Ear
Infection**

Overactive Bladder
Muscarinic Receptor
Antagonists

Paget's Disease
Bisphosphonates
Colchicine

Pain
Acetaminophen
Anti-Inflammatory Drugs,
Nonsteroidal (NSAIDs)
Anti-Inflammatory Drugs,
Nonsteroidal (NSAIDs)
COX-2 Inhibitors
Aspirin
Barbiturates, Aspirin &
Codeine
Butorphanol
Carbamazepine
Narcotic Analgesics
Narcotic Analgesics &
Acetaminophen
Narcotic Analgesics &
Aspirin
Orphenadrine, Aspirin &
Caffeine
Salicylates
Tramadol
Trazodone

Pain In Mouth
Anesthetics (Mucosal-Local)

Panic Disorder
Antidepressants, Tricyclic
Benzodiazepines
Monoamine Oxidase
Inhibitors

Parasites
Anthelmintics
Pentamidine

Parkinson's Disease
Antidyskinetics
Antihistamines
Antivirals for Influenza
Bromocriptine
Carbidopa & Levodopa
Levodopa
Monoamine Oxidase Type B
(MAO-B) Inhibitors
Orphenadrine
Tolcapone

Parkinson's Tremors
Antihistamines
Niacin

Peripheral Neuropathy
Serotonin & Norepinephrine
Reuptake Inhibitors
(SNRIs)

Peyronie's Disease
Aminobenzoate Potassium

Pneumocystis Jiroveci
Atovaquone
Dapsone
Primaquine
Trimethoprim

Pneumonia
Fluoroquinolones
Ribavirin
Sulfonamides

Pneumonia, Community Acquired
Telithromycin

Poisoning
Charcoal, Activated

Potassium Deficiency
Potassium Supplements

Premature Labor
Isoxsuprine
Ritodrine

Premenstrual Syndrome (PMS)
Antidepressants, Tricyclic
Anti-Inflammatory Drugs, Nonsteroidal (NSAIDs)
Buspirone
Calcium Supplements
Contraceptives, Oral & Skin
Danazol
Pyridoxine (Vitamin B-6)
Selective Serotonin Reuptake Inhibitors (SSRIs)
Vitamin E

Pressure Sores
Benzoyl Peroxide

Prostate Hyperplasia, Benign
5-Alpha Reductase Inhibitors
Alpha Adrenergic Receptor Blockers

Psoriasis
Adrenocorticoids (Topical)
Anthralin (Topical)
Biologics for Psoriasis
Coal Tar
Cyclosporine
Keratolytics
Methotrexate
Psoralens
Retinoids (Oral)
Retinoids (Topical)
Tumor Necrosis Factor Blockers
Vitamin D (Topical)

Psychotic Disorders
Aripiprazole
Carbamazepine
Clozapine
Haloperidol
Loxapine
Molindone
Olanzapine
Phenothiazines
Quetiapine

Serotonin-Dopamine Antagonists
Thiothixene
Ziprasidone

Pulmonary Arterial Hypertension (PAH)
Endothelin Receptor Antagonists

Rashes – See Skin Disorders

Rectal Fissures
Anesthetics (Rectal)

Respiratory Syncytial Virus (RSV)
Ribavirin

Restless Legs Syndrome
Antidyskinetics
Benzodiazepines
Carbidopa & Levodopa
Clonidine
Narcotic Analgesics

Rheumatoid Arthritis – See Arthritis

Rickets
Vitamin D

Ringworm – See Fungal Infections

Rosacea
Antibacterials (Topical)
Antibacterials for Acne (Topical)
Azelaic Acid
Benzoyl Peroxide
Nitroimidazoles
Tetracyclines

Scabies
Pediculicides

Schizophrenia
Aripiprazole
Carbamazepine
Clozapine
Haloperidol
Molindone
Olanzapine
Phenothiazines
Quetiapine
Serotonin-Dopamine Antagonists

Scleroderma
Aminobenzoate Potassium

Seasonal Affective Disorder (SAD)
Bupropion
Selective Serotonin Reuptake Inhibitors (SSRIs)

Seizures – See Convulsions

Shingles
Antivirals (Topical)
Antivirals for Herpes Virus
Capsaicin

Sickle Cell Disease
Hydroxyurea

Sinusitis
Cephalosporins
Erythromycins
Macrolide Antibiotics
Penicillins
Penicillins & Beta-Lactamase Inhibitors
Sulfonamides
Tetracyclines
Trimethoprim
Xylometazoline

Skin Cancer – See Cancer of the Skin

Skin Disorders
Anesthetics (Topical)
Antibacterials (Topical)
Antibacterials, Antifungals (Topical)
Cyclophosphamide
Condyloma Acuminatum Agents
Fluorouracil (Topical)
Isotretinoin
Neomycin (Topical)
Retinoids (Topical)

Skin Lines and Wrinkles
Botulinum Toxin Type A

Sleep Apnea
Antidepressants, Tricyclic
Progestins
Stimulants, Amphetamine-Related
Theophylline

Smoking Cessation
Bupropion
Central Alpha Agonists
Nicotine
Varenicline

Sore Throat
Anesthetics (Mucosal-Local)
See also – Bacterial Infections

Stroke Prevention
Platelet Inhibitors

Sunburn
Adrenocorticoids (Topical)
Anesthetics (Topical)

Swelling – See Fluid Retention

Thyroid Disorders – See Hyperthyroidism; Hypothyroidism

Tonsillitis
Cephalosporins
Macrolide Antibiotics

Tourette's Syndrome
Antidyskinetics
Haloperidol

Toxoplasmosis
Atovaquone

Transplantation, Organ (Antirejection)
Azathioprine
Cyclosporine
Immunosuppressive Agents

Tremors
Benzodiazepines
Beta-Adrenergic Blocking Agents

Trichomoniasis
Nitroimidazoles

Trigeminal Neuralgia
Baclofen
Carbamazepine

Tuberculosis
Cycloserine
Ethionamide
Isoniazid
Nitroimidazoles
Rifamycins

Ulcers
Antacids
Anticholinergics
Bismuth Salts
Glycopyrrolate
Histamine H_2 Receptor Antagonists
Nitroimidazoles
Proton Pump Inhibitors
Sodium Bicarbonate
Sucralfate
Tetracyclines

Ulcers, Skin
Becaplermin

Ulcerative Colitis
Olsalazine
Sulfasalazine

Urethra Spasms
Clidinium
Propantheline

Urethritis
Erythromycins
Fluoroquinolones
Macrolide Antibiotics
Phenazopyridine
Sulfonamides & Phenazopyridine
Tetracyclines

Urinary Frequency
Muscarinic Receptor Antagonists

Urinary Retention
Antimyasthenics
Bethanechol

Urinary Tract Infection
Acetohydroxamic Acid (AHA)
Atropine, Hyoscyamine, Methenamine
Cephalosporins
Cinoxacin
Cycloserine
Flavoxate
Fluoroquinolones
Methenamine
Penicillins
Penicillins & Beta-Lactamase Inhibitors
Phenazopyridine
Sulfonamides
Tetracyclines
Trimethoprim

Urine Acidity
Citrates
Vitamin C

Uveitis
Anti-Inflammatory Drugs, Steroidal (Ophthalmic)

Vaginal Infections or Irritation
Clindamycin
Estrogens
Nitroimidazoles
Progestins

Vaginal Yeast Infections
Antifungals (Vaginal)

Vertigo
Antihistamines, Piperazine
Niacin

Virus Infections Of The Eye
Antivirals (Ophthalmic)

Vitamin Deficiency
Pantothenic Acid
Riboflavin
Vitamin A
Vitamin B-12
Vitamin C
Vitamin D
Vitamin E
Vitamin K

Vitiligo
Psoralens

Vomiting – See Nausea & Vomiting

Warts
Keratolytics
Retinoids (Topical)

Wilson's Disease
Penicillamine
Zinc Supplements

Worms
Anthelmintics

Zinc Deficiency
Zinc Supplements

DRUG CHARTS

5-ALPHA REDUCTASE INHIBITORS

GENERIC AND BRAND NAMES

FINASTERIDE
  Propecia
  Proscar

DUTASTERIDE
  Avodart
  Duagen
  Neulasta

BASIC INFORMATION

Habit forming? No
Prescription needed? Yes
Available as generic? Yes, for some
Drug class: Dihydrotestosterone inhibitor

USES

- Treats noncancerous enlargement of the prostate gland in men (benign prostatic hypertrophy or BPH).
- Theoretically, may prevent the development of prostate cancer. Studies are ongoing.
- Treatment of male pattern hair loss in men.

DOSAGE & USAGE INFORMATION

How to take:
Tablet or capsule—Swallow with liquid. If you can't swallow whole, crumble tablet and take with liquid or food.

When to take:
Once a day or as directed, with or without meals.

If you forget a dose:
Take as soon as you remember up to 2 hours late. If more than 2 hours, wait for next scheduled dose (don't double this dose).

What drug does:
Inhibits the enzyme needed for the conversion of testosterone to dihydrotestosterone. Dihydrotestosterone is required for the development of benign prostatic hypertrophy.

Continued next column

 OVERDOSE

SYMPTOMS:
Effects unknown.
WHAT TO DO:
Overdose unlikely to threaten life. If person uses much larger amount than prescribed or if accidentally swallowed, call doctor or poison control center 1-800-222-1222 for help.

Time lapse before drug works:
- May require up to 6 months for full therapeutic effect for BPH.
- For treatment of hair loss, may not see any benefit for 3 months or more.

Don't take with:
Any other medicine or dietary supplement without consulting your doctor or pharmacist, especially nonprescription decongestants.

 POSSIBLE ADVERSE REACTIONS OR SIDE EFFECTS

SYMPTOMS	WHAT TO DO
Life-threatening: None expected.	
Common: None expected.	
Infrequent: Decreased volume of ejaculation, back or stomach pain, headache.	Continue. Call doctor when convenient.
Rare:	
• Impotence, decreased libido, breast enlargement and tenderness.	Continue. Call doctor when convenient.
• Allergic reaction (skin rash, swelling of lips).	Discontinue. Call doctor right away.

WARNINGS & PRECAUTIONS

Don't take if:
* You are allergic to dutasteride or finasteride.
* You are a female, are pregnant, or a child.

Before you start, consult your doctor if:
* You have not had a blood test to check for prostate cancer.
* Your sexual partner is pregnant or may become pregnant.
* You have a liver disorder.
* You have reduced urinary flow.
* You have large residual urinary volume.

Over age 60:
No special problems expected.

Pregnancy:
* Not recommended for women.
* Pregnant women should not handle the crushed tablets.
* Ask your doctor if you should avoid exposure to mate's semen if he takes these drugs.
* Risk category X (see page xviii).

Breast-feeding:
Not recommended for women.

Infants & children:
Not recommended.

Prolonged use:
Talk to your doctor about the need for follow-up medical examinations or laboratory studies to check the effectiveness of the treatment.

Skin & sunlight:
No special problems expected.

Driving, piloting or hazardous work:
No special problems expected.

Discontinuing:
Don't discontinue without medical advice.

Others:
* Advise any doctor or dentist whom you consult that you take this medicine.
* May affect results of some medical tests (especially prostate specific antigen [PSA] which is a test for prostate cancer).
* For those who respond well, the drug must be continued indefinitely.

 ## POSSIBLE INTERACTION WITH OTHER DRUGS

GENERIC NAME OR DRUG CLASS	COMBINED EFFECT
None expected.	

 ## POSSIBLE INTERACTION WITH OTHER SUBSTANCES

INTERACTS WITH	COMBINED EFFECT
Alcohol:	No proven problems.
Beverages:	Grapefruit juice may increase effect of finasteride.
Cocaine:	No proven problems.
Foods:	No proven problems.
Marijuana:	No proven problems.
Tobacco:	No proven problems.

*See Glossary

ACAMPROSATE

BRAND NAMES

Campral

BASIC INFORMATION

Habit forming? No
Prescription needed? Yes
Available as generic? No
Drug class: Alcohol-abuse deterrent

 ## USES

Treatment for alcohol dependence. It is used after alcohol withdrawal to help maintain abstinence by reducing cravings. The drug should be part of a complete treatment plan (e.g., counseling, behavior therapy and support of family and friends). The drug does not diminish or eliminate withdrawal symptoms.

 ## DOSAGE & USAGE INFORMATION

How to take:
Tablet—Swallow whole with liquid. May be taken with or without food.

When to take:
Usually three times a day at the same time each day (such as at mealtimes).

If you forget a dose:
Take as soon as you remember. If it is almost time for the next dose, wait for that dose (don't double this dose) and resume regular schedule.

What drug does:
Action is not fully understood. It appears to affect chemicals (called neurotransmitters) in the brain and reduces the craving for alcohol.

Time lapse before drug works:
About one week.

Don't take with:
Any other medicine or any dietary supplement without consulting your doctor or pharmacist.

 ## OVERDOSE

SYMPTOMS:
Diarrhea and possibly other symptoms.
WHAT TO DO:
Overdose unlikely to threaten life. If person uses much larger amount than prescribed or if accidentally swallowed, call doctor or poison control center 1-800-222-1222 for help.

 ## POSSIBLE ADVERSE REACTIONS OR SIDE EFFECTS

SYMPTOMS	WHAT TO DO
Life-threatening: None expected.	
Common: Diarrhea, dizziness, itching, nausea, gas, bloating, vomiting, abdominal pain, headache, insomnia.	Continue. Call doctor when convenient.
Infrequent: Depression, anxiety, increase or decrease in sexual desire, rash or other skin reaction, heart palpitations, fainting, muscle pain, swelling (face, feet or ankles).	Continue. Call doctor when convenient.
Rare: • Thoughts of suicide or patient talks of suicide.	Discontinue. Get emergency help.
• Low blood pressure, increased heart rate, other symptoms that may occur (can be due to the drug or are a result of alcohol abuse or alcohol withdrawal symptoms).	Continue. Call doctor when convenient.

WARNINGS & PRECAUTIONS

Don't take if:
You are allergic to acamprosate.

Before you start, consult your doctor if:
- You have kidney (renal) disease or severe kidney impairment.
- You suffer from depression or have thoughts about suicide.

Over age 60:
No special problems expected.

Pregnancy:
Decide with your doctor if drug benefits justify risk to unborn child. Risk category C. (See page xviii).

Breast-feeding:
It is unknown if drug passes into milk. Avoid drug or discontinue nursing until you finish medicine. Consult doctor for advice on maintaining milk supply.

Infants & children:
Safety and effectiveness of use in children under age 18 not established.

Prolonged use:
Talk to your doctor about the need for follow-up medical examinations or laboratory studies to determine drug's effectiveness and to monitor for symptoms and suicidal thoughts.

Skin & sunlight:
No problems expected.

Driving, piloting or hazardous work:
- Avoid if the drug makes you feel dizzy, otherwise no problems expected.
- If you start drinking alcohol again, avoid driving, piloting or hazardous work.

Discontinuing:
Do not stop taking acamprosate without talking to your doctor. Continue taking acamprosate even if you start drinking alcohol again.

Others:
- Advise any doctor or dentist whom you consult that you take this medicine.
- Drug may affect the accuracy of some medical tests.
- Contact your doctor if you develop symptoms of depression, have suicidal thoughts or start drinking alcohol again.

POSSIBLE INTERACTION WITH OTHER DRUGS

GENERIC NAME OR DRUG CLASS	COMBINED EFFECT
None expected.	

POSSIBLE INTERACTION WITH OTHER DRUGS

INTERACTS WITH	COMBINED EFFECT
Alcohol:	None expected, but all alcohol should be avoided.
Beverages:	None expected.
Cocaine:	Effects unknown. Avoid.
Foods:	None expected. Avoid foods that contain alcohol.
Marijuana:	Effects unknown. Avoid.
Tobacco:	None expected.

ACARBOSE

BRAND NAMES

Precose

BASIC INFORMATION

Habit forming? No
Prescription needed? Yes
Available as generic? Yes
Drug class: Antihyperglycemic, antidiabetic

 ## USES

Treatment for hyperglycemia (excess sugar in the blood) that cannot be controlled by diet alone in patients with type 2 diabetes. It may be used alone or in combination with other antidiabetic drugs.

 ## DOSAGE & USAGE INFORMATION

How to take:
Tablet—Swallow with liquid. Take at the very beginning of a meal.

When to take:
Usually 3 times a day or as directed by doctor. Dosage may be increased at 4- to 8-week intervals until maximum benefits are achieved.

Continued next column

 ## OVERDOSE

SYMPTOMS:
* Symptoms of lactic acidosis (acid in the blood)—chills, diarrhea, severe muscle pain, sleepiness, slow heartbeat, breathing difficulty, unusual weakness.
* Symptoms of hypoglycemia (not a problem with acarbose used alone)—stomach pain, anxious feeling, cold sweats, chills, confusion, convulsions, cool pale skin, excessive hunger, nausea or vomiting, rapid heartbeat, nervousness, shakiness, unsteady walk, unusual weakness or tiredness, vision changes, unconsciousness.

WHAT TO DO:
* For mild low blood sugar symptoms, drink or eat something containing sugar right away.
* For more severe symptoms, dial 911 (emergency) for medical help or call doctor or poison control center 1-800-222-1222 for instructions.
* See emergency information on last 3 pages of this book.

If you forget a dose:
Take as soon as you remember. If it is almost time for the next dose, then skip the missed dose and wait for your next scheduled dose (don't double this dose).

What drug does:
Impedes the digestion and absorption of carbohydrates and their subsequent conversion into glucose, improving control of blood glucose, and may reduce the complications of diabetes. However, acarbose does not cure diabetes.

Time lapse before drug works:
May take several weeks for full effectiveness.

Don't take with:
Any other medicine or any dietary supplement without consulting your doctor or pharmacist.

 ## POSSIBLE ADVERSE REACTIONS OR SIDE EFFECTS

SYMPTOMS	WHAT TO DO
Life-threatening:	
In case of overdose or low blood sugar, see previous column.	
Common:	
Diarrhea, stomach cramps, gas, bloating, feeling of fullness in stomach, nausea.	Continue. Call doctor when convenient.
Infrequent:	
None expected.	
Rare:	
Lactic acidosis or severe low blood sugar (see symptoms under Overdose).	Discontinue. Call doctor right away or seek emergency help.

WARNINGS & PRECAUTIONS

Don't take if:
You are allergic to acarbose.

Before you start, consult your doctor if:
- You have any kidney or liver disease or any heart or blood vessel disorder.
- You have any chronic health problem.
- You have an infection, illness or any condition that can cause low blood sugar.
- You have a history of acid in the blood (metabolic acidosis or ketoacidosis).
- You have inflammatory bowel disease or any other intestinal disorder.
- You are allergic to any medication, food or other substance.

Over age 60:
No special problems expected. A lower starting dosage may be recommended by your doctor.

Pregnancy:
Decide with your doctor if drug benefits justify risks to unborn child. Risk category B (see page xviii).

Breast-feeding:
It is unknown if drug passes into milk. Avoid drug or discontinue nursing until you finish medicine. Consult doctor for advice on maintaining milk supply.

Infants & children:
Safety and efficacy have not been established. Use only under close medical supervision.

Prolonged use:
- Schedule regular doctor visits to determine if the drug is continuing to be effective in controlling the diabetes and to check for any problems in kidney function.
- You will most likely require an antidiabetic medicine for the rest of your life.
- You will need to test your blood glucose levels several times a day, or for some, once to several times a week.
- Acarbose may reduce absorption of iron, causing anemia. Discuss with your doctor.

Skin & sunlight:
No special problems expected.

Driving, piloting or hazardous work:
No special problems expected.

Discontinuing:
Don't discontinue without consulting your doctor even if you feel well. You can have diabetes without feeling any symptoms. Untreated diabetes can cause serious problems.

Others:
- Advise any doctor or dentist whom you consult that you take this medicine. Drug may interfere with the accuracy of some medical tests.
- Follow any special diet your doctor may prescribe. It can help control diabetes.
- Consult doctor if you become ill with vomiting or diarrhea.
- Use caution when exercising. Ask your doctor about an appropriate exercise program.
- Wear medical identification stating that you have diabetes and take this medication.
- Learn to recognize the symptoms of low blood sugar. You and your family need to know what to do if these symptoms occur.
- Have a glucagon kit and syringe in the event severe low blood sugar occurs.
- High blood sugar (hyperglycemia) may occur with diabetes. Ask your doctor about symptoms to watch for and treatment steps to take.
- Educate yourself about diabetes.

POSSIBLE INTERACTION WITH OTHER DRUGS

GENERIC NAME OR DRUG CLASS	COMBINED EFFECT
Amylase (Pancreatic enzyme)	Decreased acarbose effect.
Charcoal, activated	Decreased acarbose effect.
Hyperglycemia-causing medications*	Increased risk of hyperglycemia.
Metformin	Decreased acarbose effect. Increased risk of side effects.
Pancreatin (Pancreatic enzyme)	Decreased acarbose effect.
Pramlintide	Decreased absorption of nutrients.

POSSIBLE INTERACTION WITH OTHER SUBSTANCES

INTERACTS WITH	COMBINED EFFECT
Alcohol:	May increase effect of acarbose. Avoid excessive amounts.
Beverages:	No special problems.
Cocaine:	No special problems.
Foods:	No special problems.
Marijuana:	No special problems.
Tobacco:	No special problems.

ACETAMINOPHEN

BRAND NAMES

See full list of brand names in the *Generic and Brand Name Directory*, page 864.

BASIC INFORMATION

Habit forming? No
Prescription needed? No
Available as generic? Yes
Drug class: Analgesic, fever reducer

 ## USES

Treatment of mild to moderate pain and fever. Acetaminophen does not relieve redness, stiffness or swelling of joints or tissue inflammation. Use other drugs for inflammation.

 ## DOSAGE & USAGE INFORMATION

How to take:
- Note—Acetaminophen comes in several dosage forms and is also an ingredient in many cold, cough and flu remedies. Read labels carefully. Do not use, or give, more than the dosage recommended for adults or children. Too much acetaminophen can result in liver or kidney damage.
- Tablet or capsule—Swallow with liquid. Do not open, crush or chew tablet or capsule.
- Chewable tablet—Chew and swallow.
- Liquid drops—Follow package instructions.
- Liquid—Follow instructions on label.
- Powder—Mix as instructed with water or other liquid and swallow. May be mixed with small amount of food and eaten.
- Granules—Mix with a small amount of apple-sauce, ice cream or jam and eat.
- Rectal suppository—Remove wrapper and moisten suppository with water. Gently insert into rectum. Push well into rectum with finger.

Continued next column

 ## OVERDOSE

SYMPTOMS:
Stomach upset, irritability, sweating, diarrhea, loss of appetite, abdominal cramps, convulsions, coma.
WHAT TO DO:
- **Call your doctor or poison control center 1-800-222-1222 for help if you suspect overdose, even if not sure. Symptoms may not appear until damage has occurred.**
- **See emergency information on last 3 pages of this book.**

When to take:
As needed, depending on the dosage. May range from 3-8 hours between dosages.

If you forget a dose:
Take as soon as you remember. Wait 3-8 hours for next dose (depending on dosage used).

What drug does:
Exact mechanism is not fully known. Blocks pain impulses in central nervous system. Reduces fever by acting on the hypothalamic heat regulating center.

Time lapse before drug works:
15 to 30 minutes. May last 4 or more hours.

Don't take with:
- Other drugs that contain acetaminophen. An overdose may occur.
- Any other medicine or any dietary supplement without consulting your doctor or pharmacist.

 ## POSSIBLE ADVERSE REACTIONS OR SIDE EFFECTS

SYMPTOMS	WHAT TO DO
Life-threatening: In case of overdose, see previous column.	
Common: None expected.	
Infrequent: None expected.	
Rare: Extreme fatigue; rash, itch, hives; sore throat and fever; unexplained bleeding or bruising; blood in urine; painful, decreased or frequent urination; yellow skin or eyes, black or tarry stools, illness symptoms not present before taking drug (sore throat, pain, fever).	Discontinue. Call doctor right away.

ACETAMINOPHEN

 **WARNINGS &
PRECAUTIONS**

Don't take if:
You are allergic to acetaminophen or aspirin.

Before you start, consult your doctor if:
• You have kidney or liver disease.
• You drink 3 or more alcoholic drinks a day.

Over age 60:
No problems expected as long as proper dosage is taken.

Pregnancy:
No proven harm to unborn child. Avoid if possible. Consult doctor. Risk category B (see page xviii).

Breast-feeding:
No proven harm to nursing infant.

Infants & children:
Read the label on the product to see if it is approved for your child's age. Always follow the directions on product's label about how to use. If unsure, ask your doctor or pharmacist.

Prolonged use:
• May affect blood system and cause anemia. Limit use to 5 days for children 12 and under, and 10 days for adults.
• Talk to your doctor about the need for follow-up medical examinations or laboratory studies to check liver function, kidney function.

Skin & sunlight:
No problems expected.

Driving, piloting or hazardous work:
Avoid if you feel drowsy. Otherwise, no restrictions.

Discontinuing:
Discontinue in 3-10 days if symptoms don't improve.

Others:
• May interfere with the accuracy of some medical tests.
• Advise any doctor or dentist whom you consult that you take this medicine (if you take it regularly).
• Diabetic patients may get false blood glucose results while taking this drug. Check with the doctor if any changes occur.
• If the sore throat or fever symptoms don't improve after 2-3 days use, or if pain symptoms continue more than 5-10 days, call your doctor.

 **POSSIBLE INTERACTION
WITH OTHER DRUGS**

GENERIC NAME OR DRUG CLASS	COMBINED EFFECT
Anticoagulants, oral*	May increase anticoagulant effect. If combined frequently, prothrombin time should be monitored.
Anti-inflammatory drugs, nonsteroidal (NSAIDs)	Increased risk of adverse effects of both drugs.
Aspirin and other salicylates*	Increased risk of adverse effects of both drugs.
Caffeine-containing products	May increase stimulant effect. Take 8-12 hours apart.
Enzyme inducers*	Increased risk of liver damage.
Hepatotoxic medications*	Increased risk of liver damage.

 **POSSIBLE INTERACTION
WITH OTHER SUBSTANCES**

INTERACTS WITH	COMBINED EFFECT
Alcohol:	Drowsiness; long-term use may cause toxic effect in liver.
Beverages:	None expected.
Cocaine:	None expected. However, cocaine may slow body's recovery. Avoid.
Foods:	None expected.
Marijuana:	Increased pain relief. However, marijuana may slow body's recovery. Avoid.
Tobacco:	None expected.

ACETOHYDROXAMIC ACID (AHA)

BRAND NAMES

Lithostat

BASIC INFORMATION

Habit forming? No
Prescription needed? Yes
Available as generic? No
Drug class: Antibacterial (antibiotic), antiurolithic

 USES

- Treatment for chronic urinary tract infections.
- Prevents formation of urinary tract stones. Will not dissolve stones already present.

 DOSAGE & USAGE INFORMATION

How to take:
Tablet—Swallow with liquid. If you can't swallow whole, crumble tablet and take with liquid or food.

When to take:
At the same time each day, according to instructions on prescription label.

If you forget a dose:
Take as soon as you remember up to 2 hours late. If more than 2 hours, wait for next scheduled dose (don't double this dose).

What drug does:
Stops enzyme action that makes urine too alkaline. Alkaline urine favors bacterial growth and stone formation and growth.

Time lapse before drug works:
1 to 3 weeks.

Don't take with:
- Alcohol or iron supplement.
- Any other medicine or any dietary supplement without consulting your doctor or pharmacist.

 OVERDOSE

SYMPTOMS:
Loss of appetite, tremor, nausea, vomiting.
WHAT TO DO:
Overdose unlikely to threaten life. If person uses much larger amount than prescribed or if accidentally swallowed, call doctor or poison control center 1-800-222-1222 for help.

 POSSIBLE ADVERSE REACTIONS OR SIDE EFFECTS

SYMPTOMS	WHAT TO DO
Life-threatening: In case of overdose, see previous column.	
Common: Appetite loss, nausea, vomiting, anxiety, depression, mild headache, unusual tiredness.	Continue. Call doctor when convenient.
Infrequent:	
• Loss of coordination, slurred speech, severe headache, sudden change in vision, shortness of breath, clot or pain over a blood vessel, sudden chest pain, leg pain in calf (deep vein blood clot).	Discontinue. Seek emergency treatment.
• Rash on arms and face.	Continue. Call doctor when convenient.
Rare:	
• Sore throat, fever, unusual bleeding, bruising.	Discontinue. Call doctor right away.
• Hair loss.	Continue. Call doctor when convenient.

ACETOHYDROXAMIC ACID (AHA)

WARNINGS & PRECAUTIONS

Don't take if:
You have severe chronic kidney disease.

Before you start, consult your doctor if:
- You are anemic.
- You have or have had phlebitis or thrombophlebitis.

Over age 60:
Adverse reactions and side effects may be more frequent and severe than in younger persons.

Pregnancy:
Studies inconclusive on harm to unborn child. Animal studies show fetal abnormalities. Don't use. Risk category X (see page xviii).

Breast-feeding:
Studies inconclusive. May have a potential for adverse reactions in nursing children. Avoid drug or discontinue nursing until you finish medicine. Consult doctor on maintaining milk supply.

Infants & children:
Not recommended. Safety and dosage have not been established.

Prolonged use:
Talk to your doctor about the need for follow-up medical examinations or laboratory studies to check blood pressure, liver function, kidney function, urinary pH.

Skin & sunlight:
No problems expected.

Driving, piloting or hazardous work:
Don't drive or pilot aircraft until you learn how medicine affects you. Don't work around dangerous machinery. Don't climb ladders or work in high places. Danger increases if you drink alcohol or take medicine affecting alertness and reflexes, such as antihistamines, tranquilizers, sedatives, pain medicines, narcotics and mind-altering drugs.

Discontinuing:
Don't discontinue without consulting doctor. Dose may require gradual reduction if you have taken drug for a long time. Doses of other drugs may also require adjustment.

Others:
No problems expected.

POSSIBLE INTERACTION WITH OTHER DRUGS

GENERIC NAME OR DRUG CLASS	COMBINED EFFECT
Iron	Decreased effects of both drugs.

POSSIBLE INTERACTION WITH OTHER SUBSTANCES

INTERACTS WITH	COMBINED EFFECT
Alcohol:	Severe skin rash common in many patients within 30 to 45 minutes after drinking alcohol.
Beverages:	None expected.
Cocaine:	None expected.
Foods:	None expected.
Marijuana:	None expected.
Tobacco:	None expected.

ADRENOCORTICOIDS (Nasal Inhalation)

GENERIC AND BRAND NAMES

BECLOMETHASONE
(nasal)
Beconase
Beconase AQ
Vancenase
Vancenase AQ
BUDESONIDE
(nasal)
Rhinocort Aqua
Rhinocort Nasal
Inhaler
Rhinocort Turbuhaler
CICLESONIDE
(nasal)
Omnaris
DEXAMETHASONE
(nasal)
Dexacort Turbinaire

FLUNISOLIDE
(nasal)
Nasalide
Nasarel
Rhinalar
FLUTICASONE
(nasal)
Flonase
Veramyst
MOMETASONE
(nasal)
Asmanex
Nasonex
Nasonex Aqueous
Nasal Spray
TRIAMCINOLONE
(nasal)
AllerNaze
Nasacort AQ
Nasacort HFA
Tri-Nasal

BASIC INFORMATION

Habit forming? No
Prescription needed? Yes
Available as generic? Yes, for some
Drug class: Adrenocorticoid (nasal); anti-inflammatory (steroidal), nasal

 ## USES

- Treats allergic conditions such as hay fever (seasonal rhinitis).
- Treats nasal polyps and noninfectious-inflammatory nasal conditions.

Continued next column

 ## OVERDOSE

SYMPTOMS:
None expected.
WHAT TO DO:
Overdose unlikely to threaten life. If person uses much larger amount than prescribed or if accidentally swallowed, call doctor or poison control center 1-800-222-1222 for help.

 ## DOSAGE & USAGE INFORMATION

How to take:
Spray—Read patient instruction sheet supplied with your prescription. Usually 1 or 2 sprays into each nostril every 12 hours. Save container for possible refills.

When to take:
At the same time each day, according to instructions on prescription label.

If you forget a dose:
Use as soon as you remember up to an hour late. If you remember more than an hour late, skip this dose. Don't double the next dose.

What drug does:
- Subdues inflammation by decreasing secretion of prostaglandins in cells of the lining of the nose and by inhibiting release of histamine.
- Very little, if any, of the nasal adrenocorticoid gets absorbed into the bloodstream.

Time lapse before drug works:
Usually 5 to 7 days, but may be as long as 2 to 3 weeks.

Don't take with:
Any other medicine or any dietary supplement without consulting your doctor or pharmacist.

 ## POSSIBLE ADVERSE REACTIONS OR SIDE EFFECTS

SYMPTOMS	WHAT TO DO
Life-threatening: None expected.	
Common: Burning or dryness of nose, sneezing.	Continue. Call doctor when convenient.
Infrequent: Crusting inside the nose, nosebleed, sore throat, ulcers in nose, cough, dizziness, headache, hoarseness, nausea, runny nose, bloody mucus.	Discontinue. Call doctor right away.
Rare: • White patches in nose or throat.	Discontinue. Call doctor right away.
• Eye pain, wheezing respiration.	Discontinue. Seek emergency treatment.

ADRENOCORTICOIDS (Nasal Inhalation)

 ## WARNINGS & PRECAUTIONS

Don't take if:
You are allergic to cortisone or any cortisone-like medication.

Before you start, consult your doctor if:
- You are allergic to any of the propellants in the spray. These include benzalkonium chloride, disodium acetate, phenylethanol, fluorocarbons and propylene glycol.
- You have sores in the nose, have had recent surgery or injury involving the nose.
- You have amebiasis, asthma, type 2 diabetes, glaucoma, herpes eye infection, liver disease, tuberculosis, underactive thyroid, any heart condition or any infection.

Over age 60:
No special problems expected.

Pregnancy:
Risk factors vary for drugs in this group. See category list on page xviii and consult doctor.

Breast-feeding:
Drug may pass into milk. Avoid drug or discontinue nursing until you finish medicine. Consult doctor on maintaining milk supply.

Infants & children:
- Approval for use in children varies for these drugs (ranging from ages over 2, 4 and 6).
- Adrenocorticoids taken by mouth may slow or decrease growth rate or cause reduced adrenal gland function. The nasal form is generally considered safer than the oral form. Be sure you and your child's doctor discuss all benefits and risks of the drug.

Prolonged use:
Not recommended.

Skin & sunlight:
No special problems expected.

Driving, piloting or hazardous work:
Don't drive or pilot aircraft until you learn how medicine affects you. Don't work around dangerous machinery. Don't climb ladders or work in high places. Danger increases if you drink alcohol or take medicine affecting alertness and reflexes.

Discontinuing:
No special problems expected.

Others:
Advise any doctor or dentist whom you consult that you use this medicine.

 ## POSSIBLE INTERACTION WITH OTHER DRUGS

GENERIC NAME OR DRUG CLASS	COMBINED EFFECT
Ephedrine	Decreased effect of nasal adrenocorticoid.
Phenobarbital	Decreased effect of nasal adrenocorticoid.
Rifampin	Decreased effect of nasal adrenocorticoid.
Ritonavir	Increased effect of fluticasone.

 ## POSSIBLE INTERACTION WITH OTHER SUBSTANCES

INTERACTS WITH	COMBINED EFFECT
Alcohol:	None expected.
Beverages:	None expected.
Cocaine:	None expected.
Foods:	None expected.
Marijuana:	None expected.
Tobacco:	None expected.

ADRENOCORTICOIDS (Oral Inhalation)

GENERIC AND BRAND NAMES

BECLOMETHASONE
(oral inhalation)
Beclodisk
Becloforte
Qvar
Vanceril
BUDESONIDE
(oral inhalation)
Pulmicort Flexhaler
Pulmicort Respules
Symbicort
CICLESONIDE
(oral inhalation)
Alvesco Inhalation
DEXAMETHASONE
(oral inhalation)
Decadron Respihaler

FLUNISOLIDE
(oral inhalation)
Aerobid
Aerobid-M
Aerospan
Bronalide
FLUTICASONE
(oral inhalation)
Advair Diskus
Advair HFA
Flovent
Flovent HFA
TRIAMCINOLONE
(oral inhalation)
Azmacort

BASIC INFORMATION

Habit forming? No
Prescription needed? Yes
Available as generic? No
Drug class: Anti-inflammatory (inhalation), antiasthmatic

 ## USES

Treatment for prevention of symptoms in patients with chronic bronchial asthma. Does not relieve the symptoms of an acute asthma attack.

 ## DOSAGE & USAGE INFORMATION

How to take:
Oral inhaler—Follow instructions that come with your prescription or take as directed by your doctor. If you don't understand the instructions or have any questions, consult your doctor or pharmacist. Most effective if taken regularly. More effective if taken with a spacer. Talk with your doctor or pharmacist.

Continued next column

 ## OVERDOSE

SYMPTOMS:
None expected.
WHAT TO DO:
Overdose unlikely to threaten life. If person uses much larger amount than prescribed or if accidentally swallowed, call doctor or poison control center 1-800-222-1222 for help.

When to take:
Your doctor will determine the dosage amount and schedule that will help control the asthma symptoms and lessen risks of side effects. Usually 1 to 2 inhaled puffs 3 to 4 times a day is sufficient.

If you forget a dose:
Take as soon as you remember. Then spread out the remaining doses for that day at regularly spaced intervals.

What drug does:
Helps prevent inflammation in the lungs and breathing passages. May decrease progression of severe disease.

Time lapse before drug works:
1 to 4 weeks for the initial response and up to several months for full benefits.

Don't take with:
Any other medicine or any dietary supplement without consulting your doctor or pharmacist.

 ## POSSIBLE ADVERSE REACTIONS OR SIDE EFFECTS

SYMPTOMS	WHAT TO DO
Life-threatening: None expected.	
Common: Dry mouth, cough, throat irritation, hoarseness or other voice changes.	Continue. Call doctor when convenient.
Infrequent: Dry throat, headache, nausea, skin bruising, unpleasant taste, white curd-like patches in mouth or throat, pain when eating or swallowing (thrush).	Continue. Call doctor when convenient.
Rare: Increased wheezing; difficulty in breathing; pain, tightness or burning in chest; behavior changes (restlessness, nervousness, depression) with budesonide.	Continue, but call doctor right away.

14

ADRENOCORTICOIDS (Oral Inhalation)

WARNINGS & PRECAUTIONS

Don't use if:
You are allergic to any corticosteroids.*

Before you start, consult your doctor if:
* You have osteoporosis.
* You have or have had tuberculosis.
* You are taking oral corticosteroid drugs.

Over age 60:
No special problems expected.

Pregnancy:
Risk factors may vary for drugs in this group. See category list on page xviii and consult doctor.

Breast-feeding:
Unknown effect. Decide with your doctor if you should continue breast-feeding while using this drug.

Infants & children:
* Should be safe with regular low-dosage regimen. These drugs may slow or decrease growth rate or cause reduced adrenal gland function. Be sure you and your child's doctor discuss all benefits and risks of the drug.
* Children using large doses of this drug are more susceptible to infectious disease (chicken pox, measles). Avoid exposure to infected people and keep all immunizations up to date.

Prolonged use:
* Talk to your doctor about the need for follow-up medical examinations or laboratory studies to check adrenal function, growth and development in children, pulmonary function, and inhalation technique.
* The drug may lose its effectiveness. If this occurs, consult your doctor.

Skin & sunlight:
No special problems expected.

Driving, piloting or hazardous work:
No special problems expected.

Discontinuing:
Don't discontinue this drug after prolonged use without consulting doctor. Dosage may require a gradual reduction before stopping to avoid any withdrawal symptoms.

Others:
* Advise any doctor or dentist whom you consult that you use this medicine.
* Carry or wear identification to state that you use this medicine.
* Call your doctor if you have any injury, infection or other stress to your body.
* Take medicine only as directed. Do not increase or reduce dosage without doctor's approval.

POSSIBLE INTERACTION WITH OTHER DRUGS

GENERIC NAME OR DRUG CLASS	COMBINED EFFECT
None significant.	

POSSIBLE INTERACTION WITH OTHER SUBSTANCES

INTERACTS WITH	COMBINED EFFECT
Alcohol:	None expected.
Beverages:	None expected.
Cocaine:	Effects not known. Best to avoid.
Foods:	None expected.
Marijuana:	Effects not known. Best to avoid.
Tobacco:	Asthma patients should avoid.

*See Glossary

ADRENOCORTICOIDS (Systemic)

GENERIC AND BRAND NAMES

See full list of generic and brand names in the *Generic and Brand Name Directory*, page 866.

BASIC INFORMATION

Habit forming? No
Prescription needed? Yes
Available as generic? Yes
Drug class: Corticosteroid, anti-inflammatory (steroidal), immunosuppressant

USES

- Used for their anti-inflammatory and immuno-suppressive effect in the treatment of many medical problems including some cancers.
- Treatment for some allergic diseases, blood disorders, kidney diseases, asthma and emphysema.
- Treats mild to moderate Crohn's disease.
- Replaces corticosteroid lost due to adrenal deficiencies.

DOSAGE & USAGE INFORMATION

How to take:
- Tablet, capsule or liquid—Swallow with liquid or food to lessen stomach irritation. If you can't swallow whole, crumble tablet or open capsules.
- Oral disintegrating tablet—Let tablet dissolve in mouth. Do not chew or swallow tablet.
- Oral suspension—Follow instructions on label.
- Enema—Follow package instructions.

When to take:
At the same times each day. Take once-a-day or once-every-other-day doses in mornings.

If you forget a dose:
Take as soon as you remember up to 2 hours late. If more than 2 hours, wait for next scheduled dose (don't double this dose).

Continued next column

OVERDOSE

SYMPTOMS:
Severe headache, retained fluids, convulsions, heart failure.
WHAT TO DO:
- **Dial 911 (emergency) for medical help or call poison control center 1-800-222-1222 for instructions.**
- **See emergency information on last 3 pages of this book.**

What drug does:
Decreases inflammatory responses. Suppresses immune response. Stimulates bone marrow.

Time lapse before drug works:
2 to 4 days.

Don't take with:
Any other medicine or any dietary supplement without consulting your doctor or pharmacist.

POSSIBLE ADVERSE REACTIONS OR SIDE EFFECTS

SYMPTOMS	WHAT TO DO
Life-threatening: Hives, rash, intense itching, faintness, swelling soon after a dose (anaphylaxis).	Seek emergency treatment immediately.
Common: Acne, indigestion, nausea, vomiting, gaseousness, headache, insomnia, dizziness, increased appetite, weight gain, poor wound healing, swollen legs or feet.	Continue. Call doctor when convenient.
Infrequent: • Black, bloody or tarry stool; various infections; decreased or blurred vision; fever.	Continue. Call doctor right away.
• Mood or emotional changes, insomnia, restlessness, frequent urination, round face, irregular menstrual periods, euphoria, muscle cramps or weakness, stomach or hip or shoulder pain, thirstiness, fatigue, loss of appetite (with triamcinolone).	Continue. Call doctor when convenient.
Rare: • Irregular heartbeat, convulsions, leg or thigh pain.	Continue. Call doctor right away.
• Skin rash, joint pain, unusual hair growth on face or body, hallucinations, confusion, excitement, darkened or lightened skin color, rectal problems with use of rectal products (irritation, blisters, bleeding).	Continue. Call doctor when convenient.

WARNINGS & PRECAUTIONS

Don't take if:
- You are allergic to any cortisone* drug.
- You have an active case of tuberculosis, systemic fungal infection, herpes infection of eyes or peptic ulcer disease.

Before you start, consult your doctor if:
You have, or have had, heart disease, congestive heart failure, diabetes, AIDS, HIV infection, glaucoma, underactive or overactive thyroid, high blood pressure, myasthenia gravis, blood clots in legs or lungs, peptic ulcer disease, tuberculosis, recent or current chickenpox or measles, kidney or liver disease, esophagitis, cold sores, osteoporosis, systemic lupus erythematosus or hyperlipidemia.

Over age 60:
Adverse reactions and side effects may be more frequent and severe than in younger persons. Likely to aggravate edema, diabetes or ulcers. Likely to cause cataracts and osteoporosis (softening of the bones) with long term use.

Pregnancy:
Decide with your doctor if drug benefits justify risk to unborn child. Risk category C (see page xviii).

Breast-feeding:
Drug passes into milk. Avoid drug or discontinue nursing until you finish medicine. Consult doctor for advice on maintaining milk supply.

Infants & children:
- Use only under close medical supervision. These drugs may slow or decrease growth rate or cause reduced adrenal gland function. Be sure you and your child's doctor discuss all benefits and risks of the drug.
- Children using large doses of this drug are more susceptible to infectious disease.

Prolonged use:
- May lead to glaucoma, cataracts, diabetes, fragile bones and thin skin, growth retardation in children, functional dependence.*
- Talk to your doctor about the need for follow-up medical exams or laboratory studies.

Skin & sunlight:
No problems expected.

Driving, piloting or hazardous work:
No problems expected.

Discontinuing:
- Don't discontinue without doctor's advice until you complete prescribed dose, even though symptoms diminish or disappear.
- Drug dose needs to be gradually reduced after long-term therapy. Don't stop drug suddenly.
- Drug can affect your response to surgery, illness, injury or stress for 2 years after discontinuing. Tell anyone who takes medical care of you within 2 years about use of this drug.

Others:
- Avoid immunizations if possible.
- Resistance to infection is less while taking this medicine. Consult doctor if infection occurs.
- Call doctor about swelling or rapid weight gain.
- Advise any doctor or dentist whom you consult that you take this medicine.
- May cause recurrence of tuberculosis.
- Can interfere with the accuracy of some medical tests.
- Wear or carry medical identification that indicates use of this drug.

POSSIBLE INTERACTION WITH OTHER DRUGS

GENERIC NAME OR DRUG CLASS	COMBINED EFFECT
Antacids*	Decreased effect of prednisone and dexamethasone.
Anticholinergics*	Possible glaucoma.
Anticoagulants,* oral	Decreased anti-coagulant effect.
Anticonvulsants, hydantoin*	Decreased adreno-corticoid effect.
Antidepressants, tricyclic*	Increased risk of mental side effects.
Antidiabetics,* oral	Decreased anti-diabetic effect.
Antihistamines*	Decreased adreno-corticoid effect.
Anti-inflammatory drugs, nonsteroidal (NSAIDs)*	Increased risk of ulcers. Increased adrenocorticoid effect.
Aspirin	Increased adreno-corticoid effect.

Continued on page 899

POSSIBLE INTERACTION WITH OTHER SUBSTANCES

INTERACTS WITH	COMBINED EFFECT
Alcohol:	Stomach ulcer risk.
Beverages: Grapefruit juice.	Risk of toxicity with methylprednisolone or budesonide. Avoid.
Cocaine:	Unknown. Avoid.
Foods:	No proven problems.
Marijuana:	Decreased immunity.
Tobacco:	Increased adreno-corticoid effect.

*See Glossary

GENERIC AND BRAND NAMES

See full list of generic and brand names in the *Generic and Brand Name Directory*, page 866.

BASIC INFORMATION

Habit forming? No
Prescription needed? For some
Available as generic? Yes
Drug class: Adrenocorticoid (topical)

USES

Relieves redness, swelling, itching, skin discomfort of hemorrhoids; insect bites; poison ivy, oak, sumac; soaps, cosmetics; jewelry; burns; sunburn; numerous skin rashes; eczema; discoid lupus erythematosus; swimmer's ear; sun poisoning; hair loss; scars; pemphigus; psoriasis; pityriasis rosea.

DOSAGE & USAGE INFORMATION

How to use:
• Cream, lotion, ointment, gel—Apply small amount and rub in gently.
• Foam—Follow directions on container. Don't breathe vapors.
• Other forms—Follow directions on container.

When to use:
When needed or as directed. Don't use more often than directions allow.

If you forget an application:
Use as soon as you remember.

What drug does:
Reduces inflammation by affecting enzymes that produce inflammation.

Time lapse before drug works:
15 to 20 minutes.

Don't use with:
Any other topical medicine without consulting your doctor or pharmacist.

OVERDOSE

SYMPTOMS:
None expected.
WHAT TO DO:
If person swallows or inhales drug, call doctor, poison control center 1-800-222-1222 or hospital emergency room for help.

POSSIBLE ADVERSE REACTIONS OR SIDE EFFECTS

SYMPTOMS	WHAT TO DO
Life-threatening: None expected.	
Common: None expected.	
Infrequent: Infection on skin with pain, redness, blisters, pus; skin irritation with burning, itching, blistering or peeling; acne-like skin eruptions.	Continue. Call doctor when convenient.
Rare: None expected.	

Note: Side effects are unlikely if topical adrenocorticoids are used in low doses for short periods of time. High doses for long periods can possibly cause the adverse reactions of cortisone, listed under ADRENOCORTICOIDS (Systemic).

ADRENOCORTICOIDS (Topical)

 ## WARNINGS & PRECAUTIONS

Don't take if:
You are allergic to any topical adrenocorticoid (cortisone) preparation.

Before you start, consult your doctor if:
- You plan pregnancy within medication period.
- You have diabetes.
- You have infection at treatment site.
- You have stomach ulcer.
- You have tuberculosis.

Over age 60:
Adverse reactions and side effects may be more frequent and severe than in younger persons, especially thinning of the skin.

Pregnancy:
Decide with your doctor whether drug benefits justify risk to unborn child. Risk category C (see page xviii).

Breast-feeding:
No problems expected.

Infants & children:
- Use only under medical supervision. Too much for too long can be absorbed into blood stream through skin and retard growth.
- For infants in diapers, avoid plastic pants or tight diapers.

Prolonged use:
- Increases chance of absorption into blood stream to cause side effects of oral cortisone drugs.
- May thin skin where used.
- Talk to your doctor about the need for follow-up medical examinations or laboratory studies to check complete blood counts (white blood cell count, platelet count, red blood cell count, hemoglobin, hematocrit), adrenal function.

Skin & sunlight:
Desoximetasone may cause rash or intensify sunburn in areas exposed to sun or ultraviolet light (photosensitivity reaction). Avoid over-exposure. Notify doctor if reaction occurs.

Driving, piloting or hazardous work:
No problems expected.

Discontinuing:
May be unnecessary to finish medicine. Follow doctor's instructions.

Others:
- Don't use a plastic dressing longer than 2 weeks.
- Aerosol spray—Store in cool place. Don't use near heat or open flame or while smoking. Don't puncture, break or burn container.
- Don't use for acne or gingivitis.

 ## POSSIBLE INTERACTION WITH OTHER DRUGS

GENERIC NAME OR DRUG CLASS	COMBINED EFFECT
Antibacterials* (topical)	Decreased antibiotic effect.
Antifungals* (topical)	Decreased antifungal effect.

 ## POSSIBLE INTERACTION WITH OTHER SUBSTANCES

INTERACTS WITH	COMBINED EFFECT
Alcohol:	None expected.
Beverages:	None expected.
Cocaine:	None expected.
Foods:	None expected.
Marijuana:	None expected.
Tobacco:	None expected.

*See Glossary

ALPHA ADRENERGIC RECEPTOR BLOCKERS

GENERIC AND BRAND NAMES

ALFUZOSIN
  UroXatral
DOXAZOSIN
  Cardura
  Cardura XL
PRAZOSIN
  Minipress
  Minizide

SILODOSIN
  Rapaflo
TAMSULOSIN
  Flomax
TERAZOSIN
  Hytrin

BASIC INFORMATION

Habit forming? No
Prescription needed? Yes
Available as generic? Yes, for some
Drug class: Antihypertensive

USES

* Treatment for high blood pressure.
* May improve congestive heart failure.
* Treatment for Raynaud's disease.
* Treatment for benign prostatic hyperplasia.

DOSAGE & USAGE INFORMATION

How to take:
* Tablet (doxazosin)—Swallow with liquid. If you can't swallow whole, crush or crumble tablet and take with liquid or food.
* Tablet or capsule or extended-release tablet—Swallow whole with liquid. Do not crumble or crush or chew tablet or open capsule.

Continued next column

OVERDOSE

SYMPTOMS:
Extreme weakness; rapid or irregular heart-beat; loss of consciousness; cold, sweaty skin; weak, rapid pulse; coma.
WHAT TO DO:
* Dial 911 (emergency) for medical help or call poison control center 1-800-222-1222 for instructions.
* If person is unconscious, check breathing and pulse. If not breathing, begin mouth-to-mouth rescue breathing. If heart is not beating, begin chest compressions.
* See emergency information on last 3 pages of this book.

When to take:
At the same times each day.

If you forget a dose:
Take as soon as you remember up to 2 hours late. If more than 2 hours, wait for next scheduled dose (don't double this dose).

What drug does:
Expands and relaxes blood vessel walls to lower blood pressure.

Time lapse before drug works:
30 minutes; may take days or weeks for full effect.

Don't take with:
Any other medicine or any dietary supplement without consulting your doctor or pharmacist.

POSSIBLE ADVERSE REACTIONS OR SIDE EFFECTS

SYMPTOMS	WHAT TO DO
Life-threatening: In case of overdose, see previous column.	
Common: Headache, dizziness.	Continue. Call doctor when convenient.
Infrequent:	
• Rash or itchy skin, blurred vision, shortness of breath, difficulty breathing, chest pain, rapid heartbeat.	Discontinue. Call doctor right away.
• Appetite loss, constipation or diarrhea, abdominal pain, nausea, vomiting, fluid retention, joint or muscle aches, tiredness, weakness and faintness when arising from bed or chair, little or no semen when ejaculating.	Continue. Call doctor when convenient.
• Headache, irritability, depression, dry mouth, stuffy nose, increased urination, drowsiness.	Continue. Tell doctor at next visit.
Rare: Decreased sexual function, numbness or tingling in hands or feet.	Continue. Call doctor when convenient.

ALPHA ADRENERGIC RECEPTOR BLOCKERS

WARNINGS & PRECAUTIONS

Don't take if:
You are allergic to alpha adrenergic receptor blockers.

Before you start, consult your doctor if:
* You experience lightheadedness or fainting with other antihypertensive drugs.
* You are easily depressed.
* You have impaired brain circulation or have had a stroke.
* You will have surgery within 2 months, including dental surgery, requiring general or spinal anesthesia.
* You have coronary heart disease (with or without angina).
* You have kidney disease or impaired liver function.

Over age 60:
Begin with no more than 1 mg. per day for first 3 days. Increases should be gradual and supervised by your doctor. Don't stand while taking. Sudden changes in position may cause falls. Sit or lie down promptly if you feel dizzy. If you have impaired brain circulation or coronary heart disease, excessive lowering of blood pressure should be avoided. Report problems to your doctor immediately.

Pregnancy:
Risk factors vary for drugs in this group. See category page xviii and consult doctor.

Breast-feeding:
It is unknown if drug passes into milk. Avoid drug or discontinue nursing until you finish medicine. Consult doctor for advice on maintaining milk supply.

Infants & children:
Not recommended.

Prolonged use:
Talk to your doctor about the need for follow-up medical examinations or laboratory studies.

Skin & sunlight:
No problems expected.

Driving, piloting or hazardous work:
Don't drive or pilot aircraft until you learn how medicine affects you. Don't work around dangerous machinery. Don't climb ladders or work in high places.

Discontinuing:
Don't discontinue without doctor's advice until you complete prescribed dose, even though symptoms diminish or disappear.

Others:
* First dose likely to cause dizziness or light-headedness. Take drug at night and get out of bed slowly next morning.
* Advise any doctor or dentist whom you consult that you take this medicine.
* May affect the results in some medical tests.

POSSIBLE INTERACTION WITH OTHER DRUGS

GENERIC NAME OR DRUG CLASS	COMBINED EFFECT
Amphetamines*	Decreased alpha adrenergic blocker effect.
Antihypertensives, other*	Increased anti-hypertensive effect. Dosages may require adjustments.
Anti-inflammatory drugs, nonsteroidal (NSAIDs)*	Decreased effect of alpha adrenergic blocker.
Enzyme inhibitors*	Increased effect of alpha adrenergic blocker.
Estrogen	Decreased effect of alpha adrenergic blocker.
Ritonavir	Increased effect of alfuzosin.
Sympathomimetics*	Decreased effect of alpha adrenergic blocker.

POSSIBLE INTERACTION WITH OTHER SUBSTANCES

INTERACTS WITH	COMBINED EFFECT
Alcohol:	Excessive blood pressure drop.
Beverages:	Grapefruit juice may increase effect of one or more of these drugs.
Cocaine:	Increased risk of heart block and high blood pressure.
Foods:	None expected.
Marijuana:	Fainting. Avoid.
Tobacco:	Possible spasm of coronary arteries. Avoid.

*See Glossary

ALPROSTADIL

BRAND NAMES

Caverject   Muse
Edex

BASIC INFORMATION

Habit forming? No
Prescription needed? Yes
Available as generic? No
Drug class: Impotence therapy

USES

Treatment for impotence in some men who have erectile dysfunction due to neurologic, vascular, psychological or mixed causes.

DOSAGE & USAGE INFORMATION

How to use:
- Injection—The first injection will be given in the doctor's office to determine proper dosage and to train you in preparing and self-injecting the drug. When using it at home, follow the instructions provided with the prescription or use as directed by your doctor to inject drug into the penis.
- Intraurethral—Use as a single dose suppository 10 to 30 minutes prior to intercourse.

When to take:
Usually 10 to 30 minutes prior to sexual intercourse. Do not use injection more than 3 times in one week, and do not use more than once in a 24-hour period. Do not use more than 2 suppositories in one 24-hour period.

If you forget a dose:
Not used on a scheduled basis.

What drug does:
Increases the blood flow into the penis and decreases the blood flow from the penis. The change in blood flow causes the penis to swell and elongate.

Continued next column

OVERDOSE

SYMPTOMS:
Prolonged penile erection.
WHAT TO DO:
Overdose unlikely to threaten life. If person uses much larger amount than prescribed or if accidentally swallowed, call doctor or poison control center 1-800-222-1222 for help.

Time lapse before drug works:
5 to 20 minutes. Erections may last up to 60 minutes.

Don't take with:
Any other medicine or any dietary supplement without consulting your doctor or pharmacist.

POSSIBLE ADVERSE REACTIONS OR SIDE EFFECTS

SYMPTOMS	WHAT TO DO
Life-threatening: None expected.	
Common:	
• Pain at site of injection, aching or burning pain during erection.	Discontinue. Call doctor when convenient.
• Pinching sensation at injection site.	Continue. Tell doctor at next visit.
Infrequent: None expected.	
Rare:	
• Erection lasting more than 4 hours is not priapism; (priapism is defined as an erection lasting more than 6 hours). Could cause permanent damage to the penis.	Call doctor right away or seek emergency care.
• Bruising or bleeding at site of injection; redness, swelling, tenderness, lumpiness, itching, rash, irritation, strange feeling, numbness or curving of the erect penis; slight bleeding from urethra, swelling of leg veins, dizziness, fainting, rapid pulse. Female partners may have mild vaginal itching or burning.	Discontinue. Call doctor when convenient.

WARNINGS & PRECAUTIONS

Don't use if:
You are allergic to alprostadil or you have been advised not to have sex.

Before you start, consult your doctor if:
- You have liver disease.
- You have sickle cell anemia or trait.
- You have multiple myeloma or leukemia.
- You have a penile implant or any type of penile malformation.
- You are allergic to any other medications.
- You have a history of priapism (prolonged penile erection).

Over age 60:
Effects on this age group are variable. Consult doctor.

Pregnancy:
Not used by females. Men should not use the product to have sexual intercourse with a pregnant woman unless the couple uses a condom barrier.

Breast-feeding:
Not used by females.

Infants & children:
Not used in this age group.

Prolonged use:
Have regular checkups with your doctor while using this drug to determine the effectiveness of the treatment and to check for any penile problems.

Skin & sunlight:
No special problems expected.

Driving, piloting or hazardous work:
No special problems expected.

Discontinuing:
No special problems expected.

Others:
- Don't increase dosage or frequency of use without your doctor's approval.
- Follow label instructions, and dispose of all needles properly after use. Do not reuse or share needles.
- The injection of this drug provides no protection from sexually transmitted diseases. Other protective measures, such as condoms, should be used when necessary to prevent the spread of sexually transmitted diseases.
- Slight bleeding may occur at injection site. Apply pressure if this occurs. If bleeding persists, consult doctor.

POSSIBLE INTERACTION WITH OTHER DRUGS

GENERIC NAME OR DRUG CLASS	COMBINED EFFECT
None significant.	

POSSIBLE INTERACTION WITH OTHER SUBSTANCES

INTERACTS WITH	COMBINED EFFECT
Alcohol:	No special problems expected.
Beverages:	No special problems expected.
Cocaine:	No special problems expected.
Foods:	No special problems expected.
Marijuana:	No special problems expected.
Tobacco:	No special problems expected.

AMINOGLUTETHIMIDE

BRAND NAMES

Cytadren

BASIC INFORMATION

Habit forming? No
Prescription needed? Yes
Available as generic? No
Drug class: Antiadrenal, antineoplastic

 ## USES

- Treats Cushing's syndrome.
- Treats breast malignancies.

 ## DOSAGE & USAGE INFORMATION

How to take:
Tablet—Swallow with liquid. If you can't swallow whole, crumble tablet and take with liquid or food. Instructions to take on empty stomach mean 1 hour before or 2 hours after eating.

When to take:
Follow doctor's instructions exactly.

If you forget a dose:
Take as soon as you remember up to 2 hours late. If more than 2 hours, wait for next scheduled dose (don't double this dose).

What drug does:
Suppresses adrenal cortex.

Time lapse before drug works:
1 to 2 hours.

Don't take with:
Any other medicines (including over-the-counter drugs such as cough and cold medicines, laxatives, antacids, diet pills, caffeine, nose drops, vitamins or other diet supplements) without consulting your doctor or pharmacist.

 ## OVERDOSE

SYMPTOMS:
None expected.
WHAT TO DO:
Overdose unlikely to threaten life. If person uses much larger amount than prescribed or if accidentally swallowed, call doctor or poison control center 1-800-222-1222 for help.

 ## POSSIBLE ADVERSE REACTIONS OR SIDE EFFECTS

SYMPTOMS	WHAT TO DO
Life-threatening: None expected.	
Common: Skin rash on face and hands.	Continue. Tell doctor at next visit.
Infrequent: • Dizziness, drowsiness, unexplained fatigue, low back pain, pain on urinating, clumsiness, unusual eye movements, appetite loss.	Discontinue. Call doctor right away.
• Vomiting, skin darkening, depression, headache, muscle pain.	Continue. Call doctor when convenient.
Rare: Unusual bleeding or bruising.	Discontinue. Call doctor right away.

WARNINGS & PRECAUTIONS

Don't take if:
* You have recently been exposed to chicken pox.
* You have shingles (herpes zoster).

Before you start, consult your doctor if:
* You have decreased thyroid function (hypothyroidism).
* You have any form of infection.

Over age 60:
Adverse reactions and side effects may be more frequent and severe than in younger persons. You may need smaller doses for shorter periods of time.

Pregnancy:
Risk category D (see page xviii).

Breast-feeding:
Effect not documented. Consult your doctor.

Infants & children:
Effect not documented. Consult your doctor.

Prolonged use:
Talk to your doctor about the need for follow-up medical examinations or laboratory studies to check thyroid function, liver function, serum electrolytes (sodium, potassium, chloride) and blood pressure.

Skin & sunlight:
No problems expected.

Driving, piloting or hazardous work:
No problems expected.

Discontinuing:
No special problems expected.

Others:
* Advise any doctor or dentist whom you consult that you take this medicine.
* May affect results in some medical tests.
* May cause decreased thyroid function.

POSSIBLE INTERACTION WITH OTHER DRUGS

GENERIC NAME OR DRUG CLASS	COMBINED EFFECT
Anticoagulants*	Decreased anti-coagulant effect.
Clozapine	Toxic effect on the central nervous system.
Cortisone-like drugs*	Decreased cortisone effects.
Dexamethasone	Dexamethasone effect decreased by half.
Trilostane	Too much decrease in adrenal function.

POSSIBLE INTERACTION WITH OTHER SUBSTANCES

INTERACTS WITH	COMBINED EFFECT
Alcohol:	Increased stomach irritation.
Beverages: Coffee, tea, cocoa.	Increased stomach irritation.
Cocaine:	No proven problems.
Foods:	No proven problems.
Marijuana:	No proven problems.
Tobacco:	No proven problems.

AMIODARONE

BRAND NAMES

Cordarone

BASIC INFORMATION

Habit forming? No
Prescription needed? Yes
Available as generic? Yes
Drug class: Antiarrhythmic

 USES

Prevents and treats life-threatening heartbeat irregularities.

 DOSAGE & USAGE INFORMATION

How to take:
Tablet—Swallow whole with liquid or food to lessen stomach irritation. If you can't swallow whole, crumble tablet and take with liquid or food.

When to take:
According to prescription instructions.

If you forget a dose:
Skip this dose and resume regular schedule. Do not double the next dose. If you forget 2 doses or more, consult your doctor.

What drug does:
• Slows nerve impulses in the heart.
• Makes heart muscle fibers less responsive to abnormal electrical impulses arising in the electrical regulatory system of the heart.

Time lapse before drug works:
About 10 days but may take 2 to 3 months for full effectiveness.

Don't take with:
Any other medicine or any dietary supplement without consulting your doctor or pharmacist.

 OVERDOSE

SYMPTOMS:
Irregular heartbeat, loss of consciousness, seizures.
WHAT TO DO:
• **Dial 911 (emergency) for medical help or call poison control center 1-800-222-1222 for instructions.**
• **If person is unconscious, check breathing and pulse. If not breathing, begin mouth-to-mouth rescue breathing. If heart is not beating, begin chest compressions.**
• **See emergency information on last 3 pages of this book.**

 POSSIBLE ADVERSE REACTIONS OR SIDE EFFECTS

SYMPTOMS	WHAT TO DO
Life-threatening: Shortness of breath, difficulty breathing, cough.	Discontinue. Seek emergency treatment.
Common: • Walking difficulty, fever, numbness or tingling in hands or feet, shakiness, weakness in arms and legs.	Discontinue. Call doctor right away.
• Constipation, headache, appetite loss, nausea, vomiting.	Continue. Call doctor when convenient.
Infrequent: • Skin color change to blue-gray, blurred vision, cold feeling, dry eyes, nervousness, scrotum swelling or pain, insomnia, swollen feet and ankles, fast or slow heartbeat, eyes hurt in light, weight gain or loss, sweating.	Discontinue. Call doctor right away.
• Bitter or metallic taste, diminished sex drive, dizziness, flushed face, coldness and unusual tiredness.	Continue. Call doctor when convenient.
Rare: Jaundice, skin rash.	Discontinue. Call doctor right away.

 WARNINGS & PRECAUTIONS

Don't take if:
You are allergic to amiodarone.

Before you start, consult your doctor if:
• You have liver, kidney or thyroid disease.
• You have heart disease other than coronary artery disease.

Over age 60:
• Adverse reactions and side effects may be more frequent and severe than in younger persons. Ask about smaller doses.
• Pain in legs (while walking) much more likely.

Pregnancy:
Risk category D (see page xviii). Consult doctor.

Breast-feeding:
Drug passes into milk. Avoid drug or discontinue nursing until you finish medicine. Consult doctor for advice on maintaining milk supply.

Infants & children:
Safety not established. Use only under close medical supervision.

Prolonged use:
* Blue-gray discoloration of skin may appear.
* Don't discontinue without consulting doctor. Dose may require gradual reduction if you have taken drug for a long time. Doses of other drugs may also require adjustment.
* Talk to your doctor about the need for follow-up medical examinations or laboratory studies.

Skin & sunlight:
May cause rash or intensify sunburn in areas exposed to sun or ultraviolet light (photosensitivity reaction). Avoid overexposure. Notify doctor if reaction occurs.

Driving, piloting or hazardous work:
Avoid if you feel dizzy or lightheaded. Otherwise, no problems expected.

Discontinuing:
* Don't discontinue without consulting doctor. Dose may require gradual reduction if you have taken drug for a long time. Doses of other drugs may also require adjustment.
* Notify doctor if cough, fever, breathing difficulty or shortness of breath occur after discontinuing medicine.

Others:
* Call doctor right away if you have symptoms of lung toxicity (cough, fever or painful breathing) or liver toxicity (swollen and painful abdomen, weight loss and appetite loss).
* Learn to check your own pulse. If it drops to lower than 50 or rises to higher than 100 beats per minute, don't take amiodarone until you consult your doctor.
* Advise any doctor or dentist whom you consult that you take this medicine.
* May interfere with the accuracy of some medical tests.

 POSSIBLE INTERACTION WITH OTHER DRUGS

GENERIC NAME OR DRUG CLASS	COMBINED EFFECT
Antiarrhythmics, other*	Increased likelihood of heartbeat irregularity.
Anticoagulants*	Increased anti-coagulant effect.
Beta-adrenergic blocking agents*	Increased likelihood of slow heartbeat.
Calcium channel blockers*	Possible heart block.
Cholestyramine	May decrease amiodarone blood levels.

Dextromethorphan	Unknown effect. Avoid.
Digitalis	Increased digitalis effect.
Diltiazem	Increased likelihood of slow heartbeat.
Diuretics*	Increased risk of heartbeat irregularity due to low potassium level.
Encainide	Increased effect of toxicity on the heart muscle.
Flecainide	Increased flecainide effect.
HMG-CoA reductase inhibitors	Risk of muscle injury and kidney failure.
Isoniazid	Increased risk of liver damage.
Nicardipine	Possible increased effect and toxicity of each drug.
Nifedipine	Increased likelihood of slow heartbeat.
Phenytoin	Increased effect of phenytoin.
Procainamide	Increased procainamide effect.
Propafenone	Increased effect of both drugs and increased risk of toxicity.
Quinidine	Increased quinidine effect.

 POSSIBLE INTERACTION WITH OTHER SUBSTANCES

INTERACTS WITH	COMBINED EFFECT
Alcohol:	Increased risk of heartbeat irregularity. Avoid.
Beverages: Grapefruit juice.	Risk of toxicity. Avoid.
Cocaine:	Increased risk of heartbeat irregularity. Avoid.
Foods:	None expected.
Marijuana:	Possible irregular heartbeat. Avoid.
Tobacco:	Possible irregular heartbeat. Avoid.

AMLEXANOX

BRAND NAMES

Aphthasol   **OraDisc**

BASIC INFORMATION

Habit forming? No
Prescription needed? Yes
Available as generic? No
Drug class: Antiaphthous ulcer agent

 USES

Treatment for severe canker sores (aphthous ulcers) in the mouth.

 DOSAGE & USAGE INFORMATION

How to use:
- Oral paste—Use fingertips to apply paste directly to each canker sore following oral hygiene.
- Patch—Apply to affected area in the mouth. The drug will dissolve slowly.

When to use:
Use as soon as symptoms of a canker sore appear. Apply four times a day—after meals and before bedtime. Wash hands after application.

If you forget a dose:
Use as soon as you remember. If it is almost time for the next dose, wait for the next dose (don't double this dose).

What drug does:
Exact healing mechanism is unknown. Appears to stop the inflammatory process and hypersensitivity reaction.

Time lapse before drug works:
Pain relief may occur within hours or up to 24 hours. Complete healing time will take several days.

Don't use with:
Any other medicine for mouth ulcers without consulting your doctor or pharmacist.

 OVERDOSE

SYMPTOMS:
None expected.
WHAT TO DO:
If person accidentally swallows drug, call doctor, poison control center 1-800-222-1222 or hospital emergency room for help.

 POSSIBLE ADVERSE REACTIONS OR SIDE EFFECTS

SYMPTOMS	WHAT TO DO
Life-threatening: None expected.	
Common: None expected.	
Infrequent: Slight pain, stinging or burning at site of application.	No action necessary.
Rare: Diarrhea, nausea, rash.	Discontinue. Call doctor when convenient.

WARNINGS & PRECAUTIONS

Don't take if:
You are allergic to amlexanox.

Before you start, consult your doctor if:
- You are allergic to any medication, food or other substance.
- You have weak immune system due to drugs or illness.

Over age 60:
No problems expected.

Pregnancy:
Decide with your doctor if drug benefits outweigh risks to unborn child. Risk category B (see page xviii).

Breast-feeding:
It is unknown if drug passes into milk. Absorption into the body has occurred with this drug. Avoid drug or discontinue nursing until you finish medicine. Consult doctor for advice on maintaining milk supply.

Infants & children:
Safety and efficacy have not been established. Use only under close medical supervision.

Prolonged use:
Normally only used for up to 10 days of treatment.

Skin & sunlight:
No problems expected.

Driving, piloting or hazardous work:
No problems expected.

Discontinuing:
May be unnecessary to finish medicine. Discontinue when canker sores heal.

Others:
- If canker sores do not heal after 10 days, consult your dentist or health-care provider.
- Advise any doctor or dentist whom you consult that you take this medicine.

 ## POSSIBLE INTERACTION WITH OTHER DRUGS

GENERIC NAME OR DRUG CLASS	COMBINED EFFECT
None expected.	

 ## POSSIBLE INTERACTION WITH OTHER SUBSTANCES

INTERACTS WITH	COMBINED EFFECT
Alcohol:	None expected.
Beverages:	None expected.
Cocaine:	None expected.
Foods:	None expected.
Marijuana:	None expected.
Tobacco:	None expected.

AMPHETAMINES

GENERIC AND BRAND NAMES

**AMPHETAMINE &
   DEXTRO-
      AMPHETAMINE**
   Adderall
   Adderall XR
DEXTROAMPHETAMINE
   Dexedrine
   Dexedrine Spansule
   Liquadd
   Oxydess
   Spancap

LISDEXAMFETAMINE
   Vyvanse
METHAMPHETAMINE
   Desoxyn
   Desoxyn Gradumet

BASIC INFORMATION

Habit forming? Yes
Prescription needed? Yes
Available as generic? Yes
**Drug class: Central nervous system
   stimulant**

USES

- Treats narcolepsy (sleep attacks).
- Treats attention deficit hyperactivity disorder in adults, adolescents and children.

DOSAGE & USAGE INFORMATION

How to take:
- Tablet—Swallow with liquid.
- Extended-release capsule or tablet—Swallow each dose whole with liquid; do not crush.
- Solution—Follow instructions on prescription.

When to take:
- Short-acting form—Don't take later than 6 hours before bedtime.
- Long-acting form—Take on awakening.

If you forget a dose:
Take as soon as you remember. If it is almost time for the next dose, wait for that dose (don't double this dose) and resume regular schedule.

Continued next column

OVERDOSE

SYMPTOMS:
Rapid heartbeat, hyperactivity, high fever, hallucinations, suicidal or homicidal feelings, convulsions, coma.
WHAT TO DO:
- **Dial 911 (emergency) for medical help or call poison control center 1-800-222-1222 for instructions.**
- **See emergency information on last 3 pages of this book.**

What drug does:
- Hyperactivity—Decreases motor restlessness and increases ability to pay attention.
- Narcolepsy—Increases motor activity and mental alertness; diminishes drowsiness.

Time lapse before drug works:
Take several weeks to see if drug is effective.

Don't take with:
Any other medicine or any diet supplement without consulting your doctor or pharmacist.

POSSIBLE ADVERSE REACTIONS OR SIDE EFFECTS

SYMPTOMS	WHAT TO DO
Life-threatening:	
In case of overdose, see previous column.	
Common:	
• Irritability, nervousness, insomnia, euphoria. signs of addiction.*	Continue. Call doctor when convenient.
• Dry mouth.	Continue. Tell doctor at next visit.
• Fast, pounding heartbeat.	Discontinue. Call doctor right away.
Infrequent:	
• Dizziness, reduced alertness, blurred vision, unusual sweating.	Discontinue. Call doctor right away.
• Headache, diarrhea or constipation, appetite loss, stomach pain, nausea, vomiting, weight loss, diminished sex drive, impotence.	Continue. Call doctor when convenient.
Rare:	
• Rash, hives, chest pain, irregular heart-beat, trouble breathing, fainting, hallucinations, becoming suspicious, manic behavior, uncontrollable movements (head, neck, arms, legs).	Discontinue. Call doctor right away.
• Mood changes, swollen breasts.	Continue. Call doctor when convenient.

WARNINGS & PRECAUTIONS

Don't take if:
You are allergic to any amphetamine.

Before you start, consult your doctor if:
- You plan to become pregnant.
- You have glaucoma.
- You have diabetes, overactive thyroid, anxiety or tension.
- You have a history of substance abuse.

- You will have surgery within 2 months, requiring general or spinal anesthesia.
- Adult or child patient has a mental illness.

Over age 60:
Adverse reactions and side effects may be more frequent and severe than in younger persons.

Pregnancy:
Decide with your doctor if drug benefits justify risk to unborn child. Consult doctor. Risk category C (see page xviii).

Breast-feeding:
Drugs pass into breast milk. Consult your doctor.

Infants & children:
- Amphetamine-dextroamphetamine is used to treat attention deficit disorder in children age 3 and older. Do not use this drug in children under the age of 12 years for weight loss.
- Reports of sudden unexplained death (SUD) in children has been associated with amphetamine abuse and reported in children with underlying heart defects taking amphetamines. A very small number of cases of SUD have been reported in children without heart defects taking amphetamines. Talk to your child's doctor about this risk.

Prolonged use:
- Drug can be habit forming. Ask your doctor about the risks involved.
- Talk to your doctor about the need for follow-up medical examinations or laboratory studies to check blood pressure, growth charts in children, and need for continued treatment.

Skin & sunlight:
No problems expected.

Driving, piloting or hazardous work:
Don't drive or pilot aircraft until you learn how medicine affects you. Don't work around dangerous machinery. Don't climb ladders or work in high places. Danger increases if you drink alcohol or take medicine affecting alertness and reflexes.

Discontinuing:
May be unnecessary to finish medicine, but don't suddenly stop. Follow doctor's instructions.

Others:
- Use of this drug must be closely supervised. Don't use for appetite control or depression.
- Advise any doctor or dentist whom you consult that you take this medicine.
- During a withdrawal phase, may cause prolonged sleep of several days.
- Don't use for fatigue or to replace rest.
- Drug may cause serious heart and psychiatric (mental) problems, including sudden death. Read warning information provided with prescription. Call doctor right away if symptoms develop (e.g., chest pain, shortness of breath, fainting, or hallucinations).

 POSSIBLE INTERACTION WITH OTHER DRUGS

GENERIC NAME OR DRUG CLASS	COMBINED EFFECT
Antidepressants, tricyclic*	Decreased amphetamine effect.
Antihypertensives*	Decreased antihypertensive effect.
Beta-adrenergic blocking agents*	High blood pressure, slow heartbeat.
Carbonic anhydrase inhibitors*	Increased amphetamine effect.
Central nervous system (CNS) stimulants,* other	Excessive CNS stimulation.
Doxazosin	Decreased doxazosin effect.
Furazolidone	Sudden and severe high blood pressure.
Haloperidol	Decreased amphetamine effect.
Monoamine oxidase (MAO) inhibitors*	Severe increase in blood pressure.
Phenothiazines*	Decreased amphetamine effect.
Prazosin	Decreased prazosin effect.
Sodium bicarbonate	Increased amphetamine effect.

Continued on page 899

 POSSIBLE INTERACTION WITH OTHER SUBSTANCES

INTERACTS WITH	COMBINED EFFECT
Alcohol:	Decreased amphetamine effect. Avoid.
Beverages: Caffeine drinks.	Overstimulation. Avoid.
Cocaine:	Dangerous risk to body's nervous system. Avoid.
Foods:	None expected.
Marijuana:	Frequent use— Severely impaired mental function.
Tobacco:	None expected.

*See Glossary

ANAGRELIDE

BRAND NAMES

Agrylin

BASIC INFORMATION

Habit forming? No
Prescription needed? Yes
Available as generic? Yes
Drug class: Platelet count–reducing agent, antithrombocythemia

 ## USES

Reduces elevated platelet counts and the risk of thrombosis (formation of a blood clot); also makes symptoms more tolerable in patients with essential thrombocythemia.

 ## DOSAGE & USAGE INFORMATION

How to take:
Capsule—Swallow with liquid. Take with or without food.

When to take:
At the same time each day. Dose may be adjusted to maintain proper platelet count.

If you forget a dose:
Take as soon as you remember. If it is almost time for the next dose, then skip the missed dose and wait for your next scheduled dose (don't double this dose).

What drug does:
Exact mechanism is unknown.

Time lapse before drug works: .
One to two weeks.

Don't take with:
Any other medicine or any dietary supplement without consulting your doctor or pharmacist.

 ## OVERDOSE

SYMPTOMS:
None expected immediately. May lower platelet count, leading to increased bleeding.
WHAT TO DO:
Overdose unlikely to threaten life. If person uses much larger amount than prescribed or if accidentally swallowed, call doctor or poison control center 1-800-222-1222 for help.

 ## POSSIBLE ADVERSE REACTIONS OR SIDE EFFECTS

SYMPTOMS	WHAT TO DO
Life-threatening: Severe headache or weakness; pain or pressure in chest, jaw, neck, back or arms; swelling of feet or legs; severe tiredness or weakness; increased heart rate; difficulty breathing or shortness of breath.	Seek emergency treatment immediately.
Common: • Abdominal pain, weakness, dizziness palpitations, shortness of breath.	Continue. Call doctor right away.
• Diarrhea, heartburn, gas, bloating, headache, loss of appetite, general feeling of discomfort or illness, nausea, pain.	Continue. Call doctor if symptoms persist.
Infrequent: • Blurred or double vision, painful or difficult urination, blood in urine, tingling in hands or feet, unusual bruising or bleeding, flushing, faintness.	Discontinue. Call doctor right away.
• Canker sore, joint pain, back pain, confusion, constipation, fever or chills, insomnia, leg cramps, depression, nervousness, runny nose, ringing in ears, skin rash, itching, sleepiness, sensitivity to light, vomiting.	Continue. Call doctor if symptoms persist.
Rare: Hair loss.	Tell doctor at next visit.

WARNINGS & PRECAUTIONS

Don't take if:
You are allergic to anagrelide.

Before you start, consult your doctor if:
* You have any kidney or liver disease or any heart or blood vessel disorder.
* You have any chronic health problem.
* You are pregnant or nursing.

Over age 60:
No problems expected.

Pregnancy:
Decide with your doctor if drug benefits justify risk to unborn child. Risk category C (see page xviii).

Breast-feeding:
It is unknown if drug passes into milk. Avoid drug or discontinue nursing until you finish medicine. Consult doctor for advice on maintaining milk supply.

Infants & children:
Safety and efficacy have not been established in patients under 16. Use only under close medical supervision.

Prolonged use:
Schedule regular visits with your doctor for laboratory examinations to monitor the continued effectiveness of the medication.

Skin & sunlight:
No problems expected.

Driving, piloting or hazardous work:
No problems expected.

Discontinuing:
Don't discontinue without consulting your doctor even if you feel well.

Others:
* Close medical supervision, including frequent platelet counts, required at start of therapy with this drug.
* Advise any doctor or dentist whom you consult that you are using this medicine.

POSSIBLE INTERACTION WITH OTHER DRUGS

GENERIC NAME OR DRUG CLASS	COMBINED EFFECT
Sucralfate	May interfere with anagrelide absorption. Don't take at the same time.

POSSIBLE INTERACTION WITH OTHER SUBSTANCES

INTERACTS WITH	COMBINED EFFECT
Alcohol:	None expected.
Beverages:	None expected.
Cocaine:	Effects unknown. Avoid.
Foods:	None expected.
Marijuana:	Effects unknown. Avoid.
Tobacco:	None expected.

ANAKINRA

BRAND NAMES

Kineret

BASIC INFORMATION

Habit forming? No
Prescription needed? Yes
Available as generic? No
Drug class: Antirheumatic; biological
   response modifier

USES

Treatment of moderately to severely active
rheumatoid arthritis. Used for patients who have
not responded to one or more disease modifying
antirheumatic drugs (DMARDs). May be used
alone or in combination with certain other
arthritis drugs.

DOSAGE & USAGE INFORMATION

How to take:
Injection—The drug is self-injected under the
skin (subcutaneously). Follow your doctor's
instructions and the directions provided with the
prescription on how and where to inject. Do not
use the medication unless you are sure about
the proper method for injection. Store
medication in the refrigerator (do not freeze)
until you plan to use it. After each use, throw
away the syringe and any medicine left in it (ask
your pharmacist about disposal methods). Never
reuse the needle or syringe.

When to take:
Inject every day at the same time each day.

If you forget a dose:
Inject as soon as possible. If it is almost time for
your next dose, skip the missed dose and go
back to your regular dosing schedule. Do not
double doses.

What drug does:
Reduces the actions of chemicals in the body
that cause inflammatory and immune responses.
It helps prevent progressive joint destruction.

Continued next column

OVERDOSE

SYMPTOMS:
None expected.
WHAT TO DO:
If an overdose is suspected, call doctor or
poison control center 1-800-222-1222 for
help.

Time lapse before drug works:
It will take several weeks before full benefits of
the drug are noticeable.

Don't use with:
Any other medicine or any dietary supplement
without consulting your doctor or pharmacist.

POSSIBLE ADVERSE REACTIONS OR SIDE EFFECTS

SYMPTOMS	WHAT TO DO
Life-threatening: None expected.	
Common: Diarrhea, headache, nausea, mild stomach pain.	Continue. Call doctor when convenient.
Infrequent: Reaction at injection site (pain, purple discoloration, inflammation), pain in bones or joints, fever or chills, chest pain, skin symptoms (itching, redness, swelling, hot), cold or flu symptoms (sneezing, cough, sore throat, muscle aches, runny or stuffy nose), trouble with breathing, insomnia, unusual tiredness, vomiting, other signs or symptoms of an infection.	Discontinue. Call doctor right away.
Rare: Allergic reaction (itching, rash, hives, swelling of face or lips, wheezing).	Discontinue. Call doctor right away.

WARNINGS & PRECAUTIONS

Don't take if:
You are allergic to anakinra or the components of the drug (including proteins made from bacterial cells such as *E coli*).

Before you start, consult your doctor if:
* You have a chronic disorder or infection or are immunosuppressed.
* You have asthma (increases risk of infections).
* You have a kidney disorder.
* You have an active infection.
* You are allergic or sensitive to latex.

Over age 60:
Used with caution in elderly patients, since infections are more common in this age group.

Pregnancy:
Usually safe, but decide with your doctor if drug benefits justify any possible risk to unborn child. Risk category B (see page xviii).

Breast-feeding:
It is unknown if drug passes into milk. Consult doctor for advice on breast-feeding if you use this medication.

Infants & children:
Not recommended for children under age 18.

Prolonged use:
* No specific problems expected, but medical studies are ongoing.
* Talk to your doctor about the need for follow-up medical examinations or laboratory studies to check effectiveness of the drug and to monitor for infections.

Skin & sunlight:
No problems expected.

Driving, piloting or hazardous work:
No problems expected.

Discontinuing:
No problems expected. Consult doctor.

Others:
* Advise any doctor or dentist whom you consult that you take this medicine.
* Using this drug increases the risk of infections. Consult your doctor if any signs or symptoms of infection occur.
* Avoid immunizations unless approved by your doctor.

 ## POSSIBLE INTERACTION WITH OTHER DRUGS

GENERIC NAME OR DRUG CLASS	COMBINED EFFECT
Tumor necrosis factor blockers	Increased risk of infections. Use only with close medical supervision.
Vaccines, live	Vaccines may not be effective.

 ## POSSIBLE INTERACTION WITH OTHER SUBSTANCES

INTERACTS WITH	COMBINED EFFECT
Alcohol:	None expected.
Beverages:	None expected.
Cocaine:	None expected. However, cocaine may slow body's recovery. Avoid.
Foods:	None expected.
Marijuana:	None expected. However, marijuana may slow body's recovery. Avoid.
Tobacco:	None expected.

ANDROGENS

GENERIC AND BRAND NAMES

See full list of generic and brand names in the *Generic and Brand Name Directory*, page 867.

BASIC INFORMATION

Habit forming? No
Prescription needed? Yes
Available as generic? Yes
Drug class: Androgen

USES

- Corrects male hormone deficiency. Reduces "male menopause" symptoms (loss of sex drive, depression, anxiety).
- Decreases calcium loss of osteoporosis (softened bones).
- Blocks breast cancer cell growth in women.
- Stimulates beginning of puberty in certain boys.
- Augments treatment of aplastic anemia.
- Stimulates weight gain after illness, injury or for chronically underweight persons.
- Stimulates growth in treatment of dwarfism.

DOSAGE & USAGE INFORMATION

How to take:
- Tablet or capsule—Take with food to lessen stomach irritation.
- Injection—Once or twice a month.
- Gel—Follow instructions with prescription.
- Buccal system—Follow instructions provided with prescription.
- Transdermal (skin patch)—Follow instructions provided with prescription.

When to take:
At the same time each day.

If you forget a dose:
Take as soon as you remember up to 2 hours late. If more than 2 hours, wait for next scheduled dose (don't double this dose). For gel or patch, usually wait for next scheduled time.

Continued next column

OVERDOSE

SYMPTOMS:
None expected.
WHAT TO DO:
Overdose unlikely to threaten life. If person uses much larger amount than prescribed or if accidentally swallowed, call doctor or poison control center 1-800-222-1222 for help.

What drug does:
- Stimulates cells that produce male sex characteristics.
- Replaces hormone deficiencies.
- Stimulates red-blood-cell production.
- Suppresses production of estrogen (female sex hormone).

Time lapse before drug works:
Varies with problems treated. May require 2 or 3 months of regular use for desired effects.

Don't take with:
Any other medicine or any dietary supplement without consulting your doctor or pharmacist.

POSSIBLE ADVERSE REACTIONS OR SIDE EFFECTS

SYMPTOMS	WHAT TO DO
Life-threatening: Intense itching, weakness, loss of consciousness.	Seek emergency treatment immediately.
Common: Acne or oily skin, deep voice, enlarged clitoris in females; frequent or continuing erections, sore or swollen breasts in men, pain or sores under patch.	Discontinue. Call doctor right away.
Infrequent: • Yellow skin or eyes, depression or confusion, other changes in moods, flushed face, rash or itch, nausea, vomiting, diarrhea, swollen feet or legs, headache, rapid weight gain, difficult or frequent urination, unusual bleeding, scrotum pain.	Discontinue. Call doctor right away.
• Sore mouth, higher or lower sex drive, decreased testicle size, impotence in men, mild redness or itching at site of patch, hair loss, pubic hair growth.	Continue. Call doctor when convenient
Rare: Black stools, ongoing symptoms at patch, site, vomiting blood, fever, chills, hives or spots on body.	Discontinue. Call doctor right away.

WARNINGS & PRECAUTIONS

Don't take if:
You are allergic to any male hormone.

Before you start, consult your doctor if:
* You might be pregnant.
* You have cancer of- or enlarged prostate.
* You have heart disease or arteriosclerosis.
* You have kidney or liver disease.
* You have breast cancer (male or female).
* You have high blood pressure.
* You have diabetes (drug can affect blood sugar).

Over age 60:
* May stimulate sexual activity.
* In males, can enlarge prostate, worsen prostate cancer, and cause urinary retention. Have a prostate exam before starting this medication.

Pregnancy:
Risk to unborn child outweighs drug benefits. Don't use. Risk category X (see page xviii).

Breast-feeding:
Drug passes into milk. Avoid drug or discontinue nursing until you finish medicine. Consult doctor for advice on maintaining milk supply.

Infants & children:
Use with children only under close medical supervision.

Prolonged use:
* May cause liver cancer, possible kidney stones. In women may cause unnatural hair growth and deep voice.
* Talk to your doctor about the need for follow-up medical examinations or laboratory studies to check effectiveness or unwanted effects of the drug.

Skin & sunlight:
No problems expected.

Driving, piloting or hazardous work:
No problems expected.

Discontinuing:
No problems expected.

Others:
* Reduces sperm count and volume of semen. This effect is usually temporary.
* With patch or gel, drug can pass to sexual partner. Consult doctor if partner starts getting any of the side effects listed.
* Wash hands carefully after applying gel and cover area where gel applied.
* Children and women need to avoid contact with areas of skin where men have applied the gel. It can cause serious side effects, especially in children. Consult doctor if symptoms occur.
* Will not increase strength in athletes.
* Advise any doctor or dentist whom you consult that you take this medicine.
* In women, may cause changes such as deepened voice, increased hair growth, enlarged clitoris. Some changes may not go away after drug is discontinued.

POSSIBLE INTERACTION WITH OTHER DRUGS

GENERIC NAME OR DRUG CLASS	COMBINED EFFECT
Anticoagulants*	Increased anticoagulant effect.
Antidiabetic agents*	Increased antidiabetic effect.
Chlorzoxazone	Decreased androgen effect.
Cyclosporine	Increased cyclosporine effect.
Hepatotoxic drugs* (other)	Increased liver toxicity.
Insulin	Increased antidiabetic effect.
Oxyphenbutazone	Decreased androgen effect.
Phenobarbital	Decreased androgen effect.
Phenylbutazone	Decreased androgen effect.

POSSIBLE INTERACTION WITH OTHER SUBSTANCES

INTERACTS WITH	COMBINED EFFECT
Alcohol:	None expected.
Beverages:	None expected.
Cocaine:	No proven problems.
Foods: Salt.	Excessive fluid retention (edema). Decrease salt intake while taking male hormones.
Marijuana:	Decreased blood levels of androgens.
Tobacco:	No proven problems.

*See Glossary

ANESTHETICS (Mucosal-Local)

GENERIC AND BRAND NAMES

BENZOCAINE
 Anbesol Baby Gel
 Anbesol Maximum
  Strength Gel
 Anbesol Maximum
  Strength Liquid
 Baby Anbesol
 Baby Orabase
 Baby Oragel
 Baby Oragel
  Nighttime Formula
 Benzodent
 Children's
  Chloraseptic
  Lozenges
 Dentapaine
 Dentocaine
 Dent-Zel-Ite
 Hurricaine
 Numzident
 Num-Zit Gel
 Num-Zit Lotion
 Orabase-B with
  Benzocaine
 Orajel Extra
  Strength
 Orajel Liquid
 Orajel Maximum
  Strength
 Oratect Gel
 Rid-A-Pain
 SensoGARD Canker
  Sore Relief
 Spec-T Sore Throat
  Anesthetic
 Topicaine

BENZOCAINE &
 MENTHOL
 Chloraseptic
  Lozenges
  Cherry Flavor
BENZOCAINE &
 PHENOL
 Anbesol Gel
 Anbesol Liquid
 Anbesol Regular
  Strength Gel
 Anbesol Regular
  Strength Liquid
DYCLONINE
 Children's Sucrets
 Sucrets Maximum
  Strength
 Sucrets Regular
  Strength
LIDOCAINE
 Xylocaine
 Xylocaine Viscous
 Zilactin-L
TETRACAINE
 Supracaine

BASIC INFORMATION

Habit forming? No
Prescription needed? Yes, for some
Available as generic? Yes, for some
Drug class: Anesthetic (mucosal-local)

 OVERDOSE

SYMPTOMS:
Overabsorption by body—Dizziness, blurred
vision, seizures, drowsiness.
WHAT TO DO:
- **Dial 911 (emergency) for medical help or**
  call poison control center 1-800-222-1222
  for instructions.
- **Not for internal use. If child accidentally**
  swallows, call numbers above.
- **See emergency information on last 3**
  pages of this book.

 USES

Relieves pain or irritation in mouth caused by
toothache, teething, mouth sores, dentures,
braces, dental appliances. Also relieves pain of
sore throat for short periods of time.

 DOSAGE & USAGE
INFORMATION

How to use:
- For mouth problems—Apply to sore places
  with cotton-tipped applicator. Don't swallow.
- For throat—Gargle, but don't swallow.
- For aerosol spray—Don't inhale.

When to use:
As directed by physician or label on package.

If you forget a dose:
Use as soon as you remember.

What drug does:
Blocks pain impulses to the brain.

Time lapse before drug works:
Immediately.

Don't use with:
Any other medicine for your mouth without
consulting your doctor or pharmacist.

 POSSIBLE
ADVERSE REACTIONS
OR SIDE EFFECTS

SYMPTOMS	WHAT TO DO
Life-threatening: Unusual anxiety, excitement, nervousness, irregular or slow heartbeat.	Discontinue. Seek emergency treatment.
Common: None expected.	
Infrequent: Redness, irritation, sores not present before treatment, rash, itchy skin, hives.	Discontinue. Call doctor right away.
Rare: None expected.	

WARNINGS & PRECAUTIONS

Don't take if:
You are allergic to any of the products listed.

Before you start, consult your doctor if:
- You are allergic to anything.
- You have infection, canker sores or other sores in your mouth.
- You take medicine for myasthenia gravis, eye drops for glaucoma or any sulfa medicine.

Over age 60:
Adverse reactions and side effects may be more frequent and severe than in younger persons. Ask doctor about smaller doses.

Pregnancy:
Risk factors vary for drugs in this group. See category list on page xviii and consult doctor.

Breast-feeding:
No problems expected, but check with doctor.

Infants & children:
No problems expected, but check with doctor.

Prolonged use:
Not intended for prolonged use.

Skin & sunlight:
No problems expected.

Driving, piloting or hazardous work:
Wait to see if causes dizziness, sweating, drowsiness or blurred vision. If not, no problems expected.

Discontinuing:
No problems expected.

Others:
- Keep cool, but don't freeze.
- Don't puncture, break or burn aerosol containers.
- Don't eat, drink or chew gum for 1 hour after use.
- Heat and moisture in bathroom medicine cabinet can cause breakdown of medicine. Store someplace else.
- Before anesthesia, tell dentist about any medicines you take or use.

POSSIBLE INTERACTION WITH OTHER DRUGS

GENERIC NAME OR DRUG CLASS	COMBINED EFFECT
So remote, they are not considered clinically significant.	

POSSIBLE INTERACTION WITH OTHER SUBSTANCE

INTERACTS WITH	COMBINED EFFECT
Alcohol:	Adverse reactions more common.
Beverages:	None expected.
Cocaine:	May cause too much nervousness and trembling. Avoid.
Foods:	None expected.
Marijuana:	None expected.
Tobacco:	Avoid. Tobacco makes mouth problems worse.

ANESTHETICS (Rectal)

GENERIC AND BRAND NAMES

BENZOCAINE
  Americaine
    Hemorrhoidal
  Ethyl
    Aminobenzoate
DIBUCAINE
  Nupercainal
LIDOCAINE
  Anamantle HC
    Cream Kit
  Peranex HC Cream
  Xyralid RC
PRAMOXINE
  Fleet Relief
  Proctofoam
  Tronolane
  Tronothane

TETRACAINE
  Pontocaine Cream
TETRACAINE &
  MENTHOL
  Pontocaine
  Ointment

BASIC INFORMATION

Habit forming? No
Prescription needed? Yes, for some
Available as generic? Yes
Drug class: Anesthetic (rectal)

 ## USES

- Relieves pain, itching and swelling of hemorrhoids (piles).
- Relieves pain of rectal fissures (breaks in lining membrane of the anus).

 ## DOSAGE & USAGE INFORMATION

How to use:
- Rectal cream or ointment—Apply to surface of rectum with fingers. Insert applicator into rectum no farther than 1/2 and apply inside. Wash applicator with warm soapy water or discard.
- Aerosol foam—Read patient instructions. Don't insert into rectum. Use the special applicator and wash carefully after using.

Continued next column

 ## OVERDOSE

SYMPTOMS:
None expected.
WHAT TO DO:
Not intended for internal use. If child accidentally swallows, call doctor or poison control center 1-800-222-1222 for help.

- Suppository—Remove wrapper and moisten with water. Lie on side. Push blunt end of suppository into rectum with finger. If suppository is too soft, run cold water over wrapper or put in refrigerator for 15 to 45 minutes before using.
- Pads—For external use only. Follow instructions on label. Do not use for more than 1 week without doctor's approval.

When to use:
As directed on the product's label.

If you forget a dose:
Use as soon as you remember.

What drug does:
Deadens nerve endings to pain and touch.

Time lapse before drug works:
5 to 15 minutes.

Don't use with:
Any other topical rectal medicine without consulting your doctor or pharmacist.

 ## POSSIBLE ADVERSE REACTIONS OR SIDE EFFECTS

SYMPTOMS	WHAT TO DO
Life-threatening: None expected.	
Common: None expected.	
Infrequent:	
• Nervousness, trembling, hives, rash, itch, inflammation or tenderness not present before application, slow heartbeat.	Discontinue. Call doctor right away.
• Dizziness, blurred vision, swollen feet.	Continue. Call doctor when convenient.
Rare:	
• Blood in urine.	Discontinue. Call doctor right away.
• Increased or painful urination.	Continue. Call doctor when convenient.

WARNINGS & PRECAUTIONS

Don't use if:
You are allergic to any topical anesthetic.

Before you start, consult your doctor if:
- You have skin infection at site of treatment.
- You have had severe or extensive skin disorders such as eczema or psoriasis.
- You have bleeding hemorrhoids.

Over age 60:
Adverse reactions and side effects may be more frequent and severe than in younger persons.

Pregnancy:
Risk factors vary for drugs in this group. See category list on page xviii and consult doctor.

Breast-feeding:
No problems expected. Consult doctor.

Infants & children:
Use caution. More likely to be absorbed through skin and cause adverse reactions.

Prolonged use:
Possible excess absorption. Don't use longer than 3 days for any one problem.

Skin & sunlight:
No problems expected.

Driving, piloting or hazardous work:
No problems expected.

Discontinuing:
May be unnecessary to finish medicine. Follow doctor's instructions.

Others:
- Report any rectal bleeding to your doctor.
- Keep cool, but don't freeze.

POSSIBLE INTERACTION WITH OTHER DRUGS

GENERIC NAME OR DRUG CLASS	COMBINED EFFECT
Sulfa drugs*	Decreased anti-infective effect of sulfa drugs.

POSSIBLE INTERACTION WITH OTHER SUBSTANCE

INTERACTS WITH	COMBINED EFFECT
Alcohol:	None expected.
Beverages:	None expected.
Cocaine:	Possible nervous system toxicity. Avoid.
Foods:	None expected.
Marijuana:	None expected.
Tobacco:	None expected.

*See Glossary

ANESTHETICS (Topical)

GENERIC AND BRAND NAMES

See full list of generic and brand names in the *Generic and Brand Name Directory*, page 868.

BASIC INFORMATION

Habit forming? No
Prescription needed?
   High strength: Yes
   Low strength: No
Available as generic? Yes
Drug class: Anesthetic (topical)

 ## USES

Relieves pain and itch of sunburn, insect bites, scratches and other minor skin irritations.

 ## DOSAGE & USAGE INFORMATION

How to use:
All forms—Use only enough to cover irritated area. Follow instructions on label or use as directed by doctor. Avoid using on large areas of skin.

When to use:
When needed for discomfort, no more often than every hour.

If you forget an application:
Use as needed.

What drug does:
Blocks pain impulses from skin to brain.

Time lapse before drug works:
3 to 15 minutes.

Don't take with:
Any other topical medicine without consulting your doctor or pharmacist.

 ## OVERDOSE

SYMPTOMS:
If swallowed or inhaled—Dizziness, nervousness, trembling, seizures.
WHAT TO DO:
- **Dial 911 (emergency) for medical help or call poison control center 1-800-222-1222 for instructions.**
- **See emergency information on last 3 pages of this book.**

 ## POSSIBLE ADVERSE REACTIONS OR SIDE EFFECTS

SYMPTOMS	WHAT TO DO
Life-threatening: None expected.	
Common: None expected.	
Infrequent: Hives-like swellings on skin or in mouth or throat; skin problems not present before treatment (rash, burning, stinging, tenderness, redness).	Discontinue. Call doctor right away.
Rare: If too much of drug absorbed into body (very rare)—Nervousness, slow heartbeat, dizziness, blurred or double vision, confusion, convulsions, noises in ears, feeling hot or cold, numbness, trembling, anxiety, paleness, tiredness or weakness.	Discontinue. Call doctor right away.

WARNINGS & PRECAUTIONS

Don't use if:
You are allergic to any topical anesthetic.

Before you start, consult your doctor if:
- You have skin infection at site of treatment.
- You have had severe or extensive skin disorders such as eczema or psoriasis.
- You have bleeding hemorrhoids.

Over age 60:
Adverse reactions and side effects may be more frequent and severe than in younger persons.

Pregnancy:
Risk factors vary for drugs in this group. See category list on page xviii and consult doctor.

Breast-feeding:
No problems expected. Consult doctor.

Infants & children:
Use caution. More likely to be absorbed through skin and cause adverse reactions.

Prolonged use:
Possible excess absorption. Don't use longer than 3 days for any one problem.

Skin & sunlight:
May cause rash or intensify sunburn in areas exposed to sun or ultraviolet light (photosensitivity reaction). Avoid overexposure. Notify doctor if reaction occurs.

Driving, piloting or hazardous work:
No problems expected.

Discontinuing:
May be unnecessary to finish medicine. Follow doctor's instructions.

Others:
- Contact doctor if condition being treated doesn't improve within a week. Call sooner if new symptoms develop or pain worsens.
- Wash hands carefully after use.

POSSIBLE INTERACTION WITH OTHER DRUGS

GENERIC NAME OR DRUG CLASS	COMBINED EFFECT
Sulfa drugs*	Decreased effect of sulfa drugs for infection.

POSSIBLE INTERACTION WITH OTHER SUBSTANCE

INTERACTS WITH	COMBINED EFFECT
Alcohol:	None expected.
Beverages:	None expected.
Cocaine:	Possible nervous system toxicity. Avoid.
Foods:	None expected.
Marijuana:	None expected.
Tobacco:	None expected.

ANGIOTENSIN II RECEPTOR ANTAGONISTS

GENERIC AND BRAND NAMES

CANDESARTAN
Atacand
EPROSARTAN
Teveten
Teveten HCT
IRBESARTAN
Avalide
Avapro
LOSARTAN
Cozaar
Hyzaar

OLMESARTAN
Azor
Benicar
Benicar HCT
TELMISARTAN
Micardis
Micardis HCT
Micardis Plus
VALSARTAN
Diovan
Diovan HCT
Diovan Oral
Exforge

BASIC INFORMATION

Habit forming? No
Prescription needed? Yes
Available as generic? No
Drug class: Antihypertensive, angiotensin II receptor antagonist

USES

- Treatment for hypertension (high blood pressure) and heart failure. May be used alone or in combination with other antihypertensive medications.
- Reduces risk of stroke in certain patients.

DOSAGE & USAGE INFORMATION

How to take:
Tablet—Swallow with liquid. May be taken with or without food.

When to take:
Once or twice daily as directed.

If you forget a dose:
Take as soon as you remember. If it is almost time for the next dose, wait for that dose (don't double this dose) and resume regular schedule.

Continued next column

OVERDOSE

SYMPTOMS:
Slow or irregular heartbeat, faintness, dizziness, lightheadedness.
WHAT TO DO:
Overdose unlikely to threaten life. If person uses much larger amount than prescribed or if accidentally swallowed, call doctor or poison control center 1-800-222-1222 for help.

What drug does:
Lowers blood pressure by relaxing the blood vessels to allow improved blood flow in the body.

Time lapse before drug works:
May take several weeks for full effectiveness.

Don't take with:
Any other medicine or any dietary supplement without consulting your doctor or pharmacist.

POSSIBLE ADVERSE REACTIONS OR SIDE EFFECTS

SYMPTOMS	WHAT TO DO
Life-threatening: None expected.	
Common: Headache.	Continue. Call doctor when convenient.
Infrequent:	
• Dizziness, fever or sore throat (upper respiratory infection).	Continue, but call doctor right away.
• Diarrhea, back pain, cough, fatigue, stuffy nose.	Continue. Call doctor when convenient.
Rare: Dry cough, trouble sleeping, muscle cramps, leg pain.	Continue. Call doctor when convenient.

ANGIOTENSIN II RECEPTOR ANTAGONISTS

 ## WARNINGS & PRECAUTIONS

Don't take if:
You are allergic to angiotensin II receptor antagonists.

Before you start, consult your doctor if:
- You have any kidney or liver disease.
- You are allergic to any medication, food or other substance.

Over age 60:
No special problems expected.

Pregnancy:
Decide with your doctor if drug benefits justify risks to unborn child. Risk category C for first trimester and category D for second and third trimesters (see page xviii).

Breast-feeding:
One or more of these drugs may pass into milk. Avoid drug or discontinue nursing until you finish medicine. Consult doctor for advice.

Infants & children:
Valsartan is approved to treat high blood pressure in children 6 to 16. For other angiotensin II receptor antagonists, consult doctor.

Prolonged use:
- No special problems expected. Hypertension usually requires life-long treatment.
- Schedule regular doctor visits to determine if drug is continuing to be effective in controlling the hypertension and to check for any kidney problems.

Skin & sunlight:
No special problems expected.

Driving, piloting or hazardous work:
Don't drive or pilot aircraft until you learn how medicine affects you. Don't work around dangerous machinery. Don't climb ladders or work in high places. Danger increases if you drink alcohol or take other medicines affecting alertness and reflexes.

Discontinuing:
Don't discontinue without consulting your doctor, even if you feel well. You can have hypertension without feeling any symptoms. Untreated high blood pressure can cause serious problems.

Others:
- Advise any doctor or dentist whom you consult that you take this medicine. May interfere with the accuracy of some medical tests.
- Follow any special diet your doctor may prescribe. It can help control hypertension.
- Consult doctor if you become ill with vomiting or diarrhea.
- Use caution when exercising or performing activities in hot weather and with excessive sweating. You may experience dizziness, lightheadedness or faintness.

 ## POSSIBLE INTERACTION WITH OTHER DRUGS

GENERIC NAME OR DRUG CLASS	COMBINED EFFECT
Anti-inflammatory drugs, nonsteroidal (NSAIDs)*	Decreased anti-hypertensive effect.
Cyclosporine	Excess potassium levels in the body.
Diuretics*	Increased anti-hypertensive effect.
Diuretics, potassium-sparing*	Excess potassium levels in the body.
Hypotension-causing drugs,* other	Increased anti-hypertensive effect.
Indomethacin	Decreased anti-hypertensive effect.
Potassium-containing medications	Excess potassium levels in the body.
Potassium supplements*	Excess potassium levels in the body.
Sympathomimetics*	Decreased anti-hypertensive effect.

POSSIBLE INTERACTION WITH OTHER SUBSTANCES

INTERACTS WITH	COMBINED EFFECT
Alcohol:	Unknown effect. Consult doctor.
Beverages: Low-salt milk.	Possible excess potassium in the body.
Grapefruit juice	Decreased effect of losartan.
Cocaine:	Unknown effect. Avoid.
Foods: Salt substitutes containing potassium.	Excess potassium in the body.
Marijuana:	Increased sedation. Avoid.
Tobacco:	None expected.

*See Glossary

ANGIOTENSIN-CONVERTING ENZYME (ACE) INHIBITORS

GENERIC AND BRAND NAMES

See full list of generic and brand names in the *Generic and Brand Name Directory*, page 868.

BASIC INFORMATION

Habit forming? No
Prescription needed? Yes
Available as generic? Yes, for some
Drug class: Antihypertensive, angiotensin converting enzyme (ACE) inhibitor

 ## USES

- Treatment for hypertension (high blood pressure) and congestive heart failure.
- Used for kidney disease in diabetic patients.
- Helps prevent complications in patients with stable coronary artery disease.
- Treatment for acute myocardial infarction.

 ## DOSAGE & USAGE INFORMATION

How to take:
Capsule, tablet, long-acting tablet, liquid—Follow directions provided with your prescription.

When to take:
At the same times each day, usually 2-3 times daily. Captopril should be taken on an empty stomach 1 hour before or 2 hours after eating.

If you forget a dose:
Take as soon as you remember. If it is almost time for the next dose, wait for that dose (don't double this dose) and resume regular schedule.

What drug does:
Relaxes artery walls and lowers blood pressure.

Time lapse before drug works:
60 to 90 minutes.

Don't take with:
Any other medicine or any dietary supplement without consulting your doctor or pharmacist.

 ## OVERDOSE

SYMPTOMS:
Low blood pressure, fever, chills, sore throat, fainting, convulsions, coma.
WHAT TO DO:
- **Dial 911 (emergency) for medical help or call poison control center 1-800-222-1222 for instructions.**
- **See emergency information on last 3 pages of this book.**

 ## POSSIBLE ADVERSE REACTIONS OR SIDE EFFECTS

SYMPTOMS	WHAT TO DO
Life-threatening	
Hives, rash, intense itching, faintness soon after a dose (anaphylaxis); difficulty breathing.	Seek emergency treatment immediately.
Common:	
Rash, loss of taste.	Discontinue. Call doctor right away.
Infrequent:	
• Swelling of mouth, face, hands or feet.	Discontinue. Seek emergency treatment.
• Dizziness, fainting, chest pain, fast or irregular heartbeat, confusion, nervousness, numbness and tingling in hands or feet.	Discontinue. Call doctor right away.
• Diarrhea, headache, tiredness, cough.	Continue. Call doctor when convenient.
Rare:	
• Sore throat, cloudy urine, fever, chills.	Discontinue. Call doctor right away.
• Nausea, vomiting, indigestion, abdominal pain.	Continue. Call doctor when convenient.

 ## WARNINGS & PRECAUTIONS

Don't take if:
- You are allergic to any ACE inhibitor.*
- You are receiving blood from a blood bank.
- You will have surgery within 2 months, including dental surgery, requiring general or spinal anesthesia.

Before you start, consult your doctor if:
- You have had a stroke.
- You have angina or heart or blood vessel disease.
- You have any autoimmune disease, including AIDS or lupus.
- You have high level of potassium in blood.
- You have kidney or liver disease.
- You are on severe salt-restricted diet.
- You have a bone marrow disorder.

Over age 60:
Adverse reactions and side effects may be more frequent and severe than in younger persons.

Pregnancy:
Drugs increase risk of birth defects. Risk factors vary for drugs in this group. See category list on page xviii and consult doctor.

Breast-feeding:
Drug passes into milk. Avoid drug or discontinue nursing until you finish medicine. Consult doctor for advice on maintaining milk supply.

Infants & children:
Under close medical supervision only.

Prolonged use:
Request periodic laboratory blood counts and urine tests.

Skin & sunlight:
One or more drugs in this group may cause rash or intensify sunburn in areas exposed to sun or ultraviolet light (photosensitivity reaction). Avoid overexposure. Notify doctor if reaction occurs.

Driving, piloting or hazardous work:
Avoid if you become dizzy or faint. Otherwise, no problems expected.

Discontinuing:
Don't discontinue without consulting doctor. Dose may require gradual reduction if you have taken drug for a long time. Doses of other drugs may also require adjustment.

Others:
- Avoid exercising in hot weather.
- May affect results in some medical tests.
- Advise any doctor or dentist whom you consult that you take this medicine.

POSSIBLE INTERACTION WITH OTHER DRUGS

GENERIC NAME OR DRUG CLASS	COMBINED EFFECT
Amiloride	Possible excessive potassium in blood.
Antihypertensives, other*	Increased antihypertensive effect. Dosage of each may require adjustment.
Anti-inflammatory drugs nonsteroidal (NSAIDs), cox-2 inhibitors	May decrease ACE inhibitor effect.
Beta-adrenergic blocking agents*	Increased antihypertensive effect. Dosage of each may require adjustment.

Carteolol	Increased antihypertensive effects of both drugs. Dosages may require adjustment.
Chloramphenicol	Possible blood disorders.
Diuretics*	Possible severe blood pressure drop with first dose.
Diclofenac	May decrease ACE inhibitor effect.
Guanfacine	Increased effect of both drugs.
Meloxicam	Decreased effect of ACE inhibitor.
Nicardipine	Possible excessive potassium in blood. Dosages may require adjustment.
Nimodipine	Possible excessive potassium in blood. Dangerous blood pressure drop.
Nitrates*	Possible excessive blood pressure drop.
Pentamidine	May increase bone marrow depression or make kidney damage more likely.

Continued on page 900

POSSIBLE INTERACTION WITH OTHER SUBSTANCES

INTERACTS WITH	COMBINED EFFECT
Alcohol:	Possible excessive blood pressure drop.
Beverages: Low-salt milk.	Possible excessive potassium in blood.
Cocaine	Increased risk of heart block and high blood pressure.
Foods: Salt substitutes.	Possible excessive potassium.
Marijuana:	Increased dizziness.
Tobacco:	May decrease ACE inhibitor effect.

*See Glossary

47

ANGIOTENSIN-CONVERTING ENZYME (ACE) INHIBITORS & HYDROCHLOROTHIAZIDE

GENERIC AND BRAND NAMES

See full list of generic and brand names in the *Generic and Brand Name Directory*, page 868.

BASIC INFORMATION

Habit forming? No
Prescription needed? Yes
Available as generic? Yes, for some
Drug class: Antihypertensive, diuretic (thiazide), ACE inhibitor

USES

- Treatment for high blood pressure and congestive heart failure.
- Reduces fluid retention.

DOSAGE & USAGE INFORMATION

How to take:
Tablet—Swallow with liquid. Instructions to take on empty stomach mean 1 hour before or 2 hours after eating.

When to take:
At the same times each day, usually 2 to 3 times daily. Take first dose at bedtime and lie down immediately.

If you forget a dose:
Take as soon as you remember up to 2 hours late. If more than 2 hours, wait for next scheduled dose (don't double this dose).

What drug does:
- Forces sodium and water excretion, thereby reducing body fluid.
- Relaxes muscle cells of small arteries.
- Reduced body fluid and relaxed arteries lower blood pressure.
- Reduces resistance in arteries.
- Strengthens heartbeat.

Continued next column

OVERDOSE

SYMPTOMS:
Cramps, weakness, drowsiness, weak pulse, low blood pressure.
WHAT TO DO:
- **Dial 911 (emergency) for medical help or call poison control center 1-800-222-1222 for instructions.**
- **See emergency information on last 3 pages of this book.**

Don't take with:
Any other medicine or any dietary supplement without consulting your doctor or pharmacist.

POSSIBLE ADVERSE REACTIONS OR SIDE EFFECTS

SYMPTOMS	WHAT TO DO
Life-threatening:	
Irregular heartbeat (fast or uneven); hives, rash, intense itching, faintness soon after a dose (anaphylaxis).	Discontinue. Seek emergency treatment.
Common:	
• Dry mouth, thirst, tiredness, weakness, muscle cramps, vomiting, chest pain, skin rash, coughing, weak pulse.	Discontinue. Call doctor right away.
• Taste loss, dizziness.	Continue. Call doctor when convenient.
Infrequent:	
• Face, mouth, hands swell.	Discontinue. Call doctor right away.
• Nausea, diarrhea.	Continue. Call doctor when convenient.
Rare:	
Jaundice (yellow eyes and skin), bruising, back pain.	Discontinue. Call doctor right away.

WARNINGS & PRECAUTIONS

Don't take if:
- You are allergic to any ACE inhibitor or any thiazide diuretic drug.
- You are receiving blood from a blood bank.
- If you will have surgery within 2 months, including dental surgery, requiring general or spinal anesthesia.

Before you start, consult your doctor if:
- You have had a stroke.
- You have angina, heart or blood vessel disease, a high level of potassium in blood, lupus, gout, liver, pancreas or kidney disorder.
- You have any autoimmune disease, including AIDS or lupus.
- You are on severe salt-restricted diet.
- You are allergic to any sulfa drug.
- You have a bone marrow disorder.

Over age 60:
Adverse reactions and side effects may be more frequent and severe than in younger persons, such as dizziness and excessive potassium loss.

ANGIOTENSIN-CONVERTING ENZYME (ACE) INHIBITORS & HYDROCHLOROTHIAZIDE

Pregnancy:
Drugs increase risk of birth defects. Risk factors vary for drugs in this group. See category list on page xviii and consult doctor.

Breast-feeding:
Drug passes into milk. Avoid drug or discontinue nursing until you finish medicine. Consult doctor for advice on maintaining milk supply.

Infants & children:
Not recommended.

Prolonged use:
Talk to your doctor about the need for follow-up medical examinations or laboratory studies to check blood pressure, ECG,* liver function, kidney function.

Skin & sunlight:
One or more drugs in this group may cause rash or intensify sunburn in areas exposed to sun or ultraviolet light (photosensitivity reaction). Avoid overexposure. Notify doctor if reaction occurs.

Driving, piloting or hazardous work:
Don't drive or pilot aircraft until you learn how medicine affects you. Don't work around dangerous machinery. Don't climb ladders or work in high places. Danger increases if you drink alcohol or take medicine affecting alertness and reflexes, such as antihistamines, tranquilizers, sedatives, pain medicine, narcotics and mind-altering drugs.

Discontinuing:
Don't discontinue without consulting doctor. Dose may require gradual reduction if you have taken drug for a long time. Doses of other drugs may also require adjustment.

Others:
- Hot weather and fever may cause dehydration and drop in blood pressure. Dose may require temporary adjustment. Weigh daily and report any unexpected weight decreases to your doctor.
- May cause rise in uric acid, leading to gout.
- May cause blood-sugar rise in diabetics.

 POSSIBLE INTERACTION WITH OTHER DRUGS

GENERIC NAME OR DRUG CLASS	COMBINED EFFECT
Allopurinol	Decreased allopurinol effect.
Amiloride	Possible excessive potassium in blood.

Antidepressants, tricyclic*	Dangerous drop in blood pressure. Avoid combination unless under medical supervision.
Antihypertensives, other*	Increased antihypertensive effect. Dosage of each may require adjustment.
Anti-inflammatory drugs nonsteroidal (NSAIDs)*	Decreased captopril effect.
Barbiturates*	Increased hydrochlorothiazide effect.
Beta-adrenergic blocking agents*	Increased antihypertensive effect. Dosage of each may require adjustments.
Carteolol	Increased antihypertensive effects of both drugs. Dosages may require adjustment.
Chloramphenicol	Possible blood disorders.
Cholestyramine	Decreased hydrochlorothiazide effect.
Digitalis preparations*	Excessive potassium loss that causes dangerous heart rhythms.

Continued on page 900

 POSSIBLE INTERACTION WITH OTHER SUBSTANCES

INTERACTS WITH	COMBINED EFFECT
Alcohol:	Dangerous blood pressure drop. Avoid.
Beverages: Low-salt milk.	Possible excessive potassium in blood.
Cocaine	Increased risk of heart block and high blood pressure.
Foods: Salt substitutes.	Possible excessive potassium.
Marijuana:	Increased dizziness; may increase blood pressure.
Tobacco:	May decrease blood pressure lowering effect.

*See Glossary

ANTACIDS

GENERIC AND BRAND NAMES

See full list of generic and brand names in the *Generic and Brand Name Directory*, page 868.

BASIC INFORMATION

Habit forming? No
Prescription needed? No
Available as generic? Yes, for some
Drug class: Antacid

 ## USES

Treatment for hyperacidity in upper gastrointestinal tract, including stomach and esophagus. Symptoms may be heartburn or acid indigestion. Diseases include peptic ulcer, gastritis, esophagitis, hiatal hernia.

 ## DOSAGE & USAGE INFORMATION

How to take:
Follow package instructions.

When to take:
1 to 3 hours after meals unless directed otherwise by your doctor.

If you forget a dose:
Take as soon as you remember, but not simultaneously with any other medicine.

What drug does:
• Neutralizes some of the hydrochloric acid in the stomach.
• Reduces action of pepsin, a digestive enzyme.

Time lapse before drug works:
15 minutes for antacid effect.

Continued next column

 ## OVERDOSE

SYMPTOMS:
Dry mouth, shallow breathing, diarrhea or constipation, headache, mental confusion, weakness, fatigue, stupor, bone pain.
WHAT TO DO:
• Overdose unlikely to threaten life. Depending on severity of symptoms and amount taken, dial 911 (emergency) for medical help or call poison control center 1-800-222-1222 for instructions.
• See emergency information on last 3 pages of this book.

Don't take with:
• Any other medicine or any dietary supplement without consulting your doctor or pharmacist.
• Other drugs at the same time. Decreases absorption of that drug. Wait 2 hours.

 ## POSSIBLE ADVERSE REACTIONS OR SIDE EFFECTS

SYMPTOMS	WHAT TO DO
Life-threatening: None expected.	
Common: Chalky taste.	Continue. Tell doctor at next visit.
Infrequent: Mild constipation, increased thirst, laxative effect, unpleasant taste in mouth, stomach cramps, stool color changes (whitish or speckling).	Continue. Call doctor when convenient.
Rare: Bone pain, frequent or urgent urination, muscle weakness or pain, nausea, weight gain, severe constipation, dizziness, headache, appetite loss, mood changes, vomiting, nervousness, swollen feet and ankles, tiredness or weakness.	Discontinue. Call doctor right away.

Note: Side effects are rare unless too much medicine is taken for a long time.

 ## WARNINGS & PRECAUTIONS

Don't take if:
• You are allergic to any antacid.
• You have a high blood-calcium level.

Before you start, consult your doctor if:
You have kidney disease, chronic constipation, colitis, diarrhea, symptoms of appendicitis, stomach or intestinal bleeding, irregular heartbeat.

Over age 60:
Adverse reactions and side effects may be more frequent and severe than in younger persons. Diarrhea or constipation particularly likely.

Pregnancy:
Risk factors vary for drugs in this group. See category list on page xviii and consult doctor.

Breast-feeding:
Drug passes into milk. Consult doctor.

Infants & children:
Use only under medical supervision.

Prolonged use:
- High blood level of calcium (if your antacid contains calcium) which disturbs electrolyte balance.
- Kidney stones, impaired kidney function.
- Talk to your doctor about the need for follow-up medical examinations or laboratory studies to check kidney function, serum calcium, serum potassium.

Skin & sunlight:
No problems expected.

Driving, piloting or hazardous work:
No problems expected.

Discontinuing:
May be unnecessary to finish medicine. Follow doctor's instructions.

Others:
- Don't take longer than 2 weeks unless under medical supervision.
- Advise any doctor or dentist whom you consult that you take this medicine. May affect results in some medical tests.

POSSIBLE INTERACTION WITH OTHER DRUGS

GENERIC NAME OR DRUG CLASS	COMBINED EFFECT
Alendronate	Decreased alendronate effect. Take antacid 30 minutes after alendronate.
Antifungals, azoles	Decreased azole absorption.
Anti-inflammatory drugs nonsteroidal (NSAIDs), COX-2 inhibitors	Decreased pain relief.
Capecitabine	Increased risk of capecitabine toxicity.
Chlorpromazine	Decreased chlorpromazine effect.
Ciprofloxacin	May cause kidney dysfunction.
Dexamethasone	Decreased dexamethasone effect.
Digitalis preparations*	Decreased digitalis effect.
Iron supplements*	Decreased iron effect.
Isoniazid	Decreased isoniazid effect.
Levodopa	Increased levodopa effect.
Mecamylamine	Increased mecamylamine effect.
Meperidine	Increased meperidine effect.
Methenamine	Reduced methenamine effect.
Nalidixic acid	Decreased nalidixic acid effect.
Nicardipine	Possible decreased nicardipine effect.
Nizatidine	Decreased nizatidine absorption.
Ofloxacin	Decreased ofloxacin effect.
Oxyphenbutazone	Decreased oxyphenbutazone effect.
Para-aminosalicylic acid (PAS)	Decreased PAS effect.
Penicillins*	Decreased penicillin effect.
Prednisone	Decreased prednisone effect.
Pseudoephedrine	Increased pseudoephedrine effect.
Salicylates*	Increased salicylate effect.
Tetracyclines	Decreased tetracycline effect.
Ticlopidine	Decreased ticlopidine effect.

POSSIBLE INTERACTION WITH OTHER SUBSTANCES

INTERACTS WITH	COMBINED EFFECT
Alcohol:	Decreased antacid effect.
Beverages:	No proven problems.
Cocaine:	No proven problems.
Foods:	Decreased antacid effect. Wait 1 hour after eating.
Marijuana:	Decreased antacid effect.
Tobacco:	Decreased antacid effect.

*See Glossary

ANTHELMINTICS

GENERIC AND BRAND NAMES

ALBENDAZOLE
  Albenza
IVERMECTIN
  Stromectol
MEBENDAZOLE
  Mebendacin
  Mebutar
  Nemasole
  Vermox

PYRANTEL
  Antiminth
  Aut
  Cobantril
  Helmex
  Lombriareu
  Reese's Pinworm
    Medicine
  Trilombrin
PYRVINIUM
  Vanquin
  Viprynium
THIABENDAZOLE
  Foldan
  Mintezol
  Mintezol Topical
  Minzolum
  Triasox

BASIC INFORMATION

Habit forming? No
Prescription needed? Yes
Available as generic? Yes
Drug class: Anthelmintics, antiparasitic

 ## USES

- Treatment of roundworms, pinworms, whipworms, hookworms and other intestinal parasites.
- Treatment of hydatid disease and neurocysticercosis; strongyloidiasis and onchocerciasis.

 ## OVERDOSE

SYMPTOMS:
Increased severity of adverse reactions and side effects.
WHAT TO DO:
Overdose unlikely to threaten life. If person uses much larger amount than prescribed or if accidentally swallowed, call doctor or poison control center 1-800-222-1222 for help.

 ## DOSAGE & USAGE INFORMATION

How to take or apply:
- Tablet—Swallow with liquid or food to lessen stomach irritation.
- Topical suspension—Apply to end of each tunnel or burrow made by worm.
- Chewable tablet—Chew thoroughly before swallowing.
- Oral suspension—Follow package instructions.

When to take:
Morning and evening with food to increase uptake.

If you forget a dose:
Skip dose and begin treatment again. Often only one or two doses are needed to complete treatment.

What drug does:
Kills or paralyzes the parasites. They then pass out of the body in the feces. Usually the type of worm parasite must be identified so the appropriate drug can be prescribed.

Time lapse before drug works:
Some take only hours; others, 1-3 days.

Don't take with:
Any other medicine or any dietary supplement without consulting your doctor or pharmacist.

 ## POSSIBLE ADVERSE REACTIONS OR SIDE EFFECTS

SYMPTOMS	WHAT TO DO
Life-threatening: None expected.	
Common: None expected.	
Infrequent:	
• Abdominal pain, diarrhea, dizziness, fever, nausea, rectal itching.	Continue. Call doctor when convenient.
• Red stools, asparagus-like urine smell, bad taste in mouth.	No action necessary.
Rare: Skin rash, itching, sore throat and fever, weakness (severe), hair loss, headache, blurred vision, seizures.	Discontinue. Call doctor right away.

WARNINGS & PRECAUTIONS

Don't take if:
You are allergic to any anthelmintics.

Before you start, consult your doctor if:
- You have liver disease.
- You have Crohn's disease.
- You have ulcerative colitis.

Over age 60:
Adverse reactions and side effects may be more frequent and severe than in younger persons. You may need smaller doses for shorter periods of time.

Pregnancy:
Risk factors vary for drugs in this group. See category list on page xviii and consult doctor.

Breast-feeding:
Unknown effect. Consult your doctor.

Infants & children:
No problems expected. Don't give to a child under age 2 without doctor's approval.

Prolonged use:
- Not intended for long-term use.
- Talk to your doctor about the need for follow-up medical examinations or laboratory studies to check stools, cellophane tape swabs pressed against rectal area to check for parasite eggs, complete blood counts (white blood cell count, platelet count, red blood cell count, hemoglobin, hematocrit).

Skin & sunlight:
Thiabendazole may cause rash or intensify sunburn in areas exposed to sun or ultraviolet light (photosensitivity reaction). Avoid overexposure. Notify doctor if reaction occurs.

Driving, piloting or hazardous work:
Use caution if the medicine causes you to feel dizzy or weak. Otherwise, no problems expected.

Discontinuing:
No problems expected.

Others:
- Take full course of treatment. Repeat course may be necessary if follow-up examinations reveal persistent infection.
- Advise any doctor or dentist whom you consult that you take this medicine.
- Wash all bedding after treatment to prevent re-infection.

POSSIBLE INTERACTION WITH OTHER DRUGS

GENERIC NAME OR DRUG CLASS	COMBINED EFFECT
Carbamazepine	Decreased effect of mebendazole.
Phenytoin	Decreased effect of mebendazole.
Piperazine	Decreased effect of each drug.
Theophylline	Increased effect of theophylline (with thiabendazole use).

POSSIBLE INTERACTION WITH OTHER SUBSTANCES

INTERACTS WITH	COMBINED EFFECT
Alcohol:	Decreased mebendazole effect. Avoid.
Beverages: Grapefruit juice.	Increased effect of albendazole. Avoid.
Cocaine:	None expected.
Foods:	None expected.
Marijuana:	None expected.
Tobacco:	None expected.

ANTHRALIN (Topical)

BRAND NAMES

Anthra-Derm
Anthraforte
Anthranol
Anthrascalp
Dithranol
Drithocreme
Drithocreme HP

Dritho-Scalp
Lasan
Lasan HP
Lasan Pomade
Lasan Unguent
Micanol

BASIC INFORMATION

Habit forming? No
Prescription needed? Yes
Available as generic? No
Drug class: Antipsoriatic, hair growth stimulant

USES

- Treats quiescent or chronic psoriasis.
- Stimulates hair growth in some people (not an approved use by the FDA).

DOSAGE & USAGE INFORMATION

How to use:
- Wear plastic gloves for all applications.
- If directed, apply at night.
- Cream, lotion, ointment—Bathe and dry area before use. Apply small amount and rub gently.
- If for short contact, same as above for cream.
- Leave on 20 to 30 minutes. Then remove medicine by bathing or shampooing.
- If for scalp overnight—Shampoo before use to remove scales or medicine. Dry hair. Part hair several times and apply to scalp. Wear plastic cap on head. Clean off next morning with petroleum jelly, then shampoo.

When to use:
As directed.

If you forget a dose:
Use as soon as you remember.

Continued next column

OVERDOSE

SYMPTOMS:
None expected.
WHAT TO DO:
Not for internal use. If child accidentally swallows, call doctor or poison control center 1-800-222-1222 for help.

What drug does:
Reduces growth activity within abnormal cells by inhibiting enzymes.

Time lapse before drug works:
May require several weeks or more.

Don't use with:
Any other medicine or any dietary supplement without consulting your doctor or pharmacist.

POSSIBLE ADVERSE REACTIONS OR SIDE EFFECTS

SYMPTOMS	WHAT TO DO
Life-threatening: None expected.	
Common: None expected.	
Infrequent: Redness or irritation of skin not present before application, rash.	Discontinue. Call doctor when convenient.
Rare: None expected.	

WARNINGS & PRECAUTIONS

Don't use if:
* You are allergic to anthralin.
* You have infected skin.

Before you start, consult your doctor if:
* You have chronic kidney disease.
* You are allergic to anything.

Over age 60:
No problems expected, but check with doctor.

Pregnancy:
Studies in animals and humans have not been done. Consult doctor. Risk category C (see page xviii).

Breast-feeding:
No problems expected, but check with doctor.

Infants & children:
No problems expected, but check with doctor.

Prolonged use:
No problems expected, but check with doctor.

Skin & sunlight:
May cause rash or intensify sunburn in areas exposed to sun or ultraviolet light (photosensitivity reaction). Avoid overexposure. Notify doctor if reaction occurs.

Driving, piloting or hazardous work:
No problems expected.

Discontinuing:
No problems expected.

Others:
* Keep cool, but don't freeze.
* Apply petroleum jelly to normal skin or scalp to protect areas not being treated.
* Will stain hair, clothing, shower, bathtub or sheets. Wash as soon as possible.
* Advise any doctor or dentist whom you consult that you take this medicine.
* Heat and moisture in bathroom medicine cabinet can cause breakdown of medicine. Store someplace else.

 ## POSSIBLE INTERACTION WITH OTHER DRUGS

GENERIC NAME OR DRUG CLASS	COMBINED EFFECT
Antidiabetic agents*	Increased sensitivity to sun exposure.
Coal tar preparations*	Increased sensitivity to sun exposure.
Diuretics, thiazide*	Increased sensitivity to sun exposure.
Griseofulvin	Increased sensitivity to sun exposure.
Methoxsalen	Increased sensitivity to sun exposure.
Nalidixic acid	Increased sensitivity to sun exposure.
Phenothiazines*	Increased sensitivity to sun exposure.
Sulfa drugs*	Increased sensitivity to sun exposure.
Tetracyclines*	Increased sensitivity to sun exposure.
Trioxsalen	Increased sensitivity to sun exposure.

 ## POSSIBLE INTERACTION WITH OTHER SUBSTANCES

INTERACTS WITH	COMBINED EFFECT
Alcohol:	None expected.
Beverages:	None expected.
Cocaine:	None expected.
Foods:	None expected.
Marijuana:	None expected.
Tobacco:	None expected.

*See Glossary

ANTIACNE, CLEANSING (Topical)

GENERIC AND BRAND NAMES

ALCOHOL &
  ACETONE
  Seba-Nil
ALCOHOL &
  SULFUR
  Liquimat
  Postacne

SULFURATED LIME
  Vlemasque
  Vleminckx Solution

BASIC INFORMATION

Habit forming? No
Prescription needed? No
Available as generic? Yes
Drug class: Antiacne agent, Cleansing agent

USES

Treats acne or oily skin.

DOSAGE & USAGE INFORMATION

How to use:
* Lotion, gel or pledget—Start with small amount and wipe over face to remove dirt and surface oil. Don't apply to wounds or burns. Don't rinse with water and avoid contact with eyes. Skin may be more sensitive in dry or cold climates.
* Plaster—Follow package instructions.

When to use:
As directed. May increase frequency up to 3 or more times daily as tolerated. Warm, humid weather may allow more frequent use.

If you forget a dose:
Use as soon as you remember and then go back to regular schedule.

Continued next column

OVERDOSE

SYMPTOMS:
None expected.
WHAT TO DO:
* Not for internal use. If child accidentally swallows, call numbers below.
* Dial 911 (emergency) for medical help or call poison control center 1-800-222-1222 for instructions.
* See emergency information on last 3 pages of this book.

What drug does:
Helps remove oil from skin's surface.

Time lapse before drug works:
Works immediately.

Don't use with:
Other topical acne treatments unless directed by doctor.

POSSIBLE ADVERSE REACTIONS OR SIDE EFFECTS

SYMPTOMS	WHAT TO DO
Life-threatening: None expected.	
Common: None expected.	
Infrequent:	
• Skin infection, pustules or rash; unusual pain, swelling or redness of treated skin.	Discontinue. Call doctor right away.
• Burning, dryness, stinging, peeling of skin.	Continue. Call doctor when convenient.
Rare: None expected.	

WARNINGS & PRECAUTIONS

Don't use if:
You have to apply over a wounded or burned area.

Before you start, consult your doctor if:
You use benzoyl peroxide, resorcinol, salicylic acid, sulfur or tretinoin (vitamin A acid).

Over age 60:
No problems expected.

Pregnancy:
Risk category not assigned to this drug group. Consult doctor about use.

Breast-feeding:
No problems expected, but check with doctor.

Infants & children:
No problems expected, but check with doctor. Use only under close medical supervision.

Prolonged use:
Excessive drying of skin.

Skin & sunlight:
No special problems expected.

Driving, piloting or hazardous work:
No problems expected, but check with doctor.

Discontinuing:
No problems expected, but check with doctor.

Others:
Some antiacne agents are flammable. Don't use near fire or while smoking.

 POSSIBLE INTERACTION WITH OTHER DRUGS

GENERIC NAME OR DRUG CLASS	COMBINED EFFECT
Abrasive or medicated soaps	Irritation or too much drying.
After-shave lotions	Irritation or too much drying.
Antiacne topical preparations (other)	Irritation or too much drying.
"Cover-up" cosmetics	Irritation or too much drying.
Drying cosmetic soaps	Irritation or too much drying.
Isotretinoin	Irritation or too much drying.
Mercury compounds	May stain skin black and smell bad.
Perfumed toilet water	Irritation or too much drying.
Preparations containing skin-peeling agents such as benzoyl peroxide, resorcinol, salicylic acid, sulfur, tretinoin	Irritation or too much drying.

 POSSIBLE INTERACTION WITH OTHER SUBSTANCES

INTERACTS WITH	COMBINED EFFECT
Alcohol:	None expected.
Beverages:	None expected.
Cocaine:	None expected.
Foods:	None expected.
Marijuana:	None expected.
Tobacco:	None expected.

ANTIALLERGIC AGENTS (Ophthalmic)

GENERIC AND BRAND NAMES

AZELASTINE
  (ophthalmic)
  Optivar
EMEDASTINE
  Emadine
EPINASTINE
  Elestat
KETOTIFEN
  Alaway
  Refresh Eye Itch
  Relief
  Zaditor

LEVOCABASTINE
  Livostin
LODOXAMIDE
  Alomide
NEDOCROMIL
  Alocril
OLOPATADINE
  Pataday
  Patanol
PEMIROLAST
  Alamast

BASIC INFORMATION

Habit forming? No
Prescription needed? Yes
Available as generic? Yes, for some
Drug class: Ophthalmic antiallergic agents, antihistaminic

 USES

Prevention and treatment of seasonal allergic (hay fever) eye disorders. May be referred to as seasonal conjunctivitis, vernal conjunctivitis, vernal keratitis and vernal keratoconjunctivitis.

 DOSAGE & USAGE INFORMATION

How to use:
Eye solution
• Wash hands.
• Apply pressure to inside corner of eye with middle finger.
• Continue pressure for 1 minute after placing medicine in eye.
• Tilt head backward. Pull lower lid away from eye with index finger of the same hand.
• Drop eye drops into pouch and close eye. Don't blink.
• Keep eyes closed for 1 to 2 minutes.

Continued next column

 OVERDOSE

SYMPTOMS:
None expected.
WHAT TO DO:
Not intended for internal use. If child accidentally swallows, call doctor or poison control center 1-800-222-1222 for help.

When to use:
1 to 2 drops 4 times a day or as directed by doctor.

If you forget a dose:
Use as soon as you remember, then return to regular schedule.

What drug does:
Prevents a hypersensitivity reaction to certain allergens such as pollen.

Time lapse before drug works:
Relief of symptoms may begin immediately, but full benefit might take a few days.

Don't use with:
Any other eye medications without consulting your doctor or pharmacist.

 POSSIBLE ADVERSE REACTIONS OR SIDE EFFECTS

SYMPTOMS	WHAT TO DO
Life-threatening: None expected.	
Common: Brief and mild burning or stinging when drops are administered.	No action necessary.
Infrequent: Blurred vision, feeling that something is in the the eye, redness of eye, eye irritation not present before, eye tearing or discharge.	Discontinue. Call doctor right away.
Rare: • Aching in eye, crusting in corner of eye or eyelid, dryness of eyes or nose, drowsiness or sleepiness, feeling of heat in eye or body, nausea, stomach discomfort, sneezing, sticky or tired feeling of eye.	Continue. Call doctor when convenient.
• Redness or irritation of eyelid, swelling of eye, pain in eye, sensitivity to light, headache, dizziness, skin rash.	Discontinue. Call doctor right away.

WARNINGS & PRECAUTIONS

Don't use if:
You are allergic to any of the antiallergic ophthalmic drugs.

Before you start, consult your doctor if:
* You wear soft contact lenses.
* You are allergic to any other medications, foods or other substances.

Over age 60:
No special problems expected.

Pregnancy:
Risk category B for azelastine, emedastine, levocabastine, lodoxamide, nedocromil and pemirolast. Risk category C for epinastine, olopatadine and ketotifen. See page xviii for category information. Consult doctor about use.

Breast-feeding:
It is unknown if these drugs placed in the eyes then pass into milk. Consult your doctor.

Infants & children:
No information available on safety or effectiveness for children under age 2 for lodoxamide and under age 12 for levocabastine. Consult doctor. Azelastine approved for children 3 years and older.

Prolonged use:
No special problems expected.

Skin & sunlight:
No special problems expected.

Driving, piloting or hazardous work:
Avoid if you feel dizzy or side effects cause vision problems.

Discontinuing:
No special problems expected.

Others:
* Don't use leftover medicine for other eye problems without your doctor's approval.
* If symptoms don't improve after a few days of use, call your doctor.

POSSIBLE INTERACTION WITH OTHER DRUGS

GENERIC NAME OR DRUG CLASS	COMBINED EFFECT
None significant.	

POSSIBLE INTERACTION WITH OTHER SUBSTANCES

INTERACTS WITH	COMBINED EFFECT
Alcohol:	None expected.
Beverages:	None expected.
Cocaine	None expected.
Foods:	None expected.
Marijuana:	None expected.
Tobacco:	None expected.

ANTIANDROGENS, NONSTEROIDAL

GENERIC AND BRAND NAMES

BICALUTAMIDE
  Casodex
FLUTAMIDE
  Euflex
  Eulexin

NILUTAMIDE
  Amandron
  Nilandron

BASIC INFORMATION

Habit forming? No
Prescription needed? Yes
Available as generic? No
Drug class: Antineoplastic

 USES

Treatment for prostate cancer. Used in combination with a testosterone lowering measure such as surgery (removal of the testicles) or use of a special monthly injection of luteinizing hormone-releasing hormone (LHRH).

 DOSAGE & USAGE INFORMATION

How to take:
Tablet or capsule—Swallow with liquid. May be taken with or without food.

When to take:
According to doctor's instructions. Normally at the same times each day.

If you forget a dose:
Take as soon as you remember. If it is almost time for your next dose, skip the missed dose and return to your regular dosing schedule (don't double this dose).

What drug does:
Interferes with utilization of androgen (male hormone) testosterone by body cells. Prostate cancer cells require testosterone in order to grow and reproduce.

Continued next column

 OVERDOSE

SYMPTOMS:
Diarrhea, nausea, vomiting, tiredness, headache, dizziness, breast tenderness.
WHAT TO DO:
Overdose unlikely to threaten life. If person uses much larger amount than prescribed or if accidentally swallowed, call doctor or poison control center 1-800-222-1222 for help.

Time lapse before drug works:
Starts working within two hours, but may take several weeks to be effective.

Don't take with:
Any other medicine or any dietary supplement without consulting your doctor or pharmacist.

 POSSIBLE ADVERSE REACTIONS OR SIDE EFFECTS

SYMPTOMS	WHAT TO DO
Life-threatening: None expected.	
Common: • Decreased sex drive, diarrhea, appetite loss, nausea, vomiting, cough or hoarseness, fever, runny nose, sneezing, sore throat, tightness in chest or wheezing, constipation, insomnia.	Continue. Call doctor when convenient.
• Hot flashes with mild sweating.	No action necessary.
Infrequent: • Hands and feet tingling or numb, painful or swollen breasts, swollen feet and legs, chest pain, shortness of breath.	Continue. Call doctor right away.
• Bloody or black tarry stools, itching, back or side pain, depression, muscle weakness, unusual tiredness, skin rash, bloated feeling, confusion, dry mouth, nervousness, color vision changes (with nilutamide).	Continue. Call doctor when convenient.
Rare: • Jaundice (yellow eyes and skin), pain or tenderness in the stomach.	Continue. Call doctor right away.
• Bluish colored lips, skin or nails; dark urine; dizziness or fainting; unusual bleeding or bruising.	Continue. Call doctor when convenient.

Note: Adverse effects that occur may also be due to use of LHRH or symptoms of prostate cancer.

WARNINGS & PRECAUTIONS

Don't take if:
- You are allergic to any of the antiandrogens.
- You are female.

Before you start, consult your doctor if:
- You have liver disease.
- You use tobacco.
- You have lung disease or other breathing problems.
- You have glucose-6-phosphate dehydrogenase (G6PD) deficiency or hemoglobin M disease.
- You are planning on starting a family. May decrease sperm count.

Over age 60:
Adverse reactions and side effects may be more frequent and severe than in younger persons. You may need smaller doses for shorter periods of time.

Pregnancy:
These drugs are not intended for use in women. Risk categories vary for each drug. Bicalutamide is risk category X, flutamide is risk category D and nilutamide is risk category C (see page xviii).

Breast-feeding:
Not intended for use in women.

Infants & children:
Not intended for use in infants and children.

Prolonged use:
Talk to your doctor about the need for follow-up medical examinations or laboratory studies to check liver and pulmonary functions, PSA levels, chest x-rays, and other tests as recommended.

Skin & sunlight:
May cause rash or intensify sunburn in areas exposed to sun or ultraviolet light (photosensitivity reaction). Avoid overexposure. Notify doctor if reaction occurs.

Driving, piloting or hazardous work:
You may experience vision problems when going from a dark area to a lighted area and vice versa (such as driving in and out of tunnels). Use caution.

Discontinuing:
No special problems expected. Don't discontinue drug without doctor's approval.

Others:
- Advise any doctor or dentist whom you consult that you take this medicine.
- May affect results in some medical tests.
- May decrease sperm count.

POSSIBLE INTERACTION WITH OTHER DRUGS

GENERIC NAME OR DRUG CLASS	COMBINED EFFECT
Anticoagulants*	Increased effect of anticoagulant.
Phenytoin	Increased effect of phenytoin with nilutamide.
Theophylline	Increased effect of theophylline.

POSSIBLE INTERACTION WITH OTHER SUBSTANCES

INTERACTS WITH	COMBINED EFFECT
Alcohol:	Nilutamide may cause alcohol intolerance reaction. Avoid alcohol while on this drug.
Beverages:	None expected.
Cocaine:	None expected. Best to avoid.
Foods:	None expected.
Marijuana:	None expected. Best to avoid.
Tobacco:	Increased risk of toxicity. Avoid.

ANTIBACTERIALS, ANTIFUNGALS (Topical)

GENERIC AND BRAND NAMES

CLIOQUINOL &
HYDROCORTISONE
Vioform Hydro-
cortisone Cream
Vioform Hydro-
cortisone Lotion
Vioform Hydro-
cortisone Mild
Cream
Vioform Hydro-
cortisone Mild
Ointment
Vioform Hydro-
cortisone Ointment

SULFADIAZINE
Flamazine
Flint SSD
Sildamac
Silvadene
SSD
SSD AF
Thermazene

BASIC INFORMATION

Habit forming? No
Prescription needed? Yes
Available as generic? Yes, some are
Drug class: Antibacterial (topical),
antifungal (topical)

USES

Treats eczema, other inflammatory skin
conditions, athlete's foot, skin infections.

DOSAGE & USAGE INFORMATION

How to use:
- Cream, lotion, ointment—Bathe and dry area
  before use. Apply small amount and rub
  gently.
- Keep away from eyes.

When to use:
2 to 4 times a day.

If you forget a dose:
Use as soon as you remember.

Continued next column

OVERDOSE

SYMPTOMS:
Severe nausea, vomiting, diarrhea.
WHAT TO DO:
- Not for internal use. If child accidentally
  swallows, call numbers below.
- Dial 911 (emergency) for medical help or
  call poison control center 1-800-222-1222
  for instructions.
- See emergency information on last 3
  pages of this book.

What drug does:
Kills some types of fungus and bacteria on
contact.

Time lapse before drug works:
2 to 4 weeks, sometimes longer.

Don't use with:
Other skin ointments, creams or lotions without
consulting your doctor or pharmacist.

POSSIBLE ADVERSE REACTIONS OR SIDE EFFECTS

SYMPTOMS	WHAT TO DO
Life-threatening: None expected.	
Common: May stain skin around nails.	Continue. Tell doctor at next visit.
Infrequent: Stomach cramps; hives; itching, burning, peeling, red, stinging, swelling skin.	Discontinue. Call doctor right away.
Rare: None expected.	

WARNINGS & PRECAUTIONS

Don't use if:
You are allergic to clioquinol, iodine or any iodine-containing preparation.

Before you start, consult your doctor if:
You are allergic to anything that touches your skin.

Over age 60:
No problems expected.

Pregnancy:
Risk factors vary for drugs in this group. See category list on page xviii and consult doctor.

Breast-feeding:
No problems expected, but check with doctor.

Infants & children:
No problems expected, but check with doctor.

Prolonged use:
No problems expected, but check with doctor.

Skin & sunlight:
No special problems expected.

Driving, piloting or hazardous work:
No problems expected, but check with doctor.

Discontinuing:
No problems expected, but check with doctor.

Others:
* If not improved in 2 weeks, check with doctor.
* May stain clothing or bed linens.
* May stain hair, skin and nails yellow.
* If accidentally gets into eyes, flush with clear water immediately.
* Tests of thyroid function may yield inaccurate results if you use clioquinol within 1 month before testing.

POSSIBLE INTERACTION WITH OTHER DRUGS

GENERIC NAME OR DRUG CLASS	COMBINED EFFECT
None expected.	

POSSIBLE INTERACTION WITH OTHER SUBSTANCES

INTERACTS WITH	COMBINED EFFECT
Alcohol:	None expected.
Beverages:	None expected.
Cocaine:	None expected.
Foods:	None expected.
Marijuana:	None expected.
Tobacco:	None expected.

*See Glossary

ANTIBACTERIALS FOR ACNE (Topical)

GENERIC AND BRAND NAMES

CHLORTETRACYCLINE
(topical)
Aureomycin
CLINDAMYCIN
(topical)
Acanya
Benzaclin
Cleocin T Gel
Cleocin T Lotion
Cleocin T Topical
Solution
Clinda-Derm
ClindaReach
Dalacin T Topical
Solution
DUAC Topical Gel
Evoclin Foam
Ziana Gel
DOXYCYCLINE
(topical)
Adoxa
Adoxa Pak

ERYTHROMYCIN
(topical)
Akne-Mycin
A/T/S
Benzamycin
Erycette
EryDerm
EryGel
EryMax
ErySol
Erythro-statin
ETS
Sans-Acne
Staticin
Theramycin Z
T-Stat
MECLOCYCLINE
(topical)
Meclan
TETRACYCLINE
(topical)
Achromycin
Topicycline

BASIC INFORMATION

Habit forming? No
Prescription needed? Yes
Available as generic? Yes
Drug class: Antibacterial (topical)

 ## USES

Treats acne by killing skin bacteria that may be part of the cause of acne.

 ## OVERDOSE

SYMPTOMS:
None expected.
WHAT TO DO:
Not for internal use. If child accidentally swallows, call doctor or poison control center 1-800-222-1222 for help.

 ## DOSAGE & USAGE INFORMATION

How to use:
- Pledgets and solutions are flammable. Use away from flame or heat.
- Apply drug to entire area, not just to pimples.
- If you use other acne medicines on skin, wait an hour after using erythromycin before applying other medicine.
- Cream, lotion, ointment—Wash and dry area Then apply small amount and rub gently.

When to use:
2 times a day, morning and evening, or as directed by your doctor.

If you forget a dose:
Use as soon as you remember.

What drug does:
Kills bacteria on skin, skin glands or in hair follicles.

Time lapse before drug works:
3 to 4 weeks to begin improvement.

Don't use with:
Other skin medicine without consulting your doctor or pharmacist.

 ## POSSIBLE ADVERSE REACTIONS OR SIDE EFFECTS

SYMPTOMS	WHAT TO DO
Life-threatening: None expected.	
Common: Stinging or burning of skin for a few minutes after application; faint yellow skin color, especially around hair roots (with chlortetracycline, meclocycline or tetracycline).	Continue. Tell doctor at next visit.
Infrequent: Red, peeling, itching, irritated or dry skin.	Continue. Call doctor when convenient.
Rare (extremely): Symptoms of excess medicine absorbed by body—Abdominal pain, diarrhea, fever, nausea, vomiting, bloating, thirst, weakness, weight loss.	Discontinue. Call doctor right away.

WARNINGS & PRECAUTIONS

Don't use if:
You are allergic to erythromycins, clindamycins or tetracyclines.

Before you start, consult your doctor if:
* You are allergic to any substance that touches your skin.
* You use benzoyl peroxide, resorcinol, salicylic acid, sulfur or tretinoin (vitamin A acid).

Over age 60:
No problems expected.

Pregnancy:
Risk factors vary for drugs in this group. See category list on page xviii and consult doctor.

Breast-feeding:
No problems expected, but check with doctor.

Infants & children:
No problems expected, but check with doctor.

Prolonged use:
Excess irritation to skin.

Skin & sunlight:
No special problems expected.

Driving, piloting or hazardous work:
No problems expected, but check with doctor.

Discontinuing:
No problems expected, but check with doctor.

Others:
* Use water-base cosmetics.
* Keep medicine away from mouth or eyes.
* If accidentally gets into eyes, flush immediately with clear water.
* Keep away from heat or flame.
* Keep cool, but don't freeze.

POSSIBLE INTERACTION WITH OTHER DRUGS

GENERIC NAME OR DRUG CLASS	COMBINED EFFECT
Abrasive or medicated soaps	Irritation or too much drying.
After-shave lotions	Irritation or too much drying.
Antiacne topical preparations (other)	Irritation or too much drying.
"Cover-up" cosmetics	Irritation or too much drying.
Drying cosmetic soaps	Irritation or too much drying.
Isotretinoin	Irritation or too much drying.
Mercury compounds	May stain skin black and smell bad.
Perfumed toilet water	Irritation or too much drying.
Preparations containing skin peeling agents such as benzoyl peroxide, resorcinol, salicylic acid, sulfur, tretinoin	Irritation or too much drying.

POSSIBLE INTERACTION WITH OTHER SUBSTANCES

INTERACTS WITH	COMBINED EFFECT
Alcohol:	None expected.
Beverages:	None expected.
Cocaine:	None expected.
Foods:	None expected.
Marijuana:	None expected.
Tobacco:	None expected.

*See Glossary

ANTIBACTERIALS (Ophthalmic)

GENERIC AND BRAND NAMES

See full list of generic and brand names in the *Generic and Brand Name Directory*, page 869.

BASIC INFORMATION

Habit forming? No
Prescription needed? Yes
Available as generic? Yes, for some
Drug class: Antibacterial (ophthalmic)

 ## USES

• Helps body overcome eye infections on surface tissues of the eye.
• Treatment for corneal ulcers.

 ## DOSAGE & USAGE INFORMATION

How to use:
Eye drops
• Wash hands.
• Apply pressure to inside corner of eye with middle finger.
• Continue pressure for 1 minute after placing medicine in eye.
• Tilt head backward. Pull lower lid away from eye with index finger of the same hand.
• Drop eye drops into pouch and close eye. Don't blink.
• Keep eyes closed for 1 to 2 minutes.

Eye ointment
• Wash hands.
• Pull lower lid down from eye to form a pouch.
• Squeeze tube to apply thin strip of ointment into pouch.
• Close eye for 1 to 2 minutes.
• Don't touch applicator tip to any surface (including the eye). If you accidentally touch tip, clean with warm soap and water.
• Keep container tightly closed.
• Keep cool, but don't freeze.
• Wash hands immediately after using.

Continued next column

 ## OVERDOSE

SYMPTOMS:
None expected.
WHAT TO DO:
Not intended for internal use. If child accidentally swallows, call doctor or poison control center 1-800-222-1222 for help.

When to use:
As directed. Don't miss doses.

If you forget a dose:
Use as soon as you remember.

What drug does:
Penetrates bacterial cell membrane and prevents cells from multiplying.

Time lapse before drug works:
Begins in 1 hour. May require 7 to 10 days to control infection.

Don't use with:
Any other eye drops or ointment without checking with your doctor or pharmacist.

 ## POSSIBLE ADVERSE REACTIONS OR SIDE EFFECTS

SYMPTOMS	WHAT TO DO
Life-threatening: None expected.	
Common: Ointments cause blurred vision for a few minutes.	Continue. Tell doctor at next visit.
Infrequent: • Signs of irritation not present before drug use.	Discontinue. Call doctor right away.
• Burning or stinging of the eye.	Continue. Call doctor when convenient.
Rare (with chloramphenicol): Sore throat, pale skin, fever, unusual bleeding or bruising.	Discontinue. Call doctor right away.

WARNINGS & PRECAUTIONS

Don't use if:
You are allergic to any antibiotic used on skin, ears, vagina or rectum.

Before you start, consult your doctor if:
You have had an allergic reaction to any medicine, food or other substances.

Over age 60:
No problems expected.

Pregnancy:
Risk factors vary for drugs in this group. See category list on page xviii and consult doctor.

Breast-feeding:
No problems expected, but check with doctor.

Infants & children:
No problems expected. Use only under medical supervision.

Prolonged use:
Sensitivity reaction may develop.

Skin & sunlight:
No problems expected.

Driving, piloting or hazardous work:
No problems expected.

Discontinuing:
Possible rare adverse reaction of bone marrow depression that leads to aplastic anemia may occur after discontinuing chloramphenicol.

Others:
* Notify doctor if symptoms fail to improve in 2 to 4 days.
* Keep medicine cool, but don't freeze.

POSSIBLE INTERACTION WITH OTHER DRUGS

GENERIC NAME OR DRUG CLASS	COMBINED EFFECT
Clinically significant interactions with oral or injected medicines unlikely.	

POSSIBLE INTERACTION WITH OTHER SUBSTANCES

INTERACTS WITH	COMBINED EFFECT
Alcohol:	None expected.
Beverages:	None expected.
Cocaine:	None expected.
Foods:	None expected.
Marijuana:	None expected.
Tobacco:	None expected.

*See Glossary

ANTIBACTERIALS (Otic)

GENERIC AND BRAND NAMES

ACETIC ACID
  VoSol
ACETIC ACID &
  ALUMINUM
  ACETATE
  Domeboro
ACETIC ACID &
  HYDROCORTISONE
  Acetasol HC
  VoSol HC
CIPROFLOXACIN &
  DEXAMETHASONE
  Ciprodex
CIPROFLOXACIN &
  HYDROCORTISONE
  Cipro HC
NEOMYCIN, COLISTIN
  & HYDRO-
  CORTISONE
  Coly-Mycin S

NEOMYCIN,
  POLYMIXIN B &
  HYDROCORTI-
  SONE (otic)
  Antibiotic Ear
  Cortatrigen
  Cort-Biotic
  Drotic
  Ear-Eze
  LazerSporin
  Masporin Otic
  Oticair
  Octigen
  Otimar
  Otocidin
  Otocort
  Pediotic
OFLOXACIN (otic)
  Floxin Otic

BASIC INFORMATION

Habit forming? No
Prescription needed? Yes
Available as generic? Yes, for some
Drug class: Antibacterial (otic)

USES

- Treatment for outer ear infection (called swimmer's ear or otitis externa).
- Treats certain acute or chronic middle ear infections (e.g., otitis media).
- Most of these drugs contain an antibacterial to fight the infection and an anti-inflammatory to help provide relief from redness, irritation and discomfort.

OVERDOSE

SYMPTOMS:
None expected.
WHAT TO DO:
Not intended for internal use. If child accidentally swallows, call doctor or poison control center 1-800-222-1222 for help.

DOSAGE & USAGE INFORMATION

How to use:
As directed by your doctor or pharmacist. The following are general instructions.

How to use ear drops:
- Wash and dry hands.
- Warm drops by holding container in your hand for a few minutes.
- Lie down with affected ear up.
- Adults—Pull ear lobe back and up.
- Children—Pull ear lobe down and back.
- Put the correct number of drops into the ear. Do not allow dropper to touch the ear.
- Wipe away any spilled drops.
- Stay lying down for 2 to 5 minutes.

When to use:
As directed on label. The number of daily doses will vary depending on the specific drug.

If you forget a dose:
Use as soon as you remember. If it is almost time for the next dose, wait for next scheduled dose (don't double this dose).

What drug does:
Antibacterials destroy the bacteria causing the infection. Anti-inflammatories reduce symptoms of inflammation.

Time lapse before drug works:
Symptoms should improve within a few days. Complete healing of the infection will take longer.

Don't use with:
Other ear medications unless directed by your doctor or pharmacist.

POSSIBLE ADVERSE REACTIONS OR SIDE EFFECTS

SYMPTOMS	WHAT TO DO
Life-threatening: None expected.	
Common: None expected.	
Infrequent: Burning or stinging of the ear.	Continue. Call doctor if symptoms persist.
Rare: • Itching, redness, hives, swelling (allergic reaction), hearing changes, bleeding from ear.	Discontinue. Call doctor right away.
• Headache, fever, sore throat, runny or stuffy nose, taste changes, ear ringing.	Continue. Call doctor when convenient.

WARNINGS & PRECAUTIONS

Don't use if:
You are allergic to any of the drugs listed or other antibiotics, fluoroquinolones or steroid medications.

Before you start, consult your doctor if:
• Your eardrum is punctured.
• You have tendonitis (if ofloxacin prescribed).
• You have a viral infection such as chickenpox (varicella) or herpes simplex.

Over age 60:
No problems expected.

Pregnancy:
Decide with your doctor if drug benefits justify risk to unborn child. Risk category C for most of these drugs (see page xviii).

Breast-feeding:
Drugs may be absorbed into the body and into milk. Avoid drugs or discontinue nursing until you finish medicine. Consult doctor for advice on maintaining milk supply.

Infants & children:
Follow instructions provided by your doctor. Use the correct dosage for your infant or child's age and weight.

Prolonged use:
• Not intended for prolonged use. Don't use longer than prescribed by your doctor.
• Overuse or unnecessary use of the drug can lead to its decreased effectiveness in fighting infections.

Skin & sunlight:
No problems expected.

Driving, piloting or hazardous work:
Avoid if you experience dizziness or balance problems caused by the ear infection.

Discontinuing:
Don't discontinue without doctor's advice until you complete prescribed dosage.

Others:
• Follow your doctor's instructions for additional ear care at home.
• Call your doctor if ear symptoms worsen or don't improve after a few days of treatment.
• There is a slight risk of a secondary infection (one that occurs during or after treatment of another infection). Consult doctor if new, unexpected symptoms develop.
• Rarely, some of these drugs may increase the risk of hearing or balance problems. Discuss the drug's benefits and risks with your doctor.
• Advise any doctor or dentist whom you consult that you are using this drug.

 ## POSSIBLE INTERACTION WITH OTHER DRUGS

GENERIC NAME OR DRUG CLASS	COMBINED EFFECT
None expected.	

 ## POSSIBLE INTERACTION WITH OTHER SUBSTANCES

INTERACTS WITH	COMBINED EFFECT
Alcohol:	None expected.
Beverages:	None expected.
Cocaine:	None expected.
Foods:	None expected.
Marijuana:	None expected.
Tobacco:	None expected.

ANTIBACTERIALS (Topical)

GENERIC AND BRAND NAMES

CHLORAMPHENICOL
  (topical)
  Chloromycetin
GENTAMICIN
  Garamycin
  Gentamar
  G-Myticin
  Antibiotic
MUPIROCIN
  Bactroban
  Bactroban Nasal
NEOMYCIN &
  POLYMIXIN B
  Neosporin Cream

NEOMYCIN,
  POLYMIXIN B &
  BACITRACIN
  Bactine First Aid
  Foille
  Mycitracin
  Neo-Polycin
  Neosporin
  Ointment
  Topisporin
  Triple Antibiotic
RETAPAMULIN
  Altabax

BASIC INFORMATION

Habit forming? No
Prescription needed? Yes, for some
Available as generic? Yes, for some
Drug class: Antibacterial (topical)

 USES

Treats skin infections that may accompany burns, superficial boils, insect bites or stings, skin ulcers, impetigo, minor surgical wounds.

 DOSAGE & USAGE INFORMATION

How to use:
- Cream, lotion, ointment—Bathe and dry area before use. Apply small amount and rub gently. May cover with gauze or bandage if desired.
- Nasal ointment—Follow instructions provided with prescription.

Continued next column

 OVERDOSE

SYMPTOMS:
None expected.
WHAT TO DO:
Not for internal use. If child accidentally swallows, call numbers below.
- Dial 911 (emergency) for medical help or call poison control center 1-800-222-1222 for instructions.
- See emergency information on last 3 pages of this book.

When to use:
3 or 4 times daily, or as directed by doctor.

If you forget a dose:
Use as soon as you remember.

What drug does:
Kills susceptible bacteria by interfering with bacterial DNA and RNA.

Time lapse before drug works:
Begins first day. May require treatment for a week or longer to cure infection.

Don't use with:
Any other topical medicine without consulting your doctor or pharmacist.

 POSSIBLE ADVERSE REACTIONS OR SIDE EFFECTS

SYMPTOMS	WHAT TO DO
Life-threatening: None expected.	
Common: None expected.	
Infrequent: Itching, swollen or red skin; rash.	Discontinue. Call doctor right away.
Rare: Any sort of hearing loss (with neomycin products); pale skin, sore throat, fever, unusual bleeding or bruising, unusual tiredness or weakness (with chloramphenicol).	Discontinue. Call doctor right away.

WARNINGS & PRECAUTIONS

Don't use if:
You are allergic to chloramphenicol, gentamicin or related antibiotics (name usually ends with "mycin" or "micin"), mupirocin, neomycin, polymyxins.

Before you start, consult your doctor if:
Any of the lesions on the skin are open sores.

Over age 60:
No problems expected.

Pregnancy:
Risk factors vary for drugs in this group. See category list on page xviii and consult doctor.

Breast-feeding:
No problems expected, but check with doctor.

Infants & children:
No problems expected, but check with doctor.

Prolonged use:
No problems expected, but check with doctor.

Skin & sunlight:
No special problems expected.

Driving, piloting or hazardous work:
No problems expected, but check with doctor.

Discontinuing:
No problems expected, but check with doctor.

Others:
* Heat and moisture in bathroom medicine cabinet can cause breakdown of medicine. Store someplace else.
* Keep cool, but don't freeze.

 POSSIBLE INTERACTION WITH OTHER DRUGS

GENERIC NAME OR DRUG CLASS	COMBINED EFFECT
Any other topical medication	Hypersensitivity* reactions more likely to occur.

 POSSIBLE INTERACTION WITH OTHER SUBSTANCES

INTERACTS WITH	COMBINED EFFECT
Alcohol:	None expected.
Beverages:	None expected.
Cocaine:	None expected.
Foods:	None expected.
Marijuana:	None expected.
Tobacco:	None expected.

*See Glossary

ANTICHOLINERGICS

GENERIC AND BRAND NAMES

See full list of generic and brand names in the *Generic and Brand Name Directory*, page 870.

BASIC INFORMATION

Habit forming? No
Prescription needed?
   Low strength: No
   High strength: Yes
Available as generic? Yes
Drug class: Antispasmodic, anticholinergic

 ## USES

- Reduces spasms of digestive system, bladder and urethra.
- Treatment of bronchial spasms.
- Used as a component in some cough and cold preparations.
- Treatment of peptic ulcers.

 ## DOSAGE & USAGE INFORMATION

How to take:
- Tablet—Swallow with liquid or food to lessen stomach irritation.
- Aerosol—Dilute in saline and inhale as nebulizer.

When to take:
30 minutes before meals (unless directed otherwise by doctor).

If you forget a dose:
Take as soon as you remember up to 2 hours late. If more than 2 hours, wait for next scheduled dose (don't double this dose).

What drug does:
Blocks nerve impulses at parasympathetic nerve endings, preventing muscle contractions and gland secretions of organs involved.

Continued next column

 ## OVERDOSE

SYMPTOMS:
Dilated pupils, rapid pulse and breathing, dizziness, fever, hallucinations, confusion, slurred speech, agitation, flushed face, convulsions, coma.
WHAT TO DO:
- **Dial 911 (emergency) for medical help or call poison control center 1-800-222-1222 for instructions.**
- **See emergency information on last 3 pages of this book.**

Time lapse before drug works:
15 to 30 minutes.

Don't take with:
- Antacids* or antidiarrheals.*
- Any other medicine or any dietary supplement without consulting your doctor or pharmacist.

 ## POSSIBLE ADVERSE REACTIONS OR SIDE EFFECTS

SYMPTOMS	WHAT TO DO
Life-threatening:	
In case of overdose, see previous column.	
Common:	
• Confusion, delirium, rapid heartbeat.	Discontinue. Call doctor right away.
• Nausea, vomiting, decreased sweating.	Continue. Call doctor when convenient.
• Constipation.	Continue. Tell doctor at next visit.
• Dryness in ears, nose, throat, mouth.	No action necessary.
Infrequent:	
• Headache, difficult or painful urination, nasal congestion, altered taste, increased sensitivity to light.	Continue. Call doctor when convenient.
• Lightheadedness.	Discontinue. Call doctor right away.
Rare:	
Rash or hives, eye pain, blurred vision, fever.	Discontinue. Call doctor right away.

 ## WARNINGS & PRECAUTIONS

Don't take if:
- You are allergic to any anticholinergic.
- You have trouble with stomach bloating.
- You have difficulty emptying your bladder completely.
- You have narrow-angle glaucoma.
- You have severe ulcerative colitis.

Before you start, consult your doctor if:
- You have open-angle glaucoma.
- You have angina or any heart disease or heart rhythm problem.
- You have chronic bronchitis or asthma.
- You have liver, kidney or thyroid disease.
- You have hiatal hernia or esophagitis.
- You have enlarged prostate or urinary retention.
- You have myasthenia gravis.
- You have peptic ulcer.
- You will have surgery within 2 months, including dental surgery, requiring general or spinal anesthesia.

Over age 60:
Adverse reactions and side effects may be more frequent and severe than in younger persons.

Pregnancy:
Risk factors vary for drugs in this group. See category list on page xviii and consult doctor.

Breast-feeding:
Drug may pass into milk and could affect milk flow. Avoid drug or discontinue nursing until you finish medicine. Consult doctor for advice on maintaining milk supply.

Infants & children:
Use only under medical supervision.

Prolonged use:
Chronic constipation, possible fecal impaction. Consult doctor immediately.

Skin & sunlight:
No special problems expected.

Driving, piloting or hazardous work:
Use disqualifies you for piloting aircraft. Otherwise, no problems expected.

Discontinuing:
May be unnecessary to finish medicine. Follow doctor's instructions.

Others:
Advise any doctor or dentist whom you consult that you take this medicine.

POSSIBLE INTERACTION WITH OTHER DRUGS

GENERIC NAME OR DRUG CLASS	COMBINED EFFECT
Adrenocorticoids, systemic	Possible glaucoma.
Amantadine	Increased anti-cholinergic effect.
Antacids*	Space doses of the drugs 2 to 3 hours apart.
Anticholinergics, other*	Increased anti-cholinergic effect.
Antidepressants, tricyclic*	Increased anti-cholinergic effect. Increased sedation.
Antifungals, azoles	Decreased azole absorption.
Antihistamines*	Increased anti-cholinergic effect.
Attapulgite	Decreased anti-cholinergic effect.
Haloperidol	Increased internal eye pressure.
Methylphenidate	Increased anti-cholinergic effect.
Molindone	Increased anti-cholinergic effect.
Monoamine oxidase (MAO) inhibitors*	Increased anti-cholinergic effect.
Narcotics*	Increased risk of severe constipation.
Orphenadrine	Increased anti-cholinergic effect.
Phenothiazines*	Increased anti-cholinergic effect.
Potassium supplements*	Possible intestinal ulcers with oral potassium tablets.
Quinidine	Increased anti-cholinergic effect.

POSSIBLE INTERACTION WITH OTHER SUBSTANCES

INTERACTS WITH	COMBINED EFFECT
Alcohol:	None expected.
Beverages:	None expected.
Cocaine:	Excessively rapid heartbeat. Avoid.
Foods:	None expected.
Marijuana:	Drowsiness and dry mouth.
Tobacco:	None expected.

*See Glossary

ANTICOAGULANTS (Oral)

GENERIC AND BRAND NAMES

ANISINDIONE
Miradon

WARFARIN SODIUM
Coumadin
Panwarfarin
Sofarin
Warfilone

BASIC INFORMATION

Habit forming? No
Prescription needed? Yes
Available as generic? Yes
Drug class: Anticoagulant

 USES

Reduces blood clots. Used for abnormal clotting inside blood vessels.

 DOSAGE & USAGE INFORMATION

How to take:
Tablet—Swallow with liquid. If you can't swallow whole, crumble tablet and take with liquid or food.

When to take:
At the same time each day.

If you forget a dose:
Take as soon as you remember up to 12 hours late. If more than 12 hours, wait for next scheduled dose (don't double this dose). Inform your doctor of any missed doses.

What drug does:
Blocks action of vitamin K necessary for blood clotting.

Time lapse before drug works:
36 to 48 hours.

Don't take with:
Any other medicine or any dietary supplement without consulting your doctor or pharmacist.

 OVERDOSE

SYMPTOMS:
Bloody vomit, coughing blood, bloody or black stools, red urine.
WHAT TO DO:
- **Dial 911 (emergency) for medical help or call poison control center 1-800-222-1222 for instructions.**
- **See emergency information on last 3 pages of this book.**

 POSSIBLE ADVERSE REACTIONS OR SIDE EFFECTS

SYMPTOMS	WHAT TO DO
Life-threatening:	
In case of overdose, see previous column.	
Common:	
Bloating, gas.	Continue. Tell doctor at next visit.
Infrequent:	
• Black stools or bloody vomit, coughing up blood.	Discontinue. Seek emergency treatment.
• Rash, hives, itch, blurred vision, sore throat, easy bruising, bleeding, cloudy or red urine, back pain, jaundice, fever, chills, fatigue, weakness, painful urination, decreased amount of urine, heavy menstruation, bleeding gums.	Discontinue. Call doctor right away.
• Diarrhea, cramps, nausea, vomiting, swollen feet or legs, hair loss.	Continue. Call doctor when convenient.
Rare:	
• Bleeding into and under skin.	Discontinue. Seek emergency treatment.
• Dizziness, headache, mouth sores.	Discontinue. Call doctor right away.

 WARNINGS & PRECAUTIONS

Don't take if:
- You have been allergic to any oral anticoagulant.
- You have a bleeding disorder.
- You have an active peptic ulcer.
- You have ulcerative colitis.

Before you start, consult your doctor if:
- You take any other drugs, including nonprescription drugs.
- You have high blood pressure.
- You have heavy or prolonged menstrual periods.
- You have diabetes.
- You have a bladder catheter.
- You have serious liver or kidney disease.
- You will have surgery within 2 months, including dental surgery, requiring general or spinal anesthesia.

Over age 60:
Adverse reactions and side effects may be more frequent and severe than in younger persons.

Pregnancy:
Risk factors vary for drugs in this group. See category list on page xviii and consult doctor.

Breast-feeding:
Drug filters into milk. May harm child. Avoid.

Infants & children:
Use only under doctor's supervision.

Prolonged use:
Talk to your doctor about the need for follow-up medical examinations or laboratory studies to check prothrombin time, stool and urine for blood.

Skin & sunlight:
No problems expected.

Driving, piloting or hazardous work:
Avoid hazardous activities that could cause injury. Don't drive if you feel dizzy or have blurred vision.

Discontinuing:
Don't discontinue without consulting doctor. Dose may require gradual reduction if you have taken drug for a long time. Doses of other drugs may also require adjustment.

Others:
- Carry identification to state that you take anticoagulants.
- Your genetic makeup may influence your response to warfarin. Ask your doctor about genetic testing.
- Advise any doctor or dentist whom you consult that you take this medicine.

 POSSIBLE INTERACTION WITH OTHER DRUGS

GENERIC NAME OR DRUG CLASS	COMBINED EFFECT
Acetaminophen	Increased effect of anticoagulant.
Adrenocorticoids, systemic	Decreased anticoagulant effect.
Allopurinol	Increased effect of anticoagulant.
Aminoglutethimide	Decreased effect of anticoagulant.
Amiodarone	Increased effect of anticoagulant.
Androgens*	Increased effect of anticoagulant.
Antacids* (large doses)	Decreased effect of anticoagulant.
Antibiotics*	Increased effect of anticoagulant.
Antidiabetic agents*	Increased effect of anticoagulant.

Antifungals, azoles	Increased anticoagulant effect.
Antihistamines*	Unpredictable increased or decreased effect of anticoagulant.
Anti-inflammatory drugs, nonsteroidal (NSAIDs)*	Increased risk of bleeding.
Anti-inflammatory drugs, nonsteroidal (ophthalmic)*	May increase bleeding tendency.
Aspirin	Possible spontaneous bleeding.
Barbiturates*	Decreased effect of anticoagulant.
Benzodiazepines*	Unpredictable increased or decreased effect of anticoagulant.
Bismuth subsalicylate	Increased risk of bleeding.
Calcium supplements*	Decreased effect of anticoagulant.
Carbamazepine	Decreased effect of anticoagulant.
Cefixime	Increased effect of anticoagulant.
Chloramphenicol	Increased effect of anticoagulant.
Estramustine	Decreased effect of anticoagulant.

Continued on page 900

 POSSIBLE INTERACTION WITH OTHER SUBSTANCES

INTERACTS WITH	COMBINED EFFECT
Alcohol:	Can increase or decrease effect of anticoagulant. Avoid.
Beverages:	None expected.
Cocaine:	None expected.
Foods: High in vitamin K such as fish, liver, spinach, cabbage, cauliflower, Brussels sprouts.	May decrease anticoagulant effect.
Marijuana:	None expected.
Tobacco:	Decreased effect of anticoagulant.

*See Glossary

ANTICONVULSANTS, HYDANTOIN

GENERIC AND BRAND NAMES

ETHOTOIN
  Peganone

PHENYTOIN
  Dilantin
  Dilantin 30
  Dilantin 125
  Dilantin Infatabs
  Dilantin Kapseals
  Diphenylan

BASIC INFORMATION

Habit forming? No
Prescription needed? Yes
Available as generic? Yes
Drug class: Anticonvulsant (hydantoin)

 ## USES

- Prevents some forms of epileptic seizures.
- Stabilizes irregular heartbeat.

 ## DOSAGE & USAGE INFORMATION

How to take:
- Tablet—Swallow with liquid.
- Chewable tablet—Chew well before swallowing.
- Suspension—Shake solution well before taking with liquid.

When to take:
At the same time each day.

If you forget a dose:
- If drug taken 1 time per day—Take as soon as you remember up to 12 hours late. If more than 12 hours, wait for next scheduled dose (don't double this dose).
- If taken several times per day—Take as soon as possible, then return to regular schedule.

Continued next column

 ## OVERDOSE

SYMPTOMS:
Jerky eye movements; stagger; slurred speech; imbalance; drowsiness; blood pressure drop; slow, shallow breathing; coma.
WHAT TO DO:
- **Dial 911 (emergency) for medical help or call poison control center 1-800-222-1222 for instructions.**
- **See emergency information on last 3 pages of this book.**

What drug does:
Promotes sodium loss from nerve fibers. This lessens excitability and inhibits spread of nerve impulses.

Time lapse before drug works:
7 to 10 days continual use.

Don't take with:
Any other medicine or any dietary supplement without consulting your doctor or pharmacist.

 ## POSSIBLE ADVERSE REACTIONS OR SIDE EFFECTS

SYMPTOMS	WHAT TO DO
Life-threatening: Severe allergic reaction (rash, fever, swollen glands, kidney failure).	Seek emergency help.
Common:	
• Bleeding, swollen or tender gums.	Continue, but call doctor right away.
• Mild dizziness or drowsiness, constipation.	Continue. Call doctor when convenient.
Infrequent:	
• Hallucinations, confusion, stagger, fever, uncontrolled eye movements, increase in seizures, rash, change in vision, agitation, sore throat, diarrhea, slurred speech, muscle twitching.	Continue, but call doctor right away.
• Increased body and facial hair, breast swelling, insomnia, enlargement of facial features.	Continue. Call doctor when convenient.
Rare: Nausea; vomiting; unusual bleeding or bruising; swollen lymph nodes; stomach pain; yellow skin or eyes; joint pain; light gray stools; loss of appetite; weight loss; trouble breathing; uncontrolled movements of arms, legs, hands, lips, tongue or cheeks; slowed growth; learning problems.	Continue, but call doctor right away.

WARNINGS & PRECAUTIONS

Don't take if:
You are allergic to any hydantoin anticonvulsant.

Before you start, consult your doctor if:
- You have had impaired liver function or disease.
- You will have surgery within 2 months, including dental surgery, requiring general or spinal anesthesia.
- You have diabetes.
- You have a blood disorder.

Over age 60:
Adverse reactions and side effects may be more frequent and severe than in younger persons.

Pregnancy:
Decide with your doctor if drug benefits justify risk to unborn child. Risk category C (see page xviii).

Breast-feeding:
Drug passes into milk. Avoid drug or discontinue nursing until you finish medicine. Consult doctor for advice on maintaining milk supply.

Infants & children:
Use only under medical supervision.

Prolonged use:
- Weakened bones.
- Lymph gland enlargement.
- Possible liver damage.
- Numbness and tingling of hands and feet.
- Continual back-and-forth eye movements.
- Talk to your doctor about the need for follow-up medical examinations or laboratory studies to check complete blood counts (white blood cell count, platelet count, red blood cell count, hemoglobin, hematocrit), liver function, EEG.*

Skin & sunlight:
One or more drugs in this group may cause rash or intensify sunburn in areas exposed to sun or ultraviolet light (photosensitivity reaction). Avoid overexposure. Notify doctor if reaction occurs.

Driving, piloting or hazardous work:
Don't drive or pilot aircraft until you learn how medicine affects you. Don't work around dangerous machinery. Don't climb ladders or work in high places. Danger increases if you drink alcohol or take medicine affecting alertness and reflexes.

Discontinuing:
Don't discontinue without consulting doctor. Dose may require gradual reduction if you have taken drug for a long time. Doses of other drugs may also require adjustment.

Others:
- May cause learning disability.
- Good dental care is important while using this medicine.
- Advise any doctor or dentist whom you consult about the use of this drug.
- Rarely, antiepileptic drugs may lead to suicidal thoughts and behaviors. Call doctor right away if suicidal symptoms or unusual behaviors occur.

 POSSIBLE INTERACTION WITH OTHER DRUGS

GENERIC NAME OR DRUG CLASS	COMBINED EFFECT
Adrenocorticoids, systemic	Decreased adrenocorticoid effect.
Amiodarone	Increased anticonvulsant effect.
Antacids*	Decreased anticonvulsant effect.
Antiandrogens, nonsteroidal	Increased effect of phenytoin.
Anticoagulants*	Increased effect of both drugs.
Antidepressants, tricyclic*	May need to adjust anticonvulsant dose.
Antifungals, azoles	Increased anticoagulant effect.
Antivirals, HIV/AIDS*	Increased risk of peripheral neuropathy with phenytoin.
Barbiturates*	Changed seizure pattern.
Calcium	Decreased effects of both drugs.
Carbamazepine	Possible increased anticonvulsant metabolism.
Carbonic anhydrase inhibitors*	Increased chance of bone disease.

Continued on page 902

 POSSIBLE INTERACTION WITH OTHER SUBSTANCES

INTERACTS WITH	COMBINED EFFECT
Alcohol:	Possible decreased anticonvulsant effect. Use with caution.
Beverages:	None expected.
Cocaine:	Possible seizures.
Foods:	None expected.
Marijuana:	Drowsiness, unsteadiness, decreased anticonvulsant effect.
Tobacco:	None expected.

*See Glossary

ANTICONVULSANTS, SUCCINIMIDE

GENERIC AND BRAND NAMES

ETHOSUXIMIDE
Zarontin

METHSUXIMIDE
Celontin

BASIC INFORMATION

Habit forming? No
Prescription needed? Yes
Available as generic? Yes, for some
Drug class: Anticonvulsant (succinimide)

 USES

Controls seizures in treatment of some forms of epilepsy.

 DOSAGE & USAGE INFORMATION

How to take:
Capsule or syrup—Swallow with liquid or food to lessen stomach irritation.

When to take:
Every day in regularly spaced doses, according to prescription.

If you forget a dose:
Take as soon as you remember up to 2 hours late. If more than 2 hours, wait for next scheduled dose (don't double this dose).

What drug does:
Depresses nerve transmissions in part of brain that controls muscles.

Time lapse before drug works:
3 hours.

Don't take with:
Any other medicine or any dietary supplement without consulting your doctor or pharmacist.

 OVERDOSE

SYMPTOMS:
Severe drowsiness, slow or irregular breathing, coma.
WHAT TO DO:
• Dial 911 (emergency) for medical help or call poison control center 1-800-222-1222 for instructions.
• If person is unconscious, check breathing and pulse. If not breathing, begin mouth-to-mouth rescue breathing. If heart is not beating, begin chest compressions.
• See emergency information on last 3 pages of this book.

 POSSIBLE ADVERSE REACTIONS OR SIDE EFFECTS

SYMPTOMS	WHAT TO DO
Life-threatening:	
In case of overdose, see previous column.	
Common:	
• Nausea, vomiting, appetite loss, dizziness, drowsiness, hiccups, stomach pain, headache, loss of appetite.	Continue. Call doctor when convenient.
• Muscle pain, skin rash or itching, swollen glands, sore throat, fever.	Continue, but call doctor right away.
• Change in urine color (pink, red, red-brown).	No action necessary.
Infrequent:	
Nightmares, irritability, mood changes, tiredness, difficulty concentrating.	Continue, but call doctor right away.
Rare:	
Unusual bleeding or bruising, depression, swollen glands, chills, increased seizures, shortness of breath, wheezing, chest pain, sores in mouth or on lips.	Continue, but call doctor right away.

WARNINGS & PRECAUTIONS

Don't take if:
You are allergic to any succinimide anticonvulsant.

Before you start, consult your doctor if:
- You plan to become pregnant within medication period.
- You take other anticonvulsants.
- You have blood disease.
- You have kidney or liver disease.

Over age 60:
Adverse reactions and side effects may be more frequent and severe than in younger persons.

Pregnancy:
Risk factors vary for drugs in this group. See category list on page xviii and consult doctor.

Breast-feeding:
Drug passes into milk. Avoid drug or discontinue nursing. Consult your doctor about maintaining milk supply.

Infants & children:
Use only under medical supervision.

Prolonged use:
Talk to your doctor about the need for follow-up medical examinations or laboratory studies to check complete blood counts (white blood cell count, platelet count, red blood cell count, hemoglobin, hematocrit), liver function, kidney function, urine.

Skin & sunlight:
No problems expected.

Driving, piloting or hazardous work:
Don't drive or pilot aircraft until you learn how medicine affects you. Don't work around dangerous machinery. Don't climb ladders or work in high places. Danger increases if you drink alcohol or take medicine affecting alertness and reflexes, such as antihistamines, tranquilizers, sedatives, pain medicine, narcotics and mind-altering drugs.

Discontinuing:
Don't discontinue without doctor's advice until you complete prescribed dose, even though symptoms diminish or disappear.

Others:
- Your response to medicine should be checked regularly by your doctor. Dose and schedule may have to be altered frequently to fit individual needs.
- Periodic blood cell counts, kidney and liver function studies recommended.
- May discolor urine pink to red-brown. No action necessary.

- Advise any doctor or dentist whom you consult that you use this medicine.
- Rarely, antiepileptic drugs may lead to suicidal thoughts and behaviors. Call doctor right away if suicidal symptoms or unusual behaviors occur.

POSSIBLE INTERACTION WITH OTHER DRUGS

GENERIC NAME OR DRUG CLASS	COMBINED EFFECT
Anticonvulsants, other*	Increased effect of both drugs.
Antidepressants, tricyclic*	May provoke seizures.
Antipsychotics*	May provoke seizures.
Central nervous system (CNS) depressants*	Decreased anti-convulsant effect.
Haloperidol	Decreased haloperidol effect; changed seizure pattern.
Phenytoin	Increased phenytoin effect.

POSSIBLE INTERACTION WITH OTHER SUBSTANCES

INTERACTS WITH	COMBINED EFFECT
Alcohol:	May provoke seizures.
Beverages:	None expected.
Cocaine:	May provoke seizures.
Foods:	None expected.
Marijuana:	May provoke seizures.
Tobacco:	None expected.

*See Glossary

ANTIDEPRESSANTS, TRICYCLIC

GENERIC AND BRAND NAMES

See full list of generic and brand names in the *Generic and Brand Name Directory*, page 870.

BASIC INFORMATION

Habit forming? No
Prescription needed? Yes
Available as generic? Yes
Drug class: Antidepressant (tricyclic)

USES

- Gradually relieves symptoms of depression.
- Used to decrease bedwetting in children.
- Pain relief (sometimes).
- Clomipramine is used to treat obsessive-compulsive disorder.
- Treatment for narcolepsy, bulimia, panic attacks, cocaine withdrawal, attention-deficit disorder.
- May be useful for restless leg syndrome.

DOSAGE & USAGE INFORMATION

How to take:
Tablet, capsule or syrup—Swallow with liquid.

When to take:
At the same time each day, usually at bedtime.

If you forget a dose:
Bedtime dose—If you forget your once-a-day bedtime dose, don't take it more than 3 hours late. If more than 3 hours, wait for next scheduled dose. Don't double this dose.

What drug does:
Probably affects part of brain that controls messages between nerve cells.

Continued next column

OVERDOSE

SYMPTOMS:
Hallucinations, drowsiness, enlarged pupils, respiratory failure, fever, cardiac arrhythmias, convulsions, coma.
WHAT TO DO:
- **Dial 911 (emergency) for medical help or call poison control center 1-800-222-1222 for instructions.**
- **If person is unconscious, check breathing and pulse. If not breathing, begin mouth-to-mouth rescue breathing. If heart is not beating, begin chest compressions.**
- **See emergency information on last 3 pages of this book.**

Time lapse before drug works:
2 to 4 weeks. May require 4 to 6 weeks for maximum benefit.

Don't take with:
Any other medicine or any dietary supplement without consulting your doctor or pharmacist.

POSSIBLE ADVERSE REACTIONS OR SIDE EFFECTS

SYMPTOMS	WHAT TO DO
Life-threatening:	
In case of overdose, see previous column.	
Common:	
• Tremor.	Discontinue. Call doctor right away.
• Headache, dry mouth or unpleasant taste, constipation or diarrhea, nausea, indigestion, fatigue, weakness, drowsiness, nervousness, anxiety, excessive sweating.	Continue. Call doctor when convenient.
• Insomnia, "sweet tooth."	Continue. Tell doctor at next visit.
Infrequent:	
• Convulsions.	Discontinue. Seek emergency treatment.
• Hallucinations, shakiness, dizziness, fainting, blurred vision, eye pain, vomiting, irregular heartbeat or slow pulse, inflamed tongue, abdominal pain, jaundice, hair loss, rash, fever, chills, joint pain, palpitations, hiccups, visual changes.	Discontinue. Call doctor right away.
• Difficult or frequent urination; decreased sex drive; muscle aches; abnormal dreams; nasal congestion; weakness and faintness when arising from bed or chair; back pain.	Continue. Call doctor when convenient.
Rare:	
Itchy skin; sore throat; involuntary movements of jaw, lips and tongue; nightmares; confusion; swollen breasts; swollen testicles.	Discontinue. Call doctor right away.

WARNINGS & PRECAUTIONS

Don't take if:
- You are allergic to any tricyclic antidepressant.
- You drink alcohol in excess.
- You have had a heart attack in past 6 weeks.
- You have taken MAO inhibitors* within 2 weeks.
- Patient is younger than age 12.

Before you start, consult your doctor if:
- You will have surgery within 2 months, including dental surgery, requiring anesthesia.
- You have an enlarged prostate or glaucoma.
- You have high blood pressure, heart disease or stomach or intestinal problems.
- You have an overactive thyroid.
- You have asthma or liver disease.

Over age 60:
More likely to develop urination difficulty and serious side effects such as seizures, hallucinations, shaking, dizziness, fainting, headache, insomnia.

Pregnancy:
Risk factors vary for drugs in this group. See category list on page xviii and consult doctor.

Breast-feeding:
Drug may pass into milk. Avoid drug or discontinue nursing until you finish medicine. Consult doctor about maintaining milk supply.

Infants & children:
- Not recommended for ages 12. and under.
- Carefully read information provided with prescription. Contact doctor right away if depression symptoms get worse or there is any talk of suicide or suicide behaviors. Also, read information under Others.

Prolonged use:
Talk to your doctor about the need for follow-up medical examinations or laboratory studies to check complete blood counts (white blood cell count, platelet count, red blood cell count, hemoglobin, hematocrit), blood pressure, eyes, teeth.

Skin & sunlight:
One or more drugs in this group may cause rash or intensify sunburn in areas exposed to sun or ultraviolet light (photosensitivity reaction). Avoid overexposure and use sunscreen. Notify doctor if reaction occurs.

Driving, piloting or hazardous work:
Don't drive or pilot aircraft until you learn how medicine affects you. Don't work around dangerous machinery. Don't climb ladders or work in high places. Danger increases if you drink alcohol or take medicine affecting alertness and reflexes.

Discontinuing:
- Don't discontinue without consulting doctor. Dose may require gradual reduction if you have taken drug for a long time. Doses of other drugs may also require adjustment.
- Physical or emotional withdrawal symptoms may occur once you stop drug. Contact your doctor if any symptoms cause concern.

Others:
- Adults and children taking antidepressants may experience a worsening of the depression symptoms and may display increased suicidal thoughts or behavior. Call doctor right away if these symptoms or behaviors occur.
- Advise any doctor or dentist whom you consult that you take this medicine.

POSSIBLE INTERACTION WITH OTHER DRUGS

GENERIC NAME OR DRUG CLASS	COMBINED EFFECT
Adrenocorticoids, systemic	Increased risk of mental side effects.
Anticoagulants,* oral	Possible increased anticoagulant effect.
Anticholinergics*	Increased anticholinergic effect.
Antifungals, azoles	Increased effect of antidepressant.
Antiglaucoma agents*	Decreased ocular hypertensive effect.
Antihistamines*	Increased antihistamine effect.
Barbiturates*	Decreased antidepressant effect. Increased sedation.

Continued on page 903

POSSIBLE INTERACTION WITH OTHER SUBSTANCES

Alcohol:	Sedation. Avoid.
Beverages:	Grapefruit juice may increase effect of clomipramine.
Cocaine:	Increased risk of heartbeat irregularity.
Foods:	None expected.
Marijuana:	Drowsiness. Risk of side effects. Avoid.
Tobacco:	Decreased antidepressant effect.

*See Glossary

ANTIDYSKINETICS

GENERIC AND BRAND NAMES

See full list of generic and brand names in the *Generic and Brand Name Directory*, page 871.

BASIC INFORMATION

Habit forming? No
Prescription needed? Yes
Available as generic? Yes
Drug class: Antidyskinetic, antiparkinsonism, dopamine agonists

USES

- Treatment of Parkinson's disease.
- Treatment of adverse effects of certain central nervous system drugs.
- Treatment of moderate to severe restless leg syndrome.
- Treatment for Tourette's syndrome.

DOSAGE & USAGE INFORMATION

How to take:
- Tablet—Swallow with liquid. If you can't swallow whole, crumble tablet.
- Extended-release capsule or tablet—Swallow whole with liquid.
- Elixir—Follow directions on prescription label.
- All forms—Take with, or right after, a meal to lessen stomach irritation (unless otherwise directed by doctor).

When to take:
At the same time(s) each day.

If you forget a dose:
Take as soon as you remember up to 2 hours late. If more than 2 hours, wait for next scheduled dose (don't double this dose).

Continued next column

OVERDOSE

SYMPTOMS:
Agitation, dilated pupils, hallucinations, dry mouth, rapid heartbeat, sleepiness.
WHAT TO DO:
- **Dial 911 (emergency) for medical help or call poison control center 1-800-222-1222 for instructions.**
- **If person is unconscious, check breathing and pulse. If not breathing, begin mouth-to-mouth rescue breathing. If heart is not beating, begin chest compressions.**
- **See emergency information on last 3 pages of this book.**

What drug does:
- Balances chemical reactions necessary to send nerve impulses within base of brain.
- Improves muscle control and reduces stiffness.

Time lapse before drug works:
1 to 2 hours. Full effect may take 2 to 3 days.

Don't take with:
Any other medicine or any dietary supplement without consulting your doctor or pharmacist.

POSSIBLE ADVERSE REACTIONS OR SIDE EFFECTS

SYMPTOMS	WHAT TO DO
Life-threatening: In case of overdose, see previous column.	
Common:	
• Blurred vision, light sensitivity, unusual body movements, painful or difficult or frequent urination, vomiting, hallucinations.	Continue, but call doctor right away.
• Dry mouth, tiredness, weakness, drowsiness or insomnia, constipation, nausea, lightheadedness.	Continue. Call doctor when convenient.
Infrequent: Headache, memory loss, abdominal pain, weakness and faintness when arising from bed or chair, nervousness, impotence, sore throat, cough or wheezing, viral infection, appetite loss, restlessness.	Continue. Call doctor when convenient.
Rare:	
• Rash, hives, eye pain, delusions, amnesia, paranoia, fever, swollen neck glands, vision changes, chest pain, swallowing or breathing difficulty, numbness or tingling or swelling in hands or feet, urine bloody or cloudy, ear buzzing, irregular heartbeat.	Continue. Call doctor right away.
• Confusion, dizziness, sore mouth or tongue, muscle cramps or weakness, depression.	Continue. Call doctor when convenient.

Note: Most symptoms representing side effects either disappear or decrease when dose is reduced. Consult doctor.

WARNINGS & PRECAUTIONS

Don't take if:
You are allergic to any antidyskinetic.

Before you start, consult your doctor if:
* You have glaucoma or retinal problems.
* You have had high blood pressure, heart disease, impaired liver function.
* You have hypotension or orthostatic hypotension.*
* You have had tardive dyskinesia.*
* You have had kidney disease, urination difficulty, prostatic hypertrophy or intestinal obstruction.
* You have myasthenia gravis.

Over age 60:
More sensitive to drug. Aggravates symptoms of enlarged prostate. Causes impaired thinking, hallucinations, nightmares. Consult doctor about any of these.

Pregnancy:
Decide with your doctor whether drug benefits justify risk to unborn child. Risk category C (see page xviii).

Breast-feeding:
Effects unknown. May inhibit lactation. Consult doctor.

Infants & children:
Use only under doctor's supervision.

Prolonged use:
* Possible glaucoma.
* Talk to your doctor about the need for follow-up medical examinations to assess drug's effectiveness and examination to check eye pressure.

Skin & sunlight:
No special problems expected.

Driving, piloting or hazardous work:
Don't drive or pilot aircraft until you learn how medicine affects you. Don't work around dangerous machinery. Don't climb ladders or work in high places. Danger increases if you drink alcohol or take medicine affecting alertness and reflexes, such as antihistamines, tranquilizers, sedatives, pain medicine, narcotics and mind-altering drugs.

Discontinuing:
* Don't discontinue without consulting doctor. Dose may require gradual reduction if you have taken drug for a long time. Doses of other drugs may also require adjustment.
* After discontinuing, if you experience extrapyramidal reaction* recurrence or worsening, orthostatic hypotension, fast heartbeat, trouble in sleeping, consult doctor.

Others:
* Internal eye pressure should be measured regularly.
* Avoid becoming overheated.
* Use caution when arising from a sitting or lying position.
* Advise any doctor or dentist whom you consult that you take this medicine.

POSSIBLE INTERACTION WITH OTHER DRUGS

GENERIC NAME OR DRUG CLASS	COMBINED EFFECT
Antacids*	Possible decreased absorption.
Anticholinergics, others*	Increased anticholinergic effect.
Antidepressants, tricyclic*	Increased antidyskinetic effect.
Antihistamines*	Increased antidyskinetic effect.
Carbidopa	Increased effect of carbidopa.
Central nervous system (CNS) depressants*	May add to any sedative effect.
Chlorpromazine	Decreased effect of chlorpromazine.
Ciprofloxacin	Increased effect of ropinirole.
Dopamine antagonists*	Decreased effect of pramipexole and ropinirole.
Estrogens	Increased effect of ropinirole.

Continued on page 904

POSSIBLE INTERACTION WITH OTHER SUBSTANCES

INTERACTS WITH	COMBINED EFFECT
Alcohol:	Oversedation. Avoid.
Beverages:	None expected.
Cocaine:	Decreased antidyskinetic effect. Avoid.
Foods:	None expected.
Marijuana:	None expected.
Tobacco:	Decreased effect of ropinirole.

*See Glossary

ANTIFIBRINOLYTIC AGENTS

GENERIC AND BRAND NAMES

AMINOCAPROIC ACID   **TRANEXAMIC ACID**
  Amicar   Cyklokapron

BASIC INFORMATION

Habit forming? No
Prescription needed? Yes
Available as generic? Yes
Drug class: Antifibrinolytic, antihemorrhagic

 USES

- Treats serious bleeding, especially occurring after surgery, dental or otherwise.
- Sometimes used before surgery in hopes of preventing excessive bleeding in patients with disorders that increase the chance of serious bleeding.

 DOSAGE & USAGE INFORMATION

How to take:
- Tablet—Swallow with liquid or food to lessen stomach irritation. If you can't swallow whole, crumble tablet and take with liquid or food.
- Syrup—Take as directed on label.

When to take:
As directed by your doctor.

If you forget a dose:
Take as soon as you remember. Don't double this dose.

What drug does:
Inhibits activation of plasminogen to cause blood clots to disintegrate.

Time lapse before drug works:
Within 2 hours.

Don't take with:
- Thrombolytic chemicals such as streptokinase or urokinase.
- Any other medicine or any dietary supplement without consulting your doctor or pharmacist.

 OVERDOSE

SYMPTOMS:
None expected for oral forms. Injectable forms may cause drop in blood pressure or slow heartbeat.
WHAT TO DO:
Follow doctor's instructions.

 POSSIBLE ADVERSE REACTIONS OR SIDE EFFECTS

SYMPTOMS	WHAT TO DO
Life-threatening: Shortness of breath, slurred speech, leg or arm numbness.	Seek emergency treatment.
Common: Diarrhea, nausea, vomiting, severe menstrual cramps.	Continue. Call doctor when convenient.
Infrequent: Dizziness; headache; muscular pain and weakness; red eyes; ringing in ears; skin rash; abdominal pain; stuffy nose; decreased urine; swelling of feet, face, legs; rapid weight gain.	Continue. Call doctor when convenient.
Rare: • Unusual tiredness, blurred vision, clotting of menstrual flow.	Continue. Call doctor when convenient.
• Signs of thrombosis (sudden, severe headache; pains in chest, groin or legs; loss of coordination; shortness of breath; slurred speech; vision changes; weakness or numbness in arms or leg).	Seek emergency treatment.

WARNINGS & PRECAUTIONS

Don't take if:
* You are allergic to aminocaproic acid or tranexamic acid.
* You have a diagnosis of disseminated intravascular coagulation (DIC).

Before you start, consult your doctor if:
* You have heart disease.
* You have bleeding from the kidney.
* You have had impaired liver function.
* You have had kidney disease or urination difficulty.
* You have blood clots in parts of the body.

Over age 60:
No changes from other age groups expected.

Pregnancy:
Risk factors vary for drugs in this group. See category list on page xviii and consult doctor.

Breast-feeding:
No problems documented. Consult doctor.

Infants & children:
Use for children only under doctor's supervision.

Prolonged use:
Talk to your doctor about the need for follow-up medical examinations or laboratory studies to check eyes.

Skin & sunlight:
No problems expected.

Driving, piloting or hazardous work:
Don't drive or pilot aircraft until you learn how medicine affects you. Don't work around dangerous machinery. Don't climb ladders or work in high places. Danger increases if you drink alcohol or take medicine affecting alertness and reflexes, such as antihistamines, tranquilizers, sedatives, pain medicine, narcotics and mind-altering drugs.

Discontinuing:
Don't discontinue without consulting doctor. Dose may require gradual reduction if you have taken drug for a long time. Doses of other drugs may also require adjustment.

Others:
* Should not be used in patients with disseminated intravascular coagulation.
* Advise any doctor or dentist whom you consult that you take this medicine.
* Have eyes checked frequently.

 ## POSSIBLE INTERACTION WITH OTHER DRUGS

GENERIC NAME OR DRUG CLASS	COMBINED EFFECT
Contraceptives, oral*	Increased possibility of blood clotting.
Estrogens*	Increased possibility of blood clotting.
Thrombolytic agents* (alteplase, streptokinase, urokinase)	Decreased effects of both drugs.

 ## POSSIBLE INTERACTION WITH OTHER SUBSTANCES

INTERACTS WITH	COMBINED EFFECT
Alcohol:	Decreases effectiveness. Avoid.
Beverages:	No problems expected.
Cocaine:	Combined effect unknown. Avoid.
Foods:	No problems expected.
Marijuana:	Combined effect unknown. Avoid.
Tobacco:	Combined effect unknown. Avoid.

*See Glossary

ANTIFUNGALS, AZOLES

GENERIC AND BRAND NAMES

FLUCONAZOLE
Diflucan
ITRACONAZOLE
Sporanox
KETOCONAZOLE
Nizoral

POSACONAZOLE
Noxafil
VORICONAZOLE
Vfend

BASIC INFORMATION

Habit forming? No
Prescription needed? Yes, for some
Available as generic? Yes, for some
Drug class: Antifungal

 USES

- Treatment for fungal infections.
- Treatment for meningitis.
- Treatment for prostate cancer.

 DOSAGE & USAGE INFORMATION

How to take:
- Capsule or tablet—Swallow with liquid. If you can't swallow whole, crumble tablet or open capsule and take with liquid or food.
- Oral suspension—Shake well before using; follow instructions supplied with medication.
- Shampoo or cream—Follow instructions supplied with medication.

When to take:
At the same time each day.

If you forget a dose:
- Take as soon as you remember up to 2 hours late. If more than 2 hours, wait for next scheduled dose (don't double this dose).
- Itraconazole may come in one-a-day or twice daily dosages. Follow instructions for proper usage (don't double this dose).

What drug does:
Prevents fungi from growing and reproducing. In treating prostate cancer, ketoconazole decreases male hormone (testosterone) levels.

Continued next column

 OVERDOSE

SYMPTOMS:
None expected.
WHAT TO DO:
If person is unconscious, check breathing and pulse. If not breathing, begin mouth-to-mouth rescue breathing. If heart is not beating, begin chest compressions.

Time lapse before drug works:
Several weeks or months for full benefit.

Don't take with:
Any other medicine or any dietary supplement without consulting your doctor or pharmacist.

 POSSIBLE ADVERSE REACTIONS OR SIDE EFFECTS

SYMPTOMS	WHAT TO DO
Life-threatening: None expected.	
Common: None expected.	
Infrequent:	
• Skin rash.	Discontinue. Call doctor right away.
• Diarrhea, nausea, vomiting, appetite loss, constipation, head-ache, abdominal pain.	Continue. Call doctor when convenient.
Rare:	
• Pale stools, yellow skin or eyes, dark or amber urine, unusual tiredness or weakness.	Discontinue. Call doctor right away.
• Diminished sex drive in males, swollen breasts in males, increased sensitivity to light, drowsiness, dizziness, insomnia.	Continue. Call doctor when convenient.

 WARNINGS & PRECAUTIONS

Don't take if:
You have had an allergic reaction to any of the azoles.

Before you start, consult your doctor if:
- You have impaired kidney or liver function.
- You have been diagnosed with reduced stomach acidity.

Over age 60:
Adverse reactions and side effects may be more frequent and severe than in younger persons. Dosage may need adjustment if there is age-related kidney impairment.

Pregnancy:
Decide with your doctor whether drug benefits justify risk to unborn child. Risk category C (see page xviii).

Breast-feeding:
Drug passes into milk. Avoid drug or discontinue nursing until you finish medicine. Consult doctor for advice on maintaining milk supply.

Infants & children:
Use only under close medical supervision.

Prolonged use:
Request periodic liver function studies.

Skin & sunlight:
No problems expected.

Driving, piloting or hazardous work:
Don't drive or pilot aircraft until you learn how medicine affects you. Don't work around dangerous machinery. Don't climb ladders or work in high places. Danger increases if you drink alcohol or take medicine affecting alertness and reflexes, such as antihistamines, tranquilizers, sedatives, pain medicine, narcotics and mind-altering drugs.

Discontinuing:
Don't discontinue without consulting doctor. Dose may require gradual reduction if you have taken drug for a long time. Doses of other drugs may also require adjustment.

Others:
* Advise any doctor or dentist whom you consult that you take this medicine.
* May affect the results of some medical tests.

POSSIBLE INTERACTION WITH OTHER DRUGS

GENERIC NAME OR DRUG CLASS	COMBINED EFFECT
Adrenocorticoids, systemic	Decreased azole effect.
Antacids*	Decreased azole effect.
Anticholinergics*	Decreased azole effect.
Anticoagulants, oral*	Increased effect of anticoagulant.
Antidepressants, tricyclic*	Increased effect of antidepressant.
Antidiabetics, oral*	Increased risk of hypoglycemia.
Antivirals, HIV/AIDS*	Reduced effect of both drugs. Risk of pancreatitis.
Atropine	Decreased azole effect.
Belladonna	Decreased azole effect.
Carbamazepine	Decreased azole effect.
Cimetidine	Decreased azole effect.

Clidinium	Decreased azole absorption.
Contraceptives, oral*	Decreased effect of contraceptive.
Cyclosporine	Increased risk of toxicity to kidney.
Digoxin	Possible toxic levels of digoxin.
Ergot preparations*	Can cause serious or life-threatening problems with blood circulation. Avoid.
Eszopiclone	Decreased effect of ketoconazole.
Famotidine	Reduced antifungal effect. Take 2 hours apart.
Glycopyrrolate	Decreased azole effect.
Hepatotoxic medications*	Increased risk of toxicity to kidney.
Histamine H_2 receptor antagonists	Decreased azole absorption.
HMG-CoA reductase inhibitors	Risk of muscle toxicity.
Hyoscyamine	Decreased azole effect.
Hypoglycemics, oral	Increased effect of oral hypoglycemics.
Isoniazid	Decreased azole effect.

Continued on page 904

POSSIBLE INTERACTION WITH OTHER SUBSTANCES

INTERACTS WITH	COMBINED EFFECT
Alcohol:	Liver damage risk or disulfiram reaction.*
Beverages: Grapefruit juice.	Decreased effect of drug. Avoid.
Cocaine:	Decreased azole effect. Avoid.
Foods:	None expected.
Marijuana:	Decreased azole effect. Avoid.
Tobacco:	Decreased azole effect. Avoid.

*See Glossary

ANTIFUNGALS (Topical)

GENERIC AND BRAND NAMES

See full list of generic and brand names in the *Generic and Brand Name Directory*, page 871.

BASIC INFORMATION

Habit forming? No
Prescription needed? Yes, for some
Available as generic? Yes, for some
Drug class: Antifungal (topical)

 USES

- Treats skin fungus infections such as ringworm of the scalp, athlete's foot, jock itch, "sun fungus," nail fungus and others.
- Treatment of seborrheic dermatitis (dandruff, cradle cap).

 DOSAGE & USAGE INFORMATION

How to use:
- Solution—Apply to affected area once daily for one week.
- Cream, lotion, ointment, gel—Bathe and dry area before use. Apply small amount and rub gently.
- Powder—Apply lightly to skin.
- Shampoo—Follow package instructions.
- Don't bandage or cover treated areas with plastic wrap.
- Follow other instructions from manufacturer listed on label.

When to use:
Twice a day, morning and evening, unless otherwise directed by your doctor.

If you forget a dose:
Use as soon as you remember.

What drug does:
Kills fungi by damaging the fungal cell wall.

Continued next column

 OVERDOSE

SYMPTOMS:
None expected.
WHAT TO DO:
- **Not for internal use. If child accidentally swallows, call poison control center.**
- **Dial 911 (emergency) for medical help or call poison control center 1-800-222-1222 for instructions.**
- **See emergency information on last 3 pages of this book.**

Time lapse before drug works:
May require 6 to 8 weeks or longer for cure.

Don't use with:
Other skin medicines without consulting your doctor or pharmacist.

 POSSIBLE ADVERSE REACTIONS OR SIDE EFFECTS

SYMPTOMS	WHAT TO DO
Life-threatening: None expected.	
Common: None expected.	
Infrequent: Itching, redness, swelling of treated skin not present before treatment.	Discontinue. Call doctor right away.
Rare: None expected.	

WARNINGS & PRECAUTIONS

Don't use if:
You are allergic to any topical antifungal medicine listed.

Before you start, consult your doctor if:
You are allergic to anything that touches your skin.

Over age 60:
No problems expected.

Pregnancy:
Risk factors vary for drugs in this group. See category list on page xviii and consult doctor.

Breast-feeding:
No problems expected, but check with doctor.

Infants & children:
No problems expected, but check with doctor. Some drugs in this group have not been studied in children under age 12.

Prolonged use:
No problems expected, but check with doctor.

Skin & sunlight:
No special problems expected.

Driving, piloting or hazardous work:
No problems expected, but check with doctor.

Discontinuing:
No problems expected, but check with doctor.

Others:
* Avoid contact with eyes.
* Heat and moisture in bathroom medicine cabinet can cause breakdown of medicine. Store someplace else.
* Keep medicine cool, but don't freeze.
* Store away from heat or sunlight.
* Don't use on other members of the family without consulting your doctor.
* If using for jock itch, avoid wearing tight underwear.
* If using for athlete's foot, dry feet carefully after bathing, wear clean cotton socks with sandals or well-ventilated shoes.

POSSIBLE INTERACTION WITH OTHER DRUGS

GENERIC NAME OR DRUG CLASS	COMBINED EFFECT
None expected.	

POSSIBLE INTERACTION WITH OTHER SUBSTANCES

INTERACTS WITH	COMBINED EFFECT
Alcohol:	None expected.
Beverages:	None expected.
Cocaine:	None expected.
Foods:	None expected.
Marijuana:	None expected.
Tobacco:	None expected.

ANTIFUNGALS (Vaginal)

GENERIC AND BRAND NAMES

See full list of generic and brand names in the *Generic and Brand Name Directory*, page 871.

BASIC INFORMATION

Habit forming? No
Prescription needed? Yes, for some
Available as generic? Yes, for some
Drug class: Antifungal (vaginal)

USES

Treats fungus infections of the vagina.

DOSAGE & USAGE INFORMATION

How to use:
* Vaginal cream—Insert into vagina with applicator as illustrated in patient instructions that come with prescription.
* Vaginal tablet—Insert with applicator as illustrated in instructions.
* Vaginal suppository—Insert as illustrated in instructions.

When to use:
According to instructions. Usually once or twice daily.

If you forget a dose:
Use as soon as you remember.

What drug does:
Destroys fungus cells membrane causing loss of essential elements to sustain fungus cell life.

Time lapse before drug works:
Begins immediately. May require 2 weeks of treatment to cure vaginal fungus infections. Recurrence common.

Don't use with:
Other vaginal preparations or douches unless otherwise instructed by your doctor.

OVERDOSE

SYMPTOMS:
None expected.
WHAT TO DO:
Not for internal use. If child accidentally swallows, call doctor or poison control center 1-800-222-1222 for help.

POSSIBLE ADVERSE REACTIONS OR SIDE EFFECTS

SYMPTOMS	WHAT TO DO
Life-threatening: None expected.	
Common: None expected.	
Infrequent: Vaginal burning, itching, irritation, swelling of labia, redness, increased discharge (not present before starting medicine).	Discontinue. Call doctor right away.
Rare: Skin rash, hives, irritation of sex partner's penis.	Discontinue. Call doctor right away.

WARNINGS & PRECAUTIONS

Don't use if:
* You are allergic to any of the products listed.
* You have pre-existing liver disease.

Before you start, consult your doctor if:
You are pregnant.

Over age 60:
No problems expected.

Pregnancy:
Risk factors vary for drugs in this group. See category list on page xviii and consult doctor.

Breast-feeding:
No problems expected. Consult doctor.

Infants & children:
Use only under close medical supervision.

Prolonged use:
No problems expected.

Skin & sunlight:
No problems expected.

Driving, piloting or hazardous work:
No problems expected.

Discontinuing:
Recurrence likely if you stop before time suggested.

Others:
* Gentian Violet and some of the other products can stain clothing. Sanitary napkins may protect against staining.
* Keep the genital area clean. Use plain unscented soap.
* Take showers rather than tub baths.
* Wear cotton underpants or pantyhose with a cotton crotch. Avoid underpants made from non-ventilating materials. Wear freshly laundered underpants.
* Don't sit around in wet clothing—especially a wet bathing suit.
* After urination or bowel movements, cleanse by wiping or washing from front to back (vagina to anus).
* Don't douche unless your doctor recommends it.
* If urinating causes burning, urinate through a tubular device, such as a toilet-paper roll or plastic cup with the end cut out.

POSSIBLE INTERACTION WITH OTHER DRUGS

GENERIC NAME OR DRUG CLASS	COMBINED EFFECT
Warfarin	May cause bleeding with miconazole vaginal cream.

POSSIBLE INTERACTION WITH OTHER SUBSTANCES

INTERACTS WITH	COMBINED EFFECT
Alcohol:	None expected.
Beverages:	None expected.
Cocaine:	None expected.
Foods:	None expected.
Marijuana:	None expected.
Tobacco:	None expected.

*See Glossary

GENERIC AND BRAND NAMES

APRACLONIDINE
 Iopidine
BRIMONIDINE
 Alphagan
 Alphagan P
 Combigan
DIPIVEFRIN
 AKPro
 DPE
 Ophtho-Dipivefrin
 Propine
 Propine C Cap

EPINEPHRINE
 Epifren
 Epinal
 Eppy/N
 Glaucon

BASIC INFORMATION

Habit forming? No
Prescription needed? Yes
Available as generic? Yes, for some
Drug class: Antiglaucoma

USES

Treats open-angle glaucoma, secondary glaucoma and ocular hypertension. May be used with eye surgery.

DOSAGE & USAGE INFORMATION

How to use:
Eye drops
• Wash hands.
• Apply pressure to inside corner of eye with middle finger.
• Continue pressure for 1 minute after placing medicine in eye.
• Tilt head backward. Pull lower lid away from eye with index finger of the same hand.
• Drop eye drops into pouch and close eye. Don't blink.
• Keep eyes closed for 1 to 2 minutes.
• If using more than one eye solution, wait at least 10 minutes between instillations to avoid a "wash-out" effect.

Continued next column

OVERDOSE

SYMPTOMS:
Effects unknown.
WHAT TO DO:
Overdose unlikely to threaten life. If person uses much larger amount than prescribed or if accidentally swallowed, call doctor or poison control center 1-800-222-1222 for help.

When to use:
As directed on label.

If you forget a dose:
Apply as soon as you remember. If almost time for next dose, wait and apply at regular time (don't double this dose).

What drug does:
Inactivates enzyme and facilitates movement of fluid (aqueous humor) into and out of the eye.

Time lapse before drug works:
30 minutes to 4 hours.

Don't use with:
Any other eye medicine without consulting your doctor or pharmacist.

POSSIBLE ADVERSE REACTIONS OR SIDE EFFECTS

SYMPTOMS	WHAT TO DO
Life-threatening: None expected.	
Common:	
• Allergic reaction (itching, redness, tearing of eye).	Discontinue. Call doctor right away.
• Headache, eye discomfort, dry mouth.	Continue. Call doctor when convenient.
Infrequent: Eye symptoms: pain, changes in vision, blurred vision, discharge or swelling, color change in white of eye, feeling of something in the eye, stinging, burning, watering, light sensitivity, crusting on eyelid, paleness of eye or inner eyelid.	Continue. Call doctor right away.
Rare:	
• Symptoms of too much drug absorbed in body: faintness, skin paleness, chest pain, increased or fast or irregular heartbeat, swelling (face, hands, or feet), dizziness, numbness or tingling in fingers or toes, wheezing, troubled breathing.	Discontinue. Call doctor right away.
• Other symptoms of drug absorbed in body: sore throat, muscle aches, nausea, smell or taste changes, anxiety, nervousness, depression, constipation, insomnia or drowsiness.	Continue. Call doctor when convenient.

WARNINGS & PRECAUTIONS

Don't use if:
You are allergic to any of the adrenergic agonist antiglaucoma drugs.

Before you start, consult your doctor if:
- You suffer from depression.
- You have any eye disease.
- You have heart problems, high or low blood pressure or thromboangiitis obliterans.
- You have Raynaud's disease.
- You have a history of vasovagal attacks* (if using apraclonidine).
- You have liver or kidney problems.

Over age 60:
No problems expected.

Pregnancy:
Risk factors vary for drugs in this group. See category list on page xviii and consult doctor.

Breast-feeding:
It is not known if drugs pass into milk. Avoid drugs or discontinue nursing until you finish medicine. Consult doctor for advice on maintaining milk supply.

Infants & children:
Use only under close medical supervision.

Prolonged use:
May be necessary.

Skin & sunlight:
No problems expected.

Driving, piloting or hazardous work:
Your vision may be blurred or there may be a change in your near or far vision or night vision for a short time after drug use. Don't drive or pilot aircraft until you learn how medicine affects you. Don't work around dangerous machinery. Don't climb ladders or work in high places.

Discontinuing:
Don't discontinue without consulting your doctor. Dose may require gradual reduction if you have used drug for a long time. Doses of other drugs may also require adjustment.

Others:
- Advise any doctor or dentist whom you consult that you use this medicine.
- Drugs may cause your eyes to become more sensitive to light. Wear sunglasses and avoid too much exposure to bright light.
- Brimonidine contains a preservative that could be absorbed by soft contact lenses. Wait at least 15 minutes after putting eye drops in before you put in your soft contact lenses.
- If you have any eye infection, injury or wound, consult doctor before using this medicine.
- Keep appointments for regular eye examinations to measure pressure in the eye.

POSSIBLE INTERACTION WITH OTHER DRUGS

GENERIC NAME OR DRUG CLASS	COMBINED EFFECT
Antidepressants, tricyclic	May decrease ocular hypertensive effect. Dipivefrin may cause heart rhythm problem, high blood pressure.
Antiglaucoma, beta blockers	May help decrease eye pressure.
Antihypertensives*	May decrease blood pressure.
Central nervous system (CNS) depressants*	May increase CNS depressant effect.
Digitalis preparations*	Increased risk of heart problems.
Maprotiline	Heart rhythm problems, high blood pressure.
Monoamine oxidase (MAO) inhibitors*	Separate use by at least 14 days.

POSSIBLE INTERACTION WITH OTHER SUBSTANCES

INTERACTS WITH	COMBINED EFFECT
Alcohol:	None expected.
Beverages:	None expected.
Cocaine:	None expected. Best to avoid.
Foods:	None expected.
Marijuana:	Unknown effect. Consult doctor.
Tobacco:	None expected.

*See Glossary

GENERIC AND BRAND NAMES

DEMECARIUM
Humorsol

ECHOTHIOPHATE
Phospholine Iodide

BASIC INFORMATION

Habit forming? No
Prescription needed? Yes
Available as generic? No
Drug class: Antiglaucoma

 ## USES

- Treatment for certain types of glaucoma.
- Used for diagnosis and treatment for other eye conditions.

 ## DOSAGE & USAGE INFORMATION

How to use:
Eye drops
- Wash hands. Tilt head back.
- Press finger gently on the skin right under the lower eyelid; pull the eyelid away from the eye to make a space or small pocket.
- Drop the medicine into this pocket, then let go of the skin and gently close the eyes; don't blink.
- Keep the eyes closed and apply pressure to the inner corner of the eye with your finger for 1 to 2 minutes.
- Wash hands again after using the drops.
- To keep the solution germ-free, do not allow the applicator tip to touch the skin or eye.
- If using more than one eye solution, wait at least 10 minutes between instillations to avoid a "wash-out" effect.

Continued next column

 ## OVERDOSE

SYMPTOMS:
Fast heartbeat, diarrhea, heavy sweating, breathing difficulty, unable to control bladder, shock.
WHAT TO DO:
- For overdose in the eye, flush with warm tap water and call doctor immediately.
- For accidentally ingested overdose or signs of system toxicity, dial 911 (emergency) for medical help or call poison control center 1-800-222-1222 for instructions.
- See emergency information on last 3 pages of this book.

When to use:
As directed on label.

If you forget a dose:
Apply as soon as you remember. If almost time for next dose, wait and apply at regular time (don't double this dose).

What drug does:
Inactivates an enzyme to reduce pressure inside the eye.

Time lapse before drug works:
5 to 60 minutes.

Don't use with:
Any other eye medicine without consulting your doctor or pharmacist.

 ## POSSIBLE ADVERSE REACTIONS OR SIDE EFFECTS

SYMPTOMS	WHAT TO DO
Life-threatening: None expected.	
Common: Stinging, burning watery eyes.	Continue. Call doctor when convenient.
Infrequent: Blurred vision, change in vision, change in night vision, eyelids twitch, headache, ache in brow area.	Continue. Call doctor when convenient.
Rare: Decreased vision with veil or curtain appearing in part of vision, eye redness, symptoms of too much of drug absorbed in body (loss of bladder control, slow heartbeat, increased sweating, weakness, difficult breathing, vomiting, nausea, diarrhea, stomach pain or cramping).	Discontinue. Call doctor right away.

WARNINGS & PRECAUTIONS

Don't use if:
You are allergic to demecarium or echothiophate.

Before you start, consult your doctor if:
- You have eye infection or other eye disease.
- You have ulcers in stomach or duodenum or other stomach disorder.
- You have myasthenia gravis, overactive thyroid or urinary tract blockage.
- You have asthma, epilepsy, Down syndrome, heart disease, high or low blood pressure, Parkinson's disease.

Over age 60:
Adverse reactions and side effects may be more frequent and severe than in younger persons.

Pregnancy:
Risk factors vary for drugs in this group. See category list on page xviii and consult doctor.

Breast-feeding:
It is not known if drug passes into milk. Avoid drugs or discontinue nursing until you finish medicine. Consult doctor for advice on maintaining milk supply.

Infants & children:
Use under medical supervision only. Children are more susceptible to adverse effects.

Prolonged use:
Cataracts or other eye problems may occur. Be sure to see your doctor for regular eye examinations.

Skin & sunlight:
No problems expected.

Driving, piloting or hazardous work:
Your vision may be blurred or there may be a change in your near or far vision or night vision for a short time after drug use. Don't drive or pilot aircraft until you learn how medicine affects you. Don't work around dangerous machinery. Don't climb ladders or work in high places.

Discontinuing:
Don't discontinue without consulting your doctor. Dose may require gradual reduction if you have used drug for a long time. Doses of other drugs may also require adjustment.

Others:
- Advise any doctor or dentist whom you consult that you use this medicine.
- Keep appointments for regular eye examinations to measure pressure in the eye.
- If you have any eye infection, injury or wound, consult doctor before using this medicine.

POSSIBLE INTERACTION WITH OTHER DRUGS

GENERIC NAME OR DRUG CLASS	COMBINED EFFECT
Anticholinergics*	Increased risk of toxicity.
Antimyasthenics*	Increased risk of side effects.
Cholinesterase inhibitors*	Increased risk of toxicity.
Insecticides or pesticides with organic phosphates	Increased toxic absorption of pesticides.
Topical anesthetics	Increased risk of toxic effects of antiglaucoma eye medicines.

POSSIBLE INTERACTION WITH OTHER SUBSTANCES

INTERACTS WITH	COMBINED EFFECT
Alcohol:	None expected.
Beverages:	None expected.
Cocaine:	None expected. Best to avoid.
Foods:	None expected.
Marijuana:	Unknown effect. Consult doctor.
Tobacco:	None expected.

*See Glossary

ANTIGLAUCOMA, BETA BLOCKERS

GENERIC AND BRAND NAMES

BETAXOLOL
(ophthalmic)
Betoptic
Betoptic S
CARTEOLOL
(ophthalmic)
Ocupress
LEVOBUNOLOL
(ophthalmic)
AKBeta
Betagen C Cap B.I.D.
Betagen C Cap Q.D.
Betagen Standard
Cap
METIPRANOLOL
(ophthalmic)
OptiPranolol

TIMOLOL
(ophthalmic)
Apo-Timop
Beta-Tim
Betimol
Combigan
Cosopt
Gen-Timolol
Istalol
Med Timolol
Novo-Timolol
Nu-Timolol
Timodal
Timoptic
Timoptic in
Ocudose
Timoptic-XE
Xalcom

BASIC INFORMATION

Habit forming? No
Prescription needed? Yes
Available as generic? Yes, for some
Drug class: Antiglaucoma

 ## USES

Treatment for glaucoma and ocular hypertension.
May be used in eye surgery.

 ## DOSAGE & USAGE INFORMATION

How to take:
Eye drops—Follow directions on prescription.

Continued next column

 ## OVERDOSE

SYMPTOMS:
Slow heartbeat, low blood pressure, broncho-spasm, heart failure (these symptoms are what might be expected if similar drugs were taken orally).
WHAT TO DO:
• For overdose in the eye, flush with warm tap water and call doctor immediately.
• For accidentally ingested overdose or signs of system toxicity, dial 911 (emergency) for medical help or call poison control center 1-800-222-1222 for instructions.
• See emergency information on last 3 pages of this book.

When to take:
At the same time each day usually in the morning. Follow your doctor's instructions.

If you forget a dose:
• Once-a-day dose—Apply as soon as you remember. If almost time for next dose, wait and apply at regular time (don't double this dose).
• More than once-a-day dose—Apply as soon as you remember. If close to time for next dose, wait and apply at regular time (don't double this dose).

What drug does:
Appears to reduce production of aqueous humor (fluid inside eye), thereby reducing pressure inside eye.

Time lapse before drug works:
30 minutes to 1 hour.

Don't take with:
Any other eye medicine without consulting your doctor or pharmacist.

 ## POSSIBLE ADVERSE REACTIONS OR SIDE EFFECTS

SYMPTOMS	WHAT TO DO
Life-threatening: In case of overdose, see previous column.	
Common: • Redness of eyes or inside of eyelids.	Continue. Call doctor right away.
• Temporary blurred vision, night vision decreased, eye irritation or discomfort when drug is used.	Continue. Call doctor when convenient.
Infrequent: Ongoing blurred vision, other vision changes, different size pupils, eyeball discolored, droopy eyelid, eye pain, or swelling or irritation.	Continue. Call doctor when convenient.
Rare: • Increased sensitivity to light; sensation of foreign body in eye; dryness, discharge or pain in eye; crusty eyelids; inflammation.	Continue. Call doctor when convenient.
• Symptoms of body absorbing too much of drug include problems with heart, stomach, lungs (breathing difficulties), skin, nervous system, hair loss, and others.	Discontinue. Call doctor right away.

WARNINGS & PRECAUTIONS

Don't take if:
You are allergic to any beta-adrenergic blocking agent taken orally or used in the eye.

Before you start, consult your doctor if:
- You have asthma, a bronchial disorder or pulmonary disease.
- You have any heart disease or heart problem.
- You suffer from depression.
- You have diabetes or low blood sugar, over-active thyroid or myasthenia gravis.

Over age 60:
Adverse reactions and side effects may be more frequent and severe than in younger persons.

Pregnancy:
Decide with your doctor whether drug benefits justify risk to unborn child. Risk category C (see page xviii).

Breast-feeding:
Some of these drugs pass into milk; others are unknown. Avoid drugs or discontinue nursing until you finish medicine. Consult doctor for advice on maintaining milk supply.

Infants & children:
Give only under close medical supervision. Children may be more sensitive to drug and side effects.

Prolonged use:
Talk to your doctor about the need for follow-up medical examinations to check pressure inside eye.

Skin & sunlight:
No special problems expected.

Driving, piloting or hazardous work:
Your vision may be blurred or there may be a change in your near or far vision or night vision for a short time after drug use. Don't drive or pilot aircraft until you learn how medicine affects you. Don't work around dangerous machinery. Don't climb ladders or work in high places.

Discontinuing:
- Don't discontinue without doctor's approval.
- May need to discontinue drug temporarily before major surgery. Your doctor will provide instructions.

Others:
- Advise any doctor or dentist whom you consult that you take this medicine.
- These drugs may affect blood sugar levels in diabetic patients.
- Keep appointments for regular eye examinations to measure pressure in the eye.
- If you have any eye infection, injury or wound, consult doctor before using this medicine.

POSSIBLE INTERACTION WITH OTHER DRUGS

GENERIC NAME OR DRUG CLASS	COMBINED EFFECT

Drug interactions are unlikely unless a significant amount of the eye medication is absorbed into the system. Potential interactions that may occur are similar to those listed in Possible Interactions With Other Drugs under Beta-Adrenergic Blocking Agents.

POSSIBLE INTERACTION WITH OTHER SUBSTANCES

INTERACTS WITH	COMBINED EFFECT
Alcohol:	None expected.
Beverages:	None expected.
Cocaine:	Decreased anti-glaucoma effect; heart problems. Avoid.
Foods:	None expected.
Marijuana:	Unknown effect. Consult doctor.
Tobacco:	None expected.

*See Glossary

ANTIGLAUCOMA, CARBONIC ANHYDRASE INHIBITORS

GENERIC AND BRAND NAMES

BRINZOLAMIDE
Azopt

DORZOLAMIDE
Cosopt
Trusopt

BASIC INFORMATION

Habit forming? No
Prescription needed? Yes
Available as generic? Yes, for some
Drug class: Antiglaucoma

 USES

- Treatment for open-angle glaucoma (increased pressure in the eye).
- Treatment for ocular hypertension.

 DOSAGE & USAGE INFORMATION

How to use:
Eye drops
- Wash hands. Tilt head back.
- Press finger gently on the skin right under the lower eyelid; pull the eyelid away from the eye to make a space or small pocket.
- Drop the medicine into this pocket, then let go of the skin and gently close the eyes; don't blink.
- Keep the eyes closed and apply pressure to the inner corner of the eye with your finger for 1 to 2 minutes.
- Wash hands again after using the drops.
- To keep the solution germ-free, do not allow the applicator tip to touch the skin or eye.
- If using more than one eye solution, wait at least 10 minutes between instillations to avoid a "wash-out" effect.

When to use:
Normally used 3 times a day (about 8 hours apart). Always use as directed by your doctor.

Continued next column

 OVERDOSE

SYMPTOMS:
Unknown effect.
WHAT TO DO:
Overdose unlikely to threaten life. If person uses much larger amount than prescribed or if accidentally swallowed, call doctor or poison control center 1-800-222-1222 for help.

If you forget a dose:
Use as soon as you remember. If it is almost time for the next dose, wait for next dose (don't double this dose).

What drug does:
This medicine is a topically applied carbonic anhydrase inhibitor that helps decrease production of aqueous humor (the fluid in the eye) and lowers the pressure inside the eye.

Time lapse before drug works:
30 to 60 minutes.

Don't take with:
Any other eye medicine without consulting your doctor or pharmacist.

 POSSIBLE ADVERSE REACTIONS OR SIDE EFFECTS

SYMPTOMS	WHAT TO DO
Life-threatening: None expected.	
Common:	
• Allergic reaction (redness, itching or swelling of eye or eyelid); feeling of something in the eye; continued or severe sensitivity to light.	Discontinue. Call doctor right away.
• Bitter taste; burning, stinging or discomfort when medicine is used; mild sensitivity to light.	Continue. Call doctor when convenient.
Infrequent: Blurred vision, dryness or mild tearing of eyes, tiredness or weakness, headache hair loss.	Continue. Call doctor when convenient.
Rare: Blood in urine; continued nausea or vomiting; hives; pain in chest, back, side or abdomen; eye pain; severe or continued tearing; seeing double; skin rash; shortness of breath.	Discontinue. Call doctor right away.

WARNINGS & PRECAUTIONS

Don't use if:
You are allergic to ophthalmic carbonic anhydrase inhibitors or any sulfonamide* medications.

Before you start, consult your doctor if:
* You have kidney or liver disease.
* You are allergic to any medication, food, preservatives or other substances.

Over age 60:
No special problems expected.

Pregnancy:
Decide with your doctor whether drug benefits justify risk to unborn child. Risk category C (see page xviii).

Breast-feeding:
It is not known if drug passes into milk. Avoid drugs or discontinue nursing until you finish medicine. Consult doctor for advice on maintaining milk supply.

Infants & children:
* Dorzolamide is used to treat pediatric patients.
* Safety and dosage of other drugs in this group has not been established. Use only under medical supervision.

Prolonged use:
Schedule regular appointments with your eye doctor for eye examinations to be sure the medication is controlling the glaucoma.

Skin & sunlight:
No special problems expected.

Driving, piloting or hazardous work:
Your vision may be blurred or there may be a change in your near or far vision or night vision for a short time after drug use. Don't drive or pilot aircraft until you learn how medicine affects you. Don't work around dangerous machinery. Don't climb ladders or work in high places.

Discontinuing:
Don't discontinue without consulting your doctor.

Others:
* If you have any eye infection, injury or wound, consult doctor before using this medicine.
* Advise any doctor or dentist whom you consult that you use this medicine.
* Keep appointments for regular eye examinations to measure pressure in the eye.
* Wear sunglasses when outside in sunlight.

POSSIBLE INTERACTION WITH OTHER DRUGS

GENERIC NAME OR DRUG CLASS	COMBINED EFFECT
Amphetamines	Increased risk of side effects.
Carbonic anhydrase inhibitors (oral)	Increased effect of both drugs. Avoid.
Mecamylamine	Increased risk of side effects.
Quinidine	Increased risk of side effects.
Salicylates (High doses)	Increased risk of adverse effects.

POSSIBLE INTERACTION WITH OTHER SUBSTANCES

INTERACTS WITH	COMBINED EFFECT
Alcohol:	None expected.
Beverages:	None expected.
Cocaine:	None expected. Best to avoid.
Foods:	None expected.
Marijuana:	Unknown effect. Consult doctor.
Tobacco:	None expected.

ANTIGLAUCOMA, CHOLINERGIC AGONISTS

GENERIC AND BRAND NAMES

CARBACHOL
Carbastat
Carboptic
Isopto Carbachol
Miostat

PILOCARPINE
Adsorbocarpine
Akarpine
Almocarpine
Isopto Carpine
Minims
Miocarpine
Ocu-Carpine
Ocusert Pilo
Pilocarpine Pilocar
Pilopine HS
Piloptic
Pilostat
P.V. Carpine
Liquifilm

BASIC INFORMATION

Habit forming? No
Prescription needed? Yes
Available as generic? Yes, for some
Drug class: Antiglaucoma

 ## USES

Treatment for glaucoma and other eye conditions. May be used in eye surgery.

 ## DOSAGE & USAGE INFORMATION

How to take:
• Drops—Apply to eyes. Close eyes for 1 or 2 minutes to absorb medicine.
• Eye insert system—Follow label directions.
• Gel—Follow label directions.

When to use:
As directed on label.

Continued next column

 ## OVERDOSE

SYMPTOMS:
If accidental overdose in eye, flush with water. If swallowed—nausea, vomiting, diarrhea, sweating.
WHAT TO DO:
Overdose unlikely to threaten life. If person uses much larger amount than prescribed or if accidentally swallowed, call doctor or poison control center 1-800-222-1222 for help.

If you forget a dose:
• For eye drops or gel, use as soon as possible. If it is almost time for your next dose, skip the missed dose and return to regular schedule (don't double this dose).
• For eye insert, replace it as soon as possible. Then return to your regular schedule.

What drug does:
Reduces internal eye pressure.

Time lapse before drug works:
75 minutes to 4 hours.

Don't take with:
Any other eye medicine without consulting your doctor or pharmacist.

 ## POSSIBLE ADVERSE REACTIONS OR SIDE EFFECTS

SYMPTOMS	WHAT TO DO
Life-threatening: None expected.	
Common: Blurred or altered vision (near or distant vision), eye stinging or burning.	Continue. Call doctor when convenient.
Infrequent: Headache, eye irritation, redness, of eye, eyelid twitching.	Continue. Call doctor when convenient.
Rare: Eye pain, a veil or curtain appears across part of vision, symptoms of too much of drug absorbed in the body (increased sweating, muscle trembling, nausea, vomiting, diarrhea, troubled breathing or wheezing, mouth watering, stomach cramps, fainting, flushing or redness of face, urge to urinate).	Discontinue. Call doctor right away.

WARNINGS & PRECAUTIONS

Don't take if:
You are allergic to carbachol or pilocarpine.

Before you start, consult your doctor if:
* You have other eye problems.
* You have heart disease, overactive thyroid, Parkinson's disease, ulcers, or urinary blockage problems.
* You have asthma.

Over age 60:
No special problems expected.

Pregnancy:
Decide with your doctor if drug benefits justify risk to unborn child. Risk category C (see page xviii).

Breast-feeding:
It is not known if drugs pass into milk. Avoid drugs or discontinue nursing until you finish medicine. Consult doctor for advice on maintaining milk supply.

Infants & children:
Not recommended.

Prolonged use:
* You may develop tolerance* for drug, making it ineffective. Your doctor may switch antiglaucoma drugs for a period of time to return effectiveness.
* Talk to your doctor about the need for follow-up medical examinations to check eye pressure.

Skin & sunlight:
No problems expected.

Driving, piloting or hazardous work:
Your vision may be blurred or there may be a change in your near or far vision or night vision for a short time after drug use. Don't drive or pilot aircraft until you learn how medicine affects you. Don't work around dangerous machinery. Don't climb ladders or work in high places.

Discontinuing:
Don't discontinue without consulting your doctor.

Others:
* Advise any doctor or dentist whom you consult that you use this medicine.
* Keep appointments for regular eye examinations to measure pressure in the eye.
* If you have any eye infection, injury or wound, consult doctor before using this medicine.

POSSIBLE INTERACTION WITH OTHER DRUGS

GENERIC NAME OR DRUG CLASS	COMBINED EFFECT
Belladonna (ophthalmic)	Decreased antiglaucoma effect.
Flurbiprofen (ophthalmic)	Decreased antiglaucoma effect.
Cyclopentolate	Decreased antiglaucoma effect.

POSSIBLE INTERACTION WITH OTHER SUBSTANCES

INTERACTS WITH	COMBINED EFFECT
Alcohol:	None expected.
Beverages:	None expected.
Cocaine:	None expected. Best to avoid.
Foods:	None expected.
Marijuana:	Unknown effect. Consult doctor.
Tobacco:	None expected.

*See Glossary

ANTIGLAUCOMA, PROSTAGLANDINS

GENERIC AND BRAND NAMES

BIMATOPROST
  Latisse
  Lumigan
  Xalcom
ISOPROPYL
  UNOPROSTONE
  Rescula

LATANOPROST
  Xalatan
TRAVOPROST
  Travatan
  Travatan Z

BASIC INFORMATION

Habit forming? No
Prescription needed? Yes
Available as generic? Yes, for some
Drug class: Antiglaucoma

 ## USES

* Treats diseases of the eye like glaucoma and hypertension of the eye.
* Treats hypotrichosis (reduced amount of hair) of the eyelashes.

 ## DOSAGE & USAGE INFORMATION

How to use:
Eye drops
* Wash hands.
* Apply pressure on the skin just beneath the lower eyelid. Pull the lower eyelid away from the eye to make a space.
* Drop the medicine into this space.
* Release eyelid and gently close eyes.
* Don't blink.
* Keep eyes closed for 1 to 2 minutes.
* Remove excess solution from around the eye with a clean tissue, being careful not to touch the eye.
* Don't touch applicator tip to any surface (including the eye). If you accidentally touch tip, clean with warm water and soap.
* Keep container tightly closed.
* Wash hands immediately after using.

When to use:
As directed on label.

Continued next column

 ## OVERDOSE

SYMPTOMS:
Unknown effect.
WHAT TO DO:
Overdose unlikely to threaten life. If person uses much larger amount than prescribed or if accidentally swallowed, call doctor or poison control center 1-800-222-1222 for help.

If you forget a dose:
Use as soon as you remember. If it is almost time for the next dose, wait for next dose (don't double this dose).

What drug does:
Inactivates enzyme and facilitates movement of fluid (aqueous humor) into and out of the eye.

Time lapse before drug works:
10-30 minutes.

Don't use with:
Any other eye medicine without consulting your doctor or pharmacist.

 ## POSSIBLE ADVERSE REACTIONS OR SIDE EFFECTS

SYMPTOMS	WHAT TO DO
Life-threatening: None expected.	
Common: Eye symptoms: itching, discomfort, mild pain, redness, feeling of something in eye, vision decreased.	Continue. Call doctor when convenient.
Infrequent: Eye tearing or dry, crusting on eyelid, eyes more sensitive to light, eye discharge, color vision or other vision changes, hair growth increased.	Continue. Call doctor when convenient.
Rare: • Faintness, increased sweating, irregular or fast heartbeat, chest pain or tightness, shortness of breath, wheezing, unusual tiredness, paleness, heartburn, indigestion, coughing up mucus, fainting, chills or fever, dizziness, pain and stiffness in muscles or joints, headache, urination problems, cold symptoms, back pain, mental and mood changes.	Discontinue. Call doctor right away.

• May cause changes in the treated eye only (color of the iris and eyelid). It may change eyelashes (thicker, longer, color). Changes may take months or years and may be permanent.	Continue. Call doctor when convenient.

Others:
- If you have any eye infection, injury or wound, consult doctor before using this medicine.
- Advise any doctor or dentist whom you consult that you use this medicine.
- Keep appointments for regular eye examinations to measure pressure in the eye.

WARNINGS & PRECAUTIONS

Don't take if:
You are allergic to any prostaglandin eye medicine.

Before you start, consult your doctor if:
- You plan to have eye or dental surgery.
- You have any eye disease.
- You have heart problems or high blood pressure.
- You have liver or kidney problems.

Over age 60:
Adverse reactions and side effects may be more frequent and severe than in younger persons. Ask doctor about smaller doses.

Pregnancy:
Risk factors vary for drugs in this group. See category list on page xviii and consult doctor.

Breast-feeding:
It is not known if drugs pass into milk. Avoid drugs or discontinue nursing until you finish medicine. Consult doctor for advice on maintaining milk supply.

Infants & children:
Safety and efficacy not established in this age group.

Prolonged use:
May be necessary.

Skin & sunlight:
No problems expected.

Driving, piloting or hazardous work:
Your vision may be blurred or there may be a change in your near or far vision or night vision for a short time after drug use. Don't drive or pilot aircraft until you learn how medicine affects you. Don't work around dangerous machinery. Don't climb ladders or work in high places.

Discontinuing:
Don't discontinue without consulting your doctor. Dose may require gradual reduction if you have used drug for a long time. Doses of other drugs may also require adjustment.

POSSIBLE INTERACTION WITH OTHER DRUGS

GENERIC NAME OR DRUG CLASS	COMBINED EFFECT
None specific	Other drugs may increase or decrease antiglaucoma effect. Consult doctor.

POSSIBLE INTERACTION WITH OTHER SUBSTANCES

INTERACTS WITH	COMBINED EFFECT
Alcohol:	None expected.
Beverages:	None expected.
Cocaine:	None expected. Best to avoid.
Foods:	None expected.
Marijuana:	Unknown effect. Consult doctor.
Tobacco:	None expected.

ANTIGOUT DRUGS

GENERIC AND BRAND NAMES

ALLOPURINOL
  Alloprin
  Apo-Allopurinol
  Lopurin
  Novopural
  Purinol
  Zyloprim

FEBUXOSTAT
  Uloric

BASIC INFORMATION

Habit forming? No
Prescription needed? Yes
Available as generic? Yes, for some
Drug class: Antigout

 ## USES

- Treats symptoms of chronic gout.
- Treatment for increased levels of uric acid (hyperuricemia) in the body.
- Prevention of kidney stones caused by uric acid.

 ## DOSAGE & USAGE INFORMATION

How to take:
Tablet—Swallow with liquid or food to lessen stomach irritation. Drink extra fluids each day.

When to take:
At the same time(s) each day.

If you forget a dose:
Take as soon as you remember. If it is almost time for the next dose, skip the missed dose and wait for your next scheduled dose (don't double this dose).

What drug does:
Slows formation of uric acid by inhibiting enzyme (xanthine oxidase) activity.

Continued next column

 ## OVERDOSE

SYMPTOMS:
May have nausea, vomiting and diarrhea.
WHAT TO DO:
Overdose unlikely to threaten life. If person uses much larger amount than prescribed or if accidentally swallowed, call doctor or poison control center 1-800-222-1222 for help.

Time lapse before drug works:
Reduces blood uric acid in 1 to 3 weeks. May require 6 months to prevent acute gout attacks.

Don't take with:
Any other medicine or any dietary supplement without consulting your doctor or pharmacist.

 ## POSSIBLE ADVERSE REACTIONS OR SIDE EFFECTS

SYMPTOMS	WHAT TO DO
Life-threatening: Rare allergic reaction (rash, painful urination, blood in the urine, eye irritation, swelling of mouth or lips).	Discontinue. Seek emergency help.
Common: Rash, hives, itch.	Discontinue. Call doctor right away.
Infrequent: Drowsiness, diarrhea, stomach ache or pain, nausea or vomiting without other symptoms, headache.	Continue. Call doctor when convenient.
Rare: • Sore throat, fever, unusual bleeding or bruising, black or tarry stools, mouth or lips sores, blood in urine or stools, skin problems (redness, peeling, burning, tenderness, scaly, thickened), red or itchy eyes, wheezing or shortness of breath or trouble breathing or swelling (hands, feet, lower legs, fingers), fast weight gain, unusual tiredness or weakness, yellow skin or eyes, abnormal heartbeat, chest pain, dizziness, vision problems, hearing loss, slurred speech, numbness or tingling in face or arm or legs.	Discontinue. Call doctor right away.
• Loose fingernails, pain in lower back or side, unexpected nosebleeds, hair loss.	Continue. Call doctor when convenient.

WARNINGS & PRECAUTIONS

Don't take if:
You are allergic to allopurinol or febuxostat.

Before you start, consult your doctor if:
- You have liver or kidney problems.
- You have history of heart disease or stroke.
- You have diabetes.
- You have hypertension (high blood pressure).
- You are having an acute gout attack.

Over age 60:
No problems expected.

Pregnancy:
Decide with your doctor whether drug benefits justify risk to unborn child. Risk category C (see page xviii).

Breast-feeding:
Allopurinol passes into milk. It is unknown if febuxostat passes into milk. Avoid drug or discontinue nursing. Consult doctor for advice on maintaining milk supply.

Infants & children:
Usually not recommended for ages under 18. Allopurinol may be used to treat certain rare conditions in children.

Prolonged use:
Talk to your doctor about the need for follow-up medical examinations or laboratory studies to check liver function, kidney function and serum uric-acid levels.

Skin & sunlight:
No problems expected.

Driving, piloting or hazardous work:
Avoid if you feel drowsy. Use of this drug may disqualify you for piloting aircraft.

Discontinuing:
Don't discontinue without doctor's advice, even though symptoms diminish or disappear. These drugs are usually prescribed for long-term use to prevent gout attacks.

Others:
- Acute gout attacks may increase during first weeks of use. If so, consult doctor about your symptoms.
- Consult your doctor before taking vitamin C supplement as it can increase the risk for kidney stones.
- Febuxostat may rarely increase the risk for heart attack or stroke.
- Advise any doctor or dentist whom you consult that you use this medicine.

POSSIBLE INTERACTION WITH OTHER DRUGS

GENERIC NAME OR DRUG CLASS	COMBINED EFFECT
Amoxicillin	Risk of skin rash (with allopurinol).
Ampicillin	Risk of skin rash (with allopurinol).
Anticoagulants, oral*	May increase anticoagulant effect (with allopurinol).
Antineoplastics*	Usage needs to be carefully monitored (with allopurinol).
Azathioprine	Increased effect of azathioprine. Don't use with febuxostat.
Chlorpropamide	Increased effect of chlorpropamide (with allopurinol).
Chlorthalidone	Decreased allopurinol effect.
Cyclosporine	Increased cyclosporine effect (with allopurinol).
Diuretics, thiazide*	Risk of adverse effects (with allopurinol).
Mercaptopurine	Increased mercaptopurine effect. Don't use with febuxostat.
Probenecid	Increased allopurinol effect.
Theophylline	Increased effect of theophylline . Don't use with febuxostat.

POSSIBLE INTERACTION WITH OTHER SUBSTANCES

INTERACTS WITH	COMBINED EFFECT
Alcohol:	May increase uric acid. Avoid.
Beverages:	None expected.
Cocaine:	Unknown. Avoid.
Foods:	None expected.
Marijuana:	Unknown. Avoid..
Tobacco:	None expected.

ANTIHISTAMINES

GENERIC AND BRAND NAMES

See full list of generic and brand names in the *Generic and Brand Name Directory*, page 872.

BASIC INFORMATION

Habit forming? No
Prescription needed?
    High strength: Yes
    Low strength: No
Available as generic? Yes
Drug class: Antihistamine

 ## USES

- Reduces allergic symptoms such as hay fever, hives, rash or itching.
- Prevents motion sickness, nausea, vomiting.
- Relieves symptoms associated with the common cold.
- Induces sleep.
- Reduces stiffness and tremors of Parkinson's disease.

 ## DOSAGE & USAGE INFORMATION

How to take:
Follow label directions.

When to take:
Varies with form. Follow label directions.

If you forget a dose:
Take as soon as you remember up to 2 hours late. If more than 2 hours, wait for next scheduled dose (don't double this dose).

What drug does:
- Blocks action of histamine after an allergic response triggers histamine release in sensitive cells. Histamines cause itching, sneezing, runny nose and eyes and other symptoms.
- Appears to work in the vomiting center of the brain to control nausea and vomiting and help prevent motion sickness.

Continued next column

 ## OVERDOSE

SYMPTOMS:
Convulsions, red face, hallucinations, coma.
WHAT TO DO:
- **Dial 911 (emergency) for medical help or call poison control center 1-800-222-1222 for instructions.**
- **See emergency information on last 3 pages of this book.**

Time lapse before drug works:
15 minutes to 1 hour.

Don't take with:
Any other medicine or any dietary supplement without consulting your doctor or pharmacist.

 ## POSSIBLE ADVERSE REACTIONS OR SIDE EFFECTS

SYMPTOMS	WHAT TO DO
Life-threatening: In case of overdose, see previous column.	
Common: Drowsiness; dizziness; dryness of mouth, nose or throat.	Continue. Tell doctor at next visit.
Infrequent: • Change in vision, clumsiness, rash.	Discontinue. Call doctor right away.
• Less tolerance for contact lenses, painful or difficult urination.	Continue. Call doctor when convenient.
• Appetite loss.	Continue. Tell doctor at next visit.
Rare: Nightmares, agitation, irritability, sore throat, fever, rapid heartbeat, unusual bleeding or bruising, fatigue, weakness, confusion, fainting, seizures.	Discontinue. Call doctor right away.

 ## WARNINGS & PRECAUTIONS

Don't take if:
You are allergic to any antihistamine.

Before you start, consult your doctor if:
- You have glaucoma.
- You have enlarged prostate.
- You have asthma.
- You have kidney disease.
- You have peptic ulcer.
- You will have surgery within 2 months, including dental surgery, requiring general or spinal anesthesia.

Over age 60:
Don't exceed recommended dose. Adverse reactions and side effects may be more frequent and severe than in younger persons, especially urination difficulty, diminished alertness and other brain and nervous-system symptoms.

Pregnancy:
Risk factors vary for drugs in this group. See category list on page xviii and consult doctor.

Breast-feeding:
Drug passes into milk. Avoid drug or discontinue nursing until you finish medicine. Consult doctor for advice on maintaining milk supply.

Infants & children:
* Read the label on the product to see if it is approved for your child's age. Always follow the directions on product's label about how to use. If unsure, ask your doctor or pharmacist.
* Do not use antihistamines for the purpose of making a child sleepy.

Prolonged use:
Consult your doctor.

Skin & sunlight:
May cause rash or intensify sunburn in areas exposed to sun or sunlamp.

Driving, piloting or hazardous work:
Don't drive or pilot aircraft until you learn how medicine affects you. Don't work around dangerous machinery. Don't climb ladders or work in high places. Danger increases if you drink alcohol or take medicine affecting alertness and reflexes, such as other antihistamines, tranquilizers, sedatives, pain medicine, narcotics and mind-altering drugs.

Discontinuing:
No problems expected.

Others:
* May mask symptoms of hearing damage from aspirin, other salicylates, cisplatin, paromomycin, vancomycin or anticonvulsants. Consult doctor if you use these.
* Advise any doctor or dentist whom you consult that you take this medicine.

POSSIBLE INTERACTION WITH OTHER DRUGS

GENERIC NAME OR DRUG CLASS	COMBINED EFFECT
Adrenocorticoids, systemic	Decreased adrenocorticoid effect.
Anticholinergics*	Increased anticholinergic effect.
Anticoagulants, oral*	Decreased antihistamine effect.
Antidepressants*	Excess sedation. Avoid.
Antihistamines, other*	Excess sedation. Avoid.
Carteolol	Decreased antihistamine effect.
Central nervous system (CNS) depressants*	May increase sedation.

Clozapine	Toxic effect on the central nervous system.
Dronabinol	Increased effects of both drugs. Avoid.
Hypnotics*	Excess sedation. Avoid.
Mind-altering drugs*	Excess sedation. Avoid.
Molindone	Increased sedative and antihistamine effect.
Monoamine oxidase (MAO) inhibitors*	Increased antihistamine effect.
Nabilone	Greater depression of central nervous system.
Narcotics*	Excess sedation. Avoid.
Procarbazine	May increase sedation.
Sedatives*	Excess sedation. Avoid.
Sertraline	Increased depressive effects of both drugs.
Sleep inducers*	Excess sedation. Avoid.
Sotalol	Increased antihistamine effect.
Tranquilizers*	Excess sedation. Avoid.

POSSIBLE INTERACTION WITH OTHER SUBSTANCES

INTERACTS WITH	COMBINED EFFECT
Alcohol:	Excess sedation. Avoid.
Beverages: Caffeine drinks.	Less antihistamine sedation.
Cocaine:	Decreased antihistamine effect. Avoid.
Foods:	None expected.
Marijuana:	Excess sedation. Avoid.
Tobacco:	None expected.

*See Glossary

ANTIHISTAMINES (Nasal)

GENERIC AND BRAND NAMES

AZELASTINE
Astelin
Astepro

OLOPATADINE
Patanase

BASIC INFORMATION

Habit forming? No
Prescription needed? Yes
Available as generic? No
Drug class: Antihistamine

 ## USES

- Reduces allergic symptoms caused by hay fever (seasonal allergic rhinitis), such as sneezing, itching, runny nose and other nasal symptoms of allergies.
- Azelastine is used to treat vasomotor rhinitis (also called nonallergic rhinitis) which is not caused by allergic reactions, but has similar symptoms.

 ## DOSAGE & USAGE INFORMATION

How to use:
Nasal spray—Gently blow nose before using. Prime the pump per package instructions. Use 2 sprays per nostril. Use 1 spray of azelastine in children ages 5 through 11. Avoid eyes.

When to take:
Usually twice a day or according to doctor's instructions. Effects of spray last for 12 hours.

If you forget a dose:
Use as soon as you remember. If it is almost time for next dose, wait for next scheduled dose (don't double this dose).

Continued next column

 ## OVERDOSE

SYMPTOMS:
May include extreme drowsiness, and feeling restless or agitated, but an overdose with this dosage form is unlikely to occur.
WHAT TO DO:
If person uses much larger amount than prescribed, call doctor, poison control center 1-800-222-1222 or hospital emergency room for help.

What drug does:
- Blocks action of histamines which are released in the body during an allergic reaction (such as to seasonal pollens). Histamines cause itching, swollen tissues, sneezing, runny nose and eyes and other symptoms.
- Azelastine also blocks the action of other inflammatory chemicals that cause stuffy and runny nose.

Time lapse before drug works:
Thirty minutes to 1 to 3 hours.

Don't take with:
Any other medicine or any dietary supplement without consulting your doctor or pharmacist.

 ## POSSIBLE ADVERSE REACTIONS OR SIDE EFFECTS

SYMPTOMS	WHAT TO DO
Life-threatening:	
Rare allergic reaction (hives, itching, rash, trouble breathing, tightness in chest, swelling of lips or tongue or face).	Seek emergency treatment immediately.
Common:	
• Mild drowsiness, bitter taste.	Usually no action needed. If symptoms continue, call doctor.
• Mild nosebleeds, irritation/soreness in the nose, runny nose, headache.	Discontinue. Call doctor when convenient.
Infrequent:	
Dry mouth, sore or painful throat, cough, nausea.	Discontinue. Call doctor when convenient.
Rare:	
• Extreme drowsiness, severe or frequent nosebleeds, rapid or forceful heartbeat, nasal perforation (pain and swelling).	Discontinue. Call doctor right away.
• Fatigue, flu or cold-like symptoms, post nasal drip, sinus infection, dizziness, weight gain, burning or pain when urinating, changes in urination, other unexplained symptoms.	Discontinue. Call doctor when convenient.

WARNINGS & PRECAUTIONS

Don't take if:
You are allergic to azelastine or olopatadine.

Before you start, consult your doctor if:
* You have kidney problems.
* You have any disorder or injury involving the nose (such as a deviated septum).
* You are allergic to any medication, food or other substance.

Over age 60:
No problems expected.

Pregnancy:
Decide with your doctor if drug benefits justify risks to unborn child. Risk category C (see page xviii).

Breast-feeding:
It is not known if drugs pass into milk. Avoid drug or discontinue nursing until you finish medicine. Consult doctor for advice on maintaining milk supply.

Infants & children:
* Azelastine is approved in children 12 years and older for vasomotor rhinitis and in children 5 years and older for allergic rhinitis.
* Olopatadine is approved in children 12 years and older for allergic rhinitis.

Prolonged use:
* Antihistamines are normally used during the hay fever season. They are not intended for long-term uninterrupted use.
* Consult your doctor about long-term use of azelastine for vasomotor rhinitis symptoms.

Skin & sunlight:
No problems expected.

Driving, piloting or hazardous work:
Don't drive or pilot aircraft until you learn how medicine affects you. Don't work around dangerous machinery. Don't climb ladders or work in high places. Danger increases if you drink alcohol or take other medicines affecting alertness and reflexes such as antihistamines, tranquilizers, sedatives, pain medicine, narcotics and mind-altering drugs.

Discontinuing:
No problems expected. Consult your doctor if you have been using the spray for a long time.

Others:
* Don't exceed recommended dose. It could increase the risk of adverse reactions.
* Advise any doctor or dentist whom you consult that you take this medicine.
* Consult doctor if new nasal problems occur.
* Avoid getting the spray in your eyes. Rinse eyes with water if this occurs.

POSSIBLE INTERACTION WITH OTHER DRUGS

GENERIC NAME OR DRUG CLASS	COMBINED EFFECT
Central nervous system (CNS) depressants*	May add to any sedative effect.
Cimetidine	Increased azelastine effect. May result in increased sedation.

POSSIBLE INTERACTION WITH OTHER SUBSTANCES

INTERACTS WITH	COMBINED EFFECT
Alcohol:	May cause excessive sedation. Avoid.
Beverages:	None expected.
Cocaine:	Decreased antihistamine effect. Avoid.
Foods:	None expected.
Marijuana:	May cause sedation. Avoid.
Tobacco:	None expected.

*See Glossary

ANTIHISTAMINES, NONSEDATING

GENERIC AND BRAND NAMES

CETIRIZINE
　Reactine
　Zyrtec
　Zyrtec-D
　Zyrtec Children's
　　Allergy Syrup
　Zyrtec Children's
　　Chewable
　Zyrtec Children's
　　Hives Relief Syrup
DESLORATADINE
　Clarinex
　Clarinex D 12 Hour
　Clarinex D 24 Hour
　Clarinex RediTabs
　Clarinex Syrup
FEXOFENADINE
　Allegra
　Allegra-D
　Allegra-D 24 Hour
　Allegra ODT
　Allegra Oral
　　Suspension

LEVOCETIRIZINE
　Xyzal
LORATADINE
　Alavert
　Alavert D-12
　Childrens Claritin
　　Grape Chewable
　Childrens Claritin
　　Syrup, Grape
　Claritin
　Claritin-D
　Claritin-D 12 Hour
　Claritin-D 24 Hour
　Claritin Extra
　Claritin Hives
　　Relief
　Claritin Liqui-Gels
　Claritin RediTabs
　Claritin Syrup

BASIC INFORMATION

Habit forming? No
Prescription needed? Yes, for some
Available as generic? Yes, for some
Drug class: Antihistamine

 ## USES

- Reduces allergic symptoms caused by hay fever (seasonal allergic rhinitis) and perennial rhinitis, such as sneezing, runny nose, itchy nose or throat, itchy and watery eyes.
- Treatment for urticaria (hives).
- Used to help relieve some asthma symptoms.
- Other uses as recommended by your doctor.

Continued next column

 ## OVERDOSE

SYMPTOMS:
Serious irregular heartbeat, convulsions, severe headache, nausea.
WHAT TO DO:
- Dial 911 (emergency) for medical help or call poison control center 1-800-222-1222 for instructions.
- See emergency information on last 3 pages of this book.

 ## DOSAGE & USAGE INFORMATION

How to take:
- Capsule, tablet, suspension, syrup—Swallow with liquid. Most may be taken with food or milk to lessen stomach irritation.
- Chewable tablet—Chew the tablets well before swallowing.
- Oral disintegrating tablet—Let tablet dissolve in mouth. Don't chew. No need to drink fluid.

When to take:
Varies with form and brand. Follow label directions.

If you forget a dose:
Take as soon as you remember. If it is almost time for the next dose, wait for the next scheduled dose (don't double this dose).

What drug does:
Blocks action of histamine after an allergic response triggers histamine release in sensitive cells. Histamines cause itching, sneezing, runny nose and eyes and other symptoms.

Time lapse before drug works:
1 to 2 hours.

Don't take with:
Any other medicine or any dietary supplement without consulting your doctor or pharmacist.

 ## POSSIBLE ADVERSE REACTIONS OR SIDE EFFECTS

SYMPTOMS	WHAT TO DO
Life-threatening:	
In case of overdose, see previous column.	
Common:	
Dryness of mouth, nose or throat.	Continue. Tell doctor at next visit.
Infrequent:	
Increased appetite, weight gain, mild stomach or intestinal problems, cold or flu-like symptoms.	Continue. Call doctor when convenient.
Rare:	
• Heart rhythm disturbances, fainting.	Discontinue. Call doctor right away or get emergency care.
• Allergic reaction such as mild skin rash, headache, nausea, dizziness, nervousness, fatigue, muscle aches. Drowsiness may occur even though these drugs are nonsedating.	Discontinue. Call doctor when convenient.

WARNINGS & PRECAUTIONS

Don't take if:
You are allergic to any antihistamine.

Before you start, consult your doctor if:
- You have any type of heart disorder.
- You have glaucoma.
- You have enlarged prostate or urinary retention problems.
- You have asthma or a respiratory disease.
- You have liver or kidney disease.
- You have peptic ulcer.
- You have electrolyte abnormality, such as low potassium (hypokalemia).

Over age 60:
Adverse reactions and side effects may be more frequent and severe than in younger persons.

Pregnancy:
Risk factors vary for drugs in this group. See category list on page xviii and consult doctor.

Breast-feeding:
Drug may pass into milk. Avoid drug or discontinue nursing until you finish medicine. Consult doctor for advice on maintaining milk supply.

Infants & children:
Read the label on the product to see if it is approved for your child's age. Always follow the directions on product's label about how to use. If unsure, ask your doctor or pharmacist.

Prolonged use:
Antihistamines are normally taken during the hay fever season. Longer use may be recommended by your doctor depending on the disorder being treated.

Skin & sunlight:
Rarely, may cause rash or intensify sunburn in areas exposed to sun or ultraviolet light (photosensitivity reaction). Avoid overexposure. Notify doctor if reaction occurs.

Driving, piloting or hazardous work:
No problems expected.

Discontinuing:
No problems expected.

Others:
- Don't exceed recommended dose. This can increase the risk of adverse reactions.
- Advise any doctor or dentist whom you consult that you take this medicine.

POSSIBLE INTERACTION WITH OTHER DRUGS

GENERIC NAME OR DRUG CLASS	COMBINED EFFECT
Anticholinergics	Increased anticholinergic effect.
Central nervous system (CNS) depressants*	May add to any sedative effect.
Erythromycins*	Heart rhythm problems. Avoid.
Fluvoxamine	Increased antihistamine effect.
Leukotriene modifiers	Effects unknown. Consult doctor.
Macrolide antibiotics	Increased risk of adverse reactions.
Monoamine oxidase (MAO) inhibitors	Increased sedation. Avoid.

POSSIBLE INTERACTION WITH OTHER SUBSTANCES

INTERACTS WITH	COMBINED EFFECT
Alcohol:	May cause sedation. Avoid.
Beverages:	Grapefruit juice may increase the effect of fexofenadine.
Cocaine:	Decreased antihistamine effect. Avoid.
Foods:	None expected.
Marijuana:	May cause sedation. Avoid.
Tobacco:	None expected.

*See Glossary

ANTIHISTAMINES, PHENOTHIAZINE-DERIVATIVE

GENERIC AND BRAND NAMES

See full list of generic and brand names in the *Generic and Brand Name Directory*, page 874.

BASIC INFORMATION

Habit forming? No
Prescription needed? Yes
Available as generic? Yes
Drug class: Tranquilizer (phenothiazine), antihistamine

 USES

- Relieves itching of hives, skin allergies, chickenpox.
- Treatment for hay fever, motion sickness, vertigo.
- Treatment for nausea and vomiting.

 DOSAGE & USAGE INFORMATION

How to take:
- Tablet or syrup—Swallow with liquid or food to lessen stomach irritation.
- Extended-release capsule—Swallow each dose whole. If you take regular tablets, you may chew or crush them.

When to take:
At the same times each day.

If you forget a dose:
Take as soon as you remember up to 2 hours late. If more than 2 hours, wait for next scheduled dose (don't double this dose).

Continued next column

 OVERDOSE

SYMPTOMS:
Fast heartbeat, flushed face, shortness of breath, clumsiness, drowsiness, muscle spasms, jerking movements of head and face.
WHAT TO DO:
- **Dial 911 (emergency) for medical help or call poison control center 1-800-222-1222 for instructions.**
- **See emergency information on last 3 pages of this book.**

What drug does:
- Blocks action of histamine after an allergic response triggers histamine release in sensitive cells. Histamines cause itching, sneezing, runny nose and eyes and other symptoms.
- Appears to work in the vomiting center of the brain to control nausea and vomiting and help prevent motion sickness.

Time lapse before drug works:
15 minutes to 1 hour.

Don't take with:
- Antacid or medicine for diarrhea.
- Nonprescription drug for cough, cold or allergy.
- Any other medicine or any dietary supplement without consulting your doctor or pharmacist.

 POSSIBLE ADVERSE REACTIONS OR SIDE EFFECTS

SYMPTOMS	WHAT TO DO
Life-threatening:	
In case of overdose, see previous column.	
Common:	
Drowsiness; dryness of mouth, nose or throat; nasal congestion.	Continue. Call doctor when convenient.
Infrequent:	
• Nightmares, unusual excitement, nervousness, irritability, loss of appetite, sweating.	Continue. Call doctor when convenient.
• Difficult urination; blurred or changed vision; dizziness; ringing in ears; skin rash; uncontrolled, jerky movements (with high doses); slow, snakelike movement of arms; spasm of neck muscles; stiffening of tongue; eyes rolling upward.	Discontinue. Call doctor right away.
Rare:	
Sore throat, fever, confusion, yellow skin or eyes, fast heartbeat, feeling faint, unusual tiredness or weakness, unusual bleeding or bruising.	Discontinue. Call doctor right away.

ANTIHISTAMINES, PHENOTHIAZINE-DERIVATIVE

WARNINGS & PRECAUTIONS

Don't take if:
* You are allergic to any phenothiazine.
* You have a blood or bone marrow disease.

Before you start, consult your doctor if:
* You will have surgery within 2 months, including dental surgery, requiring anesthesia.
* You have asthma, emphysema or other lung disorder.
* You take nonprescription ulcer medicine, asthma medicine or amphetamines.

Over age 60:
Adverse reactions and side effects may be more frequent and severe than in younger persons. More likely to develop tardive dyskinesia (involuntary movement of jaws, lips, tongue, chewing). Call doctor right away. Early treatment can help.

Pregnancy:
Decide with your doctor if drug benefits justify risk to unborn child. Risk category C (see page xviii).

Breast-feeding:
Drug passes into milk. Avoid drug or discontinue nursing until you finish medicine. Consult doctor for advice on maintaining milk supply.

Infants & children:
Read the label on the product to see if it is approved for your child's age. Always follow the directions on product's label about how to use. If unsure, ask your doctor or pharmacist.

Prolonged use:
* May lead to tardive dyskinesia (involuntary movement of jaws, lips, tongue, chewing).
* Talk to your doctor about the need for follow-up medical examinations or laboratory studies to check complete blood counts, liver function, and eyes.

Skin & sunlight:
One or more drugs in this group may cause rash or intensify sunburn in areas exposed to sun or ultraviolet light (photosensitivity reaction). Avoid overexposure. Notify doctor if reaction occurs.

Driving, piloting or hazardous work:
Don't drive or pilot aircraft until you learn how medicine affects you. Don't work around dangerous machinery. Don't climb ladders or work in high places. Danger increases if you drink alcohol or take medicine affecting alertness and reflexes.

Discontinuing:
May be unnecessary to finish medicine. Follow doctor's instructions.

Others:
* Advise any doctor or dentist whom you consult that you take this medicine.
* May affect results in some medical tests.

POSSIBLE INTERACTION WITH OTHER DRUGS

GENERIC NAME OR DRUG CLASS	COMBINED EFFECT
Antacids*	Decreased antihistamine effect.
Anticholinergics*	Increased anticholinergic effect.
Anticonvulsants, hydantoin*	Increased anticonvulsant effect.
Antidepressants, tricyclic*	Increased antihistamine effect.
Antihistamines,* other	Increased antihistamine effect.
Antithyroid drugs*	Increased risk of bone marrow depression.
Appetite suppressants*	Decreased appetite suppressant effect.
Barbiturates*	Oversedation.
Carteolol	Decreased antihistamine effect.
Central nervous system (CNS) depressants*	Dangerous degree of sedation.
Cisapride	Decreased antihistamine effect.

Continued on page 905

POSSIBLE INTERACTION WITH OTHER SUBSTANCES

INTERACTS WITH	COMBINED EFFECT
Alcohol:	Dangerous oversedation.
Beverages:	None expected.
Cocaine:	Decreased trimeprazine effect. Avoid.
Foods:	None expected.
Marijuana:	Drowsiness.
Tobacco:	None expected.

*See Glossary

ANTIHISTAMINES, PIPERAZINE (Antinausea)

GENERIC AND BRAND NAMES

CYCLIZINE
  Marezine

MECLIZINE
  Antivert
  Antivert/25
  Antivert/50
  Bonamine
  Bonine
  Dramamine II
  D-Vert 15
  D-Vert 30
  Meclicot
  Medivert

BASIC INFORMATION

Habit forming? No
Prescription needed? Yes, for some
Available as generic? Yes
Drug class: Antihistamine, antiemetic, anti-motion sickness

 ## USES

- Prevention and treatment of motion sickness.
- Treats nausea and vomiting after operations or radiation treatment.
- Treatment for vertigo.

 ## DOSAGE & USAGE INFORMATION

How to take:
- Tablet or capsule—Swallow with liquid or food to lessen stomach irritation. If you can't swallow whole, crumble tablet or open capsule and take with liquid or food.
- Chewable tablet—May be chewed, swallowed whole or mixed with food.

When to take:
30 minutes to 1 hour before traveling, or as directed by doctor, or follow label instructions.

Continued next column

 ## OVERDOSE

SYMPTOMS:
Drowsiness, confusion, incoordination, stupor, coma, weak pulse, blurred vision, shallow breathing, hallucinations, seizures.
WHAT TO DO:
- Dial 911 (emergency) for medical help or call poison control center 1-800-222-1222 for instructions.
- See emergency information on last 3 pages of this book.

If you forget a dose:
Take as soon as you remember. Wait 4 hours for next dose or as directed on label.

What drug does:
It is not known just how drug works. Appears to reduce sensitivity of nerve endings in inner ear, blocking messages to brain's vomiting center.

Time lapse before drug works:
30 to 60 minutes.

Don't take with:
Any other medicine or any dietary supplement without consulting your doctor or pharmacist.

 ## POSSIBLE ADVERSE REACTIONS OR SIDE EFFECTS

SYMPTOMS	WHAT TO DO
Life-threatening: In case of overdose, see previous column.	
Common: Drowsiness.	Continue. Tell doctor at next visit.
Infrequent: • Headache, diarrhea or constipation, upset stomach.	Continue. Call doctor when convenient.
• Dry mouth, nose, throat.	Continue. Tell doctor at next visit.
Rare: Restlessness, insomnia, blurred vision, frequent or difficult urination, hallucinations, dizziness, increased heartbeat, loss of appetite.	Discontinue. Call doctor if symptoms continue or are severe.

WARNINGS & PRECAUTIONS

Don't take if:
You are allergic to meclizine or cyclizine.

Before you start, consult your doctor if:
- You have glaucoma.
- You have an intestinal or bladder blockage.
- You have heart problems.
- You have chronic obstructive pulmonary disease (COPD).
- You have prostate enlargement.

Over age 60:
Adverse reactions and side effects may be more frequent and severe than in younger persons, especially impaired urination from enlarged prostate gland.

Pregnancy:
Usually safe, but decide with your doctor if drug benefits justify any possible risk to unborn child. Risk category B (see page xviii).

Breast-feeding:
Meclizine passes into milk; it is unknown if cyclizine does. Consult doctor.

Infants & children:
Follow doctor's instructions or those on the label if used in children. Children may be more sensitive to side effects. Not recommended for children under age 6.

Prolonged use:
No problems expected.

Skin & sunlight:
No problems expected.

Driving, piloting or hazardous work:
Don't drive or pilot aircraft until you learn how medicine affects you. Don't work around dangerous machinery. Don't climb ladders or work in high places. Danger increases if you drink alcohol or take medicine affecting alertness and reflexes.

Discontinuing:
No problems expected.

Others:
- Advise any doctor or dentist whom you consult that you take this medicine (if using on a regular basis).
- May interfere with some skin allergy tests.
- If you have dry mouth from using this drug, try sugarless candy or gum or small pieces of ice. If dry mouth continues longer than 2 weeks, consult doctor.

POSSIBLE INTERACTION WITH OTHER DRUGS

GENERIC NAME OR DRUG CLASS	COMBINED EFFECT
Anticholinergics*	Increased effect of both drugs.
Central nervous system (CNS) depressants*	Increased depressive effects of both drugs.

POSSIBLE INTERACTION WITH OTHER SUBSTANCES

INTERACTS WITH	COMBINED EFFECT
Alcohol:	Increased sedation. Avoid.
Beverages:	None expected.
Cocaine:	None expected. Best to avoid.
Foods:	None expected.
Marijuana:	Increased drowsiness, dry mouth.
Tobacco:	None expected.

ANTI-INFLAMMATORY DRUGS, NONSTEROIDAL (NSAIDs)

GENERIC AND BRAND NAMES

See full list of generic and brand names in the *Generic and Brand Name Directory*, page 874.

BASIC INFORMATION

Habit forming? No
Prescription needed? Yes, for some.
Available as generic? Yes, for some.
Drug class: Anti-inflammatory (nonsteroidal), analgesic, antigout agent, fever-reducer

 ## USES

- Treatment for joint pain, stiffness, inflammation and swelling of arthritis, gout, osteoarthritis, juvenile rheumatoid arthritis and others.
- Treatment for pain, fever and inflammation of a variety of disorders, illnesses and injuries.

 ## DOSAGE & USAGE INFORMATION

How to take:
- Tablet or capsule—Swallow with liquid or food to lessen stomach irritation. If you can't swallow whole, crumble tablet and take with liquid or food. Don't crumble delayed release tablet.
- Liquid—Take as directed on bottle. Don't freeze.
- Rectal suppository—Remove wrapper and moisten suppository with water. Gently insert into rectum, large end first. If suppository is too soft, chill in refrigerator or cool water before removing wrapper.

When to take:
At the same times each day.

If you forget a dose:
Take as soon as you remember up to 2 hours late. If more than 2 hours, wait for next scheduled dose (don't double this dose).

Continued next column

 ## OVERDOSE

SYMPTOMS:
Confusion, agitation, severe headache, incoherence, convulsions, possible hemorrhage from stomach or intestine, coma.
WHAT TO DO:
- Dial 911 (emergency) for medical help or call poison control center 1-800-222-1222 for instructions.
- See emergency information on last 3 pages of this book.

What drug does:
Reduces tissue concentration of prostaglandins (hormones which produce inflammation and pain).

Time lapse before drug works:
Begins in 4 to 24 hours. May require 3 weeks regular use for maximum benefit.

Don't take with:
Any other medicine or any dietary supplement without consulting your doctor or pharmacist.

 ## POSSIBLE ADVERSE REACTIONS OR SIDE EFFECTS

SYMPTOMS	WHAT TO DO
Life-threatening:	
Hives, rash, intense itching, faintness soon after a dose (anaphylaxis in aspirin-sensitive persons).	Seek emergency treatment immediately.
Common:	
• Diarrhea, skin rash, bleeding from rectum (with suppositories).	Discontinue. Call doctor right away.
• Dizziness, nausea, stomach cramps, headache.	Continue. Call doctor when convenient.
Infrequent:	
• Muscle cramps, numbness or tingling in hands or feet, mouth ulcers, rapid weight gain.	Discontinue. Call doctor right away.
• Depression; drowsiness; ringing in ears; swollen feet, face or legs; constipation or diarrhea; vomiting; gaseousness; dry mouth; tremors; insomnia.	Continue. Call doctor when convenient.
Rare:	
• Convulsions; confusion; rash, hives, itch; blurred vision; black, bloody, tarry stool; difficult breathing; tightness in chest; rapid heartbeat; unusual bleeding or bruising; blood in urine; jaundice; psychosis; frequent, painful urination; fainting; sore throat; fever; chills; diminished hearing; eye pain; nose bleeds; severe abdominal pain.	Discontinue. Call doctor right away.
• Fatigue, weakness, menstrual irregularities, skin irritation with patch.	Continue. Call doctor if symptoms persist.

WARNINGS & PRECAUTIONS

Don't take if:
- You are allergic to aspirin or any nonsteroidal, anti-inflammatory drug.
- You have gastritis, peptic ulcer, enteritis, ileitis, ulcerative colitis, asthma, heart failure, high blood pressure or bleeding problems.
- Patient is younger than 15.

Before you start, consult your doctor if:
- You have epilepsy.
- You have Parkinson's disease.
- You have been mentally ill.
- You have impaired kidney or liver function.

Over age 60:
Adverse reactions and side effects may be more frequent and severe than in younger persons.

Pregnancy:
Risk factors vary for drugs in this group. See category list on page xviii and consult doctor.

Breast-feeding:
May harm child. Avoid.

Infants & children:
Approved for treatment of juvenile rheumatoid arthritis in children over age 2.

Prolonged use:
- Eye damage.
- Reduced hearing.
- Sore throat, fever.
- Weight gain.
- Talk to your doctor about the need for follow-up medical examinations or laboratory studies to check complete blood counts (white blood cell count, platelet count, red blood cell count, hemoglobin, hematocrit), liver function, stools for blood, eyes.

Skin & sunlight:
One or more drugs in this group may cause rash or intensify sunburn in areas exposed to sun or ultraviolet light (photosensitivity reaction). Avoid overexposure. Notify doctor if reaction occurs.

Driving, piloting or hazardous work:
Don't drive or pilot aircraft until you learn how medicine affects you. Don't work around dangerous machinery. Don't climb ladders or work in high places. Danger increases if you drink alcohol or take medicine affecting alertness and reflexes, such as antihistamines, tranquilizers, sedatives, pain medicine, narcotics and mind-altering drugs.

Discontinuing:
No problems expected. If drug has been taken for a long time, consult doctor before discontinuing.

Others:
Advise any doctor or dentist whom you consult that you take this medicine.

POSSIBLE INTERACTION WITH OTHER DRUGS

GENERIC NAME OR DRUG CLASS	COMBINED EFFECT
Adrenocorticoids, systemic	Increased risk of ulcers. Increased adrenocorticoid effect.
Angiotensin-converting enzyme (ACE) inhibitors*	May decrease ACE inhibitor effect.
Antacids*	Decreased pain relief.
Anticoagulants, oral*	Increased risk of bleeding.
Anticonvulsants, hydantoin*	Increased anti-convulsant effect.
Anti-inflammatory pain relievers (any combination of)	Danger of increased side effects such as stomach bleeding.
Aspirin	Increased risk of stomach ulcer.
Beta-adrenergic blocking agents*	Decreased anti-hypertensive effect.
Carteolol	Decreased anti-hypertensive effect.
Cephalosporins*	Increased risk of bleeding.
Didanosine	Increased risk of pancreatitis (sulindac only).

Continued on page 905

POSSIBLE INTERACTION WITH OTHER SUBSTANCES

INTERACTS WITH	COMBINED EFFECT
Alcohol:	Possible stomach ulcer or bleeding.
Beverages:	None expected.
Cocaine:	None expected.
Foods:	None expected.
Marijuana:	Increased pain relief from NSAIDs.
Tobacco:	None expected.

*See Glossary

ANTI-INFLAMMATORY DRUGS, NONSTEROIDAL (NSAIDs) COX-2 INHIBITORS

GENERIC AND BRAND NAMES

CELECOXIB
  Celebrex

ROFECOXIB
VALDECOXIB

BASIC INFORMATION

Habit forming? No
Prescription needed? Yes
Available as generic? No
Drug class: Anti-inflammatory (nonsteroidal), analgesic, antigout agent, fever-reducer

USES

- Treatment for joint pain, stiffness, inflammation and swelling of rheumatoid arthritis, osteoarthritis, ankylosing spondylitis and gout.
- Treatment for pain, fever and inflammation.
- Treatment for dysmenorrhea (painful or difficult menstruation).
- Treatment for colorectal polyps.

Special note: This class of drugs has been linked to an increased risk of heart attack and stroke. Consult doctor before using.

DOSAGE & USAGE INFORMATION

How to take:
- Tablet or capsule—Swallow with liquid. If you can't swallow whole, open capsule or crumble tablet and take with liquid or food.
- Suspension—Shake the bottle well before use. Carefully measure dose with measuring spoon or cup.

When to take:
At the same times each day.

If you forget a dose:
Take as soon as you remember up to 2 hours late. If more than 2 hours, wait for next scheduled dose (don't double this dose).

Continued next column

OVERDOSE

SYMPTOMS:
Breathing problems, tightness in chest, decreased urine amount, swelling, thirst, tiredness or weakness, stomach pain, bloody or black stools, dizziness, headache, nausea or vomiting.
WHAT TO DO:
If person takes much larger amount than prescribed, call doctor or poison control center 1-800-222-1222 for help.

What drug does:
Reduces tissue concentration of prostaglandins (hormones which produce inflammation and pain).

Time lapse before drug works:
Begins in 2 to 3 hours. May require 3 weeks of regular use for maximum benefit.

Don't take with:
Any other medicine or any dietary supplement without consulting your doctor or pharmacist.

POSSIBLE ADVERSE REACTIONS OR SIDE EFFECTS

SYMPTOMS	WHAT TO DO
Life-threatening: Hives, rash, intense itching, faintness soon after a dose (anaphylaxis in aspirin-sensitive persons).	Seek emergency treatment immediately.
Common: • Cough, fever, skin rash, swelling of face, fingers, feet and/or lower legs.	Discontinue. Call doctor right away.
• Back pain, dizziness, gas, headache, nausea, heartburn, burning in throat, sleeplessness, stuffy or runny nose.	Continue. Call doctor when convenient.
Infrequent: • Bloody or tarry stools, chills, congestion, diarrhea, fatigue, loss of appetite, muscle pains, blood in urine, pale skin, shortness of breath, severe stomach pain, weight gain, vomiting.	Discontinue. Call doctor right away.
• Anxiety, vision changes, noises in ears, changes in sense of taste, difficulty swallowing, dry mouth, constipation, depression, rapid heartbeat, increased sweating, numbness in fingers or toes, sleepiness.	Continue. Call doctor when convenient.
Rare: None expected.	

WARNINGS & PRECAUTIONS

Don't take if:
* You are allergic to aspirin or any nonsteroidal, anti-inflammatory drug.
* You are in the third trimester of your pregnancy.
* You have had recent heart surgery.
* You have not read special note under Uses.

Before you start, consult your doctor if:
* You have a history of alcohol abuse.
* You have bleeding problems or ulcers.
* You have used tobacco recently.
* You have impaired kidney or liver function.
* You have anemia, asthma, dehydration or fluid retention.
* You have high blood pressure or heart disease.

Over age 60:
Adverse reactions and side effects may be more frequent and severe than in younger persons.

Pregnancy:
Decide with your doctor whether drug benefits justify risk to unborn child. Risk category C (see page xviii).

Breast-feeding:
Avoid drug or discontinue nursing until you finish medicine. Consult doctor for advice on maintaining milk supply.

Infants & children:
Celecoxib is used to treat juvenile rheumatoid arthritis (JRA) in patients age 2 years and older.

Prolonged use:
* Eye damage; reduced hearing.
* Sore throat, fever.
* Weight gain.
* Talk to your doctor about the need for follow-up medical exams or laboratory studies to check complete blood counts, liver function, stools for blood, eyes.

Skin & sunlight:
No problems expected.

Driving, piloting or hazardous work:
Don't drive or pilot aircraft until you learn how medicine affects you. Don't work around dangerous machinery. Don't climb ladders or work in high places. Danger increases if you drink alcohol or take medicine affecting alertness and reflexes, such as antihistamines, tranquilizers, sedatives, pain medicine, narcotics and mind-altering drugs.

Discontinuing:
No problems expected. If drug has been taken for a long time, consult doctor before discontinuing.

Others:
* May affect results in some medical tests.
* Advise any doctor or dentist whom you consult that you take this medicine.

POSSIBLE INTERACTION WITH OTHER DRUGS

GENERIC NAME OR DRUG CLASS	COMBINED EFFECT
Angiotensin-converting enzyme (ACE) inhibitors*	May decrease ACE inhibitor effect.
Antacids*	Decreased pain relief.
Antifungals, azole	Increased risk of side effects.
Anti-inflammatory drugs, nonsteroidal (NSAIDs)* other	Increased risk of side effects.
Aspirin	Increased risk of stomach ulcer.
Dextromethorphan	Increased effect of dextromethorphan.
Diuretics	Decreased diuretic effect.
Lithium	Increased lithium effect.
Methotrexate	Increased methotrexate effect.
Phenytoin	Decreased pain relief.
Rifampin	Decreased rifampin effect.
Warfarin	Increased risk of bleeding problems.

POSSIBLE INTERACTION WITH OTHER SUBSTANCES

INTERACTS WITH	COMBINED EFFECT
Alcohol:	Possible stomach ulcer or bleeding.
Beverages:	None expected.
Cocaine:	None expected.
Foods:	None expected.
Marijuana:	May increase pain relief.
Tobacco:	Possible stomach ulcer or bleeding.

*See Glossary

ANTI-INFLAMMATORY DRUGS, NONSTEROIDAL (NSAIDs) (Ophthalmic)

GENERIC AND BRAND NAMES

BROMFENAC
  Xibrom
DICLOFENAC
  Voltaren Ophtha
  Voltaren
    Ophthalmic
FLURBIPROFEN
  Ocufen

INDOMETHACIN
  Indocid
KETOROLAC
  Acular
  Acular LS
NEPAFENAC
  Nevanac
SUPROFEN
  Profenal

BASIC INFORMATION

Habit forming? No
Prescription needed? Yes
Available as generic? Yes, for some
Drug class: Ophthalmic anti-inflammatory agents, nonsteroidal

USES

- Used to prevent problems during and following eye surgery, such as cataract removal.
- Treatment for eye itching caused by seasonal allergic conjunctivitis.

DOSAGE & USAGE INFORMATION

How to use:
Eye solution
- Wash hands.
- Apply pressure to inside corner of eye with middle finger.
- Continue pressure for 1 minute after placing medicine in eye.
- Tilt head backward. Pull lower lid away from eye with index finger of the same hand.
- Drop eye drops into pouch and close eye. Don't blink.
- Keep eyes closed for 1 to 2 minutes.

When to use:
As directed by your doctor or on the label. Your doctor or nurse may instill the drug before an eye operation.

Continued next column

OVERDOSE

SYMPTOMS:
None expected.
WHAT TO DO:
Not intended for internal use. If child accidentally swallows, call doctor or poison control center 1-800-222-1222 for help.

If you forget a dose:
Use as soon as you remember.

What drug does:
Blocks prostaglandin production. Prostaglandins cause inflammatory responses and constriction of the pupil.

Time lapse before drug works:
Immediately.

Don't use with:
Any other medicine or any dietary supplement without consulting your doctor or pharmacist.

POSSIBLE ADVERSE REACTIONS OR SIDE EFFECTS

SYMPTOMS	WHAT TO DO
Life-threatening: None expected.	
Common: Brief and mild burning or stinging when drops are administered.	No action necessary.
Infrequent: None expected.	
Rare: Allergic reaction (itching, tearing); redness, swelling or bleeding in eye not present before; eye pain; sensitivity to light.	Discontinue. Call doctor right away.

WARNINGS & PRECAUTIONS

Don't use if:
- You are allergic to any eye medication.
- You are allergic to any nonsteroidal anti-inflammatory drugs taken orally, e.g., aspirin.

Before you start, consult your doctor if:
- You have any bleeding disorder such as hemophilia.
- You have or have had herpes simplex keratitis (an inflammation of the cornea).
- You have allergies to any medications, foods or other substances.

Over age 60:
No special problems expected.

Pregnancy:
Risk category C (see page xviii). Decide with your doctor whether drug benefit justifies risk to unborn child.

Breast-feeding:
Unknown if drug passes into breast milk after administration into the eye. Consult doctor.

Infants & children:
No information available on safety or effectiveness. Consult doctor.

Prolonged use:
Not intended for long-term use.

Skin & sunlight:
No special problems expected.

Driving, piloting or hazardous work:
No special problems expected.

Discontinuing:
No special problems expected.

Others:
Don't use leftover medicine for other eye problems without your doctor's approval. Some eye infections could be made worse.

POSSIBLE INTERACTION WITH OTHER DRUGS

GENERIC NAME OR DRUG CLASS	COMBINED EFFECT
Anticoagulants,* oral	May increase bleeding tendency.
Antiglaucoma drugs*	May decrease antiglaucoma effect (with flurbiprofen).
Carbachol	Decreased carbachol effect.

POSSIBLE INTERACTION WITH OTHER SUBSTANCES

INTERACTS WITH	COMBINED EFFECT
Alcohol:	None expected.
Beverages:	None expected.
Cocaine:	None expected.
Foods:	None expected.
Marijuana:	None expected.
Tobacco:	None expected.

*See Glossary

ANTI-INFLAMMATORY DRUGS, STEROIDAL (Ophthalmic)

GENERIC AND BRAND NAMES

See full list of generic and brand names in the *Generic and Brand Name Directory*, page 875.

BASIC INFORMATION

Habit forming? No
Prescription needed? Yes
Available as generic? Yes
Drug class: Adrenocorticoid (ophthalmic); anti-inflammatory, steroidal (ophthalmic)

USES

- Relieves redness and irritation due to allergies or other irritants.
- Prevents damage to eye.
- Treatment for anterior uveitis (a type of eye infection).

DOSAGE & USAGE INFORMATION

How to use:
Eye drops
- Wash hands.
- Apply pressure to inside corner of eye with middle finger.
- Continue pressure for 1 minute after placing medicine in eye.
- Tilt head backward. Pull lower lid away from eye with index finger of the same hand.
- Drop eye drops into pouch and close eye. Don't blink.
- Keep eyes closed for 1 to 2 minutes.

Eye ointment
- Wash hands.
- Pull lower lid down from eye to form a pouch.
- Squeeze tube to apply thin strip of ointment into pouch.
- Close eye for 1 to 2 minutes.
- Don't touch applicator tip to any surface (including the eye). If you accidentally touch tip, clean with warm water and soap.
- Keep container tightly closed.

Continued next column

OVERDOSE

SYMPTOMS:
None expected.
WHAT TO DO:
Not intended for internal use. If child accidentally swallows, call doctor or poison control center 1-800-222-1222 for help.

- Keep cool, but don't freeze.
- Wash hands immediately after using.

When to use:
As directed.

If you forget a dose:
Use as soon as you remember.

What drug does:
Affects cell membranes and decreases response to irritating substances.

Time lapse before drug works:
Immediately.

Don't use with:
Medicines for abdominal cramps or glaucoma without first consulting your doctor.

POSSIBLE ADVERSE REACTIONS OR SIDE EFFECTS

SYMPTOMS	WHAT TO DO
Life-threatening: None expected.	
Common: None expected.	
Infrequent: Watery, stinging, burning eyes.	Continue. Call doctor when convenient.
Rare:	
• Eye pain, blurred vision, drooping eyelid, halos around lights, enlarged pupils, flashes of light.	Discontinue. Call doctor right away.
• Eye symptoms (discharge, dryness, irritation, tearing, sensation of foreign body); sore throat; runny or stuffy nose.	Continue. Call doctor when convenient.

ANTI-INFLAMMATORY DRUGS, STEROIDAL
(Ophthalmic)

WARNINGS & PRECAUTIONS

Don't use if:
You are allergic to any cortisone medicine.

Before you start, consult your doctor if:
- You have or ever have had any eye infection, glaucoma, virus (herpes) or fungus infection of the eye, tuberculosis of the eye.
- You wear contact lenses (may need to discontinue wearing temporarily).

Over age 60:
No problems expected.

Pregnancy:
Risk factors vary for drugs in this group. See category list on page xviii and consult doctor.

Breast-feeding:
Safety not established. Avoid if possible. Consult doctor.

Infants & children:
Use for short periods of time only.

Prolonged use:
- Recheck with eye doctor at regular intervals.
- May develop glaucoma, hypertension of the eye, damage to optic nerve, vision changes, cataracts or infections due to suppressive effects of drug.

Skin & sunlight:
No problems expected.

Driving, piloting or hazardous work:
No problems expected.

Discontinuing:
No problems expected.

Others:
- Cortisone eye medicines should not be used for bacterial, viral, fungal or tubercular infections.
- Keep cool, but don't freeze.
- Notify doctor if condition doesn't improve within 3 days.
- Contact lens wearers have increased risk of infection.

POSSIBLE INTERACTION WITH OTHER DRUGS

GENERIC NAME OR DRUG CLASS	COMBINED EFFECT
Antiglaucoma drugs,* long- and short-acting	Decreased antiglaucoma effect.

POSSIBLE INTERACTION WITH OTHER SUBSTANCES

INTERACTS WITH	COMBINED EFFECT
Alcohol:	None expected.
Beverages:	None expected.
Cocaine:	None expected.
Foods:	None expected.
Marijuana:	None expected.
Tobacco:	None expected.

ANTI-INFLAMMATORY DRUGS, STEROIDAL (Otic)

GENERIC AND BRAND NAMES

BETAMETHASONE
   (otic)
   Betnesol

DEXAMETHASONE
   (otic)
   Decadron

BASIC INFORMATION

Habit forming? No
Prescription needed? Yes
Available as generic? Yes
Drug class: Anti-inflammatory, steroidal
   (otic); adrenocorticoid (otic)

USES

- Treats inflammation symptoms (redness, swelling, itching) of the ear due to allergies or other disorders.
- Treats seborrheic and eczematoid dermatitis involving the ear.

DOSAGE & USAGE INFORMATION

How to use:
As directed by your doctor or pharmacist. The following are general instructions.

How to use ear drops:
- Wash and dry hands.
- Warm drops by holding container in your hand for a few minutes.
- Lie down with affected ear up.
- Adults—Pull ear lobe back and up.
- Children—Pull ear lobe down and back.
- Put the correct number of drops into the ear. Do not allow dropper to touch the ear.
- Wipe away any spilled drops.
- Stay lying down for 2 to 5 minutes.

When to use:
As directed by your doctor.

Continued next column

OVERDOSE

SYMPTOMS:
None expected.
WHAT TO DO:
Not intended for internal use. If child accidentally swallows, call doctor or poison control center 1-800-222-1222 for help.

If you forget a dose:
Use as soon as you remember. If it is almost time for the next dose, wait for next scheduled dose (don't double this dose).

What drug does:
Decreases inflammation.

Time lapse before drug works:
Symptoms should improve within 5 to 7 days. Complete healing may take up to several weeks.

Don't use with:
Other ear medications unless directed by your doctor.

POSSIBLE ADVERSE REACTIONS OR SIDE EFFECTS

SYMPTOMS	WHAT TO DO
Life-threatening: None expected.	
Common: None expected.	
Infrequent: Burning or stinging of the ear.	Continue. Call doctor if symptoms persist.
Rare: New or unusual symptoms occur (may be due to drug being absorbed into the body).	Discontinue. Call doctor right away.

ANTI-INFLAMMATORY DRUGS, STEROIDAL
(Otic)

 WARNINGS & PRECAUTIONS

Don't use if:
You are allergic to any corticosteroid* drugs.

Before you start, consult your doctor if:
- Eardrum is punctured.
- You have diabetes, heart disease, epilepsy, glaucoma, high blood pressure, osteoporosis, or tuberculosis.
- You have a chronic ear infection or other ear problem.
- You have a viral or fungal infection.

Over age 60:
No problems expected.

Pregnancy:
Decide with your doctor if drug benefits justify risk to unborn child. Risk category C (see page xviii).

Breast-feeding:
It is unknown if ear medications are absorbed and then pass into breast milk. Consult doctor.

Infants & children:
Use these drops only if prescribed by your child's doctor.

Prolonged use:
Not intended for prolonged use.

Skin & sunlight:
No problems expected.

Driving, piloting or hazardous work:
No problems expected.

Discontinuing:
No problems expected.

Others:
- Do not increase or decrease dosage without doctor's approval.
- Follow your doctor's instructions for additional ear care at home.
- Call your doctor if ear symptoms worsen or don't improve after a few days of treatment.
- Advise any doctor or dentist whom you consult that you are using this drug.

 POSSIBLE INTERACTION WITH OTHER DRUGS

GENERIC NAME OR DRUG CLASS	COMBINED EFFECT
Phenytoin	May decrease effect of anti-inflammatory.

 POSSIBLE INTERACTION WITH OTHER SUBSTANCES

INTERACTS WITH	COMBINED EFFECT
Alcohol:	None expected.
Beverages:	None expected.
Cocaine:	None expected.
Foods:	None expected.
Marijuana:	None expected.
Tobacco:	None expected.

*See Glossary

ANTIMALARIAL

GENERIC AND BRAND NAMES

HALOFANTRINE
Halfan

MEFLOQUINE
Lariam

BASIC INFORMATION

Habit forming? No
Prescription needed? Yes
Available as generic? Yes, for some
Drug class: Antiprotozoal, antimalarial, antiparasitic

 USES

- Treats malaria caused by *plasmodium falciparum* (either chloroquine-sensitive or chloroquine-resistant).
- Treats malaria caused by *plasmodium vivax.*
- Mefloquine helps prevent malaria in people traveling into areas where malaria is prevalent.

 DOSAGE & USAGE INFORMATION

How to take:
- Mefloquine tablet—Swallow with food, milk or water to lessen stomach irritation.
- Halofantrine tablet—Take on an empty stomach.
- Halofantrine suspension—Varies by age and weight; follow physician's directions.

When to take:
- Mefloquine treatment is usually given as 5 tablets in a single dose, while prevention with mefloquine should start a week prior to travel.
- Halofantrine tablets and suspension are taken every 6 hours, 3 times a day for one day on an empty stomach, 1 hour before or 2 hours after a meal.

Continued next column

 OVERDOSE

SYMPTOMS:
Seizures, heart rhythm disturbances.
WHAT TO DO:
- Dial 911 (emergency) for medical help or call poison control center 1-800-222-1222 for instructions.
- Induce vomiting and see a doctor immediately because of the potential cardiotoxic effect. Treat vomiting or diarrhea with standard fluid therapy.
- See emergency information on last 3 pages of this book.

If you forget a dose:
Take as soon as you remember, then return to regular dosing schedule.

What drug does:
Exact mechanism unknown. Mefloquine kills parasite in one of its developmental stages, while halofantrine treats malaria in its acute stage.

Time lapse before drug works:
6 to 24 hours.

Don't take with:
- Sulfadoxine and pyrimethamine combination (Fansidar).
- Any other medicines (including over-the-counter drugs such as cough and cold medicines, laxatives, antacids, diet pills, caffeine, nose drops or vitamins) without consulting your doctor or pharmacist.

 POSSIBLE ADVERSE REACTIONS OR SIDE EFFECTS

SYMPTOMS	WHAT TO DO
Life-threatening:	
Seizures.	Seek emergency treatment immediately.
Common:	
• Dizziness, headache, lightheadedness, abdominal pain, diarrhea, nausea or vomiting, rash, visual disturbances.	Discontinue. Call doctor right away.
• Insomnia, appetite loss.	Continue. Call doctor when convenient.
Infrequent:	
None expected.	
Rare:	
Change in heart rate, confusion, anxiety, depression, hallucinations, psychosis, black urine or decrease in urine amount, chest or lower back pain, rapid breathing.	Discontinue. Call doctor right away.

WARNINGS & PRECAUTIONS

Don't take if:
You are allergic to mefloquine, halofantrine, quinine, quinidine or related medications.

Before you start, consult your doctor if:
* You plan to become pregnant within the medication period or 2 months after.
* You have heart trouble, especially heart block.
* You have depression or other emotional problems.
* You are giving this to a child under 40 pounds of body weight.
* You have epilepsy or a seizure disorder.

Over age 60:
Adverse reactions and side effects may be more frequent and severe than in younger persons.

Pregnancy:
Not recommended. If traveling to an area where malaria is endemic, consult your doctor about prophylaxis. Risk category C (see page xviii).

Breast-feeding:
One or more of these drugs may pass into mother's milk. Avoid drug or discontinue nursing.

Infants & children:
* For halofantrine pediatric use, consult your doctor.
* Mefloquine is not recommended for children under 2.

Prolonged use:
Not recommended.

Skin & sunlight:
No problems expected.

Driving, piloting or hazardous work:
Don't drive or pilot aircraft until you learn how medicine affects you. Don't work around dangerous machinery. Don't climb ladders or work in high places. Danger increases if you drink alcohol or take medicine affecting alertness and reflexes.

Discontinuing:
Don't discontinue without doctor's advice until you complete the prescribed dosage.

Others:
* Periodic physical (including eye) examinations and blood studies recommended.
* Resistance to one or more of these drugs by some strains of malaria has been reported, so prevention and treatment of malaria may not be uniformly effective.

POSSIBLE INTERACTION WITH OTHER DRUGS

GENERIC NAME OR DRUG CLASS	COMBINED EFFECT
Anticonvulsants*	Possible lowered seizure control.
Beta-adrenergic blocking agents*	Heartbeat irregularities or cardiac arrest. Avoid.
Calcium channel blockers*	Heartbeat irregularities.
Chloroquine	Increased chance of seizures. Avoid.
Propranolol	Heartbeat irregularities.
Quinidine	Increased chance of seizures and heart rhythm disturbances.
Quinine	Increased chance of seizures and heart rhythm disturbances.
Typhoid vaccine (oral)	Concurrent use may decrease effectiveness of vaccine.

POSSIBLE INTERACTION WITH OTHER SUBSTANCES

INTERACTS WITH	COMBINED EFFECT
Alcohol:	Possible liver toxicity. Avoid.
Beverages: Any alcoholic beverage.	Possible liver toxicity. Avoid.
Cocaine:	No problems expected.
Foods:	No problems expected.
Marijuana:	No problems expected.
Tobacco:	No problems expected.

ANTIMYASTHENICS

GENERIC AND BRAND NAMES

AMBENONIUM
  Mytelase Caplets
NEOSTIGMINE
  Prostigmin

PYRIDOSTIGMINE
  Mestinon
  Mestinon Timespans
  Regonol

BASIC INFORMATION

Habit forming? No
Prescription needed? Yes
Available as generic? Yes, for some
Drug class: Cholinergic, antimyasthenic

USES

- Diagnosis and treatment of myasthenia gravis.
- Treatment of urinary retention and abdominal distension.
- Antidote to adverse effects of muscle relaxants used in surgery.

DOSAGE & USAGE INFORMATION

How to take:
- Tablet or syrup—Swallow with liquid or food to lessen stomach irritation.
- Extended-release tablet—Swallow each dose whole. If you take regular tablets, you may chew or crush them.

When to take:
As directed, usually 3 or 4 times a day.

If you forget a dose:
Take as soon as you remember up to 2 hours late. If more than 2 hours, wait for next scheduled dose (don't double this dose).

Continued next column

OVERDOSE

SYMPTOMS:
Muscle weakness or paralysis, cramps, twitching or clumsiness; severe diarrhea, nausea, vomiting, stomach cramps or pain; breathing difficulty; confusion, irritability, nervousness, restlessness, fear; unusually slow heartbeat; seizures; blurred vision; extreme fatigue.
WHAT TO DO:
- **Dial 911 (emergency) for medical help or call poison control center 1-800-222-1222 for instructions.**
- **See emergency information on last 3 pages of this book.**

What drug does:
Inhibits the chemical activity of an enzyme (cholinesterase) so nerve impulses can cross the junction of nerves and muscles.

Time lapse before drug works:
Usually takes 10 to 14 days to determine if drug helps relieve symptoms.

Don't take with:
Any other medicine or any dietary supplement without consulting your doctor or pharmacist.

POSSIBLE ADVERSE REACTIONS OR SIDE EFFECTS

SYMPTOMS	WHAT TO DO
Life-threatening:	
In case of overdose, see previous column.	
Common:	
Excess saliva, unusual sweating, mild diarrhea, nausea, vomiting, stomach cramps or pain.	Continue. Call doctor when convenient.
Infrequent:	
Constricted pupils, watery eyes, lung congestion, frequent urge to urinate, confusion, slurred speech.	Continue. But call doctor right away.
Rare:	
Other symptoms.	Continue. Call doctor when convenient.

WARNINGS & PRECAUTIONS

Don't take if:
You are allergic to any cholinergic* or bromide.

Before you start, consult your doctor if:
- You plan to become pregnant within medication period.
- You have bronchial asthma.
- You have heartbeat irregularities.
- You have urinary obstruction or urinary tract infection.

Over age 60:
Adverse reactions and side effects may be more frequent and severe than in younger persons.

Pregnancy:
Decide with your doctor if drug benefits justify risk to unborn child. Risk category C (see page xviii).

Breast-feeding:
Pyridostigmine passes into milk. It is unknown if others pass into milk. Avoid drug or discontinue nursing until you finish medicine. Consult doctor for advice on maintaining milk supply.

Infants & children:
Use only under close medical supervision.

Prolonged use:
Medication may lose effectiveness. Ask your doctor about discontinuing drug for a few days to possibly help restore effect.

Skin & sunlight:
No problems expected.

Driving, piloting or hazardous work:
Don't drive or pilot aircraft until you learn how medicine affects you. Don't work around dangerous machinery. Don't climb ladders or work in high places. Danger increases if you drink alcohol or take medicine affecting alertness and reflexes, such as antihistamines, tranquilizers, sedatives, pain medicine, narcotics and mind-altering drugs.

Discontinuing:
Don't discontinue without doctor's advice until you complete prescribed dose, even though symptoms diminish or disappear.

Others:
- Advise any doctor or dentist whom you consult that you take this medicine.
- Be cautious about participating in hot weather activities since drug may cause excessive sweating.

POSSIBLE INTERACTION WITH OTHER DRUGS

GENERIC NAME OR DRUG CLASS	COMBINED EFFECT
Anesthetics, local or general*	Decreased effect of antimyasthenic.
Antiarrhythmics*	Decreased effect of antimyasthenic.
Anticholinergics*	May mask severe side effects.
Cholinergics,* other	Possible brain and nervous system toxicity.
Guanadrel	Decreased effect of antimyasthenic.
Guanethidine	Decreased effect of antimyasthenic.
Mecamylamine	Decreased effect of antimyasthenic.
Procainamide	Decreased effect of antimyasthenic.
Quinidine	Decreased effect of antimyasthenic.

POSSIBLE INTERACTION WITH OTHER SUBSTANCES

INTERACTS WITH	COMBINED EFFECT
Alcohol:	No proven problems with small doses.
Beverages:	None expected.
Cocaine:	Decreased antimyasthenic effect. Avoid.
Foods:	None expected.
Marijuana:	No proven problems.
Tobacco:	No proven problems.

*See Glossary

ANTIPYRINE & BENZOCAINE (Otic)

BRAND NAMES

A/B Otic
Allergen
Analgesic Ear
 Drops
Antiben
Auralgan

Aurodex
Dolotic
Earache Drops
Earocol
Otiprin
Otocalm

BASIC INFORMATION

Habit forming? No
Prescription needed?
   Yes (in US;
   No in Canada)
Available as generic? Yes
Drug class: Analgesic (otic); anesthetic

USES

* Relieves symptoms of middle ear infections (otitis media). It does not treat the infection itself.
* Used to soften earwax so it can be removed.

DOSAGE & USAGE INFORMATION

How to use ear drops:
* Wash and dry hands.
* Warm drops by holding container in your hand for a few minutes.
* Lie down with affected ear up.
* Adults—Pull ear lobe back and up.
* Children—Pull ear lobe down and back.
* Put the correct number of drops into the ear. Do not allow dropper to touch the ear.
* Wipe away any spilled drops.
* Stay lying down for 2 to 5 minutes.
* For ear wax removal, follow your doctor's instructions.

When to use:
Every 1 to 2 hours for 4 hours, then 4 times a day when needed for pain.

If you forget a dose:
Use as soon as you remember. If it is almost time for the next dose, wait for next scheduled dose (don't double this dose).

Continued next column

OVERDOSE

SYMPTOMS:
None expected.
WHAT TO DO:
Not intended for internal use. If child accidentally swallows, call doctor or poison control center 1-800-222-1222 for help.

What drug does:
Helps relieve the pain. congestion and swelling of ear infections. It does not cure the infection.

Time lapse before drug works:
10 minutes.

Don't use with:
Any other ear medicine without consulting your doctor or pharmacist.

POSSIBLE ADVERSE REACTIONS OR SIDE EFFECTS

SYMPTOMS	WHAT TO DO
Life-threatening: None expected.	
Common: None expected.	
Infrequent: Itching or burning in ear (probably represents allergic reaction).	Discontinue. Call doctor right away.
Rare: None expected.	

WARNINGS & PRECAUTIONS

Don't use if:
You are allergic to any local anesthetic (name usually ends with "caine").

Before you start, consult your doctor if:
Eardrum is ruptured.

Over age 60:
No problems expected.

Pregnancy:
Decide with your doctor if drug benefits justify risk to unborn child. Risk category C (see page xviii).

Breast-feeding:
No problems expected. Consult doctor.

Infants & children:
No problems expected.

Prolonged use:
Not intended for prolonged use.

Skin & sunlight:
No problems expected.

Driving, piloting or hazardous work:
No problems expected.

Discontinuing:
No problems expected.

Others:
* Keep cool, but don't freeze.
* Don't touch tip of dropper to any other surface.
* Don't rinse the dropper. Wipe with clean cloth and close tightly.

POSSIBLE INTERACTION WITH OTHER DRUGS

GENERIC NAME OR DRUG CLASS	COMBINED EFFECT
None expected.	

POSSIBLE INTERACTION WITH OTHER SUBSTANCES

INTERACTS WITH	COMBINED EFFECT
Alcohol:	None expected.
Beverages:	None expected.
Cocaine:	None expected.
Foods:	None expected.
Marijuana:	None expected.
Tobacco:	None expected.

ANTISEBORRHEICS (Topical)

GENERIC AND BRAND NAMES

See full list of generic and brand names in the *Generic and Brand Name Directory,* page 876.

BASIC INFORMATION

Habit forming? No
Prescription needed? Yes
Available as generic? Yes
Drug class: Antiseborrheic

 ## USES

Treats dandruff or seborrheic dermatitis of scalp.

 ## DOSAGE & USAGE INFORMATION

How to use:
- Wet hair and scalp.
- Apply enough medicine to form lather.
- Rub in well. Keep away from eyes.
- Allow to remain on scalp 3 to 5 minutes, then rinse.
- Repeat above steps once.

When to use:
As directed by doctor. Twice a week for shampoo is average.

If you forget a dose:
Use as soon as you remember.

What drug does:
Slows cell growth in scales on scalp.

Time lapse before drug works:
Varies a great deal. If no improvement in 2 weeks, notify doctor.

Don't use with:
Other hair or scalp preparations without consulting your doctor or pharmacist.

 ## OVERDOSE

SYMPTOMS:
None expected.
WHAT TO DO:
- Not for internal use. If child accidentally swallows, dial 911 (emergency) for medical help or call poison control center 1-800-222-1222 for instructions.
- See emergency information on last 3 pages of this book.

 ## POSSIBLE ADVERSE REACTIONS OR SIDE EFFECTS

SYMPTOMS	WHAT TO DO
Life-threatening: None expected.	
Common: None expected.	
Infrequent:	
• Irritation not present before using, rash.	Discontinue. Call doctor when convenient.
• Dryness or itching scalp.	Continue. Call doctor when convenient.
Rare: None expected.	

**WARNINGS &
PRECAUTIONS**

Don't use if:
* You have had an allergic reaction to chloroxine, clioquinol (iodochlorhydroxyquin), iodoquinol (diiodohydroxyquin) or edate sodium.
* Scalp is blistered or infected with oozing or raw areas.

Before you start, consult your doctor if:
You are allergic to anything.

Over age 60:
No problems expected.

Pregnancy:
Risk factors vary for drugs in this group. See category list on page xviii and consult doctor.

Breast-feeding:
No problems expected, but check with doctor.

Infants & children:
No problems expected, but check with doctor.

Prolonged use:
No problems expected, but check with doctor.

Skin & sunlight:
No special problems expected.

Driving, piloting or hazardous work:
No problems expected, but check with doctor.

Discontinuing:
No problems expected, but check with doctor.

Others:
* If medicine accidentally gets into eyes, flush them immediately with cool water.
* Heat and moisture in bathroom medicine cabinet can cause breakdown of medicine. Store someplace else.
* Keep cool, but don't freeze.

 **POSSIBLE INTERACTION
WITH OTHER DRUGS**

GENERIC NAME OR DRUG CLASS	COMBINED EFFECT
Other medicated shampoos	May increase adverse reactions of each medicine.

 **POSSIBLE INTERACTION
WITH OTHER SUBSTANCES**

INTERACTS WITH	COMBINED EFFECT
Alcohol:	None expected.
Beverages:	None expected.
Cocaine:	None expected.
Foods:	None expected.
Marijuana:	None expected.
Tobacco:	None expected.

ANTITHYROID DRUGS

GENERIC AND BRAND NAMES

METHIMAZOLE
   Tapazole
   Thiamazole

PROPYLTHIOURACIL
   Propyl-Thyracil

BASIC INFORMATION

Habit forming? No
Prescription needed? Yes
Available as generic? Yes
Drug class: Antihyperthyroid

 ## USES

- Treatment of overactive thyroid (hyperthyroidism).
- Treatment of angina in patients who have overactive thyroid.

 ## DOSAGE & USAGE INFORMATION

How to take:
Tablet—Swallow with liquid or food to lessen stomach irritation. If you can't swallow whole, crumble tablet and take with liquid or food.

When to take:
At the same times each day.

If you forget a dose:
Take as soon as you remember up to 2 hours late. If more than 2 hours, wait for next scheduled dose (don't double this dose).

What drug does:
Prevents thyroid gland from producing excess thyroid hormone.

Time lapse before drug works:
10 to 20 days.

Don't take with:
Any other medicine or any dietary supplement without consulting your doctor or pharmacist.

 ## OVERDOSE

SYMPTOMS:
Bleeding, spots on skin, jaundice (yellow eyes and skin), loss of consciousness.
WHAT TO DO:
Overdose unlikely to threaten life. If person uses much larger amount than prescribed or if accidentally swallowed, call doctor or poison control center 1-800-222-1222 for help.

 ## POSSIBLE ADVERSE REACTIONS OR SIDE EFFECTS

SYMPTOMS	WHAT TO DO
Life-threatening:	
In case of overdose, see previous column.	
Common:	
Skin rash, itching, dryness.	Continue. Call doctor right away.
Infrequent:	
• Dizziness, sore throat with chills and fever, abdominal pain.	Continue. Call doctor right away.
• Taste loss, constipation, diarrhea.	Continue. Call doctor when convenient.
Rare:	
Headache; enlarged lymph glands; irregular or rapid heartbeat; unusual bruising or bleeding; backache; numbness or tingling in toes, fingers or face; joint pain; muscle aches; menstrual irregularities; jaundice; tired, weak, sleepy, listless; swollen eyes or feet; black stools; excessive cold feeling; puffy skin; irritability.	Continue. Call doctor right away.

 ## WARNINGS & PRECAUTIONS

Don't take if:
You are allergic to antithyroid medicines.

Before you start, consult your doctor if:
- You have liver disease.
- You have blood disease.
- You have an infection.
- You take anticoagulants.

Over age 60:
Adverse reactions and side effects may be more frequent and severe than in younger persons.

Pregnancy:
Consult doctor. Risk category D (see page xviii).

Breast-feeding:
Drug filters into milk. Consult doctor.

Infants & children:
Use only under special medical supervision.

Prolonged use:
* Adverse reactions and side effects more common.
* Talk to your doctor about the need for follow-up medical examinations or laboratory studies to check thyroid function, complete blood counts (white blood cell count, platelet count, red blood cell count, hemoglobin, hematocrit).

Skin & sunlight:
No problems expected.

Driving, piloting or hazardous work:
Don't drive or pilot aircraft until you learn how medicine affects you. Don't work around dangerous machinery. Don't climb ladders or work in high places. Danger increases if you drink alcohol or take medicine affecting alertness and reflexes, such as antihistamines, tranquilizers, sedatives, pain medicine, narcotics and mind-altering drugs.

Discontinuing:
Don't discontinue without consulting doctor. Dose may require gradual reduction if you have taken drug for a long time. Doses of other drugs may also require adjustment.

Others:
* Advise any doctor or dentist whom you consult that you take this medicine.
* Ask your doctor about the symptoms of over-active or underactive thyroid and what to do if they occur.

 POSSIBLE INTERACTION WITH OTHER DRUGS

GENERIC NAME OR DRUG CLASS	COMBINED EFFECT
Amiodarone	Decreased antithyroid effect.
Anticoagulants*	Increased effect of anticoagulants.
Antineoplastic drugs*	Increased chance to suppress bone marrow.
Chloramphenicol	Increased chance to suppress bone marrow.
Clozapine	Toxic effect on bone marrow.
Digitalis preparations*	Increased digitalis effect.
Iodine	Decreased antithyroid effect.
Levamisole	Increased risk of bone marrow depression.
Lithium	Decreased thyroid activity.
Potassium iodide	Decreased antithyroid effect.
Tiopronin	Increased risk of toxicity to bone marrow.

 POSSIBLE INTERACTION WITH OTHER SUBSTANCES

INTERACTS WITH	COMBINED EFFECT
Alcohol:	Increased possibility of liver toxicity. Avoid.
Beverages:	No problems expected.
Cocaine:	Increased toxicity potential of medicines. Avoid.
Foods:	No problems expected.
Marijuana:	Increased rapid or irregular heartbeat. Avoid.
Tobacco:	Increased chance of rapid heartbeat. Avoid.

*See Glossary

ANTIVIRALS FOR HERPES VIRUS

GENERIC AND BRAND NAMES

ACYCLOVIR
Alti-Acyclovir
Avirax
Zovirax
FAMCICLOVIR
Famvir

GANCICLOVIR
Cytovene
VALACYCLOVIR
Valtrex

BASIC INFORMATION

Habit forming? No
Prescription needed? Yes
Available as generic? Yes, for some
Drug class: Antiviral

 USES

- Treatment for symptoms of herpes virus infections (does not cure the disorders). These infections include herpes simplex, genital herpes and herpes zoster (also known as shingles). Herpes infections may occur on the lips and mouth, genitals, skin and the brain.
- May be used to treat chickenpox and other viral infections as prescribed by your doctor.
- Ganciclovir is used for treatment of cytomegalovirus (CMV) eye infection in persons whose immune system is impaired.

 DOSAGE & USAGE INFORMATION

How to take:
Tablet, capsule or oral suspension—Swallow with liquid. If you can't swallow whole, open capsule or crumble tablet and take with liquid or food. Take ganciclovir with food and do not open capsule. Other drugs may be taken with or without food. Measure oral suspension with specially marked measuring device.

Continued next column

 OVERDOSE

SYMPTOMS:
Unknown effects.
WHAT TO DO:
Overdose unlikely to threaten life. If person uses much larger amount than prescribed or if accidentally swallowed, call doctor or poison control center 1-800-222-1222 for help.

When to take:
At the same times each day and night. Drugs work best if started within 48 hours of diagnosis (or when symptoms first appear).

If you forget a dose:
Take as soon as you remember up to 2 hours late. If more than 2 hours, wait for next dose (don't double this dose).

What drug does:
Inhibits the growth and spread of the virus thereby decreasing length of infection and lessening the severity of the symptoms.

Time lapse before drug works:
Begins the first day, but may take several days for symptoms (pain, burning and blisters) to improve.

Don't take with:
Any other medicine or any dietary supplement without consulting your doctor or pharmacist.

 POSSIBLE ADVERSE REACTIONS OR SIDE EFFECTS

SYMPTOMS	WHAT TO DO
Life-threatening: Hives, rash, intense itching, faintness soon after a dose (anaphylaxis); difficulty breathing.	Seek emergency treatment immediately.
Common: General feeling of illness or discomfort.	Continue. Call doctor when convenient.
Infrequent: Headache, nausea, diarrhea, vomiting, tiredness, dizziness; with ganciclovir— sore throat and fever, unusual bleeding or bruising, mood changes.	Continue. Call doctor when convenient.
Rare: Vision changes, eyes irritated, swelling agitation, confusion, fever, hallucinations, chills, fever, sore throat or mouth, skin (rash, blister, itch, peel), muscle cramps.	Discontinue. Call doctor right away.

WARNINGS & PRECAUTIONS

Don't take if:
You are allergic to antiviral agents.

Before you start, consult your doctor if:
- You have kidney disease or neurological problems.
- You have any disease of the blood.
- You are allergic to any medication, food or other substance.

Over age 60:
No special problems expected.

Pregnancy:
Risk factors vary for drugs in this group. See category page xviii and consult doctor.

Breast-feeding:
Drugs may pass into milk. Avoid nursing until you finish medicine. Consult doctor for advice on maintaining milk supply.

Infants & children:
Use only under medical supervision.

Prolonged use:
See your doctor for regular visits to check effectiveness of the drug and to check for any blood problems.

Skin & sunlight:
No special problems expected.

Driving, piloting or hazardous work:
Avoid if you experience dizziness after taking drug, otherwise no problems expected.

Discontinuing:
Don't discontinue without doctor's advice until you complete prescribed dose, even though symptoms diminish or disappear.

Others:
- Advise any doctor or dentist whom you consult that you take this medicine.
- If symptoms don't improve within a few days, or if they worsen, consult doctor.
- See your eye doctor regularly if you are taking the drug for eye infection.
- If drug is prescribed for genital herpes, be sure you use proper precautions to prevent spreading the disorder to your sexual partner. If unsure, ask your doctor for information.
- Keep affected skin area clean and dry.
- Decrease blister irritation by wearing loose-fitting clothing.

POSSIBLE INTERACTION WITH OTHER DRUGS

GENERIC NAME OR DRUG CLASS	COMBINED EFFECT
Bone marrow depressants*	Increased risk of bone marrow depression with ganciclovir.
Cimetidine	Increased antiviral effect.
Didanosine	Increased didanosine effect with ganciclovir.
Probenecid	Increased effect of antivirals.
Nephrotoxic medications*	Increased risk of nephrotoxicity.
Nucleotide reverse transcriptase inhibitors	Increased effect of nucleotide reverse transcriptase inhibitor.
Zidovudine	Increased risk of adverse effects.

POSSIBLE INTERACTION WITH OTHER SUBSTANCES

INTERACTS WITH	COMBINED EFFECT
Alcohol:	None expected.
Beverages:	None expected.
Cocaine:	None expected. Best to avoid.
Foods:	None expected.
Marijuana:	None expected. Best to avoid.
Tobacco:	None expected.

ANTIVIRALS FOR INFLUENZA

GENERIC AND BRAND NAMES

AMANTADINE
Symadine
Symmetrel

RIMANTADINE
Flumadine

BASIC INFORMATION

Habit forming? No
Prescription needed? Yes
Available as generic? Yes
Drug class: Antiviral, antiparkinsonism

 ## USES

- Prevention and treatment for Type-A flu infections.
- Relief for symptoms of Parkinson's disease (amantadine).

 ## DOSAGE & USAGE INFORMATION

How to take:
- Capsule—Swallow with liquid or food to lessen stomach irritation.
- Syrup—Dilute dose in beverage before swallowing.

When to take:
At the same times each day. For Type-A flu it is especially important to take regular doses as prescribed.

If you forget a dose:
Take as soon as you remember. Wait 4 hours for next dose. Return to schedule.

What drug does:
- Type-A flu—May block penetration of tissue cells by infectious material from virus cells.
- Parkinson's disease and drug-induced extrapyramidal* reactions—Improves muscular condition and coordination.

Continued next column

 ## OVERDOSE

SYMPTOMS:
Heart rhythm disturbances, blood pressure drop, convulsions, hallucinations, violent behavior, confusion, slurred speech, rolling eyes.
WHAT TO DO:
- Dial 911 (emergency) for medical help or call poison control center 1-800-222-1222 for instructions.
- See emergency information on last 3 pages of this book.

Time lapse before drug works:
- Type-A flu—48 hours.
- Parkinson's disease—2 days to 2 weeks.

Don't take with:
- Alcohol.
- Any other medicine or any dietary supplement without consulting your doctor or pharmacist.

 ## POSSIBLE ADVERSE REACTIONS OR SIDE EFFECTS

SYMPTOMS	WHAT TO DO
Life-threatening: In case of overdose, see previous column.	
Common: Headache, difficulty in concentrating, dizziness or lightheadedness, insomnia, irritability, nervousness, nightmares (these side effects infrequent with rimantadine).	Continue. Call doctor when convenient.
Infrequent:	
• With amantadine— Blurred or changed vision, confusion, difficult urination, hallucinations, fainting.	Discontinue. Call doctor right away.
• Constipation; dry mouth, nose or throat; vomiting, appetite loss, nausea.	Continue. Call doctor when convenient.
Rare:	
• With amantadine— Swelling or irritated eyes; depression; swelling of hands, legs or feet; skin rash.	Discontinue. Call doctor right away.
• Seizures (may occur in persons with a history of seizures).	Discontinue. Seek emergency help.

WARNINGS & PRECAUTIONS

Don't take if:
You are allergic to amantadine or rimantadine.

Before you start, consult your doctor if:
- You have had epilepsy or other seizures.
- You have had heart disease or heart failure.
- You have had liver or kidney disease.
- You have had peptic ulcers.
- You have had eczema or skin rashes.
- You have had emotional or mental disorders or taken drugs for them.

Over age 60:
Adverse reactions and side effects may be more frequent and severe than in younger persons.

Pregnancy:
Decide with your doctor whether benefits justify risk to unborn child. Risk category C (see page xviii).

Breast-feeding:
Drug may pass into milk. Avoid drug or discontinue nursing until you finish medicine. Consult doctor for advice on maintaining milk supply.

Infants & children:
Use only under medical supervision.

Prolonged use:
Skin splotches, feet swelling, rapid weight gain, shortness of breath. Consult doctor.

Skin & sunlight:
One or more drugs in this group may cause rash or intensify sunburn in areas exposed to sun or ultraviolet light (photosensitivity reaction). Avoid overexposure. Notify doctor if reaction occurs.

Driving, piloting or hazardous work:
Don't drive or pilot aircraft until you learn how medicine affects you. Don't work around dangerous machinery. Don't climb ladders or work in high places. Danger increases if you drink alcohol or take medicine affecting alertness and reflexes.

Discontinuing:
- Parkinson's disease—Don't discontinue without doctor's advice until you complete prescribed dose, even though symptoms diminish or disappear.
- Type-A flu—Discontinue 48 hours after symptoms disappear.

Others:
- Parkinson's disease—May lose effectiveness in 3 to 6 months. Consult doctor.
- These drugs are not effective for influenza-B virus.
- Drug-resistant strains of the virus may occur within the same household.

POSSIBLE INTERACTION WITH OTHER DRUGS

GENERIC NAME OR DRUG CLASS	COMBINED EFFECT
Acetaminophen	With rimantadine—Decreased antiviral effect.
Anticholinergics*	With amantadine—Increased risk of side effects.
Antidepressants, tricyclic*	With amantadine—Increased risk of side effects.
Antidyskinetics*	With amantadine—Increased risk of side effects.
Antihistamines*	With amantadine—Increased risk of side effects.
Aspirin	With rimantadine—Decreased antiviral effect.
Carbidopa & Levodopa	With amantadine—Increased effect of carbidopa & levodopa.
Central nervous system (CNS) stimulants*	With amantadine—Increased risk of adverse reactions.
Memantine	With amantadine—Adverse effects of either drug.

POSSIBLE INTERACTION WITH OTHER SUBSTANCES

INTERACTS WITH	COMBINED EFFECT
Alcohol:	Increased alcohol effect. Possible fainting.
Beverages:	None expected.
Cocaine:	Dangerous overstimulation.
Foods:	None expected.
Marijuana:	None expected.
Tobacco:	None expected.

*See Glossary

ANTIVIRALS FOR INFLUENZA, NEURAMINIDASE INHIBITORS

GENERIC AND BRAND NAMES

OSELTAMIVIR
Tamiflu

ZANAMIVIR
Relenza

BASIC INFORMATION

Habit forming? No
Prescription needed? Yes
Available as generic? No
Drug class: Anti-influenza

 USES

- Shortens the duration of influenza types A and B. It is best to start using this medicine within 2 days of onset of symptoms.
- Used to help prevent influenza types A and B.

 DOSAGE & USAGE INFORMATION

How to take:
- Capsule—Swallow with liquid. If you can't swallow whole, open capsule and take with liquid or food.
- Oral solution—Take as directed on label.
- Powder—This medication is to be used with a device called a Diskhaler. Read and carefully follow the instructions provided with the device. If you are still unsure, consult your pharmacist for detailed instructions.

When to take:
- For oseltamivir, take two doses daily at the same times.
- For zanamivir, take two doses on the first day separated by 2 hours and then two doses daily for 5 days separated by 12 hours.

Continued next column

 OVERDOSE

SYMPTOMS:
There has been very little experience with overdose; however, relatively large doses have resulted in nausea and vomiting.
WHAT TO DO:
- Dial 911 (emergency) for medical help or call poison control center 1-800-222-1222 for instructions.
- See emergency information on last 3 pages of this book.

If you forget a dose:
Take or use the missed dose as soon as possible. You can use your next dose 2 hours after taking the missed dose, then return to your normal dosing schedule. Do not double dose.

What drug does:
Inhibits the spread of the virus by preventing release of the cells within the respiratory tract.

Time lapse before drug works:
Begins in 2 to 3 days.

Don't take with:
Any other medicine or any dietary supplement without consulting your doctor or pharmacist.

 POSSIBLE ADVERSE REACTIONS OR SIDE EFFECTS

SYMPTOMS	WHAT TO DO
Life-threatening: Hives, rash, intense itching, faintness soon after a dose (anaphylaxis).	Seek emergency treatment immediately.
Common:	
• Cough, fever, skin rash, swelling (of face, fingers, feet and/or lower legs).	Discontinue. Call doctor right away.
• Back pain, dizziness, gas, headache, nausea, heartburn, burning in throat, sleeplessness, stuffy or runny nose.	Continue. Call doctor when convenient.
Infrequent:	
• Bloody or tarry stools, chills, congestion, diarrhea, fatigue, loss of appetite, muscle pains, shortness of breath, severe stomach pain, weight gain, vomiting.	Discontinue. Call doctor right away.
• Anxiety, vision changes, noises in ears, change in sense of taste, difficulty swallowing, dry mouth, constipation, depression, rapid heartbeat, increased sweating, numbness in fingers or toes, sleepiness.	Continue. Call doctor if symptoms persist.
Rare: Abnormal behaviors.	Discontinue. Call doctor right away.

WARNINGS & PRECAUTIONS

Don't take if:
You are allergic to oseltamivir or zanamivir.

Before you start, consult your doctor if:
- You have a history of asthma or chronic obstructive pulmonary disease (zanamivir).
- You have kidney disease (oseltamivir).

Over age 60:
Adverse reactions and side effects may be more frequent and severe than in younger persons.

Pregnancy:
Decide with your doctor whether drug benefits justify risk to unborn child. Risk category B for zanamivir and risk category C for oseltamivir (see page xviii).

Breast-feeding:
It is unknown if oseltamivir or zanamivir pass into milk. Avoid drug or discontinue nursing until you finish medicine. Consult doctor for advice on maintaining milk supply.

Infants & children:
- Oseltamivir is approved for children over age 1 for influenza treatment and prevention. Do not give to infants under age 1.
- Zanamivir is not recommended for children under 5 years of age.

Prolonged use:
Not intended for long-term use.

Skin & sunlight:
No problems expected.

Driving, piloting or hazardous work:
Don't drive or pilot aircraft until you learn how medicine affects you. Don't work around dangerous machinery. Don't climb ladders or work in high places. Danger increases if you drink alcohol or take medicine affecting alertness and reflexes, such as antihistamines, tranquilizers, sedatives, pain medicine, narcotics and mind-altering drugs.

Discontinuing:
Do not discontinue until you finish all of your medicine; otherwise, symptoms may return.

Others:
- You should continue receiving an annual flu shot according to guidelines on immunization practices or as recommended by your doctor.
- People with the flu (including children and adolescents) may be at increased risk shortly after taking oseltamivir of self-injury, confusion, hallucinations, delirium and abnormal behavior leading to injury which in some cases may have fatal outcomes. Watch patient's behavior closely and call doctor if symptoms develop.
- Use of the drug does not reduce the risk of transmitting influenza to others.
- Advise any doctor or dentist whom you consult that you take this medicine.

POSSIBLE INTERACTION WITH OTHER DRUGS

GENERIC NAME OR DRUG CLASS	COMBINED EFFECT
None expected.	

POSSIBLE INTERACTION WITH OTHER SUBSTANCES

INTERACTS WITH	COMBINED EFFECT
Alcohol:	None expected.
Beverages:	None expected.
Cocaine:	None expected.
Foods:	None expected.
Marijuana:	None expected.
Tobacco:	None expected.

*See Glossary

ANTIVIRALS (Ophthalmic)

GENERIC AND BRAND NAMES

IDOXURIDINE
  Herplex Eye Drops
  Stoxil Eye Ointment

TRIFLURIDINE
  Trifluorothymidine
  Viroptic

BASIC INFORMATION

Habit forming? No
Prescription needed? Yes
Available as generic? No
Drug class: Antiviral (ophthalmic)

 ## USES

Treats virus infections of the eye (usually herpes simplex virus).

 ## DOSAGE & USAGE INFORMATION

How to use:
Eye drops
- Wash hands.
- Apply pressure to inside corner of eye with middle finger.
- Continue pressure for 1 minute after placing medicine in eye.
- Tilt head backward. Pull lower lid away from eye with index finger of the same hand.
- Drop eye drops into pouch and close eye. Don't blink.
- Keep eyes closed for 1 to 2 minutes.

Eye ointment
- Wash hands.
- Pull lower lid down from eye to form a pouch.
- Squeeze tube to apply thin strip of ointment into pouch.
- Close eye for 1 to 2 minutes.
- Don't touch applicator tip to any surface (including the eye). If you accidentally touch tip, clean with warm water and soap.
- Keep container tightly closed.
- Keep cool, but don't freeze.
- Wash hands immediately after using.

Continued next column

 ## OVERDOSE

SYMPTOMS:
None expected.
WHAT TO DO:
Not intended for internal use. If child accidentally swallows, call doctor or poison control center 1-800-222-1222 for help.

When to use:
As directed. Usually 1 drop every 2 hours up to maximum of 9 drops daily.

If you forget a dose:
Use as soon as you remember.

What drug does:
Destroys reproductive capacity of virus.

Time lapse before drug works:
Begins to work immediately. Usual course of treatment is 7 days.

Don't use with:
Other eye drops, boric acid or ointment without consulting doctor or pharmacist.

 ## POSSIBLE ADVERSE REACTIONS OR SIDE EFFECTS

SYMPTOMS	WHAT TO DO
Life-threatening None expected.	
Common Stinging or burning eyes.	Continue. Tell doctor at next visit.
Infrequent Blurred vision for a few minutes (with ointment).	No action necessary.
Rare Itchy, red eyes; swollen eyelid or eye; excess flow of tears; dimming or haziness of vision.	Discontinue. Call doctor right away.

WARNINGS & PRECAUTIONS

Don't use if:
You are allergic to trifluridine or idoxuridine.

Before you start, consult your doctor if:
- You have had any other eye problems.
- You use eye drops for glaucoma.

Over age 60:
No problems expected.

Pregnancy:
Risk factors vary for drugs in this group. See category list on page xviii and consult doctor.

Breast-feeding:
No problems expected, but safety not established. Consult doctor.

Infants & children:
Use only under close medical supervision.

Prolonged use:
Avoid unless directed by your eye doctor.

Skin & sunlight:
No problems expected.

Driving, piloting or hazardous work:
No problems expected.

Discontinuing:
Don't discontinue without consulting doctor.

Others:
- Don't use more often or longer than prescribed.
- Keep cool, but don't freeze.
- If problem doesn't improve within a week, notify your doctor.

POSSIBLE INTERACTION WITH OTHER DRUGS

GENERIC NAME OR DRUG CLASS	COMBINED EFFECT
Eye products containing boric acid	Increased risk of toxicity to eye.

POSSIBLE INTERACTION WITH OTHER SUBSTANCES

INTERACTS WITH	COMBINED EFFECT
Alcohol:	None expected.
Beverages:	None expected.
Cocaine:	None expected.
Foods:	None expected.
Marijuana:	None expected.
Tobacco:	None expected.

*See Glossary

ANTIVIRALS (Topical)

GENERIC AND BRAND NAMES

ACYCLOVIR (topical)   PENCICLOVIR
  Zovirax Ointment   (topical)
DOCOSANOL (topical)   Denavir
  Abreva

BASIC INFORMATION

Habit forming? No
Prescription needed? Yes
Available as generic? No
Drug class: Antiviral

 ## USES

- Treatment of symptoms of herpes infections of the skin, mucous membranes, lips, mouth and genitals.
- May be used for other skin disorders as prescribed by your doctor.

 ## DOSAGE & USAGE INFORMATION

How to take:
- Acyclovir ointment—Apply to skin and mucous membranes every 3 hours (6 times a day) for 7 days. Use rubber glove when applying. Apply 1/2-inch strip to each sore or blister. Wash before using.
- Penciclovir cream—Use only on lips and face. Avoid eye area. Use every 2 hours, while awake, for 4 days.
- Docosanol—Apply directly to the affected area at the first sign of a cold sore. It should be used five times daily until the cold sore or fever blister is completely healed.

When to use:
Use as soon as symptoms begin to appear (burning, pain or blisters).

If you forget a dose:
Apply as soon as you remember, then continue with regular schedule.

Continued next column

 ## OVERDOSE

SYMPTOMS:
None expected.
WHAT TO DO:
If person accidentally swallows topical form of drug, call doctor, poison control center 1-800-222-1222 or hospital emergency room for help.

What drug does:
- Inhibits reproduction of virus in cells without killing normal cells.
- Does not cure. Herpes breakout often recurs.

Time lapse before drug works:
2 hours.

Don't take with:
Any other topical medicine without consulting your doctor or pharmacist.

 ## POSSIBLE ADVERSE REACTIONS OR SIDE EFFECTS

SYMPTOMS	WHAT TO DO
Life-threatening: None expected.	
Common: May cause mild pain, burning, itching or stinging.	Continue. Call doctor when convenient.
Infrequent: None expected.	
Rare: Skin rash.	Continue. Call doctor when convenient.

WARNINGS & PRECAUTIONS

Don't take if:
You are allergic to topical acyclovir, docosanol or penciclovir.

Before you start, consult your doctor if:
You are allergic to any medication, food or other substance.

Over age 60:
Adverse reactions and side effects may be more frequent and severe than in younger persons.

Pregnancy:
Decide with your doctor whether drug benefits justify risk to unborn child. Risk category C (see page xviii).

Breast-feeding:
It is unknown if topical antivirals are absorbed and then pass into breast milk. Consult doctor.

Infants & children:
Use only under special medical supervision.

Prolonged use:
Don't use longer than prescribed time.

Skin & sunlight:
No problems expected.

Driving, piloting or hazardous work:
No problems expected.

Discontinuing:
May be unnecessary to finish medicine. Follow doctor's instructions.

Others:
- Women: Get pap smear every 6 months because those with herpes infections are possibly at increased risk to develop cancer of the cervix. Avoid sexual activity until all blisters or sores heal.
- Don't get topical medicine in eyes.
- Check with doctor if no improvement in 1 week.

POSSIBLE INTERACTION WITH OTHER DRUGS

GENERIC NAME OR DRUG CLASS	COMBINED EFFECT
None expected.	

POSSIBLE INTERACTION WITH OTHER SUBSTANCES

INTERACTS WITH	COMBINED EFFECT
Alcohol:	None expected.
Beverages:	None expected.
Cocaine:	None expected.
Foods:	None expected.
Marijuana:	None expected.
Tobacco:	None expected.

APPETITE SUPPRESSANTS

GENERIC AND BRAND NAMES

See full list of generic and brand names in the *Generic and Brand Name Directory*, page 876.

BASIC INFORMATION

Habit forming? Yes
Prescription needed? Yes
Available as generic? Yes
Drug class: Appetite suppressant

 ## USES

Suppresses appetite. Temporary treatment for obesity.

 ## DOSAGE & USAGE INFORMATION

How to take:
* Tablet or capsule—Swallow with liquid. You may chew or crush tablet.
* Extended-release tablet or capsule—Swallow each dose whole with liquid; do not crush.
* Elixir—Swallow with liquid.

When to take:
* Long-acting forms—10 to 14 hours before bedtime.
* Short-acting forms—1 hour before meals. Last dose no later than 4 to 6 hours before bedtime.

If you forget a dose:
* Long-acting form—Take as soon as you remember up to 2 hours late. If more than 2 hours, wait for next scheduled dose (don't double this dose).
* Short-acting form—Wait for next scheduled dose. Don't double this dose.

Continued next column

 ## OVERDOSE

SYMPTOMS:
Irritability, overactivity, trembling, insomnia, mood changes, fever, rapid heartbeat, confusion, disorientation, hallucinations, convulsions, coma.
WHAT TO DO:
* **Dial 911 (emergency) for medical help or call poison control center 1-800-222-1222 for instructions.**
* **See emergency information on last 3 pages of this book.**

What drug does:
Apparently stimulates brain's appetite control center.

Time lapse before drug works:
Begins in 1 hour. Short-acting form lasts 4 hours. Long-acting form lasts 14 hours.

Don't take with:
Any other medicine or any dietary supplement without consulting your doctor or pharmacist.

 ## POSSIBLE ADVERSE REACTIONS OR SIDE EFFECTS

SYMPTOMS	WHAT TO DO
Life-threatening:	
In case of overdose, see previous column.	
Common:	
Irritability, nervousness, insomnia, false sense of well-being.	Continue. Call doctor when convenient.
Infrequent:	
• Irregular or pounding heartbeat, urgent or difficult urination.	Discontinue. Call doctor right away.
• Blurred vision, unpleasant taste or dry mouth, constipation or diarrhea, nausea, vomiting, cramps, changes in sex drive, increased sweating, headache, nightmares, weakness.	Continue. Call doctor when convenient.
Rare:	
• Rash or hives, breathing difficulty.	Discontinue. Call doctor right away.
• Hair loss.	Continue. Call doctor when convenient.

 ## WARNINGS & PRECAUTIONS

Don't take if:
* You are allergic to benzphetamine, diethylpropion, mazindol, phendimetrazine or phentermine.
* You have glaucoma.
* You have taken MAO inhibitors within 2 weeks.
* You plan to become pregnant within medication period.
* You have a history of drug or alcohol abuse.
* You have irregular or rapid heartbeat.

Before you start, consult your doctor if:
- You have high blood pressure or heart disease.
- You have an overactive thyroid, nervous tension or anxiety.
- You have epilepsy.
- You will have surgery within 2 months, including dental surgery, requiring general or spinal anesthesia.
- You take any other nonprescription medicine.

Over age 60:
Adverse reactions and side effects may be more frequent and severe than in younger persons.

Pregnancy:
Risk factors vary for drugs in this group. See category list on page xviii and consult doctor.

Breast-feeding:
Safety not established. Consult doctor.

Infants & children:
Don't give to children younger than 12.

Prolonged use:
- Loses effectiveness. Avoid.
- Talk to your doctor about the need for follow-up medical examinations or laboratory studies.

Skin & sunlight:
No problems expected.

Driving, piloting or hazardous work:
Don't drive or pilot aircraft until you learn how medicine affects you. Don't work around dangerous machinery. Don't climb ladders or work in high places. Danger increases if you drink alcohol or take medicine affecting alertness and reflexes, such as antihistamines, tranquilizers, sedatives, pain medicine, narcotics and mind-altering drugs.

Discontinuing:
- Don't discontinue without consulting doctor. Dose may require gradual reduction if you have taken drug for a long time. Doses of other drugs may also require adjustment.
- Consult doctor if following symptoms occur after stopping the drug—depression, nausea and vomiting, stomach cramps, insomnia, nightmares, extreme tiredness or weakness.

Others:
- Don't increase dose without doctor's approval.
- Advise any doctor or dentist whom you consult that you take this medicine.

 POSSIBLE INTERACTION WITH OTHER DRUGS

GENERIC NAME OR DRUG CLASS	COMBINED EFFECT
Antidiabetic agents,* oral or insulin	May require dosage adjustment of anti-diabetic agent.
Antihypertensives*	Decreased anti-hypertensive effect.
Appetite suppressants, other*	Dangerous overstimulation.
Caffeine	Increased stimulant effect.
Central nervous system (CNS) depressants*	Increased depressive effects of both drugs.
Central nervous system (CNS) stimulants*	Increased stimulant effects of both drugs.
Guanethidine	Decreased guanethidine effect.
Methyldopa	Decreased methyldopa effect.
Monoamine oxidase (MAO) inhibitors*	Dangerous blood pressure rise.
Phenothiazines*	Decreased appetite suppressant effect.
Rauwolfia alkaloids*	Decreased effect of rauwolfia alkaloids.

 POSSIBLE INTERACTION WITH OTHER SUBSTANCES

INTERACTS WITH	COMBINED EFFECT
Alcohol:	Increased sedation.
Beverages: Caffeine drinks.	Excessive stimulation.
Cocaine:	Convulsions or excessive nervousness.
Foods:	None expected.
Marijuana:	Frequent use— Irregular heartbeat.
Tobacco:	None expected.

ARIPIPRAZOLE

BRAND NAMES

Abilify
Abilify Oral Solution
Abilify DiscMelt

BASIC INFORMATION

Habit forming? Not expected to be
Prescription needed? Yes
Available as generic? No
Drug class: Antipsychotic

 ## USES

- Treats nervous, mental and emotional conditions. Helps in managing the signs and symptoms of schizophrenia (treats positive symptoms such as hearing voices and negative symptoms such as social withdrawal).
- Treatment for bipolar disorder.
- Treatment for major depressive disorder (MDD).
- May be used for treatment of other disorders as determined by your doctor.

 ## DOSAGE & USAGE INFORMATION

How to take:
- Tablet or capsule—Swallow with liquid. May be taken with or without food.
- Oral disintegrating tablet—Let tablet dissolve in mouth. Do not chew or swallow.
- Oral solution—Use the oral dosing cup provided with the bottle. Store open bottle in a refrigerator; can be used for up to 6 months after opening.

When to take:
Once a day at the same time each day. Always follow the advice of your doctor.

If you forget a dose:
Take as soon as you remember. If it is almost time for the next dose, wait for the next scheduled dose (don't double this dose).

Continued next column

 ## OVERDOSE

SYMPTOMS:
Unknown, possibly drowsiness and vomiting.
WHAT TO DO:
Overdose unlikely to threaten life. If person uses much larger amount than prescribed or if accidentally swallowed, call doctor or poison center control 1-800-222-1222 for help.

What drug does:
The exact mechanism is unknown. It appears to block certain nerve impulses between nerve cells.

Time lapse before drug works:
1-4 weeks. A further increase in the dosage amount may be necessary to relieve symptoms for some patients. Do not increase dosage without your doctor's approval.

Don't take with:
Any other medicine or any dietary supplement without consulting your doctor or pharmacist.

 ## POSSIBLE ADVERSE REACTIONS OR SIDE EFFECTS

SYMPTOMS	WHAT TO DO
Life-threatening: High fever, rapid pulse, profuse sweating, muscle rigidity, confusion and irritability, seizures (neuroleptic malignant syndrome – rare).	Discontinue. Seek emergency treatment.
Common: Anxiety, insomnia, headache, stomach upset, vomiting, constipation, light-headedness, restlessness (akathisia), weight loss.	Continue. Call doctor when convenient.
Infrequent: Runny nose, cough, skin rash, dry mouth, weight gain, drowsiness.	Continue. Call doctor when convenient.
Rare: • Tardive dyskinesia (involuntary movements, especially of the face, lips, jaw and tongue; sometimes involves twitching of hands or feet), high blood sugar (thirstiness, frequent urination, increased hunger, weakness).	Discontinue. Call doctor right away.
• Other symptoms causing concern, not listed above.	Continue. Call doctor when convenient.

WARNINGS & PRECAUTIONS

Don't take if:
You are allergic to aripiprazole.

Before you start, consult your doctor if:
* You have or have had liver or kidney disease, heart disease or stroke.
* You have irregular heartbeat, problems with blood pressure or a blood disorder.
* You have depression, or a history of alcohol or drug abuse.
* You have a family history of, are at risk for, or have diabetes.
* You have difficulty in swallowing.
* You are allergic to any other medications.
* You have a history of seizures.

Over age 60:
* Adverse reactions and side effects may be more likely than in younger persons.
* Use of antipsychotic drugs in elderly patients with dementia-related psychosis may increase risk of death. Consult doctor.

Pregnancy:
Decide with your doctor if drug benefits justify any possible risk to unborn child. Risk category C (see page xviii).

Breast-feeding:
It is unknown if drug passes into milk. Avoid nursing until you finish medicine.

Infants & children:
* Used in the treatment of schizophrenia in adolescents 13 to 17 years of age.
* Used for treatment of manic and mixed episodes associated with bipolar disorder in ages 10-17.

Prolonged use:
Consult with your doctor on a regular basis while taking this drug to check your progress or to discuss any increase or changes in side effects, blood sugar levels, and the need for continued treatment.

Skin & sunlight:
No problems expected.

Driving, piloting or hazardous work:
Don't drive or pilot aircraft until you learn how medicine affects you. Don't work around dangerous machinery. Don't climb ladders or work in high places. Danger increases if you drink alcohol or take medicine affecting alertness and reflexes.

Discontinuing:
Don't discontinue this drug without consulting doctor even if you feel well. Dosage may require a gradual reduction before stopping.

Others:
* Get up slowly from a sitting or lying position to avoid any dizziness, faintness or lightheadedness.
* The drug may reduce the body's ability to reduce body temperature. Avoid getting overheated or dehydrated.
* Advise any doctor or dentist whom you consult that you take this medicine.
* Take medicine as directed. Do not increase or reduce dosage without doctor's approval.
* Consult doctor if weight loss is a problem.

POSSIBLE INTERACTION WITH OTHER DRUGS

GENERIC NAME OR DRUG CLASS	COMBINED EFFECT
Enzyme inducers*	Decreased effect of aripiprazole.
Enzyme inhibitors*	Increased effect of aripiprazole.

POSSIBLE INTERACTION WITH OTHER SUBSTANCES

INTERACTS WITH	COMBINED EFFECT
Alcohol:	Increased sedative affect. Avoid.
Beverages:	None expected.
Cocaine:	Effect not known. Best to avoid.
Foods:	None expected.
Marijuana:	Effect not known. Best to avoid.
Tobacco:	None expected.

*See Glossary

ASPIRIN

BRAND NAMES

See full list of brand names in the *Generic and Brand Name Directory*, page 876.

BASIC INFORMATION

Habit forming? No
Prescription needed? No
Available as generic? Yes
Drug class: Analgesic, anti-inflammatory (nonsteroidal)

 ## USES

- Reduces pain, fever, inflammation.
- Relieves swelling, stiffness, joint pain of arthritis or rheumatism.
- Antiplatelet effect to reduce chances of heart attack and/or stroke.

 ## DOSAGE & USAGE INFORMATION

How to take:
- Tablet or capsule—Swallow with liquid or food to lessen stomach irritation.
- Extended-release tablet or capsule— Swallow each dose whole.
- Effervescent tablet—Dissolve in water.
- Chewing gum tablet—Chew completely. Don't swallow whole.
- Dispersible tablet—Dissolve in the mouth before swallowing.
- Chewable tablet—Chew before swallowing or dissolve in liquid before swallowing.

Continued next column

 ## OVERDOSE

SYMPTOMS:
- **Mild overdose–Confusion, severe diarrhea, stomach pain, increased thirst, vision problems, ringing or buzzing in ears, dizziness, lightheadedness, severe headache.**
- **Severe overdose–Bloody urine; hallucinations; severe nervousness, excitement or confusion; shortness of breath; trouble breathing; convulsions.**
- **In some children–The only symptoms may be behavior changes, severe drowsiness or tiredness, fast or deep breathing.**

WHAT TO DO:
- **Dial 911 (emergency) for medical help or call poison control center 1-800-222-1222 for instructions.**
- **See emergency information on last 3 pages of this book.**

- Suppository—Remove wrapper and moisten suppository with water. Gently insert into rectum, large end first.

When to take:
Pain, fever, inflammation—As needed, no more often than every 4 hours.

If you forget a dose:
- Pain, fever—Take as soon as you remember. Wait 4 hours for next dose.
- Arthritis—Take as soon as you remember up to 2 hours late. Return to regular schedule.

What drug does:
- Affects hypothalamus, the part of the brain which regulates temperature by dilating small blood vessels in skin.
- Prevents clumping of platelets (small blood cells) so blood vessels remain open.
- Decreases prostaglandin effect.
- Suppresses body's pain messages.

Time lapse before drug works:
30 minutes for pain, fever, arthritis.

Don't take with:
- Tetracyclines. Space doses 1 hour apart.
- Any other medicine or any dietary supplement without consulting your doctor or pharmacist.

 ## POSSIBLE ADVERSE REACTIONS OR SIDE EFFECTS

SYMPTOMS	WHAT TO DO
Life-threatening:	
Black or bloody vomit; blood in urine; difficulty breathing; hives, rash, intense itching, faintness soon after a dose (anaphylaxis).	Seek emergency treatment immediately.
Common:	
Heartburn, indigestion, mild nausea or vomiting.	Continue. Call doctor when convenient.
Infrequent:	
Trouble sleeping; rectal irritation (with suppository).	Continue. Call doctor when convenient.
Rare:	
Severe headache, convulsions, extreme drowsiness, flushing or other change in skin color, any loss of hearing, severe vomiting, swelling of face, vision problems, bloody or black stools, ringing in ears, severe stomach cramps or pain (all symptoms more likely with repeated doses for long periods since aspirin can build up in the body).	Discontinue. Call doctor right away or seek emergency treatment.

WARNINGS & PRECAUTIONS

Don't take if:
- You need to restrict sodium in your diet. Buffered effervescent tablets and sodium salicylate are high in sodium.
- You are sensitive to aspirin or aspirin has a strong vinegar-like odor, which means it has decomposed.
- You have a peptic ulcer of stomach or duodenum or a bleeding disorder.

Before you start, consult your doctor if:
- You have had stomach or duodenal ulcers.
- You have had gout.
- You have asthma or nasal polyps.
- You have kidney or liver disease.

Over age 60:
More likely to cause hidden bleeding in stomach or intestines. Watch for dark stools.

Pregnancy:
Risk category C; D in third trimester (see page xviii). Consult doctor.

Breast-feeding:
Drug passes into milk. Avoid drug or discontinue nursing until you finish medicine. Consult doctor for advice on maintaining milk supply.

Infants & children:
- Overdose frequent and severe. Keep bottles out of children's reach.
- Do not give to persons under age 18 who have fever and discomfort of viral illness, especially chicken pox and influenza. Probably increases risk of Reye's syndrome.

Prolonged use:
- Talk to your doctor about the need for follow-up medical examinations or laboratory studies to check liver function, complete blood counts (white blood cell count, platelet count, red blood cell count, hemoglobin, hematocrit).
- Kidney damage may result. Periodic kidney function tests recommended.

Skin & sunlight:
No special problems expected.

Driving, piloting or hazardous work:
No restrictions unless you feel drowsy.

Discontinuing:
For chronic illness—Don't discontinue without doctor's advice until you complete prescribed dose, even though symptoms diminish or disappear.

Others:
- Aspirin can complicate surgery, pregnancy, labor and delivery, and illness.
- For arthritis—Don't change dose without consulting doctor.
- Urine tests for blood sugar may be inaccurate.
- Don't take if pills have vinegar-like odor.

POSSIBLE INTERACTION WITH OTHER DRUGS

GENERIC NAME OR DRUG CLASS	COMBINED EFFECT
Acebutolol	Decreased anti-hypertensive effect of acebutolol.
Adrenocorticoids, systemic	Increased adreno-corticoid effect.
Alendronate	Increased risk of stomach irritation.
Allopurinol	Decreased allopurinol effect.
Angiotensin-converting enzyme (ACE) inhibitors*	Decreased ACE inhibitor effect.
Antacids*	Decreased aspirin effect.
Anticoagulants*	Increased anti-coagulant effect. Abnormal bleeding.
Antidiabetic agents, oral*	Low blood sugar.
Anti-inflammatory drugs nonsteroidal (NSAIDs)*	Risk of stomach bleeding and ulcers.
Bumetanide	Possible aspirin toxicity.
Carteolol	Decreased anti-hypertensive effect of carteolol.

Continued on page 906

 ## POSSIBLE INTERACTION WITH OTHER SUBSTANCES

INTERACTS WITH	COMBINED EFFECT
Alcohol:	Possible stomach irritation and bleeding. Avoid.
Beverages:	None expected.
Cocaine:	None expected.
Foods:	None expected.
Marijuana:	Possible increased pain relief, but marijuana may slow body's recovery. Avoid.
Tobacco:	None expected.

*See Glossary

ATOMOXETINE

BRAND NAMES

Strattera

BASIC INFORMATION

Habit forming? Not expected
Prescription needed? Yes
Available as generic? No
Drug class: Selective norepinephrine
reuptake inhibitor

 ## USES

Treatment of symptoms (inattention,
hyperactivity and impulsiveness) of attention
deficit hyperactivity disorder (ADHD) in children,
adolescents and adults. The drug is used as part
of a total treatment program for ADHD that may
include other therapy measures (psychological,
educational and social) for patients.

 ## DOSAGE & USAGE INFORMATION

How to take:
Capsule—Swallow whole with liquid. It may be
taken with or without food. Do not open capsule.

When to take:
• Once-a-day dose at the same time each day
  usually in the morning.
• Twice-a-day dose at the same times each day
  usually in the morning and then late afternoon
  or early evening.

If you forget a dose:
Take as soon as you remember. If it is almost
time for your next dose, skip the missed dose
and go back to your regular dosing schedule. Do
not double doses.

Continued next column

 ## OVERDOSE

SYMPTOMS:
Sleepiness, agitation, being hyperactive,
abnormal behavior, stomach symptoms,
blurred vision, fast heartbeat or dry mouth.
WHAT TO DO:
Overdose unlikely to threaten life. If person
uses much larger amount than prescribed or
if accidentally swallowed, call doctor or
poison center control 1-800-222-1222 for
help.

What drug does:
The exact mechanism by which the drug works
is unknown. It appears to block a chemical
(neurotransmitter) in the brain having to do with
attention and activity.

Time lapse before drug works:
1 to 2 hours, but full benefits may take up to 4
weeks with possible dosage increases. Don't
increase dosage without doctor's approval.

Don't take with:
Any other medicine or any dietary supplement
without consulting your doctor or pharmacist.

 ## POSSIBLE ADVERSE REACTIONS OR SIDE EFFECTS

SYMPTOMS	WHAT TO DO
Life-threatening: Rare allergic reaction (hives, itching, rash, trouble breathing, tightness in chest, swelling of lips or tongue or face); heart problems (chest pain, trouble breathing, fainting).	Seek emergency treatment immediately.
Common: In children—appetite loss, mood swings, nausea, vomiting, upset stomach, dizziness, tiredness, weight loss, runny nose, eyes tearing.	Continue. Call doctor when convenient.
Infrequent: In adults—insomnia, dry mouth, stomach pain, constipation, weight loss, loss of libido, impotence, ejaculatory difficulty, problems in urinating, menstrual pain; in adults and children—may feel lightheaded when getting up after sitting or lying down.	Continue. Call doctor when convenient.
Rare: Mental problems (hallucinations, manic behavior, becoming suspicious); liver problems (dark urine, itching, yellow skin or eyes, tender abdomen, flu-like symptoms); suicidal thoughts or behaviors.	Discontinue. Call doctor right away.

WARNINGS & PRECAUTIONS

Don't take if:
You are allergic to atomoxetine.

Before you start, consult your doctor if:
- You have liver or kidney disease.
- You have narrow angle glaucoma.
- You take MAO inhibitors* or have taken them in the last 14 days.
- You have heart problems, high or low blood pressure, or blood vessel disorder.
- You have history of mental disorders.
- You have history of alcohol or drug abuse.

Over age 60:
Drug has not been studied in this age group. Consult doctor.

Pregnancy:
Decide with your doctor if drug benefits justify any possible risk to unborn child. Risk category C (see page xviii).

Breast-feeding:
It is unknown if drug passes into breast milk. Avoid drug or discontinue nursing until you finish medicine. Consult doctor for advice on maintaining milk supply.

Infants & children:
- Use only under medical supervision for children 6 or older.
- Regular doctor visits are important to monitor drug's effectiveness and side effects.
- Read the warnings under Others.

Prolonged use:
It is unknown about the long term effects of taking this drug. Talk to your doctor about the need for follow-up medical examinations to check weight and height changes in children and adolescents, and to check the effectiveness of the drug in treating ADHD.

Skin & sunlight:
No problems expected.

Driving, piloting or hazardous work:
Don't drive or pilot aircraft until you learn how medicine affects you. Don't work around dangerous machinery. Don't climb ladders or work in high places. Danger increases if you drink alcohol or take other medicines affecting alertness and reflexes such as antihistamines, tranquilizers, sedatives, pain medicine, narcotics and mind-altering drugs.

Discontinuing:
No problems expected, but talk to your doctor before discontinuing the drug.

Others:
- Consult doctor if your child is not gaining weight or growing at an expected or satisfactory level.

- Will commonly cause a slight increase in blood pressure. Your doctor will monitor your blood pressure on a regular basis.
- In children and teenagers, the drug may increase suicidal thoughts or behaviors. Watch for any new or increased suicidal thoughts, mood or behavioral changes (e.g., becoming irritable or anxious). Call doctor right away if any symptoms occur.
- Rarely, the drug can cause liver damage. Call doctor if you have dark urine, itching, yellowing of skin or eyes, abdominal tenderness or flu-like symptoms.
- Rarely, use of this drug in children, teenagers and adults can lead to serious heart problems, including sudden unexplained death. Adults may have stroke or heart attack. Patients with with heart defects or serious heart problems are more at risk. Consult doctor.
- Consult doctor if new mental symptoms occur (e.g., abnormal thoughts or behaviors).
- Follow your doctor's recommendation for any additional measures for treating ADHD.
- Advise any doctor or dentist whom you consult about the use of this medicine.

POSSIBLE INTERACTION WITH OTHER DRUGS

GENERIC NAME OR DRUG CLASS	COMBINED EFFECT
Beta agonists*	Increased risk of heart problems.
Enzyme inhibitors*	May increase effect of atomoxetine.
Monoamine oxidase (MAO) inhibitors*	Serious reactions (potentially fatal). Take at least 2 weeks apart.
Vasoconstrictors* (vasopressors)	May increase heart rate and/or blood pressure.

POSSIBLE INTERACTION WITH OTHER SUBSTANCES

INTERACTS WITH	COMBINED EFFECT
Alcohol:	None expected. Best to avoid.
Beverages:	None expected.
Cocaine:	Unknown. Avoid.
Foods:	None expected.
Marijuana:	Unknown. Avoid.
Tobacco:	None expected. Best to avoid.

*See Glossary

ATOVAQUONE

BRAND NAMES

Malarone   Mepron

BASIC INFORMATION

Habit forming? No
Prescription needed? Yes
Available as generic? No
Drug class: Antiprotozoal, antimalarial.

 ## USES

- Treats mild to moderate pneumocystis carinii pneumonia.
- May be effective for other parasitic infections such as toxoplasmosis and malaria.

 ## DOSAGE & USAGE INFORMATION

How to take:
- Tablet—Swallow with liquid. Take with a meal. If you cannot swallow whole, crumble tablet and take with liquid or food.
- Suspension—Follow instructions provided with product.

When to take:
At the same times each day. Take with meals that are high in fat (eggs, cheese, butter, milk, meat, pizza, nuts) to increase absorption.

If you forget a dose:
Take as soon as you remember up to 2 hours late. If more than 2 hours, wait for next scheduled dose (don't double this dose).

What drug does:
Stops harmful growth of susceptible organisms.

Time lapse before drug works:
3 weeks.

Don't take with:
Any other medicine or any dietary supplement without consulting your doctor or pharmacist.

 ## OVERDOSE

SYMPTOMS:
None expected.
WHAT TO DO:
Overdose unlikely to threaten life. If person uses much larger amount than prescribed or if accidentally swallowed, call doctor or poison control center 1-800-222-1222 for help.

 ## POSSIBLE ADVERSE REACTIONS OR SIDE EFFECTS

SYMPTOMS	WHAT TO DO
Life-threatening: None expected.	
Common:	
• Fever, skin rash.	Discontinue. Call doctor right away.
• Nausea or vomiting, diarrhea, headache, cough, trouble sleeping.	Continue. Call doctor when convenient.
Infrequent: None expected.	
Rare: None expected.	

WARNINGS & PRECAUTIONS

Don't take if:
You are allergic to atovaquone.

Before you start, consult your doctor if:
You have any gastrointestinal disorder.

Over age 60:
No problems expected.

Pregnancy:
Discuss with your doctor whether drug benefits justify risk to unborn child. Risk category C (see page xviii).

Breast-feeding:
Not known if drug passes into breast milk. Avoid drug or discontinue nursing until you finish medicine. Consult doctor for advice on maintaining milk supply.

Infants & children:
Give only under close medical supervision.

Prolonged use:
Not intended for long-term use.

Skin & sunlight:
No problems expected.

Driving, piloting or hazardous work:
No problems expected.

Discontinuing:
No problems expected.

Others:
* Advise any doctor or dentist whom you consult that you take this medicine.
* May affect the results in some medical tests.
* Talk to your doctor about the need for follow-up medical examinations or laboratory studies to check blood counts and liver function.

POSSIBLE INTERACTION WITH OTHER DRUGS

GENERIC NAME OR DRUG CLASS	COMBINED EFFECT
None significant.	

POSSIBLE INTERACTION WITH OTHER SUBSTANCES

INTERACTS WITH	COMBINED EFFECT
Alcohol:	None expected.
Beverages:	None expected.
Cocaine:	None expected.
Foods:	None expected.
Marijuana:	None expected.
Tobacco:	None expected.

ATROPINE, HYOSCYAMINE, METHENAMINE, METHYLENE BLUE, PHENYLSALICYLATE & BENZOIC ACID

BRAND NAMES

Atrosept	Urinary
Dolsed	Antiseptic No. 2
Hexalol	Urised
Prosed/DS	Uriseptic
Trac Tabs 2X	Uritab
UAA	Uritin
Uridon Modified	Uro-Ves
Urimed	U-Tract

BASIC INFORMATION

Habit forming? No
Prescription needed? Yes
Available as generic? No
Drug class: Analgesic (urinary), anti-spasmodic, anti-infective (urinary)

 ## USES

A combination medicine to control infection, spasms and pain caused by urinary tract infections.

 ## DOSAGE & USAGE INFORMATION

How to take:
Tablet—Swallow with liquid or food to lessen stomach irritation.

When to take:
30 minutes before meals (unless directed otherwise by doctor).

If you forget a dose:
Take as soon as you remember up to 2 hours late. If more than 2 hours, wait for next scheduled dose (don't double this dose).

Continued next column

 ## OVERDOSE

SYMPTOMS:
Dilated pupils, rapid pulse and breathing, dizziness, fever, hallucinations, confusion, slurred speech, agitation, flushed face, convulsions, coma.
WHAT TO DO:
• Dial 911 (emergency) for medical help or call poison control center 1-800-222-1222 for instructions.
• See emergency information on last 3 pages of this book.

If you forget a dose:
Take as soon as you remember up to 2 hours late. If more than 2 hours, wait for next scheduled dose (don't double this dose).

What drug does:
Makes urine acid. Blocks nerve impulses at para-sympathetic nerve endings, preventing muscle contractions and gland secretions of organs involved. Methenamine destroys some germs.

Time lapse before drug works:
15 to 30 minutes.

Don't take with:
• Antacids* or antidiarrheals* at the same time.
• Any other medicine or any dietary supplement without consulting your doctor or pharmacist.

 ## POSSIBLE ADVERSE REACTIONS OR SIDE EFFECTS

SYMPTOMS	WHAT TO DO
Life-threatening:	
Heartbeat irregularity, shortness of breath or difficulty breathing.	Seek emergency treatment immediately.
Common:	
Dry mouth, throat, ears, nose.	Continue. Call doctor when convenient.
Infrequent:	
• Flushed, red face; drowsiness; difficult urination; nausea and vomiting; abdominal pain; ringing or buzzing in ears; severe drowsiness; back pain; lightheadedness.	Discontinue. Call doctor right away.
• Headache, nasal congestion, altered taste.	Continue. Call doctor when convenient.
Rare:	
Blurred vision; pain in eyes; skin rash, hives.	Discontinue. Seek emergency treatment.

 ## WARNINGS & PRECAUTIONS

Don't take if:
• You are allergic to any of the ingredients or aspirin.
• There is brain damage in a child.
• You have glaucoma.

ATROPINE, HYOSCYAMINE, METHENAMINE, METHYLENE BLUE, PHENYLSALICYLATE & BENZOIC ACID

Before you start, consult your doctor if:
- You are on any special diet such as low-sodium.
- You have had a hiatal hernia, bronchitis, asthma, liver disease, stomach or duodenal ulcers.
- You have asthma, nasal polyps, bleeding disorder, glaucoma or enlarged prostate.
- You will have any surgery within 2 months.
- You have heart disease.

Over age 60:
- Adverse reactions and side effects may be more frequent and severe than in younger persons.
- More likely to cause hidden bleeding in stomach or intestines. Watch for dark stools.

Pregnancy:
Risk factors vary for drugs in this group. See category list on page xviii and consult doctor.

Breast-feeding:
Drug passes into milk. Avoid or discontinue nursing until you finish medicine.

Infants & children:
Side effects more likely. Not recommended in children under 12.

Prolonged use:
May lead to constipation or kidney damage. Request lab studies to monitor effects of prolonged use.

Skin & sunlight:
No problems expected.

Driving, piloting or hazardous work:
May disqualify for piloting aircraft during time you take medicine.

Discontinuing:
May be unnecessary to finish medicine. Follow your symptoms and doctor's advice.

Others:
- Salicylates can complicate surgery, pregnancy, labor and delivery, and illness.
- Urine tests for blood sugar may be inaccurate.
- Drink cranberry juice or eat prunes or plums to help make urine more acid.

POSSIBLE INTERACTION WITH OTHER DRUGS

GENERIC NAME OR DRUG CLASS	COMBINED EFFECT
Allopurinol	Decreased allopurinol effect.
Amantadine	Increased atropine and belladonna effect.
Antacids*	Decreased salicylate and methenamine effect.
Anticoagulants*	Increased anti-coagulant effect. Abnormal bleeding.
Anticholinergics, other*	Increased atropine and belladonna effect.
Antidepressants, other*	Increased sedation.
Antidiabetics, oral*	Low blood sugar.
Antifungals, azoles	Reduced azole effect.
Antihistamines*	Increased atropine and hyoscyamine effect.
Anti-inflammatory drugs, nonsteroidal (NSAIDs)*	Risk of stomach bleeding and ulcers.
Aspirin	Likely salicylate toxicity.
Beta-adrenergic blocking agents*	Decreased anti-hypertensive effect.
Carbonic anhydrase inhibitors*	Decreased methenamine effect.
Cortisone drugs*	Increased internal eye pressure, increased cortisone effect. Risk of ulcers and stomach bleeding.

Continued on page 906

POSSIBLE INTERACTION WITH OTHER SUBSTANCES

INTERACTS WITH	COMBINED EFFECT
Alcohol:	Excessive sedation. Possible stomach irritation and bleeding. Avoid.
Beverages:	None expected.
Cocaine:	Excessively rapid heartbeat. Avoid.
Foods:	None expected.
Marijuana:	Drowsiness and dry mouth. May slow body's recovery.
Tobacco:	Dry mouth.

*See Glossary

ATTAPULGITE

BRAND NAMES

Diar-Aid
Diasorb
Fowlers Diarrhea
  Tablets
Kaopectate
Kaopectate Advanced
  Formula

Kaopectate
  Maximum Strength
Rheaban
St. Joseph
  Antidiarrheal

BASIC INFORMATION

Habit forming? No
Prescription needed? No
Available as generic? Yes
Drug class: Antidiarrheal

 USES

Treats diarrhea. Used in conjunction with fluids, appropriate diet and rest. Treats symptoms only. Does not cure any disorder that causes diarrhea.

 DOSAGE & USAGE INFORMATION

How to take:
* Tablet—Swallow with liquid. If you can't swallow whole, crumble tablet and take with liquid or food. Instructions to take on empty stomach mean 1 hour before or 2 hours after eating.
* Chewable tablet—Chew well before swallowing.
* Oral suspension—Follow label instructions.

When to take:
2 hours before or 3 hours after taking any other oral medications. Outside of this restriction, take a dose after each loose bowel movement until diarrhea is controlled.

If you forget a dose:
Take as soon as you remember, then resume regular schedule.

Continued next column

 OVERDOSE

SYMPTOMS:
None expected.
WHAT TO DO:
Overdose unlikely to threaten life. If person uses much larger amount than prescribed or if accidentally swallowed, call doctor or poison control center 1-800-222-1222 for help.

What drug does:
Absorbs bacteria and toxins and reduces water loss. Attapulgite does not get absorbed into the body.

Time lapse before drug works:
5 to 8 hours.

Don't take with:
Any other medicine or any dietary supplement without consulting your doctor or pharmacist.

 POSSIBLE ADVERSE REACTIONS OR SIDE EFFECTS

SYMPTOMS	WHAT TO DO
Life-threatening: None expected.	
Common: None expected.	
Infrequent: Constipation (usually mild and of short duration).	Continue. Call doctor when convenient.
Rare: None expected.	

WARNINGS & PRECAUTIONS

Don't take if:
- You are allergic to attapulgite.
- You or your doctor suspects intestinal obstruction.

Before you start, consult your doctor if:
You are dehydrated (signs are a dry mouth, loose skin, sunken eyes and parched lips).

Over age 60:
- Dehydration is more likely in this age group.
- Side effects of constipation are more likely.

Pregnancy:
Risk category not designated. See list on page xviii and consult doctor.

Breast-feeding:
No problems expected, but consult doctor.

Infants & children:
Use only under close medical supervision for children up to 3 years of age. This age group is quite susceptible to fluid and electrolyte loss.

Prolonged use:
Not intended for prolonged use.

Skin & sunlight:
No special problems expected.

Driving, piloting or hazardous work:
No special problems expected.

Discontinuing:
May be unnecessary to finish medicine. Follow doctor's instructions.

Others:
No special problems expected.

POSSIBLE INTERACTION WITH OTHER DRUGS

GENERIC NAME OR DRUG CLASS	COMBINED EFFECT
Digitalis	May decrease effectiveness of digitalis.
Lincomycins*	May decrease effectiveness of lincomycins.
Any other medicine taken by mouth	When taken at the same time, neither drug may be as effective. Take other medicines 2 hours before or 3 hours after attapulgite.

POSSIBLE INTERACTION WITH OTHER SUBSTANCES

INTERACTS WITH	COMBINED EFFECT
Alcohol:	None expected.
Beverages:	None expected.
Cocaine:	None expected.
Foods: Prunes, prune juice and other fruits or foods that may cause diarrhea.	Decreased effect of attapulgite.
Marijuana:	None expected.
Tobacco:	None expected.

AZATHIOPRINE

BRAND NAMES

Azasan   Imuran

BASIC INFORMATION

Habit forming? No
Prescription needed? Yes
Available as generic? Yes
Drug class: Immunosuppressant,
    antirheumatic

USES

- Protects against rejection of transplanted organs (e.g., kidney, heart).
- Treats severe active rheumatoid arthritis and other immunologic diseases if simpler treatment plans have been ineffective.

DOSAGE & USAGE INFORMATION

How to take:
Tablet—Swallow with liquid. If you can't swallow whole, crumble tablet and take with liquid or food. Instructions to take on empty stomach mean 1 hour before or 2 hours after eating.

When to take:
Follow your doctor's instructions. Usually once a day.

If you forget a dose:
Take as soon as you remember up to 2 hours late. If more than 2 hours, wait for next scheduled dose (don't double this dose).

What drug does:
Unknown; probably inhibits synthesis of DNA and RNA.

Time lapse before drug works:
6 to 8 weeks.

Don't take with:
Any other medicines (including over-the-counter drugs such as cough and cold medicines, laxatives, antacids, diet pills, caffeine, nose drops or vitamins) without consulting your doctor.

OVERDOSE

SYMPTOMS:
None expected.
WHAT TO DO:
Overdose unlikely to threaten life. If person uses much larger amount than prescribed or if accidentally swallowed, call doctor or poison control center 1-800-222-1222 for help.

POSSIBLE ADVERSE REACTIONS OR SIDE EFFECTS

SYMPTOMS	WHAT TO DO
Life-threatening: Rapid heart rate, sudden fever, muscle or joint pain, cough, shortness of breath.	Seek emergency treatment immediately.
Common: • Infection or low blood count causing fever and chills, back pain, cough, painful urination; anemia (tiredness or weakness); nausea; vomiting.	Discontinue. Call doctor right away.
• Appetite loss.	Continue. Call doctor when convenient.
Infrequent: Jaundice (yellow eyes, skin), skin rash.	Discontinue. Call doctor right away.
Rare: Low platelet count causing bleeding or bruising, tarry or black stools, bloody urine, red spots under skin; severe abdominal pain; mouth sores.	Discontinue. Call doctor right away.

WARNINGS & PRECAUTIONS

Don't take if:
- You are allergic to azathioprine.
- You have chicken pox.
- You have shingles (herpes zoster).

Before you start, consult your doctor if:
- You have gout.
- You have liver or kidney disease.
- You have an infection.

Over age 60:
Adverse reactions and side effects may be more frequent and severe than in younger persons. You may need smaller doses for shorter periods of time.

Pregnancy:
Risk to unborn child outweighs drug benefits. Don't use. Risk category D (see page xviii).

Breast-feeding:
Drug passes into milk. Avoid drug or discontinue nursing until you finish medicine. Consult doctor for advice on maintaining milk supply.

Infants & children:
No special problems expected.

Prolonged use:
- May increase likelihood of problems upon discontinuing.
- Talk to your doctor about the need for follow-up medical examinations or laboratory studies to check thyroid function, liver function, electrolytes (sodium, potassium, chloride), blood pressure and complete blood counts (white blood count, platelet count, red blood cell count, hemoglobin, hematocrit) every week during first two months, then once a month.

Skin & sunlight:
No special problems expected.

Driving, piloting or hazardous work:
Avoid if you feel confused, drowsy or dizzy.

Discontinuing:
May still experience symptoms of bone marrow depression, such as: blood in stools, fever or chills, blood spots under the skin, back pain, hoarseness, bloody urine. If any of these occur, call your doctor right away.

Others:
- Advise any doctor or dentist whom you consult that you take this medicine.
- May affect results in some medical tests.

POSSIBLE INTERACTION WITH OTHER DRUGS

GENERIC NAME OR DRUG CLASS	COMBINED EFFECT
Allopurinol	Greatly increased azathioprine activity.
Antivirals, HIV/AIDS*	Increased risk of pancreatitis.
Clozapine	Toxic effect on bone marrow.
Immunosuppressants, other*	Higher risk of developing infection or malignancies.
Levamisole	Increased risk of bone marrow depression.
Tiopronin	Increased risk of toxicity to bone marrow.
Vaccines	May decrease effectiveness or cause disease itself.

POSSIBLE INTERACTION WITH OTHER SUBSTANCES

INTERACTS WITH	COMBINED EFFECT
Alcohol:	No special problems expected.
Beverages:	No special problems expected.
Cocaine:	Increased likelihood of adverse reactions. Avoid.
Foods:	No special problems expected.
Marijuana:	Increased likelihood of adverse reactions. Avoid.
Tobacco:	No special problems expected.

*See Glossary

AZELAIC ACID

BRAND NAMES

Azelex   Finevin
Finacea

BASIC INFORMATION

Habit forming? No
Prescription needed? Yes
Available as generic? No
Drug class: Antiacne agent,
  hypopigmentation agent

 USES

- Topical treatment for mild to moderate acne vulgaris.
- May be used for treatment of melasma (chloasma), a skin condition in which brownish patches of pigmentation appear on the face.

 DOSAGE & USAGE INFORMATION

How to use:
Cream—Wash the affected skin area and then apply the prescribed amount of cream and rub it into the skin. Rub it in thoroughly, but gently, to avoid irritation. Wash hands after applying.

When to use:
Usually twice a day (morning and evening).

If you forget a dose:
Use as soon as you remember.

What drug does:
The drug helps prevents the development of new acne lesions (whiteheads), but the exact mechanism is unknown. It appears to have some antibacterial and anti-inflammatory effect, and also helps in skin renewal.

Time lapse before drug works:
Results should be visible in about 4 weeks, but full benefits may take months.

Don't use with:
Other topical medications without consulting your doctor or pharmacist.

 OVERDOSE

SYMPTOMS:
None expected.
WHAT TO DO:
If person accidentally swallows drug, call doctor, poison control center 1-800-222-1222 or hospital emergency room for help.

 POSSIBLE ADVERSE REACTIONS OR SIDE EFFECTS

SYMPTOMS	WHAT TO DO
Life-threatening: None expected.	
Common: Peeling, itching, redness or dryness of skin; tingling, burning or stinging may occur when medicine first used.	Continue. Call doctor when convenient.
Infrequent: None expected.	
Rare: Lightening of skin or white spots in persons with darker complexions.	Discontinue. Call doctor when. convenient.

WARNINGS & PRECAUTIONS

Don't use if:
You are sensitive to azelaic acid.

Before you start, consult your doctor if:
* You are allergic to any medicine, food or other substance, or have a family history of allergies.
* You have a dark complexion.

Over age 60:
No special problems expected, however the drug has not been tested extensively in this age group.

Pregnancy:
Consult doctor. Risk category B (see page xviii).

Breast-feeding:
No special problems expected. Consult doctor.

Infants & children:
Normally not used in this age group. Safety and effectiveness in children under age 12 has not been established.

Prolonged use:
No problems expected.

Skin & sunlight:
No problems expected.

Driving, piloting or hazardous work:
No problems expected.

Discontinuing:
No problems expected.

Others:
* Use as directed. Don't increase or decrease dosage without doctor's approval. Using more of the cream or using it more frequently than prescribed won't improve results and may cause excessive skin irritation.
* The side effects involving skin irritation usually go away with continued use. If they continue beyond 4 weeks, or are severe, consult doctor about reducing the dosage to once a day.
* You may use water-based cosmetics while undergoing treatment with this drug.

POSSIBLE INTERACTION WITH OTHER DRUGS

GENERIC NAME OR DRUG CLASS	COMBINED EFFECT
None expected.	

POSSIBLE INTERACTION WITH OTHER SUBSTANCES

INTERACTS WITH	COMBINED EFFECT
Alcohol:	None expected.
Beverages:	None expected.
Cocaine:	None expected.
Foods:	None expected.
Marijuana:	None expected.
Tobacco:	None expected.

BACLOFEN

BRAND NAMES

Kemstro   Lioresal

BASIC INFORMATION

Habit forming? No
Prescription needed? Yes
Available as generic? Yes
Drug class: Muscle relaxant for multiple
  sclerosis

 ## USES

- Relieves spasms, cramps and spasticity of muscles caused by medical problems, including multiple sclerosis and spine injuries.
- Reduces number and severity of trigeminal neuralgia attacks.

 ## DOSAGE & USAGE INFORMATION

How to take:
- Tablet—Swallow with liquid or food to lessen stomach irritation.
- Oral disintegrating tablet—Dissolves in the mouth.

When to take:
3 or 4 times daily as directed.

If you forget a dose:
Take as soon as you remember up to 2 hours late. If more than 2 hours, wait for next scheduled dose (don't double this dose).

What drug does:
Blocks body's pain and reflex messages to brain.

Time lapse before drug works:
Variable. Few hours to weeks.

Don't take with:
Any other medicine or any dietary supplement without consulting your doctor or pharmacist.

 ## OVERDOSE

SYMPTOMS:
Blurred vision, blindness, difficult breathing, vomiting, drowsiness, muscle weakness, convulsive seizures.
WHAT TO DO:
- Dial 911 (emergency) for medical help or call poison control center 1-800-222-1222 for instructions.
- If person is unconscious, check breathing and pulse. If not breathing, begin mouth-to-mouth rescue breathing. If heart is not beating, begin chest compressions.
- See emergency information on last 3 pages of this book.

 ## POSSIBLE ADVERSE REACTIONS OR SIDE EFFECTS

SYMPTOMS	WHAT TO DO
Life-threatening: In case of overdose, see previous column.	
Common: Dizziness, lightheadedness, nausea, drowsiness, confusion.	Continue. Call doctor when convenient.
Infrequent: • Rash with itching, numbness or tingling in hands or feet.	Discontinue. Call doctor right away.
• Headache, stomach pain, diarrhea or constipation, loss of appetite, muscle weakness,difficult or painful urination, sexual problems, stuffy nose, clumsiness, slurred speech, insomnia.	Continue. Call doctor when convenient.
Rare: • Fainting, weakness, hallucinations, depression, chest or muscle pain, pounding heartbeat.	Discontinue. Call doctor right away.
• Ringing in ears, lowered blood pressure, dry mouth, weight gain, taste change, overexcitement.	Continue. Call doctor when convenient.

 ## WARNINGS & PRECAUTIONS

Don't take if:
- You are allergic to any muscle relaxant.
- Muscle spasm is due to strain or sprain.

Before you start, consult your doctor if:
- You have Parkinson's disease.
- You have cerebral palsy.
- You have had a recent stroke.
- You have had a recent head injury.
- You have arthritis, diabetes or epilepsy.
- You have psychosis.
- You have kidney disease.
- You will have surgery within 2 months, including dental surgery, requiring general or spinal anesthesia.

Over age 60:
Adverse reactions and side effects may be more frequent and severe than in younger persons.

Pregnancy:
Decide with your doctor if drug benefits justify risk to unborn child. Risk category C (see page xviii).

Breast-feeding:
Avoid nursing or discontinue until you finish medicine. Consult doctor about maintaining milk supply.

Infants & children:
Not recommended.

Prolonged use:
Epileptic patients should be monitored with EEGs. Diabetics should more closely monitor blood sugar levels. Obtain periodic liver function tests.

Skin & sunlight:
No problems expected.

Driving, piloting or hazardous work:
Don't drive or pilot aircraft until you learn how medicine affects you. Don't work around dangerous machinery. Don't climb ladders or work in high places. Danger increases if you drink alcohol or take medicine affecting alertness and reflexes, such as antihistamines, tranquilizers, sedatives, pain medicine, narcotics and mind-altering drugs.

Discontinuing:
Don't discontinue without consulting doctor. Dose may require gradual reduction if you have taken drug for a long time. Doses of other drugs may also require adjustment.

Others:
Advise any doctor or dentist whom you consult that you take this medicine.

POSSIBLE INTERACTION WITH OTHER DRUGS

GENERIC NAME OR DRUG CLASS	COMBINED EFFECT
Anesthetics, general*	Increased sedation. Low blood pressure. Avoid.
Antidiabetic drugs,* insulin or oral	Need to adjust diabetes medicine dosage.
Central nervous system (CNS) depressants*	Increased sedation. Low blood pressure. Avoid.
Clozapine	Toxic effect on the central nervous system.
Ethinamate	Dangerous increased effects of ethinamate. Avoid combining.
Fluoxetine	Increased depressant effects of both drugs.
Guanfacine	May increase depressant effects of either drug.
Leucovorin	High alcohol content of leucovorin may cause adverse effects.
Methyprylon	Increased sedative effect, perhaps to dangerous level. Avoid.
Nabilone	Greater depression of the central nervous system.
Sertraline	Increased depressive effects of both drugs.

POSSIBLE INTERACTION WITH OTHER SUBSTANCES

INTERACTS WITH	COMBINED EFFECT
Alcohol:	Increased sedation. Low blood pressure. Avoid.
Beverages:	None expected.
Cocaine:	Increased spasticity. Avoid.
Foods:	None expected.
Marijuana:	Increased spasticity. Avoid.
Tobacco:	May interfere with absorption of medicine.

*See Glossary

BARBITURATES

GENERIC AND BRAND NAMES

See full list of generic and brand names in the *Generic and Brand Name Directory*, page 877.

BASIC INFORMATION

Habit forming? Yes
Prescription needed? Yes
Available as generic? Yes, for some
Drug class: Sedative-hypnotic agent, anticonvulsant

 ## USES

- Reduces likelihood of seizures (tonic-clonic seizure pattern and simple partial) in epilepsy.
- Preventive treatment for febrile seizures.
- Reduces anxiety or nervous tension.
- Used in combination drugs to treat gastro-intestinal disorders, headaches and asthma.
- Aids sleep at night (on a short-term basis).

 ## DOSAGE & USAGE INFORMATION

How to take:
- Capsule—Swallow with liquid. If you can't swallow whole, open capsule and take with liquid or food. Take on empty stomach (1 hour before or 2 hours after eating).
- Elixir—Swallow with liquid.
- Rectal suppository—Remove wrapper and moisten suppository with water. Gently insert into rectum, pointed end first. If suppository is too soft, chill first in refrigerator or cool water.
- Tablet—Swallow with liquid or food to lessen stomach irritation. If you can't swallow whole, crumble tablet and take with liquid or food

When to take:
At the same times each day.

Continued next column

 ## OVERDOSE

SYMPTOMS:
Deep sleep, trouble breathing, weak pulse, coma.
WHAT TO DO:
- **Dial 911 (emergency) for medical help or call poison control center 1-800-222-1222 for instructions.**
- **If person is unconscious, check breathing and pulse. If not breathing, begin mouth-to-mouth rescue breathing. If heart is not beating, begin chest compressions.**
- **See emergency information on last 3 pages of this book.**

If you forget a dose:
Take as soon as you remember up to 2 hours late. If more than 2 hours, wait for next scheduled dose (don't double this dose).

What drug does:
They block the transmission of nerve impulses from the brain to other parts of the body.

Time lapse before drug works:
60 minutes, but will take several weeks for maximum antiepilepsy effect.

Don't take with:
Any other medicine or any dietary supplement without consulting your doctor or pharmacist.

 ## POSSIBLE ADVERSE REACTIONS OR SIDE EFFECTS

SYMPTOMS	WHAT TO DO
Life-threatening:	
Rare allergic reaction—may have hives, rash, itching, swelling, trouble breathing, wheezing, chest pain, dizziness, faintness.	Seek emergency treatment immediately.
Common:	
Dizziness, drowsiness, clumsiness, unsteadiness, signs of addiction.*	Continue. Call doctor when convenient.
Infrequent:	
Confusion, headache, irritability, feeling faint, nausea, vomiting, depression, nightmares, trouble sleeping.	Continue, but call doctor right away.
Rare:	
Agitation, slow heartbeat, difficult breathing, bleeding sores on lips, fever, chest pain, unexplained bleeding or bruising, muscle or joint pain, skin rash or hives, thickened or scaly skin, white spots in mouth, tightness in chest, face swelling, sore throat, yellow eyes or skin, hallucinations, unusual tiredness or weakness, sleep-related behaviors.*	Continue, but call doctor right away.

 ## WARNINGS & PRECAUTIONS

Don't take if:
- You are allergic to any barbiturate.
- You have porphyria.

Before you start, consult your doctor if:
- You have epilepsy, kidney or liver problems, asthma, anemia or chronic pain.
- You will have surgery within 2 months, including dental surgery, requiring anesthesia.

Over age 60:
Adverse reactions and side effects may be more frequent and severe than in younger persons. Use small doses.

Pregnancy:
Risk to unborn child outweighs drug benefits. Don't use. Risk category D (see page xviii).

Breast-feeding:
Drug passes into milk. Avoid drug or discontinue nursing until you finish medicine. Consult doctor for advice on maintaining milk supply.

Infants & children:
Use only under doctor's supervision.

Prolonged use:
- May cause addiction, anemia, chronic intoxication. Unlikely to occur with the usual anticonvulsant or sedative dosage levels.
- May lower body temperature, making exposure to cold temperatures hazardous.
- Talk to your doctor about the need for follow-up medical examinations or laboratory studies to check blood sugar, kidney function.

Skin and sunlight:
No problems expected.

Driving, piloting or hazardous work:
Don't drive or pilot aircraft until you learn how medicine affects you. Don't work around dangerous machinery. Don't climb ladders or work in high places. Danger increases if you drink alcohol or take medicine affecting alertness and reflexes.

Discontinuing:
If you become addicted, don't stop taking barbiturates suddenly. Seek medical help for safe withdrawal.

Others:
- May affect results in some medical tests.
- Barbiturate addiction is common. Withdrawal effects may be fatal.
- Advise any doctor or dentist whom you consult that you take this medicine.

POSSIBLE INTERACTION WITH OTHER DRUGS

GENERIC NAME OR DRUG CLASS	COMBINED EFFECT
Adrenocorticoids, systemic	Decreased effect of prednisone.
Anticoagulants, oral*	Decreased effect of anticoagulant.
Anticonvulsants*	Changed seizure patterns.

Antidepressants, tricyclic*	Decreased antidepressant effect. Possible dangerous oversedation.
Antidiabetic, agents, oral*	Increased effect of barbiturate.
Antihistamines*	Dangerous sedation. Avoid.
Aspirin	Decreased aspirin effect.
Beta-adrenergic blocking agents*	Decreased effect of beta-adrenergic blocker.
Carbamazepine	Decreased carbamazepine effect.
Carteolol	Increased barbiturate effect. Dangerous sedation.
Clozapine	Toxic effect on the central nervous system.
Contraceptives, oral*	Decreased contraceptive effect.
Dextrothyroxine	Decreased barbiturate effect.
Doxycycline	Decreased doxycycline effect.
Griseofulvin	Decreased griseofulvin effect.
Lamotrigine	Decreased lamotrigine effect.
Leukotriene modifiers	Decreased montelukast effect.

Continued on page 907

POSSIBLE INTERACTION WITH OTHER SUBSTANCES

INTERACTS WITH	COMBINED EFFECT
Alcohol:	Possible fatal oversedation. Avoid.
Beverages:	None expected.
Cocaine:	Decreased barbiturate effect.
Foods:	None expected.
Marijuana:	Excessive sedation. Avoid.
Tobacco:	None expected.

*See Glossary

BARBITURATES, ASPIRIN & CODEINE
(Also contains caffeine)

GENERIC AND BRAND NAMES

See full list of generic and brand names in the *Generic and Brand Name Directory*, page 878.

BASIC INFORMATION

Habit forming? Yes
Prescription needed? Yes
Available as generic? Yes
Drug class: Narcotic, analgesic

 ## USES

- Reduces anxiety or nervous tension (low dose).
- Reduces pain, fever, inflammation.

 ## DOSAGE & USAGE INFORMATION

How to take:
- Tablet or capsule—Swallow with liquid or food to lessen stomach irritation. If you can't swallow whole, crumble tablet or open capsule and take with liquid or food.
- Extended-release tablet or capsule— Swallow each dose whole. Do not crush, open or chew,

When to take:
When needed. No more often than every 4 hours.

If you forget a dose:
Take as soon as you remember. Wait 4 hours for next dose.

Continued next column

 ## OVERDOSE

SYMPTOMS:
Deep sleep, slow and weak pulse, ringing in ears, nausea, vomiting, dizziness, fever, deep and rapid breathing, hallucinations, convulsions, coma.
WHAT TO DO:
- **Dial 911 (emergency) for medical help or call poison control center 1-800-222-1222 for instructions.**
- **If person is unconscious, check breathing and pulse. If not breathing, begin mouth-to-mouth rescue breathing. If heart is not beating, begin chest compressions.**
- **See emergency information on last 3 pages of this book.**

What drug does:
- May partially block nerve impulses at nerve-cell connections.
- Affects hypothalamus, the part of the brain which regulates temperature by dilating small blood vessels in skin.
- Prevents clumping of platelets (small blood cells) so blood vessels remain open.
- Decreases prostaglandin effect.
- Blocks pain messages to brain and spinal cord.
- Reduces sensitivity of brain's cough-control center.

Time lapse before drug works:
30 minutes.

Don't take with:
Any other medicine or any dietary supplement without consulting your doctor or pharmacist.

 ## POSSIBLE ADVERSE REACTIONS OR SIDE EFFECTS

SYMPTOMS	WHAT TO DO
Life-threatening: Rare allergic reaction (hives, itching, rash, wheezing, tightness in chest, swelling of lips or tongue or throat).	Seek emergency treatment immediately.
Common: Dizziness, drowsiness, heartburn, flushed face, depression, false sense of well-being, increased urination.	Continue. Call doctor when convenient.
Infrequent: Jaundice; vomiting blood; easy bruising; skin rash, hives; confusion; depression; sore throat, fever, mouth sores; difficult urination; hearing loss; slurred speech; blood in urine; decreased vision.	Discontinue. Call doctor right away.
Rare: Insomnia, nightmares, constipation, headache, nervousness, flushed face, increased sweating, unusual tiredness, sleep-related behaviors.*	Continue. Call doctor when convenient.

BARBITURATES, ASPIRIN & CODEINE
(Also contains caffeine)

 ## WARNINGS & PRECAUTIONS

Don't take if:
You are allergic to any barbiturate or narcotic or aspirin.

Before you start, consult your doctor if:
* You have had stomach or duodenal ulcers.
* You have asthma, epilepsy, kidney or liver damage, anemia, chronic pain, gout.
* You will have surgery within 2 months, including dental surgery, requiring general or spinal anesthesia.

Over age 60:
* Adverse reactions and side effects may be more frequent and severe than in younger persons.
* More likely to cause hidden bleeding in stomach or intestines. Watch for dark stools.
* More likely to be drowsy, dizzy, unsteady or constipated. Use only if absolutely necessary.

Pregnancy:
Risk factors vary for drugs in this group. See category list on page xviii and consult doctor.

Breast-feeding:
Drug passes into milk. Avoid drug or discontinue nursing until you finish medicine. Consult doctor for advice on maintaining milk supply.

Infants & children:
* Overdose frequent and severe. Keep bottles out of children's reach.
* Use only under doctor's supervision.
* Do not give to persons under age 18 who have fever and discomfort of viral illness, especially chicken pox and influenza. May increase risk of Reye's syndrome.*

Prolonged use:
* Kidney damage. Periodic kidney function test recommended.
* May cause addiction, anemia, chronic intoxication.
* May lower body temperature, making exposure to cold temperatures hazardous.

Skin & sunlight:
One or more drugs in this group may cause rash or intensify sunburn in areas exposed to sun or ultraviolet light (photosensitivity reaction). Avoid overexposure. Notify doctor if reaction occurs.

Driving, piloting or hazardous work:
Don't drive or pilot aircraft until you learn how medicine effects you. Don't work around dangerous machinery. Don't climb ladders or work in high places. Danger increases if you drink alcohol or take medicine affecting alertness and reflexes, such as antihistamines, tranquilizers, sedatives, pain medicine, narcotics and mind-altering drugs.

Discontinuing:
May be unnecessary to finish medicine. Follow doctor's instructions. If you develop withdrawal symptoms of hallucinations, agitation or sleeplessness after discontinuing, call doctor right away.

Others:
* Aspirin can complicate surgery, illness, pregnancy, labor and delivery.
* For arthritis—Don't change dose without consulting doctor.
* Advise any doctor or dentist whom you consult that you take this medicine.
* Urine tests for blood sugar may be inaccurate.
* Great potential for abuse.

 ## POSSIBLE INTERACTION WITH OTHER DRUGS

GENERIC NAME OR DRUG CLASS	COMBINED EFFECT
Adrenocorticoids, systemic	Increased risk of ulcers.
Allopurinol	Decreased allopurinol effect.
Analgesics, other*	Increased analgesic effect.
Antacids*	Decreased aspirin effect.

Continued on page 908

 ## POSSIBLE INTERACTION WITH OTHER SUBSTANCES

INTERACTS WITH	COMBINED EFFECT
Alcohol:	Possible stomach irritation and bleeding, possible fatal oversedation. Avoid.
Beverages:	None expected.
Cocaine:	Increased cocaine toxic effects. Avoid.
Foods:	None expected.
Marijuana:	Possible increased pain relief, but marijuana may slow body's recovery. Impairs physical and mental performance. Avoid.
Tobacco:	None expected.

*See Glossary

BECAPLERMIN

BRAND NAMES

Regranex

BASIC INFORMATION

Habit forming? No
Prescription needed? Yes
Available as generic? No
Drug class: Platelet-derived growth factor

 USES

Treatment of skin ulcers in patients with diabetes.

 DOSAGE & USAGE INFORMATION

How to use:
Gel—Apply to the affected area. Follow all instructions provided with the prescription. Dosage may change as wound heals.

When to use:
At the same time each day. Change the wound dressing between applications of the medication.

If you forget a dose:
Apply it as soon as possible. If it is almost time for your next dose, skip the missed dose and go back to your regular dosing schedule. Do not double doses.

What drug does:
Stimulates growth of cells involved in wound repair.

Time lapse before drug works:
Up to six months.

Don't use with:
Any other medicine or any dietary supplement without consulting your doctor or pharmacist.

 OVERDOSE

SYMPTOMS:
None expected.
WHAT TO DO:
Overdose unlikely to threaten life. If person uses much larger amount than prescribed, call doctor, poison control center 1-800-222-1222 or hospital emergency room for help.

POSSIBLE ADVERSE REACTIONS OR SIDE EFFECTS

SYMPTOMS	WHAT TO DO
Life-threatening: None expected.	
Common: None expected.	
Infrequent: Rash in area of skin ulcer.	Discontinue. Call doctor right away.
Rare: None expected.	

WARNINGS & PRECAUTIONS

Don't take if:
- You are allergic to becaplermin, parabens or metacresol.
- You have any new growths or wounds in the application area.

Before you start, consult your doctor if:
- You have any other medical problem.
- You are allergic to any other substances, such as food preservatives or dyes.
- You have a malignancy or cancer.

Over age 60:
No problems expected.

Pregnancy:
Decide with your doctor if drug benefits justify risk to unborn child. Risk category C (see page xviii).

Breast-feeding:
It is not known if drug passes into milk. Avoid drug or discontinue nursing until you finish medicine. Consult doctor for advice on maintaining milk supply.

Infants & children:
Safety and efficacy in children under age 16 has not been established.

Prolonged use:
No problems expected. Your doctor should periodically evaluate your response to the drug and adjust the dose according to the rate of change in the width and length of the diabetic ulcer.

Skin & sunlight:
No problems expected.

Driving, piloting or hazardous work:
No problems expected.

Discontinuing:
Don't discontinue without consulting doctor.

Others:
- There is an increased risk of cancer death in patients who use 3 or more tubes of this drug. Consult your doctor about your risks.
- Do not place tip of tube onto ulcer or any other object; it may contaminate the medication.
- Be sure you follow application instructions carefully.
- Avoid bearing weight on the affected extremity.
- Wash hands carefully before preparing your dose.
- Keep this medication in refrigerator; do not freeze.
- Advise any doctor or dentist whom you consult that you take this medicine.

POSSIBLE INTERACTION WITH OTHER DRUGS

GENERIC NAME OR DRUG CLASS	COMBINED EFFECT
None expected.	

POSSIBLE INTERACTION WITH OTHER SUBSTANCES

INTERACTS WITH	COMBINED EFFECT
Alcohol:	None expected.
Beverages:	None expected.
Cocaine:	Effects unknown. Avoid.
Foods:	None expected.
Marijuana:	Effects unknown. Avoid.
Tobacco:	None expected.

BELLADONNA ALKALOIDS & BARBITURATES

GENERIC AND BRAND NAMES

See full list of generic and brand names in the *Generic and Brand Name Directory*, page 878.

BASIC INFORMATION

Habit forming? Yes
Prescription needed? Yes
Available as generic? Some yes, some no
Drug class: Antispasmodic, anticholinergic, sedative

USES

• Reduces spasms of digestive system, bladder and urethra.
• Reduces anxiety or nervous tension.
• Relieves insomnia.

DOSAGE & USAGE INFORMATION

How to take:
• Tablet, liquid or capsule—Swallow with liquid or food to lessen stomach irritation. If you can't swallow whole, crumble tablet or open capsule and take with liquid or food.
• Extended-release tablet or capsule— Swallow each dose whole. Don't crush, open or chew.
• Chewable tablets—Chew well before swallowing.
• Elixir—Take by mouth. Follow directions on the product label. Measure the dose with the special dropper or spoon provided. Take 30 to 60 minutes before meals.
• Drops—Dilute dose in beverage before swallowing.

When to take:
At the same times each day.

Continued next column

OVERDOSE

SYMPTOMS:
Blurred vision, confusion, convulsions, irregular heartbeat, hallucinations, coma.
WHAT TO DO:
• **Dial 911 (emergency) for medical help or call poison control center 1-800-222-1222 for instructions.**
• **See emergency information on last 3 pages of this book.**

If you forget a dose:
Take as soon as you remember up to 2 hours late. If more than 2 hours, wait for next scheduled dose (don't double this dose).

What drug does:
• May partially block nerve impulses at nerve cell connections.
• Blocks nerve impulses at parasympathetic nerve endings, preventing muscle contractions and gland secretions of organs involved.

Time lapse before drug works:
15 to 30 minutes.

Don't take with:
• Antacids* or antidiarrheals* at the same time.
• Any other medicine or any dietary supplement without consulting your doctor or pharmacist.

POSSIBLE ADVERSE REACTIONS OR SIDE EFFECTS

SYMPTOMS	WHAT TO DO
Life-threatening:	
Rare allergic reaction (hives, itching, rash, wheezing, tightness in chest, swelling (lips, tongue or throat).	Seek emergency treatment immediately.
Common:	
• Dry mouth, throat, nose; drowsiness; constipation; dizziness; nausea; vomiting; "hangover" effect; depression; confusion.	Discontinue. Call doctor right away.
• Reduced sweating, slurred speech, agitation, nasal congestion, altered taste.	Continue. Call doctor when convenient.
Infrequent:	
Difficult urination; difficult swallowing; rash or hives; face, lip or eyelid swelling; joint or muscle pain; lightheadedness.	Discontinue. Call doctor right away.
Rare:	
Jaundice; unusual bruising or bleeding; hives, skin rash; pain in eyes; blurred vision; sore throat, fever, mouth sores, sleep-related behaviors.*	Discontinue. Call doctor right away.

172

WARNINGS & PRECAUTIONS

Don't take if:
- You are allergic to any barbiturate or any anticholinergic.
- You have porphyria, trouble with stomach bloating, difficulty emptying your bladder completely, narrow-angle glaucoma, severe ulcerative colitis.

Before you start, consult your doctor if:
- You have open-angle glaucoma, angina, chronic bronchitis or asthma, hiatal hernia, liver disease, enlarged prostate, myasthenia gravis, peptic ulcer, epilepsy, kidney or liver damage, anemia, chronic pain, thyroid disease.
- You will have surgery within 2 months, including dental surgery, requiring general or spinal anesthesia.

Over age 60:
Adverse reactions and side effects may be more frequent and severe than in younger persons. Ask your doctor about small doses.

Pregnancy:
Risk factors vary for drugs in this group. See category list on page xviii and consult doctor.

Breast-feeding:
Drug passes into milk. Avoid drug or discontinue nursing until you finish medicine.

Infants & children:
Use only under doctor's supervision.

Prolonged use:
- May cause addiction, anemia, chronic intoxication.
- May lower body temperature, making exposure to cold temperatures hazardous.

Skin & sunlight:
One or more drugs in this group may cause rash or intensify sunburn in areas exposed to sun or ultraviolet light (photosensitivity reaction). Avoid overexposure. Notify doctor if reaction occurs.

Driving, piloting or hazardous work:
Don't drive or pilot aircraft until you learn how medicine affects you. Don't work around dangerous machinery. Don't climb ladders or work in high places. Danger increases if you drink alcohol or take medicine affecting alertness and reflexes.

Discontinuing:
May be unnecessary to finish medicine. Follow doctor's instructions. If you develop withdrawal symptoms of hallucinations, agitation or sleeplessness after discontinuing, call doctor right away.

Others:
- Great potential for abuse.
- Advise any doctor or dentist whom you consult that you take this medicine.

POSSIBLE INTERACTION WITH OTHER DRUGS

GENERIC NAME OR DRUG CLASS	COMBINED EFFECT
Acetaminophen	Possible decreased barbiturate effect.
Adrenocorticoids, systemic	Possible glaucoma.
Amantadine	Increased belladonna effect.
Antacids*	Decreased belladonna effect.
Anticholinergics, other*	Increased belladonna effect.
Anticoagulants, oral*	Decreased anti-coagulant effect.
Anticonvulsants*	Changed seizure patterns.
Antidepressants, tricyclic*	Possible dangerous oversedation. Avoid.
Antidiabetics, oral*	Increased barbiturate effect.
Antihistamines*	Dangerous sedation. Avoid.
Anti-inflammatory drugs nonsteroidal (NSAIDs)*	Decreased anti-inflammatory effect.
Aspirin	Decreased aspirin effect.

Continued on page 909

POSSIBLE INTERACTION WITH OTHER SUBSTANCES

INTERACTS WITH	COMBINED EFFECT
Alcohol:	Possible fatal oversedation. Avoid.
Beverages:	None expected.
Cocaine:	Excessively rapid heartbeat. Avoid.
Foods:	None expected.
Marijuana:	Drowsiness and dry mouth. Avoid.
Tobacco:	Decreased effectiveness of acid reduction in stomach.

*See Glossary

BENZODIAZEPINES

GENERIC AND BRAND NAMES

See full list of generic and brand names in the *Generic and Brand Name Directory*, page 878.

BASIC INFORMATION

Habit forming? Yes
Prescription needed? Yes
Available as generic? Yes, for most
Drug class: Tranquilizer (benzodiazepine), anticonvulsant

 USE

- Treatment for anxiety disorders and panic disorders.
- Treatment for muscle spasm.
- Treatment for seizure disorders.
- Treatment for alcohol withdrawal.
- Treatment for insomnia (short-term).

 DOSAGE & USAGE INFORMATION

How to take:
- Tablet or capsule—Swallow with liquid. If you can't swallow whole, crumble tablet or open capsule and take with liquid or a bite of food.
- Extended-release capsule—Swallow capsule whole. Do not open or chew.
- Oral suspension—Dilute dose in water, soda or sodalike beverage or small amount of food such as applesauce or pudding.
- Sublingual tablet—Do not chew or swallow. Place under tongue until dissolved.
- Disintegrating tablet—Let dissolve on tongue.
- Rectal gel—Follow instructions provided with prescription or as directed by the doctor.

When to take:
At the same time each day, according to instructions on prescription label.

Continued next column

 OVERDOSE

SYMPTOMS:
Drowsiness, weakness, tremor, stupor, coma.
WHAT TO DO:
- Dial 911 (emergency) for medical help or call poison control center 1-800-222-1222 for instructions.
- If person is unconscious, check breathing and pulse. If not breathing, begin mouth-to-mouth rescue breathing. If heart is not beating, begin chest compressions.
- See emergency information on last 3 pages of this book.

If you forget a dose:
Take as soon as you remember. If it is almost time for the next dose, wait for that dose (don't double this dose) and resume regular schedule.

What drug does:
Affects limbic system of brain, the part that controls emotions.

Time lapse before drug works:
May take 6 weeks for full benefit; depends on drug when treating anxiety.

Don't take with:
Any other medicine or any dietary supplement without consulting your doctor or pharmacist.

 POSSIBLE ADVERSE REACTIONS OR SIDE EFFECTS

SYMPTOMS	WHAT TO DO
Life-threatening: Rare allergic reaction—may have hives, rash, itching, swelling, trouble breathing, wheezing, chest pain, dizziness, faintness.	Seek emergency treatment immediately.
Common: Clumsiness, unsteadiness, dizziness, light-headed, drowsiness, slurred speech.	Continue. Call doctor when convenient.
Infrequent: • Memory loss, anxiety, confusion, depression, fast heartbeat.	Discontinue. Call doctor right away.
• Constipation or diarrhea, nausea, vomiting, urination problems, stomach pain, headache, mouth is dry or watering, muscle spasm, changes in sexual function.	Continue. Call doctor when convenient.
Rare: Behavior changes (may be bizarre), confusion, delusions, outbursts of anger, loss of reality, infection symptoms (fever, chills), unusual tiredness or weakness, unusual bleeding or bruising, skin rash or itching, sores in mouth, body movements uncontrolled, hallucinations, yellow skin or eyes, sleep-related behaviors.*	Discontinue. Call doctor right away.

WARNINGS & PRECAUTIONS

Don't take if:
You are allergic to any benzodiazepine.

Before you start, consult your doctor if:
- You have myasthenia gravis.
- You have a history of drug or alcohol abuse, or severe depression or mental disorder.
- You have liver, kidney or lung disease.
- You have diabetes, seizure disorder, a swallowing problem (in children), or porphyria.
- You have sleep apnea.
- You have glaucoma.

Over age 60:
Adverse reactions and side effects may be more frequent and severe than in younger persons. May need smaller doses for shorter period.

Pregnancy:
Risk factors vary for drugs in this group. See category list on page xviii and consult doctor.

Breast-feeding:
Drug passes into milk. Avoid drug or discontinue nursing until you finish medicine. Consult doctor for advice on maintaining milk supply.

Infants & children:
Use only under medical supervision.

Prolonged use:
Risk of physical or psychological dependence.

Skin & sunlight:
One or more drugs in this group may cause rash or intensify sunburn in areas exposed to sun or ultraviolet light (photosensitivity reaction). Avoid overexposure and use sunscreen. Notify doctor if reaction occurs.

Driving, piloting or hazardous work:
Don't drive or pilot aircraft until you learn how medicine affects you. Don't work around dangerous machinery. Don't climb ladders or work in high places. Danger increases if you drink alcohol or take medicine affecting alertness and reflexes.

Discontinuing:
- Don't discontinue without consulting doctor. Adverse effects can occur (may be life-threatening) if the drug has been taken for longer periods. Dose may require gradual reduction. Doses of other drugs may also require adjustment.
- If withdrawal symptoms (emotional or physical) occur after stopping the drug, call doctor.

Others:
- Don't use for insomnia more than 4-7 days.
- Hot weather, heavy exercise and sweating may increase risk of heat stroke.
- Advise any doctor or dentist whom you consult that you take this drug.

- Rarely, anticonvulsant (antiepileptic) drugs may lead to suicidal thoughts and behaviors. Call doctor right away if suicidal symptoms or unusual behaviors occur.

POSSIBLE INTERACTION WITH OTHER DRUGS

GENERIC NAME OR DRUG CLASS	COMBINED EFFECT
Antidepressants, tricyclic*	Increased sedative effect of both drugs.
Carbamazepine	Decreased effect of benzodiazepine.
Central nervous system (CNS) depressants*	Increased sedative effect.
Cimetidine	Increased effect of benzodiazepine.
Clozapine	Toxic effect on the central nervous system.
Contraceptives, oral*	Increased effect of benzodiazepine.
Enzyme inhibitors*	Increased effect of benzodiazepine.
Erythromycins*	Increased effect of benzodiazepine.
Fluoxetine	Increased effect of benzodiazepine.
Fluvoxamine	Increased effect of benzodiazepine.
Isoniazid	Increased effect of benzodiazepine.

Continued on page 910

POSSIBLE INTERACTION WITH OTHER SUBSTANCES

INTERACTS WITH	COMBINED EFFECT
Alcohol:	Sedation. Avoid.
Beverages: Grapefruit juice.	Increased effect of benzodiazepine.
Cocaine:	Unknown effect. Avoid.
Foods:	None expected.
Marijuana:	Sedation. Avoid.
Tobacco:	Decreased effect of benzodiazepine.

*See Glossary

BENZOYL PEROXIDE

BRAND NAMES

See full list of brand names in the *Generic and Brand Name Directory*, page 878.

BASIC INFORMATION

Habit forming? No
Prescription needed? No
Available as generic? Yes
Drug class: Antiacne (topical)

USES

- Treatment for acne.
- Treats pressure sores.

DOSAGE & USAGE INFORMATION

How to use:
Cream, gel, pads, sticks, lotion, cleansing bar or facial mask—Wash affected area with plain soap and water. Dry gently with towel. Rub medicine into affected areas. Keep away from eyes, nose, mouth. Wash hands after using.

When to use:
Apply 1 or more times daily. If you have a fair complexion, start with single application at bedtime.

If you forget an application:
Use as soon as you remember.

What drug does:
Slowly releases oxygen from skin, which controls some skin bacteria. Also causes peeling and drying, helping control blackheads and whiteheads.

Time lapse before drug works:
1 to 2 weeks.

Don't use with:
Any other topical medicine without consulting your doctor or pharmacist.

OVERDOSE

SYMPTOMS:
None expected.
WHAT TO DO:
- If person swallows drug, call doctor, poison control center 1-800-222-1222 or hospital emergency room for help.
- See emergency information on last 3 pages of this book.

POSSIBLE ADVERSE REACTIONS OR SIDE EFFECTS

SYMPTOMS	WHAT TO DO
Life-threatening: None expected.	
Common: Mild redness and chapping of skin during first few weeks of use.	No action necessary.
Infrequent: • Rash, excessive dryness, peeling skin.	Discontinue. Call doctor right away.
• Painful skin irritation.	Continue. Call doctor when convenient.
Rare: None expected.	

WARNINGS & PRECAUTIONS

Don't take if:
You are allergic to benzoyl peroxide.

Before you start, consult your doctor if:
* You plan to become pregnant within medication period.
* You take oral contraceptives.
* You are using any other prescription or nonprescription medicine for acne.
* You are using abrasive skin cleansers or medicated cosmetics.

Over age 60:
No problems expected.

Pregnancy:
Consult doctor. Risk category C (see page xviii).

Breast-feeding:
No proven problems. Consult doctor.

Infants & children:
Not recommended.

Prolonged use:
Permanent rash or scarring.

Skin & sunlight:
May cause rash or intensify sunburn in areas exposed to sun or ultraviolet light (photosensitivity reaction). Avoid overexposure. Notify doctor if reaction occurs.

Driving, piloting or hazardous work:
No problems expected.

Discontinuing:
* May be unnecessary to finish medicine. Discontinue when acne improves.
* If acne doesn't improve in 2 weeks, call doctor.

Others:
* Drug may bleach hair or dyed fabrics, including clothing or carpet.
* Store away from heat in cool, dry place.
* Avoid contact with eyes, lips, nose and sensitive areas of the neck.

POSSIBLE INTERACTION WITH OTHER DRUGS

GENERIC NAME OR DRUG CLASS	COMBINED EFFECT
Antiacne topical preparations, other	Excessive skin irritation.
Skin-peeling agents (salicylic acid, sulfur, resorcinol, tretinoin)	Excessive skin irritation.

POSSIBLE INTERACTION WITH OTHER SUBSTANCES

INTERACTS WITH	COMBINED EFFECT
Alcohol:	None expected.
Beverages:	None expected.
Cocaine:	None expected.
Foods: Cinnamon, foods with benzoic acid.	Skin rash.
Marijuana:	None expected.
Tobacco:	None expected.

BETA CAROTENE

BRAND NAMES

Solatene
Numerous multiple vitamin and mineral
supplements. Check labels.

BASIC INFORMATION

Habit forming? No
Prescription needed? No
Available as generic? Yes
Drug class: Nutritional supplement

 ## USES

- Used as a nutritional supplement.
- Used as an adjunct to the treatment of
  steatorrhea, chronic fever, obstructive
  jaundice, pancreatic insufficiency, protein
  deficiency, total parenteral nutrition and photosensitivity in photo porphyria.

 ## DOSAGE & USAGE INFORMATION

How to take:
Tablet or capsule—Swallow with liquid. If you
can't swallow whole, crumble tablet or open
capsule and take with liquid or food.

When to take:
At the same time each day, according to
directions on package or prescription label.

If you forget a dose:
Take as soon as you remember (don't double
this dose).

What drug does:
Enables the body to manufacture vitamin A,
which is essential for the normal functioning of
the retina, normal growth and development and
normal testicular and ovarian function.

Time lapse before drug works:
Total effect may take several weeks.

Don't take with:
No restrictions unless advised by doctor.

 ## OVERDOSE

SYMPTOMS:
Yellow skin.
WHAT TO DO:
Overdose unlikely to threaten life. If person
takes much larger amount than prescribed,
call doctor, poison control center
1-800-222-1222 or hospital emergency room
for help.

 ## POSSIBLE ADVERSE REACTIONS OR SIDE EFFECTS

SYMPTOMS	WHAT TO DO
Life-threatening: None expected.	
Common: Yellow palms, hands, soles of feet.	Continue. Call doctor when convenient.
Infrequent: None expected.	
Rare:	
• Joint pain, unusual bleeding or bruising.	Discontinue. Call doctor right away.
• Diarrhea, dizziness.	Continue. Call doctor when convenient.

WARNINGS & PRECAUTIONS

Don't take if:
You are hypersensitive to beta carotene.

Before you start, consult your doctor if:
* You have liver or kidney disease.
* You have hypervitaminosis.*

Over age 60:
No problems expected.

Pregnancy:
Consult doctor. Risk category C (see page xviii).

Breast-feeding:
No problems expected.

Infants & children:
No problems expected.

Prolonged use:
No problems expected.

Skin & sunlight:
No special problems expected.

Driving, piloting or hazardous work:
No special problems expected.

Discontinuing:
No special problems expected.

Others:
* Some researchers claim that beta carotene may reduce the occurrence of some cancers. There is insufficient data to substantiate this claim.
* Advise any doctor or dentist whom you consult that you take this medicine.
* May affect results of some medical tests.

POSSIBLE INTERACTION WITH OTHER DRUGS

GENERIC NAME OR DRUG CLASS	COMBINED EFFECT
Cholestyramine	Decreased absorption of beta carotene.
Colestipol	Decreased absorption of beta carotene.
Mineral oil	Decreased absorption of beta carotene.
Neomycin	Decreased absorption of beta carotene.

POSSIBLE INTERACTION WITH OTHER SUBSTANCES

INTERACTS WITH	COMBINED EFFECT
Alcohol:	None expected.
Beverages:	None expected.
Cocaine:	None expected.
Foods:	None expected.
Marijuana:	None expected.
Tobacco:	None expected.

*See Glossary

BETA-ADRENERGIC BLOCKING AGENTS

GENERIC AND BRAND NAMES

See full list of generic and brand names in the *Generic and Brand Name Directory*, page 879.

BASIC INFORMATION

Habit forming? No
Prescription needed? Yes
Available as generic? Yes, for some.
Drug class: Antiadrenergic, antianginal, antiarrhythmic, antihypertensive

USES

- Treats high blood pressure (hypertension).
- Some beta-blockers are used to relieve angina (chest pain).
- May be used to treat irregular heartbeat.
- May be used to treat anxiety disorders and other conditions as determined by your doctor.
- Treats tremors (some types).
- Reduces frequency of vascular headaches (does not relieve headache pain).

DOSAGE & USAGE INFORMATION

How to take:
Tablet, liquid, extended-release caplet or extended-release tablet—Swallow with liquid. If you can't swallow whole, crumble tablet or open capsule and take with liquid or food. Don't crush or open extended-release forms.

When to take:
With meals or immediately after.

If you forget a dose:
Take as soon as you remember. Return to regular schedule, but allow 3 hours between doses.

Continued next column

OVERDOSE

SYMPTOMS:
Weakness, slow or weak pulse, blood pressure drop, fainting, difficulty breathing, convulsions, cold and sweaty skin.
WHAT TO DO:
- **Dial 911 (emergency) for medical help or call poison control center 1-800-222-1222 for instructions.**
- **See emergency information on last 3 pages of this book.**

What drug does:
- Blocks certain actions of sympathetic nervous system.
- Lowers heart's oxygen requirements.
- Slows nerve impulses through heart.
- Reduces blood vessel contraction in heart, scalp and other body parts.

Time lapse before drug works:
1 to 4 hours.

Don't take with:
Any other medicine or any dietary supplement without consulting your doctor or pharmacist.

POSSIBLE ADVERSE REACTIONS OR SIDE EFFECTS

SYMPTOMS	WHAT TO DO
Life-threatening:	
Congestive heart failure (severe shortness of breath, rapid heartbeat); severe asthma.	Discontinue. Seek emergency treatment.
Common:	
• Pulse slower than 50 beats per minute.	Discontinue. Call doctor right away.
• Drowsiness, fatigue, numbness or tingling of fingers or toes, dizziness, diarrhea, nausea, weakness.	Continue. Call doctor when convenient.
• Cold hands or feet; dry mouth, eyes and skin.	Continue. Tell doctor at next visit.
Infrequent:	
• Hallucinations, nightmares, insomnia, headache, difficult breathing, joint pain, anxiety, chest pain.	Discontinue. Call doctor right away.
• Confusion, reduced alertness, depression, impotence, abdominal pain.	Continue. Call doctor when convenient.
• Constipation.	Continue. Tell doctor at next visit.
Rare:	
• Rash, sore throat, fever.	Discontinue. Call doctor right away.
• Unusual bleeding and bruising; dry, burning eyes.	Continue. Call doctor when convenient.

WARNINGS & PRECAUTIONS

Don't take if:
- You are allergic to any beta-adrenergic blocker.
- You have asthma.
- You have hay fever symptoms.
- You have taken a monoamine oxidase (MAO) inhibitor* in the past 2 weeks.

Before you start, consult your doctor if:
- You have heart disease or poor circulation to the extremities.
- You have hay fever, asthma, chronic bronchitis, emphysema.
- You have overactive thyroid function.
- You have impaired liver or kidney function.
- You will have surgery within 2 months, including dental surgery, requiring general or spinal anesthesia.
- You have diabetes or hypoglycemia.

Over age 60:
Adverse reactions and side effects may be more frequent and severe than in younger persons.

Pregnancy:
Risk factors vary for drugs in this group. See category list on page xviii and consult doctor.

Breast-feeding:
Drug passes into milk. Avoid drug or discontinue nursing until you finish medicine. Consult doctor for advice on maintaining milk supply.

Infants & children:
Not recommended.

Prolonged use:
Talk to your doctor about the need for follow-up medical examinations or laboratory studies to check blood pressure, ECG,* kidney function, blood sugar.

Skin & sunlight:
No problems expected.

Driving, piloting or hazardous work:
Don't drive or pilot aircraft until you learn how medicine affects you. Don't work around dangerous machinery. Don't climb ladders or work in high places. Danger increases if you drink alcohol or take medicine affecting alertness and reflexes.

Discontinuing
Don't discontinue without consulting doctor. Dose may require gradual reduction if you have taken drug for a long time. Doses of other drugs may also require adjustment. Angina may result from abrupt discontinuing.

Others:
- May mask diabetic hypoglycemia symptoms.
- May affect results in some medical tests.
- Advise any doctor or dentist whom you consult that you take this medicine.

POSSIBLE INTERACTION WITH OTHER DRUGS

GENERIC NAME OR DRUG CLASS	COMBINED EFFECT
Angiotensin-converting (ACE) inhibitors*	Increased antihypertensive effects of both drugs. Dosages may require adjustment.
Antidiabetics*	Increased antidiabetic effect.
Antihistamines*	Decreased antihistamine effect.
Antihypertensives*	Increased antihypertensive effect.
Anti-inflammatory drugs, nonsteroidal (NSAIDs)*	Decreased antihypertensive effect of beta blocker.
Betaxolol eyedrops	Possible increased beta blocker effect.
Calcium channel blockers*	Additional blood pressure drop.
Clonidine	Additional blood pressure drop. High blood pressure if clonidine stopped abruptly.
Dextrothyroxine	Possible decreased beta blocker effect.

Continued on page 910

POSSIBLE INTERACTION WITH OTHER SUBSTANCES

INTERACTS WITH	COMBINED EFFECT
Alcohol:	Excessive blood pressure drop. Avoid.
Beverages:	None expected.
Cocaine:	Irregular heartbeat; decreased beta-adrenergic effect. Avoid.
Foods:	None expected.
Marijuana:	Daily use—Impaired circulation to hands and feet.
Tobacco:	Possible irregular heartbeat.

*See Glossary

BETA-ADRENERGIC BLOCKING AGENTS & THIAZIDE DIURETICS

GENERIC AND BRAND NAMES

See full list of generic and brand names in the *Generic and Brand Name Directory*, page 879.

BASIC INFORMATION

Habit forming? No
Prescription needed? Yes
Available as generic? Yes
Drug class: Beta-adrenergic blocker, diuretic (thiazide)

USES

- Controls, but doesn't cure, high blood pressure.
- Reduces fluid retention (edema).
- Reduces angina attacks.
- Stabilizes irregular heartbeat.
- Reduces frequency of migraine headaches. (Does not relieve headache pain.)
- Other uses as determined by your doctor.

DOSAGE & USAGE INFORMATION

How to take:
- Tablet—Swallow with liquid.
- Extended-release capsule—Swallow with liquid. Do not open or chew capsule.

When to take:
At the same time each day.

If you forget a dose:
Take as soon as you remember. If it is almost time for the next dose, wait for next scheduled dose (don't double this dose).

What drug does:
- Forces sodium and water excretion, reducing body fluid.
- Relaxes muscle cells of small arteries.

Continued next column

OVERDOSE

SYMPTOMS:
Irregular heartbeat (usually too slow), seizures, confusion, fainting, convulsions, coma.
WHAT TO DO:
- **Dial 911 (emergency) for medical help or call poison control center 1-800-222-1222 for instructions.**
- **See emergency information on last 3 pages of this book.**

- Reduced body fluid and relaxed arteries lower blood pressure.
- Blocks some of the actions of sympathetic nervous system.
- Lowers heart's oxygen requirements.
- Slows nerve impulses through heart.
- Reduces blood vessel contraction in heart, scalp and other body parts.

Time lapse before drug works:
- 1 to 4 hours for beta-blocker effect.
- May require several weeks to lower blood pressure.

Don't take with:
Any other medicines, even over-the-counter drugs such as cough/cold medicines, diet pills, nose drops, or caffeine, without consulting your doctor or pharmacist.

POSSIBLE ADVERSE REACTIONS OR SIDE EFFECTS

SYMPTOMS	WHAT TO DO
Life-threatening: Wheezing, chest pain, seizures, irregular heartbeat.	Seek emergency treatment immediately.
Common:	
• Dry mouth, weak pulse, vomiting, muscle cramps, increased thirst, mood changes, nausea.	Discontinue. Call doctor right away.
• Weakness, tiredness, dizziness, mental depression, diminished sex drive, constipation, nightmares, insomnia.	Continue. Call doctor when convenient.
Infrequent:	
• Cold feet and hands, chest pain, breathing difficulty, anxiety, nervousness, headache, appetite loss, abdominal pain, numbness and tingling in fingers and toes, slow heartbeat.	Discontinue. Call doctor right away.
• Confusion, diarrhea.	Continue. Call doctor when convenient.
Rare:	
• Hives, skin rash; joint pain; jaundice; fever, sore throat, mouth ulcers.	Discontinue. Call doctor right away.
• Impotence, back pain.	Continue. Call doctor when convenient.

BETA-ADRENERGIC BLOCKING AGENTS & THIAZIDE DIURETICS

WARNINGS & PRECAUTIONS

Don't take if:
- You are allergic to any beta-adrenergic blocker or any thiazide diuretic drug.
- You have asthma or hay fever symptoms.
- You have taken MAO inhibitors in past two weeks.

Before you start, consult your doctor if:
- You have heart disease or poor circulation to the extremities.
- You have hay fever, asthma, chronic bronchitis, emphysema, overactive thyroid function, impaired liver or kidney function, gout, diabetes, hypoglycemia, pancreas disorder, systemic lupus erythematosus.
- You are allergic to any sulfa drug or tartrazine dye.
- You will have surgery within 2 months, including dental surgery, requiring general or spinal anesthesia.

Over age 60:
Adverse reactions and side effects may be more frequent and severe than in younger persons, especially dizziness and excessive potassium loss.

Pregnancy:
Risk factors vary for drugs in this group. See category list on page xviii and consult doctor.

Breast-feeding:
Drug passes into milk. Avoid drug or discontinue nursing until you finish medicine. Consult doctor for advice on maintaining milk supply.

Infants & children:
Not recommended.

Prolonged use:
- Weakens heart muscle contractions.
- You may need medicine to treat high blood pressure for the rest of your life.
- Talk to your doctor about the need for follow-up medical examinations or laboratory studies.

Skin & sunlight:
One or more drugs in this group may cause rash or intensify sunburn in areas exposed to sun or ultraviolet light (photosensitivity reaction). Avoid overexposure. Notify doctor if reaction occurs.

Driving, piloting or hazardous work:
Don't drive or pilot aircraft until you learn how medicine affects you. Don't work around dangerous machinery. Don't climb ladders or work in high places. Danger increases if you drink alcohol or take medicine affecting alertness and reflexes, such as antihistamines, tranquilizers, sedatives, pain medicine, narcotics and mind-altering drugs.

Discontinuing:
Don't discontinue without consulting doctor. Dose may require gradual reduction if you have taken drug for a long time. Doses of other drugs may also require adjustment.

Others:
- May mask hypoglycemia symptoms.
- Hot weather and fever may cause dehydration and drop in blood pressure. Dose may require temporary adjustment. Weigh daily and report any unexpected weight decreases to your doctor.
- May cause rise in uric acid, leading to gout.
- May cause blood sugar rise in diabetics.

POSSIBLE INTERACTION WITH OTHER DRUGS

GENERIC NAME OR DRUG CLASS	COMBINED EFFECT
Allopurinol	Decreased allopurinol effect.
Aminophylline	Decreased effectiveness of both.
Antidepressants, tricyclic*	Dangerous drop in blood pressure. Avoid combination unless under medical supervision.

Continued on page 911

POSSIBLE INTERACTION WITH OTHER SUBSTANCES

INTERACTS WITH	COMBINED EFFECT
Alcohol:	Dangerous blood pressure drop. Avoid.
Beverages:	None expected.
Cocaine:	Irregular heartbeat, decreased beta blocker effect. Avoid.
Foods: Licorice.	Excessive potassium loss that causes dangerous heart rhythms.
Marijuana:	May increase blood pressure.
Tobacco:	May increase blood pressure and make heart work harder. Avoid.

*See Glossary

BETHANECHOL

BRAND NAMES

Duvoid   Urecholine
Urabeth

BASIC INFORMATION

Habit forming? No
Prescription needed? Yes
Available as generic? Yes
Drug class: Cholinergic

 USES

- Helps initiate urination following surgery, or for persons with urinary infections or enlarged prostate.
- Treats reflux esophagitis.

 DOSAGE & USAGE INFORMATION

How to take:
Tablet—Swallow with liquid, 1 hour before or 2 hours after eating.

When to take:
At the same times each day.

If you forget a dose:
Take as soon as you remember up to 2 hours late. If more than 2 hours, wait for next scheduled dose (don't double this dose).

What drug does:
Affects chemical reactions in the body that strengthen bladder muscles.

Time lapse before drug works:
30 to 90 minutes.

Don't take with:
Any other medicine or any dietary supplement without consulting your doctor or pharmacist.

 OVERDOSE

SYMPTOMS:
Shortness of breath, wheezing or chest tightness, unconsciousness, coma.
WHAT TO DO:
- Dial 911 (emergency) for medical help or call poison control center 1-800-222-1222 for instructions.
- If person is unconscious, check breathing and pulse. If not breathing, begin mouth-to-mouth rescue breathing. If heart is not beating, begin chest compressions.
- See emergency information on last 3 pages of this book.

 POSSIBLE ADVERSE REACTIONS OR SIDE EFFECTS

SYMPTOMS	WHAT TO DO
Life-threatening: In case of overdose, see previous column.	
Common: None expected.	
Infrequent: Dizziness, headache, faintness, blurred or changed vision, diarrhea, nausea, vomiting, stomach discomfort, belching, excessive urge to urinate.	Continue. Call doctor when convenient.
Rare: Shortness of breath, wheezing, tightness in chest.	Discontinue. Call doctor right away.

WARNINGS & PRECAUTIONS

Don't take if:
You are allergic to any cholinergic.

Before you start, consult your doctor if:
* You plan to become pregnant within medication period.
* You have asthma.
* You have epilepsy.
* You have heart or blood vessel disease.
* You have high or low blood pressure.
* You have overactive thyroid.
* You have intestinal blockage.
* You have Parkinson's disease.
* You have stomach problems (including ulcer).
* You have had bladder or intestinal surgery within 1 month.

Over age 60:
Adverse reactions and side effects may be more frequent and severe than in younger persons.

Pregnancy:
Decide with your doctor if drug benefits justify risk to unborn child. Risk category C (see page xviii).

Breast-feeding:
Unknown effect. Consult doctor.

Infants & children:
Use only under medical supervision.

Prolonged use:
No problems expected.

Skin & sunlight:
No problems expected.

Driving, piloting or hazardous work:
Don't drive or pilot aircraft until you learn how medicine effects you. Don't work around dangerous machinery. Don't climb ladders or work in high places. Danger increases if you drink alcohol or take medicine affecting alertness and reflexes, such as antihistamines, tranquilizers, sedatives, pain medicine, narcotics and mind-altering drugs.

Discontinuing:
May be unnecessary to finish medicine. Follow doctor's instructions.

Others:
* Be cautious about standing up suddenly.
* Advise any doctor or dentist whom you consult that you take this medicine.
* Interferes with laboratory studies of liver and pancreas function.

POSSIBLE INTERACTION WITH OTHER DRUGS

GENERIC NAME OR DRUG CLASS	COMBINED EFFECT
Cholinergics, other*	Increased effect of both drugs. Possible toxicity.
Ganglionic blockers*	Decreased blood pressure.
Nitrates*	Decreased bethanechol effect.
Procainamide	Decreased bethanechol effect.
Quinidine	Decreased bethanechol effect.

POSSIBLE INTERACTION WITH OTHER SUBSTANCES

INTERACTS WITH	COMBINED EFFECT
Alcohol:	None expected.
Beverages:	None expected.
Cocaine:	None expected.
Foods:	None expected.
Marijuana:	None expected.
Tobacco:	None expected.

BIOLOGICS FOR PSORIASIS

GENERIC AND BRAND NAMES

ALEFACEPT
  Amevive

BASIC INFORMATION

Habit forming? No
Prescription needed? Yes
Available as generic? No
Drug class: Immunosuppressive;
  antipsoriatic

 ## USES

Treatment for adult patients with moderate to severe, chronic, plaque psoriasis. It helps treat the cause of psoriasis as well as treating the symptoms.

 ## DOSAGE & USAGE INFORMATION

How to take:
Injection—It is injected weekly by a health care provider for 12-24 weeks.

When to take:
Once a week on the same day each week.

If you forget a dose:
For an injection given by a health care provider, call the medical office.

What drug does:
The exact mechanism is unknown. The drug blocks certain cells in the body's immune system to help prevent skin inflammation that leads to psoriasis.

Time lapse before drug works:
Improvement may be seen in 4 weeks, but it may take 3 months for maximum benefits.

Don't take with:
Any other medicine or any dietary supplement without consulting your doctor or pharmacist.

 ## OVERDOSE

SYMPTOMS:
Unknown effects.
WHAT TO DO:
If person takes much larger amount than prescribed, call doctor, poison control center 1-800-222-1222 or hospital emergency room for help.

 ## POSSIBLE ADVERSE REACTIONS OR SIDE EFFECTS

SYMPTOMS	WHAT TO DO
Life-threatening: Rare allergic reaction— Breathing difficulty; swelling of hands, feet, face, mouth, neck; skin rash.	Discontinue. Seek emergency treatment.
Common: • Chills, fever, cough, urination painful or difficult, lower back or side pain, hoarseness.	Discontinue. Call doctor right away.
• Injection site problems (pain, swelling, rash, bleeding, lumps).	Continue. Call doctor when convenient.
Infrequent: • Congestion, dry or sore throat, body aches or pain, runny nose, swollen or tender neck glands, signs of infection, swallowing difficulty, voice changes.	Discontinue. Call doctor right away.
• Dizziness, itching skin, painful or swollen joints, muscle aches or stiffness, difficulty in moving, headache.	Continue. Call doctor when convenient.
Rare: Chest symptoms (pain, heaviness, tightness, discomfort), arm or jaw pain, fast or irregular heartbeat, shortness of breath, nausea or vomiting, sweating, bloating, dark urine, tiredness or weakness, light color stools, loss of appetite, yellow eyes or skin, flu-like symptoms.	Discontinue. Call doctor right away.

WARNINGS & PRECAUTIONS

Don't take if:
You are allergic to alefacept.

Before you start, consult your doctor if:
- You have kidney or liver problems.
- You have heart or blood vessel disorders.
- You have or have had cancer.
- You have any type of infection or have recurrent or chronic infections.
- You have a weak (suppressed) immune system due to illness or drugs.
- You are getting phototherapy treatment.
- You are allergic to any medication, food or other substance.

Over age 60:
Unknown effect. Adverse reactions and side effects may be more frequent and severe.

Pregnancy:
Decide with your doctor if drug benefits justify risks to unborn child. Risk category B. (see page xviii).

Breast-feeding:
It is unknown if drug passes into milk. Avoid drug or discontinue nursing until you finish medicine. Consult doctor for advice on maintaining milk supply.

Infants & children:
Not recommended for ages under 18.

Prolonged use:
- Long-term use has not been established. Alefacept may be given for two 12 week periods. Discuss continued use with the doctor.
- Visit the doctor regularly to see if the drug continues to be effective and to monitor your blood and platelet counts. If they get too low, the drug may be stopped on a temporary or permanent basis.

Skin & sunlight:
No special problems expected.

Driving, piloting or hazardous work:
Avoid if you feel dizzy, otherwise no special problems expected.

Discontinuing:
Consult doctor about discontinuing.

Others:
- Advise any doctor or dentist whom you consult about the use of this medicine.
- The drug may increase the risk of developing cancer.
- Because the drug affects the immune system, you are at risk for new infections or reactivation of a chronic infection that has not been active. These include bacterial, viral and fungal infections that can be serious, possibly fatal. Call your doctor right away if symptoms of an infection develop.
- Avoid people with infections and people who have recently had a live virus vaccine.

POSSIBLE INTERACTION WITH OTHER DRUGS

GENERIC NAME OR DRUG CLASS	COMBINED EFFECT
Immunosuppressants,* other	Increased risk of infections or cancer.
Other drugs	Unknown. Consult doctor or pharmacist.
Vaccines, live virus	Unknown. May decrease effect of vaccine or may be harmful.

POSSIBLE INTERACTION WITH OTHER SUBSTANCES

INTERACTS WITH	COMBINED EFFECT
Alcohol:	None expected. Best to avoid.
Beverages:	None expected.
Cocaine:	Unknown. Best to avoid.
Foods:	None expected.
Marijuana:	Unknown. Best to avoid.
Tobacco:	None expected.

*See Glossary

BISMUTH SALTS

GENERIC AND BRAND NAMES

BISKALCITRATE
  Pylera

BISMUTH SUB-
  SALICYLATE
  Bismatrol
  Helidac
  Maalox Total
    Stomach Relief
  Pepto-Bismol

BASIC INFORMATION

Habit forming? No
Prescription needed? No
Available as generic? Yes
Drug class: Antidiarrheal; antacid

 USES

- Treats symptoms of diarrhea, heartburn, nausea, acid indigestion.
- Helps prevent traveler's diarrhea.
- Treats ulcers.
- Used with other medications to treat a stomach infected by the bacteria *H. Pylori*.

 DOSAGE & USAGE INFORMATION

How to take:
- Tablet—Swallow with water.
- Chewable tablet—Chew well before swallowing.
- Liquid—Take as directed on label.

When to take:
As directed on label or by your doctor.

If you forget a dose:
Take as soon as you remember. Don't double this dose.

Continued next column

 OVERDOSE

SYMPTOMS:
Hearing loss, ringing or buzzing in the ears, severe drowsiness or tiredness, severe excitement or nervousness, fast or deep breathing, unconsciousness or death.
WHAT TO DO:
- **Dial 911 (emergency) for medical help or call poison control center 1-800-222-1222 for instructions.**
- **See emergency information on last 3 pages of this book.**

What drug does:
- Decreases inflammation and increased motility of the intestinal muscles and lining.
- In combination with other drugs, it works to destroy certain bacterial infections.

Time lapse before drug works:
30 minutes to 1 hour.

Don't take with:
Any other medicine or any dietary supplement without consulting your doctor or pharmacist.

 POSSIBLE ADVERSE REACTIONS OR SIDE EFFECTS

SYMPTOMS	WHAT TO DO
Life-threatening: In case of overdose, see previous column.	
Common: Black stools, dark tongue. (These symptoms are normal and medically insignificant.)	No action necessary.
Infrequent: None expected.	
Rare: Abdominal pain, increased sweating, muscle weakness, drowsiness, anxiety, trembling, hearing loss, ringing or buzzing in ears, confusion, dizziness, headache, increased thirst, vision problems, severe constipation, continuing diarrhea, trouble breathing (all more likely to occur with high doses or chronic use).	Discontinue. Call doctor right away.

WARNINGS & PRECAUTIONS

Don't take if:
- You are allergic to aspirin, salicylates or other nonsteroidal anti-inflammatory drugs.
- You have stomach ulcers that have ever bled.
- The patient is a child with fever.

Before you start, consult your doctor if:
- You are on a low-sodium, low-sugar or other special diet.
- You have had diarrhea for more than 24 hours. This is especially applicable to infants, children and those over 60.
- You have had kidney disease.

Over age 60:
- Consult doctor before using.
- May cause severe constipation.

Pregnancy:
Decide with your doctor if drug benefits justify risk to unborn child. Risk category C; D in third trimester (see page xviii).

Breast-feeding:
Drug passes into milk. Avoid or discontinue nursing until you finish medicine. Consult doctor about maintaining milk supply.

Infants & children:
Not recommended for children 3 and younger. May cause constipation.

Prolonged use:
May cause constipation.

Skin & sunlight:
No problems expected.

Driving, piloting or hazardous work:
Don't drive or pilot aircraft if you take high or prolonged dose until you learn how medicine affects you. Don't work around dangerous machinery. Don't climb ladders or work in high places. Danger increases if you drink alcohol or take medicine affecting alertness and reflexes, such as antihistamines, tranquilizers, sedatives, pain medicine, narcotics and mind-altering drugs.

Discontinuing:
No problems expected.

Others:
- Pepto-Bismol contains salicylates. When given to children with flu or chicken pox, salicylates may cause a serious illness called Reye's syndrome.* An overdose in children can cause the same problems as aspirin poisoning.
- May cause false urine sugar tests.
- Dehydration can develop if too much body fluid has been lost. Consult doctor if any of the following symptoms occur: decreased urination, dizziness or lightheadedness, dryness of mouth, increased thirst, wrinkled skin.

- Don't store tablet form of drug in bathroom or near kitchen sink. Heat and moisture can cause it to break down.
- Consult doctor if diarrhea doesn't improve within 2 days.
- Read labels of any other drugs being used, such as for pain or inflammation. They may contain salicylates* and can lead to increased risk of side effects and overdose.

POSSIBLE INTERACTION WITH OTHER DRUGS

GENERIC NAME OR DRUG CLASS	COMBINED EFFECT
Anticoagulants*	Increased risk of bleeding.
Insulin or oral antidiabetic drugs*	Increased insulin effect. May require dosage adjustment.
Probenecid	Decreased effect of probenecid.
Salicylates,* other	Increased risk of salicylate toxicity.
Sulfinpyrazone	Decreased effect of sulfinpyrazone.
Tetracyclines*	Decreased absorption of tetracycline.
Thrombolytic agents*	Increased risk of bleeding.

POSSIBLE INTERACTION WITH OTHER SUBSTANCES

INTERACTS WITH	COMBINED EFFECT
Alcohol:	None expected.
Beverages:	None expected.
Cocaine:	Decreased bismuth subsalicylate effect. Avoid.
Foods:	None expected.
Marijuana:	None expected.
Tobacco:	None expected.

*See Glossary

BISPHOSPHONATES

GENERIC AND BRAND NAMES

ALENDRONATE
  Fosamax
  Fosamax Plus D
  Fosavance
ETIDRONATE
  Didronel
IBANDRONATE
  Boniva
PAMIDRONATE
  Aredia

RISEDRONATE
  Actonel
  Actonel with
    Calcium
TILUDRONATE
  Skelid
ZOLEDRONIC ACID
  Reclast
  Zometa

BASIC INFORMATION

Habit forming? No
Prescription needed? Yes
Available as generic? Yes, for some
**Drug class: Osteoporosis therapy,
    bisphosphonate; osteopenia therapy**

USES

- Prevention and treatment of postmenopausal osteopenia and osteoporosis (thinning of bones). Treatment for osteoporosis in men.
- Treats osteoporosis caused by certain drugs.
- May be used to treat other bone disease or bone cancer as determined by your doctor.
- Treatment for Paget's disease of bone.
- Treatment for hypercalcemia (high calcium).

DOSAGE & USAGE INFORMATION

How to take:
- Tablet (alendronate or risedronate)—Swallow with a full glass of water (6 to 8 oz.). To help the medicine reach your stomach faster and to prevent throat irritation, stay upright for 30 minutes after you take it. Don't lie down.
- Tablet (etidronate or tiludronate)—Take morning, midday or evening 2 hours before or after any food.

Continued next column

OVERDOSE

SYMPTOMS:
May rarely increase the severity of heartburn, stomach cramps, throat irritation.
WHAT TO DO:
Overdose unlikely to threaten life. If person takes much larger amount than prescribed, call doctor, poison control center 1-800-222-1222 or hospital emergency room for help.

- Tablet (ibandronate)—Take before first meal of the day. Swallow whole with water (6 to 8 oz). Do not lie down for 60 minutes.
- Injection—Etidronate, pamidronate or zoledronic acid are given by a medical person.

When to take:
- Daily dose (alendronate or risedronate), take first thing in the morning at least 30 to 60 minutes before eating, drinking or taking any other medications.
- Daily dose (etidronate or tiludronate), take anytime during the day 2 hours before or 2 hours after eating.
- Once-a-week dose, take on the same day each week. Follow instructions as daily dose.
- Once a month dose (ibandronate), take on the same date each month.

If you forget a dose:
- Daily dose taken first thing in morning: skip the missed dose entirely, then resume schedule the next day. Do not double this dose.
- For weekly dose: take the next morning and then return to your regular weekly schedule.
- Daily dose taken anytime: take as soon as you remember. If it is almost time for the next dose, wait for the next scheduled dose (don't double this dose).

What drug does:
Slows down the loss of bone tissue and increases bone mass. Osteoporosis and osteopenia are progressive diseases in which bone breakdown increases faster than bone formation.

Time lapse before drug works:
Up to 6 months or longer.

Don't take with:
- Any other medicine or any dietary supplement without consulting your doctor or pharmacist.
- Any other medication at the same time as the bisphosphonate. Follow doctor's instructions.

POSSIBLE ADVERSE REACTIONS OR SIDE EFFECTS

SYMPTOMS	WHAT TO DO
Life-threatening: None expected.	
Common: Stomach pain.	Continue. Call doctor when convenient.
Infrequent: Mild bone or muscle pain, nausea, diarrhea, constipation, gas, leg cramps, bloated feeling, anxiety, depression, throat pain or irritation, mild heartburn, swallowing difficulty, headache, weak muscles.	Continue. Call doctor when convenient.

Rare:

• Skin rash, ankle or leg swelling, eye or dental problems, cold or flu symptoms.	Continue. Call doctor when convenient.
• Chest pain, severe throat pain, severe heartburn, severe muscle pain.	Discontinue. Call doctor right away.

WARNINGS & PRECAUTIONS

Don't take if:
You are allergic to any bisphosphonate.

Before you start, consult your doctor if:
• You currently have a gastrointestinal problem or serious esophageal disease.
• You have low blood levels of calcium (hypocalcemia) or vitamin D deficiency.
• You have asthma or heart disease.
• You have dental disease or plan dental surgery. Consult your dentist also.
• You have kidney problems.

Over age 60:
No special problems expected.

Pregnancy:
Risk factors vary for drugs in this group. See category list on page xviii and consult doctor.

Breast-feeding:
Unknown if drugs pass into milk. Avoid drug or discontinue nursing until you finish medicine. Consult doctor for advice on maintaining milk supply.

Infants & children:
Not recommended for this age group.

Prolonged use:
Visit your doctor regularly to determine if the drug is continuing to control bone loss.

Skin & sunlight:
No special problems expected.

Driving, piloting or hazardous work:
No special problems expected.

Discontinuing:
No problems expected, but don't discontinue without your doctor's approval. After stopping the drug, it still remains in the body bound to the bone for as long as 10 years in some patients.

Others:
• In addition to taking the drug, weight-bearing exercise and adequate dietary intake of calcium and vitamin D are essential in preventing bone loss. Your doctor may prescribe calcium and vitamin D supplements.
• May affect the results of some medical tests.
• To avoid throat (esophagus) problems, carefully follow directions for taking the drug.

• Advise any doctor and especially any dentist whom you consult that you take this medicine.
• Though rare, bisphosphonates can increase the risk for osteonecrosis (bone destruction), especially of the jaw. Dental disease, oral surgery or tooth removal add to the risk. Talk to your doctor and dentist about your risks.

POSSIBLE INTERACTION WITH OTHER DRUGS

GENERIC NAME OR DRUG CLASS	COMBINED EFFECT
Antacids*	Decreased effect of bisphosphonate. Take 30 minutes after bisphosphonate.
Aspirin-containing products	Increased risk of stomach irritation.
Calcium supplements*	Decreased effect of bisphosphonate. Take 30 minutes after bisphosphonate.
Mineral or vitamin supplements	Decreased effect of bisphosphonate. Take 30 minutes after bisphosphonate.

POSSIBLE INTERACTION WITH OTHER SUBSTANCES

INTERACTS WITH	COMBINED EFFECT
Alcohol:	None expected. Alcohol will increase risk for osteoporosis. Try to avoid.
Beverages: Any beverage other than plain water.	Decreased effect of drug. Wait 30 minutes after you take drug.
Cocaine:	No special problems expected.
Foods: Any food.	Decreased effect of drug. Wait 30 minutes to 2 hours after you take drug.
Marijuana:	No special problems expected.
Tobacco:	None expected. Smoking will increase risk for osteoporosis. Try to avoid.

*See Glossary

BONE FORMATION AGENTS

GENERIC AND BRAND NAMES

TERIPARATIDE
 Forteo

BASIC INFORMATION

Habit forming? No
Prescription needed? Yes
Available as generic? No
Drug class: Osteoporosis therapy

USES

- Treatment of advanced postmenopausal osteoporosis (thinning of bones) in females. Osteoporosis is a cause of bone fractures.
- Treatment for hypogonadal osteoporosis in men at high risk for fracture.

DOSAGE & USAGE INFORMATION

How to take:
Injection—Inject under the skin (subcutaneously) with the pen device provided. Follow your doctor's instructions and the directions provided with the prescription on how, when and where to inject. Do not use the medication unless you are sure about the proper method for injection. Store medication in the refrigerator (do not freeze) until you plan to use it.

When to take:
At the same time each day.

If you forget a dose:
Inject as soon as possible. If it is almost time for your next dose, skip the missed dose and go back to your regular dosing schedule. Do not double doses.

What drug does:
Increases the action of osteoblasts, the body's bone building cells. The bones become more dense and more resistant to fractures.

Time lapse before drug works:
Up to 3 months or longer.

Don't take with:
Any other medicine or any dietary supplement without consulting your doctor or pharmacist.

OVERDOSE

SYMPTOMS:
None expected.
WHAT TO DO:
If an overdose is suspected, call doctor or call poison control center 1-800-222-1222 for help.

POSSIBLE ADVERSE REACTIONS OR SIDE EFFECTS

SYMPTOMS	WHAT TO DO
Life-threatening: None expected.	
Common: None expected.	
Infrequent: Injection site discomfort or redness, nausea, headache, stomach cramps, dizziness.	Continue. Call doctor when convenient.
Rare: Leg cramps, light-headedness when rising after sitting or lying down, syncope (fainting), vertigo.	Continue. Call doctor when convenient.

WARNINGS & PRECAUTIONS

Don't take if:
You are allergic to teriparatide or its components.

Before you start, consult your doctor if:
- You have had radiation treatment on the skeleton (bones).
- You have excess calcium in blood (hypercalcemia) or urine (hypercalcuria).
- You have or have had bone cancer/disease.
- You have Paget's disease.
- You have urolithiasis.
- You are allergic to any medication, food or other substance or latex.

Over age 60:
No special problems expected, but caution should be used in the elderly.

Pregnancy:
Normally not used in premenopausal women. Risk category C (see page xviii).

Breast-feeding:
Normally not used in premenopausal women.

Infants & children:
Not recommended for this age group.

Prolonged use:
- Long-term use after 2 years has not been established. Discuss with your doctor.
- Visit your doctor regularly to determine if the drug is continuing to be effective and to monitor your calcium levels.

Skin & sunlight:
No special problems expected.

Driving, piloting or hazardous work:
No special problems expected.

Discontinuing:
No problems expected. Consult doctor.

Others:
- In medical studies on rats injected with teriparatide, a few developed bone cancer (osteosarcoma). Risk in humans is unknown. To date, no women taking the drug have developed the cancer.
- Too much calcium in the blood (hypercalcemia) occurs in some patients using this drug. Consult your doctor about blood tests.
- Other therapies and nondrug routines (e.g., weight-bearing exercise), for treating osteo-porosis may be recommended by your doctor. Teriparatide works effectively with certain other drugs for osteoporosis because the drugs work by different mechanisms.
- Advise any doctor or dentist whom you consult that you take this medicine.
- Smoking and alcohol consumption are risk factors for osteoporosis and should be discontinued.

POSSIBLE INTERACTION WITH OTHER DRUGS

GENERIC NAME OR DRUG CLASS	COMBINED EFFECT
Other drugs	Consult doctor or pharmacist.

POSSIBLE INTERACTION WITH OTHER SUBSTANCES

INTERACTS WITH	COMBINED EFFECT
Alcohol:	No special problems expected, but alcohol is a risk factor for osteoporosis.
Beverages:	No special problems expected.
Cocaine:	No special problems expected.
Foods:	No special problems expected.
Marijuana:	No special problems expected.
Tobacco:	No special problems expected, but smoking is a risk factor for osteoporosis.

*See Glossary

BOTULINUM TOXIN TYPE A

BRAND NAMES

Botox   Botox Cosmetic

BASIC INFORMATION

Habit forming? No
Prescription needed? Yes
Available as generic? No
Drug class: Neuromuscular blocking agent

 ## USES

- Provides temporary improvement in appearance in the frown lines between the eyebrows (glabellar lines). May also be used for lines and wrinkles in the forehead, around the eyes, in the lower face area and the neck.
- Treats strabismus (lazy eye) and blepharospasm (uncontrolled eye blinking).
- Treats certain facial nerve disorders and cervical dystonia (neck and shoulder tightness).
- May be used for treatment of other disorders as determined by your doctor (such as headaches, writer's cramp, excessive sweating, tremor, muscle-related disorders, pain and effects of a stroke). Research is ongoing for use in treating a variety of medical disorders.

 ## DOSAGE & USAGE INFORMATION

How to take:
Injection—The medicine is administered by your doctor or a qualified health professional. It is injected into the muscle in or around the area being treated.

When to take:
As directed by your doctor.

If you forget a dose:
Injection is done only by scheduled appointment.

What drug does:
It paralyzes, weakens or relaxes the injected muscle by blocking the release of a chemical that normally signals the muscle to contract or tighten. The effect is temporary and most patients will require repeat treatments.

Continued next column

 ## OVERDOSE

SYMPTOMS:
Unknown. May possibly cause body weakness.
WHAT TO DO:
If accidentally injected or swallowed, call doctor or call poison control center 1-800-222-1222 for help.

Time lapse before drug works:
Improvement may be seen in 1-3 days and lasts up to 3-6 months. The degree of improvement will vary from person to person and will depend on the disorder being treated.

Don't take with:
Any other medicine or any dietary supplement without consulting your doctor or pharmacist.

 ## POSSIBLE ADVERSE REACTIONS OR SIDE EFFECTS

SYMPTOMS	WHAT TO DO
Life-threatening: None expected.	
Common:	
• With blepharospasm (dry eyes, eyelid does not close completely).	Call doctor right away.
• With blepharospasm or strabismus (eye irritation or watering, eyelid drooping or bruised, light sensitivity).	Call doctor if you are concerned or symptoms continue.
Infrequent:	
• With blepharospasm or strabismus (blinking decreased, cornea irritation, eyelid edge turns in or out, skin rash, eyelid swelling, vision changes, eye pointing up or down).	Call doctor right away.
• With lines/wrinkles (injection site numb, burning or swelling).	Call doctor if you are concerned or symptoms continue.
Rare:	
• Any problems with speech, breathing or swallowing or heart symptoms occur or allergic reaction occurs.	Call doctor right away or seek emergency treatment if symptoms severe.
• With lines/wrinkles (drooping eyelids, redness or bruising at injection site, facial pain, skin rash or itching, headache, nausea, flu or cold symptoms).	Call doctor if you are concerned or symptoms continue.
• Other side effects or adverse reactions may occur depending on the disorder being treated. Drugs injected into muscles can be absorbed by the body and cause symptoms.	Call doctor if you are concerned or symptoms continue or they are severe.

WARNINGS & PRECAUTIONS

Don't take if:
You are allergic to botulinum toxin type A.

Before you start, consult your doctor if:
- You have heart problems.
- You have a nerve or muscle disorder, or a problem with swallowing.
- You have inflammation in the muscle area to be treated.
- You are allergic to any medication, food or other substance.
- You have a history of infection involving botulism poisoning.

Over age 60:
No special problems expected. Currently, for wrinkle treatment, the drug is approved for people between ages 18 and 65.

Pregnancy:
Decide with your doctor if drug benefits justify any possible risk to unborn child. Risk category C (see page xviii). Consult doctor if you become pregnant and have had a botulinum injection.

Breast-feeding:
It is unknown if drug passes into milk. Avoid nursing if you use this medicine. Consult doctor for advice on maintaining milk supply.

Infants & children:
Not approved for children under age 12 for strabismus or blepharospasm treatment, or under age 18 for facial lines or wrinkle treatment.

Prolonged use:
- Long term effects are unknown. Discuss with you doctor about long term use. Benefits and risks will differ depending on the problem being treated.
- Benefits may decrease with continued use.
- For facial lines and wrinkles, the injections should be at least 3 months apart.

Skin & sunlight:
No special problems expected.

Driving, piloting or hazardous work:
Since this medicine may be used for treatment of a variety of disorders (including eye muscle disorders, muscle contraction problems and muscle spasms), always consult your doctor about your individual circumstances.

Discontinuing:
Symptoms and signs of the problem being treated will most likely return.

Others:
- This treatment is given in a medical office and the risks and benefits will be explained to you. The information provided in this topic does not replace the information or special instructions provided by your doctor.
- Patients who have been inactive (sedentary) should resume activities gradually after receiving an injection.
- Advise any doctor or dentist whom you consult (within the few months following the injection) that you have used this medicine.

POSSIBLE INTERACTION WITH OTHER DRUGS

GENERIC NAME OR DRUG CLASS	COMBINED EFFECT
Aminoglycosides*	Increased effect of botulinum toxin type A.

POSSIBLE INTERACTION WITH OTHER SUBSTANCES

INTERACTS WITH	COMBINED EFFECT
Alcohol:	None expected.
Beverages:	None expected.
Cocaine:	None expected. Best to avoid.
Foods:	None expected.
Marijuana:	May contribute to facial lines. Avoid.
Tobacco:	May contribute to facial lines. Avoid.

*See Glossary

BROMOCRIPTINE

BRAND NAMES

Alti-Bromocriptine   Parlodel
Apo-Bromocriptine   Parlodel Snaptabs

BASIC INFORMATION

Habit forming? No
Prescription needed? Yes
Available as generic? Yes
Drug class: Antiparkinsonism

 ## USES

- Controls Parkinson's disease symptoms such as rigidity, tremors and unsteady gait.
- Treats male and female infertility.
- Treats acromegaly (an overproduction of growth hormone).
- Treats some pituitary tumors.

 ## DOSAGE & USAGE INFORMATION

How to take:
Tablet or capsule—Swallow with liquid or food to lessen stomach irritation. If you can't swallow whole, crumble tablet or open capsule and take with liquid or food.

When to take:
At the same times each day.

If you forget a dose:
Take as soon as you remember up to 2 hours late. If more than 2 hours, wait for next scheduled dose (don't double this dose).

What drug does:
Restores chemical balance necessary for normal nerve impulses.

Continued next column

 ## OVERDOSE

SYMPTOMS:
Muscle twitch, spastic eyelid closure, nausea, vomiting, diarrhea, irregular and rapid pulse, weakness, fainting, confusion, agitation, hallucination, coma.
WHAT TO DO:
- **Dial 911 (emergency) for medical help or call poison control center 1-800-222-1222 for instructions.**
- **If person is unconscious, check breathing and pulse. If not breathing, begin mouth-to-mouth rescue breathing. If heart is not beating, begin chest compressions.**
- **See emergency information on last 3 pages of this book.**

Time lapse before drug works:
2 to 3 weeks to improve; several months or longer for maximum benefit.

Don't take with:
Any other medicine or any dietary supplement without consulting your doctor or pharmacist.

 ## POSSIBLE ADVERSE REACTIONS OR SIDE EFFECTS

SYMPTOMS	WHAT TO DO
Life-threatening:	
In case of overdose, see previous column.	
Common:	
Dizziness, mild nausea, lightheadedness when getting up, headache.	Continue. Call doctor when convenient.
Infrequent:	
Constipation, diarrhea, tiredness, drowsiness, dry mouth, depression, tingling and numbness of hands and feet.	Continue. Call doctor when convenient.
Rare:	
• Severe nausea and vomiting (may be bloody), vision changes, nervousness, sudden weakness, unusual headache, excess sweating, seizures, fainting, chest pain, black or tarry stools, uncontrollable body movements.	Discontinue. Call doctor right away.
• Stomach or back pain, runny nose, urinary frequency.	Continue. Call doctor when convenient.

WARNINGS & PRECAUTIONS

Don't take if:
- You are allergic to bromocriptine or ergotamine.
- You have taken a monoamine oxidase (MAO) inhibitor* in the past 2 weeks.
- You have glaucoma (narrow-angle type).

Before you start, consult your doctor if:
- You have diabetes or epilepsy.
- You have had high blood pressure, heart or lung disease.
- You have had liver or kidney disease.
- You have a peptic ulcer.
- You have a history of mental problems.
- You will have surgery within 2 months, requiring general or spinal anesthesia.

Over age 60:
Adverse reactions and side effects may be more frequent and severe than in younger persons.

Pregnancy:
Decide with your doctor if drug benefits justify risk to unborn child. Risk category B (see page xviii).

Breast-feeding:
Drug inhibits milk production. Avoid.

Infants & children:
Not recommended if under 15 years old.

Prolonged use:
- May lead to uncontrolled movements of head, face, mouth, tongue, arms or legs.
- Changes in lung tissue and excess fluid in chest cavity may occur.
- Talk to your doctor about the need for follow-up medical examinations or laboratory studies to check blood pressure, x-rays, growth hormone levels.

Skin & sunlight:
No problems expected.

Driving, piloting or hazardous work:
Don't drive or pilot aircraft until you learn how medicine effects you. Don't work around dangerous machinery. Don't climb ladders or work in high places. Danger increases if you drink alcohol or take medicine affecting alertness and reflexes, such as antihistamines, tranquilizers, sedatives, pain medicine, narcotics and mind-altering drugs.

Discontinuing:
Don't discontinue without doctor's advice until you complete prescribed dose, even though symptoms diminish or disappear.

Others:
- Expect to start with small doses and increase gradually to lessen frequency and severity of adverse reactions.
- Advise any doctor or dentist whom you consult that you take this medicine.

POSSIBLE INTERACTION WITH OTHER DRUGS

GENERIC NAME OR DRUG CLASS	COMBINED EFFECT
Antihypertensives*	May decrease blood pressure.
Antiparkinsonism drugs, other*	Increased bromocriptine effect.
Ergot alkaloids, other	Increased risk of high blood pressure.
Erythromycin	Increased bromocriptine effect.
Haloperidol	Decreased bromocriptine effect.
Levodopa	Decreased antiparkinson effect.
Methyldopa	Decreased bromocriptine effect.
Papaverine	Decreased bromocriptine effect.
Phenothiazines*	Decreased bromocriptine effect.
Risperidone	Increased bromocriptine effect.
Ritonavir	Increased bromocriptine effect.

POSSIBLE INTERACTION WITH OTHER SUBSTANCES

INTERACTS WITH	COMBINED EFFECT
Alcohol:	Decreased alcohol tolerance. Avoid.
Beverages:	None expected.
Cocaine:	Decreased bromocriptine effect. Avoid.
Foods:	None expected.
Marijuana:	Increased fatigue, lethargy, fainting. Avoid.
Tobacco:	Interferes with absorption. Avoid.

BRONCHODILATORS, ADRENERGIC

GENERIC AND BRAND NAMES

See full list of generic and brand names in the *Generic and Brand Name Directory*, page 880.

BASIC INFORMATION

Habit forming? No
Prescription needed? Yes, for most
Available as generic? Yes, for some
Drug class: Sympathomimetic

 ## USES

- Relieves bronchial asthma.
- Decreases congestion of breathing passages.
- Suppresses allergic reactions.
- Treats bronchoconstriction in COPD.*
- Relieves exercise-induced bronchospasm.

 ## DOSAGE & USAGE INFORMATION

How to take:
- Tablet or capsule—Swallow with liquid. You may chew or crush tablet.
- Extended-release tablet—Swallow each dose whole.
- Syrup—Take as directed on bottle.
- Drops—Dilute dose in beverage.
- Inhaler—Follow directions in package.

When to take:
As directed by your doctor.

If you forget a dose:
Take up to 2 hours late. If more than 2 hours, wait for next dose (don't double this dose).

What drug does:
- Prevents cells from releasing allergy-causing chemicals (histamines).
- Relaxes muscles of bronchial tubes.
- Decreases blood-vessel size and blood flow, thus causing decongestion.

Continued next column

 ## OVERDOSE

SYMPTOMS:
Severe anxiety, confusion, delirium, muscle tremors, rapid and irregular pulse, severe weakness.
WHAT TO DO:
- **Dial 911 (emergency) for medical help or call poison control center 1-800-222-1222 for instructions.**
- **See emergency information on last 3 pages of this book.**

Time lapse before drug works:
30 to 60 minutes.

Don't take with:
- Nonprescription drugs with ephedrine, pseudoephedrine or epinephrine.
- Nonprescription drugs for cough, cold, allergy or asthma without consulting doctor.
- Any other medicine or any dietary supplement without consulting your doctor or pharmacist.

 ## POSSIBLE ADVERSE REACTIONS OR SIDE EFFECTS

SYMPTOMS	WHAT TO DO
Life-threatening:	
In case of overdose, see previous column.	
Common:	
• Nervousness, restlessness, trembling.	Continue. Call doctor when convenient.
• Dry mouth or throat.	Continue. Tell doctor at next visit.
Infrequent:	
• Fast heartbeat, nausea, vomiting, headache, dizziness, lightheadedness.	Discontinue. Call doctor right away.
• Trouble sleeping, appetite loss, coughing.	Continue. Call doctor when convenient.
Rare:	
• Increased wheezing, difficulty breathing, chest discomfort or pain, irregular heartbeat, painful or difficult urination, allergic reaction (bluish, reddish or flushed skin; rash; itching; hives; swelling of face area; wheezing).	Discontinue. Call doctor right away or seek emergency treatment.
• Smell or taste changes.	No action necessary.

 ## WARNINGS & PRECAUTIONS

Don't take if:
You are allergic to ephedrine, any bronchodilator* drug or sulfites used in some preparations.

Before you start, consult your doctor if:
- You have high blood pressure.
- You have diabetes.
- You have cardiovascular disease.
- You have overactive thyroid gland.
- You have difficulty urinating.
- You have taken any monoamine oxidase (MAO) inhibitor* in past 2 weeks.
- You have taken digitalis preparations* in the last 7 days.

- If you will have surgery within 2 months, including dental surgery, requiring anesthesia.
- If you have pheochromocytoma.

Over age 60:
More likely to develop high blood pressure, heart rhythm disturbances, angina and to feel drug's stimulant effects.

Pregnancy:
Risk factors vary for drugs in this group. See category list on page xviii and consult doctor.

Breast-feeding:
Drug passes into milk. Avoid drug or discontinue nursing until you finish medicine. Consult doctor for advice on maintaining milk supply.

Infants & children:
No problems expected for most. Use only under close medical supervision. Xopenex is not recommended for children under 12.

Prolonged use:
- Excessive doses—Rare toxic psychosis.
- Men with enlarged prostate gland may have more urination difficulty.
- Talk to your doctor about the need for follow-up medical examinations or laboratory studies.

Skin & sunlight:
No problems expected.

Driving, piloting or hazardous work:
Avoid if you feel dizzy. Otherwise, no problems expected.

Discontinuing:
- May be unnecessary to finish medicine. Follow doctor's instructions.
- Don't suddenly discontinue the drug without medical advice.

Others:
- May affect results in some medical tests.
- Advise any doctor or dentist whom you consult that you take this medicine.
- Ask your doctor about specific risks that may involve the drug salmeterol.
- Some of these drugs may increase the chance of severe asthma episodes, and death when those episodes occur. Ask your doctor about your risk for the drug you are using.
- Complications increase if you use more than prescribed. If you need to use the drug more frequently, consult your doctor.

POSSIBLE INTERACTION WITH OTHER DRUGS

GENERIC NAME OR DRUG CLASS	COMBINED EFFECT
Antidepressants, tricyclic*	Increased effect of bronchodilator. Heart and blood pressure problems.
Antihypertensives*	Decreased anti-hypertensive effect.
Beta-adrenergic blocking agents*	Decreased effects of both drugs.
Digitalis preparations*	Serious heart rhythm disturbances.
Epinephrine	Increased bronchodilator effect.
Ergot preparations*	Serious blood-pressure rise.
Finasteride	Decreased finasteride effect.
Furazolidone	Increased risk of heart problems.
Maprotiline	Increased risk of heart problems.
Methyldopa	Increased risk of heart problems.
Monoamine oxidase (MAO) inhibitors*	Increased broncho-dilator effect. Increased risk of heart problems.
Nicotine	Decreased effect of isoproterenol.
Nitrates*	Decreased effect of both drugs.
Phenothiazines*	Increased risk of heart problems.
Pseudoephedrine	Increased effect of bronchodilator.

Continued on page 912

POSSIBLE INTERACTION WITH OTHER SUBSTANCES

INTERACTS WITH	COMBINED EFFECT
Alcohol:	None expected.
Beverages: Caffeine drinks.	Nervousness or insomnia.
Grapefruit juice	Risk of toxicity of theophylline. Avoid.
Cocaine:	Irregular heartbeat and high blood pressure. Avoid.
Foods:	None expected.
Marijuana:	Rapid heartbeat or heart rhythm problem. Avoid.
Tobacco:	None expected.

BRONCHODILATORS, XANTHINE

GENERIC AND BRAND NAMES

See full list of generic and brand names in the *Generic and Brand Name Directory*, page 880.

BASIC INFORMATION

Habit forming? No
Prescription needed? Yes
Available as generic? Yes
Drug class: Bronchodilator (xanthine)

 USES

- Treatment for bronchial asthma symptoms.
- Treatment for chronic bronchitis, emphysema and other pulmonary diseases.

 DOSAGE & USAGE INFORMATION

How to take:
- Tablet or capsule—Swallow with liquid.
- Extended-release tablet or capsule—Swallow each dose whole. If you take regular tablets, you may chew or crush them.
- Suppository—Remove wrapper and moisten suppository with water. Gently insert larger end into rectum. Push well into rectum with finger.
- Syrup, elixir or oral solution—Take as directed on bottle.
- Enema—Use as directed on label.

When to take:
Most effective taken on empty stomach 1 hour before or 2 hours after eating. However, may take with food to lessen stomach upset.

If you forget a dose:
Take as soon as you remember up to 2 hours late. If more than 2 hours, wait for next scheduled dose (don't double this dose).

What drug does:
Relaxes and expands bronchial tubes.

Continued next column

 OVERDOSE

SYMPTOMS:
Restlessness, irritability, confusion, black or tarry stool, breathing difficulty, pounding and irregular heartbeat, vomiting blood, delirium, convulsions, rapid pulse, coma.
WHAT TO DO:
- **Dial 911 (emergency) for medical help or call poison control center 1-800-222-1222 for instructions.**
- **See emergency information on last 3 pages of this book.**

Time lapse before drug works:
15 to 30 minutes.

Don't take with:
Any other medicine or any dietary supplement without consulting your doctor or pharmacist.

 POSSIBLE ADVERSE REACTIONS OR SIDE EFFECTS

SYMPTOMS	WHAT TO DO
Life-threatening:	
In case of overdose, see previous column.	
Common:	
Headache, irritability, nervousness, nausea, restlessness, insomnia, vomiting, stomach pain.	Continue. Call doctor when convenient.
Infrequent:	
• Rash or hives, flushed face, diarrhea, rapid breathing, irregular heartbeat.	Discontinue. Call doctor right away.
• Dizziness or light-headedness, appetite loss, trembling, fatigue, weakness.	Continue. Call doctor when convenient.
Rare:	
Frequent urination.	Continue. Call doctor when convenient.

 WARNINGS & PRECAUTIONS

Don't take if:
- You are allergic to any bronchodilator.
- You have an active peptic ulcer.

Before you start, consult your doctor if:
- You have had impaired kidney or liver function.
- You have gastritis.
- You have a peptic ulcer.
- You have high blood pressure or heart disease.
- You take medication for gout.

Over age 60:
Adverse reactions and side effects may be more frequent and severe than in younger persons.

Pregnancy:
Decide with your doctor if drug benefits justify risk to unborn child. Risk category C (see page xviii).

Breast-feeding:
Drug passes into milk. Avoid drug or discontinue nursing until you finish medicine. Consult doctor for advice on maintaining milk supply.

Infants & children:
Use only under medical supervision.

Prolonged use:
Stomach irritation may occur.

Skin & sunlight:
No problems expected.

Driving, piloting or hazardous work:
Avoid if lightheaded or dizzy. Otherwise, no problems expected.

Discontinuing:
May be unnecessary to finish medicine. Follow doctor's instructions.

Others:
Advise any doctor or dentist whom you consult that you take this medicine.

 POSSIBLE INTERACTION WITH OTHER DRUGS

GENERIC NAME OR DRUG CLASS	COMBINED EFFECT
Allopurinol	Increased theophylline effect.
Aminoglutethimide	Possible decreased bronchodilator effect.
Beta-agonists*	Increased effect of both drugs.
Beta-adrenergic blocking agents*	Decreased bronchodilator effect.
Cimetidine	Increased bronchodilator effect.
Clarithromycin	Increased concentration of theophylline.
Clindamycin	May increase bronchodilator effect.
Corticosteroids*	Possible increased bronchodilator effect.
Erythromycin	Increased bronchodilator effect.
Finasteride	Decreased finasteride effect.
Fluoroquinolones	Increased xanthine bronchodilator in blood. May need dose adjustment.
Fluvoxamine	Increased theophylline effect.
Furosemide	Increased furosemide effect.
Lansoprazole	May require dosage adjustment of theophylline.
Leukotriene modifiers	Unknown effects. Consult doctor.
Lincomycins*	May increase bronchodilator effect.
Lithium	Decreased lithium effect.
Modafinil	Decreased bronchodilator effect.
Moricizine	Decreased bronchodilator effect.
Nicotine	Possible increased bronchodilator effect.
Phenobarbital	Decreased bronchodilator effect.
Phenytoin	Decreased effect of both drugs.
Probenecid	Increased effect of dyphylline.
Ranitidine	Possible increased bronchodilator effect and toxicity.
Rauwolfia alkaloids*	Rapid heartbeat.
Rifampin	Decreased bronchodilator effect.
Sulfinpyrazone	Increased effect of dyphylline.
Sympathomimetics*	Possible increased bronchodilator effect
Tacrine	Increased bronchodilator effect.

Continued on page 912

 POSSIBLE INTERACTION WITH OTHER SUBSTANCES

INTERACTS WITH	COMBINED EFFECT
Alcohol:	None expected.
Beverages: Caffeine drinks.	Nervousness and insomnia.
Grapefruit juice	Toxicity risk with theophylline. Avoid.
Cocaine:	Excess stimulation. Avoid.
Foods:	None expected.
Marijuana:	Slightly increased antiasthmatic effect of bronchodilator. Decreased effect with chronic use.
Tobacco:	Decreased bronchodilator effect.

*See Glossary

BUPRENORPHINE & NALOXONE

BRAND NAMES

Suboxone   Subutex

BASIC INFORMATION

Habit forming? Yes
Prescription needed? Yes
Available as generic? No
Drug class: Narcotic

USES

- Treatment for dependence on narcotic (opioid) painkillers including prescription drugs and illicit drugs such as heroin. Should be used in conjunction with an addiction treatment program that involves counseling and/or behavioral therapy. Only certain qualified doctors are able to start in-office treatment and provide prescriptions for ongoing medication.
- Subutex (buprenorphine only) is used in the first few days of treatment. Suboxone (buprenorphine plus naloxone) is then used for the maintenance phase of treatment.

DOSAGE & USAGE INFORMATION

How to take:
Sublingual tablet—Put under your tongue until it dissolves (melts). This may take 2-10 minutes. Do not chew or swallow. Chewing or swallowing the tablet will make it ineffective and may cause withdrawal symptoms. If 2 or more tablets are prescribed, follow your doctor's instructions on how to take. Do not attempt to inject this drug. Read the product information carefully.

When to take:
Once a day at the same time every day. Do not take more or less tablets than prescribed. Dosage may be adjusted only by your doctor.

Continued next column

OVERDOSE

SYMPTOMS:
Especially if injected—slowed breathing, dizziness, faintness, confusion, pinpoint pupils, low blood pressure (an untreated overdose can lead to death).
WHAT TO DO:
- **Dial 911 (emergency) for medical help or call poison control center 1-800-222-1222 for instructions.**
- **See emergency information on last 3 pages of this book.**

If you forget a dose:
Take as soon as you remember. If it is almost time for your next dose, skip the missed dose and go back to your regular dosing schedule. Do not double doses (unless advised by doctor).

What drug does:
- Reduces withdrawal symptoms and blocks the craving without producing a strong narcotic high.
- Naloxone is combined with buprenorphine to guard against the intravenous abuse of buprenorphine. It can produce intense withdrawal symptoms if misused that way. When used as prescribed, naloxone has no effect.

Time lapse before drug works:
Within 30-60 minutes of taking the dose. May take 3-7 days for the effects of the drug to become stable in the body.

Don't take with:
Any other medicine or any dietary supplement without consulting your doctor or pharmacist.

POSSIBLE ADVERSE REACTIONS OR SIDE EFFECTS

SYMPTOMS	WHAT TO DO
Life-threatening: Allergic reaction (hives, facial swelling, sweating, wheezing, loss of blood pressure, and consciousness).	Seek emergency treatment immediately.
Common: Constipation, nausea, headache, appetite loss, drowsiness, pain, insomnia, mood swings, cold or flu symptoms, sweating.	Continue. Call doctor when convenient.
Infrequent: • Liver problems (yellow skin or eyes, dark urine, stools light in color, stomach pain).	Discontinue. Call doctor right away.
• Withdrawal syndrome (nausea or vomiting, muscle aches, runny nose, teary eyes, enlarged pupils, diarrhea, yawning, fever, insomnia).	Continue, but call doctor right away.
Rare: Other unexplained symptoms occur that cause concern.	Continue. Call doctor when convenient.

BUPRENORPHINE & NALOXONE

WARNINGS & PRECAUTIONS

Don't take if:
You are allergic to buprenorphine or naloxone.

Before you start, consult your doctor if:
- You have liver or kidney disease.
- You have gallbladder problems, adrenal gland problems, low thyroid (hypothyroidism) or pancreatitis.
- You have severe mental problems or suffer from hallucinations.
- You are an alcoholic.
- You have respiratory (lung) problems.
- You have problems with urination or constipation, or bowel obstruction.
- You have a head injury or brain problem.
- You have enlarged prostate (males).
- You have scoliosis (causing breathing problems).

Over age 60:
No special problems expected, but caution should be used in the elderly.

Pregnancy:
Decide with your doctor whether drug benefits justify risk to unborn child. Risk category C (see page xviii).

Breast-feeding:
Drug passes into milk. Avoid drug or discontinue nursing until you finish medicine. Consult doctor for advice on maintaining milk supply.

Infants & children:
Not recommended for children under age 16.

Prolonged use:
Talk to your doctor about the need for follow-up medical examinations or laboratory studies to check liver function.

Skin & sunlight:
No problems expected.

Driving, piloting or hazardous work:
Don't drive or pilot aircraft until you learn how medicine affects you. Don't work around dangerous machinery. Don't climb ladders or work in high places. Danger increases if you drink alcohol or take medicine affecting alertness and reflexes.

Discontinuing:
Don't discontinue without consulting doctor. Withdrawal syndrome can occur. Dose may require gradual reduction. Doses of other drugs may also require adjustment.

Others:
- This drug treatment must be given and followed up closely by a specially trained doctor. Be sure to see your doctor as scheduled for office visits. Be compliant with your treatment plan. The information in this chart does not take the place of talking to your doctor.
- Withdrawal syndrome may occur as you are transferred (or switched) from the addicting drug or methadone treatment to this drug. Consult your doctor if symptoms occur.
- Be sure your family members are aware of your drug dependence and that you are taking this drug. They will need to advise medical professionals if an emergency occurs.
- Keep the tablets in a safe place, protect from theft and don't let anyone else use them.
- Use only as directed. Deaths have been reported in addicts who have intravenously misused this drug.
- Advise any doctor or dentist whom you consult that you take this medicine.
- Your doctor will discuss the possibility of discontinuing the drug therapy once you are on a maintenance dose or are stabilized.

POSSIBLE INTERACTION WITH OTHER DRUGS

GENERIC NAME OR DRUG CLASS	COMBINED EFFECT
Benzodiazepines	Serious overdose may occur.
CNS depressants,* other	Increased risk of adverse effects.
Enzyme inhibitors*	Increased effect of buprenorphine.
Phenothiazines	Decreased effect of buprenorphine.

POSSIBLE INTERACTION WITH OTHER SUBSTANCES

INTERACTS WITH	COMBINED EFFECT
Alcohol:	Increased adverse effects including diminished breathing and death. Avoid.
Beverages:	None expected.
Cocaine:	Unpredictable effects. Avoid.
Foods:	None expected.
Marijuana:	Unpredictable effects. Avoid.
Tobacco:	None expected.

*See Glossary

BUPROPION

BRAND NAMES

Aplenzin

Wellbutrin

Wellbutrin SR

Wellbutrin XL

Zyban

BASIC INFORMATION

Habit forming? No
Prescription needed? Yes
Available as generic? Yes
Drug class: Antidepressant

 ## USES

- Relieves severe depression. (Has less effect on sexual functioning than some other antidepressants and may be more acceptable to some patients.)
- May be used in combination with other therapy for smoking cessation.
- Prevention of major depressive episodes in those with seasonal affective disorder (SAD).
- Treatment for other disorders as determined by your doctor.

 ## DOSAGE & USAGE INFORMATION

How to take:
- Tablet—Swallow with liquid. If you can't swallow whole, crumble tablet and take with liquid or food (but drug does have a bitter taste). May take with food to lessen stomach irritation.
- Sustained-release tablet or extended release tablet—Swallow with liquid. Do not crush or crumble tablet.

When to take:
At the same time(s) each day, according to instructions on prescription label.

If you forget a dose:
Take as soon as you remember. If it is almost time for the next dose, wait for the next scheduled dose (don't double this dose).

Continued next column

 ## OVERDOSE

SYMPTOMS:
Confusion, agitation, seizures, coma.
WHAT TO DO:
- Dial 911 (emergency) for medical help or call poison control center 1-800-222-1222 for instructions.
- See emergency information on last 3 pages of this book.

What drug does:
Blocks certain chemicals that are necessary for nerve transmission in the brain. Boosts dopamine and norepinephrine (two brain chemicals) that are also boosted by nicotine.

Time lapse before drug works:
For depression symptoms, about 3 to 4 weeks. For smoking cessation, may take 7-12 weeks.

Don't take with:
Any other medicine or any dietary supplement without consulting your doctor or pharmacist.

 ## POSSIBLE ADVERSE REACTIONS OR SIDE EFFECTS

SYMPTOMS	WHAT TO DO
Life-threatening:	
In case of overdose, see previous column.	
Common:	
• Dry mouth, dizziness, insomnia, loss of appetite, constipation, stomach or muscle pain, nausea or vomiting, sore throat, unusual weight loss, trembling, increased sweating.	Continue. Call doctor when convenient.
• Agitation, anxiety.	Discontinue. Call doctor right away.
Infrequent:	
• Skin rash or hives or itching, severe headache, hearing noises in ears.	Discontinue. Call doctor right away.
• Drowsiness, change in taste, blurred vision, frequent urination, euphoria.	Continue. Call doctor when convenient.
Rare:	
Fainting, seizures, confusion, delusions, hallucinations, feeling paranoid, unable to concentrate, fast or irregular heartbeat, increase in blood pressure.	Discontinue. Call doctor right away.

 ## WARNINGS & PRECAUTIONS

Don't take if:
You are allergic to bupropion.

Before you start, consult your doctor if:
- You have or have had any mental illness.
- You have a seizure disorder.
- You have anorexia nervosa or bulimia.
- You have a history of alcohol or drug abuse.

- You have liver, kidney or heart disease.
- You have had recent head injury.
- You have a brain or spinal cord tumor.

Over age 60:
Adverse reactions and side effects may be more frequent and severe than in younger persons. You may need smaller doses for shorter periods of time.

Pregnancy:
Decide with your doctor whether drug benefits justify risk to unborn child. Risk category B (see page xviii).

Breast-feeding:
Drug passes into milk. May cause adverse reactions. Avoid drug or stop breast-feeding. Consult doctor about maintaining milk supply.

Infants & children:
If prescribed for age under 18, carefully read information provided with prescription. Contact doctor right away if depression symptoms get worse or there is any talk of suicide or suicide behaviors. Also, read information under Others.

Prolonged use:
Talk to your doctor about the need for follow-up medical examinations or laboratory studies to check kidney function, liver function, blood pressure and levels of bupropion in your blood.

Skin & sunlight:
No problems expected.

Driving, piloting or hazardous work:
Don't drive or pilot aircraft until you learn how medicine affects you. Don't work around dangerous machinery. Don't climb ladders or work in high places. Danger increases if you drink alcohol or take drugs affecting alertness and reflexes.

Discontinuing:
Don't discontinue without doctor's advice. Dose may require gradual reduction.

Others:
- If drug is taken to help stop smoking, be sure to follow all medical instructions.
- Adults and children taking antidepressants may experience a worsening of the depression symptoms and may display increased suicidal thoughts or behavior. Call doctor right away if these symptoms or behaviors occur.
- Advise any doctor or dentist whom you consult that you take this medicine.

 ## POSSIBLE INTERACTION WITH OTHER DRUGS

GENERIC NAME OR DRUG CLASS	COMBINED EFFECT
Adrenocorticoids (systemic)	Increased risk of seizures.
Antidepressants, tricyclic*	Increased risk of seizures.
Clozapine	Increased risk of seizures.
Enzyme inducers*	Decreased effect of bupropion.
Enzyme inhibitors*	Increased effect of bupropion.
Fluoxetine	Increased risk of seizures.
Haloperidol	Increased risk of seizures.
Levodopa	Increased risk of side effects.
Lithium	Increased risk of seizures.
Loxapine	Increased risk of seizures.
Maprotiline	Increased risk of seizures.
Molindone	Increased risk of seizures.
Monoamine oxidase (MAO) inhibitors*	Increased risk of toxicity. Take at least 14 days apart.
Nicotine	May increase blood pressure.
Phenothiazines*	Increased risk of seizures.
Phenytoin	Increased phenytoin effect and risk of seizures.
Ritonivir	Increased risk of seizures.
Thioxanthenes*	Increased risk of seizures.
Trazodone	Increased risk of seizures.

 ## POSSIBLE INTERACTION WITH OTHER SUBSTANCES

INTERACTS WITH	COMBINED EFFECT
Alcohol:	Seizure risk. Avoid.
Beverages: Grapefruit juice.	Toxicity risk. Avoid.
Cocaine:	Unknown. Avoid.
Foods:	None expected.
Marijuana:	Unknown. Avoid.
Tobacco:	None expected.

*See Glossary

BUSPIRONE

BRAND NAMES

BuSpar

BASIC INFORMATION

Habit forming? Probably not
Prescription needed? Yes
Available as generic? Yes
Drug class: Antianxiety agent

USES

- Treats chronic anxiety disorders with nervousness or tension. Not intended for treatment of ordinary stress of daily living. Causes less sedation than some antianxiety drugs. Not useful for acute anxiety.
- Useful in agitation associated with dementia.
- Reduces aggression and irritability in patients with dementia, brain injury, mental retardation.
- Used for anxiety in alcoholics or substance abusers (buspirone has low abuse potential).
- Reduces frequency of vascular headaches (does not relieve headache pain).
- Not useful in withdrawal from sedatives.

DOSAGE & USAGE INFORMATION

How to take:
Tablet—Swallow with water. Take with or without food, but be consistent and always take it the same way.

When to take:
As directed. Usually 3 times daily. Food increases absorption.

If you forget a dose:
Take as soon as you remember. If it is almost time for your next dose, skip the missed dose and go back to your regular dosing schedule. Do not double doses.

Continued next column

OVERDOSE

SYMPTOMS:
Severe drowsiness or nausea, vomiting, small pupils, unconsciousness.
WHAT TO DO:
- Dial 911 (emergency) for medical help or call poison control center 1-800-222-1222 for instructions.
- See emergency information on last 3 pages of this book.

What drug does:
Affects certain chemicals in the brain and causes a calming effect.

Time lapse before drug works:
1 to 2 weeks before beneficial effects may be observed.

Don't take with:
- Alcohol, other tranquilizers, antihistamines, muscle relaxants, sedatives or narcotics.
- Any other medicine or any dietary supplement without consulting your doctor or pharmacist.

POSSIBLE ADVERSE REACTIONS OR SIDE EFFECTS

SYMPTOMS	WHAT TO DO
Life-threatening: Chest pain; pounding, fast heartbeat (rare).	Discontinue. Seek emergency treatment.
Common: Lightheadedness, headache, nausea, restlessness, dizziness.	Continue. Call doctor when convenient.
Infrequent: Drowsiness, dry mouth, ringing in ears, nightmares or vivid dreams, unusual fatigue.	Continue. Call doctor when convenient.
Rare: Numbness or tingling in feet or hands; sore throat; fever; depression or confusion; uncontrollable movements of tongue, lips, arms and legs; slurred speech; psychosis; blurred vision.	Discontinue. Call doctor right away.

WARNINGS & PRECAUTIONS

Don't take if:
You are allergic to buspirone.

Before you start, consult your doctor if:
- You have ever been addicted to any substance.
- You have chronic kidney or liver disease.
- You are already taking any medicine.

Over age 60:
Adverse reactions and side effects may be more frequent and severe than in younger persons.

Pregnancy:
No problems expected, but better to avoid if possible. Consult doctor. Risk category B (see page xviii).

Breast-feeding:
Unknown if drug passes into milk. Avoid nursing until you finish medicine. Consult doctor for advice on maintaining milk supply.

Infants & children:
Safety and efficacy not established for children under 18 years old.

Prolonged use:
- Not recommended for prolonged use. Adverse side effects more likely.
- Request follow-up studies to check kidney function, blood counts, and platelet counts.

Skin & sunlight:
No problems expected.

Driving, piloting or hazardous work:
Don't drive or pilot aircraft until you learn how medicine affects you. Don't work around dangerous machinery. Don't climb ladders or work in high places. Danger increases if you drink alcohol or take medicine affecting alertness and reflexes, such as antihistamines, tranquilizers, sedatives, pain medicine, narcotics and mind-altering drugs.

Discontinuing:
No problems expected.

Others:
- Before elective surgery requiring local or general anesthesia, tell your dentist, surgeon or anesthesiologist that you take buspirone.
- Advise any doctor or dentist whom you consult that you take this medicine.

POSSIBLE INTERACTION WITH OTHER DRUGS

GENERIC NAME OR DRUG CLASS	COMBINED EFFECT
Antihistamines*	Increased sedative effect of both drugs.
Barbiturates*	Excessive sedation. Sedative effect of both drugs may be increased.
Benzodiazepines*	Recent use of benzodiazepines may lessen effect of buspirone.
Central nervous system (CNS) depressants*	Increased sedative effect.
Monoamine oxidase MAO inhibitors*	May increase blood pressure.
Narcotics*	Excessive sedation. Sedative effect of both drugs may be increased.

POSSIBLE INTERACTION WITH OTHER SUBSTANCES

INTERACTS WITH	COMBINED EFFECT
Alcohol:	Excess sedation. Use caution.
Beverages: Caffeine-containing drinks.	Avoid. Decreased antianxiety effect of buspirone.
Grapefruit juice	Toxicity risk. Avoid.
Cocaine:	Avoid. Decreased antianxiety effect of buspirone.
Foods:	None expected.
Marijuana:	Avoid. Decreased antianxiety effect of buspirone.
Tobacco:	Avoid. Decreased antianxiety effect of buspirone.

BUSULFAN

BRAND NAMES

Myleran

BASIC INFORMATION

Habit forming? No
Prescription needed? Yes
Available as generic? No
Drug class: Antineoplastic, immunosuppressant

 USES

- Treatment for some kinds of cancer.
- Suppresses immune response after transplant and in immune disorders.

 DOSAGE & USAGE INFORMATION

How to take:
Tablet—Swallow with liquid after light meal. Don't drink fluids with meals. Drink extra fluids between meals. Avoid sweet or fatty foods.

When to take:
At the same time each day.

If you forget a dose:
Take as soon as you remember. Never double dose.

What drug does:
Inhibits abnormal cell reproduction. May suppress immune system.

Time lapse before drug works:
Up to 6 weeks for full effect.

Don't take with:
Any other medicine or any dietary supplement without consulting your doctor or pharmacist.

 OVERDOSE

SYMPTOMS:
Bleeding, chills, fever, collapse, stupor, seizure.
WHAT TO DO:
- Dial 911 (emergency) for medical help or call poison control center 1-800-222-1222 for instructions.
- If person is unconscious, check breathing and pulse. If not breathing, begin mouth-to-mouth rescue breathing. If heart is not beating, begin chest compressions.
- See emergency information on last 3 pages of this book.

 POSSIBLE ADVERSE REACTIONS OR SIDE EFFECTS

SYMPTOMS	WHAT TO DO
Life-threatening:	
In case of overdose, see previous column.	
Common:	
• Unusual bleeding or bruising, mouth sores with sore throat, chills and fever, black stools, lip sores, menstrual irregularities.	Discontinue. Call doctor right away.
• Hair loss.	Continue. Call doctor when convenient.
• Nausea, vomiting, diarrhea (almost always occurs), tiredness, weakness.	Continue. Tell doctor at next visit.
Infrequent:	
• Mental confusion, shortness of breath.	Continue. Call doctor when convenient.
• Cough, joint pain, dizziness, appetite loss.	Continue. Tell doctor at next visit.
Rare:	
• Jaundice, cataracts, symptoms of myasthenia gravis.*	Discontinue. Call doctor right away.
• Swollen breasts.	Continue. Call doctor when convenient.

WARNINGS & PRECAUTIONS

Don't take if:
- You have had hypersensitivity to alkylating antineoplastic drugs.
- Your physician has not explained the serious nature of your medical problem and risks of taking this medicine.

Before you start, consult your doctor if:
- You have gout.
- You have had kidney stones.
- You have active infection.
- You have impaired kidney or liver function.
- You have taken other antineoplastic drugs or had radiation treatment in last 3 weeks.

Over age 60:
Adverse reactions and side effects may be more frequent and severe than in younger persons.

Pregnancy:
Consult doctor. Risk to child is significant. Risk category D (see page xviii).

Breast-feeding:
Drug passes into milk. Don't nurse.

Infants & children:
Use only under care of medical supervisors who are experienced in anticancer drugs.

Prolonged use:
- Adverse reactions more likely the longer drug is required.
- Talk to your doctor about the need for follow-up medical examinations or laboratory studies to check complete blood counts (white blood cell count, platelet count, red blood cell count, hemoglobin, hematocrit), serum uric acid.

Skin & sunlight:
No problems expected.

Driving, piloting or hazardous work:
No problems expected.

Discontinuing:
Don't discontinue without doctor's advice until you complete prescribed dose, even though symptoms diminish or disappear. Some side effects may follow discontinuing. Report to doctor blurred vision, convulsions, confusion, persistent headache.

Others:
- Advise any doctor or dentist whom you consult that you take this medicine.
- May increase chance of developing lung or blood problems.

 POSSIBLE INTERACTION WITH OTHER DRUGS

GENERIC NAME OR DRUG CLASS	COMBINED EFFECT
Antigout drugs*	Decreased antigout effect.
Antineoplastic drugs, other*	Increased effect of all drugs (may be beneficial).
Chloramphenicol	Increased likelihood of toxic effects of both drugs.
Clozapine	Toxic effect on bone marrow.
Lovastatin	Increased heart and kidney damage.
Tiopronin	Increased risk of toxicity to bone marrow.
Vaccines, live or killed	Increased risk of toxicity or reduced effectiveness of vaccine.

 POSSIBLE INTERACTION WITH OTHER SUBSTANCES

INTERACTS WITH	COMBINED EFFECT
Alcohol:	May increase chance of intestinal bleeding.
Beverages:	None expected.
Cocaine:	Increases chance of toxicity.
Foods:	Reduces irritation in stomach.
Marijuana:	None expected.
Tobacco:	Increases lung toxicity.

*See Glossary

BUTORPHANOL

BRAND NAMES

**Butorphanol Tartrate   Stadol NS
Nasal Spray**

BASIC INFORMATION

**Habit forming? Yes
Prescription needed? Yes
Available as generic? No
Drug class: Narcotic analgesic**

 USES

- Treatment for migraine headache pain and postoperative pain.
- Treatment for other types of pain for which a narcotic analgesic is appropriate.

 DOSAGE & USAGE INFORMATION

How to take:
Nasal spray—Spray in one nostril using the metered-dose pump.

When to take:
For pain as directed by your doctor. Usual treatment consists of one dose in one nostril followed by a second dose in 60 to 90 minutes if pain persists. Your doctor may direct that the initial 2-dose sequence may be repeated in 3 to 4 hours as needed.

If you forget a dose:
Unlikely to be a problem since the drug is taken for pain and not routinely.

What drug does:
Blocks the pain impulses at specific sites in the brain and spinal cord.

Time lapse before drug works:
Within 15 minutes of the first dose.

Don't take with:
Any other medicine or any dietary supplement without consulting your doctor or pharmacist.

 OVERDOSE

SYMPTOMS:
Heartbeat irregularities, breathing difficulty, coma.
WHAT TO DO:
- **Dial 911 (emergency) for medical help or call poison control center 1-800-222-1222 for instructions.**
- **See emergency information on last 3 pages of this book.**

 POSSIBLE ADVERSE REACTIONS OR SIDE EFFECTS

SYMPTOMS	WHAT TO DO
Life-threatening: In case of overdose, see previous column.	
Common: Drowsiness, dizziness, nausea or vomiting, nasal congestion or irritation.	Discontinue. Call doctor when convenient.
Infrequent: Constipation (with continued use), faintness, high or low blood pressure.	Discontinue. Call doctor when convenient.
Rare:	
• Taste changes, ear ringing, dry mouth.	No action necessary.
• Difficult breathing, heart palpitations.	Discontinue. Call doctor right away.

WARNINGS & PRECAUTIONS

Don't take if:
You are allergic to butorphanol or the preservative benzethonium chloride,* which is used in the manufacture of the drug.

Before you start, consult your doctor if:
- You have a respiratory disorder or a central nervous system disease.
- You have had adverse reactions to other narcotics.*
- You have a history of emotional problems.
- You have heart, kidney or liver disease.

Over age 60:
Adverse reactions and side effects (particularly dizziness) may be more frequent and severe than in younger persons.

Pregnancy:
Risk category C (see page xviii). Decide with your doctor if drug benefits justify any possible risk to unborn child.

Breast-feeding:
Drug may pass into milk. Decide with your doctor if you should continue breast-feeding while taking this drug.

Infants & children:
Not recommended for children under age 18. Safety and effectiveness have not been established.

Prolonged use:
Long-term use effects are unknown. Probably habit forming. Consult with your doctor on a regular basis while using this drug.

Skin & sunlight:
No special problems expected.

Driving, piloting or hazardous work:
Don't drive or pilot aircraft until you learn how medicine affects you. Don't work around dangerous machinery. Don't climb ladders or work in high places. Danger increases if you drink alcohol or take medicine affecting alertness and reflexes.

Discontinuing:
Don't discontinue this drug after prolonged use without consulting doctor. Dosage may require a gradual reduction before stopping to avoid any withdrawal symptoms.

Others:
- When first using this drug, get up slowly from a sitting or lying position to avoid any dizziness, faintness or lightheadedness.
- Advise any doctor or dentist whom you consult that you take this medicine.
- Take medicine only as directed. Do not increase or reduce dosage without doctor's approval.

POSSIBLE INTERACTION WITH OTHER DRUGS

GENERIC NAME OR DRUG CLASS	COMBINED EFFECT
Central nervous system (CNS) depressants,* other	Increased sedative effect.
Oxymetazoline	Delays start of butorphanol effect.

POSSIBLE INTERACTION WITH OTHER SUBSTANCES

INTERACTS WITH	COMBINED EFFECT
Alcohol:	Increased sedative affect. Avoid.
Beverages:	None expected.
Cocaine:	Effect not known. Best to avoid.
Foods:	None expected.
Marijuana:	Effect not known. Best to avoid.
Tobacco:	None expected.

CAFFEINE

BRAND NAMES

See full list of brand names in the *Generic and Brand Name Directory*, page 881.

BASIC INFORMATION

Habit forming? Yes
Prescription needed? No
Available as generic? Yes
Drug class: Stimulant (xanthine), vasoconstrictor

 ## USES

- Treatment for drowsiness and fatigue (occasional use only).
- Treatment for migraine and other vascular headaches in combination with ergot.

 ## DOSAGE & USAGE INFORMATION

How to take:
- Tablet or liquid—Swallow with liquid or food to lessen stomach irritation. If you can't swallow whole, crumble tablet and take with liquid or food.
- Extended-release capsule—Swallow whole with liquid.
- Powder—Stir powder into water or other liquid. The powder may also be placed on the tongue and then followed by liquid.

When to take:
At the same times each day.

If you forget a dose:
Take as soon as you remember up to 2 hours late. If more than 2 hours, wait for next scheduled dose (don't double this dose).

What drug does:
- Constricts blood vessel walls.
- Stimulates central nervous system.

Continued next column

 ## OVERDOSE

SYMPTOMS:
Excitement, insomnia, rapid heartbeat (infants can have slow heartbeat), confusion, fever, hallucinations, convulsions, coma.
WHAT TO DO:
- Dial 911 (emergency) for medical help or call poison control center 1-800-222-1222 for instructions.
- See emergency information on last 3 pages of this book.

Time lapse before drug works:
30 minutes.

Don't take with:
Any other medicine or any dietary supplement without consulting your doctor or pharmacist.

 ## POSSIBLE ADVERSE REACTIONS OR SIDE EFFECTS

SYMPTOMS	WHAT TO DO
Life-threatening:	
In case of overdose, see previous column.	
Common:	
• Rapid heartbeat, low blood sugar (hunger, anxiety, cold sweats, rapid pulse) with tremor, irritability (mild).	Discontinue. Call doctor right away.
• Nervousness, insomnia.	Continue. Tell doctor at next visit.
• Increased urination.	No action necessary.
Infrequent:	
• Confusion, irritability (severe).	Discontinue. Call doctor right away.
• Nausea, indigestion, burning feeling in stomach.	Continue. Call doctor when convenient.
Rare:	
None expected.	

WARNINGS & PRECAUTIONS

Don't take if:
- You are allergic to any stimulant.
- You have heart disease.
- You have active peptic ulcer of stomach or duodenum.

Before you start, consult your doctor if:
- You have irregular heartbeat.
- You have hypoglycemia (low blood sugar).
- You have epilepsy.
- You have a seizure disorder.
- You have high blood pressure.
- You have insomnia.

Over age 60:
Adverse reactions and side effects may be more frequent and severe than in younger persons.

Pregnancy:
Decide with your doctor if drug benefits justify risk to unborn child. Risk category C (see page xviii).

Breast-feeding:
Drug passes into milk. Avoid drug or discontinue nursing until you finish medicine. Consult doctor for advice on maintaining milk supply.

Infants & children:
Not recommended.

Prolonged use:
Can affect people in different ways. Consult your doctor if you are concerned.

Skin & sunlight:
No problems expected.

Driving, piloting or hazardous work:
No problems expected.

Discontinuing:
Will cause withdrawal symptoms of headache, irritability, drowsiness. Discontinue gradually if you use caffeine for a month or more.

Others:
Consult your doctor if drowsiness or fatigue continues, recurs or is not relieved by caffeine.

POSSIBLE INTERACTION WITH OTHER DRUGS

GENERIC NAME OR DRUG CLASS	COMBINED EFFECT
Caffeine-containing drugs, other	Increased risk of overstimulation.
Central nervous system (CNS) stimulants*	Increased risk of overstimulation.
Cimetidine	Increased caffeine effect.
Contraceptives, oral*	Increased caffeine effect.
Isoniazid	Increased caffeine effect.
Monoamine oxidase (MAO) inhibitors*	Dangerous blood pressure rise.
Sympathomimetics*	Overstimulation.
Xanthines*	Increased risk of overstimulation.

POSSIBLE INTERACTION WITH OTHER SUBSTANCES

INTERACTS WITH	COMBINED EFFECT
Alcohol:	Decreased alcohol effect.
Beverages: Caffeine drinks (coffee, tea or soft drinks).	Increased caffeine effect. Use caution.
Cocaine	Convulsions or excessive nervousness.
Foods:	None expected.
Marijuana:	Increased effect of both drugs. May lead to dangerous, rapid heartbeat. Avoid.
Tobacco:	Increased heartbeat. Avoid. Decreased caffeine effect.

CALCITONIN

BRAND NAMES

Fortical   Miacalcin

BASIC INFORMATION

Habit forming? No
Prescription needed? Yes
Available as generic? No
Drug class: Osteoporosis therapy

 USES

Treatment for postmenopausal osteoporosis (thinning of bones) in females. Osteoporosis is a major cause of bone fractures.

 DOSAGE & USAGE INFORMATION

How to take:
Nasal spray—One spray per day in a nostril, alternating nostrils daily. Follow directions on label about activating and using the pump supplied with the medication.

When to take:
At the same time each day.

If you forget a dose:
Take as soon as you remember up to 12 hours late. If more than 12 hours, wait for next scheduled dose (don't double this dose).

What drug does:
The exact mechanism is not fully understood. It slows down the loss of bone tissue and increases bone mass in women with osteoporosis.

Time lapse before drug works:
Up to 6 months or longer.

Don't take with:
Any other medicine or any dietary supplement without consulting your doctor or pharmacist.

 OVERDOSE

SYMPTOMS:
None reported.
WHAT TO DO:
Overdose unlikely to threaten life. If person uses much larger amount than prescribed or if accidentally swallowed, call doctor or poison control center 1-800-222-1222 for help.

 POSSIBLE ADVERSE REACTIONS OR SIDE EFFECTS

SYMPTOMS	WHAT TO DO
Life-threatening: Rare allergic reaction—Breathing difficulty; swelling of hands, feet, face, mouth, neck; skin rash.	Discontinue. Seek emergency treatment.
Common: Nasal inflammation, dryness, crusting, sores, irritation, itching, redness; swollen, runny, stuffy nose; small amount of nasal bleeding, discomfort, tenderness.	Continue. Call doctor when convenient.
Infrequent: Back pain, joint pain, headache, mild bloody nose, flushing, nausea, sinus infection.	Continue. Call doctor when convenient.
Rare: None expected.	

WARNINGS & PRECAUTIONS

Don't take if:
You are allergic to calcitonin.

Before you start, consult your doctor if:
You are allergic to any medication, food or other substance. A skin test may be performed before beginning treatment with calcitonin.

Over age 60:
No special problems expected.

Pregnancy:
Not normally used in premenopausal women. Risk category C (see page xviii).

Breast-feeding:
Not normally used in premenopausal women.

Infants & children:
Not recommended for this age group.

Prolonged use:
* No special problems expected.
* Visit your doctor regularly to determine if the drug is continuing to control bone loss and to have periodic nasal examinations to check for ulceration or irritation.

Skin & sunlight:
No special problems expected.

Driving, piloting or hazardous work:
No special problems expected.

Discontinuing:
Don't discontinue without your doctor's approval.

Others:
* In addition to taking the drug, weight-bearing exercise and adequate dietary intake of calcium and vitamin D are essential in preventing bone loss. Dietary supplements of 1000 mg elemental calcium and 400 I.U. vitamin D daily may be recommended by your doctor.
* Advise any doctor or dentist whom you consult that you take this medicine.
* May affect the results of some medical tests.

POSSIBLE INTERACTION WITH OTHER DRUGS

GENERIC NAME OR DRUG CLASS	COMBINED EFFECT
None significant.	

POSSIBLE INTERACTION WITH OTHER SUBSTANCES

INTERACTS WITH	COMBINED EFFECT
Alcohol:	None expected.
Beverages:	None expected.
Cocaine:	None expected.
Foods:	None expected.
Marijuana:	None expected.
Tobacco:	None expected.

CALCIUM CHANNEL BLOCKERS

GENERIC AND BRAND NAMES

See full list of generic and brand names in *Generic and Brand Name Directory*, page 881.

BASIC INFORMATION

Habit forming? No
Prescription needed? Yes
Available as generic? Yes, for most
Drug class: Calcium channel blocker, antiarrhythmic, antianginal

USES

- Used for high blood pressure (hypertension) angina attacks and irregular heartbeat.
- Treats migraines and Raynaud's disease.

DOSAGE & USAGE INFORMATION

How to take:
- Tablet or capsule—Swallow with liquid. You may chew or crush tablet.
- Extended-release tablet or capsule—Swallow each dose whole with liquid; do not crush tablet or open capsule.

When to take:
At the same times each day. Take verapamil with food.

If you forget a dose:
Take as soon as you remember up to 2 hours late. If more than 2 hours, wait for next scheduled dose (don't double this dose).

What drug does:
- Reduces work that heart must perform.
- Reduces normal artery pressure.
- Increases oxygen to heart muscle.

Continued next column

OVERDOSE

SYMPTOMS:
Unusually fast or unusually slow heartbeat, loss of consciousness, cardiac arrest.
WHAT TO DO:
- **Dial 911 (emergency) for medical help or call poison control center 1-800-222-1222 for instructions.**
- **If person is unconscious, check breathing and pulse. If not breathing, begin mouth-to-mouth rescue breathing. If heart is not beating, begin chest compressions.**
- **See emergency information on last 3 pages of this book.**

Time lapse before drug works:
1 to 2 hours.

Don't take with:
Any other medicine or any dietary supplement without consulting your doctor or pharmacist.

POSSIBLE ADVERSE REACTIONS OR SIDE EFFECTS

SYMPTOMS	WHAT TO DO
Life-threatening:	
In case of overdose, see previous column.	
Common:	
Tiredness.	Continue. Tell doctor at next visit.
Infrequent:	
• Unusually fast or unusually slow heart-beat, wheezing, cough, shortness of breath.	Discontinue. Call doctor right away.
• Dizziness; numbness or tingling in hands and feet; swollen feet, ankles or legs; difficult urination.	Continue. Call doctor when convenient.
• Nausea, constipation.	Continue. Tell doctor at next visit.
Rare:	
• Fainting, depression, psychosis, rash, jaundice.	Discontinue. Call doctor right away.
• Headache, insomnia, vivid dreams, hair loss.	Continue. Tell doctor at next visit.

WARNINGS & PRECAUTIONS

Don't take if:
- You are allergic to calcium channel blockers.
- You have very low blood pressure.

Before you start, consult your doctor if:
- You have kidney or liver disease.
- You have high blood pressure.
- You have heart disease other than coronary artery disease.

Over age 60:
Adverse reactions and side effects may be more frequent and severe than in younger persons.

Pregnancy:
Decide with your doctor if drug benefits justify risk to unborn child. Risk category C (see page xviii).

Breast-feeding:
Safety not established. Avoid if possible. Consult doctor.

Infants & children:
Not recommended.

Prolonged use:
Talk to your doctor about the need for follow-up medical examinations or laboratory studies to check blood pressure, liver function, kidney function, ECG.*

Skin & sunlight:
One or more drugs in this group may cause rash or intensify sunburn in areas exposed to sun or ultraviolet light (photosensitivity reaction). Avoid overexposure. Notify doctor if reaction occurs.

Driving, piloting or hazardous work:
Avoid if you feel dizzy. Otherwise, no problems expected.

Discontinuing:
Don't discontinue without doctor's advice until you complete prescribed dose, even though symptoms diminish or disappear.

Others:
* Learn to check your own pulse rate. If it drops to 50 beats per minute or lower, don't take drug until you consult your doctor.
* Advise any doctor or dentist whom you consult that you take this medicine.

POSSIBLE INTERACTION WITH OTHER DRUGS

GENERIC NAME OR DRUG CLASS	COMBINED EFFECT
Angiotensin-converting enzyme (ACE) inhibitors*	Possible excessive potassium in blood. Dosages may require adjustment.
Antiarrhythmics*	Possible increased effect and toxicity of each drug.
Anticoagulants, oral*	Possible increased anticoagulant effect.
Anticonvulsants, hydantoin*	Increased anticonvulsant effect.
Antihypertensives*	Blood pressure drop. Dosages may require adjustment.
Beta-adrenergic blocking agents*	Possible irregular heartbeat and congestive heart failure.
Calcium (large doses)	Possible decreased effect of calcium channel blocker.
Carbamazepine	May increase carbamazepine effect and toxicity.

Cimetidine	Possible increased effect of calcium channel blocker.
Colesevelam	Unknown effect. Consult doctor.
Cyclosporine	Increased cyclosporine toxicity.
Digitalis preparations*	Increased digitalis effect. May need to reduce dose.
Disopyramide	May cause dangerously slow, fast or irregular heartbeat.
Diuretics*	Dangerous blood pressure drop. Dosages may require adjustment.
Dofetilide	Increased risk of heart problems.
Encainide	Increased effect of toxicity on heart muscle.
Fluvoxamine	Slow heartbeat (with diltiazem).
HMG-CoA reductase inhibitors	Increased effect of HMG-CoA reductase inhibitor.
Hypokalemia-causing medications*	Increased antihypertensive effect.
Leukotriene modifiers	Increased effect of calcium channel blocker.

Continued on page 912

POSSIBLE INTERACTION WITH OTHER SUBSTANCES

INTERACTS WITH	COMBINED EFFECT
Alcohol:	Very low blood pressure. Avoid.
Beverages: Grapefruit juice.	Possible increased drug effect.
Cocaine:	Possible irregular heartbeat. Avoid.
Foods: Grapefruit.	Possible increased drug effect.
Marijuana:	Possible irregular heartbeat. Avoid.
Tobacco:	Possible rapid heartbeat. Avoid.

*See Glossary

CALCIUM SUPPLEMENTS

GENERIC AND BRAND NAMES

See full list of generic and brand names in the *Generic and Brand Name Directory*, page 881.

BASIC INFORMATION

Habit forming? No
Prescription needed? For some
Available as generic? Yes
Drug class: Antihypocalcemic, dietary
    replacement

 USES

- Treats or prevents osteoporosis (thin, porous, easily fractured bones). Frequently prescribed with estrogen beginning at menopause.
- Helps heart, muscle and nervous system to work properly.
- Dietary supplement when calcium ingestion is insufficient or there is a deficiency such as osteomalacia or rickets.

 DOSAGE & USAGE INFORMATION

How to take:
- Tablet or capsule—Swallow whole with liquid.
- Chewable tablet—Chew tablet well before swallowing.
- Syrup—Take before meals.
- Powder—Follow directions on label.
- Suspension—Swallow with liquid.

When to take:
Take 1 to 1 1/2 hours after meals (except for syrup) in 3 to 4 daily doses. Try to avoid taking other medicine you take by mouth within 1 to 2 hours of taking calcium.

If you forget a dose:
Use as soon as you remember. Then return to regular schedule.

Continued next column

 OVERDOSE

SYMPTOMS:
Confusion, irregular heartbeat, depression, bone pain, coma.
WHAT TO DO:
- **Dial 911 (emergency) for medical help or call poison control center 1-800-222-1222 for instructions.**
- **See emergency information on last 3 pages of this book.**

What drug does:
Calcium helps maintain strong bones and teeth. It also helps heart function, muscle contraction, blood clotting and nerve transmission.

Time lapse before drug works:
Starts within 15 to 30 minutes, but may take months or years to improve certain conditions.

Don't take with:
- Any other oral medicine until 1 to 2 hours have passed since taking calcium.
- Any other medicine or any dietary supplement without consulting your doctor or pharmacist.

 POSSIBLE ADVERSE REACTIONS OR SIDE EFFECTS

SYMPTOMS	WHAT TO DO
Life-threatening: Irregular or very slow heart rate.	Discontinue. Seek emergency treatment.
Common: None expected.	
Infrequent: Constipation, diarrhea, drowsiness, headache, appetite loss, dry mouth, weakness.	Discontinue. Call doctor right away.
Rare: Frequent, painful or difficult urination; increased thirst; nausea, vomiting; rash; urine frequency increased and volume larger; confusion; high blood pressure; eyes sensitive to light.	Discontinue. Call doctor right away.

 WARNINGS & PRECAUTIONS

Don't take if:
- You are allergic to calcium.
- You have a high blood calcium level.

Before you start, consult your doctor if:
You have diarrhea, heart disease, kidney stones, kidney disease, sarcoidosis or malabsorption.

Over age 60:
No problems expected.

Pregnancy:
Consult doctor. Risk category C (see page xviii).

Breast-feeding:
No problems expected. Consult doctor.

Infants & children:
Use correct dose for your child's age and weight.

Prolonged use:
Talk to your doctor about the need for any follow-up laboratory studies to check calcium levels in the body.

Skin & sunlight:
No problems expected.

Driving, piloting or hazardous work:
No problems expected.

Discontinuing:
No problems expected.

Others:
* Exercise, along with vitamin D from sunshine and calcium, helps prevent osteoporosis.
* Advise any doctor or dentist whom you consult that you take this medicine.

POSSIBLE INTERACTION WITH OTHER DRUGS

GENERIC NAME OR DRUG CLASS	COMBINED EFFECT
Alendronate	Decreased alendronate effect. Take calcium 30 minutes after alendronate.
Anticoagulants, oral*	Decreased anticoagulant effect.
Calcitonin	Decreased calcitonin effect.
Calcium-containing medicines, other	Increased calcium effect.
Chlorpromazine	Decreased chlorpromazine effect.
Contraceptives, oral*	May increase absorption of calcium—frequently a desirable combined effect.
Corticosteroids*	Decreased calcium absorption and effect.
Digitalis preparations*	Decreased digitalis effect.
Diuretics, thiazide*	Increased calcium in blood.
Estrogens*	May increase absorption of calcium—frequently a desirable combined effect.
Etidronate	Decreased etidronate absorption. Take drugs 2 hours apart.
Iron supplements*	Decreased iron effect.

Meperidine	Increased meperidine effect.
Mexiletine	May slow elimination of mexiletine and cause need to adjust dosage.
Nalidixic acid	Decreased effect of nalidixic acid.
Nicardipine	Possible decreased nicardipine effect.
Nimodipine	Possible decreased nimodipine effect.
Oxyphenbutazone	Decreased oxyphenbutazone effect.
Para-aminosalicylic acid (PAS)	Decreased PAS effect.
Penicillins*	Decreased penicillin effect.
Pentobarbital	Decreased pentobarbital effect.
Phenylbutazone	Decreased effect of phenylbutazone.
Phenytoin	Decreased phenytoin effect.
Propafenone	Increased effects of both drugs and increased risk of toxicity.
Pseudoephedrine	Increased pseudoephedrine effect.

Continued on page 912

POSSIBLE INTERACTION WITH OTHER SUBSTANCES

INTERACTS WITH	COMBINED EFFECT
Alcohol:	Decreased absorption of calcium.
Beverages:	None expected.
Cocaine:	No proven problems.
Foods:	None expected.
Marijuana:	Decreased absorption of calcium.
Tobacco:	Decreased absorption of calcium.

*See Glossary

CAPECITABINE

BRAND NAMES

Xeloda

BASIC INFORMATION

Habit forming? No
Prescription needed? Yes
Available as generic? No
Drug class: Antineoplastic

 USES

Treatment of cancer of the colon after surgery and colorectal or breast cancer that has spread to other parts of the body (metastatic cancer).

 DOSAGE & USAGE INFORMATION

How to take:
Tablet—Swallow with water. If you can't swallow whole, crumble tablet and take with liquid or food.

When to take:
Take in two divided doses every 12 hours after a meal and with water.

If you forget a dose:
Do not take missed dose or double next dose. Continue your regular dosing schedule and consult your doctor.

What drug does:
Capecitabine is converted in the body to the substance 5-fluorouracil. In some patients, this substance kills cancer cells and decreases the size of the tumor.

Time lapse before drug works:
Results may not show for several months.

Don't take with:
Any other medicine or any dietary supplement without consulting your doctor or pharmacist.

 OVERDOSE

SYMPTOMS:
Nausea, vomiting, diarrhea, gastrointestinal irritation and bleeding, and bone marrow depression.
WHAT TO DO:
Overdose unlikely to threaten life. If person uses much larger amount than prescribed or if accidentally swallowed, call doctor or poison control center 1-800-222-1222 for help.

 POSSIBLE ADVERSE REACTIONS OR SIDE EFFECTS

SYMPTOMS	WHAT TO DO
Life-threatening: None expected.	
Common: • Diarrhea (if you have more than 4 bowel movements in a day or any diarrhea at night); vomiting (more than once a day); nausea; loss of appetite; stomatitis (pain, redness or swelling in mouth); hand and foot syndrome (pain, redness or swelling in hands or feet); fever (100.5 or higher).	Discontinue. Call doctor right away.
• Diarrhea, nausea and vomiting, rash, dry or itchy skin, tiredness, weakness, dizziness, headache.	Continue. Call doctor when convenient.
Infrequent: Jaundice.	Continue, but call doctor right away.
Rare: None expected.	

WARNINGS & PRECAUTIONS

Don't take if:
You are allergic to capecitabine.

Before you start, consult your doctor if:
* You have an infection or any other medical problem.
* You have heart problems.
* You are taking folic acid.
* You are pregnant or if you plan to become pregnant.
* You have had liver problems.

Over age 60:
Adverse reactions and side effects, especially gastrointestinal, may be more severe and frequent than in younger patients.

Pregnancy:
Animal studies show fetal abnormalities and increased risk of abortion. Discuss with your doctor whether drug benefits justify risk to unborn child. Risk category D (see page xviii).

Breast-feeding:
Not known if drug passes into milk. Avoid drug or discontinue nursing until you finish medicine. Consult doctor for advice on maintaining milk supply.

Infants & children:
Safety and effectiveness of use in children not established.

Prolonged use:
Talk to your doctor about the need for follow-up medical examinations or laboratory studies.

Skin & sunlight:
No problems expected.

Driving, piloting or hazardous work:
Avoid if you feel side effects such as nausea and vomiting.

Discontinuing:
Your doctor will determine the schedule.

Others:
Advise any doctor or dentist whom you consult that you take this medicine.

POSSIBLE INTERACTION WITH OTHER DRUGS

GENERIC NAME OR DRUG CLASS	COMBINED EFFECT
Antacids	Increased risk of capecitabine toxicity.
Leucovorin	Increased risk of capecitabine toxicity.

POSSIBLE INTERACTION WITH OTHER SUBSTANCES

INTERACTS WITH	COMBINED EFFECT
Alcohol:	None expected.
Beverages:	None expected.
Cocaine:	Effects unknown. Avoid.
Foods:	None expected.
Marijuana:	Effects unknown. Avoid.
Tobacco:	None expected.

CAPSAICIN

BRAND NAMES

ArthriCare
ARTH-RX
Axsain
Capsagel
Dura-Patch
Dura Patch Joint

Methacin
Sinol Nasal Spray
Sinus Buster
Zostrix
Zostrix-HP
Zostrix Neuropathy
   Cream

BASIC INFORMATION

Habit forming? No
Prescription needed? No
Available as generic? Yes
Drug class: Analgesic (topical)

 USES

- Treats neuralgias, such as pain that occurs following shingles (herpes zoster) or neuropathy of the feet, ankles and fingers (common in diabetes).
- Nasal spray helps relieves sinus, allergy, and headache symptoms, including migraines.
- Treats discomfort caused by arthritis.

 DOSAGE & USAGE INFORMATION

How to use:
- Cream—Apply a small amount and rub carefully on the affected areas. Use every day. Wash hands after applying. Don't apply to irritated skin. Don't bandage over treated areas.
- Nasal spray—Use will depend on condition being treated. Follow package instructions.
- Patch—Follow package instructions for proper application.

When to use:
Apply 3 or 4 times a day.

If you forget a dose:
Use as soon as you remember.

What drug does:
It is made from red chili peppers. When applied to the skin, it appears to decrease a chemical that causes pain.

Continued next column

 OVERDOSE

SYMPTOMS:
None expected.
WHAT TO DO:
Not intended for internal use. If child accidentally swallows, call doctor or poison control center 1-800-222-1222 for help.

Time lapse before drug works:
Begins to work immediately. Frequently takes 2 to 3 weeks for full benefit, but may take up to 6 or 8 weeks.

Don't use with:
No problems expected.

 POSSIBLE ADVERSE REACTIONS OR SIDE EFFECTS

SYMPTOMS	WHAT TO DO
Life-threatening: None expected.	
Common: Stinging or burning sensation at application site.	Nothing. It usually improves in 2 to 3 days or becomes less severe the longer you use the drug.
Infrequent: None expected.	
Rare: None expected.	

CAPSAICIN

WARNINGS & PRECAUTIONS

Don't use if:
You are allergic to capsaicin or to the fruit of capsaicin plants (for example, hot peppers).

Before you start, consult your doctor if:
You have any allergies.

Over age 60:
No problems expected.

Pregnancy:
Consult doctor. Risk category C (see page xviii).

Breast-feeding:
No problems expected. Consult doctor.

Infants & children:
Not recommended for children under age 2.

Prolonged use:
No problems expected.

Skin & sunlight:
No problems expected.

Driving, piloting or hazardous work:
No problems expected.

Discontinuing:
Discontinue if there are no signs of improvement within a month.

Others:
- Capsaicin is not a local anesthetic.*
- Although capsaicin may help relieve the pain of neuropathy, it does not cure any disorder.
- If you accidentally get some capsaicin in your eye, flush with water.

POSSIBLE INTERACTION WITH OTHER DRUGS

GENERIC NAME OR DRUG CLASS	COMBINED EFFECT
None expected.	

POSSIBLE INTERACTION WITH OTHER SUBSTANCES

INTERACTS WITH	COMBINED EFFECT
Alcohol:	None expected.
Beverages:	None expected.
Cocaine:	None expected.
Foods:	None expected.
Marijuana:	None expected.
Tobacco:	None expected.

*See Glossary

CARBAMAZEPINE

BRAND NAMES

Apo-Carbamazepine	PMS Carbamazepine
Carbatrol	Taro-Carbamazepine
Epitol	Tegretol
Equetro	Tegretol Chewtabs
Mazepine	Tegretol CR
Novocarbamaz	Tegretol XR
Nu-Carbamazepine	

BASIC INFORMATION

Habit forming? No
Prescription needed? Yes
Available as generic? Yes
Drug class: Analgesic, anticonvulsant, antimanic agent

USES

- Treatment of tic douloureux.*
- Treats bipolar (manic-depressive) disorder.
- Used to control certain types of seizures.
- Used for pain relief, restless leg syndrome, alcohol/drug withdrawal and other disorders.

DOSAGE & USAGE INFORMATION

How to take:
- Tablet—Swallow with liquid. Take with food to lessen stomach upset. For chewable tablet, chew well before swallowing.
- Extended-release capsule or tablet or controlled release tablet—Swallow with liquid. May be taken with or without food. Capsule may be opened and sprinkled on food (e.g., teaspoon of applesauce). Do not chew or crush tablet or capsule.
- Oral suspension—Follow label instructions. Do not mix it with other liquid drugs.

When to take:
At the same times each day as directed.

Continued next column

OVERDOSE

SYMPTOMS:
Abnormal movements, slurred speech, nausea and vomiting, drowsiness, high or low blood pressure, dilated pupils, flushed skin, irregular heartbeat and breathing, decreased urine, seizures, tremor, fainting, coma.
WHAT TO DO:
- **Dial 911 (emergency) for medical help or call poison control center 1-800-222-1222 for instructions.**
- **See emergency information on last 3 pages of this book.**

What drug does:
It works by decreasing impulses in nerves that cause seizures and pain.

If you forget a dose:
Take as soon as you remember. If it is almost time for the next dose, wait for that dose (don't double this dose) and resume regular schedule.

Time lapse before drug works:
- Tic douloureux—24 to 72 hours.
- Bipolar disorder—7 to 10 days.
- Seizures—Hours to days in different patients.

Don't take with:
Any other medicine or any dietary supplement without consulting your doctor or pharmacist. May inactivate other medications, such as birth control pills.

POSSIBLE ADVERSE REACTIONS OR SIDE EFFECTS

SYMPTOMS	WHAT TO DO
Life-threatening: Rare allergic reaction—Breathing difficulty; closing of the throat; swelling of hands, feet, face, lips or tongue; hives.	Discontinue. Seek emergency treatment.
Common: • Back-and-forth eye movements, double or blurred vision.	Discontinue. Call doctor right away.
• Being clumsy or unsteady, mildly dizzy or lightheaded, mild nausea or vomiting.	Continue. Call doctor when convenient.
Infrequent: • Behavior changes in a child or in the elderly (e.g., confusion or agitation), ongoing headache, severe diarrhea or nausea or vomiting or drowsiness, increase in seizures, skin rash or hives.	Discontinue. Call doctor right away.
• Mild diarrhea, dry mouth, constipation, impotence, muscle aches, sore tongue or mouth, hair loss, upset stomach, appetite loss, increased sweating.	Continue. Call doctor when convenient.
Rare: Breathing difficulty; irregular, pounding or slow heartbeat; chest pain; uncontrollable body jerks; numbness, weakness or tingling in hands and feet; swollen legs or	Discontinue. Call doctor right away.

feet or face; unusual bleeding or bruising, stool changes (black, tarry, bloody, or pale), urine changes (frequent, decreased, bloody, dark or painful), unusual pain, yellow eyes or skin, infection (fever, chills), rapid weight gain, noises in ears, slurred speech, hallucinations, unusual tiredness or weakness.

WARNINGS & PRECAUTIONS

Don't take if:
- You are allergic to carbamazepine or any tricyclic antidepressant.*
- You have taken a monoamine oxidase (MAO) inhibitor* in the past 2 weeks.

Before you start, consult your doctor if:
- You have high blood pressure, heart block, thrombophlebitis or heart disease.
- You have glaucoma.
- You have emotional or mental problems.
- You have diabetes, liver or kidney disease.
- You have a blood disorder (e.g., anemia) or bone marrow depression or disease.
- You have had reactions to other drugs.
- You are of Asian ancestry (a genetic blood test can tell if you are at increased risk of developing a rare, but serious, skin reaction).
- You drink more than 2 alcoholic drinks a day.

Over age 60:
Adverse reactions and side effects may be more frequent and severe than in younger persons.

Pregnancy:
Decide with your doctor whether drug benefits justify risk to unborn child. Risk category C (see page xviii).

Breast-feeding:
Drug passes into milk. Avoid drug or discontinue nursing until you finish medicine. Consult doctor for advice on maintaining milk supply.

Infants & children:
May be used in children. Side effects of behavior changes are more likely in this age group.

Prolonged use:
Talk to your doctor about the need for follow-up medical examinations, blood and urine studies, eye and dental exams, liver and kidney function tests, bone density tests, and others as needed.

Skin & sunlight:
May cause rash or intensify sunburn in areas exposed to sun or ultraviolet light (photosensitivity reaction). Avoid overexposure and use sunscreen. Notify doctor if reaction occurs.

Driving, piloting or hazardous work:
Don't drive or pilot aircraft until you learn how drug effects you. Don't work around dangerous machinery. Don't climb ladders or work in high places. Danger increases if you drink alcohol or take drugs affecting alertness and reflexes.

Discontinuing:
Don't discontinue without doctor's advice until you complete prescribed dose, even though symptoms diminish or disappear.

Others:
- Wear or carry medical identification that states that you take this drug.
- Periodic blood tests are needed.
- Advise any doctor or dentist whom you consult that you take this medicine.
- Rarely, anticonvulsant (antiepileptic) drugs may lead to suicidal thoughts and behaviors. Call doctor right away if suicidal symptoms or unusual behaviors behaviors occur.

POSSIBLE INTERACTION WITH OTHER DRUGS

GENERIC NAME OR DRUG CLASS	COMBINED EFFECT
Acetaminophen	Increased risk of liver problems.
Adrenocorticoids, systemic	Decreased adreno-corticoid effect.
Antibiotics, macrolide	Increased effect of carbamazepine.
Anticoagulants, oral*	Decreased anti-coagulant effect.
Anticonvulsants, hydantoin* or succinimide*	Decreased effect of both drugs.
Antidepressants, tricyclic*	Confusion. Possible psychosis.

Continued on page 913

POSSIBLE INTERACTION WITH OTHER SUBSTANCES

INTERACTS WITH	COMBINED EFFECT
Alcohol:	Increased sedative effect. Avoid.
Beverages: Grapefruit juice.	Risk of toxicity. Avoid.
Cocaine:	Increased adverse effects. Avoid.
Foods:	None expected.
Marijuana:	Increased adverse effects. Avoid.
Tobacco:	None expected.

*See Glossary

CARBIDOPA & LEVODOPA

BRAND NAMES

Parcopa	Sinemet CR
Sinemet	Stalevo

BASIC INFORMATION

Habit forming? No
Prescription needed? Yes
Available as generic? Yes
Drug class: Antiparkinsonism

 ## USES

Controls Parkinson's disease symptoms such as rigidity, tremor and unsteady gait.

 ## DOSAGE & USAGE INFORMATION

How to take:
* Tablet—Swallow with liquid or food to lessen stomach irritation. If you can't swallow whole, crumble tablet and take with liquid or food. Do not crush, break or chew Stalevo tablet.
* Extended-release tablet—Swallow each dose whole; do not crumble.

When to take:
At the same times each day.

If you forget a dose:
Take as soon as you remember up to 2 hours late. If more than 2 hours, wait for next scheduled dose (don't double this dose).

What drug does:
Restores chemical balance necessary for normal nerve impulses.

Continued next column

 ## OVERDOSE

SYMPTOMS:
Muscle twitch, spastic eyelid closure, nausea, vomiting, diarrhea, irregular and rapid pulse, weakness, fainting, confusion, agitation, hallucination, coma.
WHAT TO DO:
* **Dial 911 (emergency) for medical help or call poison control center 1-800-222-1222 for instructions.**
* **If person is unconscious, check breathing and pulse. If not breathing, begin mouth-to-mouth rescue breathing. If heart is not beating, begin chest compressions.**
* **See emergency information on last 3 pages of this book.**

Time lapse before drug works:
2 to 3 weeks to improve; 6 weeks or longer for maximum benefit.

Don't take with:
Any other medicine or any dietary supplement without consulting your doctor or pharmacist.

 ## POSSIBLE ADVERSE REACTIONS OR SIDE EFFECTS

SYMPTOMS	WHAT TO DO
Life-threatening:	
In case of overdose, see previous column.	
Common:	
• Mood changes, uncontrollable body movements, diarrhea.	Continue. Call doctor when convenient.
• Dry mouth, body odor.	No action necessary.
Infrequent:	
• Fainting, severe dizziness, headache, insomnia, nightmares, rash, itch, nausea, vomiting, irregular heartbeat.	Discontinue. Call doctor right away.
• Flushed face, blurred vision, muscle twitching, discolored or dark urine, difficult urination.	Continue. Call doctor when convenient.
• Constipation, tiredness.	Continue. Tell doctor at next visit.
Rare:	
• High blood pressure.	Discontinue. Call doctor right away.
• Upper abdominal pain, anemia.	Continue. Call doctor when convenient.

 ## WARNINGS & PRECAUTIONS

Don't take if:
* You are allergic to levodopa or carbidopa.
* You have taken MAO inhibitors in past 2 weeks.
* You have glaucoma (narrow-angle type).

Before you start, consult your doctor if:
* You have diabetes or epilepsy.
* You have had high blood pressure, heart or lung disease.
* You have had liver or kidney disease.
* You have a peptic ulcer.
* You have malignant melanoma.
* You will have surgery within 2 months, including dental surgery, requiring general or spinal anesthesia.

Over age 60:
Adverse reactions and side effects may be more frequent and severe than in younger persons.

Pregnancy:
Decide with your doctor whether drug benefits justify risk to unborn child. Risk category C (see page xviii).

Breast-feeding:
It is unknown if drug passes into milk. Avoid drug or discontinue nursing until you finish medicine. Consult doctor for advice on maintaining milk supply.

Infants & children:
Not recommended.

Prolonged use:
- May lead to uncontrolled movements of head, face, mouth, tongue, arms or legs.
- Talk to your doctor about the need for follow-up medical examinations or laboratory studies to check complete blood counts (white blood cell count, platelet count, red blood cell count, hemoglobin, hematocrit), liver function, eyes, kidney function.

Skin & sunlight:
No problems expected.

Driving, piloting or hazardous work:
Don't drive or pilot aircraft until you learn how medicine affects you. Don't work around dangerous machinery. Don't climb ladders or work in high places. Danger increases if you drink alcohol or take medicine affecting alertness and reflexes, such as antihistamines, tranquilizers, sedatives, pain medicine, narcotics and mind-altering drugs.

Discontinuing:
Don't discontinue without doctor's advice until you complete prescribed dose, even though symptoms diminish or disappear.

Others:
- Expect to start with small dose and increase gradually to lessen frequency and severity of adverse reactions.
- Advise any doctor or dentist whom you consult that you take this medicine.

POSSIBLE INTERACTION WITH OTHER DRUGS

GENERIC NAME OR DRUG CLASS	COMBINED EFFECT
Anticonvulsants,* hydantoin	Decreased effect of carbidopa and levodopa.
Antidepressants*	Weakness or faintness when arising from bed or chair.
Antihypertensives*	Decreased blood pressure and effect of carbidopa and levodopa.
Antiparkinsonism drugs, other*	Increased effect of carbidopa and levodopa.
Bupropion	Increased levodopa effect.
Haloperidol	Decreased effect of carbidopa and levodopa.
Methyldopa	Decreased effect of carbidopa and levodopa.
Monoamine oxidase (MAO) inhibitors*	Dangerous rise in blood pressure.
Papaverine	Decreased effect of carbidopa and levodopa.
Phenothiazines*	Decreased effect of carbidopa and levodopa.
Phenytoin	Decreased effect of carbidopa and levodopa.
Pyridoxine (Vitamin B-6)	Decreased effect of carbidopa and levodopa.
Rauwolfia alkaloids*	Decreased effect of carbidopa and levodopa.
Selegiline	May require adjustment in dosage of carbidopa and levodopa.

POSSIBLE INTERACTION WITH OTHER SUBSTANCES

INTERACTS WITH	COMBINED EFFECT
Alcohol:	None expected.
Beverages:	None expected.
Cocaine:	Decreased carbidopa and levodopa effect. High rise of heart-beat irregularities. Avoid.
Foods:	None expected.
Marijuana:	Increased fatigue, lethargy, fainting.
Tobacco:	None expected.

*See Glossary

CARBONIC ANHYDRASE INHIBITORS

GENERIC AND BRAND NAMES

ACETAZOLAMIDE
Acetazolam
Ak-Zol
Apo Acetazolamide
Dazamide
Diamox
Storzolamide

DICHLORPHENAMIDE
Daranide
METHAZOLAMIDE
MZM
Neptazane

BASIC INFORMATION

Habit forming? No
Prescription needed? Yes
Available as generic? Yes
Drug class: Carbonic anhydrase inhibitor

 ## USES

- Treatment of glaucoma.
- Treatment of epileptic seizures.
- Treatment of body fluid retention.
- Treatment for shortness of breath, insomnia and fatigue at high altitudes.
- Treatment for prevention of altitude illness.

 ## DOSAGE & USAGE INFORMATION

How to take:
- Sustained-release tablet—Swallow whole with liquid or food to lessen stomach irritation.
- Extended-release capsule—Swallow whole with liquid.
- Topical—1 drop in the affected eye 3 times a day.

When to take:
- 1 dose per day—At the same time each morning.
- More than 1 dose per day—Take last dose several hours before bedtime.

Continued next column

 ## OVERDOSE

SYMPTOMS:
Drowsiness, confusion, excitement, nausea, vomiting, numbness in hands and feet, coma.
WHAT TO DO:
- Dial 911 (emergency) for medical help or call poison control center 1-800-222-1222 for instructions. Symptoms may not appear until damage has occurred.
- See emergency information on last 3 pages of this book.

If you forget a dose:
Take as soon as you remember. Continue regular schedule.

What drug does:
- Inhibits action of carbonic anhydrase, an enzyme. This lowers the internal eye pressure by decreasing fluid formation in the eye.
- Forces sodium and water excretion, reducing body fluid.

Time lapse before drug works:
2 hours.

Don't take with:
Any other medicine or any dietary supplement without consulting your doctor or pharmacist.

 ## POSSIBLE ADVERSE REACTIONS OR SIDE EFFECTS

SYMPTOMS	WHAT TO DO
Life-threatening: Convulsions.	Seek emergency treatment immediately.
Common: None expected.	
Infrequent: Back pain, sedation, fatigue, weakness, tingling or burning in feet or hands.	Continue. Call doctor when convenient.
Rare: • Headache; mood changes; nervousness; clumsiness; trembling; confusion; hives, itch, rash; sores; ringing in ears; hoarseness; dry mouth; thirst; sore throat; fever; appetite change; nausea; vomiting; black, tarry stool; breathing difficulty; irregular or weak heartbeat; easy bleeding or bruising; muscle cramps; painful or frequent urination; blood in urine.	Continue. Call doctor right away.
• Depression, loss of libido.	Continue. Call doctor when convenient.

228

CARBONIC ANHYDRASE INHIBITORS

WARNINGS & PRECAUTIONS

Don't take if:
You are allergic to any carbonic anhydrase inhibitor.

Before you start, consult your doctor if:
- You have gout or lupus.
- You are allergic to any sulfa drug.
- You have liver or kidney disease.
- You have Addison's disease (adrenal gland failure).
- You have diabetes.
- You will have surgery within 2 months, including dental surgery, requiring general or spinal anesthesia.

Over age 60:
- Don't exceed recommended dose.
- If you take a digitalis preparation, eat foods high in potassium content or take a potassium supplement.

Pregnancy:
Avoid if possible, especially first 3 months. Consult doctor. Risk category C (see page xviii).

Breast-feeding:
Avoid drug or don't nurse your infant. Consult doctor about maintaining milk supply.

Infants & children:
Not recommended for children younger than 12.

Prolonged use:
May cause kidney stones, vision change, loss of taste and smell, jaundice or weight loss.

Skin & sunlight:
One or more drugs in this group may cause rash or intensify sunburn in areas exposed to sun or ultraviolet light (photosensitivity reaction). Avoid overexposure. Notify doctor if reaction occurs.

Driving, piloting or hazardous work:
Avoid if you feel drowsy or dizzy. Otherwise, no problems expected.

Discontinuing:
Don't discontinue without medical advice.

Others:
- Medicine may increase sugar levels in blood and urine. Diabetics may need insulin adjustment.
- Advise any doctor or dentist whom you consult that you take this medicine.

POSSIBLE INTERACTION WITH OTHER DRUGS

GENERIC NAME OR DRUG CLASS	COMBINED EFFECT
Adrenocorticoids, systemic	Increased loss of calcium & potassium.
Amphetamines*	Increased amphetamine effect.
Anticonvulsants*	Increased loss of bone minerals.
Antidiabetics, oral*	May need dosage adjustment.
Antiglaucoma, carbonic anhydrase inhibitors	Increased effect of both drugs. Avoid.
Ciprofloxacin	May cause kidney dysfunction.
Digitalis preparations*	Possible digitalis toxicity.
Diuretics*	Increased potassium loss.
Lithium	Decreased lithium effect.
Mecamylamine	Increased mecamylamine effect.
Memantine	Increased effect of memantine.
Methenamine	Decreased methenamine effect.
Mexiletine	May slow elimination of mexiletine and cause need to adjust dosage.
Quinidine	Increased quinidine effect.
Salicylates*	Salicylate toxicity.
Sympathomimetics*	Increased sympathomimetic effect.

POSSIBLE INTERACTION WITH OTHER SUBSTANCES

INTERACTS WITH	COMBINED EFFECT
Alcohol:	None expected.
Beverages:	None expected.
Cocaine:	Avoid. Decreased carbonic anhydrase inhibitor effect.
Foods: Potassium-rich foods.*	Eat these to decrease potassium loss.
Marijuana:	Avoid. Increased carbonic anhydrase inhibitor effect.
Tobacco:	May decrease effect of carbonic anhydrase inhibitors.

CELLULOSE SODIUM PHOSPHATE

BRAND NAMES

Calcibind

BASIC INFORMATION

Habit forming? No
Prescription needed? Yes
Available as generic? No
Drug class: Antiurolithic

USES

Prevents formation of calcium kidney stones.

DOSAGE & USAGE INFORMATION

How to take:
Oral suspension—Dissolve in full glass of liquid and swallow. Note: Drink 8 ounces of water or other liquid every hour while you are awake.

When to take:
* According to instructions on prescription label. Usually 3 times a day with meals.
* Don't take within 1-1/2 hours of taking any laxative or antacid containing magnesium.

If you forget a dose:
Take as soon as you remember up to 2 hours late. If more than 2 hours, wait for next scheduled dose (don't double this dose).

What drug does:
Combines with calcium in food to prevent absorption into the bloodstream.

Time lapse before drug works:
None. Works right away.

Don't take with:
Any other medicines (including over-the-counter drugs such as cough and cold medicines, laxatives, antacids, diet pills, caffeine, nose drops or vitamins) without consulting your doctor or pharmacist.

OVERDOSE

SYMPTOMS:
Drowsiness, mental changes, muscle spasms, seizures.
WHAT TO DO:
* Dial 911 (emergency) for medical help or call poison control center 1-800-222-1222 for instructions.
* See emergency information on last 3 pages of this book.

POSSIBLE ADVERSE REACTIONS OR SIDE EFFECTS

SYMPTOMS	WHAT TO DO
Life-threatening:	
In case of overdose, see previous column.	
Common:	
Loose bowel movements.	Continue. Call doctor when convenient.
Infrequent:	
Abdominal pain.	Discontinue. Call doctor right away.
Rare:	
None expected.	

CELLULOSE SODIUM PHOSPHATE

WARNINGS & PRECAUTIONS

Don't take if:
- You have bone disease.
- You have hyperparathyroidism.
- You have too little calcium in your blood.

Before you start, consult your doctor if:
- You have heart disease.
- You have kidney disease.

Over age 60:
No special problems expected.

Pregnancy:
Decide with your doctor if drug benefits justify risk to unborn child. Risk category C (see page xviii).

Breast-feeding:
No special problems expected. Consult doctor.

Infants & children:
Not recommended up to age 16.

Prolonged use:
Talk to your doctor about the need for follow-up medical examinations or laboratory studies to check serum calcium and magnesium concentrations (every 6 months), serum parathyroid hormone, urinary calcium and urinary oxalate levels (occasionally).

Skin & sunlight:
No problems expected.

Driving, piloting or hazardous work:
Avoid if you feel confused, drowsy or dizzy.

Discontinuing:
No special problems expected.

Others:
Advise any doctor or dentist whom you consult that you take this medicine.

POSSIBLE INTERACTION WITH OTHER DRUGS

GENERIC NAME OR DRUG CLASS	COMBINED EFFECT
Calcium-containing medications	Decreased effect of cellulose sodium phosphate.
Magnesium-containing medicines (includes many laxatives* and antacids*)	Decreased magnesium effect.
Vitamin C (ascorbic acid)	Decreased vitamin C effect.

POSSIBLE INTERACTION WITH OTHER SUBSTANCES

INTERACTS WITH	COMBINED EFFECT
Alcohol:	None expected.
Beverages: Milk or other dairy products or tea.	Decreases effectiveness of cellulose sodium phosphate.
Cocaine:	None expected.
Foods: Spinach, broccoli, rhubarb.	Decreases effectiveness of cellulose sodium phosphate.
Marijuana:	None expected.
Tobacco:	None expected.

CENTRAL ALPHA AGONISTS

GENERIC AND BRAND NAMES

CLONIDINE
  Catapres
  Catapres-TTS
  Dixarit
GUANABENZ
  Wytensin
GUANFACINE
  Tenex

METHYLDOPA
  Aldoclor
  Aldomet
  Aldoril
  Apo-Methyldopa
  Dopamet
  Novodoparil
  Novomedopa
  Nu-Medopa
  PMS Dopazide
  Supres

BASIC INFORMATION

Habit forming? No
Prescription needed? Yes
Available as generic? Yes
Drug class: Antihypertensive

 ## USES

• Control of hypertension (high blood pressure).
• May be used for symptoms of narcotic, alcohol or nicotine withdrawal.
• Prevention of migraine headaches.
• Treatment for menstrual cramps or hot flashes due to menopause.
• May be used for treatment of other disorders as determined by your doctor.

 ## DOSAGE & USAGE INFORMATION

How to take:
• Tablet—Swallow with liquid. May take with or without food.
• Transdermal patch (attaches to skin)—Apply to clean, dry, hairless skin on arm or trunk. Follow all prescription instructions carefully.

Continued next column

 ## OVERDOSE

SYMPTOMS:
Vomiting, slow heartbeat, weakness, low blood pressure, lightheadedness, cold feeling, extreme tiredness or drowsiness, coma.
WHAT TO DO:
• Dial 911 (emergency) for medical help or call poison control center 1-800-222-1222 for instructions.
• If person is unconscious, check breathing and pulse. If not breathing, begin mouth-to-mouth rescue breathing. If heart is not beating, begin chest compressions.
• See emergency information on last 3 pages of this book.

When to take:
• Tablet—One to four times a day according to the instructions on your prescription.
• Transdermal patch—Replace as directed, usually once a week.

If you forget a dose:
• Take tablet as soon as you remember. If it is almost time for the next dose, wait for the next scheduled dose (don't double this dose). If you miss 2 doses in a row, call your doctor.
• If the once-a-week patch change is 3 days late, call your doctor for advice.

What drug does:
• Hypertension—Reduces nerve stimulating impulses to the heart and blood vessels. This lowers blood pressure by relaxing and dilating (widening) blood vessels. This helps to increase the flow of blood in the body.
• Withdrawal symptoms—Thought to block nerve impulses in the area of the brain responsible for the symptoms.

Time lapse before drug works:
2 to 3 weeks for full benefit.

Don't take with:
Any other medicine or any dietary supplement without consulting your doctor or pharmacist.

 ## POSSIBLE ADVERSE REACTIONS OR SIDE EFFECTS

SYMPTOMS	WHAT TO DO
Life-threatening: Allergic reaction (difficulty breathing, closing of the throat, swelling of the lips or face or tongue, hives).	Seek emergency treatment immediately.
Common: Dizziness, constipation, drowsiness, irritated skin (with skin patch), dry mouth, tiredness, headache, insomnia, weakness, low blood pressure.	Continue. Call doctor when convenient.
Infrequent: • Darkened skin (with skin patch), light-headedness, dry or burning eyes, anxiety, decreased sex function, nervousness, appetite loss, nausea, vomiting, depression.	Continue. Call doctor when convenient.
• Swollen feet or legs, slow or fast heartbeat, fever.	Continue, but call doctor right away.

Rare:

• Joint pain, pale stools, skin rash or itching, nightmares, confusion.	Continue. Call doctor when convenient.
• Cold fingers and toes, dark urine, chills, breathing difficulty, yellow eyes or skin, stomach pain.	Continue, but call doctor right away.

WARNINGS & PRECAUTIONS

Don't take if:
You are allergic to any central alpha agonist.

Before you start, consult your doctor if:
• You will have surgery within 2 months requiring general or spinal anesthesia.
• You have heart, liver or kidney disease.
• You had a recent stroke or heart attack.
• You have a peripheral circulation disorder (intermittent claudication, Raynaud's syndrome, Buerger's disease).
• You have Parkinson's disease.
• You have a history of depression.
• You have a disorder affecting the skin or any skin irritation (with use of transdermal patch).

Over age 60:
Adverse reactions and side effects may be more frequent and severe than in younger persons.

Pregnancy:
Decide with your doctor whether drug benefits justify risk to unborn child. Risk category B for guanfacine and methyldopa; risk category C for clonidine and guanabenz (see page xviii).

Breast-feeding:
Clonidine and methyldopa pass into breast milk. It is unknown if guanabenz or guanfacine pass into breast milk. Consult your doctor.

Infants & children:
Use only with doctor's approval. Clonidine may be prescribed for attention deficit hyperactivity disorder.

Prolonged use:
Talk to your doctor about the need for follow-up medical or eye exams or laboratory tests.

Skin & sunlight:
None expected.

Driving, piloting or hazardous work:
Don't drive or pilot aircraft until you learn how medicine affects you. Don't work around dangerous machinery. Don't climb ladders or work in high places. Danger increases if you drink alcohol or take medicine affecting alertness and reflexes.

Discontinuing:
• Don't discontinue abruptly. May cause a withdrawal syndrome (anxiety, chest pain, head-ache, nausea, insomnia, irregular heart-beat, flushed face, sweating). Consult doctor if any symptoms occur after stopping the drug.
• Dose may require gradual reduction if you have taken drug for a long time. Doses of other drugs may also require adjustment.

Others:
• Advise any doctor or dentist whom you consult that you take this medicine.
• For dry mouth, suck sugarless hard candy or chew sugarless gum. If dry mouth continues, consult your dentist.

POSSIBLE INTERACTION WITH OTHER DRUGS

GENERIC NAME OR DRUG CLASS	COMBINED EFFECT
Antidepressants, tricyclic*	Decreased effect of central alpha agonist.
Antihypertensives,* other	Excessive lowering of blood pressure.
Beta-adrenergic blocking agents*	Increased risk of adverse reactions and excessive low blood pressure.

Continued on page 914

POSSIBLE INTERACTION WITH OTHER SUBSTANCES

INTERACTS WITH	COMBINED EFFECT
Alcohol:	Increased sedative effect of alcohol and very low blood pressure. Avoid.
Beverages:	None expected.
Cocaine:	Increased risk of heart problems and high blood pressure. Avoid.
Foods:	None expected.
Marijuana:	Weakness on standing. Avoid.
Tobacco:	None expected. Persons with high blood pressure should not smoke.

CEPHALOSPORINS

GENERIC AND BRAND NAMES

CEFACLOR
  Ceclor
  Ceclor CD
  Raniclor
CEFADROXIL
  Duricef
  Ultracef
CEFDINIR
  Omnicef
CEFDITOREN
  Spectracef
CEFIXIME
  Suprax
CEFOTETAN
  Cefotan
CEFPODOXIME
  Vantin

CEFPROZIL
  Cefzil
CEFTIBUTEN
  Cedax
CEFUROXIME
  Ceftin
CEPHALEXIN
  Apo-Cephalex
  Cefanex
  Ceporex
  C-Lexin
  Keflex
  Keftab
  Novolexin
  Nu-Cephalex
CEPHRADINE
  Anspor
  Velosef

BASIC INFORMATION

Habit forming? No
Prescription needed? Yes
Available as generic? Yes
Drug class: Antibacterial

 USES

Treatment of bacterial infections. Will not cure viral infections such as cold and flu.

 DOSAGE & USAGE INFORMATION

How to take:
- Tablet or capsule—Swallow with liquid. If you can't swallow whole, crumble tablet or open capsule and take with liquid or food.
- Extended-release tablet—Swallow with liquid. Do not crush or chew tablet.

Continued next column

 OVERDOSE

SYMPTOMS:
Abdominal cramps, nausea, vomiting, severe diarrhea with mucus or blood in stool, convulsions.
WHAT TO DO:
Overdose unlikely to threaten life. If person uses much larger amount than prescribed or if accidentally swallowed, call doctor or poison control center 1-800-222-1222 for help.

- Chewable tablet—Follow instructions on prescription.
- Liquid and oral suspension—Use measuring spoon. Mix according to package instructions.

When to take:
- At same times each day, 1 hour before or 2 hours after eating.
- Take until gone or as directed.

If you forget a dose:
Take as soon as you remember or double next dose. Return to regular schedule.

What drug does:
Kills susceptible bacteria.

Time lapse before drug works:
May require several days to affect infection.

Don't take with:
Any other medicine or any dietary supplement without consulting your doctor or pharmacist.

 POSSIBLE ADVERSE REACTIONS OR SIDE EFFECTS

SYMPTOMS	WHAT TO DO
Life-threatening: Hives, rash, intense itching, faintness soon after a dose (anaphylaxis); difficulty breathing.	Seek emergency treatment immediately.
Common: Mild diarrhea, nausea, vomiting, sore mouth or tongue, mild stomach cramps (all less common with some cephalosporins).	Continue. Call doctor when convenient.
Infrequent: None expected.	
Rare: • Severe stomach cramps, severe diarrhea with mucus or blood in stool, fever, unusual weakness or tiredness, weight loss, bleeding or bruising, increased thirst, decreased urine, dizziness, joint pain, appetite loss, skin symptoms (rash, itching, redness, swelling), yellow skin or eyes.	Discontinue. Call doctor right away.
• Genital itching or vaginal discharge.	Continue. Call doctor when convenient.

234

WARNINGS & PRECAUTIONS

Don't take if:
You are allergic to any cephalosporin antibiotic.

Before you start, consult your doctor if:
- You are allergic to any penicillin antibiotic.
- You have a kidney disorder.
- You have colitis or enteritis.

Over age 60:
Adverse reactions and side effects may be more frequent and severe than in younger persons. More likely to itch around rectum and genitals.

Pregnancy:
No proven harm to unborn child. Avoid if possible. Consult doctor. Risk category B (see page xviii).

Breast-feeding:
Drug passes into milk. Avoid drug or discontinue nursing until you finish medicine. Consult doctor for advice on maintaining milk supply.

Infants & children:
No special warnings.

Prolonged use:
- Kills beneficial bacteria that protect body against other germs. Unchecked germs may cause secondary infections.
- Talk to your doctor about the need for follow-up medical examinations or laboratory studies to check prothrombin time.

Skin & sunlight:
No problems expected.

Driving, piloting or hazardous work:
No problems expected.

Discontinuing:
Don't discontinue without doctor's advice until you complete prescribed dose, even though symptoms diminish or disappear.

Others:
- Don't use drug for other medical problems without doctor's approval.
- Advise any doctor or dentist whom you consult that you take this medicine.
- If diarrhea occurs, consult doctor.

POSSIBLE INTERACTION WITH OTHER DRUGS

GENERIC NAME OR DRUG CLASS	COMBINED EFFECT
Anticoagulants*	Increased anticoagulant effect.
Anti-inflammatory drugs, nonsteroidal (NSAIDs)*	Increased risk of peptic ulcer.
Chloramphenicol	Decreased antibiotic effect of cephalosporin.
Probenecid	Increased cephalosporin effect.
Tetracyclines*	Decreased antibiotic effect of cephalosporin.

POSSIBLE INTERACTION WITH OTHER SUBSTANCES

INTERACTS WITH	COMBINED EFFECT
Alcohol:	Increased kidney toxicity, likelihood of disulfiram-like* effect.
Beverages:	None expected.
Cocaine:	None expected, but cocaine may slow body's recovery. Avoid.
Foods:	Slow absorption. Take with liquid 1 hour before or 2 hours after eating.
Marijuana:	None expected, but marijuana may slow body's recovery. Avoid.
Tobacco:	None expected.

*See Glossary

CHARCOAL, ACTIVATED

BRAND NAMES

Acta-Char
Acta-Char Liquid
Actidose with Sorbitol
Actidose-Aqua
Aqueous Charcodote
Charac-50
Charac-tol 50
Charcoaid
Charcocaps

Charcodote
Charcodote TFS
Insta-Char
Liqui-Char
Pediatric Aqueous
 Charcodote
Pediatric Charcodote
SuperChar

BASIC INFORMATION

Habit forming? No
Prescription needed? No
Available as generic? Yes
Drug class: Antidote (adsorbent)

 ## USES

* Treatment of poisonings from medication.
* Treatment (infrequent) for diarrhea or excessive gaseousness.

 ## DOSAGE & USAGE INFORMATION

How to take:
* Tablet or capsule—Swallow with liquid. If you can't swallow whole, crumble tablet or open capsule and take with liquid or food.
* Liquid—Take as directed on label. Don't mix with chocolate syrup, ice cream or sherbet.

When to take:
* For poisoning—Take immediately after poisoning. If your doctor or emergency poison control center has also recommended syrup of ipecac, don't take charcoal for 30 minutes or until vomiting from ipecac stops.
* For diarrhea or gas—Take at same times each day.
* Take 2 or more hours after taking other medicines.

Continued next column

 ## OVERDOSE

SYMPTOMS:
None expected.
WHAT TO DO:
Overdose unlikely to threaten life. If person uses much larger amount than prescribed or if accidentally swallowed, call doctor or poison control center 1-800-222-1222 for help.

If you forget a dose:
* For poisonings—Not applicable.
* For diarrhea or gas—Take as soon as you remember up to 2 hours late. If more than 2 hours, wait for next scheduled dose (don't double this dose).

What drug does:
* Helps prevent poison from being absorbed from stomach and intestines.
* Helps absorb gas in intestinal tract.

Time lapse before drug works:
Begins immediately.

Don't take with:
Ice cream or sherbet.

 ## POSSIBLE ADVERSE REACTIONS OR SIDE EFFECTS

SYMPTOMS	WHAT TO DO
Life-threatening: None expected.	
Always: Black bowel movements.	No action necessary.
Infrequent: None expected.	
Rare: Unless taken with cathartic, can cause constipation when taken for overdose of other medicine.	Take a laxative after crisis is over.

WARNINGS & PRECAUTIONS

Don't take if:
The poison was lye or other strong alkali, strong acids (such as sulfuric acid), cyanide, iron, ethyl alcohol or methyl alcohol. Charcoal will not prevent these poisons from causing ill effects.

Before you start, consult your doctor if:
You are taking it as an antidote for poison.

Over age 60:
No problems expected.

Pregnancy:
Consult doctor. Risk category C (see page xviii).

Breast-feeding:
No problems expected. Consult doctor.

Infants & children:
Don't give to children for more than 3 or 4 days for diarrhea. Continuing for longer periods can interfere with normal nutrition.

Prolonged use:
No problems expected.

Skin & sunlight:
No problems expected.

Driving, piloting or hazardous work:
No problems expected.

Discontinuing:
No problems expected.

Others:
No problems expected.

POSSIBLE INTERACTION WITH OTHER DRUGS

GENERIC NAME OR DRUG CLASS	COMBINED EFFECT
Any medicine taken at the same time	May decrease absorption of medicine. Take drugs 2 hours apart.

POSSIBLE INTERACTION WITH OTHER SUBSTANCES

INTERACTS WITH	COMBINED EFFECT
Alcohol:	None expected.
Beverages:	None expected.
Cocaine:	None expected.
Foods: Chocolate syrup, ice cream or sherbet.	Decreased charcoal effect.
Marijuana:	None expected.
Tobacco:	None expected.

*See Glossary

CHLORAL HYDRATE

BRAND NAMES

Aquachloral   Novochlorhydrate
Noctec

BASIC INFORMATION

Habit forming? Yes
Prescription needed? Yes
Available as generic? Yes
Drug class: Sedative-hypnotic agent

 USES

Short term treatment to relieve insomnia.

 DOSAGE & USAGE INFORMATION

How to take:
• Syrup or capsule—Swallow with liquid or food to lessen stomach irritation.
• Suppository—Remove wrapper and moisten suppository with water. Gently insert smaller end into rectum. Push well into rectum with finger.

When to take:
At the same time each day.

If you forget a dose:
Take as soon as you remember up to 2 hours late. If more than 2 hours, wait for next scheduled dose (don't double this dose).

What drug does:
Affects brain centers that control wakefulness and alertness.

Time lapse before drug works:
30 to 60 minutes.

Continued next column

 OVERDOSE

SYMPTOMS:
Confusion, weakness, breathing difficulty, throat irritation, jaundice, stagger, slow or irregular heartbeat, unconsciousness, convulsions, coma.
WHAT TO DO:
• **Dial 911 (emergency) for medical help or call poison control center 1-800-222-1222 for instructions.**
• **If person is unconscious, check breathing and pulse. If not breathing, begin mouth-to-mouth rescue breathing. If heart is not beating, begin chest compressions.**
• **See emergency information on last 3 pages of this book.**

Don't take with:
Any other medicine or any dietary supplement without consulting your doctor or pharmacist.

 POSSIBLE ADVERSE REACTIONS OR SIDE EFFECTS

SYMPTOMS	WHAT TO DO
Life-threatening:	
In case of overdose, see previous column.	
Common:	
Nausea, stomach pain, vomiting.	Discontinue. Call doctor right away.
Infrequent:	
"Hangover" effect, clumsiness or unsteadiness, drowsiness, dizziness, lightheadedness, diarrhea.	Continue. Call doctor when convenient.
Rare:	
• Hallucinations, agitation, confusion, leukopenia (white blood cells causing sore throat and fever).	Discontinue. Call doctor right away.
• Hives, rash.	Continue. Call doctor when convenient.

 WARNINGS & PRECAUTIONS

Don't take if:
You are allergic to chloral hydrate or you have porphyria.

Before you start, consult your doctor if:
• You have had liver, kidney or heart trouble.
• You are prone to stomach upsets (if medicine is in oral form).
• You are allergic to tartrazine dye.
• You have colitis or a rectal inflammation (if medicine is in suppository form).

Over age 60:
Adverse reactions and side effects may be more frequent and severe than in younger persons. More likely to have "hangover" effect.

Pregnancy:
Decide with your doctor if drug benefits justify risk to unborn child. Risk category C (see page xviii).

Breast-feeding:
It is unknown if drug passes into milk. Avoid drug or discontinue nursing until you finish medicine. Consult doctor for advice on maintaining milk supply.

Infants & children:
Use only under medical supervision.

Prolonged use:
- Drug loses its effectiveness as an antianxiety agent or sleep aid after about 2 weeks. Not recommended for longer use.
- Addiction and possible kidney damage may result if used long-term.

Skin & sunlight:
No problems expected.

Driving, piloting or hazardous work:
Don't drive or pilot aircraft until you learn how medicine affects you. Don't work around dangerous machinery. Don't climb ladders or work in high places. Danger increases if you drink alcohol or take medicine affecting alertness and reflexes, such as antihistamines, tranquilizers, sedatives, pain medicine, narcotics and mind-altering drugs.

Discontinuing:
Don't discontinue without consulting doctor. Dose may require gradual reduction if you have taken drug for a long time. Doses of other drugs may also require adjustment.

Others:
- Frequent kidney function tests recommended when drug is used for long time.
- Advise any doctor or dentist whom you consult that you take this medicine.

POSSIBLE INTERACTION WITH OTHER DRUGS

GENERIC NAME OR DRUG CLASS	COMBINED EFFECT
Anticoagulants, oral*	Possible hemorrhaging.
Antidepressants*	Increased chloral hydrate effect.
Antihistamines*	Increased chloral hydrate effect.
Central nervous system (CNS) depressants*	Increased sedative effect.
Clozapine	Toxic effect on the central nervous system.
Fluoxetine	Increased depressant effects of both drugs.
Guanfacine	May increase depressant effects of either drug.
Leucovorin	High alcohol content of leucovorin may cause adverse effects.

Mind-altering drugs*	Increased chloral hydrate effect.
Molindone	Increased tranquilizer effect.
Monoamine oxidase (MAO) inhibitors*	Increased chloral hydrate effect.
Narcotics*	Increased chloral hydrate effect.
Phenothiazines*	Increased chloral hydrate effect.
Sertraline	Increased depressive effects of both drugs.

POSSIBLE INTERACTION WITH OTHER SUBSTANCES

INTERACTS WITH	COMBINED EFFECT
Alcohol:	Increased sedative effects of both. Avoid.
Beverages:	None expected.
Cocaine:	Decreased chloral hydrate effect. Avoid.
Foods:	None expected.
Marijuana:	May severely impair mental and physical functioning. Avoid.
Tobacco:	None expected.

CHLORAMBUCIL

BRAND NAMES

Leukeran

BASIC INFORMATION

Habit forming? No
Prescription needed? Yes
Available as generic? No
Drug class: Antineoplastic, immuno-
suppressant

 USES

- Treatment for some kinds of cancer.
- Suppresses immune response after transplant and in immune disorders.

 DOSAGE & USAGE INFORMATION

How to take:
Tablet—Swallow with liquid after light meal. Don't drink fluids with meals. Drink extra fluids between meals. Avoid sweet or fatty foods.

When to take:
At the same time each day.

If you forget a dose:
Take as soon as you remember. Never double dose.

What drug does:
Inhibits abnormal cell reproduction. May suppress immune system.

Time lapse before drug works:
Up to 6 weeks for full effect.

Don't take with:
Any other medicine or any dietary supplement without consulting your doctor or pharmacist.

 OVERDOSE

SYMPTOMS:
Bleeding, chills, fever, vomiting, abdominal pain, ataxia, collapse, stupor, seizure.
WHAT TO DO:
- Dial 911 (emergency) for medical help or call poison control center 1-800-222-1222 for instructions.
- If person is unconscious, check breathing and pulse. If not breathing, begin mouth-to-mouth rescue breathing. If heart is not beating, begin chest compressions.
- See emergency information on last 3 pages of this book.

 POSSIBLE ADVERSE REACTIONS OR SIDE EFFECTS

SYMPTOMS	WHAT TO DO
Life-threatening:	
In case of overdose, see previous column.	
Common:	
• Unusual bleeding or bruising, mouth sores with sore throat, chills and fever, black stools, mouth and lip sores, menstrual irregularities, back pain.	Discontinue. Call doctor right away.
• Hair loss, joint pain.	Continue. Call doctor when convenient.
• Nausea, vomiting, diarrhea, tiredness, weakness.	Continue. Tell doctor at next visit.
Infrequent:	
• Mental confusion, shortness of breath.	Continue. Call doctor when convenient.
• Cough, rash, foot swelling.	Continue. Tell doctor at next visit.
Rare:	
Jaundice, convulsions, hallucinations, muscle twitching.	Discontinue. Call doctor right away.

WARNINGS & PRECAUTIONS

Don't take if:
- You have had hypersensitivity to alkylating antineoplastic drugs.
- Your physician has not explained serious nature of your medical problem and risks of taking this medicine.

Before you start, consult your doctor if:
- You have gout.
- You have had kidney stones.
- You have active infection.
- You have impaired kidney or liver function.
- You have taken other antineoplastic drugs or had radiation treatment in last 3 weeks.

Over age 60:
Adverse reactions and side effects may be more frequent and severe than in younger persons.

Pregnancy:
Consult doctor. Risk to unborn child is significant. Risk category D (see page xviii).

Breast-feeding:
Safety not established. Consult doctor.

Infants & children:
Use only under care of doctors who are experienced in anticancer drugs.

Prolonged use:
- Adverse reactions more likely the longer drug is required.
- Talk to your doctor about the need for follow-up medical examinations or laboratory studies to check complete blood counts (white blood cell count, platelet count, red blood cell count, hemoglobin, hematocrit).

Skin & sunlight:
No problems expected.

Driving, piloting or hazardous work:
No problems expected.

Discontinuing:
Don't discontinue without doctor's advice until you complete prescribed dose, even though symptoms diminish or disappear. Some side effects may follow discontinuing. Report to doctor blurred vision, convulsions, confusion, persistent headache.

Others:
- May cause blood problems or cancer.
- Advise any doctor or dentist whom you consult that you take this medicine.
- Consult your doctor before you or a household member gets any immunization.

POSSIBLE INTERACTION WITH OTHER DRUGS

GENERIC NAME OR DRUG CLASS	COMBINED EFFECT
Antigout drugs*	Decreased antigout effect.
Antineoplastic drugs, other*	Increased effect of all drugs (may be beneficial).
Chloramphenicol	Increased likelihood of toxic effects of both drugs.
Clozapine	Toxic effect on bone marrow.
Cyclosporine	May increase risk of infection.
Immuno-suppressants*	Increased chance of infection.
Lovastatin	Increased heart and kidney damage.
Tiopronin	Increased risk of toxicity to bone marrow.

POSSIBLE INTERACTION WITH OTHER SUBSTANCES

INTERACTS WITH	COMBINED EFFECT
Alcohol:	May increase chance of intestinal bleeding.
Beverages:	No problems expected.
Cocaine:	Increases chance of toxicity.
Foods:	Reduces irritation in stomach.
Marijuana:	No problems expected.
Tobacco:	Increases lung toxicity.

*See Glossary

CHLORAMPHENICOL

BRAND NAMES

Chloromycetin   Novochlorocap

BASIC INFORMATION

Habit forming? No
Prescription needed? Yes
Available as generic? Yes
Drug class: Antibacterial

 ## USES

Treatment of infections susceptible to chloramphenicol. Will not treat viral infections such as cold or flu.

 ## DOSAGE & USAGE INFORMATION

How to take:
Suspension or capsule—Take with a full glass of water.

When to take:
Capsule or suspension—1 hour before or 2 hours after eating.

If you forget a dose:
Take as soon as you remember up to 2 hours late. If more than 2 hours, wait for next scheduled dose (don't double this dose).

What drug does:
Prevents bacteria from growing and reproducing. Will not kill viruses.

Time lapse before drug works:
2 to 5 days, depending on type and severity of infection.

Don't take with:
Any other medicine or any dietary supplement without consulting your doctor or pharmacist.

 ## OVERDOSE

SYMPTOMS:
Nausea, vomiting, diarrhea.
WHAT TO DO:
Overdose unlikely to threaten life. If person uses much larger amount than prescribed or if accidentally swallowed, call doctor or poison control center 1-800-222-1222 for help.

 ## POSSIBLE ADVERSE REACTIONS OR SIDE EFFECTS

SYMPTOMS	WHAT TO DO
Life-threatening: Hives, rash, intense itching, faintness soon after a dose (anaphylaxis).	Seek emergency treatment immediately.
Common: None expected.	
Infrequent: • Swollen face or extremities; diarrhea; nausea; vomiting; numbness, tingling, burning pain or weakness in hands and feet; pale skin; unusual bleeding or bruising.	Discontinue. Call doctor right away.
• Headache, confusion.	Continue. Call doctor when convenient.
Rare: • Pain, blurred vision, possible vision loss, delirium, rash, sore throat, fever, jaundice, anemia.	Discontinue. Call doctor right away.
• In babies: Bloated stomach, uneven breathing, drowsiness, low temperature, gray skin.	Discontinue. Call doctor right away.

WARNINGS & PRECAUTIONS

Don't take if:
• You are allergic to chloramphenicol.
• It is prescribed for a minor disorder such as flu, cold or mild sore throat.

Before you start, consult your doctor if:
• You have had a blood disorder or bone-marrow disease.
• You have had kidney or liver disease.
• You have diabetes.

Over age 60:
Adverse reactions and side effects may be more frequent and severe than in younger persons, particularly skin irritation around rectum.

Pregnancy:
Decide with your doctor if drug benefits justify risk to unborn child. Risk category C (see page xviii).

Breast-feeding:
Drug passes into milk. Avoid drug or discontinue nursing until you finish medicine. Consult doctor for advice on maintaining milk supply.

Infants & children:
Use only under close medical supervision, especially in infants younger than 2.

Prolonged use:
- You may become more susceptible to infections caused by germs not responsive to chloramphenicol.
- Talk to your doctor about the need for follow-up medical examinations or laboratory studies to check complete blood counts (white blood cell count, platelet count, red blood cell count, hemoglobin, hematocrit), chloramphenicol serum levels.

Skin & sunlight:
No problems expected.

Driving, piloting or hazardous work:
Don't drive or pilot aircraft until you learn how medicine affects you. Don't work around dangerous machinery. Don't climb ladders or work in high places. Danger increases if you drink alcohol or take medicine affecting alertness and reflexes.

Discontinuing:
Don't discontinue without doctor's advice until you complete prescribed dose, even though symptoms diminish or disappear.

Others:
- Chloramphenicol can cause serious anemia. Frequent laboratory blood studies, liver and kidney tests recommended.
- Advise any doctor or dentist whom you consult that you take this medicine.
- Second medical opinion recommended before starting.

 ## POSSIBLE INTERACTION WITH OTHER DRUGS

GENERIC NAME OR DRUG CLASS	COMBINED EFFECT
Anticoagulants*	Increased anti-coagulant effect.
Antidiabetics, oral*	Increased antidiabetic effect.
Anticonvulsants*	Increased chance of toxicity to bone marrow.
Antivirals, HIV/AIDS*	Increased risk of peripheral neuropathy.
Cefixime	Decreased antibiotic effect of cefixime.
Cephalosporins*	Decreased chloramphenicol effect.
Clindamycin	Decreased clindamycin effect.
Clozapine	Toxic effect on bone marrow.
Cyclophosphamide	Increased cyclophosphamide effect.
Erythromycins	Decreased erythromycin effect.
Flecainide	Possible decreased blood cell production in bone marrow.
Levamisole	Increased risk of bone marrow depression.
Lincomycin	Decreased lincomycin effect.
Lisinopril	Possible blood disorders.
Penicillins*	Decreased penicillin effect.
Phenobarbital	Increased phenobarbital effect.
Phenytoin	Increased phenytoin effect.
Rifampin	Decreased chloramphenicol effect.
Thioguanine	More likelihood of toxicity of both drugs.
Tiopronin	Increased risk of toxicity to bone marrow.
Tocainide	Possible decreased blood cell production in bone marrow.

 ## POSSIBLE INTERACTION WITH OTHER SUBSTANCES

INTERACTS WITH	COMBINED EFFECT
Alcohol:	Possible liver problems. Possible disulfiram reaction.*
Beverages:	None expected.
Cocaine:	No proven problems.
Foods:	None expected.
Marijuana:	None expected.
Tobacco:	None expected.

*See Glossary

CHLORHEXIDINE

BRAND NAMES

Peridex   Periogard
Periochip

BASIC INFORMATION

Habit forming? No
Prescription needed? Yes
Available as generic? Yes
Drug class: Antibacterial (dental)

 USES

Treatment for gingivitis (inflammation of the gums), periodontal disease and other infections of the mouth.

 DOSAGE & USAGE INFORMATION

How to use:
- Oral rinse—Swish in mouth for 30 seconds, then spit out. Do not swallow the solution, and do not rinse mouth with water after using. Use product at full strength; do not dilute.
- Implants—Inserted by dentist.

When to use:
Twice a day after brushing and flossing teeth.

If you forget a dose:
Use as soon as you remember, then return to regular schedule.

What drug does:
Kills or prevents growth of susceptible bacteria.

Time lapse before drug works:
Antibacterial action begins within an hour, but full benefit may take several weeks.

Don't use with:
Other mouthwashes without consulting your dentist or pharmacist.

 OVERDOSE

SYMPTOMS:
None expected. If a child swallows several ounces of the solution, may have slurred speech, staggering or stumbling walk, sleepiness.
WHAT TO DO:
If symptoms occur, call doctor for instructions. If child weighing under 22 pounds accidentally swallows more than 4 ounces, seek emergency help. Dial 911 (emergency) or poison control center 1-800-222-1222 for help.

 POSSIBLE ADVERSE REACTIONS OR SIDE EFFECTS

SYMPTOMS	WHAT TO DO
Life-threatening: None expected.	
Common: Staining of teeth and other oral surfaces, increased tartar, taste changes, minor mouth irritation.	Continue. Call dentist when convenient.
Infrequent: None expected.	
Rare: Allergic reaction (stuffy nose, shortness of breath, skin rash, hives, itching, face swelling); swollen glands on side of face or neck.	Discontinue. Call doctor right away.

WARNINGS & PRECAUTIONS

Don't take if:
You are allergic to chlorhexidine or skin cleaners that contain chlorhexidine.

Before you start, consult your dentist if:
* You have front tooth fillings (may become discolored).
* You have periodontitis.

Over age 60:
No special problems expected.

Pregnancy:
Consult doctor. Risk category B (see page xviii).

Breast-feeding:
It is unknown if drug passes into milk. Consult doctor.

Infants & children:
Safety in children under age 18 has not been established.

Prolonged use:
See your dentist every 6 months.

Skin & sunlight:
No special problems expected.

Driving, piloting or hazardous work:
No special problems expected.

Discontinuing:
No special problems expected.

Others:
Brush teeth with a tartar-control toothpaste, and floss daily to help reduce tartar buildup.

 POSSIBLE INTERACTION WITH OTHER DRUGS

GENERIC NAME OR DRUG CLASS	COMBINED EFFECT
None expected.	

 POSSIBLE INTERACTION WITH OTHER SUBSTANCES

INTERACTS WITH	COMBINED EFFECT
Alcohol:	None expected.
Beverages:	Avoid drinking any fluids for several hours after using mouthwash.
Cocaine:	None expected.
Foods:	Avoid eating any foods for several hours after using mouthwash.
Marijuana:	None expected.
Tobacco:	None expected.

*See Glossary

CHLOROQUINE

BRAND NAMES

Aralen

BASIC INFORMATION

Habit forming? No
Prescription needed? Yes
Available as generic? Yes
Drug class: Antiprotozoal, antirheumatic

 ## USES

- Treatment for protozoal infections, such as malaria and amebiasis.
- Treatment for some forms of arthritis and lupus.

 ## DOSAGE & USAGE INFORMATION

How to take:
Tablet—Swallow with food or milk to lessen stomach irritation.

When to take:
- Depends on condition. Is adjusted during treatment.
- Malaria prevention—Begin taking medicine 2 weeks before traveling to areas where malaria is present and until 8 weeks after return.

If you forget a dose:
- 1 or more doses a day—Take as soon as you remember up to 2 hours late. If more than 2 hours, wait for next scheduled dose (don't double this dose).
- 1 dose weekly—Take as soon as possible, then return to regular dosing schedule.

What drug does:
- Inhibits parasite multiplication.
- Decreases inflammatory response in diseased joint.

Continued next column

 ## OVERDOSE

SYMPTOMS:
Severe breathing difficulty, drowsiness, faintness, headache, seizures.
WHAT TO DO:
- Dial 911 (emergency) for medical help or call poison control center 1-800-222-1222 for instructions.
- See emergency information on last 3 pages of this book.

Time lapse before drug works:
1 to 2 hours. For treatment of arthritis symptoms, may take up to 6 months for maximum effectiveness.

Don't take with:
Any other medicine or any dietary supplement without consulting your doctor or pharmacist.

 ## POSSIBLE ADVERSE REACTIONS OR SIDE EFFECTS

SYMPTOMS	WHAT TO DO
Life-threatening: In case of overdose, see previous column.	
Common: Headache, appetite loss, abdominal pain.	Continue. Tell doctor at next visit.
Infrequent: • Blurred or changed vision.	Discontinue. Call doctor right away.
• Rash or itch, diarrhea, nausea, vomiting, decreased blood pressure, hair loss, blue-black skin or mouth, dizziness, nervousness.	Continue. Call doctor when convenient.
Rare: • Mood or mental changes, seizures, sore throat, fever, unusual bleeding or bruising, muscle weakness, convulsions.	Discontinue. Call doctor right away.
• Ringing or buzzing in ears, hearing loss.	Continue. Call doctor when convenient.

WARNINGS & PRECAUTIONS

Don't take if:
You are allergic to chloroquine or hydroxychloroquine.

Before you start, consult your doctor if:
* You plan to become pregnant within the medication period.
* You have blood disease.
* You have eye or vision problems.
* You have a G6PD deficiency.
* You have liver disease.
* You have nerve or brain disease (including seizure disorders).
* You have porphyria.
* You have psoriasis.
* You have stomach or intestinal disease.
* You drink more than 3 oz. of alcohol daily.

Over age 60:
Adverse reactions and side effects may be more frequent and severe than in younger persons.

Pregnancy:
Decide with your doctor if drug benefits justify risk to unborn child. Risk category C (see page xviii).

Breast-feeding:
Drug passes into milk. Avoid drug or discontinue nursing. Consult doctor about maintaining milk supply.

Infants & children:
Not recommended. Dangerous.

Prolonged use:
* Permanent damage to the retina (back part of the eye) or nerve deafness.
* Talk to your doctor about the need for follow-up medical examinations or laboratory studies to check complete blood counts (white blood cell count, platelet count, red blood cell count, hemoglobin, hematocrit), eyes.

Skin & sunlight:
May cause rash or intensify sunburn in areas exposed to sun or ultraviolet light (photosensitivity reaction). Avoid overexposure. Notify doctor if reaction occurs.

Driving, piloting or hazardous work:
Don't drive or pilot aircraft until you learn how medicine affects you. Don't work around dangerous machinery. Don't climb ladders or work in high places. Danger increases if you drink alcohol or take medicine affecting alertness and reflexes.

Discontinuing:
Don't discontinue without doctor's advice until you complete prescribed dose, even though symptoms diminish or disappear.

Others:
* Periodic physical and blood examinations recommended.
* Advise any doctor or dentist whom you consult that you take this medicine.
* If you are in a malaria area for a long time, you may need to change to another preventive drug every 2 years.

POSSIBLE INTERACTION WITH OTHER DRUGS

GENERIC NAME OR DRUG CLASS	COMBINED EFFECT
Penicillamine	Possible blood or kidney toxicity.

POSSIBLE INTERACTION WITH OTHER SUBSTANCES

INTERACTS WITH	COMBINED EFFECT
Alcohol:	Possible liver toxicity. Avoid.
Beverages:	None expected.
Cocaine:	None expected.
Foods:	None expected.
Marijuana:	None expected.
Tobacco:	None expected.

CHOLESTYRAMINE

BRAND NAMES

Cholybar   Questran Light
Questran

BASIC INFORMATION

Habit forming? No
Prescription needed? Yes
Available as generic? Yes
Drug class: Antihyperlipidemic, antipruritic

 ## USES

- Removes excess bile acids that occur with some liver problems. Reduces persistent itch caused by bile acids.
- Lowers cholesterol level.
- Treatment of one form of colitis (rare).

 ## DOSAGE & USAGE INFORMATION

How to take:
Powder, granules—Sprinkle into 8 oz. liquid. Let stand for 2 minutes, then mix with liquid before swallowing. Or mix with cereal, soup or pulpy fruit. Don't swallow dry.

When to take:
- 3 or 4 times a day on an empty stomach, 1 hour before or 2 hours after eating.
- If taking other medicines, take 1 hour before or 4 to 6 hours after taking cholestyramine.

If you forget a dose:
Take as soon as you remember. If it is almost time for the next dose, skip the missed dose and wait for your next scheduled dose (don't double this dose).

What drug does:
Binds with bile acids to prevent their absorption.

Time lapse before drug works:
- Cholesterol reduction—1 day.
- Bile-acid reduction—3 to 4 weeks.

Continued next column

 ## OVERDOSE

SYMPTOMS:
Increased side effects and adverse reactions.
WHAT TO DO:
Overdose unlikely to threaten life. If person uses much larger amount than prescribed or if accidentally swallowed, call doctor or poison control center 1-800-222-1222 for help.

Don't take with:
- Another medicine at the same time. Space doses 2 hours apart.
- Any other medicine or any dietary supplement without consulting your doctor or pharmacist.

 ## POSSIBLE ADVERSE REACTIONS OR SIDE EFFECTS

SYMPTOMS	WHAT TO DO
Life-threatening:	
In case of overdose, see previous column.	
Common:	
Constipation.	Continue. Call doctor when convenient.
Infrequent:	
• Belching, bloating, diarrhea, mild nausea, vomiting, stomach pain, rapid weight gain.	Discontinue. Call doctor when convenient.
• Heartburn (mild).	Continue. Call doctor when convenient.
Rare:	
• Severe stomach pain; black, tarry stool.	Discontinue. Seek emergency treatment.
• Rash, hives, hiccups.	Discontinue. Call doctor right away.
• Sore tongue.	Continue. Call doctor when convenient.

 ## WARNINGS & PRECAUTIONS

Don't take if:
You are allergic to cholestyramine.

Before you start, consult your doctor if:
- You plan to become pregnant within medication period.
- You have angina, heart or blood-vessel disease.
- You have stomach problems (including ulcer).
- You have tartrazine sensitivity.
- You have constipation or hemorrhoids.
- You have kidney disease.

Over age 60:
Adverse reactions and side effects may be more frequent and severe than in younger persons.

Pregnancy:
Decide with your doctor whether drug benefits justify risk to unborn child. Risk category C (see page xviii).

Breast-feeding:
No problems expected, but consult doctor.

Infants & children:
Not recommended.

Prolonged use:
- May decrease absorption of folic acid.
- Talk to your doctor about the need for follow-up medical examinations or laboratory studies to check serum cholesterol and triglycerides.

Skin & sunlight:
No problems expected.

Driving, piloting or hazardous work:
No problems expected.

Discontinuing:
Don't discontinue without doctor's advice until you complete prescribed dose, even though symptoms diminish or disappear.

Others:
Advise any doctor or dentist whom you consult that you take this medicine.

POSSIBLE INTERACTION WITH OTHER DRUGS

GENERIC NAME OR DRUG CLASS	COMBINED EFFECT
Adrenocorticoids, systemic	Decreased adrenocorticoid effect.
Anticoagulants, oral*	Increased anticoagulant effect.
Beta carotene	Decreased absorption of beta carotene.
Dexfenfluramine	May require dosage change as weight loss occurs.
Dextrothyroxine	Decreased dextrothyroxine effect.
Digitalis preparations*	Decreased digitalis effect.
Indapamide	Decreased indapamide effect.
Penicillins*	May decrease penicillin effect.
Raloxifene	Decreased effect of raloxifene.
Thiazides*	Decreased absorption of cholestyramine.
Thyroid hormones*	Decreased thyroid effect.

Trimethoprim	Decreased absorption of cholestyramine.
Troglitazone	Decreased effect of troglitazone. Avoid.
Ursodiol	Decreased absorption of ursodiol.
Vancomycin	Increased chance of hearing loss or kidney damage. Decreased therapeutic effect of vancomycin.
Vitamins	Decreased absorption of fat-soluble vitamins (A,D,E,K).
All other medicines	Decreased absorption, so dosages or dosage intervals may require adjustment.

POSSIBLE INTERACTION WITH OTHER SUBSTANCES

INTERACTS WITH	COMBINED EFFECT
Alcohol:	None expected.
Beverages:	None expected.
Cocaine:	None expected.
Foods:	Absorption of vitamins in foods decreased. Take vitamin supplements, particularly A, D, E & K.
Marijuana:	None expected.
Tobacco:	None expected.

CHOLINESTERASE INHIBITORS

GENERIC AND BRAND NAMES

DONEPEZIL
  Aricept
  Aricept ODT
GALANTAMINE
  Razadyne
  Razadyne ER

RIVASTIGMINE
  Exelon
  Exelon Patch
TACRINE
  Cognex

BASIC INFORMATION

Habit forming? No
Prescription needed? Yes
Available as generic? Yes, for some
Drug class: Cholinesterase inhibitor

 USES

Treats symptoms of mild to moderate dementia (such as problems with memory, judgement, reasoning and other cognitive functions) in patients with Alzheimer's disease or Parkinson's disease.

 DOSAGE & USAGE INFORMATION

How to take:
* Capsule or tablet—Swallow with liquid. If unable to swallow whole, open capsule or crumble tablet and take with liquid or food.
* Disintegrating tablet—Let dissolve on tongue.
* Patch—Always follow label instructions.
* Oral solution—Take as directed on label.

When to take:
* Donepezil—Once a day at bedtime.
* Rivastigmine, galantamine and tacrine—At the same times each day.

Continued next column

 OVERDOSE

SYMPTOMS:
Severe nausea and vomiting, excessive saliva, sweating, blood pressure decrease, slow heartbeat, collapse, convulsions, muscle weakness (including respiratory muscles, which could lead to death).
WHAT TO DO:
* **Dial 911 (emergency) for medical help or call poison control center 1-800-222-1222 for instructions.**
* **If person is unconscious, check breathing and pulse. If not breathing, begin mouth-to-mouth rescue breathing. If heart is not beating, begin chest compressions.**
* **See emergency information on last 3 pages of this book.**

What drug does:
Slows breakdown of a brain chemical (acetylcholine) that gradually disappears from the brains of people with Alzheimer's disease.

If you forget a dose:
* Donepezil—Skip missed dose. Do not double the next dose.
* Others—Take as soon as you remember up to 2 hours late. If more than 2 hours, wait for next scheduled dose (do not double this dose).

Time lapse before drug works:
May take several weeks or months before beneficial results are observed. Dosage is normally increased over a period of time to help prevent adverse reactions.

Don't take with:
Any other medicine or any dietary supplement without consulting your doctor or pharmacist.

 POSSIBLE ADVERSE REACTIONS OR SIDE EFFECTS

SYMPTOMS	WHAT TO DO
Life-threatening: In case of overdose, see previous column.	
Common: Nausea, vomiting, diarrhea, lack of coordination.	Continue. Call doctor when convenient.
Infrequent: Rash, indigestion, headache, muscle aches, loss of appetite, stomach pain, nervousness, chills, dizziness, drowsiness, dry or itching eyes, increased sweating, joint pain, runny nose, sore throat, swelling of feet or legs, insomnia, weight loss, unusual tiredness or weakness, flushing of face.	Continue. Call doctor when convenient.
Rare: Changes in liver function (yellow skin or eyes; black, very dark or light stool color); lack of coordination, convulsions, speech problems, irregular heartbeat, vision changes, increased libido, changes in blood pressure, hot flashes, breathing difficulty.	Continue. Call doctor right away.

WARNINGS & PRECAUTIONS

Don't take if:
You are allergic to cholinesterase inhibitors.

Before you start, consult your doctor if:
* You have heart rhythm problems.
* You have a history of ulcer disease or are at risk of developing ulcers.
* You have a history of liver disease.
* You have a history of urinary tract problems.
* You have epilepsy or seizure disorder.
* You have a history of asthma.
* You have had a head injury with loss of consciousness.
* You have had previous treatment with any cholinesterase inhibitor that caused jaundice (yellow skin and eyes) or elevated bilirubin.

Over age 60:
No problems expected.

Pregnancy:
Unknown effect. Drug is usually not prescribed for women of childbearing age. Risk category C (see page xviii).

Breast-feeding:
Unknown effect. Not recommended for women of childbearing age.

Infants & children:
Not used in this age group.

Prolonged use:
* Drug may lose its effectiveness.
* Talk to your doctor about the need for follow-up medical examinations or laboratory studies to check blood chemistries and liver function.

Skin & sunlight:
No problems expected.

Driving, piloting or hazardous work:
Don't drive or pilot aircraft until you learn how medicine affects you. Don't work around dangerous machinery. Don't climb ladders or work in high places. Danger increases if you drink alcohol or take other medicines affecting alertness and reflexes such as antihistamines, tranquilizers, sedatives, pain medicine, narcotics and mind-altering drugs.

Discontinuing:
Do not discontinue drug unless advised by doctor. Abrupt decreases in dosage may cause a cognitive decline.

Others:
* Advise any doctor or dentist whom you consult that you take this medicine.
* May affect the results in some medical tests.
* Do not increase dosage without doctor's approval.
* Treatment may need to be discontinued or the dosage lowered if weekly blood tests indicate a sensitivity to the drug or liver toxicity develops.

POSSIBLE INTERACTION WITH OTHER DRUGS

GENERIC NAME OR DRUG CLASS	COMBINED EFFECT
Anticholinergics*	Decreased anticholinergic effect.
Anti-inflammatories, nonsteroidal (NSAIDs)	May increase gastric acid secretions.
Cimetidine	Increased tacrine effect, especially adverse effects.
Enzyme inducers*	May decrease effect of cholinesterase inhibitor.
Ketoconazole	May interact, but effect unknown.
Quinidine	May interact, but effect unknown.
Theophylline	Increased theophylline effect or toxicity.

POSSIBLE INTERACTION WITH OTHER SUBSTANCES

INTERACTS WITH	COMBINED EFFECT
Alcohol:	None expected.
Beverages:	None expected.
Cocaine:	None expected.
Foods:	None expected.
Marijuana:	None expected.
Tobacco:	May decrease tacrine effect.

*See Glossary

CINOXACIN

BRAND NAMES

Cinobac

BASIC INFORMATION

Habit forming? No
Prescription needed? Yes
Available as generic? Yes
Drug class: Anti-infective (urinary)

 USES

Treatment for urinary tract infections.

 DOSAGE & USAGE INFORMATION

How to take:
Capsule—Swallow with liquid. May be taken with or without food, but be consistent and take it the same way each day.

When to take:
At the same times each day.

If you forget a dose:
Take as soon as you remember up to 2 hours late. If more than 2 hours, wait for next scheduled dose (don't double this dose).

What drug does:
Destroys bacteria susceptible to cinoxacin.

Time lapse before drug works:
1 to 2 weeks.

Don't take with:
Any other medicine or any dietary supplement without consulting your doctor or pharmacist.

 OVERDOSE

SYMPTOMS:
Lethargy, stomach upset, behavioral changes, convulsions and stupor.
WHAT TO DO:
- Dial 911 (emergency) for medical help or call poison control center 1-800-222-1222 for instructions.
- If person is unconscious, check breathing and pulse. If not breathing, begin mouth-to-mouth rescue breathing. If heart is not beating, begin chest compressions.
- See emergency information on last 3 pages of this book.

 POSSIBLE ADVERSE REACTIONS OR SIDE EFFECTS

SYMPTOMS	WHAT TO DO
Life-threatening: Hives, rash, intense itching, faintness soon after a dose (anaphylaxis).	Seek emergency treatment immediately.
Common: Rash; itch; decreased, blurred or double vision; halos around lights or excess brightness; changes in color vision; nausea; vomiting; diarrhea.	Discontinue. Call doctor right away.
Infrequent: Dizziness, drowsiness, headache, ringing in ears, insomnia, appetite loss.	Continue. Call doctor when convenient.
Rare: Severe stomach pain, seizures, psychosis, joint pain, numbness or tingling in hands or feet (infants and children).	Discontinue. Call doctor right away.

WARNINGS & PRECAUTIONS

Don't take if:
- You are allergic to cinoxacin or nalidixic acid.
- You have a seizure disorder (epilepsy, convulsions).

Before you start, consult your doctor if:
- You plan to become pregnant during medication period.
- You have or have had kidney or liver disease.
- You have impaired circulation to the brain (hardened arteries).

Over age 60:
Adverse reactions and side effects may be more frequent and severe than in younger persons.

Pregnancy:
Decide with your doctor if drug benefits justify risk to unborn child. Risk category C (see page xviii).

Breast-feeding:
Unknown effect. Avoid drug or discontinue nursing until you finish medicine. Consult doctor for advice on maintaining milk supply.

Infants & children:
Give only under close medical supervision.

Prolonged use:
Talk to your doctor about the need for follow-up medical examinations or laboratory studies to check kidney function, liver function.

Skin & sunlight:
No special problems expected.

Driving, piloting or hazardous work:
Avoid if you feel drowsy, dizzy or have vision problems. Otherwise, no problems expected.

Discontinuing:
Don't discontinue without consulting doctor. Dose may require gradual reduction if you have taken drug for a long time. Doses of other drugs may also require adjustment.

Others:
- May interfere with the accuracy of some medical tests.
- Advise any doctor or dentist whom you consult that you take this medicine.

POSSIBLE INTERACTION WITH OTHER DRUGS

GENERIC NAME OR DRUG CLASS	COMBINED EFFECT
Probenecid	Decreased cinoxacin effect.

POSSIBLE INTERACTION WITH OTHER SUBSTANCES

INTERACTS WITH	COMBINED EFFECT
Alcohol:	Impaired alertness, judgment and coordination.
Beverages:	None expected.
Cocaine:	Impaired judgment and coordination.
Foods:	None expected.
Marijuana:	Impaired alertness, judgment and coordination.
Tobacco:	None expected.

CITRATES

GENERIC AND BRAND NAMES

POTASSIUM CITRATE
  Citra Forte
  Urocit-K
**POTASSIUM CITRATE
  & CITRIC ACID**
  Polycitra-K
**POTASSIUM CITRATE
  & SODIUM CITRATE**
  Citrolith
**SODIUM CITRATE &
  CITRIC ACID**
  Albright's Solution
  Bicitra
  Modified Shohl's
    Solution
  Oracit
  Tussirex with
    Codeine Liquid
TRICITRATES
  Polycitra
  Polycitra LC

BASIC INFORMATION

Habit forming? No
Prescription needed? Yes
Available as generic? No
Drug class: Urinary alkalizer, antiurolithic

 USES

- To make urine more alkaline (less acid).
- To treat or prevent recurrence of some types of kidney stones.

 DOSAGE & USAGE INFORMATION

How to take:
- Tablet—Take right after a meal or with a bedtime snack. Swallow tablet whole (do not crush or chew). Take with a full glass of water.
- Solution—Dilute with 6 ounces of water or juice and drink all of the mixture.
- Crystals—Stir into 6 ounces of water or juice and drink all of the mixture.

When to take:
On full stomach, usually after meals or with food.

Continued next column

 OVERDOSE

SYMPTOMS:
Listlessness, weakness, confusion, tingling in arms or legs, irregular heartbeat, chest pain.
WHAT TO DO:
- Dial 911 (emergency) for medical help or call poison control center 1-800-222-1222 for instructions.
- See emergency information on last 3 pages of this book.

If you forget a dose:
Take as soon as you remember. If it is almost time for the next dose, skip the missed dose and wait for your next scheduled dose (don't double this dose).

What drug does:
Increases urinary alkalinity by excretion of bicarbonate ions.

Time lapse before drug works:
1 hour.

Don't take with:
Any other medicine or any dietary supplement without consulting your doctor or pharmacist.

 POSSIBLE ADVERSE REACTIONS OR SIDE EFFECTS

SYMPTOMS	WHAT TO DO
Life-threatening: None expected.	
Common: Nausea or mild vomiting, diarrhea, mild stomach cramps.	Continue. Call doctor when convenient.
Infrequent: None expected.	
Rare: • Black or tarry stools, vomiting (may be bloody), severe stomach cramps.	Discontinue. Seek emergency treatment.
• Confusion, dizziness, swollen feet and ankles, irritability, depression, muscle pain, nervousness, numbness or tingling in hands or feet, unpleasant taste, unusual weakness or tiredness.	Discontinue. Call doctor right away.

WARNINGS & PRECAUTIONS

Don't take if:
You are allergic to any citrate.

Before you start, consult your doctor if:
You have any disease involving the adrenal glands, diabetes, chronic diarrhea, heart problems, hypertension, kidney disease, stomach ulcer or gastritis, urinary tract infection, intestinal or esophageal blockage or toxemia of pregnancy.

Over age 60:
Adverse reactions and side effects may be more frequent and severe than in younger persons. Ask doctor about smaller doses.

Pregnancy:
Avoid if possible. Consult doctor. Risk category C (see page xviii).

Breast-feeding:
Drug passes into milk. Avoid drug or discontinue nursing until you finish medicine. Consult doctor for advice on maintaining milk supply.

Infants & children:
Use only under close medical supervision.

Prolonged use:
- Adverse reactions more likely.
- Talk to your doctor about the need for follow-up medical examinations or laboratory studies.

Skin & sunlight:
No problems expected.

Driving, piloting or hazardous work:
Don't drive or pilot aircraft until you learn how medicine affects you. Don't work around dangerous machinery. Don't climb ladders or work in high places. Danger increases if you drink alcohol or take medicine affecting alertness and reflexes, such as antihistamines, tranquilizers, sedatives, pain medicine, narcotics and mind-altering drugs.

Discontinuing:
Don't discontinue without consulting doctor. Dose may require gradual reduction if you have taken drug for a long time. Doses of other drugs may also require adjustment.

Others:
- Liquid may be chilled (don't freeze) to improve taste.
- Advise any doctor or dentist whom you consult that you take this medicine.
- Monitor potassium in blood with frequent laboratory studies.

POSSIBLE INTERACTION WITH OTHER DRUGS

GENERIC NAME OR DRUG CLASS	COMBINED EFFECT
Antacids*	Increased risk of side effects.
Angiotensin-converting enzyme (ACE) inhibitors*	Increased risk of side effects.
Anti-inflammatories, nonsteroidal (NSAIDs)	Increased risk of side effects.
Digitalis preparations*	Increased risk of too much potassium in blood.
Diuretics, potassium sparing*	Increased risk of too much potassium in blood.
Potassium supplements	Increased risk of too much potassium in blood.
Methenamine	Decreased effects of methenamine.
Pseudoephedrine	Urinary retention. Increased effect of pseudoephedrine.
Quinidine	Prolonged quinidine effect.

POSSIBLE INTERACTION WITH OTHER SUBSTANCES

INTERACTS WITH	COMBINED EFFECT
Alcohol:	Decreased alertness.
Beverages: Salt-free milk.	Increased risk of side effects.
Cocaine:	None expected.
Foods: Salt substitutes, low salt foods.	Increased risk of side effects.
Marijuana:	None expected.
Tobacco:	Increased risk of stomach irritation.

*See Glossary

CLIDINIUM

BRAND NAMES

Apo-Chlorax
Clindex
Clinoxide
Corium
Librax

Lidox
Lodoxide
Quarzan
Zebrax

BASIC INFORMATION

Habit forming? No
Prescription needed?
    Low strength: No
    High strength: Yes
Available as generic? No
Drug class: Antispasmodic, anticholinergic

USES

Reduces spasms of digestive system, bladder and urethra.

DOSAGE & USAGE INFORMATION

How to take:
Capsule—Swallow with liquid or food to lessen stomach irritation.

When to take:
30 minutes before meals (unless directed otherwise by doctor).

If you forget a dose:
Take as soon as you remember up to 2 hours late. If more than 2 hours, wait for next scheduled dose (don't double this dose).

What drug does:
Blocks nerve impulses at parasympathetic nerve endings, preventing muscle contractions and gland secretions of organs involved.

Time lapse before drug works:
15 to 30 minutes.

Continued next column

OVERDOSE

SYMPTOMS:
Dilated pupils, rapid pulse and breathing, dizziness, fever, hallucinations, confusion, slurred speech, agitation, flushed face, convulsions, coma.
WHAT TO DO:
• **Dial 911 (emergency) for medical help or call poison control center 1-800-222-1222 for instructions.**
• **See emergency information on last 3 pages of this book.**

Don't take with:
Any other medicine or any dietary supplement without consulting your doctor or pharmacist.

POSSIBLE ADVERSE REACTIONS OR SIDE EFFECTS

SYMPTOMS	WHAT TO DO
Life-threatening:	
In case of overdose, see previous column.	
Common:	
• Confusion, delirium, rapid heartbeat.	Discontinue. Call doctor right away.
• Nausea, vomiting, decreased sweating.	Continue. Call doctor when convenient.
• Constipation.	Continue. Tell doctor at next visit.
• Dryness in ears, nose, throat, mouth.	No action necessary.
Infrequent:	
• Nasal congestion, altered taste, difficult urination, headache, impotence.	Continue. Call doctor when convenient.
• Lightheadedness.	Discontinue. Call doctor right away.
Rare:	
Rash or hives, eye pain, blurred vision.	Discontinue. Call doctor right away.

WARNINGS & PRECAUTIONS

Don't take if:
• You are allergic to any anticholinergic.
• You have trouble with stomach bloating.
• You have difficulty emptying your bladder completely (enlarged prostate).
• You have narrow-angle glaucoma.
• You have severe ulcerative colitis.

Before you start, consult your doctor if:
• You have open-angle glaucoma.
• You have angina, chronic bronchitis or asthma, kidney or thyroid disease, hiatal hernia, liver disease, enlarged prostate, myasthenia gravis, peptic ulcer.
• You will have surgery within 2 months, including dental surgery, requiring general or spinal anesthesia.

Over age 60:
Adverse reactions and side effects may be more frequent and severe than in younger persons.

Pregnancy:
Decide with your doctor whether drug benefits justify risk to unborn child. Risk category C (see page xviii).

CLIDINIUM

Breast-feeding:
Drug passes into milk and decreases milk flow. Avoid drug or discontinue nursing until you finish medicine. Consult doctor for advice on maintaining milk supply.

Infants & children:
Use only under medical supervision.

Prolonged use:
Chronic constipation, possible fecal impaction. Consult doctor immediately.

Skin & sunlight:
No problems expected.

Driving, piloting or hazardous work:
Don't drive or pilot aircraft until you learn how medicine affects you. Don't work around dangerous machinery. Don't climb ladders or work in high places. Danger increases if you drink alcohol or take medicine affecting alertness and reflexes, such as antihistamines, tranquilizers, sedatives, pain medicine, narcotics, or mind-altering drugs.

Discontinuing:
May be unnecessary to finish medicine. Follow doctor's instructions.

Others:
Advise any doctor or dentist whom you consult that you take this medicine.

 POSSIBLE INTERACTION WITH OTHER DRUGS

GENERIC NAME OR DRUG CLASS	COMBINED EFFECT
Amantadine	Increased clidinium effect.
Antacids*	Decreased clidinium effect.
Anticholinergics, other*	Increased clidinium effect.
Antidepressants, tricyclic*	Increased clidinium effect. Increased sedation.
Antidiarrheals*	Increased clidinium effect.
Antihistamines*	Increased clidinium effect.
Attapulgite	Decreased clidinium effect.
Haloperidol	Increased internal eye pressure.
Ketoconazole	Decreased ketoconazole effect.
Meperidine	Increased clidinium effect.
Methylphenidate	Increased clidinium effect.
Molindone	Increased anticholinergic effect.
Monoamine oxidase (MAO) inhibitors*	Increased clidinium effect.
Nitrates*	Increased internal eye pressure.
Nizatidine	Increased nizatidine effect.
Orphenadrine	Increased clidinium effect.
Pilocarpine	Loss of pilocarpine effect in glaucoma treatment.
Potassium supplements*	Possible intestinal ulcers with oral potassium tablets.
Tranquilizers*	Increased clidinium effect.
Vitamin C	Decreased clidinium effect. Avoid large doses of vitamin C.

 POSSIBLE INTERACTION WITH OTHER SUBSTANCES

INTERACTS WITH	COMBINED EFFECT
Alcohol:	None expected.
Beverages:	None expected.
Cocaine:	Excessively rapid heartbeat. Avoid.
Foods:	None expected.
Marijuana:	Drowsiness and dry mouth.
Tobacco:	None expected.

*See Glossary

CLINDAMYCIN

BRAND NAMES

Cleocin
Cleocin Pediatric
Cleocin (Vaginal)
Clindesse Vaginal
  Cream

Dalacin C
Dalacin C Palmitate
Dalacin C Phosphate

BASIC INFORMATION

Habit forming? No
Prescription needed? Yes
Available as generic? Yes
Drug class: Antibacterial

 ## USES

Treatment of bacterial infections that are
susceptible to clindamycin.

 ## DOSAGE & USAGE INFORMATION

How to take:
- Capsule or liquid—Swallow with liquid. Take
  with a full glass of water or a meal to avoid
  gastric irritation.
- Vaginal cream—Use applicator supplied with
  product to insert cream into vagina. Wash
  hands immediately after using.

When to take:
- Oral—At the same times each day.
- Vaginal cream—Apply at bedtime unless
  directed differently by your doctor.

If you forget a dose:
Take as soon as you remember up to 2 hours
late. If more than 2 hours, wait for next
scheduled dose (don't double this dose).

What drug does:
Destroys susceptible bacteria. Does not kill
viruses.

Time lapse before drug works:
3 to 5 days.

Continued next column

 ## OVERDOSE

SYMPTOMS:
Severe nausea, vomiting, diarrhea.
WHAT TO DO:
Overdose unlikely to threaten life. If person
uses much larger amount than prescribed or
if accidentally swallowed, call doctor or
poison control center 1-800-222-1222 for help.

Don't take with:
Any other medicine or any dietary supplement
without consulting your doctor or pharmacist.

 ## POSSIBLE ADVERSE REACTIONS OR SIDE EFFECTS

SYMPTOMS	WHAT TO DO
Life-threatening:	
Hives, wheezing, faintness, itching, coma.	Seek emergency treatment immediately.
Common:	
Bloating.	Discontinue. Call doctor right away.
Infrequent:	
• Unusual thirst; vomiting; stomach cramps; severe and watery diarrhea with blood or mucus; painful, swollen joints; fever; jaundice; tiredness; weakness.	Discontinue. Call doctor right away.
• White patches in mouth; rash, itch around groin, rectum or armpits; vaginal discharge; itching; dizziness; nausea; mild diarrhea; pain during intercourse.	Continue. Call doctor when convenient.
Rare:	
None expected.	

WARNINGS & PRECAUTIONS

Don't take if:
* You are allergic to lincomycins, clindamycin or doxorubicin.
* You have had ulcerative colitis.

Before you start, consult your doctor if:
* You have had yeast infections of mouth, skin or vagina.
* You will have surgery within 2 months, including dental surgery, requiring general or spinal anesthesia.
* You have kidney or liver disease.
* You have allergies of any kind.
* You have a history of gastrointestinal disorders.

Over age 60:
Adverse reactions and side effects may be more frequent and severe than in younger persons.

Pregnancy:
Decide with your doctor if drug benefits justify risk to unborn child. Risk category B (see page xviii).

Breast-feeding:
Drug passes into milk. Avoid drug or discontinue nursing until you finish medicine. Consult doctor for advice on maintaining milk supply.

Infants & children:
Don't give to infants younger than 1 month. Use for children only under medical supervision.

Prolonged use:
* Severe colitis with diarrhea and bleeding.
* You may become more susceptible to infections caused by germs not responsive to clindamycin.
* Talk to your doctor about the need for follow-up medical examinations or laboratory studies to check stools and perform proctosigmoidoscopy.

Skin & sunlight:
No problems expected.

Driving, piloting or hazardous work:
No problems expected.

Discontinuing:
* Don't discontinue without doctor's advice until you complete prescribed dose, even though symptoms diminish or disappear.
* If vaginal discharge, itching or pain occurs after discontinuing medicine, consult doctor.

Others:
* May interfere with the accuracy of some medical tests. Advise any doctor or dentist whom you consult that you take this medicine.
* Vaginal cream product may decrease the effectiveness of condoms, cervical caps or diaphragms. Wait 72 hours after treatment to use any of these devices.

POSSIBLE INTERACTION WITH OTHER DRUGS

GENERIC NAME OR DRUG CLASS	COMBINED EFFECT
Antidiarrheal preparations*	Decreased clindamycin effect.
Antimyasthenics*	Decreased antimyasthenic effect.
Chloramphenicol	Decreased clindamycin effect.
Erythromycins*	Decreased clindamycin effect.
Muscle blockers*	Increased actions of muscle blockers to unsafe degree. Avoid.
Narcotics*	Increased risk of respiratory problems.

POSSIBLE INTERACTION WITH OTHER SUBSTANCES

INTERACTS WITH	COMBINED EFFECT
Alcohol:	None expected.
Beverages:	None expected.
Cocaine:	None expected.
Foods:	None expected.
Marijuana:	None expected.
Tobacco:	None expected.

*See Glossary

CLOMIPHENE

BRAND NAMES

Clomid   Serophene
Milophene

BASIC INFORMATION

Habit forming? No
Prescription needed? Yes
Available as generic? Yes
Drug class: Gonad stimulant

 ## USES

- Treatment for men with low sperm counts.
- Treatment for ovulatory failure in women who wish to become pregnant.

 ## DOSAGE & USAGE INFORMATION

How to take:
Tablet—Swallow with liquid.

When to take:
- Men—Take at the same time each day.
- Women—Follow your doctor's instructions.

If you forget a dose:
Take as soon as you remember. If you forget a day, double next dose. If you miss 2 or more doses, consult doctor.

What drug does:
Antiestrogen effect stimulates ovulation and sperm production.

Time lapse before drug works:
Usually 3 to 6 months. Ovulation may occur 6 to 10 days after last day of treatment in any cycle.

Don't take with:
Any other medicine or any dietary supplement without consulting your doctor or pharmacist.

 ## OVERDOSE

SYMPTOMS:
Increased severity of adverse reactions and side effects.
WHAT TO DO:
Overdose unlikely to threaten life. If person uses much larger amount than prescribed or if accidentally swallowed, call doctor or poison control center 1-800-222-1222 for help.

 ## POSSIBLE ADVERSE REACTIONS OR SIDE EFFECTS

SYMPTOMS	WHAT TO DO
Life-threatening:	
Sudden shortness of breath.	Seek emergency treatment.
Common:	
• Bloating, abdominal pain, pelvic pain.	Discontinue. Call doctor right away.
• Hot flashes.	Continue. Tell doctor at next visit.
Infrequent:	
• Rash, itch, vomiting, jaundice.	Discontinue. Call doctor right away.
• Constipation, diarrhea, increased appetite, heavy menstrual flow, frequent urination, breast discomfort, weight change, hair loss, nausea, eyes sensitive to light.	Continue. Call doctor when convenient.
Rare:	
• Vision changes.	Discontinue. Call doctor right away.
• Dizziness, headache, tiredness, depression, nervousness.	Continue. Call doctor when convenient.

WARNINGS & PRECAUTIONS

Don't take if:
You are allergic to clomiphene.

Before you start, consult your doctor if:
* You have an ovarian cyst, fibroid uterine tumors or unusual vaginal bleeding.
* You have inflamed veins caused by blood clots.
* You have liver disease.
* You are depressed.

Over age 60:
Not recommended.

Pregnancy:
Stop taking at first sign of pregnancy. Consult doctor. Risk category C (see page xviii).

Breast-feeding:
Not used.

Infants & children:
Not used.

Prolonged use:
* Not recommended.
* Talk to your doctor about the need for follow-up medical examinations or laboratory studies to check basal body temperature, endometrial biopsy, kidney function, eyes.

Skin & sunlight:
No special problems expected.

Driving, piloting or hazardous work:
* Avoid if you feel dizzy.
* May cause blurred vision.

Discontinuing:
May be unnecessary to finish medicine. Follow doctor's instructions.

Others:
* Have a complete pelvic examination before treatment.
* Advise any doctor or dentist whom you consult that you take this medicine.
* If you become pregnant, twins or triplets are possible.

POSSIBLE INTERACTION WITH OTHER DRUGS

GENERIC NAME OR DRUG CLASS	COMBINED EFFECT
Thyroglobulin	May increase serum thyroglobulin.
Thyroxine (T-4)	May increase serum thyroxine.

POSSIBLE INTERACTION WITH OTHER SUBSTANCES

INTERACTS WITH	COMBINED EFFECT
Alcohol:	None expected.
Beverages:	None expected.
Cocaine:	None expected.
Foods:	None expected.
Marijuana:	None expected.
Tobacco:	None expected.

*See Glossary

CLONIDINE & CHLORTHALIDONE

BRAND NAMES

Combipres

BASIC INFORMATION

Habit forming? No
Prescription needed? Yes
Available as generic? Yes
Drug class: Antihypertensive, diuretic

USES

- Treatment of high blood pressure.
- Reduces fluid retention (edema) caused by conditions such as heart disorders and liver disease.

DOSAGE & USAGE INFORMATION

How to take:
Tablet—Swallow with liquid. If you can't swallow whole, crumble tablet and take with liquid or food. Don't exceed dose.

When to take:
At the same time each day.

If you forget a dose:
Take as soon as you remember up to 2 hours late. If more than 2 hours, wait for next scheduled dose (don't double this dose).

What drug does:
- Relaxes and allows expansion of blood vessel walls.
- Forces sodium and water excretion, reducing body fluid.
- Reduces body fluid and relaxes arteries to lower blood pressure.

Continued next column

OVERDOSE

SYMPTOMS:
Vomiting; fainting; rapid, irregular, slow heartbeat; diminished reflexes; cramps; shortness of breath; weakness; drowsiness; weak pulse; coma.
WHAT TO DO:
- **Dial 911 (emergency) for medical help or call poison control center 1-800-222-1222 for instructions.**
- **If person is unconscious, check breathing and pulse. If not breathing, begin mouth-to-mouth rescue breathing. If heart is not beating, begin chest compressions.**
- **See emergency information on last 3 pages of this book.**

Time lapse before drug works:
4 to 6 hours. May require several weeks to lower blood pressure.

Don't take with:
Any other medicine or any dietary supplement without consulting your doctor or pharmacist.

POSSIBLE ADVERSE REACTIONS OR SIDE EFFECTS

SYMPTOMS	WHAT TO DO
Life-threatening: Irregular heartbeat, weak pulse.	Discontinue. Seek emergency treatment.
Common: Dry mouth, increased thirst, muscle cramps, nausea or vomiting, mood changes, drowsiness.	Discontinue. Call doctor right away.
Infrequent: Vomiting, diminished sex desire and performance, insomnia, dizziness, diarrhea, constipation, appetite loss.	Continue. Call doctor when convenient.
Rare: • Jaundice; easy bruising or bleeding; sore throat, fever, mouth ulcers; rash or hives; joint pain; flank pain; abdominal pain.	Discontinue. Call doctor right away.
• Cold fingers and toes, nightmares.	Continue. Call doctor when convenient.

WARNINGS & PRECAUTIONS

Don't take if:
- You are allergic to any thiazide diuretic drug or alpha-adrenergic blocker.*
- You are under age 12.

Before you start, consult your doctor if:
- You are allergic to any sulfa drug.
- You have gout, liver, pancreas or kidney disorder, a peripheral circulation disorder (intermittent claudication, Buerger's disease), history of depression, heart disease.
- You will have surgery within 2 months, including dental surgery, requiring general or spinal anesthesia.

CLONIDINE & CHLORTHALIDONE

Over age 60:
Adverse reactions and side effects may be more frequent and severe than in younger persons, especially dizziness and excessive potassium loss.

Pregnancy:
Decide with your doctor if drug benefits justify risk to unborn child. Risk category C (see page xviii).

Breast-feeding:
Drug passes into milk. Avoid drug or discontinue nursing until you finish medicine. Consult doctor for advice on maintaining milk supply.

Infants & children:
Use only under careful medical supervision after age 12.

Prolonged use:
- Don't discontinue without consulting doctor. Dose may require gradual reduction if you have taken drug for a long time. Doses of other drugs may also require adjustment.
- Request yearly eye examinations.
- Talk to your doctor about the need for follow-up medical examinations or laboratory studies.

Skin & sunlight:
No special problems expected.

Driving, piloting or hazardous work:
Don't drive or pilot aircraft until you learn how medicine affects you. Don't work around dangerous machinery. Don't climb ladders or work in high places. Danger increases if you drink alcohol or take medicine affecting alertness and reflexes.

Discontinuing:
Don't discontinue abruptly. May cause rebound high blood pressure, anxiety, chest pain, insomnia, headache, nausea, irregular heartbeat, flushed face, sweating.

Others:
- Hot weather and fever may cause dehydration and drop in blood pressure. Dose may require temporary adjustment. Weigh daily and report any unexpected weight decreases to your doctor.
- Advise any doctor or dentist whom you consult that you take this medicine.
- May cause rise in uric acid, leading to gout.
- May cause blood-sugar rise in diabetics.

 POSSIBLE INTERACTION WITH OTHER DRUGS

GENERIC NAME OR DRUG CLASS	COMBINED EFFECT
Allopurinol	Decreased allopurinol effect.
Angiotensin-converting enzyme (ACE) inhibitors*	Possible excessive potassium in blood.

	COMBINED EFFECT
Antidepressants, tricyclic*	Dangerous drop in blood pressure. Avoid combination unless under medical supervision.
Antihypertensives, other*	Excessive blood pressure drop.
Appetite suppressants*	Decreased clonidine effect.
Barbiturates*	Increased chlorthalidone effect.
Beta-adrenergic blocking agents*	Possible precipitous change in blood pressure.
Carteolol	Increased anti-hypertensive effect.
Central nervous system (CNS) depressants*	Increased sedative effect.
Cholestyramine	Decreased chlorthalidone effect.
Digitalis preparations*	Excessive potassium loss that causes dangerous heart rhythms.

Continued on page 914

 POSSIBLE INTERACTION WITH OTHER SUBSTANCES

INTERACTS WITH	COMBINED EFFECT
Alcohol:	Increased sensitivity to sedative effect of alcohol and very low blood pressure. Avoid.
Beverages: Caffeine-containing drinks.	Decreased clonidine effect.
Cocaine:	Increased risk of heart block and high blood pressure.
Foods: Licorice.	Excessive potassium loss that causes dangerous heart rhythm.
Marijuana:	Weakness on standing. May increase blood pressure.
Tobacco:	None expected.

*See Glossary

263

CLOTRIMAZOLE (Oral-Local)

BRAND NAMES

Mycelex Troches

BASIC INFORMATION

Habit forming? No
Prescription needed? Yes
Available as generic? Yes
Drug class: Antifungal

 USES

* Treats thrush, white mouth (candidiasis).
* Used primarily in immunosuppressed patients to treat and prevent mouth infection.

 DOSAGE & USAGE INFORMATION

How to take:
Lozenge—Dissolve slowly and completely in the mouth, 5 times a day (usually for 14 days or longer). Swallow saliva during this time. Don't swallow lozenge whole and don't chew.

When to take:
At the same times each day.

If you forget a dose:
Take as soon as you remember up to 2 hours late. If more than 2 hours, wait for next scheduled dose (don't double this dose).

What drug does:
Kills fungus by interfering with cell wall membrane and its permeability.

Time lapse before drug works:
1 to 3 hours.

Don't take with:
Any other medicine for your mouth without consulting your doctor or pharmacist.

 OVERDOSE

SYMPTOMS:
None expected, but if large dose has been taken, follow instructions below.
WHAT TO DO:
* Dial 911 (emergency) for medical help or call poison control center 1-800-222-1222 for instructions.
* See emergency information on last 3 pages of this book.

 POSSIBLE ADVERSE REACTIONS OR SIDE EFFECTS

SYMPTOMS	WHAT TO DO
Life-threatening: None expected.	
Common: None expected.	
Infrequent: Abdominal pain, diarrhea, nausea, vomiting.	Discontinue. Call doctor right away.
Rare: None expected.	

CLOTRIMAZOLE (Oral-Local)

WARNINGS & PRECAUTIONS

Don't take if:
You have severe liver disease.

Before you start, consult your doctor if:
You have had a recent organ transplant.

Over age 60:
Adverse reactions and side effects may be more frequent and severe than in younger persons. You may need smaller doses for shorter periods of time.

Pregnancy:
Decide with your doctor if drug benefits justify risk to unborn child. Risk category C (see page xviii).

Breast-feeding:
Unknown effect. Consult doctor.

Infants & children:
Use only under medical supervision for children younger than 4 or 5 years.

Prolonged use:
No problems expected.

Skin & sunlight:
No problems expected.

Driving, piloting or hazardous work:
Don't drive or pilot aircraft until you learn how medicine affects you. Don't work around dangerous machinery. Don't climb ladders or work in high places. Danger increases if you drink alcohol or take medicine affecting alertness and reflexes.

Discontinuing:
Don't discontinue without consulting doctor. Dose may require gradual reduction if you have taken drug for a long time. Doses of other drugs may also require adjustment.

Others:
* Continue for full term of treatment. May require several months.
* Check with physician if not improved in 1 week.

POSSIBLE INTERACTION WITH OTHER DRUGS

GENERIC NAME OR DRUG CLASS	COMBINED EFFECT
None expected.	

POSSIBLE INTERACTION WITH OTHER SUBSTANCES

INTERACTS WITH	COMBINED EFFECT
Alcohol:	Decreased effects of clotrimazole.
Beverages:	None expected.
Cocaine:	Decreased effects of clotrimazole.
Foods:	None expected.
Marijuana:	Decreased effects of clotrimazole.
Tobacco:	Decreased effects of clotrimazole.

*See Glossary

CLOZAPINE

BRAND NAMES

Clozaril   Leponex
FazaClo

BASIC INFORMATION

Habit forming? No
Prescription needed? Yes, prescribed only
through a special program.
Available as generic? Yes
Drug class: Antipsychotic

 ## USES

- Treats severe schizophrenia in patients not helped by other medicines.
- Reduces the risk of recurrent suicide behavior in patients with schizophrenia or schizoaffective disorder.

 ## DOSAGE & USAGE INFORMATION

How to take:
- Tablet—Swallow with liquid. If you can't swallow whole, crumble tablet and take with liquid or food.
- Orally disintegrating tablet—Let tablet dissolve in your mouth. Do not chew or swallow it whole.

When to take:
Once or twice daily as directed.

If you forget a dose:
Take as soon as you remember up to 2 hours late. If more than 2 hours, wait for next scheduled dose (don't double this dose).

What drug does:
Interferes with binding of dopamine. May produce significant improvement, but may at times also make schizophrenia worse.

Continued next column

 ## OVERDOSE

SYMPTOMS:
Heartbeat fast, slow, irregular; hallucinations; restlessness; excitement; drowsiness; breathing difficulty.
WHAT TO DO:
- Dial 911 (emergency) for medical help or call poison control center 1-800-222-1222 for instructions.
- See emergency information on last 3 pages of this book.

Time lapse before drug works:
Weeks to months before improvement is evident. Your doctor may increase the dosage to obtain optimal effectiveness.

Don't take with:
Any other medicine or any dietary supplement without consulting your doctor or pharmacist.

 ## POSSIBLE ADVERSE REACTIONS OR SIDE EFFECTS

SYMPTOMS	WHAT TO DO
Life-threatening: High fever, rapid pulse, profuse sweating, muscle rigidity, confusion and irritability, seizures; fever, chills, mouth sores.	Discontinue. Seek emergency treatment.
Common: Dry mouth, blurred vision, constipation, difficulty urinating; sedation, low blood pressure, dizziness.	Continue. Call doctor when convenient.
Infrequent: None expected.	
Rare: • Jerky or involuntary movements (especially of the face, lips, jaw, tongue) slow-frequency tremor of head or limbs, (especially while moving), muscle rigidity, lack of facial expression and slow inflexible movements, seizures, high blood sugar (thirstiness, frequent urination, increased hunger, weakness).	Discontinue. Call doctor right away.
• Pacing or restlessness; (akathisia); intermittent spasms of muscles of face, eyes, tongue, jaw, neck, body or limbs.	Continue. Call doctor when convenient.

WARNINGS & PRECAUTIONS

Don't take if:
You are allergic to clozapine.

Before you start, consult your doctor if:
* You are significantly mentally depressed.
* You have bone marrow depression.
* You have a family history of, or have diabetes.
* You have glaucoma or an enlarged prostate.
* You have ever had seizures from any cause.
* You have liver, heart or gastrointestinal disease or any type of blood disorder.

Over age 60:
* May be more at risk of weakness or dizziness upon standing after sitting or lying down and of excitement, confusion or urination difficulty.
* Use of antipsychotic drugs in elderly patients with dementia-related psychosis may increase risk of death. Consult doctor.

Pregnancy:
Risk category B (see page xviii).

Breast-feeding:
May cause sedation, restlessness or irritability in the nursing infant. Avoid.

Infants & children:
Safety not established. Consult doctor.

Prolonged use:
Effects unknown.

Skin & sunlight:
No problems expected.

Driving, piloting or hazardous work:
Don't drive or pilot aircraft until you learn how medicine affects you. Don't work around dangerous machinery. Don't climb ladders or work in high places. Danger increases if you drink alcohol or take medicine affecting alertness and reflexes.

Discontinuing:
Don't discontinue without consulting doctor. Dose may require gradual reduction if you have taken drug for a long time. Doses of other drugs may also require adjustment.

Others:
* This medicine is available only through a special management program for monitoring and distributing this drug.
* You will need laboratory studies each week for white blood cell and differential counts.

POSSIBLE INTERACTION WITH OTHER DRUGS

GENERIC NAME OR DRUG CLASS	COMBINED EFFECT
Antihypertensives*	Risk of low blood pressure.
Bone marrow depressants*	Toxic bone marrow depression.
Bupropion	Increased risk of seizures.
Carbamazepine	Decreased clozapine effect.
Central nervous system (CNS) depressants*	Toxic effects on the central nervous system.
Fluoxetine	Increased risk of adverse reactions.
Fluvoxamine	Increased risk of adverse reactions.
Haloperidol	Increased risk of seizures.
Lithium	Increased risk of seizures.
Phenytoin	Decreased clozapine effect.
Risperidone	Increased risperidone effect.

POSSIBLE INTERACTION WITH OTHER SUBSTANCES

INTERACTS WITH	COMBINED EFFECT
Alcohol:	Avoid. Increases toxic effect on the central nervous system.
Beverages: Caffeine drinks.	Excess (more than 3 cups of coffee or equivalent) increases risk of heartbeat irregularities.
Cocaine:	Heartbeat irregularities. Avoid.
Foods:	None expected.
Marijuana:	Heartbeat irregularities. Avoid.
Tobacco:	Decreased effect of clozapine. Avoid.

*See Glossary

COAL TAR (Topical)

BRAND NAMES

See full list of brand names in the *Generic and Brand Name Directory*, page 882.

BASIC INFORMATION

Habit forming? No
Prescription needed? No (for most)
Available as generic? Yes
Drug class: Antiseborrheic, antipsoriatic, keratolytic

 USES

Applied to the skin to treat dandruff, seborrhea, dermatitis, eczema and other skin diseases.

 DOSAGE & USAGE INFORMATION

How to use:
• Follow package instructions.
• Don't apply to blistered, oozing, infected or raw skin.
• Keep away from eyes.
• Protect treated area from sunshine for 72 hours.

When to use:
According to package instructions.

If you forget a dose:
Use as soon as you remember.

What drug does:
• Kills bacteria and fungus organisms on contact.
• Suppresses overproduction of skin cells.

Time lapse before drug works:
None. Works immediately. May take several days before maximum effect.

Don't use with:
Any other topical medicine without consulting your doctor or pharmacist.

 OVERDOSE

SYMPTOMS:
None expected.
WHAT TO DO:
Overdose unlikely to threaten life. If person uses much larger amount than prescribed or if accidentally swallowed, call doctor or poison control center 1-800-222-1222 for help.

 POSSIBLE ADVERSE REACTIONS OR SIDE EFFECTS

SYMPTOMS	WHAT TO DO
Life-threatening: None expected.	
Common: Skin stinging.	Continue. Call doctor when convenient.
Infrequent: Skin more irritated.	Continue. Call doctor when convenient.
Rare: Pus forms in lesions on skin.	Continue. Call doctor when convenient.

WARNINGS & PRECAUTIONS

Don't use if:
You have intolerance to coal tar.

Before you start, consult your doctor if:
You have infected skin or open wounds.

Over age 60:
No special problems expected.

Pregnancy:
Consult doctor. Risk category C (see page xviii).

Breast-feeding:
No special problems expected. Consult doctor.

Infants & children:
Don't use on infants.

Prolonged use:
No special problems expected.

Skin & sunlight:
One or more drugs in this group may cause rash or intensify sunburn in areas exposed to sun or ultraviolet light (photosensitivity reaction). Avoid overexposure. Notify doctor if reaction occurs.

Driving, piloting or hazardous work:
No problems expected.

Discontinuing:
No special problems expected.

Others:
- May affect results in some medical tests.
- Protect treated area from direct sunlight for 72 hours.

POSSIBLE INTERACTION WITH OTHER DRUGS

GENERIC NAME OR DRUG CLASS	COMBINED EFFECT
Psoralens (methoxsalen, trioxsalen)	Excess sensitivity to sun.

POSSIBLE INTERACTION WITH OTHER SUBSTANCES

INTERACTS WITH	COMBINED EFFECT
Alcohol:	None expected.
Beverages:	None expected.
Cocaine:	None expected.
Foods:	None expected.
Marijuana:	None expected.
Tobacco:	None expected.

*See Glossary

COLCHICINE

GENERIC NAMES

COLCHICINE

BASIC INFORMATION

Habit forming? No
Prescription needed? Yes
Available as generic? Yes
Drug class: Antigout

 USES

- Relieves joint pain, inflammation, swelling of gout.
- Also used for familial Mediterranean fever, dermatitis herpetiformis, calcium pyrophosphate deposition disease, amyloidosis, Paget's disease of bone, recurrent pericarditis, Behcet's syndrome.

 DOSAGE & USAGE INFORMATION

How to take:
Tablet—Swallow with liquid or food to lessen stomach irritation.

When to take:
- As prescribed. Stop taking when pain stops or at first sign of digestive upset. Wait at least 3 days between treatments.
- Don't take more than 8 doses.

If you forget a dose:
Don't double next dose. Consult doctor.

What drug does:
Decreases acidity of joint tissues and prevents deposits of uric-acid crystals.

Time lapse before drug works:
12 to 48 hours.

Don't take with:
Any other medicine or any dietary supplement without consulting your doctor or pharmacist.

 OVERDOSE

SYMPTOMS:
Bloody urine; diarrhea; burning feeling in the throat, skin or stomach; nausea or vomiting; muscle weakness; fever; shortness of breath; stupor; convulsions; coma.
WHAT TO DO:
- Dial 911 (emergency) for medical help or call poison control center 1-800-222-1222 for instructions.
- See emergency information on last 3 pages of this book.

 POSSIBLE ADVERSE REACTIONS OR SIDE EFFECTS

SYMPTOMS	WHAT TO DO
Life-threatening:	
In case of overdose, see previous column.	
Common:	
Diarrhea, nausea, vomiting, abdominal pain.	Discontinue. Call doctor right away.
Infrequent:	
Hair loss with long-term use.	Continue. Call doctor when convenient.
Rare:	
Jaundice, black or tarry stool, blood in urine, breathing difficulty, fever, chills, headache, hives, mouth or lip sores, sore throat, unusual bruising or bleeding, unusual tiredness or weakness.	Discontinue. Call doctor right away.

WARNINGS & PRECAUTIONS

Don't take if:
You are allergic to colchicine.

Before you start, consult your doctor if:
- You have had peptic ulcers or ulcerative colitis.
- You have heart, liver or kidney disease.
- You will have surgery within 2 months, including dental surgery, requiring general or spinal anesthesia.
- You have a gastrointestinal disorder.
- You drink large amounts of alcohol.

Over age 60:
Adverse reactions and side effects may be more frequent and severe than in younger persons. Colchicine has a narrow margin of safety for people in this age group.

Pregnancy:
Consult doctor. Risk category D (see page xviii).

Breast-feeding:
Drug passes into breast milk. Effect unknown. Consult doctor.

Infants & children:
Not recommended.

Prolonged use:
- Hair loss.
- Numbness or tingling in hands and feet.
- Talk to your doctor about the need for follow-up medical examinations or laboratory studies to check complete blood counts (white blood cell count, platelet count, red blood cell count, hemoglobin, hematocrit).

Skin & sunlight:
No problems expected.

Driving, piloting or hazardous work:
Don't drive or pilot aircraft until you learn how medicine affects you. Don't work around dangerous machinery. Don't climb ladders or work in high places. Danger increases if you drink alcohol or take medicine affecting alertness and reflexes, such as antihistamines, tranquilizers, sedatives, pain medicine, narcotics and mind-altering drugs.

Discontinuing:
- May be unnecessary to finish medicine. Follow doctor's instructions.
- Stop taking if digestive upsets occur before symptoms are relieved.

Others:
- Limit each course of treatment to 8 mg. Don't exceed 3 mg. per 24 hours.
- May cause decreased sperm production in males.
- May interfere with the accuracy of some medical tests.

POSSIBLE INTERACTION WITH OTHER DRUGS

GENERIC NAME OR DRUG CLASS	COMBINED EFFECT
Anticoagulants*	Increased anticoagulant effect.
Anti-inflammatory drugs, nonsteroidal (NSAIDs)*	Increased risk of gastrointestinal problems.
Blood dyscrasia-causing medications*	Increased bone marrow depressant effect.
Bone marrow depressants,* other	Increased bone marrow depressant effect.
Phenylbutazone	Increased chance of ulcers in gastrointestinal tract.
Thioguanine	May need increased dosage of colchicine.
Vitamin B-12	Decreased absorption of vitamin B-12.

POSSIBLE INTERACTION WITH OTHER SUBSTANCES

INTERACTS WITH	COMBINED EFFECT
Alcohol:	Increased risk of gastrointestinal toxicity.
Beverages: Herbal teas.	Increased colchicine effect. Avoid.
Cocaine:	Overstimulation Avoid.
Foods:	None expected.
Marijuana:	Decreased colchicine effect.
Tobacco:	None expected.

*See Glossary

COLESEVELAM

BRAND NAMES

Welchol

BASIC INFORMATION

Habit forming? No
Prescription needed? Yes
Available as generic? No
Drug class: Antihyperlipidemic

 USES

* Reduces low density lipoprotein (LDL) cholesterol. Should be used in addition to diet and exercise.
* Helps lower blood sugar levels in adults with type 2 diabetes.

 DOSAGE & USAGE INFORMATION

How to take:
Tablet—Take with food and a full glass of water. If you can't swallow whole, crumble tablet and take with liquid and food.

When to take:
As directed by your doctor. Usually once or twice daily with meals.

If you forget a dose:
Skip the missed dose and go back to your regular dosing schedule (don't double this dose).

What drug does:
Attaches to cholesterol and bile fluid in the intestine and passes out of the body without being absorbed.

Time lapse before drug works:
2 to 4 weeks.

Don't take with:
Any other medicine or any dietary supplement without consulting your doctor or pharmacist.

 OVERDOSE

SYMPTOMS:
None expected.
WHAT TO DO:
Overdose unlikely to threaten life. If person uses much larger amount than prescribed or if accidentally swallowed, call doctor or poison control center 1-800-222-1222 for help.

 POSSIBLE ADVERSE REACTIONS OR SIDE EFFECTS

SYMPTOMS	WHAT TO DO
Life-threatening: None expected.	
Common: Acid or sour stomach, belching, constipation, indigestion, stomach upset or pain.	Continue. Call doctor if condition persists.
Infrequent: Congestion, cough, dry or sore throat, hoarseness, muscle aches or pain, trouble swallowing.	Continue. Call doctor when convenient.
Rare: None expected.	

WARNINGS & PRECAUTIONS

Don't take if:
You are allergic to colesevelam.

Before you start, consult your doctor if:
* You have been diagnosed with a bowel obstruction.
* You have had recent gastrointestinal surgery.
* You have had gastrointestinal motility disorders.
* You have a vitamin deficiency.
* You have difficulty swallowing.

Over age 60:
Colesevelam has not been shown to cause different side effects in older adults.

Pregnancy:
Decide with your doctor if drug benefits justify risk to unborn child. Risk category B. (see page xviii).

Breast-feeding:
Drug may pass into milk. Avoid drug or discontinue nursing until you finish medicine. Consult doctor for advice on maintaining milk supply.

Infants & children:
Safety and efficacy not established.

Prolonged use:
Talk to your doctor about the need for follow-up medical examinations to determine the effect of colesevelam on your body.

Skin & sunlight:
No problems expected.

Driving, piloting or hazardous work:
No problems expected.

Discontinuing:
Don't discontinue without consulting your doctor.

Others:
* Advise any doctor or dentist whom you consult that you take this medicine.
* May affect the results in some medical tests.

POSSIBLE INTERACTION WITH OTHER DRUGS

GENERIC NAME OR DRUG CLASS	COMBINED EFFECT
Verapamil	May decrease effect of verapamil.

POSSIBLE INTERACTION WITH OTHER SUBSTANCES

INTERACTS WITH	COMBINED EFFECT
Alcohol:	Unknown effect Avoid.
Beverages:	None expected.
Cocaine:	Unknown effect. Avoid.
Foods:	None expected.
Marijuana:	Unknown effect. Avoid.
Tobacco:	None expected.

*See Glossary

COLESTIPOL

BRAND NAMES

Colestid

BASIC INFORMATION

Habit forming? No
Prescription needed? Yes
Available as generic? Yes
Drug class: Antihyperlipidemic

 ## USES

- Reduces cholesterol level in blood in patients with type IIa hyperlipidemia.
- Treats overdose of digitalis.
- Reduces skin itching associated with some forms of liver disease.
- Treats diarrhea after some surgical operations.
- Treatment of one form of colitis (rare).

 ## DOSAGE & USAGE INFORMATION

How to take:
Oral suspension—Mix well with 6 ounces or more or water or liquid, or in soups, pulpy fruits, with milk or in cereals. Will not dissolve.

When to take:
- Before meals.
- If taking other medicine, take it 1 hour before or 4 to 6 hours after taking colestipol.

If you forget a dose:
Take as soon as you remember up to 2 hours late. If more than 2 hours, wait for next scheduled dose (don't double this dose).

What drug does:
Binds with bile acids in intestines, preventing reabsorption.

Time lapse before drug works:
3 to 12 months.

Don't take with:
Any other medicine or any dietary supplement without consulting your doctor or pharmacist.

 ## OVERDOSE

SYMPTOMS:
Fecal impaction.
WHAT TO DO:
Overdose unlikely to threaten life. If person uses much larger amount than prescribed or if accidentally swallowed, call doctor or poison control center 1-800-222-1222 for help.

 ## POSSIBLE ADVERSE REACTIONS OR SIDE EFFECTS

SYMPTOMS	WHAT TO DO
Life-threatening: None expected.	
Common: None expected.	
Infrequent:	
• Black, tarry stools from gastrointestinal bleeding.	Discontinue. Seek emergency treatment.
• Severe abdominal pain.	Discontinue. Call doctor right away.
• Constipation, belching, diarrhea, nausea, unexpected weight loss.	Continue. Call doctor when convenient.
Rare: Hives, skin rash, hiccups.	Discontinue. Call doctor right away.

 ## WARNINGS & PRECAUTIONS

Don't take if:
You are allergic to colestipol.

Before you start, consult your doctor if:
- You have liver disease such as cirrhosis.
- You are jaundiced.
- You will have surgery within 2 months, including dental surgery, requiring general or spinal anesthesia.
- You are constipated.
- You have peptic ulcer.
- You have coronary artery disease.

Over age 60:
Constipation more likely. Other adverse effects more likely.

Pregnancy:
Safety not established. Consult doctor. Risk category C (see page xviii).

Breast-feeding:
Unknown if drug passes into milk. Avoid nursing until you finish medicine. Consult doctor for advice on maintaining milk supply.

Infants & children:
Only under expert medical supervision.

Prolonged use:
- Request lab studies to determine serum cholesterol and serum triglycerides.
- May decrease absorption of folic acid.

Skin & sunlight:
No problems expected.

Driving, piloting or hazardous work:
No problems expected.

Discontinuing:
Don't discontinue without consulting doctor. Dose may require gradual reduction if you have taken drug for a long time. Doses of other drugs may also require adjustment, particularly digitalis.

Others:
- This medicine does not cure disorders, but helps to control them.
- May interfere with the accuracy of some medical tests.

POSSIBLE INTERACTION WITH OTHER DRUGS

GENERIC NAME OR DRUG CLASS	COMBINED EFFECT
Anticoagulants, oral*	Decreased anticoagulant effect.
Beta carotene	Decreased absorption of beta carotene.
Dexfenfluramine	May require dosage change as weight loss occurs.
Dextrothyroxine	Decreased dextrothyroxine effect.
Digitalis preparations*	Decreased absorption of digitalis preparations.
Diuretics, thiazide*	Decreased absorption of thiazide diuretics.
Penicillins*	Decreased absorption of penicillins.
Tetracyclines*	Decreased absorption of tetracyclines.
Thiazides*	Decreased absorption of colestipol.
Thyroid hormones*	Decreased thyroid effect.
Trimethoprim	Decreased absorption of colestipol.

Ursodiol	Decreased absorption of ursodiol.
Vancomycin	Increased chance of hearing loss or kidney damage. Decreased therapeutic effect of vancomycin.
Vitamins	Decreased absorption of fat-soluble vitamins (A,D,E,K).
Other medicines	May delay or reduce absorption.

POSSIBLE INTERACTION WITH OTHER SUBSTANCES

INTERACTS WITH	COMBINED EFFECT
Alcohol:	None expected.
Beverages:	None expected.
Cocaine:	None expected.
Foods:	Interferes with absorption of vitamins. Take supplements.
Marijuana:	None expected.
Tobacco:	None expected.

CONDYLOMA ACUMINATUM AGENTS

GENERIC AND BRAND NAMES

IMIQUIMOD
  Aldara
PODOFILOX
  Condylox

PODOPHYLLUM
  Podofin

BASIC INFORMATION

Habit forming? No
Prescription needed? Yes
Available as generic? No
Drug class: Cytotoxic (topical)

 ## USES

- Treatment for *condylomata acuminata*—external genital and perianal warts.
- Treatment of superficial basal cell carcinoma.
- May be used for other skin disorders as prescribed by your doctor.

 ## DOSAGE & USAGE INFORMATION

How to use:
For all treatments—Always follow instructions provided with prescription. Wash hands before and after applying medicine. Let the solution dry before allowing other skin surfaces to touch the treated area.
- Imiquimod—Apply a thin film of cream to the wart and rub in well. Leave cream on the treated skin 6 to 10 hours, then wash with soap and water.

Continued next column

 ## OVERDOSE

SYMPTOMS:
- Imiquimod: Overdose unlikely. It may increase adverse skin reactions.
- Podofilox or podophyllum: The following symptoms may occur when the body absorbs too much—painful urination, breathing difficulty, dizziness, severe nausea or vomiting, fever, heartbeat irregularity, numbness and tingling of hands and feet, abdominal pain, excitement, irritability, seizures, coma.

WHAT TO DO:
- Dial 911 (emergency) for medical help or call poison control center 1-800-222-1222 for instructions.
- See emergency information on last 3 pages of this book.

- Podofilox—Apply drug to warts with cotton applicator (supplied with drug). Allow drug to remain on warts for 1 to 6 hours, then remove with soap and water.
- Podophyllum—Apply petroleum jelly on normal skin surrounding warts. With a glass applicator or cotton swab, carefully apply podophyllum to the warts. Allow drug to remain on warts for 1 to 6 hours after application, then remove with soap and water.

When to use:
- Imiquimod cream—Once every other day 3 times a week. Apply at bedtime for up to 16 weeks.
- Podofilox topical solution—Apply twice a day (12 hours apart) for 3 consecutive days, then discontinue use for 4 consecutive days. May repeat this cycle of treatment 4 times (4 weeks).
- Podophyllum topical solution—Once at 1 week intervals for up to 6 weeks.

If you forget a dose:
Apply it as soon as you remember, then return to regular schedule.

What drug does:
Kills cells and erodes tissue.

Time lapse before drug works:
Several weeks.

Don't use with:
Any other topical medicine without consulting your doctor or pharmacist.

 ## POSSIBLE ADVERSE REACTIONS OR SIDE EFFECTS

SYMPTOMS	WHAT TO DO
Life-threatening: In case of overdose, see previous column.	
Common: Mild skin reactions (slight stinging, mild redness, tenderness or slight swelling in treated area).	No action necessary. If they continue, call doctor.
Infrequent: Skin rash, burning, red skin, severe skin reaction. If too much of drug absorbed into body: hallucinations, diarrhea, nausea and vomiting, unusual bleeding, fever, muscle pain, flu-like symptoms.	Discontinue. Call doctor right away.
Rare: Lightening of normal skin at application site.	Continue. Call doctor when convenient.

WARNINGS & PRECAUTIONS

Don't use if:
- Warts are crumbled and bleeding.
- If warts have just been biopsied or had other surgery performed on them.
- If you are allergic to condyloma acuminatum agents.

Before you start, consult your doctor if:
You have used one of these drugs previously and have a new outbreak of warts.

Over age 60:
No special problems expected.

Pregnancy:
Consult doctor. Pregnancy risk factor not designated for podophyllum. Imiquimod is risk category B and podofilox is risk category C. See category list on page xviii.

Breast-feeding:
It is not known if drugs pass into milk. Avoid drugs or discontinue nursing until you finish medicine. Consult doctor for advice on maintaining milk supply.

Infants & children:
Efficacy and safety have not been established for all these drugs. Imiquimod is approved for patients 12 and over.

Prolonged use:
Increased risk of adverse reactions.

Skin & sunlight:
No problems expected.

Driving, piloting or hazardous work:
No problems expected.

Discontinuing:
No problems expected. Discontinue medicine once warts are healed.

Others:
- Advise any doctor whom you consult that you are using this medicine.
- Keep medicine away from unaffected skin, eyes, nose and mouth. Wash hands before and after using.
- Don't bandage or cover the treated warts with material that is occlusive. If covering is needed, use cotton gauze or cotton underwear.
- Don't use medicine on moles or birthmarks.
- Don't use near heat or open flame.
- Do not apply more of the medicine than prescribed. It will increase risk of side effects.
- Avoid sexual contact while medicine is on the warts.
- Imiquimod may weaken contraceptive devices such as cervical caps, condoms and diaphragms and reduce their contraceptive effect.
- Recurrence of genital warts is common after treatment.

POSSIBLE INTERACTION WITH OTHER DRUGS

GENERIC NAME OR DRUG CLASS	COMBINED EFFECT
Other topical medicines used in same skin area.	Increases risk of side effects. Avoid.

POSSIBLE INTERACTION WITH OTHER SUBSTANCES

INTERACTS WITH	COMBINED EFFECT
Alcohol:	None expected.
Beverages:	None expected.
Cocaine:	None expected.
Foods:	None expected.
Marijuana:	None expected.
Tobacco:	None expected.

CONTRACEPTIVES, ORAL & SKIN

GENERIC AND BRAND NAMES

See full list of generic and brand names in the *Generic and Brand Name Directory*, page 882.

BASIC INFORMATION

Habit forming? No
Prescription needed? Yes
Available as generic? Yes, for some
Drug class: Female sex hormone, contraceptive (oral & skin)

 USES

- Prevents pregnancy.
- Helps regulates menstrual periods.
- Treats premenstrual dysphoric disorder.
- May be used to treat acne vulgaris in females.

 DOSAGE & USAGE INFORMATION

How to take:
- Tablet—Swallow with liquid or food.
- Chewable tablet—May be swallowed whole or chewed and swallowed. If pill is chewed, drink a full glass of liquid right afterwards.
- Extended-cycle tablet—Take as directed.
- Skin patch—Follow instructions on package.

When to take:
- Tablet—At same time each day, usually for 21 days of 28-day cycle.
- Other forms—Take or use as directed.

If you forget a dose:
Follow instructions provided with your product. May want to call doctor for advice about other protection against pregnancy.

What drug does:
Blocks release of eggs from the ovaries. Alters cervix mucus to resist sperm entry. Alters uterus lining to resist implantation of fertilized egg.

Time lapse before drug works:
10 days or more to provide contraception.

Don't take with:
Any other medicine or any dietary supplement without consulting your doctor or pharmacist.

 OVERDOSE

SYMPTOMS:
Drowsiness, nausea, vomiting, bleeding.
WHAT TO DO:
Overdose unlikely to threaten life. If person uses much larger amount than prescribed or if accidentally swallowed, call doctor or poison control center 1-800-222-1222 for help.

 POSSIBLE ADVERSE REACTIONS OR SIDE EFFECTS

SYMPTOMS	WHAT TO DO
Life-threatening:	
Blood clot (sudden and severe pain in leg, chest stomach or groin; severe headache; shortness of breath; coughing blood; sudden weakness or numbness or vision changes or slurring speech).	Seek emergency treatment immediately.
Common:	
• Menstrual bleeding changes (during first 3 months of drug use).	Continue, but call doctor right away.
• Cramping or bloating, breast tenderness or swelling, dizziness, fluid retention, acne, nausea or vomiting, feeling tired or weak.	Continue. Call doctor when convenient.
Infrequent:	
• Headache or migraine(increase in number), vaginal discharge or itching or irritation, high blood pressure, higher blood sugar (nausea, sweating, pale skin, faintness).	Continue, but call doctor right away.
• Brown blotches on skin, gain or loss of body hair, weight gain or loss, increase or decrease in sexual desire, skin sensitive to sun, dizziness.	Continue. Call doctor when convenient.
Rare:	
• Breast lumps, pain in stomach or side, yellow eyes or skin, pain or swelling in upper abdomen, depression.	Continue, but call doctor right away.
• Irritated skin from patch, swelling or bleeding gums, increased or decreased appetite, problem wearing contact lenses, other unexplained symptoms.	Continue. Call doctor when convenient.

WARNINGS & PRECAUTIONS

Don't take if:
- You are allergic to any female hormone.
- You have cancer of breast, uterus or ovaries.
- You have or have had a stroke, a history of (or risk of) blood clots, sickle-cell disease, heart attack or heart disease, blood circulation problems, jaundice, liver disease, adrenal problems (Yasmin brand), or unexplained vaginal bleeding.

Before you start, consult your doctor if:
- You have or have had benign breast problems or family history of breast cancer, medical problems in pregnancy, epilepsy, asthma, migraines or other headaches, kidney or gallbladder disease, high cholesterol, high blood pressure, diabetes or other medical disorders.
- You will have surgery in the near future.
- You are over age 35 or smoke cigarettes.

Over age 60:
Not used in this age group.

Pregnancy:
Stop drug at first sign of pregnancy. See doctor right away. Risk category X (see page xviii).

Breast-feeding:
Drug passes into milk. Avoid drug or discontinue nursing. Consult your doctor.

Infants & children:
Not recommended.

Prolonged use:
- Possibly cause gallstones or gradual blood pressure rise and possible difficulty becoming pregnant after discontinuing.
- Talk to your doctor about the need for follow-up medical examinations or laboratory studies to check blood pressure, liver function, pap smear.

Skin & sunlight:
One or more drugs in this group may cause rash or intensify sunburn in areas exposed to sun or ultraviolet light (photosensitivity reaction). Avoid overexposure. Notify doctor if reaction occurs.

Driving, piloting or hazardous work:
No problems expected.

Discontinuing:
- Use another form of birth control if you want to avoid unintended pregnancy.
- Fertility returns rapidly after discontinuing, but there may be a delay in getting pregnant.

Others:
- Failure to take drug for 1 day may reduce birth control effect. Use backup type of birth control.
- Advise any doctor you consult that you take this drug. Drug use may interfere with the accuracy of some medical tests.
- Risk of severe adverse effects is higher in smokers and in women using the skin patch.

- Use of the skin patch exposes you to about 60% more estrogen than typical birth control pills and puts you at higher risk of blood clots and other serious side effects. Consult doctor.

POSSIBLE INTERACTION WITH OTHER DRUGS

GENERIC NAME OR DRUG CLASS	COMBINED EFFECT
Ampicillin	Decreased contraceptive effect.
Antibacterials*	Decreased contraceptive effect.
Anticoagulants*	Decreased anticoagulant effect.
Anticonvulsants, hydantoin*	Decreased contraceptive effect.
Antidepressants, tricyclic*	Increased toxicity of antidepressants.
Antidiabetics* oral	Decreased antidiabetic effect.
Antifibrinolytic agents*	Increased possibility of blood clotting.
Anti-inflammatory drugs nonsteroidal (NSAIDs)*	Decreased contraceptive effect.
Antihistamines*	Decreased contraceptive effect.
Barbiturates*	Decreased contraceptive effect.
Chloramphenicol	Decreased contraceptive effect.

Continued on page 914

POSSIBLE INTERACTION WITH OTHER SUBSTANCES

INTERACTS WITH	COMBINED EFFECT
Alcohol:	None expected.
Beverages:	None expected.
Cocaine:	None expected.
Foods: Salt.	Fluid retention.
Marijuana:	Bleeding risk between periods. Avoid.
Tobacco:	Possible heart attack, blood clots and stroke. *Don't smoke.*

CONTRACEPTIVES, VAGINAL

GENERIC AND BRAND NAMES

See full list of generic and brand names in the *Generic and Brand Name Directory,* page 883.

BASIC INFORMATION

Habit forming? No
Prescription needed? Not for most
Available as generic? Many are available
Drug class: Contraceptive (vaginal)

 USES

- Provides a degree of protection against pregnancy.
- Spermicides used alone are not recommended for prevention of sexually transmitted diseases including human immunodeficiency virus (HIV).

 DOSAGE & USAGE INFORMATION

How to take:
Read package insert carefully. Some cautions to remember:
- Do not douche for 6 to 8 hours after intercourse.
- Do not remove sponge, cervical cap or diaphragm for 6 to 8 hours after intercourse.
- Follow product label instructions for storage.
- Plastic ring device—Follow special patient brochure instructions.

When to take:
For barrier forms, use consistently with every sexual exposure. The plastic ring device is replaced every month.

If you forget to use:
Contact your doctor to consider using another form of pregnancy protection, such as the "morning-after" pill.

Continued next column

 OVERDOSE

SYMPTOMS:
None expected.
WHAT TO DO:
Not intended for internal use. If child accidentally swallows, call doctor or poison control center 1-800-222-1222 for help.

What drug does:
- Spermicides form a chemical barrier between sperm in semen and the mucous membranes in the vagina. The chemical acts to inactivate viable sperm and also kills some bacteria, viruses, yeast and fungus.
- The plastic ring device releases hormones that go into the bloodstream and provide the same protection as birth control pills.

Time lapse before vaginal contraceptive works:
- Immediate for foam, gels, jellies and sponges.
- 5 to 15 minutes for film and suppositories.
- Plastic ring device takes 7 days to be effective. Use another form of birth control during that time.

Don't use with:
Other vaginal products without consulting your doctor or pharmacist.

 POSSIBLE ADVERSE REACTIONS OR SIDE EFFECTS

SYMPTOMS	WHAT TO DO
Life-threatening:	
Toxic shock syndrome (chills; fever; skin rash; muscle aches; extreme weakness; confusion; redness of vagina, inside of mouth, nose, throat or eyes). (Very rare).	Seek emergency treatment immediately.
Common: None expected.	
Infrequent: None expected.	
Rare: Vaginal discharge, irritation or rash; painful urination; cloudy or bloody urine.	Discontinue. Call doctor right away.

WARNINGS & PRECAUTIONS

Don't take if:
You are allergic to any form of octoxynol, nonoxynol or benzalkonium chloride or female hormones.

Before you start, consult your doctor if:
You desire complete protection against pregnancy. A combination of methods gives better protection than vaginal contraceptives alone.

Over age 60:
Not used in this age group.

Pregnancy:
Risk factor not designated. See categories on page xviii and consult doctor.

Breast-feeding:
Safety not established. Consult doctor.

Infants & children:
Not recommended.

Prolonged use:
Allergic reactions and irritation more likely.

Skin & sunlight:
No problems expected.

Driving, piloting or hazardous work:
No special problems expected.

Discontinuing:
No special problems expected.

Others:
- Failure rate when used alone is relatively high. Therefore a vaginal cream, sponge, suppository, foam, gel, jelly or other product should be used with a mechanical barrier, such as a condom, cervical cap, vaginal diaphragm or other form of pregnancy protection.
- Spermicidal products containing the chemical ingredient nonoxynol 9 (N9) do not provide protection against infection from HIV or other sexually transmitted diseases.
- Nonoxynol 9 (N9) in stand-alone vaginal contraceptives and spermicides can irritate the vagina and rectum, which may increase the risk of contracting HIV/AIDS from an infected partner.
- Don't use a cervical cap, sponge or diaphragm during menstruation. Consider using a condom instead if additional protection is desired.

POSSIBLE INTERACTION WITH OTHER DRUGS

GENERIC NAME OR DRUG CLASS	COMBINED EFFECT
Topical vaginal medications that include any of the following: sulfa drugs, soaps or disinfectants, nitrates,* permanganates, lanolin, hydrogen peroxide, iodides, cotton dressings, aluminum citrates, salicylates*	Spermicidal activity may be reduced or negated. Avoid combinations.
Vaginal douche products	May prevent spermicidal effect. Avoid until 8 hours following intercourse.

POSSIBLE INTERACTION WITH OTHER SUBSTANCES

INTERACTS WITH	COMBINED EFFECT
Alcohol:	None expected.
Beverages:	None expected.
Cocaine:	None expected.
Foods:	None expected.
Marijuana:	None expected.
Tobacco:	None expected.

CROMOLYN

BRAND NAMES

Crolom
Fivent
Gastrocrom
Nalcrom
Nasalcrom
Novo-Cromolyn

Opticrom
PMS-Sodium
  Cromoglycate
Rynacrom
Sodium
  Cromoglycate
Vistacrom

BASIC INFORMATION

Habit forming? No
Prescription needed? Yes, for some
Available as generic? Yes, for some
Drug class: Nasal decongestant,
    anti-inflammatory (nonsteroidal)

 USES

- Powdered form and nebulizer solution prevent asthma attacks. Will not stop an active asthma attack.
- Eye drops treat inflammation of covering to eye and cornea.
- Nasal spray reduces nasal allergic symptoms.
- Capsules may help prevent allergic symptoms.

 DOSAGE & USAGE INFORMATION

How to take:
Inhaler
Follow instructions enclosed with inhaler. Don't swallow cartridges for inhaler. Gargle and rinse mouth after inhalations.
Eye drops
- Wash hands.
- Apply pressure to inside corner of eye with middle finger.
- Continue pressure for 1 minute after placing medicine in eye.
- Tilt head backward. Pull lower lid away from eye with index finger of the same hand.
- Drop eye drops into pouch and close eye. Don't blink.

Continued next column

 OVERDOSE

SYMPTOMS:
Increased side effects and adverse reactions listed.
WHAT TO DO:
Overdose unlikely to threaten life. If person uses much larger amount than prescribed or if accidentally swallowed, call doctor or poison control center 1-800-222-1222 for help.

- Keep eyes closed for 1 to 2 minutes.
- Don't touch applicator tip to any surface (including the eye). If you accidentally touch tip, clean with warm water and soap.
- Keep container tightly closed.
- Keep cool, but don't freeze.
- Wash hands immediately after using.

Nasal solution
Follow prescription instructions.
Capsules
Open capsule and dissolve contents in 4 ounces of hot water, then add equal amount of cold water. Drink all the liquid.

When to take:
At the same times each day. If you also use a bronchodilator inhaler, use the bronchodilator before the cromolyn.

If you forget a dose:
Take as soon as you remember up to 2 hours late. If more than 2 hours, wait for next scheduled dose (don't double this dose).

What drug does:
Blocks histamine release from mast cells.

Time lapse before drug works:
- For inhaler forms: 4 weeks for prevention of asthma attacks. However, if taken 10-15 minutes before exercise or exposure to known allergens, may prevent wheezing.
- 1 to 2 weeks for nasal symptoms; only a few days for eye symptoms.

Don't take with:
Any other medicine or any dietary supplement without consulting your doctor or pharmacist.

 POSSIBLE ADVERSE REACTIONS OR SIDE EFFECTS

SYMPTOMS	WHAT TO DO
Life-threatening: Hives, rash, intense itching, faintness soon after a dose (anaphylaxis).	Seek emergency treatment immediately.
Common: Inhaler—cough, stuffy nose, dry mouth or throat; nasal—burning or stinging inside nose, increased sneezing; oral—diarrhea, headache.	Continue. Call doctor when convenient.
Infrequent: Inhaler—hoarseness, watery eyes; nasal—headache, bad taste, postnasal drip; oral—stomach pain, nausea, insomnia, rash.	Continue. Call doctor when convenient.

Rare:

Inhaler—rash, hives, swallowing difficulty, increased wheezing, joint pain or swelling, weakness, muscle pain, difficult or painful urination, difficulty breathing; nasal—difficulty swallowing, hives, itching, skin rash, facial swelling, wheezing, nosebleed; oral—cough, difficulty swallowing, facial swelling, wheezing, breathing difficulty.

Discontinue. Call doctor right away.

Others:
* Inhaler must be cleaned and work well for drug to be effective.
* Treatment with inhalation cromolyn does not stop an acute asthma attack and may aggravate it.
* Advise any doctor or dentist whom you consult about the use of this medicine.
* Be sure you and the doctor discuss benefits and risks of this drug before starting.
* Call doctor if symptoms worsen or new symptoms develop with use of this medicine.
* Wear a medical identification that indicates the use of this medicine.
* Use medicine only as directed. Don't increase or decrease dosage without doctor's approval.

WARNINGS & PRECAUTIONS

Don't take if:
You use the dry powder form of cromolyn and if you are allergic to cromolyn, lactose, milk or milk products.

Before you start, consult your doctor if:
* You plan to become pregnant within medication period.
* You have kidney or liver disease.

Over age 60:
Adverse reactions and side effects may be more frequent and severe than in younger persons.

Pregnancy:
No proven harm to unborn child, but avoid if possible. Consult doctor. Risk category B (see page xviii).

Breast-feeding:
Effects unknown. Confer with your doctor.

Infants & children:
Do not use for children under age two.

Prolonged use:
Consult doctor on a regular basis while using this drug.

Skin & sunlight:
No problems expected.

Driving, piloting or hazardous work:
No problems expected.

Discontinuing:
Don't discontinue without doctor's approval if drug is used to prevent asthma symptoms. Dosages of other drugs may need to be adjusted.

POSSIBLE INTERACTION WITH OTHER DRUGS

GENERIC NAME OR DRUG CLASS	COMBINED EFFECT
None significant.	

POSSIBLE INTERACTION WITH OTHER SUBSTANCES

INTERACTS WITH	COMBINED EFFECT
Alcohol:	None expected.
Beverages:	None expected.
Cocaine:	None expected.
Foods:	None expected.
Marijuana:	None expected.
Tobacco:	None expected, but tobacco smoke aggravates asthma and eye irritation. Avoid.

*See Glossary

CYCLANDELATE

BRAND NAMES

Cyclospasmol   Cyraso-400

BASIC INFORMATION

Habit forming? No
Prescription needed?
   U.S.: Yes
   Canada: No
Available as generic? Yes
Drug class: Vasodilator

 ## USES

May improve poor blood flow to extremities.

 ## DOSAGE & USAGE INFORMATION

How to take:
Tablet or capsule—Swallow with liquid. If you can't swallow whole, crumble tablet or open capsule and take with liquid or food.

When to take:
At the same time each day.

If you forget a dose:
Take as soon as you remember up to 2 hours late. If more than 2 hours, wait for next scheduled dose (don't double this dose).

What drug does:
Increases blood flow by relaxing and expanding blood-vessel walls.

Time lapse before drug works:
3 weeks.

Don't take with:
Any other medicine or any dietary supplement without consulting your doctor or pharmacist.

 ## OVERDOSE

SYMPTOMS:
Severe headache, dizziness; nausea, vomiting; flushed, hot face.
WHAT TO DO:
Overdose unlikely to threaten life. If person uses much larger amount than prescribed or if accidentally swallowed, call doctor or poison control center 1-800-222-1222 for help.

 ## POSSIBLE ADVERSE REACTIONS OR SIDE EFFECTS

SYMPTOMS	WHAT TO DO
Life-threatening: None expected.	
Common: None expected.	
Infrequent:	
• Rapid heartbeat.	Discontinue. Call doctor right away.
• Dizziness; headache; weakness; flushed face; tingling in face, fingers or toes; unusual sweating.	Continue. Call doctor when convenient.
• Belching, heartburn, nausea or stomach pain.	Continue. Tell doctor at next visit.
Rare: None expected.	

WARNINGS & PRECAUTIONS

Don't take if:
You have had an allergic reaction to cyclandelate.

Before you start, consult your doctor if:
• You have glaucoma.
• You have had a heart attack or stroke.

Over age 60:
Adverse reactions and side effects may be more frequent and severe than in younger persons.

Pregnancy:
Consult doctor. Risk category C (see page xviii).

Breast-feeding:
No proven problems. Consult doctor.

Infants & children:
Not recommended.

Prolonged use:
No problems expected.

Skin & sunlight:
No problems expected.

Driving, piloting or hazardous work:
Avoid if you feel dizzy or weak. Otherwise, no problems expected.

Discontinuing:
Don't discontinue without doctor's advice until you complete prescribed dose, even though symptoms diminish or disappear.

Others:
Response to drug varies. If your symptoms don't improve after 3 weeks of use, consult doctor.

POSSIBLE INTERACTION WITH OTHER DRUGS

GENERIC NAME OR DRUG CLASS	COMBINED EFFECT
None expected.	

POSSIBLE INTERACTION WITH OTHER SUBSTANCES

INTERACTS WITH	COMBINED EFFECT
Alcohol:	None expected.
Beverages:	None expected.
Cocaine:	Decreased cyclandelate effect. Avoid.
Foods:	None expected.
Marijuana:	None expected.
Tobacco:	May decrease cyclandelate effect.

*See Glossary

CYCLOBENZAPRINE

BRAND NAMES

Amrix   Flexeril
Cycoflex

BASIC INFORMATION

Habit forming? No
Prescription needed? Yes
Available as generic? Yes
Drug class: Muscle relaxant

USES

Treatment for pain and limited motion caused by spasms in voluntary muscles.

DOSAGE & USAGE INFORMATION

How to take:
- Tablet—Swallow with liquid. Take with food if stomach upset occurs.
- Extended-release tablet—Swallow whole with liquid.

When to take:
Take as directed on label.

If you forget a dose:
Take as soon as you remember. If it is almost time for the next dose, wait for that dose (don't double this dose) and resume regular schedule.

What drug does:
Blocks body's pain messages to brain.

Time lapse before drug works:
30 to 60 minutes.

Don't take with:
Any other medicine or any dietary supplement without consulting your doctor or pharmacist.

OVERDOSE

SYMPTOMS:
Drowsiness, confusion, difficulty concentrating, visual problems, vomiting, blood pressure drop, low body temperature, weak and rapid pulse, convulsions, coma.
WHAT TO DO:
- **Dial 911 (emergency) for medical help or call poison control center 1-800-222-1222 for instructions.**
- **If person is unconscious, check breathing and pulse. If not breathing, begin mouth-to-mouth rescue breathing. If heart is not beating, begin chest compressions.**
- **See emergency information on last 3 pages of this book.**

POSSIBLE ADVERSE REACTIONS OR SIDE EFFECTS

SYMPTOMS	WHAT TO DO
Life-threatening:	
In case of overdose, see previous column.	
Common:	
Drowsiness, dizziness, dry mouth.	Continue. Call doctor when convenient.
Infrequent:	
• Blurred vision, fast heartbeat.	Discontinue. Call doctor right away.
• Insomnia, numbness in extremities, bad taste in mouth, fatigue, nausea, sweating.	Continue. Call doctor when convenient.
Rare:	
• Unsteadiness, confusion, depression, hallucinations, rash, itch, swelling, breathing difficulty.	Discontinue. Call doctor right away.
• Difficult urination, rash.	Continue. Call doctor when convenient.

WARNINGS & PRECAUTIONS

Don't take if:
- You are allergic to any skeletal muscle relaxant.*
- You have taken a monoamine oxidase (MAO) inhibitor* in last 2 weeks.
- You have had a heart attack within 6 weeks, or suffer from congestive heart failure.
- You have an overactive thyroid.

Before you start, consult your doctor if:
- You have a heart problem.
- You have reacted to tricyclic antidepressants.
- You have glaucoma.
- You have a prostate condition and urination difficulty.
- You intend to pilot aircraft.

Over age 60:
Adverse reactions and side effects may be more frequent and severe than in younger persons. Avoid extremes of heat and cold.

Pregnancy:
No problems expected. Consult doctor. Risk category B (see page xviii).

Breast-feeding:
Drug may pass into milk. Avoid drug or discontinue nursing until you finish medicine. Consult doctor for advice on maintaining milk supply.

CYCLOBENZAPRINE

Infants & children:
Don't use for children younger than 15.

Prolonged use:
Do not take for longer than 2 to 3 weeks.

Skin & sunlight:
No special problems expected.

Driving, piloting or hazardous work:
Don't drive or pilot aircraft until you learn how medicine affects you. Don't work around dangerous machinery. Don't climb ladders or work in high places. Danger increases if you drink alcohol or take medicine affecting alertness and reflexes.

Discontinuing:
May be unnecessary to finish medicine. Follow doctor's instructions.

Others:
No problems expected.

 POSSIBLE INTERACTION WITH OTHER DRUGS

GENERIC NAME OR DRUG CLASS	COMBINED EFFECT
Anticholinergics*	Increased anticholinergic effect.
Antidepressants*	Increased sedation.
Antihistamines*	Increased antihistamine effect.
Barbiturates*	Increased sedation.
Central nervous system (CNS) depressants*	Increased sedation.
Cimetidine	Possible increased cyclobenzaprine effect.
Cisapride	Decreased cyclobenzaprine effect.
Clonidine	Decreased clonidine effect.
Dronabinol	Increased effect of dronabinol on central nervous system. Avoid combination.
Guanethidine	Decreased guanethidine effect.
Methyldopa	Decreased methyldopa effect.
Mind-altering drugs*	Increased mind-altering effect.

Monoamine oxidase (MAO) inhibitors*	High fever, convulsions, possible death.
Narcotics*	Increased sedation.
Pain relievers*	Increased pain reliever effect.
Procainamide	Possible increased conduction disturbance.
Quinidine	Possible increased conduction disturbance.
Rauwolfia alkaloids*	Decreased effect of rauwolfia alkaloids.
Sedatives*	Increased sedative effect.
Sleep inducers*	Increased sedation.
Tranquilizers*	Increased tranquilizer effect.

 POSSIBLE INTERACTION WITH OTHER SUBSTANCES

INTERACTS WITH	COMBINED EFFECT
Alcohol:	Depressed brain function. Avoid.
Beverages:	None expected.
Cocaine:	Decreased cyclobenzaprine effect.
Foods:	None expected.
Marijuana:	Occasional use—Drowsiness. Frequent use—Severe mental and physical impairment.
Tobacco:	None expected.

*See Glossary

287

CYCLOPENTOLATE (Ophthalmic)

BRAND NAMES

Ak-Pentolate
Cyclogyl
I-Pentolate
Minims
  Cyclopentolate

Ocu-Pentolate
Pentolair
Spectro-Pentolate

BASIC INFORMATION

Habit forming? No
Prescription needed? Yes
Available as generic? Yes
Drug class: Cycloplegic, mydriatic

 ## USES

- Enlarges (dilates) pupil.
- Temporarily paralyzes the normal pupil accommodation to light before eye examinations and to treat some eye conditions.

 ## DOSAGE & USAGE INFORMATION

How to use:
Eye drops
- Wash hands.
- Apply pressure to inside corner of eye with middle finger.
- Continue pressure for 1 minute after placing medicine in eye.
- Tilt head backward. Pull lower lid away from eye with index finger of the same hand.
- Drop eye drops into pouch and close eye. Don't blink.
- Keep eyes closed for 1 to 2 minutes.
- Don't touch applicator tip to any surface (including the eye). If you accidentally touch tip, clean with warm water and soap.
- Keep container tightly closed.
- Keep cool, but don't freeze.
- Wash hands immediately after using.

When to use:
As directed on bottle.

Continued next column

 ## OVERDOSE

SYMPTOMS:
None expected.
WHAT TO DO:
Not intended for internal use. If child accidentally swallows, call doctor or poison control center 1-800-222-1222 for help.

If you forget a dose:
Use as soon as you remember.

What drug does:
Blocks sphincter muscle of the iris and ciliary body.

Time lapse before drug works:
Within 30 to 60 minutes. Effects usually disappear in 24 hours.

Don't use with:
Other eye medicines such as carbachol, demecarium, echothiophate, isoflurophate, physostigmine, pilocarpine without doctor's approval.

 ## POSSIBLE ADVERSE REACTIONS OR SIDE EFFECTS

SYMPTOMS	WHAT TO DO
Life-threatening: None expected.	
Common: • Increased sensitivity to light.	Continue. Call doctor when convenient.
• Burning eyes.	Continue. Tell doctor at next visit.
Infrequent: None expected.	
Rare (extremely): Symptoms of excess medicine absorbed by the body—Clumsiness, confusion, fever, flushed face, hallucinations, rash, slurred speech, swollen stomach (children), drowsiness, fast heartbeat.	Discontinue. Call doctor right away.

CYCLOPENTOLATE (Ophthalmic)

WARNINGS & PRECAUTIONS

Don't use if:
You are allergic to cyclopentolate.

Before you start, consult your doctor if:
* Medicine is for a brain-damaged child or child with Down syndrome.
* Prescribed for a child with spastic paralysis.

Over age 60:
No problems expected.

Pregnancy:
Avoid if possible. Consult doctor. Risk category C (see page xviii).

Breast-feeding:
Safety not established. Avoid if possible. Consult doctor.

Infants & children:
Use only under close medical supervision.

Prolonged use:
Avoid. May increase absorption into body.

Skin & sunlight:
No special problems expected.

Driving, piloting or hazardous work:
Don't drive or pilot aircraft until you learn how medicine affects you. Don't work around dangerous machinery. Don't climb ladders or work in high places. Danger increases if you drink alcohol or take medicine affecting alertness and reflexes, such as antihistamines, tranquilizers, sedatives, pain medicine, narcotics and mind-altering drugs.

Discontinuing:
If effects last longer than 36 hours after last drops, consult doctor.

Others:
Wear sunglasses to protect eyes from sunlight and bright light.

POSSIBLE INTERACTION WITH OTHER DRUGS

GENERIC NAME OR DRUG CLASS	COMBINED EFFECT
Antiglaucoma agents*	Decreased antiglaucoma effect.

POSSIBLE INTERACTION WITH OTHER SUBSTANCES

INTERACTS WITH	COMBINED EFFECT
Alcohol:	None expected.
Beverages:	None expected.
Cocaine:	None expected.
Foods:	None expected.
Marijuana:	None expected.
Tobacco:	None expected.

*See Glossary

CYCLOPHOSPHAMIDE

BRAND NAMES

Neosar   Procytox

BASIC INFORMATION

Habit forming? No
Prescription needed? Yes
Available as generic? Yes
Drug class: Immunosuppressant, anti-
neoplastic

 ## USES

* Treatment for cancer.
* Treatment for severe rheumatoid arthritis,
  blood-vessel disease and for skin disease.

 ## DOSAGE & USAGE INFORMATION

How to take:
Tablet—Swallow with liquid. If you can't swallow
tablet whole, crumble tablet and take with liquid
or food.

When to take:
Works best if taken first thing in morning. Should
be taken on an empty stomach. However, may
take with food to lessen stomach irritation. Don't
take at bedtime.

If you forget a dose:
Take as soon as you remember up to 12 hours
late. If more than 12 hours, wait for next
scheduled dose (don't double this dose).

What drug does:
* Kills cancer cells.
* Suppresses spread of cancer cells.
* Suppresses immune system.

Time lapse before drug works:
7 to 10 days continual use.

Don't take with:
Any other medicine or any dietary supplement
without consulting your doctor or pharmacist.

 ## OVERDOSE

SYMPTOMS:
**Bloody urine, water retention, weight gain,
severe infection.**
WHAT TO DO:
**Overdose unlikely to threaten life. If person
uses much larger amount than prescribed or
if accidentally swallowed, call doctor or
poison control center 1-800-222-1222 for help.**

 ## POSSIBLE ADVERSE REACTIONS OR SIDE EFFECTS

SYMPTOMS	WHAT TO DO
Life-threatening:	
Hives, rash, intense itching, faintness soon after a dose (anaphylaxis).	Seek emergency treatment immediately.
Common:	
• Sore throat, fever.	Continue, but call doctor right away.
• Dark skin, nails; nausea; appetite loss; vomiting; missed menstrual period.	Continue. Call doctor when convenient.
Infrequent:	
• Rash, hives, itch; shortness of breath; rapid heartbeat; cough; blood in urine, painful urination; pain in side; bleeding, bruising; increased sweating; hoarseness; foot or ankle swelling.	Continue, but call doctor right away.
• Confusion, agitation, headache, dizziness, flushed face, stomach pain, joint pain, fatigue, weakness, diarrhea.	Continue. Call doctor when convenient.
Rare:	
• Mouth, lip sores; black stool; unusual thirst; jaundice.	Continue, but call doctor right away.
• Blurred vision, increased urination, hair loss.	Continue. Call doctor when convenient.

 ## WARNINGS & PRECAUTIONS

Don't take if:
* You are allergic to any alkylating agent.
* You have an infection.
* You have bloody urine.
* You will have surgery within 2 months,
  including dental surgery, requiring general or
  spinal anesthesia.

Before you start, consult your doctor if:
* You have impaired liver or kidney function.
* You have impaired bone marrow or blood cell
  production.
* You have had chemotherapy or x-ray therapy.

- You have taken cortisone drugs in the past year.
- You plan to become pregnant.

Over age 60:
Adverse reactions and side effects may be more frequent and severe than in younger persons. To reduce risk of chemical bladder inflammation, drink 8 to 10 glasses of water daily.

Pregnancy:
Risk to unborn child outweighs drug benefits. Don't use. Risk category D (see page xviii).

Breast-feeding:
Drug passes into milk. Avoid drug or discontinue nursing until you finish medicine. Consult doctor for advice on maintaining milk supply.

Infants & children:
Use only under medical supervision.

Prolonged use:
- Development of fibrous lung tissue.
- Possible jaundice.
- Swelling of feet, lower legs.
- Cancer.
- Infertility in men.
- Talk to your doctor about the need for follow-up medical examinations or laboratory studies to check complete blood counts (white blood cell count, platelet count, red blood cell count, hemoglobin, hematocrit), urine, liver function.

Skin & sunlight:
No problems expected.

Driving, piloting or hazardous work:
Avoid if you feel dizzy or have blurred vision. Otherwise, no problems expected.

Discontinuing:
Don't discontinue without consulting doctor. Dose may require gradual reduction if you have taken drug for a long time. Doses of other drugs may also require adjustment.

Others:
- Frequently causes hair loss. After treatment ends, hair should grow back.
- Avoid vaccinations.
- You will need to drink extra fluids so you will pass more urine. Follow doctor's instructions.

 ## POSSIBLE INTERACTION WITH OTHER DRUGS

GENERIC NAME OR DRUG CLASS	COMBINED EFFECT
Allopurinol or other medicines to treat gout	Possible anemia; decreased antigout effect.
Antidiabetics, oral*	Increased antidiabetic effect.
Bone marrow depressants,* other	Increased bone marrow depressant effect.
Clozapine	Toxic effect on bone marrow.
Cyclosporine	May increase risk of infection.
Digoxin	Possible decreased digoxin absorption.
Immuno-suppressants,* other	Increased risk of infection.
Insulin	Increased insulin effect.
Levamisole	Increased risk of bone marrow depression.
Lovastatin	Increased heart and kidney damage.
Phenobarbital	Increased cyclophosphamide effect.
Probenecid	Increased blood uric acid.
Sulfinpyrazone	Increased blood uric acid.
Tiopronin	Increased risk of toxicity to bone marrow.

 ## POSSIBLE INTERACTION WITH OTHER SUBSTANCES

INTERACTS WITH	COMBINED EFFECT
Alcohol:	None expected.
Beverages:	None expected. Drink plenty of fluids every day.
Cocaine:	Increased danger of brain damage.
Foods:	None expected.
Marijuana:	Increased impairment of immunity.
Tobacco:	None expected.

*See Glossary

CYCLOPLEGIC, MYDRIATIC (Ophthalmic)

GENERIC AND BRAND NAMES

ATROPINE
(ophthalmic)
Atropair
Atropine Care Eye
Drops & Ointment
Atropine Sulfate
S.O.P.
Atropisol
Atrosulf
Isopto Atropine
I-Tropine
Minims Atropine
Ocu-Tropine

HOMATROPINE
(ophthalmic)
AK Homatropine
I-Homatrine
I-Homatropine
Isopto
Homatropine
Minims
Homatropine
Spectro-
Homatropine
SCOPOLAMINE
(ophthalmic)
Isopto Hyoscine

BASIC INFORMATION

Habit forming? No
Prescription needed? Yes
Available as generic? Yes, for some
Drug class: Cycloplegic, mydriatic

 ## USES

- Dilates pupil of the eye.
- Used before some eye examinations, before and after some eye surgical procedures and, rarely, to treat some eye problems such as glaucoma.

 ## DOSAGE & USAGE INFORMATION

How to use:
Eye drops
- Wash hands.
- Apply pressure to inside corner of eye with middle finger.
- Continue pressure for 1 minute after placing medicine in eye.
- Tilt head backward. Pull lower lid away from eye with index finger of the same hand.
- Drop eye drops into pouch and close eye. Don't blink.
- Keep eyes closed for 1 to 2 minutes.

Continued next column

 ## OVERDOSE

SYMPTOMS:
None expected.
WHAT TO DO:
Not intended for internal use. If child accidentally swallows, call doctor or poison control center 1-800-222-1222 for help.

Eye ointment
- Wash hands.
- Pull lower lid down from eye to form a pouch.
- Squeeze tube to apply thin strip of ointment into pouch.
- Close eye for 1 to 2 minutes.
- Don't touch applicator tip to any surface (including the eye). If you accidentally touch tip, clean with warm water and soap.
- Keep container tightly closed.
- Keep cool, but don't freeze.
- Wash hands immediately after using.

When to use:
As directed on label.

If you forget a dose:
Use as soon as you remember.

What drug does:
Blocks normal response to sphincter muscle of the iris of the eye and the accommodative muscle of the ciliary body.

Time lapse before drug works:
Begins within 1 minute. Residual effects may last up to 14 days.

Don't use with:
Other eye medicines such as carbachol, demecarium, echothiophate, isoflurophate, physostigmine, pilocarpine.

 ## POSSIBLE ADVERSE REACTIONS OR SIDE EFFECTS

SYMPTOMS	WHAT TO DO
Life-threatening: None expected.	
Common:	
• Increased sensitivity to light.	Continue. Call doctor when convenient.
• Burning eyes.	Continue. Tell doctor at next visit.
Infrequent: None expected.	
Rare (extremely): Symptoms of excess medicine absorbed by the body—Clumsiness, confusion, fever, flushed face, hallucinations, rash, slurred speech, swollen stomach (children), unusual drowsiness, fast heartbeat.	Discontinue. Call doctor right away.

CYCLOPLEGIC MYDRIATIC (Ophthalmic)

 ## WARNINGS & PRECAUTIONS

Don't use if:
You are allergic to any mydriatic cycloplegic drug.

Before you start, consult your doctor if:
• Medicine is for a brain-damaged child or child with Down syndrome.
• Prescribed for a child with spastic paralysis.

Over age 60:
No problems expected.

Pregnancy:
Decide with your doctor if drug benefits justify risk to unborn child. Risk category C (see page xviii).

Breast-feeding:
Safety not established. Avoid if possible.

Infants & children:
Use only under close medical supervision.

Prolonged use:
Avoid. May increase absorption into body.

Skin & sunlight:
No special problems expected.

Driving, piloting or hazardous work:
Don't drive or pilot aircraft until you learn how medicine affects you. Don't work around dangerous machinery. Don't climb ladders or work in high places. Danger increases if you drink alcohol or take medicine affecting alertness and reflexes, such as antihistamines, tranquilizers, sedatives, pain medicine, narcotics and mind-altering drugs.

Discontinuing:
Effects may last up to 14 days later.

Others:
Wear sunglasses to protect eyes from sunlight and bright light.

 ## POSSIBLE INTERACTION WITH OTHER DRUGS

GENERIC NAME OR DRUG CLASS	COMBINED EFFECT
Clinically significant interactions with oral or injected medicines unlikely.	

 ## POSSIBLE INTERACTION WITH OTHER SUBSTANCES

INTERACTS WITH	COMBINED EFFECT
Alcohol:	None expected.
Beverages:	None expected.
Cocaine:	None expected.
Foods:	None expected.
Marijuana:	None expected.
Tobacco:	None expected.

*See Glossary

CYCLOSERINE

BRAND NAMES

Seromycin

BASIC INFORMATION

Habit forming? No
Prescription needed? Yes
Available as generic? No
Drug class: Antibacterial

 ## USES

• Treats urinary tract infections.
• Treats tuberculosis.

 ## DOSAGE & USAGE INFORMATION

How to take:
Capsule—Swallow with liquid or food to lessen stomach irritation. If you can't swallow whole, open capsule and take with liquid or food.

When to take:
• Once or twice daily as prescribed.
• At the same times each day after meals to prevent stomach irritation.

If you forget a dose:
Take as soon as you remember up to 2 hours late. If more than 2 hours, wait for next scheduled dose (don't double this dose).

What drug does:
Interferes with bacterial wall synthesis and keeps germs from multiplying.

Time lapse before drug works:
3 to 4 hours.

Don't take with:
Any other medicine or any dietary supplement without consulting your doctor or pharmacist.

 ## OVERDOSE

SYMPTOMS:
Seizures.
WHAT TO DO:
• Dial 911 (emergency) for medical help or call poison control center 1-800-222-1222 for instructions.
• See emergency information on last 3 pages of this book.

 ## POSSIBLE ADVERSE REACTIONS OR SIDE EFFECTS

SYMPTOMS	WHAT TO DO
Life-threatening: Seizures, muscle twitching or trembling.	Seek emergency treatment immediately.
Common: Gum inflammation, pale skin, depression, confusion, dizziness, restlessness, anxiety, nightmares, severe headache, drowsiness.	Continue, but call doctor right away.
Infrequent: Visual changes; skin rash; numbness, tingling or burning in hands and feet; jaundice; eye pain.	Continue. Call doctor when convenient.
Rare: Seizures, thoughts of suicide.	Discontinue. Seek emergency treatment.

WARNINGS & PRECAUTIONS

Don't take if:
- You are a frequent user of alcohol.
- You have a convulsive disorder.

Before you start, consult your doctor if:
- You are depressed.
- You have kidney disease.
- You have severe anxiety.

Over age 60:
Adverse reactions and side effects may be more frequent and severe than in younger persons. You may need smaller doses for shorter periods of time.

Pregnancy:
Decide with your doctor if drug benefits justify risk to unborn child. Risk category C (see page xviii).

Breast-feeding:
Drug passes into milk. Avoid drug or discontinue nursing until you finish medicine. Consult doctor for advice on maintaining milk supply.

Infants & children:
Use only under close medical supervision.

Prolonged use:
- May cause liver or kidney damage.
- May cause anemia.

Skin & sunlight:
No special problems expected.

Driving, piloting or hazardous work:
Don't drive or pilot aircraft until you learn how medicine affects you. Don't work around dangerous machinery. Don't climb ladders or work in high places. Danger increases if you drink alcohol or take medicine affecting alertness and reflexes.

Discontinuing:
Don't discontinue without consulting doctor. Dose may require gradual reduction if you have taken drug for a long time. Doses of other drugs may also require adjustment.

Others:
- May have to take anticonvulsants, sedatives and/or pyridoxine to prevent or minimize toxic effects on the brain.
- If you must take more than 500 mg per day, toxicity is much more likely to occur.
- Talk to your doctor about taking pyridoxine as a supplement.

POSSIBLE INTERACTION WITH OTHER DRUGS

GENERIC NAME OR DRUG CLASS	COMBINED EFFECT
Ethionamide	Increased risk of seizures.
Isoniazid	Increased risk of central nervous system effects.
Pyridoxine	Reduces effects of pyridoxine. Since pyridoxine is a vital vitamin, patients on cycloserine require pyridoxine supplements to prevent anemia or peripheral neuritis.

POSSIBLE INTERACTION WITH OTHER SUBSTANCES

INTERACTS WITH	COMBINED EFFECT
Alcohol:	Toxic. May increase risk of seizures. Avoid.
Beverages:	None expected. All beverages except those with alcohol.
Cocaine:	Toxic. Avoid.
Foods:	None expected.
Marijuana:	May increase risk of seizures.
Tobacco:	May decrease effect of cycloserine.

CYCLOSPORINE

BRAND NAMES

Neoral   **Sandimmune**

BASIC INFORMATION

Habit forming? No
Prescription needed? Yes
Available as generic? Yes
Drug class: Immunosuppressant

 USES

- Suppresses the immune response in patients who have transplants of the heart, lung, kidney, liver, pancreas. Cyclosporine treats rejection as well as helps prevent it.
- Treatment for severe psoriasis when regular treatment is ineffective or not appropriate.

 DOSAGE & USAGE INFORMATION

How to take:
- Oral solution—Take after meals with liquid to decrease stomach irritation. May mix with milk, chocolate milk or orange juice. Don't mix in Styrofoam cups. Use special dropper for exact dosage.
- Capsule—Take with water or other fluid. Don't break capsule open.

When to take:
At the same time each day, according to instructions on prescription label.

If you forget a dose:
Take as soon as you remember up to 2 hours late. If more than 2 hours, wait for next scheduled dose (don't double this dose).

What drug does:
Exact mechanism is unknown, but believed to inhibit interleuken II to affect T-lymphocytes.

Time lapse before drug works:
3 to 3-1/2 hours.

Don't take with:
Any other medicine or any dietary supplement without consulting your doctor or pharmacist.

 OVERDOSE

SYMPTOMS:
Irregular heartbeat, seizures, coma.
WHAT TO DO:
- Dial 911 (emergency) for medical help or call poison control center 1-800-222-1222 for instructions.
- See emergency information on last 3 pages of this book.

 POSSIBLE ADVERSE REACTIONS OR SIDE EFFECTS

SYMPTOMS	WHAT TO DO
Life-threatening:	
Seizures, wheezing with shortness of breath, convulsions.	Discontinue. Seek emergency treatment.
Common:	
• Gum inflammation, blood in urine, jaundice, tremors.	Continue. Call doctor when convenient.
• Increased hair growth.	Continue. Tell doctor at next visit.
Infrequent:	
• Fever, chills, sore throat, shortness of breath.	Continue, but call doctor right away.
• Frequent urination, headache, leg cramps.	Continue. Call doctor when convenient.
Rare:	
• Confusion, irregular heartbeat, numbness of hands and feet, nervousness, face flushing, severe abdominal pain, weakness.	Continue, but call doctor right away.
• Acne, headache.	Continue. Call doctor when convenient.

 WARNINGS & PRECAUTIONS

Don't take if:
- You have chicken pox.
- You have shingles (herpes zoster).

Before you start, consult your doctor if:
- You have liver problems.
- You have an infection.
- You have kidney disease.

Over age 60:
No special problems expected.

Pregnancy:
Decide with your doctor if drug benefits justify risk to unborn child. Risk category C (see page xviii).

Breast-feeding:
Drug passes into milk. Avoid drug or discontinue nursing until you finish medicine. Consult doctor for advice on maintaining milk supply.

Infants & children:
No problems expected.

Prolonged use:
- Can cause reduced function of kidney.
- Talk to your doctor about the need for follow-up medical examinations or laboratory studies to check blood pressure, kidney function, liver function.

Skin & sunlight:
No problems expected.

Driving, piloting or hazardous work:
Don't drive or pilot aircraft until you learn how medicine affects you. Don't work around dangerous machinery. Don't climb ladders or work in high places. Danger increases if you drink alcohol or take medicine affecting alertness and reflexes.

Discontinuing:
Don't discontinue without consulting doctor. You probably will require this medicine for the remainder of your life.

Others:
- Request regular laboratory studies to measure levels of potassium and cyclosporine in blood and to evaluate liver and kidney function.
- Check blood pressure. Cyclosporine sometimes causes hypertension.
- Don't store solution in the refrigerator.
- Avoid any immunizations except those specifically recommended by your doctor.
- Maintain good dental hygiene. Cyclosporine can cause gum problems.
- Kidney toxicity occurs commonly after 12 months of taking cyclosporine.
- Don't mix in Styrofoam cups.

 ## POSSIBLE INTERACTION WITH OTHER DRUGS

GENERIC NAME OR DRUG CLASS	COMBINED EFFECT
Androgens	Increased effect of cyclosporine.
Anticonvulsants*	Decreased effect of cyclosporine.
Cimetidine	Increased effect of cyclosporine.
Danazol	Increased effect of cyclosporine.
Diltiazem	Increased effect of cyclosporine.
Diuretics, potassium-sparing	Increased effect of cyclosporine.
Erythromycin	Increased effect of cyclosporine.
Estrogens	Increased effect of cyclosporine.

Fluconazole	Increased effect of cyclosporine. Cyclosporine dosage must be adjusted.
HMG-CoA reductase inhibitors	Increased risk of muscle and kidney problems.
Imatinib	Increased effect of cyclosporine.
Immuno-suppressants* (adrenocorticoids, azathioprine, chlorambucil, cyclophosphamide, mercaptopurine, muromonab-CD3)	May increase risk of infection.
Itraconazole	Increased cyclosporine toxicity.
Ketoconazole	Increased risk of toxicity to kidney.
Leukotriene modifiers	Increased effect of cyclosporine.
Losartan	Increased potassium levels.
Lovastatin	Increased heart and kidney damage.
Medicines that may be toxic to kidneys (gold,* NSAIDs,* sulfonamides*)	Increased risk of toxicity to kidneys.

Continued on page 915

 ## POSSIBLE INTERACTION WITH OTHER SUBSTANCES

INTERACTS WITH	COMBINED EFFECT
Alcohol:	May increase possibility of toxic effects. Avoid.
Beverages: Grapefruit juice.	Increased cyclosporine effect.
Cocaine:	May increase possibility of toxic effects. Avoid.
Foods:	None expected.
Marijuana:	May increase possibility of toxic effects. Avoid.
Tobacco:	May increase possibility of toxic effects. Avoid.

*See Glossary

DANAZOL

BRAND NAMES

Cyclomen
Danocrine

BASIC INFORMATION

Habit forming? No
Prescription needed? Yes
Available as generic? Yes
Drug class: Gonadotropin inhibitor

 ## USES

Treatment of endometriosis, fibrocystic breast disease, angioneurotic edema except in pregnant women, gynecomastia, infertility, excessive menstruation, precocious puberty.

 ## DOSAGE & USAGE INFORMATION

How to take:
Capsule—Swallow with liquid or food to lessen stomach irritation. If you can't swallow whole, open capsule and take with liquid or food.

When to take:
At the same times each day.

If you forget a dose:
Take as soon as you remember (don't double dose).

What drug does:
Partially prevents output of pituitary follicle-stimulating hormone and leuteinizing hormone reducing estrogen production.

Time lapse before drug works:
* 2 to 3 months to treat endometriosis.
* 1 to 2 months to treat other disorders.

Don't take with:
* Birth control pills.
* Any other medicine or any dietary supplement without consulting your doctor or pharmacist.

 ## OVERDOSE

SYMPTOMS:
None expected.
WHAT TO DO:
Overdose unlikely to threaten life. If person uses much larger amount than prescribed or if accidentally swallowed, call doctor or poison control center 1-800-222-1222 for help.

 ## POSSIBLE ADVERSE REACTIONS OR SIDE EFFECTS

SYMPTOMS	WHAT TO DO
Life-threatening: None expected.	
Common: Menstrual irregularities.	Continue. Call doctor when convenient.
Infrequent: • Unnatural hair growth in women, nosebleeds, bleeding gums, sore throat and chills.	Discontinue. Call doctor right away.
• Dizziness; deepened voice; hoarseness; flushed or red skin; muscle cramps; enlarged clitoris; decreased testicle size; vaginal burning, itching; swollen feet; decreased breast size; increased or decreased sex drive.	Continue. Call doctor when convenient.
• Headache, acne, weight gain, vision changes.	Continue. Tell doctor at next visit.
Rare: Jaundice, flushing, sweating, vaginitis, rash, nausea, vomiting, constipation, abdominal pain.	Discontinue. Call doctor right away.

WARNINGS & PRECAUTIONS

Don't take if:
* You become pregnant.
* You have breast cancer.

Before you start, consult your doctor if:
* You take birth control pills.
* You have diabetes.
* You have heart disease.
* You have epilepsy.
* You have kidney disease.
* You have liver disease.
* You have migraine headaches.

Over age 60:
Adverse reactions and side effects may be more frequent and severe than in younger persons.

Pregnancy:
Risk to unborn child outweighs drug benefits. Don't use. Stop if you get pregnant. Risk category X (see page xviii).

Breast-feeding:
Unknown whether medicine filters into milk. Consult doctor.

Infants & children:
Not recommended.

Prolonged use:
* Required for full effect. Don't discontinue without consulting doctor.
* Talk to your doctor about the need for follow-up medical examinations or laboratory studies to check liver function; mammogram.

Skin & sunlight:
No problems expected.

Driving, piloting or hazardous work:
No problems expected.

Discontinuing:
Don't discontinue without consulting doctor. Menstrual periods may be absent for 2 to 3 months after discontinuation.

Others:
* May alter blood sugar levels in persons with diabetes.
* Advise any doctor or dentist whom you consult that you take this medicine.
* May interfere with the accuracy of some medical tests.

POSSIBLE INTERACTION WITH OTHER DRUGS

GENERIC NAME OR DRUG CLASS	COMBINED EFFECT
Anticoagulants, oral*	Increased anticoagulant effect.
Antidiabetic agents, oral*	Decreased antidiabetic effect.
Cyclosporine	Increased risk of kidney damage.
Insulin	Decreased insulin effect.

POSSIBLE INTERACTION WITH OTHER SUBSTANCES

INTERACTS WITH	COMBINED EFFECT
Alcohol:	Excessive nervous system depression. Avoid.
Beverages: Caffeine.	Rapid, irregular heartbeat. Avoid.
Cocaine:	May interfere with expected action of danazol. Avoid.
Foods:	None expected.
Marijuana:	May interfere with expected action of danazol. Avoid.
Tobacco:	Rapid, irregular heartbeat. Avoid. Increased leg cramps.

DANTROLENE

BRAND NAMES

Dantrium

BASIC INFORMATION

Habit forming? No
Prescription needed? Yes
Available as generic? Yes
Drug class: Muscle relaxant, antispastic

 ## USES

- Relieves muscle spasticity caused by diseases such as multiple sclerosis, cerebral palsy, stroke.
- Relieves muscle spasticity caused by injury to spinal cord.
- Relieves or prevents excess body temperature brought on by some surgical procedures.

 ## DOSAGE & USAGE INFORMATION

How to take:
Capsule—Swallow with liquid.

When to take:
One to 4 times a day as prescribed for muscle spasticity. For excess body temperature, follow label instructions.

If you forget a dose:
Take as soon as you remember up to 2 hours late. If more than 2 hours, wait for next scheduled dose (don't double this dose).

What drug does:
Acts directly on muscles to prevent excess contractions.

Time lapse before drug works:
1 or more weeks.

Continued next column

 ## OVERDOSE

SYMPTOMS:
Shortness of breath, bloody urine, chest pain, convulsions.
WHAT TO DO:
- Dial 911 (emergency) for medical help or call poison control center 1-800-222-1222 for instructions.
- If person is unconscious, check breathing and pulse. If not breathing, begin mouth-to-mouth rescue breathing. If heart is not beating, begin chest compressions.
- See emergency information on last 3 pages of this book.

Don't take with:
Any other medicine or any dietary supplement without consulting your doctor or pharmacist.

 ## POSSIBLE ADVERSE REACTIONS OR SIDE EFFECTS

SYMPTOMS	WHAT TO DO
Life-threatening:	
Seizure.	Seek emergency treatment immediately.
Common:	
Drowsiness, dizziness, weakness.	Discontinue. Call doctor right away.
Infrequent:	
• Rash, hives; black or bloody stools; chest pain; fast heartbeat; backache; blood in urine; painful, swollen feet; chills; fever; shortness of breath.	Discontinue. Call doctor right away.
• Depression, confusion, headache, slurred speech, insomnia, nervousness, diarrhea, blurred vision, difficult swallowing, appetite loss, difficult urination, decreased sexual function in males.	Continue. Call doctor when convenient.
Rare:	
• Jaundice, abdominal cramps, double vision.	Discontinue. Call doctor right away.
• Constipation.	Continue. Call doctor when convenient.

WARNINGS & PRECAUTIONS

Don't take if:
You are allergic to dantrolene or any muscle relaxant or antispastic medication.

Before you start, consult your doctor if:
- You have liver disease.
- You have heart disease.
- You have lung disease (especially emphysema).
- You are over age 35.
- You will have surgery within 2 months, including dental surgery, requiring general or spinal anesthesia.

Over age 60:
Adverse reactions and side effects may be more frequent and severe than in younger persons.

Pregnancy:
Decide with your doctor if drug benefits justify risk to unborn child. Risk category C (see page xviii).

Breast-feeding:
Avoid nursing or discontinue until you finish drug. Consult doctor.

Infants & children:
Use only under close medical supervision.

Prolonged use:
Recommended periodically during prolonged use—Blood counts, G6PD* tests, liver function studies.

Skin & sunlight:
No special problems expected.

Driving, piloting or hazardous work:
Don't drive or pilot aircraft until you learn how medicine affects you. Don't work around dangerous machinery. Don't climb ladders or work in high places. Danger increases if you drink alcohol or take medicine affecting alertness and reflexes, such as antihistamines, tranquilizers, sedatives, pain medicine, narcotics and mind-altering drugs.

Discontinuing:
Don't discontinue without consulting doctor. Dose may require gradual reduction if you have taken drug for a long time. Doses of other drugs may also require adjustment.

Others:
- No problems expected.
- Advise any doctor or dentist whom you consult that you take this medicine.

 POSSIBLE INTERACTION WITH OTHER DRUGS

GENERIC NAME OR DRUG CLASS	COMBINED EFFECT
Central nervous system (CNS) depressants *	Increased risk of side effects.
Estrogens	Increased dantrolene effect.

 POSSIBLE INTERACTION WITH OTHER SUBSTANCES

INTERACTS WITH	COMBINED EFFECT
Alcohol:	Increased sedation, low blood pressure. Avoid.
Beverages:	None expected.
Cocaine:	Increased spasticity. Avoid.
Foods:	None expected.
Marijuana:	Increased spasticity. Avoid.
Tobacco:	May interfere with absorption of medicine.

*See Glossary

DAPSONE

BRAND NAMES

Aczone   DDS
Avlosulfon

BASIC INFORMATION

Habit forming? No
Prescription needed? Yes
Available as generic? Yes
**Drug class: Antibacterial (antileprosy),
sulfone**

USES

- Treatment of dermatitis herpetiformis.
- Treatment of leprosy.
- Prevention and treatment of *Pneumocystis carinii* pneumonia.
- Gel form of the drug treats acne vulgaris.
- Other uses include granuloma annulare, pemphigoid, pyoderma gangrenosum, polychondritis, eye ulcerations, systemic lupus erythematosus.

DOSAGE & USAGE INFORMATION

How to take:
- Tablet—Swallow with liquid or food to lessen stomach irritation.
- Topical gel—Follow directions provided with prescription.

When to take:
Once a day at same time.

If you forget a dose:
Take as soon as you remember up to 2 hours late. If more than 2 hours, wait for next scheduled dose (don't double this dose).

Continued next column

OVERDOSE

SYMPTOMS:
Bleeding, vomiting, seizures, cyanosis, coma.
WHAT TO DO:
- **Dial 911 (emergency) for medical help or call poison control center 1-800-222-1222 for instructions.**
- **If person is unconscious, check breathing and pulse. If not breathing, begin mouth-to-mouth rescue breathing. If heart is not beating, begin chest compressions.**
- **See emergency information on last 3 pages of this book.**

What drug does:
It helps destroy or inhibit the growth of bacteria that causes leprosy. It is unknown how it works to help dermatitis herpetiformis.

Time lapse before drug works:
- 3 years for leprosy.
- 1 to 2 weeks for dermatitis herpetiformis.

Don't take with:
Any other medicine or any dietary supplement without consulting your doctor or pharmacist.

POSSIBLE ADVERSE REACTIONS OR SIDE EFFECTS

SYMPTOMS	WHAT TO DO
Life-threatening:	
In case of overdose, see previous column.	
Common:	
• Rash, abdominal pain.	Discontinue. Call doctor right away.
• Appetite loss.	Continue. Call doctor when convenient.
Infrequent:	
Pale skin.	Discontinue. Call doctor right away.
Rare:	
• Dizziness; mental changes; sore throat; fever; difficult breathing; bleeding; jaundice; numbness, tingling, pain or burning in hands or feet; swelling of feet, hands, eyelids; blurred vision; anemia; peeling skin.	Discontinue. Call doctor right away.
• Headache, itching, nausea, vomiting, blue fingernails or lips. Gel form of the drug may cause skin symptoms (oily, peeling dryness, redness).	Continue. Call doctor when convenient.

WARNINGS & PRECAUTIONS

Don't take if:
* You have G6PD* deficiency.
* You are allergic to furosemide, thiazide diuretics, sulfonylureas, carbonic anhydrase inhibitors, sulfonamides.

Before you start, consult your doctor if:
* You take any other medicine.
* You are anemic.
* You have liver or kidney disease.
* You are of Mediterranean heritage.
* You will have surgery within 2 months, including dental surgery, requiring general or spinal anesthesia.

Over age 60:
Adverse reactions and side effects may be more frequent and severe than in younger persons.

Pregnancy:
Decide with your doctor if drug benefits justify risk to unborn child. Risk category C (see page xviii).

Breast-feeding:
Drug passes into breast milk. Avoid drug or discontinue nursing until you finish medicine. Consult doctor for advice.

Infants & children:
Use under close medical supervision only.

Prolonged use:
* Request liver function studies.
* Talk to your doctor about the need for follow-up medical examinations or laboratory studies to check complete blood counts (white blood cell count, platelet count, red blood cell count, hemoglobin, hematocrit).

Skin & sunlight:
May cause rash or intensify sunburn in areas exposed to sun or ultraviolet light (photosensitivity reaction). Avoid overexposure. Notify doctor if reaction occurs.

Driving, piloting or hazardous work:
Don't drive or pilot aircraft until you learn how medicine affects you. Don't work around dangerous machinery. Don't climb ladders or work in high places. Danger increases if you drink alcohol or take medicine affecting alertness and reflexes, such as antihistamines, tranquilizers, sedatives, pain medicine, narcotics and mind-altering drugs.

Discontinuing:
Don't discontinue without consulting doctor. Dose may require gradual reduction if you have taken drug for a long time. Doses of other drugs may also require adjustment.

Others:
* This drug has been associated with serious, and sometimes fatal blood or liver problems.
* Contact your doctor right away if you develop a rash while using the gel. In rare cases it has been associated with serious, and sometimes fatal, skin reactions.
* For full effect you may need to take dapsone for many months or years.

POSSIBLE INTERACTION WITH OTHER DRUGS

GENERIC NAME OR DRUG CLASS	COMBINED EFFECT
Aminobenzoic acid (PABA)	Decreased dapsone effect. Avoid.
Antivirals, HIV/AIDS*	Increased risk of peripheral neuropathy. Reduced absorption of both drugs.
Dideoxyinosine (ddl)	Decreased dapsone effect.
Hemolytics*	May increase adverse effects on blood cells.
Methotrexate	May increase blood toxicity.
Probenecid	Increased toxicity of dapsone.
Pyrimethamine	May increase blood toxicity.
Rifampin	Decreased effect of dapsone.
Trimethoprim	May increase blood toxicity.

POSSIBLE INTERACTION WITH OTHER SUBSTANCES

INTERACTS WITH	COMBINED EFFECT
Alcohol:	Increased chance of toxicity to liver.
Beverages:	None expected.
Cocaine:	Increased chance of toxicity. Avoid.
Foods:	None expected.
Marijuana:	Increased chance of toxicity. Avoid.
Tobacco:	May interfere with absorption of medicine.

DECONGESTANTS (Ophthalmic)

GENERIC AND BRAND NAMES

ANTAZOLINE
Vasocon-A
NAPHAZOLINE
Ak-Con
Albalon
Albalon Liquifilm
Allerest
Clear Eyes
Comfort Eye Drops
Degest 2
Estivin II
I-Naphline
Murine Plus
Muro's Opcon
Nafazair
Naphcon
Naphcon A
Naphcon Forte
Ocu-Zoline
Vasoclear
Vasoclear A
Vasocon
Vasocon Regular

OXYMETAZOLINE
OcuClear
Visine L.R.
TETRAHYDROZOLINE
Visine

BASIC INFORMATION

Habit forming? No
Prescription needed? Yes, for some
Available as generic? Yes
Drug class: Decongestant (ophthalmic)

USES

Treats eye redness, itching, burning or other irritation due to dust, colds, allergies, rubbing eyes, wearing contact lenses, swimming or eye strain from close work, watching TV, reading.

OVERDOSE

SYMPTOMS:
None expected.
WHAT TO DO:
Not intended for internal use. If child accidentally swallows, call poison control center 1-800-222-1222 for help.

DOSAGE & USAGE INFORMATION

How to use:
Eye drops
* Wash hands.
* Apply pressure to inside corner of eye with middle finger.
* Tilt head backward. Pull lower lid away from eye with index finger of the same hand.
* Drop eye drops into pouch and close eye. Don't blink.
* Keep eyes closed for 1 to 2 minutes.
* Continue pressure for 1 minute after placing medicine in eye.
* Don't touch applicator tip to any surface (including the eye). If you accidentally touch tip, clean with warm water and soap.
* Keep container tightly closed.
* Keep cool, but don't freeze.
* Wash hands immediately after using.

When to use:
As directed. Usually every 3 or 4 hours.

If you forget a dose:
Use as soon as you remember.

What drug does:
Acts on small blood vessels to make them constrict or become smaller.

Time lapse before drug works:
2 to 10 minutes.

Don't use with:
Other eye drops without consulting your doctor.

POSSIBLE ADVERSE REACTIONS OR SIDE EFFECTS

SYMPTOMS	WHAT TO DO
Life-threatening: None expected.	
Common: Increased eye irritation.	Discontinue. Call doctor right away.
Infrequent: None expected.	
Rare: Blurred vision, large pupils, weakness, drowsiness, decreased body temperature, slow heartbeat, dizziness, headache, nervousness, nausea.	Discontinue. Call doctor right away.

DECONGESTANTS (Ophthalmic)

 WARNINGS & PRECAUTIONS

Don't use if:
You are allergic to any decongestant eye drops.

Before you start, consult your doctor if:
- You take antidepressants or maprotiline.
- You have glaucoma, eye disease, infection or injury.
- You have heart disease, high blood pressure, thyroid disease.

Over age 60:
No problems expected.

Pregnancy:
Decide with your doctor if drug benefits justify risk to unborn child. Risk category C (see page xviii).

Breast-feeding:
No problems expected, but check with doctor.

Infants & children:
Don't use.

Prolonged use:
Don't use for more than 3 or 4 days.

Skin & sunlight:
No problems expected.

Driving, piloting or hazardous work:
No problems expected.

Discontinuing:
May not need all the medicine in container. If symptoms disappear, stop using.

Others:
Check with your doctor if eye irritation continues or becomes worse.

 POSSIBLE INTERACTION WITH OTHER DRUGS

GENERIC NAME OR DRUG CLASS	COMBINED EFFECT
Clinically significant interactions with oral or injected medicines unlikely.	

POSSIBLE INTERACTION WITH OTHER SUBSTANCES

INTERACTS WITH	COMBINED EFFECT
Alcohol:	None expected.
Beverages:	None expected.
Cocaine:	None expected.
Foods:	None expected.
Marijuana:	None expected.
Tobacco:	Smoke may increase eye irritation. Avoid.

DEHYDROEPIANDROSTERONE (DHEA)

BRAND NAMES

Numerous brand names are available

BASIC INFORMATION

Habit forming? No
Prescription needed? No
Available as generic? Yes
Drug class: Adrenal steroid

 ## USES

DHEA is a steroid produced in the human body by the adrenal glands (which sit on top of each kidney). DHEA concentration peaks at about age 20 and then decreases progressively with age. Supplements are sold as an antiaging remedy claimed by some to improve energy, strength, and immunity. DHEA is also said to increase muscle and decrease fat. Studies to date do not provide a clear picture of the risks and benefits of DHEA.

 ## DOSAGE & USAGE INFORMATION

How to take:
For tablet or capsule—Follow instructions on the label or consult your doctor or pharmacist. Different brands supply different doses. DHEA, as a product, is marketed as a dietary supplement and is not reviewed by the U.S. Food & Drug Administration (FDA) for effectiveness and safety. The best dosage amounts are unknown. Use with caution.

When to take:
At the same times each day according to label directions.

If you forget a dose:
Follow label instructions for your particular brand of DHEA. Usually you can take a medication as soon as you remember up to 2 hours late. If more than 2 hours, wait for the next scheduled dose (don't double this dose).

Continued next column

 ## OVERDOSE

SYMPTOMS:
It is unknown what symptoms may occur.
WHAT TO DO:
If person takes much larger amount than prescribed, call doctor, poison control center 1-800-222-1222 or hospital emergency room for help.

What drug does:
- Although it is not known whether DHEA itself causes hormonal effects, the body breaks DHEA down into two hormones—estrogen and testosterone. Some people's bodies make large amounts of estrogen and testosterone from DHEA, while others make smaller amounts.
- Hormone supplements may not have the same effects on the body as naturally produced hormones have, because the body processes them differently. Higher doses of supplements may result in higher amounts of hormones in the blood than are healthy.

Time lapse before drug works:
Effectiveness will vary from person to person and will also depend on the reason for taking DHEA, such as for a chronic health problem.

Don't take with:
Any other medicine or any dietary supplement without consulting your doctor or pharmacist.

 ## POSSIBLE ADVERSE REACTIONS OR SIDE EFFECTS

SYMPTOMS	WHAT TO DO
Life-threatening: None expected.	
Common: Unknown.	
Infrequent: In women: acne, hair loss, facial hair growth (hirsutism), deepening of voice (the last two may be irreversible).	Discontinue. Call doctor when convenient.
Rare: Unknown. If symptoms occur that you are concerned about, talk to your doctor or pharmacist. Further research may uncover other side effects.	

DEHYDROEPIANDROSTERONE (DHEA)

 WARNINGS & PRECAUTIONS

Don't use if:
You are allergic to DHEA.

Before you start, consult your doctor if:
* You have any chronic health problem.
* You have a family history of cancer.
* You are allergic to any medication, food or other substance.
* You have or have had prostate, ovarian, breast, cervical or uterine cancer.

Over age 60:
A lower starting dosage may be recommended until a response is determined.

Pregnancy:
Decide with your doctor if any possible benefits of DHEA justify risk to unborn child. Risk category is unknown since DHEA is not regulated by the FDA (see page xviii).

Breast-feeding:
It is unknown if DHEA passes into milk. Avoid it or discontinue nursing until you finish medicine. Consult doctor for advice on maintaining milk supply.

Infants & children:
Not recommended for children.

Prolonged use:
Effects are unknown. More research is needed to determine long-term effects of DHEA use.

Skin & sunlight:
No problems expected.

Driving, piloting or hazardous work:
No problems expected.

Discontinuing:
No problems expected, but effects after long-term use are unknown.

Others:
* Advise any doctor or dentist whom you consult that you take DHEA.
* DHEA is not researched carefully as yet for use in humans. Most research has been performed on animals. Studies are ongoing to find more definite answers about its effect on aging, muscles, and the immune system. Studies in men and women have shown an improvement in the feeling of well being. Studies in AIDS patients and those with multiple sclerosis also have shown improvement in well being, but without an outcome change.
* Researchers are concerned that DHEA supplements may cause high levels of estrogen or testosterone in some people. The body's own testosterone plays a role in prostate cancer and high levels of naturally produced estrogen are suspected of increasing breast cancer risk. The effect of DHEA is unknown.

 POSSIBLE INTERACTION WITH OTHER DRUGS

GENERIC NAME OR DRUG CLASS	COMBINED EFFECT
All medications	Effects are unknown. Talk to your doctor or pharmacist.

POSSIBLE INTERACTION WITH OTHER SUBSTANCES

INTERACTS WITH	COMBINED EFFECT
Alcohol:	Unknown.
Beverages:	None expected.
Cocaine:	Problems not known. Best to avoid.
Foods:	None expected.
Marijuana:	Problems not known. Best to avoid.
Tobacco:	Unknown.

DESMOPRESSIN

BRAND NAMES

DDAVP   **Stimate**

BASIC INFORMATION

Habit forming? No
Prescription needed? Yes
Available as generic? Yes
Drug class: Antidiuretic, antihemorrhagic

USES

- Prevents and controls symptoms associated with central diabetes insipidus.
- The tablet form (not the nasal spray) of the drug is used to treat primary nocturnal enuresis (bedwetting during sleep).

DOSAGE & USAGE INFORMATION

How to take:
- Tablet—Swallow with liquid.
- Nasal spray—Fill the rhinyle (a flexible, calibrated catheter) with a measured dose of the nasal spray. Blow on the other end of the catheter to deposit the solution deep in the nasal cavity.

When to take:
At the same time each day, according to instructions on prescription label. Be sure to restrict fluid intake from 1 hour before to 8 hours after taking drug.

If you forget a dose:
Take as soon as you remember up to 2 hours late. If more than 2 hours, wait for next scheduled dose. Don't double this dose.

What drug does:
Increases water reabsorption in the kidney and decreases urine output.

Time lapse before drug works:
Within 1 hour. Effect may last from 6 to 24 hours.

Don't take with:
Any other medicine or any dietary supplement without consulting your doctor or pharmacist.

OVERDOSE

SYMPTOMS:
Confusion, coma, seizures.
WHAT TO DO:
Overdose unlikely to threaten life. If person uses much larger amount than prescribed or if accidentally swallowed, call doctor or poison control center 1-800-222-1222 for help.

POSSIBLE ADVERSE REACTIONS OR SIDE EFFECTS

SYMPTOMS	WHAT TO DO
Life-threatening: None expected.	
Common: None expected.	
Infrequent: Flushing or redness of skin, headache, nausea, nasal congestion.	Continue. Call doctor when convenient.
Rare: Water intoxication—confusion, drowsiness, headache, seizures, rapid weight gain, decreased urination (very rare); low sodium level in the body (symptoms include nausea, vomiting, muscle cramps, fatigue, weakness).	Discontinue. Seek emergency treatment.

WARNINGS & PRECAUTIONS

Don't take if:
You or your child is allergic to desmopressin.

Before you start, consult your doctor if:
- You have allergic rhinitis.
- You have nasal congestion.
- You have a cold or other upper respiratory infection or are dehydrated.
- You have heart disease or high blood pressure.
- You have a history of hyponatremia, which is low sodium (salt) levels in the body.
- You have polydipsia (excessive or abnormal thirstiness).
- You have cystic fibrosis.

Over age 60:
Increased risk of water intoxication.

Pregnancy:
No proven harm to unborn child, but avoid if possible. Consult doctor. Risk category B (see page xviii).

Breast-feeding:
Drug passes into milk. Avoid drug or discontinue nursing until you finish medicine. Consult doctor for advice on maintaining milk supply.

Infants & children:
More sensitive to effect. Use only under close medical supervision.

Prolonged use:
May require increasing dosage for same effect.

Skin & sunlight:
No special problems expected.

Driving, piloting or hazardous work:
Don't drive or pilot aircraft until you learn how medicine affects you. Don't work around dangerous machinery. Don't climb ladders or work in high places. Danger increases if you drink alcohol or take medicine affecting alertness and reflexes.

Discontinuing:
No special problems expected.

Others:
- Advise any doctor or dentist whom you consult that you take this medicine.
- Be sure to carefully follow all instructions for use of intranasal desmopressin.
- Consult doctor if the amount of water the patient is drinking changes.
- Treatment with desmopressin tablets for primary nocturnal enuresis should be stopped during illnesses with symptoms of fever, recurrent vomiting, or diarrhea that may lead to fluid and/or electrolyte imbalance.
- If sodium levels fall too much causing hyponatremia, the patient could have seizures and in extreme cases, may die.

- The drug should be used cautiously in patients who may be drinking a lot of fluids (such as during hot weather or when doing vigorous exercising) due to a higher risk of hyponatremia.

POSSIBLE INTERACTION WITH OTHER DRUGS

GENERIC NAME OR DRUG CLASS	COMBINED EFFECT
Antidepressants, tricyclic (TCA)*	Increased risk of thirstiness which may lead to drinking excess fluids.
Carbamazepine	May increase desmopressin effect.
Chlorpropamide	May increase desmopressin effect.
Clofibrate	May increase desmopressin effect.
Demeclocycline	May decrease desmopressin effect.
Lithium	May decrease desmopressin effect.
Norepinephrine	May decrease desmopressin effect.
Selective serotonin reuptake inhibitors (SSRIs)	Increased risk of thirstiness which may lead to drinking excess fluids.

POSSIBLE INTERACTION WITH OTHER SUBSTANCES

INTERACTS WITH	COMBINED EFFECT
Alcohol:	May decrease desmopressin effect.
Beverages: Caffeine drinks.	May decrease desmopressin effect.
Cocaine:	May decrease desmopressin effect.
Foods:	None expected.
Marijuana:	May decrease desmopressin effect.
Tobacco:	May decrease desmopressin effect.

*See Glossary

DEXTROMETHORPHAN

BRAND NAMES

See full list of brand names in the *Generic and Brand Name Directory*, page 883.

BASIC INFORMATION

Habit forming? No
Prescription needed? No
Available as generic? Yes
Drug class: Cough suppressant, antitussive

 ## USES

Suppresses cough associated with allergies or infections such as colds, bronchitis, flu and lung disorders. Used in many cough, cold and allergy combination medicines.

 ## DOSAGE & USAGE INFORMATION

How to take:
* Chewable tablet—Chew well, then swallow.
* Oral suspension, lozenge or syrup—Take as directed on label.
* Thin strip—Allow strips to dissolve on the tongue. Water or other fluid is not needed.
* Capsule—Swallow with liquid.

When to take:
As needed, no more often than every 4 hours or as directed on label.

If you forget a dose:
Take as soon as you remember. If it is almost time for the next dose, wait for the next scheduled dose (don't double this dose).

What drug does:
Reduces sensitivity of brain's cough control center, suppressing urge to cough.

Continued next column

 ## OVERDOSE

SYMPTOMS:
Euphoria, overactivity, sense of intoxication, hallucinations, lack of coordination, stagger, stupor, shallow breathing.
WHAT TO DO:
* **Dial 911 (emergency) for medical help or call poison control center 1-800-222-1222 for instructions.**
* **See emergency information on last 3 pages of this book.**

Time lapse before drug works:
15 to 30 minutes.

Don't take with:
Any other medicine or any dietary supplement without consulting your doctor or pharmacist.

 ## POSSIBLE ADVERSE REACTIONS OR SIDE EFFECTS

SYMPTOMS	WHAT TO DO
Life-threatening: None expected.	
Common: None expected.	
Infrequent: Mild dizziness or drowsiness, nausea or vomiting, stomach cramps, constipation, headache.	Discontinue. Call doctor if symptoms persist.
Rare: None expected.	

WARNINGS & PRECAUTIONS

Don't take if:
You are allergic to dextromethorphan.

Before you start, consult your doctor if:
* You have asthma attacks.
* You have impaired liver function.

Over age 60:
Adverse reactions and side effects may be more frequent and severe than in younger persons. You may require smaller doses for shorter periods of time.

Pregnancy:
Decide with your doctor if drug benefits justify risk to unborn child. Risk category C (see page xviii).

Breast-feeding:
No proven problems. Consult doctor.

Infants & children:
Read the label on the product to see if it is approved for your child's age. Always follow the directions on product's label about how to use. If unsure, ask your doctor or pharmacist.

Prolonged use:
No problems expected.

Skin & sunlight:
No problems expected.

Driving, piloting or hazardous work:
Don't drive or pilot aircraft until you learn how medicine affects you. Don't work around dangerous machinery. Don't climb ladders or work in high places. Danger increases if you drink alcohol or take medicine affecting alertness and reflexes, such as antihistamines, tranquilizers, sedatives, pain medicine, narcotics and mind-altering drugs.

Discontinuing:
May be unnecessary to finish medicine. Follow doctor's instructions.

Others:
* If cough persists or if you cough blood or brown-yellow, thick mucus, call your doctor.
* Excessive use may lead to functional dependence.

POSSIBLE INTERACTION WITH OTHER DRUGS

GENERIC NAME OR DRUG CLASS	COMBINED EFFECT
Doxepin (topical)	Increased risk of toxicity of both drugs.
Memantine	May lead to adverse effects of either drug.
Monoamine oxidase (MAO) inhibitors*	Disorientation, high fever, drop in blood pressure and loss of consciousness.
Sedatives* and other central nervous system (CNS) depressants*	Increased sedative effect of both drugs.

POSSIBLE INTERACTION WITH OTHER SUBSTANCES

INTERACTS WITH	COMBINED EFFECT
Alcohol:	None expected.
Beverages: Grapefruit juice.	Risk of toxicity. Avoid.
Cocaine:	Decreased dextromethorphan effect. Avoid.
Foods:	None expected.
Marijuana:	None expected.
Tobacco:	Smoking increases mucus in lungs. Avoid.

*See Glossary

DICLOFENAC (Topical)

BRAND NAMES

Flector Patch   Voltaren Gel

BASIC INFORMATION

Habit forming? No
Prescription needed? Yes
Available as generic? No
Drug class: Nonsteroidal anti-inflammatory
    drug (NSAID), topical

 USES

- Topical gel is used for joint pain in the hands, wrists, elbows, knees, ankles or feet caused by osteoarthritis.
- Patch is used to treat pain due to minor strains, sprains and bruises.
- Both may be used for treatment of other disorders as determined by your doctor.
- A brand named Solaraze is used to treat actinic keratoses. It is not covered in this topic.

 DOSAGE & USAGE INFORMATION

How to use:
- Gel—Follow instructions provided with the prescription. The gel comes with dosing cards that show you how much to use for a 2-gram- or a 4-gram dose. Do not use more than 4 times a day on a single joint. Do not wear gloves for at least 10 minutes after applying gel to the hands. Wait at least 10 minutes before dressing. Do not bathe or shower for at least 1 hour after application. Don't use drug on wounded or sore skin. Don't cover treated area with bandage.
- Patch—Apply to most painful area twice daily. Wash hands after applying patch. Do not wear patch in bath or shower.
- Both gel and patch—Do not apply to wounded or broken skin. Follow product instructions for proper disposal of gel dose cards and patches.

When to take:
Follow your doctor's or label's instructions.

Continued next column

 OVERDOSE

SYMPTOMS:
None expected.
WHAT TO DO:
If person uses much larger amount than prescribed or if accidentally swallowed, call doctor or poison control center 1-800-222-1222 for help.

If you forget a dose:
Apply as soon as you remember. If it is almost time for next treatment, wait and apply at regular time (don't double this dose).

What drug does:
It is applied to and absorbed by the affected joint. It works by reducing certain hormones that cause inflammation and pain in the body.

Time lapse before drug works:
It may take several weeks or more of treatment to determine full benefit of the drug.

Don't take with:
- Any other medicine or diet supplement without consulting your doctor or pharmacist.
- Other skin products (cosmetics, sunscreen, lotions, insect repellant or other topical drugs) not prescribed by your doctor.

 POSSIBLE ADVERSE REACTIONS OR SIDE EFFECTS

SYMPTOMS	WHAT TO DO
Life-threatening:	
Rare allergic reaction if too much absorbed by body (hives; difficulty breathing; swelling of face, lips, tongue, throat).	Seek emergency treatment immediately.
Common:	
Skin reaction where gel or patch is applied.	Continue. Call doctor when convenient.
Infrequent:	
None expected.	
Rare:	
These side effects may occur if drug is absorbed into blood-stream: chest pain, shortness of breath, weakness, slurred speech, vision changes loss of balance, stool changes (black, bloody, tarry or clay-color), vomiting blood or what looks like coffee grounds, swelling, rapid weight gain, change in urination, dark urine, nausea, stomach pain, appetite loss, yellow skin or eyes, sore throat and headache, severe skin rash (blistering, red, peeling), bruising, severe tingling, numbness, fever, muscle weakness, any skin rash.	Discontinue. Call doctor right away.

DICLOFENAC (Topical)

WARNINGS & PRECAUTIONS

Don't take if:
You are allergic to diclofenac or have had an allergic reaction after taking aspirin or any non-steroidal anti-inflammatory drug (NSAID).

Before you start, consult your doctor if:
* You have had or will have heart bypass surgery.
* You have a history of asthma.
* You have a history of stomach ulcer or gastrointestinal bleeding.
* You have kidney or liver disease.
* You have high blood pressure, congestive heart failure or other heart or blood vessel disorder.

Over age 60:
Adverse reactions and side effects may be more frequent and severe than in younger persons.

Pregnancy:
Decide with your doctor if drug benefits justify risk to unborn child. Risk category C (see page xviii).

Breast-feeding:
Drug may be absorbed into body and pass into breast milk. Consult doctor.

Infants & children:
Not approved for children under age 18.

Prolonged use:
* Talk to your doctor about the need for follow-up medical exams and/or blood tests and liver and kidney function studies.
* Long-term continuous use may increase the risk of heart attack or stroke. Consult doctor.

Skin & sunlight:
Avoid exposure of treated skin areas to sunlight or artificial UV rays (sunlamps or tanning beds).

Driving, piloting or hazardous work:
No special problems expected.

Discontinuing:
No special problems expected.

Others:
* Though rare, the drug may be absorbed into your bloodstream and increase the risk of life-threatening heart or circulation problems, including heart attack or stroke. There is also increased risk of serious gastrointestinal problems (e.g., bleeding, ulcers and perforation of the stomach or intestines) which may be fatal.
* Advise any doctor or dentist whom you consult that you use this medicine.
* Avoid getting the drug in your mouth or eyes. If it does get into these areas, rinse with water.

* Do not expose treated areas to heat from a hot tub, heating pad, sauna, or heated water bed. Heat can increase the amount of drug absorbed through the skin and may cause adverse effects.

POSSIBLE INTERACTION WITH OTHER DRUGS

GENERIC NAME OR DRUG CLASS	COMBINED EFFECT
Angiotensin-converting enzyme (ACE) inhibitors*	May decrease ACE inhibitor effect.
Anticoagulants*	May increase risk of internal bleeding.
Anti-inflammatory drugs, nonsteroidal (NSAIDs)* oral	May increase risk of side effects.
Aspirin	May increase risk of side effects.
Cyclosporine	May increase effect of cyclosporine.
Diuretics*	May decrease effect of diuretic.
Lithium	May increase effect of lithium.
Methotrexate	May increase effect of methotrexate.
Topical skin products	Unknown effect. Consult doctor

POSSIBLE INTERACTION WITH OTHER SUBSTANCES

INTERACTS WITH	COMBINED EFFECT
Alcohol:	May increase risk of side effects.
Beverages:	None expected.
Cocaine:	Unknown effect. Avoid.
Foods:	None expected.
Marijuana:	Unknown effect. Avoid.
Tobacco:	May increase risk of side effects.

*See Glossary

DICYCLOMINE

BRAND NAMES

See full list of brand names in the *Generic and Brand Name Directory*, page 885.

BASIC INFORMATION

Habit forming? No
Prescription needed? Yes
Available as generic? Yes
Drug class: Antispasmodic, anticholinergic

 USES

* Reduces spasms of digestive system, bladder and urethra.
* Treats irritable bowel syndrome.

 DOSAGE & USAGE INFORMATION

How to take:
Tablet, syrup or capsule—Swallow with liquid or food to lessen stomach irritation.

When to take:
30 minutes before meals (unless directed otherwise by doctor).

If you forget a dose:
Take as soon as you remember up to 2 hours late. If more than 2 hours, wait for next scheduled dose (don't double this dose).

What drug does:
Blocks nerve impulses at parasympathetic nerve endings, preventing muscle contractions and gland secretions of organs involved.

Time lapse before drug works:
15 to 30 minutes.

Don't take with:
Any other medicine or any dietary supplement without consulting your doctor or pharmacist.

 OVERDOSE

SYMPTOMS:
Dilated pupils, blurred vision, rapid pulse and breathing, dizziness, fever, hallucinations, confusion, slurred speech, agitation, flushed face, convulsions, coma.
WHAT TO DO:
* **Dial 911 (emergency) for medical help or call poison control center 1-800-222-1222 for instructions.**
* **See emergency information on last 3 pages of this book.**

 POSSIBLE ADVERSE REACTIONS OR SIDE EFFECTS

SYMPTOMS	WHAT TO DO
Life-threatening:	
Hives, rash, intense itching, faintness soon after a dose (anaphylaxis).	Seek emergency treatment immediately.
Common:	
• Confusion, delirium, rapid heartbeat.	Discontinue. Call doctor right away.
• Nausea, vomiting.	Discontinue. Call doctor when convenient.
• Constipation, loss of taste, decreased sweating.	Continue. Tell doctor at next visit.
• Dry ears, nose, throat, mouth.	No action necessary.
Infrequent:	
• Headache, difficult urination, nasal congestion, altered taste.	Continue. Call doctor when convenient.
• Lightheadedness.	Discontinue. Call doctor right away.
Rare:	
Rash or hives, eye pain, blurred vision.	Discontinue. Call doctor right away.

 WARNINGS & PRECAUTIONS

Don't take if:
* You are allergic to any anticholinergic.
* You have trouble with stomach bloating.
* You have difficulty emptying your bladder completely.
* You have narrow-angle glaucoma.
* You have severe ulcerative colitis.

Before you start, consult your doctor if:
* You have open-angle glaucoma.
* You have angina, chronic bronchitis or asthma.
* You have hiatal hernia, liver disease, kidney or thyroid disease, enlarged prostate, myasthenia gravis, peptic ulcer.
* You will have surgery within 2 months, including dental surgery, requiring general or spinal anesthesia.

Over age 60:
Adverse reactions and side effects may be more frequent and severe than in younger persons.

Pregnancy:
Decide with your doctor whether drug benefits justify risk to unborn child. Risk category C (see page xviii).

Breast-feeding:
Drug passes into milk and decreases milk flow. Avoid drug or discontinue nursing until you finish medicine. Consult doctor for advice on maintaining milk supply.

Infants & children:
Use only under medical supervision.

Prolonged use:
Chronic constipation, possible fecal impaction. Consult doctor immediately.

Skin & sunlight:
No problems expected.

Driving, piloting or hazardous work:
Use disqualifies you for piloting aircraft. Otherwise, no problems expected.

Discontinuing:
May be unnecessary to finish medicine. Follow doctor's instructions.

Others:
Advise any doctor or dentist whom you consult that you take this medicine.

 POSSIBLE INTERACTION WITH OTHER DRUGS

GENERIC NAME OR DRUG CLASS	COMBINED EFFECT
Adrenocorticoids, systemic	Possible glaucoma.
Amantadine	Increased dicyclomine effect.
Antacids*	Decreased dicyclomine effect.
Anticholinergics, other*	Increased dicyclomine effect.
Antidepressants, tricyclic*	Increased dicyclomine effect. Increased sedation.
Antidiarrheals*	Decreased dicyclomine effect.
Antihistamines*	Increased dicyclomine effect.
Attapulgite	Decreased dicyclomine effect.
Buclizine	Increased dicyclomine effect.
Digitalis	Possible decreased absorption of digitalis.
Haloperidol	Increased internal eye pressure.
Ketoconazole	Decreased ketoconazole effect.
Meperidine	Increased dicyclomine effect.
Methylphenidate	Increased dicyclomine effect.
Monoamine oxidase (MAO) inhibitors*	Increased dicyclomine effect.
Nitrates*	Increased internal eye pressure.
Nizatidine	Increased nizatidine effect.
Orphenadrine	Increased dicyclomine effect.
Phenothiazines*	Increased dicyclomine effect.
Pilocarpine	Loss of pilocarpine effect in glaucoma treatment.
Potassium supplements*	Possible intestinal ulcers with oral potassium tablets.
Quinidine	Increased dicyclomine effect.
Sedatives* or central nervous system (CNS) depressants*	Increased sedative effect of both drugs.
Vitamin C	Decreased dicyclomine effect. Avoid large doses of vitamin C.

 POSSIBLE INTERACTION WITH OTHER SUBSTANCES

INTERACTS WITH	COMBINED EFFECT
Alcohol:	None expected.
Beverages:	None expected.
Cocaine:	Excessively rapid heartbeat. Avoid.
Foods:	None expected.
Marijuana:	Drowsiness and dry mouth.
Tobacco:	None expected.

*See Glossary

DIFENOXIN & ATROPINE

BRAND NAMES

Motofen

BASIC INFORMATION

Habit forming? Yes
Prescription needed? Yes
Available as generic? No
Drug class: Antidiarrheal

 USES

- Reduces spasms of digestive system.
- Treats severe diarrhea.

 DOSAGE & USAGE INFORMATION

How to take:
Tablet—Swallow with liquid or food to lessen stomach irritation.

When to take:
After each loose stool or every 3 to 4 hours. No more than 5 tablets in 12 hours.

If you forget a dose:
Take as soon as you remember. Don't double this dose.

What drug does:
- Blocks nerve impulses at parasympathetic nerve endings, preventing muscle contractions and gland secretions of organs involved.
- Acts on brain to decrease spasm of smooth muscle.

Time lapse before drug works:
40 to 60 minutes.

Continued next column

 OVERDOSE

SYMPTOMS:
Dilated pupils, rapid pulse and breathing, dizziness, fever, hallucinations, confusion, slurred speech, agitation, flushed face, convulsions, coma.
WHAT TO DO:
- **Dial 911 (emergency) for medical help or call poison control center 1-800-222-1222 for instructions.**
- **See emergency information on last 3 pages of this book.**

Don't take with:
Any medicine that will decrease mental alertness or reflexes, such as alcohol, other mind-altering drugs, cough/cold medicines, antihistamines, allergy medicine, sedatives, tranquilizers (sleeping pills or "downers") barbiturates, seizure medicine, narcotics, other prescription medicines for pain, muscle relaxants, anesthetics.

 POSSIBLE ADVERSE REACTIONS OR SIDE EFFECTS

SYMPTOMS	WHAT TO DO
Life-threatening: Shortness of breath, agitation, nervousness.	Discontinue. Seek emergency treatment.
Common: Dizziness, drowsiness.	Continue. Call doctor when convenient.
Infrequent: • Bloating; constipation; appetite loss; abdominal pain; blurred vision; warm, flushed skin; fast heartbeat; dry mouth.	Discontinue. Call doctor right away.
• Frequent urination, lightheadedness, dry skin, headache, insomnia.	Continue. Call doctor when convenient.
Rare: Weakness, confusion, fever.	Continue. Call doctor when convenient.

 WARNINGS & PRECAUTIONS

Don't take if:
- You are allergic to any anticholinergic.
- You have trouble with stomach bloating, difficulty emptying your bladder completely, narrow-angle glaucoma, severe ulcerative colitis.
- You are dehydrated.

Before you start, consult your doctor if:
- You have open-angle glaucoma, angina, chronic bronchitis, asthma, liver disease, hiatal hernia, enlarged prostate, myasthenia gravis, peptic ulcer.
- You will have surgery within 2 months, including dental surgery, requiring general or spinal anesthesia.

Over age 60:
Adverse reactions and side effects may be more frequent and severe than in younger persons.

Pregnancy:
Decide with your doctor whether drug benefits justify risk to unborn child. Risk category C (see page xviii).

Breast-feeding:
Drug passes into milk. Avoid drug or discontinue nursing until you finish medicine. Consult doctor for advice on maintaining milk supply.

Infants & children:
Use only under medical supervision.

Prolonged use:
* Chronic constipation, possible fecal impaction. Consult doctor immediately.
* Talk to your doctor about the need for follow-up medical examinations or laboratory studies to check liver function.

Skin & sunlight:
No problems expected.

Driving, piloting or hazardous work:
Use disqualifies you for piloting aircraft. Don't drive until you learn how medicine affects you. Don't work around dangerous machinery. Don't climb ladders or work in high places. Danger increases if you drink alcohol or take medicine affecting alertness and reflexes, such as antihistamines, tranquilizers, sedatives, pain medicine, narcotics and mind-altering drugs.

Discontinuing:
May be unnecessary to finish medicine. Follow doctor's instructions.

Others:
Atropine included at doses below therapeutic level to prevent abuse.

POSSIBLE INTERACTION WITH OTHER DRUGS

GENERIC NAME OR DRUG CLASS	COMBINED EFFECT
Addictive substances (narcotics,* others)	Increased chance of abuse.
Amantadine	Increased atropine effect.
Anticholinergics, other*	Increased atropine effect.
Antidepressants, tricyclic (TCA)*	Increased atropine effect. Increased sedation.
Antihistamines*	Increased atropine effect.
Antihypertensives*	Increased sedation.
Clozapine	Toxic effect on the central nervous system.
Cortisone drugs*	Increased internal eye pressure.
Ethinamate	Dangerous increased effects of ethinamate. Avoid combining.
Fluoxetine	Increased depressant effects of both drugs.
Guanfacine	May increase depressant effects of either drug.
Haloperidol	Increased internal eye pressure.
Leucovorin	High alcohol content of leucovorin may cause adverse effects.
Meperidine	Increased atropine effect.
Methylphenidate	Increased atropine effect.
Methyprylon	Increased sedative effect, perhaps to dangerous level. Avoid.
Monoamine oxidase (MAO) inhibitors*	Increased atropine effect.
Nabilone	Greater depression of central nervous system.
Naltrexone	Triggers withdrawal symptoms.
Narcotics*	Increased sedation. Avoid.

Continued on page 915

POSSIBLE INTERACTION WITH OTHER SUBSTANCES

INTERACTS WITH	COMBINED EFFECT
Alcohol:	Increased sedation. Avoid.
Beverages:	None expected.
Cocaine:	Excessively rapid heartbeat. Avoid.
Foods:	None expected.
Marijuana:	Drowsiness and dry mouth.
Tobacco:	May increase diarrhea. Avoid.

*See Glossary

DIGITALIS PREPARATIONS
(Digitalis Glycosides)

GENERIC AND BRAND NAMES

DIGITOXIN
Crystodigin

DIGOXIN
Lanoxicaps
Lanoxin
Novodigoxin

BASIC INFORMATION

Habit forming? No
Prescription needed? Yes
Available as generic? Yes
Drug class: Digitalis preparation

 USES

- Strengthens weak heart muscle contractions to prevent congestive heart failure.
- Corrects irregular heartbeat.

 DOSAGE & USAGE INFORMATION

How to take:
- Tablet or capsule—Swallow with liquid. If you can't swallow whole, crumble tablet or open capsule and take with liquid or food.
- Liquid—Dilute dose in beverage before swallowing.

When to take:
At the same time each day.

If you forget a dose:
Take as soon as you remember up to 12 hours late. If more than 12 hours, wait for next scheduled dose (don't double this dose).

What drug does:
- Strengthens heart muscle contraction.
- Delays nerve impulses to heart.

Time lapse before drug works:
May require regular use for a week or more.

Continued next column

 OVERDOSE

SYMPTOMS:
Nausea, vomiting, diarrhea, vision disturbances, halos around lights, fatigue, irregular heartbeat, confusion, hallucinations, convulsions.
WHAT TO DO:
- **Dial 911 (emergency) for medical help or call poison control center 1-800-222-1222 for instructions.**
- **See emergency information on last 3 pages of this book.**

Don't take with:
Any other medicine or any dietary supplement without consulting your doctor or pharmacist.

 POSSIBLE ADVERSE REACTIONS OR SIDE EFFECTS

SYMPTOMS	WHAT TO DO
Life-threatening:	
In case of overdose, see previous column.	
Common:	
Appetite loss, diarrhea.	Continue. Call doctor when convenient.
Infrequent:	
Extreme drowsiness, lethargy, disorientation, headache, fainting.	Discontinue. Call doctor right away.
Rare:	
• Rash, hives, cardiac arrhythmias, hallucinations, psychosis.	Discontinue. Call doctor right away.
• Double or yellow-green vision; enlarged, sensitive male breasts; tiredness; weakness; depression; decreased sex drive.	Continue. Call doctor when convenient.

 WARNINGS & PRECAUTIONS

Don't take if:
- You are allergic to any digitalis preparation.
- Your heartbeat is slower than 50 beats per minute.

Before you start, consult your doctor if:
- You have taken another digitalis preparation in past 2 weeks.
- You have taken a diuretic within 2 weeks.
- You have liver or kidney disease.
- You have a thyroid disorder.
- You will have surgery within 2 months, including dental surgery, requiring general or spinal anesthesia.

Over age 60:
Adverse reactions and side effects may be more frequent and severe than in younger persons.

Pregnancy:
Decide with your doctor if drug benefits justify risk to unborn child. Risk category C (see page xviii).

Breast-feeding:
Drug filters into milk. May harm child. Avoid.

Infants & children:
Use only under medical supervision.

Prolonged use:
Talk to your doctor about the need for follow-up medical examinations or laboratory studies to check ECG*, liver function, kidney function, serum electrolytes.

Skin & sunlight:
No problems expected.

Driving, piloting or hazardous work:
Possible vision disturbances. Otherwise, no problems expected.

Discontinuing:
Don't stop without doctor's advice.

Others:
Some digitalis products contain tartrazine dye. Avoid, especially if you are allergic to aspirin.

POSSIBLE INTERACTION WITH OTHER DRUGS

GENERIC NAME OR DRUG CLASS	COMBINED EFFECT
Adrenocorticoids, systemic	Dangerous potassium depletion. Possible digitalis toxicity.
Amiodarone	Increased digitalis effect.
Amphotericin B	Decreased potassium. Increased toxicity of amphotericin B.
Antacids*	Decreased digitalis effect.
Anticonvulsants, hydantoin*	Increased digitalis effect at first, then decreased.
Anticholinergics*	Possible increased digitalis effect.
Attapulgite	May decrease effectiveness of digitalis.
Beta-adrenergic blocking agents*	Increased digitalis effect.
Beta-agonists*	Increased risk of heartbeat irregularity.
Calcium supplements*	Decreased digitalis effects.
Carteolol	Can either increase or decrease heart rate. Improves irregular heartbeat.
Cholestyramine	Decreased digitalis effect.
Colestipol	Decreased digitalis effect.

Dextrothyroxine	Decreased digitalis effect.
Disopyramide	Possible decreased digitalis effect.
Diuretics*	Excessive potassium loss that may cause irregular heartbeat.
DPP-4 inhibitors	Digoxin dosage may need to be adjusted.
Ephedrine	Disturbed heart rhythm. Avoid.
Epinephrine	Disturbed heart rhythm. Avoid.
Erythromycins*	May increase digitalis absorption.
Flecainide	May increase digitalis blood level.
Fluoxetine	Confusion, agitation, convulsions and high blood pressure. Avoid combining.
Hydroxychloroquine	Possible increased digitalis toxicity.
Itraconazole	Possible toxic levels of digitalis.
Laxatives*	Decreased digitalis effect.
Metformin	Increased metformin effect.

Continued on page 915

POSSIBLE INTERACTION WITH OTHER SUBSTANCES

INTERACTS WITH	COMBINED EFFECT
Alcohol:	None expected.
Beverages: Caffeine drinks.	Irregular heartbeat. Avoid.
Cocaine:	Irregular heartbeat. Avoid.
Foods: Prune juice, bran cereals, foods high in fiber.	Decreased digitalis effect.
Marijuana:	Decreased digitalis effect.
Tobacco:	Irregular heartbeat. Avoid.

*See Glossary

DIPHENIDOL

BRAND NAMES

Vontrol

BASIC INFORMATION

Habit forming? No
Prescription needed? Yes
Available as generic? No
Drug class: Antiemetic, antivertigo

 USES

- Prevents motion sickness.
- Controls nausea and vomiting (do not use during pregnancy).

 DOSAGE & USAGE INFORMATION

How to take:
Tablet—Swallow with liquid or food to lessen stomach irritation. If you can't swallow whole, crumble tablet and chew or take with liquid or food.

When to take:
30 to 60 minutes before traveling.

If you forget a dose:
Take as soon as you remember. Wait 4 hours for next dose.

What drug does:
Reduces sensitivity of nerve endings in inner ear, blocking messages to brain's vomiting center.

Time lapse before drug works:
30 to 60 minutes.

Don't take with:
Any other medicine or any dietary supplement without consulting your doctor or pharmacist.

 OVERDOSE

SYMPTOMS:
Drowsiness, confusion, incoordination, weak pulse, shallow breathing, stupor, coma.
WHAT TO DO:
- **Dial 911 (emergency) for medical help or call poison control center 1-800-222-1222 for instructions.**
- **See emergency information on last 3 pages of this book.**

 POSSIBLE ADVERSE REACTIONS OR SIDE EFFECTS

SYMPTOMS	WHAT TO DO
Life-threatening:	
In case of overdose, see previous column.	
Common:	
Drowsiness.	Continue. Tell doctor at next visit..
Infrequent:	
• Headache, diarrhea or constipation, heartburn.	Continue. Call doctor when convenient.
• Dry mouth, nose or throat; dizziness.	Continue. Tell doctor at next visit.
Rare:	
• Hallucinations, confusion.	Discontinue. Seek emergency treatment.
• Rash or hives, depression, jaundice.	Discontinue. Call doctor right away.
• Restlessness; excitement; insomnia; blurred vision; urgent, painful or difficult urination.	Continue. Call doctor when convenient.
• Appetite loss, nausea, weakness.	Continue. Tell doctor at next visit.

WARNINGS & PRECAUTIONS

Don't take if:
- You have severe kidney disease.
- You are allergic to diphenidol or meclizine.

Before you start, consult your doctor if:
- You have prostate enlargement.
- You have glaucoma.
- You have heart disease.
- You have intestinal obstruction or ulcers in the gastrointestinal tract.
- You have kidney disease.
- You have low blood pressure.
- You will have surgery within 2 months, including dental surgery, requiring general or spinal anesthesia.

Over age 60:
Adverse reactions and side effects may be more frequent and severe than in younger persons.

Pregnancy:
Decide with your doctor whether drug benefits justify risk to unborn child. Risk category C (see page xviii).

Breast-feeding:
Drug passes into milk. Avoid drug or discontinue nursing until you finish medicine. Consult doctor for advice on maintaining milk supply.

Infants & children:
No problems expected.

Prolonged use:
No problems expected.

Skin & sunlight:
No problems expected.

Driving, piloting or hazardous work:
Don't fly aircraft. Don't drive until you learn how medicine affects you. Don't work around dangerous machinery. Don't climb ladders or work in high places. Danger increases if you drink alcohol or take medicine affecting alertness and reflexes, such as antihistamines, tranquilizers, sedatives, pain medicine, narcotics and mind-altering drugs.

Discontinuing:
No problems expected.

Others:
Advise any doctor or dentist whom you consult that you use this medicine.

POSSIBLE INTERACTION WITH OTHER DRUGS

GENERIC NAME OR DRUG CLASS	COMBINED EFFECT
Anticonvulsants*	Increased effect of both drugs.
Antidepressants, tricyclic*	Increased sedative effect of both drugs.
Antihistamines*	Increased sedative effect of both drugs.
Atropine	Increased chance of toxic effect of atropine and atropine-like medicines.
Narcotics*	Increased sedative effect of both drugs.
Sedatives*	Increased sedative effect of both drugs.
Tranquilizers*	Increased sedative effect of both drugs.

POSSIBLE INTERACTION WITH OTHER SUBSTANCES

INTERACTS WITH	COMBINED EFFECT
Alcohol:	Increased sedation. Avoid.
Beverages: Caffeine.	May decrease drowsiness.
Cocaine:	Increased chance of toxic effects of cocaine. Avoid.
Foods:	None expected.
Marijuana:	Increased drowsiness, dry mouth.
Tobacco:	None expected.

DIPHENOXYLATE & ATROPINE

BRAND NAMES

Diphenatol
Lofene
Logen
Lomanate

Lomotil
Lonox
Lo-Trol
Nor-Mil

BASIC INFORMATION

Habit forming? Yes
Prescription needed? Yes
Available as generic? Yes
Drug class: Antidiarrheal

 USES

Relieves diarrhea and intestinal cramps.

 DOSAGE & USAGE INFORMATION

How to take:
- Tablet—Swallow with liquid or food to lessen stomach irritation.
- Drops or liquid—Follow label instructions and use marked dropper.

When to take:
No more often than directed on label.

If you forget a dose:
Take as soon as you remember up to 2 hours late. If more than 2 hours, wait for next scheduled dose (don't double this dose).

What drug does:
Blocks digestive tract's nerve supply, which reduces propelling movements.

Time lapse before drug works:
May require 12 to 24 hours of regular doses to control diarrhea.

Continued next column

 OVERDOSE

SYMPTOMS:
Excitement, constricted pupils, shallow breathing, coma.
WHAT TO DO:
- **Dial 911 (emergency) for medical help or call poison control center 1-800-222-1222 for instructions.**
- **If person is unconscious, check breathing and pulse. If not breathing, begin mouth-to-mouth rescue breathing. If heart is not beating, begin chest compressions.**
- **See emergency information on last 3 pages of this book.**

Don't take with:
Any other medicine or any dietary supplement without consulting your doctor or pharmacist.

 POSSIBLE ADVERSE REACTIONS OR SIDE EFFECTS

SYMPTOMS	WHAT TO DO
Life-threatening: Hives, rash, intense itching, faintness soon after a dose (anaphylaxis).	Seek emergency treatment immediately.
Common: None expected.	
Infrequent: Dry mouth or skin, numbness of hands or feet, dizziness, depression, rash or itch, blurred vision, decreased urination, drowsiness, headache, swollen gums (these symptoms usually mean too much of the drug has been taken).	Discontinue. Call doctor right away.
Rare: Severe stomach pain, nausea, vomiting, constipation, bloating, loss of appetite.	Discontinue. Call doctor right away.

 WARNINGS & PRECAUTIONS

Don't take if:
- You are allergic to diphenoxylate and atropine or any narcotic or anticholinergic.
- You have jaundice.
- You have infectious diarrhea or antibiotic-associated diarrhea.
- Patient is younger than 2.

Before you start, consult your doctor if:
- You have had liver problems.
- You have ulcerative colitis.
- You plan to become pregnant within medication period.
- You have any medical disorder.
- You take any medication, including nonprescription drugs.

Over age 60:
Adverse reactions and side effects may be more frequent and severe than in younger persons.

Pregnancy:
Decide with your doctor if drug benefits justify risk to unborn child. Risk category C (see page xviii).

Breast-feeding:
Drug passes into milk. Avoid drug or discontinue nursing until you finish medicine. Consult doctor for advice on maintaining milk supply.

Infants & children:
Don't give to children under 2 years of age. Use only under doctor's supervision for children older than 2.

Prolonged use:
- May be habit forming if larger doses than recommended are taken for a long period of time.
- Talk to your doctor about the need for follow-up medical examinations or laboratory studies to check liver function.

Skin & sunlight:
No problems expected.

Driving, piloting or hazardous work:
Don't drive or pilot aircraft until you learn how medicine affects you. Don't work around dangerous machinery. Don't climb ladders or work in high places. Danger increases if you drink alcohol or take medicine affecting alertness and reflexes.

Discontinuing:
- May be unnecessary to finish medicine. Follow doctor's instructions.
- After discontinuing, consult doctor if you experience muscle cramps, nausea, vomiting, trembling, stomach cramps or unusual sweating.

Others:
If diarrhea lasts longer than 2 days, discontinue and call doctor.

POSSIBLE INTERACTION WITH OTHER DRUGS

GENERIC NAME OR DRUG CLASS	COMBINED EFFECT
Barbiturates*	Increased effect of both drugs.
Clozapine	Toxic effect on the central nervous system.
Ethinamate	Dangerous increased effects of ethinamate. Avoid combining.
Fluoxetine	Increased depressant effects of both drugs.
Guanfacine	May increase depressant effects of either drug.

Leucovorin	High alcohol content of leucovorin may cause adverse effects.
Methyprylon	Increased sedative effect, perhaps to dangerous level. Avoid.
Monoamine oxidase (MAO) inhibitors*	May increase blood pressure excessively.
Naltrexone	Triggers withdrawal symptoms.
Narcotics*	Increased sedation. Avoid.
Sedatives*	Increased effect of both drugs.
Sertraline	Increased depressive effects of both drugs.
Tranquilizers*	Increased effect of both drugs.

POSSIBLE INTERACTION WITH OTHER SUBSTANCES

INTERACTS WITH	COMBINED EFFECT
Alcohol:	Depressed brain function. Avoid.
Beverages:	None expected.
Cocaine:	Decreased effect of diphenoxylate and atropine.
Foods:	None expected.
Marijuana:	None expected.
Tobacco:	None expected.

DIPYRIDAMOLE

BRAND NAMES

Aggrenox
Apo-Dipyridamole
Dipimol
Dipridacot

Novodipiradol
Persantine
Pyridamole

BASIC INFORMATION

Habit forming? No
Prescription needed?
  U.S.: Yes
  Canada: No
Available as generic? Yes
Drug class: Platelet aggregation inhibitor

 ## USES

* May reduce frequency and intensity of angina attacks.
* May reduce the risk of blood clots after heart surgery.

 ## DOSAGE & USAGE INFORMATION

How to take:
Tablet—Swallow with a full glass of water. If you can't swallow whole, crumble tablet and take with liquid.

When to take:
1 hour before or 2 hours after meals.

If you forget a dose:
Take as soon as you remember up to 2 hours late. If more than 2 hours, wait for next scheduled dose (don't double this dose).

Continued next column

 ## OVERDOSE

SYMPTOMS:
Decreased blood pressure; weak, rapid pulse; cold, clammy skin; collapse.
WHAT TO DO:
* Dial 911 (emergency) for medical help or call poison control center 1-800-222-1222 for instructions.
* If person is unconscious, check breathing and pulse. If not breathing, begin mouth-to-mouth rescue breathing. If heart is not beating, begin chest compressions.
* See emergency information on last 3 pages of this book.

What drug does:
* Probably dilates blood vessels to increase oxygen to heart.
* May reduce platelet clumping, which causes blood clots.

Time lapse before drug works:
3 months of continual use.

Don't take with:
Any other medicine or any dietary supplement without consulting your doctor or pharmacist.

 ## POSSIBLE ADVERSE REACTIONS OR SIDE EFFECTS

SYMPTOMS	WHAT TO DO
Life-threatening:	
In case of overdose, see previous column.	
Common:	
Dizziness.	Continue. Call doctor when convenient.
Infrequent:	
• Fainting, headache.	Discontinue. Call doctor right away.
• Red flush, rash, nausea, vomiting, cramps, weakness.	Continue. Call doctor when convenient.
Rare:	
Chest pain.	Discontinue. Call doctor right away.

WARNINGS & PRECAUTIONS

Don't take if:
• You are allergic to dipyridamole.
• You are recovering from a heart attack.

Before you start, consult your doctor if:
• You have low blood pressure.
• You have liver disease.

Over age 60:
Begin treatment with small doses.

Pregnancy:
No proven harm to unborn child. Avoid if possible. Consult doctor. Risk category B (see page xviii).

Breast-feeding:
No proven problems. Consult doctor.

Infants & children:
Not recommended.

Prolonged use:
Talk to your doctor about the need for follow-up medical examinations or laboratory studies.

Skin & sunlight:
No problems expected.

Driving, piloting or hazardous work:
Avoid if you feel dizzy. Otherwise, no problems expected.

Discontinuing:
Don't discontinue without doctor's advice until you complete prescribed dose, even though symptoms diminish or disappear.

Others:
• Drug increases your ability to be active without angina pain. Avoid excessive physical exertion that might injure heart.
• Advise any doctor or dentist whom you consult that you take this medicine.

POSSIBLE INTERACTION WITH OTHER DRUGS

GENERIC NAME OR DRUG CLASS	COMBINED EFFECT
Anticoagulants, oral*	Increased anti-coagulant effect. Bleeding tendency.
Aspirin and combination drugs containing aspirin	Increased dipyridamole effect. Dose may need adjustment.

POSSIBLE INTERACTION WITH OTHER SUBSTANCES

INTERACTS WITH	COMBINED EFFECT
Alcohol:	May lower blood pressure excessively.
Beverages:	None expected.
Cocaine:	No proven problems.
Foods:	Decreased dipyridamole absorption unless taken 1 hour before eating.
Marijuana:	Daily use— Decreased dipyridamole effect.
Tobacco: Nicotine.	May decrease dipyridamole effect.

DISOPYRAMIDE

BRAND NAMES

Norpace
Norpace CR
Rythmodan
Rythmodan-LA

BASIC INFORMATION

Habit forming? No
Prescription needed? Yes
Available as generic? Yes
Drug class: Antiarrhythmic

 USES

Corrects heart rhythm disorders.

 DOSAGE & USAGE INFORMATION

How to take:
• Extended-release tablet or capsule—Swallow with liquid. Do not crush tablet or open capsule.
• Capsule—Swallow with liquid. If you can't swallow whole, ask your pharmacist to prepare a liquid suspension for your use.

When to take:
At the same times each day.

If you forget a dose:
Take as soon as you remember up to 2 hours late. If more than 2 hours, wait for next scheduled dose (don't double this dose).

What drug does:
Delays nerve impulses to heart to regulate heartbeat.

Time lapse before drug works:
Begins in 30 to 60 minutes. Must use for 5 to 7 days to determine effectiveness.

Continued next column

 OVERDOSE

SYMPTOMS:
Blood-pressure drop, irregular heartbeat, apnea, loss of consciousness.
WHAT TO DO:
• Dial 911 (emergency) for medical help or call poison control center 1-800-222-1222 for instructions.
• If person is unconscious, check breathing and pulse. If not breathing, begin mouth-to-mouth rescue breathing. If heart is not beating, begin chest compressions.
• See emergency information on last 3 pages of this book.

Don't take with:
Any other medicine or any dietary supplement without consulting your doctor or pharmacist.

 POSSIBLE ADVERSE REACTIONS OR SIDE EFFECTS

SYMPTOMS	WHAT TO DO
Life-threatening:	
Hives, rash, intense itching, faintness soon after a dose (anaphylaxis).	Seek emergency treatment immediately.
Common:	
• Hypoglycemia (cold sweats, fast heartbeat, extreme hunger, shakiness and nervousness, anxiety, cool and pale skin, drowsiness, headache).	Discontinue. Call doctor right away.
• Dry mouth, constipation, painful or difficult urination, rapid weight gain, blurred vision.	Continue. Call doctor when convenient.
Infrequent:	
• Dizziness, fainting, confusion, chest pain, nervousness, depression, slow or fast heartbeat.	Discontinue. Call doctor right away.
• Swollen feet.	Continue. Call doctor when convenient.
Rare:	
• Shortness of breath, psychosis.	Discontinue. Seek emergency treatment.
• Rash, sore throat, fever, headache, jaundice, muscle weakness.	Discontinue. Call doctor right away.
• Eye pain, diminished sex drive, numbness or tingling of hands and feet, bleeding tendency.	Continue. Call doctor when convenient.

 WARNINGS & PRECAUTIONS

Don't take if:
• You are allergic to disopyramide or any antiarrhythmic.
• You have second- or third-degree heart block.
• You have heart failure.

Before you start, consult your doctor if:
- You react unfavorably to other antiarrhythmic drugs.
- You have had heart disease.
- You have low blood pressure.
- You have liver disease.
- You have glaucoma.
- You have enlarged prostate.
- You have myasthenia gravis.
- You take digitalis preparations or diuretics.

Over age 60:
- May require reduced dose.
- More likely to have difficulty urinating or be constipated.
- More likely to have blood pressure drop.

Pregnancy:
Decide with your doctor if drug benefits justify risk to unborn child. Risk category C (see page xviii).

Breast-feeding:
Drug passes into milk. Avoid drug or discontinue nursing until you finish medicine. Consult doctor for advice on maintaining milk supply.

Infants & children:
Safety not established. Don't use.

Prolonged use:
Talk to your doctor about the need for follow-up medical examinations or laboratory studies to check liver function, kidney function, ECG*, blood pressure, serum potassium.

Skin & sunlight:
May cause rash or intensify sunburn in areas exposed to sun or ultraviolet light (photosensitivity reaction). Avoid overexposure. Notify doctor if reaction occurs.

Driving, piloting or hazardous work:
Don't drive or pilot aircraft until you learn how medicine affects you. Don't work around dangerous machinery. Don't climb ladders or work in high places. Danger increases if you drink alcohol or take medicine affecting alertness and reflexes, such as antihistamines, tranquilizers, sedatives, pain medicine, narcotics, or mind-altering drugs.

Discontinuing:
Don't discontinue without doctor's advice until you complete prescribed dose, even though symptoms diminish or disappear.

Others:
If new illness, injury or surgery occurs, tell doctors of disopyramide use.

 POSSIBLE INTERACTION WITH OTHER DRUGS

GENERIC NAME OR DRUG CLASS	COMBINED EFFECT
Antiarrhythmics*	May increase effect and toxicity of each drug.
Anticholinergics*	Increased anticholinergic effect.
Anticoagulants, oral*	Possible increased anticoagulant effect.
Antihypertensives*	Increased antihypertensive effect.
Cisapride	Decreased disopyramide effect.
Encainide	Increased effect of toxicity on the heart muscle.
Flecainide	Possible irregular heartbeat.
Nicardipine	May cause dangerously slow, fast or irregular heartbeat.
Nimodipine	May cause dangerous irregular, slow or fast heartbeat.
Phenobarbital	Increased metabolism, decreased disopyramide effect.
Phenytoin	Increased metabolism, decreased disopyramide effect.
Propafenone	Increased effect of both drugs and increased risk of toxicity.
Rifampin	Increased metabolism, decreased disopyramide effect.
Tocainide	Increased likelihood of adverse reactions with either drug.

 POSSIBLE INTERACTION WITH OTHER SUBSTANCES

INTERACTS WITH	COMBINED EFFECT
Alcohol:	Decreased blood pressure and blood sugar. Use caution.
Beverages:	None expected.
Cocaine:	Irregular heartbeat.
Foods:	None expected.
Marijuana:	Unpredictable. May decrease disopyramide effect.
Tobacco:	May decrease disopyramide effect.

*See Glossary

DISULFIRAM

BRAND NAMES

Antabuse

BASIC INFORMATION

Habit forming? No
Prescription needed? Yes
Available as generic? Yes
Drug class: None

USES

Treatment for alcoholism. Will not cure alcoholism, but is a powerful deterrent to drinking.

DOSAGE & USAGE INFORMATION

How to take:
Tablet—Swallow with liquid.

When to take:
Morning or bedtime. Avoid if you have used *any* alcohol, tonics, cough syrups, fermented vinegar, after-shave lotion or backrub solutions within 12 hours.

If you forget a dose:
Take as soon as you remember up to 12 hours late. If more than 12 hours, wait for next scheduled dose (don't double this dose).

What drug does:
In combination with alcohol, produces a metabolic change that causes severe, temporary toxicity.

Time lapse before drug works:
3 to 12 hours.

Continued next column

OVERDOSE

SYMPTOMS:
Memory loss, behavior disturbances, lethargy, confusion and headaches; nausea, vomiting, stomach pain and diarrhea; weakness and unsteady walk; temporary paralysis.
WHAT TO DO:
• **Dial 911 (emergency) for medical help or call poison control center 1-800-222-1222 for instructions.**
• **See emergency information on last 3 pages of this book.**

Don't take with:
• Nonprescription drugs that contain *any* alcohol.
• Any other medicine or any dietary supplement without consulting your doctor or pharmacist.
• Any other central nervous system (CNS) depressant drugs.*

POSSIBLE ADVERSE REACTIONS OR SIDE EFFECTS

SYMPTOMS	WHAT TO DO
Life-threatening:	
In case of overdose, see previous column.	
Common:	
Drowsiness.	Continue. Tell doctor at next visit.
Infrequent:	
• Eye pain, vision changes, abdominal discomfort, throbbing headache, numbness in hands and feet.	Continue. Call doctor when convenient.
• Mood change, decreased sexual ability in men, tiredness.	Continue. Tell doctor at next visit.
• Bad taste in mouth (metal or garlic).	No action necessary.
Rare:	
Rash, jaundice.	Discontinue. Call doctor right away.

WARNINGS & PRECAUTIONS

Don't take if:
• You are allergic to disulfiram (alcohol-disulfiram combination is not an allergic reaction).
• You have used alcohol in any form or amount within 12 hours.
• You have taken paraldehyde within 1 week.
• You have heart disease.

Before you start, consult your doctor if:
• You have allergies.
• You plan to become pregnant within medication period.
• No one has explained to you how disulfiram reacts with alcohol.
• You think you cannot avoid drinking.
• You have diabetes, epilepsy, liver or kidney disease.
• You take other drugs.

328

Over age 60:
Adverse reactions and side effects may be more frequent and severe than in younger persons.

Pregnancy:
Decide with your doctor if drug benefits justify risk to unborn child. Risk category C (see page xviii).

Breast-feeding:
Studies inconclusive. Consult your doctor.

Infants & children:
Not recommended.

Prolonged use:
Periodic blood cell counts and liver function tests recommended if you take this drug a long time.

Skin & sunlight:
No problems expected.

Driving, piloting or hazardous work:
Avoid if you feel drowsy or have vision side effects. Otherwise, no restrictions.

Discontinuing:
Don't discontinue without consulting doctor. Dose may require gradual reduction if you have taken drug for a long time. Doses of other drugs may also require adjustment. Avoid alcohol at least 14 days following last dose.

Others:
- Check all liquids that you take or rub on for presence of alcohol.
- Advise any doctor or dentist whom you consult that you take this medicine.

POSSIBLE INTERACTION WITH OTHER DRUGS

GENERIC NAME OR DRUG CLASS	COMBINED EFFECT
Anticoagulants*	Possible unexplained bleeding.
Anticonvulsants*	Excessive sedation.
Barbiturates*	Excessive sedation.
Central nervous system (CNS) depressants*	Increased depressive effect.
Clozapine	Toxic effect on the central nervous system.
Guanfacine	May increase depressant effects of either drug.
Isoniazid	Unsteady walk and disturbed behavior.

Leucovorin	High alcohol content of leucovorin may cause disulfiram reaction.*
Methyprylon	Increased sedative effect, perhaps to dangerous level. Avoid.
Metronidazole	Disulfiram reaction.*
Nabilone	Greater depression of central nervous system.
Sedatives*	Excessive sedation.
Theophylline	Increased theophylline effect; possibly toxic levels.

POSSIBLE INTERACTION WITH OTHER SUBSTANCES

INTERACTS WITH	COMBINED EFFECT
Alcohol: *Any* form or amount.	Possible life-threatening toxicity. See disulfiram reaction.*
Beverages: Punch or fruit drink that may contain alcohol.	Disulfiram reaction.*
Cocaine:	Increased disulfiram effect.
Foods: Sauces, fermented vinegar, marinades, desserts or other foods prepared with *any* alcohol.	Disulfiram reaction.*
Marijuana:	None expected.
Tobacco:	None expected.

DIURETICS, LOOP

GENERIC AND BRAND NAMES

BUMETANIDE
Bumex
ETHACRYNIC ACID
Edecrin

FUROSEMIDE
Apo-Furosemide
Furoside
Lasix
Lasix Special
Myrosemide
Novosemide
Uritol
TORSEMIDE
Demadex

BASIC INFORMATION

Habit forming? No
Prescription needed? Yes
Available as generic? Yes
Drug class: Diuretic (loop), antihypertensive

 USES

- Lowers high blood pressure.
- Decreases fluid retention.

 DOSAGE & USAGE INFORMATION

How to take:
Tablet or liquid—Swallow with liquid. If you can't swallow tablet whole, crumble tablet and take with liquid or food.

When to take:
- 1 dose a day—Take after breakfast.
- More than 1 dose a day—Take last dose no later than 6 p.m. unless otherwise directed.

If you forget a dose:
- 1 dose a day—Take as soon as you remember up to 12 hours late. If more than 12 hours, wait for next scheduled dose (don't double this dose).

Continued next column

 OVERDOSE

SYMPTOMS:
Weakness, lethargy, dizziness, confusion, nausea, vomiting, leg muscle cramps, thirst, stupor, deep sleep, weak and rapid pulse, cardiac arrest.
WHAT TO DO:
- **Dial 911 (emergency) for medical help or call poison control center 1-800-222-1222 for instructions.**
- **See emergency information on last 3 pages of this book.**

- More than 1 dose a day—Take as soon as you remember up to 2 hours late. If more than 2 hours, wait for next scheduled dose (don't double this dose).

What drug does:
Increases elimination of sodium, potassium and water from body. Decreased body fluid reduces blood pressure.

Time lapse before drug works:
1 hour to increase water loss. Requires 2 to 3 weeks to lower blood pressure.

Don't take with:
- Nonprescription drugs with aspirin.
- Any other medicine or any dietary supplement without consulting your doctor or pharmacist.

 POSSIBLE ADVERSE REACTIONS OR SIDE EFFECTS

SYMPTOMS	WHAT TO DO
Life-threatening:	
In case of overdose, see previous column.	
Common:	
Dizziness.	Continue. Call doctor when convenient.
Infrequent:	
Mood change, fatigue, appetite loss, diarrhea, irregular heartbeat, muscle cramps, low blood pressure, pain in abdomen, weakness.	Discontinue. Call doctor right away.
Rare:	
Rash or hives, yellow vision, ringing in ears, hearing loss, sore throat, fever, dry mouth, thirst, side or stomach pain, nausea, vomiting, unusual bleeding or bruising, joint pain, jaundice, numbness or tingling in hands or feet.	Discontinue. Call doctor right away.

 WARNINGS & PRECAUTIONS

Don't take if:
You are allergic to loop diuretics.

Before you start, consult your doctor if:
- You are taking any other prescription or nonprescription medicine.
- You are allergic to any sulfa drug.
- You have liver or kidney disease.
- You have gout, diabetes or impaired hearing.
- You will have surgery within 2 months, including dental surgery, requiring general or spinal anesthesia.

Over age 60:
Adverse reactions and side effects may be more frequent and severe than in younger persons.

Pregnancy:
Risk factors vary for drugs in this group. See category list on page xviii and consult doctor.

Breast-feeding:
Drug filters into milk. May harm child. Avoid.

Infants & children:
Use only under medical supervision.

Prolonged use:
- Impaired balance of water and salt, with low potassium level in blood and body tissues.
- Possible diabetes.

Skin & sunlight:
One or more drugs in this group may cause rash or intensify sunburn in areas exposed to sun or ultraviolet light (photosensitivity reaction). Avoid overexposure. Notify doctor if reaction occurs.

Driving, piloting or hazardous work:
Avoid if you feel dizzy; otherwise no problems expected.

Discontinuing:
Don't discontinue without doctor's advice until you complete prescribed dose, even though symptoms diminish or disappear.

Others:
Frequent laboratory studies to monitor potassium level in blood recommended. Eat foods rich in potassium or take potassium supplements. Consult doctor.

 POSSIBLE INTERACTION WITH OTHER DRUGS

GENERIC NAME OR DRUG CLASS	COMBINED EFFECT
Adrenocorticoids, systemic	Potassium depletion.
Allopurinol	Decreased allopurinol effect.
Amiodarone	Increased risk of heartbeat irregularity due to low potassium.
Angiotensin-converting enzyme (ACE) inhibitors*	Possible excessive potassium in blood.
Anticoagulants*	Abnormal clotting.
Antidepressants, tricyclic*	Excessive blood pressure drop.
Antidiabetics, oral*	Decreased antidiabetic effect.

Antihypertensives*	Increased anti-hypertensive effect. Dosages may require adjustment.
Anti-inflammatory drugs, nonsteroidal (NSAIDs)*	Decreased diuretic effect.
Antivirals, HIV/AIDS*	Increased risk of pancreatitis with furosemide.
Barbiturates*	Low blood pressure.
Beta-adrenergic blocking agents*	Increased anti-hypertensive effect. Dosages may require adjustment.
Corticosteroids*	Decreased potassium.
Digitalis preparations*	Excessive potassium loss could lead to serious heart rhythm disorders.
Diuretics, other*	Increased diuretic effect.
Hypokalemia-causing medicines*	Increased risk of excessive potassium loss.
Insulin	Decreased insulin effect.
Lithium	Increased lithium toxicity.
Metformin	Increased metformin effect with furosemide.
Narcotics*	Dangerous low blood pressure. Avoid.

Continued on page 916

 POSSIBLE INTERACTION WITH OTHER SUBSTANCES

INTERACTS WITH	COMBINED EFFECT
Alcohol:	Blood pressure drop. Avoid.
Beverages:	None expected.
Cocaine:	Dangerous blood pressure drop. Avoid.
Foods:	None expected.
Marijuana:	Increased thirst and urinary frequency, fainting.
Tobacco:	Decreased furosemide effect.

*See Glossary

DIURETICS, POTASSIUM-SPARING

GENERIC AND BRAND NAMES

AMILORIDE
Midamor
SPIRONOLACTONE
Aldactone
Novospiroton

TRIAMTERENE
Dyrenium

BASIC INFORMATION

Habit forming? No
Prescription needed? Yes
Available as generic? Yes
Drug class: Diuretic, antihypertensive, antihypokalemic

 USES

- Treatment for high blood pressure (hypertension) and congestive heart failure. Decreases fluid retention and prevents potassium loss.
- Treatment for hypokalemia (low potassium), polycystic ovary syndrome and hirsutism in women.

 DOSAGE & USAGE INFORMATION

How to take:
Capsule or tablet—Swallow with liquid. If you can't swallow whole, open capsule or crush tablet and take with liquid or food. May take with meal to lessen stomach irritation.

When to take:
At the same times each day. May interfere with sleep if taken after 6 p.m.

Continued next column

 OVERDOSE

SYMPTOMS:
Rapid, irregular heartbeat; confusion; shortness of breath; nervousness; extreme weakness; stupor; coma.
WHAT TO DO:
- **Dial 911 (emergency) for medical help or call poison control center 1-800-222-1222 for instructions.**
- **If person is unconscious, check breathing and pulse. If not breathing, begin mouth-to-mouth rescue breathing. If heart is not beating, begin chest compressions.**
- **See emergency information on last 3 pages of this book.**

If you forget a dose:
Take as soon as you remember. If it is almost time for the next dose, wait for next scheduled dose (don't double this dose).

What drug does:
- Blocks exchange of certain chemicals in the kidneys so sodium and water are excreted. Conserves potassium.
- In polycystic ovary syndrome and hirsutism, blocks androgen hormones.

Time lapse before drug works:
2 to 4 hours.

Don't take with:
Any other medicine or any dietary supplement without consulting your doctor or pharmacist.

 POSSIBLE ADVERSE REACTIONS OR SIDE EFFECTS

SYMPTOMS	WHAT TO DO
Life-threatening: In case of overdose, see previous column.	
Common: Headache, nausea, appetite loss, vomiting, mild diarrhea.	Continue. Call doctor when convenient.
Infrequent: Dizziness, muscle cramps, dry mouth, decreased sexual drive, constipation.	Continue. Call doctor when convenient.
Rare: Shortness of breath, skin rash or itch (with amiloride); cough or hoarseness, painful urination, back or side pain (with triamterene and spironolactone); potassium changes (confusion, dry mouth, breathing difficulty, irregular heartbeat, unusual tiredness or weakness, mood or mental changes, muscle cramps, tingling in body); red, burning, inflamed feeling of tongue (with triamterene).	Discontinue. Call doctor right away.

 WARNINGS & PRECAUTIONS

Don't take if:
- You are allergic to potassium-sparing diuretics.
- Your serum potassium level is high.

DIURETICS, POTASSIUM-SPARING

Before you start, consult your doctor if:
- You have diabetes.
- You have heart disease, kidney or liver disease or gout.

Over age 60:
Adverse reactions and side effects may be more frequent and severe than in younger persons. More likely to exceed safe potassium blood levels.

Pregnancy:
Avoid if possible. Consult doctor. Risk category B (see page xviii).

Breast-feeding:
Drug may pass into milk. Avoid drug or discontinue nursing until you finish medicine. Consult doctor for advice on maintaining milk supply.

Infants & children:
No special problems expected.

Prolonged use:
Talk to your doctor about the need for follow-up medical examinations or laboratory studies to check blood pressure, kidney function, ECG* and serum electrolytes.

Skin & sunlight:
One or more of these drugs may cause increased sensitivity to sunlight (photosensitivity reaction). Avoid overexposure. If reaction occurs, notify doctor.

Driving, piloting or hazardous work:
Don't drive or pilot aircraft until you learn how medicine affects you. Don't work around dangerous machinery. Don't climb ladders or work in high places. Danger increases if you drink alcohol or take medicine affecting alertness and reflexes.

Discontinuing:
Don't discontinue without doctor's advice until you complete prescribed dose, even though symptoms diminish or disappear.

Others:
- Periodic physical checkups and potassium-level tests recommended.
- Advise any doctor or dentist whom you consult that you take this medicine.
- If you experience an illness with severe vomiting and diarrhea, consult doctor.
- A special diet may be recommended in addition to this medicine. Follow doctor's advice.

 POSSIBLE INTERACTION WITH OTHER DRUGS

GENERIC NAME OR DRUG CLASS	COMBINED EFFECT
Amantadine	Increased effect of amantadine (with triamterene).
Angiotensin-converting enzyme (ACE) inhibitors*	Possible excessive potassium in blood.
Anticoagulants*, oral	Decreased anticoagulant effect.
Antigout drugs*	Decreased antigout effect.
Antihypertensives*	Increased effect of both drugs.
Anti-inflammatory drugs, nonsteroidal (NSAIDs)*	Increased potassium levels.
Cyclosporine	Increased potassium levels.
Digoxin	Increased digoxin effect (with spironolactone).
Diuretics*, other	Increased effect of both drugs.
Dofetilide	Increased risk of heart problems.
Folic acid	Decreased effect of folic acid.
Lithium	Possible lithium toxicity.
Memantine	Increased effect of memantine or triamterene.
Metformin	Increased metformin effect.
Potassium supplements*	Increased potassium levels.

 POSSIBLE INTERACTION WITH OTHER SUBSTANCES

INTERACTS WITH	COMBINED EFFECT
Alcohol:	Increased blood pressure drop. Avoid.
Beverages: Low-salt milk.	Possible excess potassium levels. Low-salt milk has extra potassium.
Cocaine:	Blood pressure rise. Avoid.
Foods: Salt substitutes.	Possible excess potassium levels.
Marijuana:	None expected.
Tobacco:	None expected.

DIURETICS, POTASSIUM-SPARING & HYDROCHLOROTHIAZIDE

GENERIC AND BRAND NAMES

AMILORIDE &
  HYDROCHLORO-
    THIAZIDE
Moduret
Moduretic

SPIRONOLACTONE
  & HYDROCHLORO-
  THIAZIDE
Aldactazide
Spirozide

TRIAMTERENE &
  HYDROCHLORO-
    THIAZIDE
Apo-Triazide
Diazide
Maxzide
Novo-Triamzide

BASIC INFORMATION

Habit forming? No
Prescription needed? Yes
Available as generic? Yes
Drug class: Diuretic, antihypertensive,
  antihypokalemic

 ## USES

- Treats, but does not cure, high blood pressure (hypertension) and congestive heart failure. Decreases fluid retention and prevents potassium loss.
- Treatment for hypokalemia (low potassium).

 ## DOSAGE & USAGE INFORMATION

How to take:
Capsule or tablet—Swallow with liquid. Take with meals or milk if stomach irritation occurs.

When to take:
At the same time or times each day. May interfere with sleep if taken after 6 p.m.

Continued next column

 ## OVERDOSE

SYMPTOMS: Rapid, irregular heartbeat; confusion; shortness of breath; nervousness; extreme weakness.
WHAT TO DO:
- **Dial 911 (emergency) for medical help or call poison control center 1-800-222-1222 for instructions.**
- **If person is unconscious, check breathing and pulse. If not breathing, begin mouth-to-mouth rescue breathing. If heart is not beating, begin chest compressions.**
- **See emergency information on last 3 pages of this book.**

If you forget a dose:
Take as soon as you remember. If it is almost time for the next dose, wait for next scheduled dose (don't double this dose).

What drug does:
This is a combination of 2 diuretics that blocks exchange of certain chemicals in the kidneys so sodium and water are excreted. Conserves potassium.

Time lapse before drug works:
Starts in 2 to 4 hours; several days for full effect.

Don't take with:
Any other medicine or any dietary supplement without consulting your doctor or pharmacist. This includes any nonprescription medicines for colds, coughs, hay fever, sinus problems, appetite control or asthma.

 ## POSSIBLE ADVERSE REACTIONS OR SIDE EFFECTS

SYMPTOMS	WHAT TO DO
Life-threatening: In case of overdose, see previous column.	
Common: Nausea or mild vomiting, appetite loss, stomach cramps, mild diarrhea, constipation (with amiloride).	Continue. Call doctor when convenient.
Infrequent: Dizziness, muscle cramps, headache, skin sensitive to sun, dry mouth, decreased interest in sex. With spironolactone—tender breasts, deepening of voice, menstrual changes, and increased hair growth in females; breast enlargement in males; increased sweating in both sexes.	Continue. Call doctor when convenient.
Rare: Black, tarry or bloody stools; blood in urine; pain or difficulty in urinating; fever or chills; pain in back, side or joints; spots, rash or hives on skin; severe stomach pain; unusual bleeding or bruising; yellow skin or eyes; potassium changes (confusion, dry mouth, breathing difficulty,	Discontinue. Call doctor right away.

irregular heartbeat, unusual tiredness or weakness, mood or mental changes, muscle cramps, tingling in body); red, burning, inflamed feeling of tongue (with triamterene).

WARNINGS & PRECAUTIONS

Don't take if:
- You are allergic to potassium-sparing or thiazide diuretics* or sulfa drugs.*
- Your serum potassium level is high.

Before you start, consult your doctor if:
- You have diabetes or lupus erythematosus.
- You have menstrual problems (in females) or enlarged breast (in males).
- You have heart or blood vessel disease, kidney or liver disease, pancreatitis or gout.

Over age 60:
Adverse reactions and side effects may be more frequent and severe than in younger persons. More likely to exceed safe potassium blood levels.

Pregnancy:
Does not control pregnancy symptoms of swollen hands and feet. Avoid if possible. Consult doctor. Risk category B (see page xviii).

Breast-feeding:
Drug passes into milk. Avoid drug or discontinue nursing until you finish medicine. Consult doctor for advice on maintaining milk supply.

Infants & children:
Unknown effect. Use only with doctor's approval.

Prolonged use:
Talk to your doctor about the need for follow-up medical examinations or laboratory studies to check blood pressure, kidney function, ECG* and serum electrolytes.

Skin & sunlight:
One or more of these drugs may cause increased sensitivity to sunlight (photosensitivity reaction). Avoid overexposure. If reaction occurs, notify doctor.

Driving, piloting or hazardous work:
Don't drive or pilot aircraft until you learn how medicine affects you. Don't work around dangerous machinery. Don't climb ladders or work in high places. Danger increases if you drink alcohol or take medicine affecting alertness and reflexes, such as antihistamines, tranquilizers, sedatives, pain medicine, narcotics and mind-altering drugs.

Discontinuing:
Don't discontinue without doctor's approval, even though symptoms diminish or disappear.

Others:
- Your doctor may prescribe a special diet.
- Advise any doctor or dentist whom you consult that you take this medicine.
- If you experience an illness with severe vomiting or diarrhea, consult doctor.

POSSIBLE INTERACTION WITH OTHER DRUGS

GENERIC NAME OR DRUG CLASS	COMBINED EFFECT
Amantadine	Increased effect of amantadine (with triamterene).
Angiotensin-converting enzyme (ACE) inhibitors*	Possible excessive potassium in blood.
Anticoagulants*, oral	Decreased anticoagulant effect.
Antigout drugs*	Decreased antigout effect.
Antihypertensives*	Increased effect of both drugs.
Anti-inflammatory drugs, nonsteroidal (NSAIDs)*	Increased potassium levels.

Continued on page 916

POSSIBLE INTERACTION WITH OTHER SUBSTANCES

INTERACTS WITH	COMBINED EFFECT
Alcohol:	Increased blood pressure drop. Avoid.
Beverages: Low-salt milk.	Possible excess potassium levels. Low-salt milk has extra potassium.
Cocaine:	Blood pressure rise. Avoid.
Foods: Salt substitutes.	Possible excess potassium levels.
Marijuana:	None expected.
Tobacco:	None expected.

---

*See Glossary

DIURETICS, THIAZIDE

GENERIC AND BRAND NAMES

See full list of generic and brand names in the *Generic and Brand Name Directory*, page 885.

BASIC INFORMATION

Habit forming? No
Prescription needed? Yes
Available as generic? Yes, for some.
Drug class: Antihypertensive, diuretic (thiazide)

 ## USES

- Controls, but doesn't cure, high blood pressure.
- Reduces fluid retention (edema) caused by conditions such as heart disorders and liver disease.

 ## DOSAGE & USAGE INFORMATION

How to take:
Tablet, capsule or liquid—Swallow with liquid. If you can't swallow whole, crumble tablet or open capsule and take with liquid or food. Don't exceed dose.

When to take:
At the same time each day.

If you forget a dose:
Take as soon as you remember up to 2 hours late. If more than 2 hours, wait for next scheduled dose (don't double this dose).

What drug does:
- Forces sodium and water excretion, reducing body fluid.
- Relaxes muscle cells of small arteries.
- Reduced body fluid and relaxed arteries lower blood pressure.

Continued next column

 ## OVERDOSE

SYMPTOMS:
Cramps, weakness, drowsiness, weak pulse, coma.
WHAT TO DO:
- Dial 911 (emergency) for medical help or call poison control center 1-800-222-1222 for instructions.
- See emergency information on last 3 pages of this book.

Time lapse before drug works:
4 to 6 hours. May require several weeks to lower blood pressure.

Don't take with:
Any other medicine or any dietary supplement without consulting your doctor or pharmacist.

 ## POSSIBLE ADVERSE REACTIONS OR SIDE EFFECTS

SYMPTOMS	WHAT TO DO
Life-threatening:	
In case of overdose, see previous column.	
Common:	
Muscle cramps.	Discontinue. Call doctor right away.
Infrequent:	
• Blurred vision, severe abdominal pain, nausea, vomiting, irregular heartbeat, weak pulse.	Discontinue. Call doctor right away.
• Dizziness, mood changes, headaches, weakness, tiredness, weight changes, decreased sex drive, diarrhea.	Continue. Call doctor when convenient.
• Dry mouth, thirst.	Continue. Tell doctor at next visit.
Rare:	
• Rash or hives.	Discontinue. Seek emergency treatment.
• Jaundice, joint pain, black stools.	Discontinue. Call doctor right away.
• Sore throat, fever.	Continue. Tell doctor at next visit.

 ## WARNINGS & PRECAUTIONS

Don't take if:
You are allergic to any thiazide diuretic drug.

Before you start, consult your doctor if:
- You are allergic to any sulfa drug or tartrazine dye.
- You have systemic lupus erythematosus.
- You have gout, diabetes or a liver, pancreas or kidney disorder.

Over age 60:
Adverse reactions and side effects may be more frequent and severe than in younger persons, especially dizziness and excessive potassium loss.

Pregnancy:
Risk factors vary for drugs in this group. See category list on page xviii and consult doctor.

Breast-feeding:
Drug passes into milk. Avoid drug or discontinue nursing.

Infants & children:
No problems expected.

Prolonged use:
* You may need medicine to treat high blood pressure for the rest of your life.
* Talk to your doctor about the need for follow-up medical examinations or laboratory studies to check blood sugar, kidney function, blood pressure, serum electrolytes.

Skin & sunlight:
One or more drugs in this group may cause rash or intensify sunburn in areas exposed to sun or ultraviolet light (photosensitivity reaction). Avoid overexposure. Notify doctor if reaction occurs.

Driving, piloting or hazardous work:
Don't drive or pilot aircraft until you learn how medicine affects you. Don't work around dangerous machinery. Don't climb ladders or work in high places. Danger increases if you drink alcohol or take medicine affecting alertness and reflexes, such as antihistamines, tranquilizers, sedatives, pain medicine, narcotics and mind-altering drugs.

Discontinuing:
Don't discontinue without medical advice.

Others:
* Hot weather and fever may cause dehydration and drop in blood pressure. Dose may require temporary adjustment. Weigh daily and report any unexpected weight decreases to your doctor.
* May cause rise in uric acid, leading to gout.
* May cause blood-sugar rise in diabetics.
* May affect results in some medical tests.
* Advise any doctor or dentist whom you consult that you take this medicine.

 POSSIBLE INTERACTION WITH OTHER DRUGS

GENERIC NAME OR DRUG CLASS	COMBINED EFFECT
Adrenocorticoids, systemic	Potassium depletion.
Allopurinol	Decreased allopurinol effect.
Amiodarone	Increased risk of heartbeat irregularity due to low potassium.
Amphotericin B	Increased potassium.
Angiotensin-converting enzyme (ACE) inhibitors*	Decreased blood pressure.

Antidepressants, tricyclic*	Dangerous drop in blood pressure. Avoid combination unless under medical supervision.
Antidiabetic agents, oral*	Increased blood sugar.
Antihypertensives*	Increased hypertensive effect.
Antivirals, HIV/AIDS*	Increased risk of pancreatitis.
Barbiturates*	Increased anti-hypertensive effect.
Beta-adrenergic blocking agents*	Increased anti-hypertensive effect. Dosages of both drugs may require adjustments.
Calcium supplements*	Increased calcium in blood.
Carteolol	Increased anti-hypertensive effect.
Cholestyramine	Decreased anti-hypertensive effect.
Colestipol	Decreased anti-hypertensive effect.
Digitalis preparations*	Excessive potassium loss that causes dangerous heart rhythms.
Diuretics, thiazide*, other	Increased effect of other thiazide diuretics.

Continued on page 917

 POSSIBLE INTERACTION WITH OTHER SUBSTANCES

INTERACTS WITH	COMBINED EFFECT
Alcohol:	Dangerous blood pressure drop.
Beverages:	None expected.
Cocaine	Increased risk of heart block and high blood pressure.
Foods: Licorice.	Excessive potassium loss that causes dangerous heart rhythms.
Marijuana:	May increase blood pressure.
Tobacco:	None expected.

*See Glossary

DIVALPROEX

BRAND NAMES

Depakote
Depakote ER

Depakote Sprinkle
Epival

BASIC INFORMATION

Habit forming? No
Prescription needed? Yes
Available as generic? Yes
Drug class: Anticonvulsant

 USES

- Treatment of epilepsy.
- Treatment of bipolar disorder.
- Treats migraine headaches.

 DOSAGE & USAGE INFORMATION

How to take:
Delayed-release tablet/capsule or extended-release tablet—Swallow whole with liquid or food to lessen stomach irritation. Do not crush or chew capsule or tablets. You may open capsule and sprinkle contents on food (such as a teaspoon of applesauce), then swallow right away.

When to take:
Delayed form 2-3 times each day; extended form one time a day. The two different forms (delayed or extended) have different actions in the body.

If you forget a dose:
Take as soon as you remember. If it is almost time for the next dose, wait for the next scheduled dose (don't double this dose).

What drug does:
It helps stabilize electrical activity in the brain.

Time lapse before drug works:
1 to 4 hours, but full effect may take weeks.

Don't take with:
Any other medicine or any dietary supplement without consulting your doctor or pharmacist.

 OVERDOSE

SYMPTOMS:
Extreme drowsiness, heart problems, loss of consciousness.
WHAT TO DO:
- **Dial 911 (emergency) for medical help or call poison control center 1-800-222-1222 for instructions.**
- **See emergency information on last 3 pages of this book.**

 POSSIBLE ADVERSE REACTIONS OR SIDE EFFECTS

SYMPTOMS	WHAT TO DO
Life-threatening: Rare allergic reaction (hives, itching, rash, wheezing, tightness in chest, swelling of lips or tongue or throat).	Seek emergency treatment immediately.
Common: Loss of appetite, indigestion, nausea, vomiting, stomach cramps, diarrhea, tremor, headache, weight gain or loss, menstrual changes.	Continue. Call doctor when convenient.
Infrequent: Clumsiness or unsteadiness, constipation, mild skin rash, dizziness, drowsiness, irritable or excited, hair loss.	Continue. Call doctor when convenient.
Rare: Mood or behavior changes; continued nausea, vomiting and appetite loss; increase in number of seizures; swelling of face, feet or legs; yellow skin or eyes; tiredness or weakness; back-and-forth eye movements (nystagmus); seeing spots/seeing double; unusual bleeding or bruising; dark urine; clay-colored stools; low fever; severe stomach cramps; confusion.	Continue, but call doctor right away.

WARNINGS & PRECAUTIONS

Don't take if:
You are allergic to divalproex or valproic acid.

Before you start, consult your doctor if:
- You have liver, kidney, blood or brain disorder or pancreatitis or urea cycle disorder.
- Drug is to be used for a young child.
- You have a history of depression or suicide thoughts or suicidal behavior.
- You are a woman of childbearing age.

Over age 60:
Adverse reactions and side effects may be more frequent and severe than in younger persons.

Pregnancy:
Risk of birth defects to unborn child exists. Use only if benefits of drug greatly exceed fetal risk. Risk category D (see page xviii).

Breast-feeding:
Unknown effect. Consult doctor.

Infants & children:
Increased risk for side effects and adverse reactions. Use under close medical supervision only.

Prolonged use:
Request periodic blood tests, liver and kidney function tests. These tests are necessary for safe and effective use.

Skin & sunlight:
No problems expected.

Driving, piloting or hazardous work:
Don't drive or pilot aircraft until you learn how medicine affects you. Don't work around dangerous machinery. Don't climb ladders or work in high places. Danger increases if you drink alcohol or take medicine affecting alertness and reflexes.

Discontinuing:
Don't discontinue without consulting doctor. Dose may require gradual reduction if you have taken drug for a long time. Doses of other drugs may also require adjustment.

Others:
- Advise any doctor or dentist whom you consult that you take this medicine.
- Be sure you and your doctor discuss benefits and risks of this drug before starting.
- Wear a medical identification that indicates your disorder and the use of this medicine.
- Read and carefully follow the prescription instructions. Use as directed. Don't increase or decrease dosage without doctor's approval.
- In rare cases, the drug can cause life-threatening liver failure (especially in children under age 2) or life-threatening pancreatitis (inflammation of the pancreas).
- Rarely, antiepileptic (anticonvulsant) drugs may lead to suicidal thoughts and behaviors. Call doctor right away if suicidal symptoms or unusual behaviors occur.

 POSSIBLE INTERACTION WITH OTHER DRUGS

GENERIC NAME OR DRUG CLASS	COMBINED EFFECT
Anticoagulants*, oral	Increased risk of bleeding problems.
Anticonvulsants*, other	Each drug may need dosage adjusted.
Anti-inflammatory drugs, nonsteroidal* (NSAIDs)	Increased risk of bleeding problems.

Aspirin	Increased effect of divalproex.
Carbamazepine	Decreased effect of divalproex.
Central nervous system (CNS) depressants*	Increased sedative effect.
Clonazepam	May prolong seizure.
Diazepam	Increased effect of diazepam.
Enzyme inducers*	May Increase effect of some enzyme inducers and decrease effect of divalproex.
Felbamate	Increased effect of divalproex.
Hepatotoxics*	Increased risk of liver problems.
Lamotrigine	Increased effect of lamotrigine and risk of life-threatening rash.
Phenobarbital	Increased effect of phenobarbital and decreased effect of divalproex.
Phenytoin	Increased phenytoin effect; decreased divalproex effect.
Primidone	Increased effect of primidone.
Rifampin	Decreased effect of divalproex.
Salicylates*	Increased effect of divalproex.
Zidovudine	Increased effect of zidovudine.

 POSSIBLE INTERACTION WITH OTHER SUBSTANCES

INTERACTS WITH	COMBINED EFFECT
Alcohol:	Deep sedation. Avoid.
Beverages:	None expected.
Cocaine:	Unknown. Avoid.
Foods:	None expected.
Marijuana:	Unknown. Avoid.
Tobacco:	None expected.

*See Glossary

DOFETILIDE

BRAND NAMES

Tikosyn

BASIC INFORMATION

Habit forming? No
Prescription needed? Yes
Available as generic? No
Drug class: Antiarrhythmic

 ## USES

Corrects irregular heartbeats to a normal rhythm.

 ## DOSAGE & USAGE INFORMATION

How to take:
Capsule—This drug is first used in a hospital or other setting where the patient can be monitored for any heart problems. Read the information provided with the prescription.

When to take:
At the same times each day.

If you forget a dose:
Skip the missed dose and go back to your regular dosing schedule (don't double this dose).

What drug does:
Slows the nerve impulses in the heart.

Time lapse before drug works:
2 to 3 hours.

Don't take with:
Any other medicine or any dietary supplement without consulting your doctor or pharmacist.

 ## OVERDOSE

SYMPTOMS:
Cardiac arrest, irregular heartbeat, fainting, shortness of breath, unusual tiredness or weakness.
WHAT TO DO:
Dial 911 (emergency) for medical help or call poison control center 1-800-222-1222 for instructions.

 ## POSSIBLE ADVERSE REACTIONS OR SIDE EFFECTS

SYMPTOMS	WHAT TO DO
Life-threatening: In case of overdose, see previous column.	
Common: Dizziness, fainting, fast or irregular heartbeat.	Discontinue. Seek emergency evaluation right away.
Infrequent: • Unusual swelling of, the extremities, chest pain, slow heartbeat, sudden numbness or tingling (hands, feet or face), paralysis, confusion, weakness, slurred speech, shortness of breath, yellow eyes or skin.	Discontinue. Call doctor right away.
• Abdominal pain, back pain, diarrhea, chills, cough, fever, general feeling of illness, joint pain, headache, nausea, runny nose, sore throat, vomiting, sleeplessness, rash.	Continue. Call doctor if symptoms persist.
Rare: None expected.	

 ## WARNINGS & PRECAUTIONS

Don't take if:
You are allergic to dofetilide.

Before you start, consult your doctor if:
• You are using any other medication.
• You have electrolyte disorders, such as low potassium or magnesium levels.
• You have been diagnosed with kidney or liver disease.

Over age 60:
Side effects or problems experienced with this medication appear to be the same in older people as in younger adults; however, older patients are more likely to have kidney problems and should be monitored regularly for possible dosage adjustment.

Pregnancy:
Decide with your doctor if drug benefits justify risk to unborn child. Risk category C (see page xviii).

Breast-feeding:
Drug may pass into milk. Avoid drug or discontinue nursing until you finish medicine. Consult doctor for advice on maintaining milk supply.

Infants & children:
Studies on this medicine have been done only in adult patients. Consult doctor before giving this medicine to persons under age 18.

Prolonged use:
Talk to your doctor about the need for follow up laboratory studies to determine the effect of the medicine on your body.

Skin & sunlight:
None expected.

Driving, piloting or hazardous work:
Don't drive or pilot aircraft until you learn how medicine affects you. Don't work around dangerous machinery. Don't climb ladders or work in high places. Danger increases if you drink alcohol or take medicine affecting alertness and reflexes.

Discontinuing:
Don't discontinue without consulting doctor.

Others:
Advise any doctor or dentist whom you consult that you take this medicine.

POSSIBLE INTERACTION WITH OTHER DRUGS

GENERIC NAME OR DRUG CLASS	COMBINED EFFECT
Antiarrhythmics, other*	Increased dofetilide effect.
Antidepressants, tricyclic*	Increased risk of heart problems.
Calcium channel blockers*	Increased risk of heart problems.
Cimetidine	Increased risk of heart problems.
Diuretics*	Increased risk of heart problems.
Enzyme inhibitors*	Increased dofetilide effect.
Ketoconazole	Increased risk of heart problems.
Macrolides, oral*	Increased risk of heart problems.
Megestrol	Increased dofetilide effect.
Metformin	Increased dofetilide effect.

Norfloxacin	Increased dofetilide effect.
Phenothiazines*	Increased risk of heart problems.
Progestins*	Increased risk of heart problems.
Selective serotonin reuptake inhibitors*	Increased dofetilide effect.
Trimethoprim	Increased dofetilide effect.
Zafirlukast	Increased dofetilide effect.

POSSIBLE INTERACTION WITH OTHER SUBSTANCES

INTERACTS WITH	COMBINED EFFECT
Alcohol:	Increases the chance of liver problems.
Beverages: Grapefruit juice	May increase effect of dofetilide.
Cocaine:	Effect unknown. Avoid.
Foods:	None expected.
Marijuana:	Effect unknown. Avoid.
Tobacco:	None expected.

DOXEPIN (Topical)

BRAND NAMES

Prudoxin   Zonalon

BASIC INFORMATION

Habit forming? No
Prescription needed? Yes
Available as generic? No
Drug class: Antipruritic (topical)

 USES

- Treats itching of the skin caused by certain types of eczema (an inflammation of the skin).
- Treatment of moderate itching of atopic dermatitis and lichen simplex chronicus in adult patients.

 DOSAGE & USAGE INFORMATION

How to use:
Cream—Apply a thin layer to the affected area of skin and gently rub it in. Do not cover the treated area with a bandage or other dressing.

When to use:
Up to 4 times a day. Allow 3 to 4 hours between applications. Not to be used longer than 8 days.

If you forget a dose:
Use as soon as you remember. If it is almost time for the next dose, wait for the next scheduled dose (don't double this dose).

Continued next column

 OVERDOSE

SYMPTOMS:
An overdose of topical medicine is unlikely to occur, but if too much is applied, it can be absorbed into the system.
- Mild effects include blurred vision, drowsiness, very dry mouth, decreased awareness or responsiveness.
- More severe effects include irregular or fast heartbeat, enlarged pupils, jerking movements, dizziness, fainting, abdominal pain or swelling, weak or feeble pulse, high fever or low temperature, vomiting, incurable constipation, seizures, breathing difficulty, unconsciousness.

WHAT TO DO:
- Dial 911 (emergency) for medical help or call poison control center 1-800-222-1222 for instructions.
- See emergency information on last 3 pages of this book.

What drug does:
The exact mechanism is unknown. It appears to block histamine* reactions, which can cause the itching. The drug also has a sedating effect on some people, which can help to relieve the itching symptoms. Variable and sometimes significant amounts of the drug are absorbed through the skin.

Time lapse before drug works:
May take up to 8 days for maximum benefit.

Don't take with:
Any other oral or topical medication without consulting your doctor or pharmacist. This includes nonprescription drugs such as cold or allergy remedies that may contain alcohol or antihistamines. They increase the risk of drowsiness.

 POSSIBLE ADVERSE REACTIONS OR SIDE EFFECTS

SYMPTOMS	WHAT TO DO
Life-threatening:	
In case of overdose, see previous column.	
Common:	
• Swelling of the skin where drug is applied; worsening of the itching; burning, tingling or crawling feeling in the skin.	Discontinue. Call doctor right away.
• Stinging of skin where drug is applied, dryness or tightness of skin, taste changes, dizziness, drowsiness, dry mouth or lips, thirst, emotional changes, fatigue, headache.	Continue. Call doctor when convenient.
Infrequent:	
Scaling or cracking of the skin, nausea, anxiety, irritation.	Continue. Call doctor when convenient.
Rare:	
Fever.	Discontinue. Call doctor right away.

Note: Though the drug is applied topically, it is absorbed into the bloodstream and can cause systemic reactions. Adverse reactions are more likely in patients who use the drug on more than 10% of their body surface.

WARNINGS & PRECAUTIONS

Don't use if:
You are allergic to doxepin.

Before you start, consult your doctor if:
• You have narrow-angle glaucoma.
• You are allergic to any other medications.
• You have a problem with urinary retention.

Over age 60:
No special problems expected.

Pregnancy:
Consult doctor. Risk category B (page xviii).

Breast-feeding:
Drug passes into milk. Avoid drug or discontinue nursing until you finish medicine. Consult doctor for advice on maintaining milk supply.

Infants & children:
Safety in children has not been established. Use only under close medical supervision.

Prolonged use:
Don't use for more than 8 days unless directed by doctor. Longer use can increase the risk of side effects or adverse reactions.

Skin & sunlight:
No special problems expected.

Driving, piloting or hazardous work:
Don't drive or pilot aircraft until you learn how medicine affects you. Don't work around dangerous machinery. Don't climb ladders or work in high places. Danger increases if you drink alcohol or take medicine affecting alertness and reflexes.

Discontinuing:
To be sure of maximum benefit, don't discontinue this medicine before the treatment has been completed unless advised to do so by your doctor.

Others:
• Use medicine only on affected area. It is not to be used in the mouth, the eyes or the vagina.
• Advise any doctor or dentist whom you consult that you are using this medicine.
• If your skin condition doesn't improve within 8 days, consult doctor.
• Use medicine only as directed. Do not increase or reduce dosage without doctor's approval.

POSSIBLE INTERACTION WITH OTHER DRUGS

GENERIC NAME OR DRUG CLASS	COMBINED EFFECT
Antidepressants*	Increased risk of toxicity of both drugs.
Carbamazepine	Increased risk of toxicity of both drugs.
Central nervous system (CNS) depressants*	Increased sedation. May need dosage adjustment.
Cimetidine	Increased risk of doxepin toxicity.
Dextromethorphan	Increased risk of toxicity of both drugs.
Flecainide	Increased risk of toxicity of both drugs.
Monoamine oxidase (MAO) inhibitors*	Potentially life-threatening. Allow 14 days between use of the 2 drugs.
Phenothiazines*	Increased risk of toxicity of both drugs.
Propafenone	Increased risk of toxicity of both drugs.
Quinidine	Increased risk of toxicity of both drugs.

POSSIBLE INTERACTION WITH OTHER SUBSTANCES

INTERACTS WITH	COMBINED EFFECT
Alcohol:	Increased sedative effect. Avoid.
Beverages:	None expected.
Cocaine:	Problems not known. Best to avoid.
Foods:	None expected.
Marijuana:	Problems not known. Best to avoid.
Tobacco:	None expected.

*See Glossary

DPP-4 INHIBITORS

GENERIC AND BRAND NAMES

SITAGLIPTIN
  Janumet
  Januvia

BASIC INFORMATION

Habit forming? No
Prescription needed? Yes
Available as generic? No
Drug class: Antidiabetic; incretin enhancer

 ## USES

Used in addition to diet and exercise to improve blood sugar levels in patients with type 2 diabetes. It may be prescribed alone or along with other oral diabetes drugs. (Note: This drug is not used for treating type 1 diabetes or diabetic ketoacidosis.)

 ## DOSAGE & USAGE INFORMATION

How to take:
Tablet—Swallow with liquid. May be taken with or without food or as directed by your doctor.

When to take:
Usually taken once a day at the same time each day.

If you forget a dose:
Take tablet as soon as you remember. If it is almost time for the next dose, wait for the next scheduled dose (don't double this dose).

Continued next column

 ## OVERDOSE

SYMPTOMS:
Rarely may cause hypoglycemia (low blood sugar)—See list of symptoms in next column under Rare.
WHAT TO DO:
* Eat some type of sugar immediately, such as glucose product, orange juice (add some sugar), nondiet sodas, candy (such as 5 Lifesavers), honey.
* If patient loses consciousness, give glucagon if you have it and know how to use it.
* Dial 911 (emergency) for medical help or call poison control center 1-800-222-1222 for instructions.
* See emergency information on last 3 pages of this book.

What drug does:
It works by increasing incretins. Incretins increase insulin release when blood sugar levels are high, especially after meals. They also decrease the amount of sugar made by the liver.

Time lapse before drug works:
One to four hours.

Don't take with:
Any other medicine or diet supplement without consulting your doctor or pharmacist.

 ## POSSIBLE ADVERSE REACTIONS OR SIDE EFFECTS

SYMPTOMS	WHAT TO DO
Life-threatening:	
Rare allergic reaction (hives, itching, rash, trouble breathing, tightness in chest, swelling of lips or tongue or throat).	Seek emergency treatment immediately.
Common:	
Sore throat, headache, runny or stuffy nose, upper respiratory infection (e.g., cold).	Continue. Call doctor if symptoms persist.
Infrequent:	
Nausea, mild stomach pain, diarrhea, joint pain.	Continue. Call doctor if symptoms persist.
Rare:	
• Symptoms of low blood sugar— nervousness, hunger (excessive), cold sweats, rapid pulse, anxiety, cold skin, chills, confusion, drowsiness, loss of concentration, headache, nausea, weakness, shakiness, vision changes.	Seek treatment (eat some form of quick-acting sugar— glucose tablets, sugar, fruit juice, corn syrup, honey).
• Symptoms of high blood sugar— increased urination, unusual thirst, dry mouth, drowsiness, flushed or dry skin, fruit-like breath odor, appetite loss, stomach pain or vomiting, tiredness, trouble breathing, increased blood sugar level.	Check your blood sugar immediately. Call doctor right away.
• Other symptoms that cause concern.	Continue. Call doctor when convenient.

WARNINGS & PRECAUTIONS

Don't take if:
You are allergic to DPP-4 inhibitors.

Before you start, consult your doctor if:
• You have any kidney problems.
• You are pregnant or plan to become pregnant.
• You are an alcoholic.

Over age 60:
A reduced drug dosage may be recommended for patients with decreased kidney function.

Pregnancy:
Decide with your doctor if drug benefits justify risk to unborn child. Risk category B (see page xviii).

Breast-feeding:
Drug may pass into milk. Consult your doctor for advice.

Infants & children:
Safety and effectiveness in children under age 18 has not been established. Consult doctor.

Prolonged use:
Talk to your doctor about the need for follow-up medical examinations and/or laboratory studies to determine continued effectiveness of drug.

Skin & sunlight:
No problems expected.

Driving, piloting or hazardous work:
No problems expected. You do need to be cautious for symptoms of hypoglycemia.

Discontinuing:
Don't discontinue without doctor's advice, even though symptoms diminish or disappear.

Others:
• Along with taking drugs for diabetes, be sure to follow your doctor's instructions for lifestyle changes such as a proper diet, weight control measures and a regular exercise program.
• Notify your doctor if you have a fever, infection, diarrhea, or experience vomiting.
• Advise any doctor or dentist whom you consult that you take this medicine.
• Wear or carry medical identification that indicates you have type 2 diabetes and the drugs you take.
• See your diabetes doctor regularly to review your treatment and check for complications.
• You and your family should educate yourselves about diabetes; learn to recognize the symptoms of hypoglycemia and how to treat it. Hypoglycemia may occur in the treatment of diabetes as a result of skipped meals, excessive exercise, or alcohol consumption. Carry non-dietetic candy or glucose tablets to treat episodes of low blood sugar.

 POSSIBLE INTERACTION WITH OTHER DRUGS

GENERIC NAME OR DRUG CLASS	COMBINED EFFECT
Digoxin	Digoxin dosage may need to be adjusted.
Hypoglycemia-causing medications*	May increase risk of low blood sugar.

 POSSIBLE INTERACTION WITH OTHER SUBSTANCES

INTERACTS WITH	COMBINED EFFECT
Alcohol:	May cause severe low blood sugar. Avoid.
Beverages:	None expected.
Cocaine:	Unknown. Avoid.
Foods:	None expected.
Marijuana:	Unknown. Avoid.
Tobacco:	No drug interaction. Tobacco use does raise risk of diabetes complications. Avoid smoking.

*See Glossary

DRONABINOL (THC, Marijuana)

BRAND NAMES

Marinol

BASIC INFORMATION

Habit forming? Yes
Prescription needed? Yes
Available as generic? Yes
Drug class: Antiemetic

 ## USES

- Prevents nausea and vomiting that may accompany taking anticancer medication (cancer chemotherapy). Should not be used unless other antinausea medicines fail.
- Appetite stimulant. Used to treat appetite loss in AIDS patients.

 ## DOSAGE & USAGE INFORMATION

How to take:
Capsule—Swallow with liquid.

When to take:
Under supervision, a total of no more than 4 to 6 doses per day, every 2 to 4 hours after cancer chemotherapy for prescribed number of days.

If you forget a dose:
Take as soon as you remember up to 2 hours late. If more than 2 hours, wait for next scheduled dose (don't double this dose).

What drug does:
Affects nausea and vomiting center in brain to make it less irritable following cancer chemotherapy. Exact mechanism is unknown.

Time lapse before drug works:
2 to 4 hours.

Don't take with:
Any other medicine or any dietary supplement without consulting your doctor or pharmacist.

 ## OVERDOSE

SYMPTOMS:
Pounding, rapid heart rate; high or low blood pressure; confusion; hallucinations; drastic mood changes; nervousness or anxiety.
WHAT TO DO:
Overdose unlikely to threaten life. If person uses much larger amount than prescribed or if accidentally swallowed, call doctor or poison control center 1-800-222-1222 for help.

 ## POSSIBLE ADVERSE REACTIONS OR SIDE EFFECTS

SYMPTOMS	WHAT TO DO
Life-threatening:	
In case of overdose, see previous column.	
Common:	
• Rapid, pounding heartbeat.	Discontinue. Call doctor right away.
• Dizziness, irritability, drowsiness, euphoria, decreased coordination.	Continue. Call doctor when convenient.
• Red eyes, dry mouth.	No action necessary.
Infrequent:	
Depression, anxiety, nervousness, headache, hallucinations, dramatic mood changes, blurred or changed vision.	Discontinue. Call doctor right away.
Rare:	
• Rapid heartbeat, fainting, frequent or difficult urination, convulsions, shortness of breath, paranoia.	Discontinue. Call doctor right away.
• Nausea, loss of appetite, dizziness when standing after sitting or lying down, diarrhea.	Continue. Call doctor when convenient.

 ## WARNINGS & PRECAUTIONS

Don't take if:
- Your nausea and vomiting is caused by anything other than cancer chemotherapy.
- You are sensitive or allergic to any form of marijuana or sesame oil.
- Your cycle of chemotherapy is longer than 7 consecutive days. Harmful side effects may occur.

Before you start, consult your doctor if:
- You have heart disease or high blood pressure.
- You are an alcoholic or drug addict.
- You are pregnant or intend to become pregnant.
- You are nursing an infant.
- You have schizophrenia or a manic-depressive disorder.

DRONABINOL (THC, Marijuana)

Over age 60:
Adverse reactions and side effects may be more frequent and severe than in younger persons.

Pregnancy:
Decide with your doctor if drug benefits justify risk to unborn child. Risk category C (see page xviii).

Breast-feeding:
Drug passes into milk. Avoid drug or discontinue nursing until you finish medicine. Consult doctor about maintaining milk supply.

Infants & children:
Not recommended.

Prolonged use:
* Avoid. Habit forming.
* Talk to your doctor about the need for follow-up medical examinations or laboratory studies to check heart function.

Skin & sunlight:
No problems expected.

Driving, piloting or hazardous work:
Don't drive or pilot aircraft until you learn how medicine affects you. Don't work around dangerous machinery. Don't climb ladders or work in high places. Danger increases if you drink alcohol or take medicine affecting alertness and reflexes, such as antihistamines, tranquilizers, sedatives, pain medicine, narcotics and mind-altering drugs.

Discontinuing:
Withdrawal effects such as irritability, insomnia, restlessness, sweating, diarrhea, hiccups, loss of appetite and hot flashes may follow abrupt withdrawal within 12 hours. Should they occur, these symptoms will probably subside within 96 hours.

Others:
* Store in refrigerator.
* Advise any doctor or dentist whom you consult that you take this medicine.

 POSSIBLE INTERACTION WITH OTHER DRUGS

GENERIC NAME OR DRUG CLASS	COMBINED EFFECT
Anesthetics*	Oversedation.
Anticonvulsants*	Oversedation.
Antidepressants, tricyclic*	Oversedation.
Antihistamines*	Oversedation.
Barbiturates*	Oversedation.
Clozapine	Toxic effect on the central nervous system.
Ethinamate	Dangerous increased effects of ethinamate. Avoid combining.
Fluoxetine	Increased depressant effects of both drugs.
Guanfacine	May increase depressant effects of either drug.
Leucovorin	High alcohol content of leucovorin may cause adverse effects.
Methyprylon	Increased sedative effect, perhaps to dangerous level. Avoid.
Molindone	Increased effects of both drugs. Avoid.
Muscle relaxants*	Oversedation.
Nabilone	Greater depression of central nervous system.
Narcotics*	Oversedation.
Sedatives*	Oversedation.
Sertraline	Increased depressive effects of both drugs.
Tranquilizers*	Oversedation.

 POSSIBLE INTERACTION WITH OTHER SUBSTANCES

INTERACTS WITH	COMBINED EFFECT
Alcohol:	Oversedation.
Beverages:	None expected.
Cocaine:	None expected.
Foods:	None expected.
Marijuana:	Oversedation.
Tobacco:	None expected.

*See Glossary

347

EFLORNITHINE (Topical)

BRAND NAMES

Vaniqa

BASIC INFORMATION

Habit forming? No
Prescription needed? Yes
Available as generic? No
Drug class: Enzyme inhibitor (topical)

 USES

Treatment for unwanted facial hair (hirsutism is the medical term) on women.

 DOSAGE & USAGE INFORMATION

How to take:
Cream—Follow directions on package label. Usually requires twice-daily application. Limit application to facial area and avoid getting medication in eyes, nose or mouth. Apply at least five minutes after hair removal technique (shaving). Do not apply cosmetics until the medication dries. Do not wash face for at least four hours after applying medication.

When to take:
At the same times each day at least 8 hours apart.

If you forget a dose:
Use as soon as possible. Do not use if it is almost time for your next application. Do not double dose.

What drug does:
Inhibits an enzyme that encourages hair growth.

Time lapse before drug works:
4-8 weeks for improvement to be seen.

Don't take with:
Any other medicine or any dietary supplement without consulting your doctor or pharmacist.

 OVERDOSE

SYMPTOMS:
None expected.
WHAT TO DO:
Not intended for internal use. If child accidentally swallows, call doctor or poison control center 1-800-222-1222 for help.

 POSSIBLE ADVERSE REACTIONS OR SIDE EFFECTS

SYMPTOMS	WHAT TO DO
Life-threatening: None expected.	
Common: Stinging skin, acne breakout.	Continue. Call doctor if condition persists.
Infrequent: Skin symptoms (tingling, redness, chapped, swollen, burning, bleeding, rash, hair bumps, continued acne).	Continue. Call doctor when convenient.
Rare: None expected.	

WARNINGS & PRECAUTIONS

Don't take if:
You are allergic to eflornithine.

Before you start, consult your doctor if:
You have facial abrasions, cuts or scrapes.

Over age 60:
No problems expected.

Pregnancy:
Consult doctor. Risk category C (see page xviii).

Breast-feeding:
It is unknown if eflornithine passes into breast milk. Avoid drug or discontinue nursing until you finish medicine. Consult doctor for advice on maintaining milk supply.

Infants & children:
Safety and efficacy has not been established in children under 12 years of age.

Prolonged use:
If no improvement is seen after six months of using this medicine, consult doctor.

Skin & sunlight:
No problems expected. However, if skin irritation occurs after prolonged exposure to sun, consult doctor.

Driving, piloting or hazardous work:
No problems expected.

Discontinuing:
• Consult doctor before discontinuing.
• In about 8 weeks, your hair growth will probably return to the same as it was before you started the medication.

Others:
Advise any doctor or dentist whom you consult that you use this drug.

 ## POSSIBLE INTERACTION WITH OTHER DRUGS

GENERIC NAME OR DRUG CLASS	COMBINED EFFECT
None significant.	

 ## POSSIBLE INTERACTION WITH OTHER SUBSTANCES

INTERACTS WITH	COMBINED EFFECT
Alcohol:	None expected.
Beverages:	None expected.
Cocaine:	None expected.
Foods:	None expected.
Marijuana:	None expected.
Tobacco:	None expected.

ENDOTHELIN RECEPTOR ANTAGONIST

GENERIC AND BRAND NAMES

AMBRISENTAN
Letairis

BOSENTAN
Tracleer

BASIC INFORMATION

Habit forming? No
Prescription needed? Yes
Available as generic? No
Drug class: Antihypertensive (pulmonary)

 ## USES

Treats the symptoms of pulmonary arterial hypertension (PAH), which is high blood pressure in the lungs. It improves the breathing and exercise capacity of patients with PAH. The drug does not cure the disorder. These drugs are available only through restricted programs which will be explained by your doctor.

 ## DOSAGE & USAGE INFORMATION

How to take:
Tablet—Swallow with liquid. Take with or without food. Do not break, crush or chew the tablet.

When to take:
Usually once or twice daily at the same times each day. Follow your doctor's instructions.

If you forget a dose:
Take as soon as you remember. If it is almost time for the next dose, wait for next scheduled dose (don't double this dose).

What drug does:
It works by blocking the effect of endothelin (a substance made by the body). In patients with PAH, the blood vessels become narrowed (constricted) due to an excess production of endothelin.

Continued next column

 ## OVERDOSE

SYMPTOMS:
Dizziness or faintness, confusion, blurred vision, sweating, increased heart rate, unusual tiredness or weakness, vomiting.
WHAT TO DO:
Overdose unlikely to threaten life. If person uses much larger amount than prescribed or if accidentally swallowed, call doctor or poison control center 1-800-222-1222 for help.

Time lapse before drug works:
It may take 1 to 2 months or longer to notice effects. The dosage may be increased after 4 weeks if there are no problems in taking the drug.

Don't take with:
Any other medicine or any dietary supplement without consulting your doctor or pharmacist.

 ## POSSIBLE ADVERSE REACTIONS OR SIDE EFFECTS

SYMPTOMS	WHAT TO DO
Life-threatening: Rare allergic reaction (hives, itching, rash, trouble breathing, tightness in chest, swelling of lips or tongue or throat).	Seek emergency treatment immediately.
Common: Feeling of warmth, flushing, stuffy or sore nose, sore throat, stomach upset, swelling of legs and ankles, mild dizziness.	Continue. Call doctor when convenient.
Infrequent: • Difficult breathing, irregular heartbeat, unusual tiredness or weakness, on-going dizziness or lightheadedness, wheezing or unusual coughing.	Discontinue. Call doctor right away.
• Stomach pain, heartburn, mild heart palpitations, constipation, hoarseness, head-ache, low blood pressure.	Continue. Call doctor when convenient.
Rare: Liver problems (symptoms include loss of appetite, nausea, vomiting, light colored stools, fever, extreme tiredness, right upper stomach pain, yellow skin or eyes, dark urine, itching).	Discontinue. Call doctor right away.

ENDOTHELIN RECEPTOR ANTAGONISTS

WARNINGS & PRECAUTIONS

Don't take if:
- You are allergic to endothelin receptor antagonists.
- You have moderate or severe liver (hepatic) impairment.
- You are pregnant or plan to become pregnant.
- You are of childbearing age and have not had a negative pregnancy test or you are not willing to use two reliable methods of birth control.

Before you start, consult your doctor if:
- You have mild liver impairment.
- You have not had a liver function test.
- You have anemia or edema (swelling in hands, lower legs or feet).

Over age 60:
Adverse reactions and side effects may be more frequent and severe than in younger persons.

Pregnancy:
- Using this drug while you are pregnant can cause very serious birth defects. Risk category X (see page xviii).
- If this drug is used during pregnancy, or if you become pregnant while taking this drug, you need to talk to your doctor about the potential hazard to the fetus.

Breast-feeding:
It is unknown if drug passes into milk. Avoid drug or discontinue nursing. Consult doctor.

Infants & children:
Not approved for ages under 18.

Prolonged use:
- Your doctor will check your progress at regular visits to make sure this drug is working properly and to check for unwanted effects.
- It is important that your doctor does a blood test to check your liver function before you start the drug and each month after that.

Skin & sunlight:
No problems expected.

Driving, piloting or hazardous work:
Use caution if you experience dizziness.

Discontinuing:
Consult doctor before discontinuing. The dosage may need to be slowly reduced before stopping.

Others:
- Females of childbearing age will be required to have a pregnancy test every month during treatment. If you miss a menstrual period while using this drug, call your doctor right away. Use two forms of effective birth control to keep from getting pregnant while you are using this drug (even if the drug is temporarily stopped), and for at least one month after you stop taking the drug.

- Use of these drugs may lead to liver problems or decreased hemoglobin.* Be sure to follow your doctor's advice about periodic liver function studies and blood tests. Call doctor right away if any symptoms of liver problems develop (see list in Possible Adverse Reactions or Side Effects).
- Advise any doctor or dentist whom you consult that you take this drug.
- The drug may decrease the amount of sperm men make and affect their ability to have children. Consult doctor.

POSSIBLE INTERACTION WITH OTHER DRUGS

GENERIC NAME OR DRUG CLASS	COMBINED EFFECT
Cyclosporine A	Increased endothelin receptor antagonist effect; decreased cyclosporine effect. Avoid use with bosentan.
Enzyme inducers*	Decreased endothelin receptor antagonist effect.
Enzyme inhibitors*	Increased endothelin receptor antagonist effect.
Glyburide	Decreased effect of both glyburide and endothelin receptor antagonist. May increase risk of liver problems. Avoid with bosentan.
Contraceptives, hormonal*	Decreased birth control effect.

POSSIBLE INTERACTION WITH OTHER SUBSTANCES

INTERACTS WITH	COMBINED EFFECT
Alcohol:	No interaction, but patients should avoid heavy alcohol use.
Beverages:	No proven problems.
Cocaine:	Unknown. Avoid.
Foods:	No proven problems.
Marijuana:	Unknown. Avoid.
Tobacco:	No interaction, but patients with PAH should not smoke.

*See Glossary

EPHEDRINE

BRAND NAMES

Ami-Rax

Broncholate

Marax

Marax D.F.

Rynatuss

Rynatuss Pediatric

 BASIC INFORMATION

Habit forming? No

Prescription needed? Yes

Available as generic? Yes, for some

Drug class: Sympathomimetic

 USES

• Relieves bronchial asthma.
• Decreases congestion of breathing passages.
• Suppresses allergic reactions.

DOSAGE & USAGE INFORMATION

How to take:
• Tablet or capsule—Swallow with liquid. You may chew or crush tablet.
• Extended-release tablet or capsule— Swallow each dose whole.
• Syrup—Take as directed on bottle.
• Drops—Dilute dose in beverage.

When to take:
As needed, no more often than every 4 hours. To prevent insomnia, take last dose at least 2 hours before bedtime.

If you forget a dose:
Take up to 2 hours late. If more than 2 hours, wait for next dose (don't double this dose).

What drug does:
• Prevents cells from releasing allergy-causing chemicals (histamines).
• Relaxes muscles of bronchial tubes.
• Decreases blood vessel size and blood flow, thus causing decongestion.

Continued next column

 OVERDOSE

SYMPTOMS:
Severe anxiety, confusion, delirium, muscle tremors, rapid and irregular pulse.
WHAT TO DO:
• Dial 911 (emergency) for medical help or call poison control center 1-800-222-1222 for instructions.
• See emergency information on last 3 pages of this book.

Time lapse before drug works:
30 to 60 minutes.

Don't take with:
• Nonprescription drugs with ephedrine, pseudoephedrine or epinephrine.
• Any other medicine or any dietary supplement without consulting your doctor or pharmacist.

 POSSIBLE ADVERSE REACTIONS OR SIDE EFFECTS

SYMPTOMS	WHAT TO DO
Life-threatening:	
In case of overdose, see previous column.	
Common:	
• Nervousness, headache, paleness, rapid heartbeat.	Continue. Call doctor when convenient.
• Insomnia.	Continue. Tell doctor at next visit.
Infrequent:	
• Irregular heartbeat.	Discontinue. Call doctor right away.
• Dizziness, appetite loss, nausea, vomiting, painful or difficult urination.	Continue. Call doctor when convenient.
Rare:	
None expected.	

 WARNINGS & PRECAUTIONS

Don't take if:
You are allergic to ephedrine or any sympathomimetic* drug.

Before you start, consult your doctor if:
• You have high blood pressure.
• You have diabetes.
• You have overactive thyroid gland.
• You have difficulty urinating.
• You have taken any MAO inhibitor in past 2 weeks.
• You have taken digitalis preparations in the last 7 days.
• You will have surgery within 2 months, including dental surgery, requiring general or spinal anesthesia.

Over age 60:
More likely to develop high blood pressure, heart-rhythm disturbances, angina and to feel drug's stimulant effects.

Pregnancy:
Decide with your doctor if drug benefits justify risk to unborn child. Risk category C (see page xviii).

Breast-feeding:
Drug passes into milk. Avoid drug or discontinue nursing until you finish medicine. Consult doctor for advice on maintaining milk supply.

Infants & children:
Read label on product to determine if it is approved for your child's age.

Prolonged use:
* Excessive doses—Rare toxic psychosis.
* Men with enlarged prostate gland may have more urination difficulty.

Skin & sunlight:
No problems expected.

Driving, piloting or hazardous work:
Avoid if you feel dizzy. Otherwise, no problems expected.

Discontinuing:
May be unnecessary to finish medicine. Follow doctor's instructions.

Others:
No problems expected.

POSSIBLE INTERACTION WITH OTHER DRUGS

GENERIC NAME OR DRUG CLASS	COMBINED EFFECT
Adrenocorticoids, systemic	Decreased adrenocorticoid effect.
Antidepressants, tricyclic*	Increased effect of ephedrine. Excessive stimulation of heart and blood pressure.
Antihypertensives*	Decreased antihypertensive effect.
Beta-adrenergic blocking agents*	Decreased effects of both drugs.
Dextrothyroxine	Increased ephedrine effect.
Digitalis preparations*	Serious heart rhythm disturbances.
Epinephrine	Increased epinephrine effect.
Ergot preparations*	Serious blood pressure rise.
Furazolidone	Sudden, severe increase in blood pressure.
Guanadrel	Decreased effect of both drugs.
Guanethidine	Decreased effect of both drugs.

Methyldopa	Possible increased blood pressure.
Monoamine oxidase (MAO) inhibitors*	Increased ephedrine effect. Dangerous blood pressure rise.
Nitrates*	Possible decreased effects of both drugs.
Phenothiazines*	Possible increased ephedrine toxicity. Possible decreased ephedrine effect.
Pseudoephedrine	Increased pseudoephedrine effect.
Rauwolfia	Decreased rauwolfia effect.
Sympathomimetics*	Increased ephedrine effect.
Terazosin	Decreases effectiveness of terazosin.
Theophylline	Increased gastrointestinal intolerance.

POSSIBLE INTERACTION WITH OTHER SUBSTANCES

INTERACTS WITH	COMBINED EFFECT
Alcohol:	None expected.
Beverages: Caffeine drinks.	Nervousness or insomnia.
Cocaine:	High risk of heartbeat irregularities and high blood pressure.
Foods:	None expected.
Marijuana:	Rapid heartbeat, possible heart rhythm disturbance.
Tobacco:	None expected.

*See Glossary

EPLERENONE

BRAND NAMES

Inspra

BASIC INFORMATION

Habit forming? No
Prescription needed? Yes
Available as generic? Yes
Drug class: Antihypertensive; selective aldosterone blocker

 USES

- Treatment for hypertension (high blood pressure). May be used alone or along with other antihypertensive medications.
- Used to treat further complications after a myocardial infarction.
- May be used for treatment of other disorders as determined by your doctor.

 DOSAGE & USAGE INFORMATION

How to take:
Tablet—Swallow with liquid. May be taken with or without food.

When to take:
Once or twice daily as directed by your doctor.

If you forget a dose:
Take as soon as you remember. If it is almost time for the next dose, then skip the missed dose and wait for your next scheduled dose (don't double this dose).

What drug does:
It blocks aldosterone, a hormone in the body that increases blood pressure by causing fluid and salt retention. The drug causes the kidneys to remove the excess water and salt from the body.

Time lapse before drug works:
May take several weeks for full effectiveness.

Don't take with:
Any other medicine or any dietary supplement without consulting your doctor or pharmacist.

 OVERDOSE

SYMPTOMS:
Unknown. Could cause very low blood pressure (hypotension).
WHAT TO DO:
Overdose unlikely to threaten life. If person uses much larger amount than prescribed or if accidentally swallowed, call doctor or poison control center 1-800-222-1222 for help.

 POSSIBLE ADVERSE REACTIONS OR SIDE EFFECTS

SYMPTOMS	WHAT TO DO
Life-threatening: None expected.	
Common: Dizziness.	Continue. Call doctor when convenient.
Infrequent: Diarrhea, flu-like, symptoms, cough, fatigue, headache, stomach pain.	Continue. Call doctor when convenient.
Rare: • Abnormal vaginal bleeding in women, enlarged breasts or breast pain in men.	Continue. Call doctor when convenient.
• Hyperkalemia (too much potassium in the body; symptoms include confusion, shortness of breath, feeling very weak and tired, numbness and tingling, irregular heartbeat, nervousness, low blood pressure).	Discontinue. Call doctor right away or seek emergency help if symptoms are severe.

 WARNINGS & PRECAUTIONS

Don't take if:
You are allergic to eplerenone.

Before you start, consult your doctor if:
- You have any kidney or liver disease.
- You have high blood potassium levels or low blood sodium levels.
- You are on any special diet using low salt or salt substitutes.
- You have diabetes.
- You have high cholesterol or heart disease.
- You are allergic to any medication, food or other substance.

Over age 60:
No special problems expected.

Pregnancy:
Usually safe, but decide with your doctor if drug benefits justify any possible risk to unborn child. Risk category B (see page xviii).

Breast-feeding:
It is unknown if drug passes into milk. Avoid nursing until you finish medicine. Consult doctor for advice on maintaining milk supply.

Infants & children:
Not approved for children under age 18.

Prolonged use:
- No special problems expected. Hypertension usually requires life-long treatment.
- Schedule regular doctor visits to determine if drug is continuing to be effective in controlling the hypertension and to check your potassium levels and kidney function.

Skin & sunlight:
No special problems expected.

Driving, piloting or hazardous work:
Use caution if you feel dizzy or are experiencing other side effects.

Discontinuing:
Don't discontinue without consulting your doctor, even if you feel well. You can have hypertension without feeling any symptoms. Untreated high blood pressure can cause serious problems.

Others:
- Advise any doctor or dentist whom you consult that you take this medicine. May interfere with the accuracy of some medical tests.
- See your doctor regularly, especially when you first start taking this drug.
- Follow any diet or exercise plan your doctor prescribes. It can help control hypertension.
- Get up slowly from a sitting or lying position to avoid any dizziness, faintness or lightheadedness.
- Can elevate triglycerides and cholesterol; these may need to be monitored regularly.
- Consult doctor if you become ill with vomiting or diarrhea.

POSSIBLE INTERACTION WITH OTHER DRUGS

GENERIC NAME OR DRUG CLASS	COMBINED EFFECT
Angiotensin-converting enzyme (ACE) inhibitors*	Decreased anti-hypertensive effect.
Angiotensin II receptor antagonists	Decreased anti-hypertensive effect.
Diuretics, potassium-sparing*	Excess potassium levels in the body.
Enzyme inhibitors*	Increased effect of eplerenone.
Potassium supplements*	Excess potassium levels in the body.
St. Johns Wort	Decreased antihypertensive effect.

POSSIBLE INTERACTION WITH OTHER SUBSTANCES

INTERACTS WITH	COMBINED EFFECT
Alcohol:	Increased risk of side effects. Avoid.
Beverages: Grapefruit juice.	Increased effect of eplerenone.
Cocaine:	Unknown effect. Avoid.
Foods: Salt substitutes containing potassium or foods high in potassium (e.g., bananas).	Excess potassium in the body. Avoid.
Marijuana:	Unknown effect. Avoid.
Tobacco:	None expected. Best to avoid.

ERECTILE DYSFUNCTION AGENTS

GENERIC AND BRAND NAMES

SILDENAFIL
Revatio
Viagra

TADALAFIL
Cialis
VARDENAFIL
Levitra

BASIC INFORMATION

Habit forming? No
Prescription needed? Yes
Available as generic? No
Drug class: Impotence therapy

 USES

- Treats male sexual function (erection) problems.
- The brand name Revatio is for treatment of pulmonary arterial hypertension (a rare fatal lung disorder).

 DOSAGE & USAGE INFORMATION

How to take:
Tablet—Swallow with water. If you can't swallow whole, crumble tablet and take with liquid or food.

When to take:
- Take about an hour before sexual activity (or as directed). Use only once daily.
- Daily dose tadalafil, take as directed on label.

If you forget a dose:
- Does not apply for the tablet taken before sexual activity.
- For once daily tadalafil, take as soon as you remember. If it is almost time for the next dose, wait for the next scheduled dose (don't double this dose).

Continued next column

 OVERDOSE

SYMPTOMS:
May include nausea, irregular heartbeat, chest pain, faintness, lightheadedness.
WHAT TO DO:
If person takes much larger amount than prescribed, dial 911 (emergency) for medical help or call poison control center 1-800-222-1222 for instructions.

What drug does:
- Increases blood flow to the penis that may help men develop and sustain an erection. Sexual stimulation is still needed for these drugs to be effective.
- In pulmonary arterial hypertension, the drug works by dilating (widening) blood vessels, thereby lowering blood pressure in the lungs.

Time lapse before drug works:
- Sildenafil, 30-60 minutes, lasts up to 4 hours.
- Vardenafil, 25-30 minutes, lasts up to 4-5 hours.
- Tadalafil, 16-60 minutes, lasts up to 36 hours.

Don't take with:
Any other medicine or any dietary supplement without consulting your doctor or pharmacist.

 POSSIBLE ADVERSE REACTIONS OR SIDE EFFECTS

SYMPTOMS	WHAT TO DO
Life-threatening: Fatalities have been reported when used with nitrate medications.	
Common: Headache, flushing, stomach upset, stuffy or runny nose, back pain, muscle aches.	Continue. Call doctor if symptoms persist.
Infrequent: • Urination problems, blurred vision, changes in color perception, light sensitivity, skin rash, dizziness, prolonged erection (lasting more than 4 hours).	Discontinue. Call doctor right away.
• Diarrhea, stuffy nose.	Continue. Call doctor if symptoms persist.
Rare: • Chest pain, fainting, foot or ankle swelling, allergic reaction, (shortness of breath, skin rash, hives, itching, face swelling), changes in hearing, ringing or buzzing in the ears.	Discontinue. Call doctor right away.
• Unexpected symptoms occur while having sexual intercourse.	Discontinue. Call doctor when convenient.

WARNINGS & PRECAUTIONS

Don't take if:
You are allergic to sildenafil, vardenafil, or tadalafil.

Before you start, consult your doctor if:
- You have any other medical problem.
- You have or have had heart, blood pressure or blood cell problems or have had a stroke.
- You have a stomach ulcer.
- You have vision problems.
- You have retinitis pigmentosa.
- You have a deformed shape of the penis or have had an erection last more than 4 hours.
- You use drugs like amyl nitrate or butyl nitrate recreationally.
- You have liver or kidney disease.

Over age 60:
No problems expected unless person has an increased sensitivity to medications.

Pregnancy:
Not indicated for use in females. Risk category B (see page xviii).

Breast-feeding:
Not indicated for use in females.

Infants & children:
Safety and effectiveness of use in children not established. Not recommended or indicated.

Prolonged use:
Talk to your doctor about the need for follow-up medical examinations or laboratory studies to determine drug's effectiveness.

Skin & sunlight:
No problems expected.

Driving, piloting or hazardous work:
No problems expected.

Discontinuing:
No problems expected.

Others:
- Advise any doctor or dentist whom you consult that you take this medicine.
- Do not increase dose without doctor's approval.
- Consult doctor if there are any significant changes in your vision. A small number of men taking one or more of these drugs have developed NAION (non-arteritic ischemic optic neuropathy) a loss of vision that is frequently irreversible. Ask your doctor about your risks.
- Do not combine the drug with any other impotence therapy unless approved by your doctor.
- These drugs do not protect against sexually transmitted diseases.
- There are many causes of impotence. Your doctor should perform a complete exam before prescribing this medication.

- Call doctor right away in the event of sudden decrease or loss of hearing. You may be also experience tinnitus (ringing/buzzing in the ears) and dizziness.

POSSIBLE INTERACTION WITH OTHER DRUGS

GENERIC NAME OR DRUG CLASS	COMBINED EFFECT
Alpha adrenergic receptor blockers	Sudden drop in blood pressure. Do not use together.
Enzyme inhibitors*	Increased effect of erectile dysfunction agent.
Protease inhibitors	Increased effect of erectile dysfunction agent.
Nitrates	Sudden drop in blood pressure. Do not use together.
Rifampin	Decreased effect of erectile dysfunction agent.

POSSIBLE INTERACTION WITH OTHER SUBSTANCES

INTERACTS WITH	COMBINED EFFECT
Alcohol:	May decrease effect of erectile dysfunction agents.
Beverages:	Grapefruit juice may increase blood levels of erectile dysfunction agents.
Cocaine:	Effects unknown. Avoid.
Foods:	None expected.
Marijuana:	Effects unknown. Avoid.
Tobacco:	None expected.

*See Glossary

ERGOLOID MESYLATES

BRAND NAMES

Gerimal
Hydergine

Hydergine LC
Niloric

BASIC INFORMATION

Habit forming? No
Prescription needed? Yes
Available as generic? Yes
Drug class: Ergot preparation

 USES

Treatment for reduced alertness, poor memory, confusion, depression or lack of motivation in the elderly.

 DOSAGE & USAGE INFORMATION

How to take:
* Tablet or capsule—Swallow with liquid. If you can't swallow whole, crumble tablet or open capsule and take with liquid or food.
* Liquid—Take as directed on label.
* Sublingual tablet—Dissolve tablet under tongue.

When to take:
At the same times each day.

If you forget a dose:
Take as soon as you remember up to 2 hours late. If more than 2 hours, wait for next scheduled dose (don't double this dose).

What drug does:
Stimulates brain-cell metabolism to increase use of oxygen and nutrients.

Time lapse before drug works:
Gradual improvements over 3 to 4 months.

Continued next column

 OVERDOSE

SYMPTOMS:
Headache, flushed face, nasal congestion, nausea, vomiting, blood pressure drop, blurred vision, weakness, collapse, coma.
WHAT TO DO:
* Dial 911 (emergency) for medical help or call poison control center 1-800-222-1222 for instructions.
* See emergency information on last 3 pages of this book.

Don't take with:
* Nonprescription drugs containing alcohol without consulting doctor.
* Any other medicine or any dietary supplement without consulting your doctor or pharmacist.

 POSSIBLE ADVERSE REACTIONS OR SIDE EFFECTS

SYMPTOMS	WHAT TO DO
Life-threatening:	
In case of overdose, see previous column.	
Common:	
Runny nose, skin flushing, headache.	Continue. Tell doctor at next visit.
Infrequent:	
Slow heartbeat, tingling fingers, blurred vision.	Discontinue. Call doctor right away.
Rare:	
• Fainting.	Discontinue. Seek emergency treatment.
• Rash, nausea, vomiting, stomach cramps, dizziness when getting up, drowsiness, soreness under tongue, appetite loss.	Continue. Call doctor when convenient.

358

WARNINGS & PRECAUTIONS

Don't use if:
- If you are allergic to any ergot preparation.
- Your heartbeat is less than 60 beats per minute.
- Your systolic blood pressure is consistently below 100.

Before you start, consult your doctor if:
- You have had low blood pressure.
- You have liver disease.
- You have severe mental illness.

Over age 60:
Primarily used in persons older than 60. Results unpredictable, but many patients show improved brain function.

Pregnancy:
Generally not used in this age group.

Breast-feeding:
Risk to nursing child outweighs drug benefits. Don't use.

Infants & children:
Not recommended.

Prolonged use:
Talk to your doctor about the need for follow-up medical examinations or laboratory studies.

Skin & sunlight:
No problems expected.

Driving, piloting or hazardous work:
Avoid if you feel dizzy, faint or have blurred vision. Otherwise, no problems expected.

Discontinuing:
No problems expected.

Others:
- May lessen your body's ability to adjust to cold temperatures.
- Advise any doctor or dentist whom you consult that you use this medicine.

POSSIBLE INTERACTION WITH OTHER DRUGS

GENERIC NAME OR DRUG CLASS	COMBINED EFFECT
Ergot preparations,* other	May cause serious side effects. Avoid.
Sympathomimetics*	May cause decreased circulation to arms, legs, feet and hands. Avoid.

POSSIBLE INTERACTION WITH OTHER SUBSTANCES

INTERACTS WITH	COMBINED EFFECT
Alcohol:	Use caution. May drop blood pressure excessively.
Beverages:	None expected.
Cocaine:	Overstimulation. Avoid.
Foods:	None expected.
Marijuana:	Decreased effect of ergot alkaloids.
Tobacco:	Decreased ergoloid effect. Don't smoke.

*See Glossary

ERGONOVINE

BRAND NAMES

Ergometrine   Ergotrate Maleate
Ergotrate

BASIC INFORMATION

Habit forming? No
Prescription needed? Yes
Available as generic? Yes
Drug class: Ergot preparation (uterine
   stimulant)

 ## USES

Retards excessive post-delivery bleeding.

 ## DOSAGE & USAGE INFORMATION

How to take:
Tablet—Swallow with liquid or food to lessen
stomach irritation.

When to take:
At the same times each day.

If you forget a dose:
Don't take missed dose and don't double next
one. Wait for next scheduled dose.

What drug does:
Causes smooth muscle cells of uterine wall to
contract and surround bleeding blood vessels of
relaxed uterus.

Time lapse before drug works:
20 to 30 minutes.

Don't take with:
Any other medicine or any dietary supplement
without consulting your doctor or pharmacist.

 ## OVERDOSE

SYMPTOMS:
**Vomiting, diarrhea, weak pulse, low blood
pressure, difficult breathing, angina,
convulsions.**
WHAT TO DO:
- **Dial 911 (emergency) for medical help or
  call poison control center 1-800-222-1222
  for instructions.**
- **If person is unconscious, check breathing
  and pulse. If not breathing, begin mouth-
  to-mouth rescue breathing. If heart is not
  beating, begin chest compressions.**
- **See emergency information on last 3 pages
  of this book.**

 ## POSSIBLE ADVERSE REACTIONS OR SIDE EFFECTS

SYMPTOMS	WHAT TO DO
Life-threatening: In case of overdose, see previous column.	
Common: Nausea, vomiting, severe lower abdominal menstrual-like cramps.	Discontinue. Call doctor right away.
Infrequent: • Confusion, ringing in ears, diarrhea, muscle cramps.	Discontinue. Call doctor right away.
• Unusual sweating.	Continue. Call doctor when convenient.
Rare: Sudden, severe headache; shortness of breath; chest pain; numb, cold hands and feet.	Discontinue. Seek emergency treatment.

WARNINGS & PRECAUTIONS

Don't take if:
You are allergic to any ergot preparation.

Before you start, consult your doctor if:
- You have coronary artery or blood vessel disease.
- You have liver or kidney disease.
- You have high blood pressure.
- You have postpartum infection.

Over age 60:
Not used in this age group.

Pregnancy:
Consult doctor.

Breast-feeding:
Drug passes into milk. Avoid drug or discontinue nursing until you finish medicine. Consult doctor for advice on maintaining milk supply.

Infants & children:
Not recommended.

Prolonged use:
Talk to your doctor about the need for follow-up medical examinations or laboratory studies to check blood pressure, ECG.*

Skin & sunlight:
No problems expected.

Driving, piloting or hazardous work:
No problems expected.

Discontinuing:
May be unnecessary to finish medicine. Follow doctor's instructions.

Others:
Drug should be used for short time only following childbirth or miscarriage.

POSSIBLE INTERACTION WITH OTHER DRUGS

GENERIC NAME OR DRUG CLASS	COMBINED EFFECT
Antifungals, azoles	Can cause serious or life-threatening problems with blood circulation. Avoid.
Beta-adrenergic blocking agents*	Possible vasospasm (peripheral and cardiac).
Ergot preparations,* other	May cause serious side effects. Avoid.
Macrolide antibiotics	Can cause serious or life-threatening problems with blood circulation. Avoid.
Protease Inhibitors	Can cause serious or life-threatening problems with blood circulation. Avoid.
Sympathomimetics*	May cause decreased circulation to arms, legs, feet and hands. Avoid.
Triptans	May cause serious side effects if taken within 24 hours of ergonovine.

POSSIBLE INTERACTION WITH OTHER SUBSTANCES

INTERACTS WITH	COMBINED EFFECT
Alcohol:	None expected.
Beverages:	None expected.
Cocaine:	None expected.
Foods:	None expected.
Marijuana:	None expected.
Tobacco:	Decreased ergonovine effect. Don't smoke.

ERGOTAMINE

BRAND NAMES

Cafergot	Ergostat
Cafergot-PB	Gotamine
Cafertine	Gynergen
Cafetrate	Medihaler
Ercaf	Ergotamine
Ergo-Caff	Migergot
Ergomar	Wigraine

BASIC INFORMATION

Habit forming? No
Prescription needed? Yes
Available as generic? Yes
**Drug class: Vasoconstrictor, ergot
    preparation**

 ## USES

Relieves pain of migraines and other headaches caused by dilated blood vessels. May be used to abort or prevent vascular headache.

 ## DOSAGE & USAGE INFORMATION

How to take:
- Tablet—Swallow with liquid. If you can't swallow whole, crumble tablet and take with liquid or food.
- Sublingual tablet—Don't swallow whole. Let dissolve under tongue. Don't eat or drink while tablet is dissolving.
- Suppository—Remove wrapper and moisten suppository with water. Gently insert larger end into rectum. Push well into rectum with finger.
- Aerosol inhaler—Use only as directed on prescription label.

Continued next column

 ## OVERDOSE

SYMPTOMS:
Tingling, cold extremities and muscle pain. Progresses to nausea, vomiting, diarrhea, cold skin, rapid and weak pulse, severe numbness of extremities, confusion, convulsions, coma.
WHAT TO DO:
- **Dial 911 (emergency) for medical help or call poison control center 1-800-222-1222 for instructions.**
- **See emergency information on last 3 pages of this book.**

When to take:
- At first sign of vascular or migraine headache.
- Lie down in quiet, dark room after taking.

If you forget a dose:
Take as soon as you remember. Wait 4 hours for next dose.

What drug does:
Constricts blood vessels in the head.

Time lapse before drug works:
30 to 60 minutes.

Don't take with:
Any other medicine or any dietary supplement without consulting your doctor or pharmacist.

 ## POSSIBLE ADVERSE REACTIONS OR SIDE EFFECTS

SYMPTOMS	WHAT TO DO
Life-threatening:	
In case of overdose, see previous column.	
Common:	
• Dizziness, nausea, diarrhea, vomiting, increased frequency or severity of headaches.	Continue. Call doctor when convenient.
• Feet and ankle swelling.	Discontinue. Call doctor right away.
Infrequent:	
Itchy or swollen skin; cold, pale hands or feet; pain or weakness in arms, legs, back.	Discontinue. Call doctor right away.
Rare:	
Anxiety or confusion; red or purple blisters, especially on hands, feet; change in vision; extreme thirst; stomach pain or bloating; unusually fast or slow heartbeat; chest pain; numbness or tingling in face, fingers, toes.	Discontinue. Call doctor right away.

WARNINGS & PRECAUTIONS

Don't take if:
You are allergic to any ergot preparation.

Before you start, consult your doctor if:
- You plan to become pregnant within medication period.
- You have an infection.
- You have angina, heart problems, high blood pressure, hardening of the arteries or vein problems.
- You have kidney or liver disease.
- You are allergic to other spray inhalants.

Over age 60:
Adverse reactions and side effects may be more frequent and severe than in younger persons.

Pregnancy:
Risk to unborn child outweighs drug benefits. Don't use. Risk category X (see page xviii).

Breast-feeding:
Drug filters into milk. May harm child. Avoid.

Infants & children:
Studies inconclusive on use in children. Consult your doctor.

Prolonged use:
Cold skin, muscle pain, gangrene of hands and feet. This medicine not intended for uninterrupted use.

Skin & sunlight:
No problems expected.

Driving, piloting or hazardous work:
Don't drive or pilot aircraft until you learn how medicine affects you. Don't work around dangerous machinery. Don't climb ladders or work in high places. Danger increases if you drink alcohol or take medicine affecting alertness and reflexes, such as antihistamines, tranquilizers, sedatives, pain medicine, narcotics and mind-altering drugs.

Discontinuing:
May be unnecessary to finish medicine. Follow doctor's instructions.

Others:
- Impaired blood circulation can lead to gangrene in intestines or extremities. Never exceed recommended dose.
- May affect results in some medical tests.

POSSIBLE INTERACTION WITH OTHER DRUGS

GENERIC NAME OR DRUG CLASS	COMBINED EFFECT
Amphetamines*	Dangerous blood pressure rise.
Beta-adrenergic blocking agents*	Narrowed arteries in heart if ergotamine is taken in high doses.
Ephedrine	Dangerous blood pressure rise.
Epinephrine	Dangerous blood pressure rise.
Ergot preparations, other	May cause decreased circulation to arms, legs, feet and hands. Avoid.
Erythromycin	Decreased ergotamine effect.
Nitroglycerin	Decreased nitroglycerin effect.
Pseudoephedrine	Dangerous blood pressure rise.
Sumatriptan	Increased vasoconstriction. Delay 24 hours between drugs.
Sympathomimetics*	May cause decreased circulation to arms, legs, feet and hands. Avoid.
Troleandomycin	Decreased ergotamine effect.

POSSIBLE INTERACTION WITH OTHER SUBSTANCES

INTERACTS WITH	COMBINED EFFECT
Alcohol:	Dilates blood vessels. Makes headache worse.
Beverages: Caffeine drinks.	May help relieve headache.
Cocaine:	Decreased ergotamine effect.
Foods: Any to which you are allergic.	May make headache worse. Avoid.
Marijuana:	Occasional use— Cool extremities. Regular use— Persistent chill.
Tobacco:	Decreased effect of ergotamine. Makes headache worse.

*See Glossary

ERYTHROMYCINS

GENERIC AND BRAND NAMES

See full list of generic and brand names in the *Generic and Brand Name Directory*, page 885.

BASIC INFORMATION

Habit forming? No
Prescription needed? Yes
Available as generic? Yes
Drug class: Antibacterial; antiacne agent

 USES

- Treatment of a variety of bacterial infections.
- Treatment for acne.
- May be used to treat other disorders as determined by your doctor.

 DOSAGE & USAGE INFORMATION

How to take:

- Tablet or capsule—Swallow with liquid. You may chew or crush.
- Extended-release tablet or capsule—Swallow each dose whole.
- Oral suspension or pediatric drop—Shake well before using. Use dropper supplied with prescription or use a special measuring device to measure dose.
- Chewable tablet—Crush or chew completely and then swallow.

When to take:
At the same times each day, 1 hour before or 2 hours after eating. May be taken with food if stomach upset occurs. Enteric-coated tablets may be taken with or without food.

If you forget a dose:
Take as soon as you remember. If it is almost time for the next dose, wait for that dose (don't double this dose) and resume regular schedule.

Continued next column

 OVERDOSE

SYMPTOMS:
Nausea, vomiting, abdominal discomfort, diarrhea.
WHAT TO DO:
Overdose unlikely to threaten life. If person uses much larger amount than prescribed or if accidentally swallowed, call doctor or poison control center 1-800-222-1222 for help.

What drug does:
Prevents growth and reproduction of susceptible bacteria.

Time lapse before drug works:
Depends on the type of infection or acne symptoms; may take 7-21 days or longer.

Don't take with:
Any other medicine or any dietary supplement without consulting your doctor or pharmacist.

 POSSIBLE ADVERSE REACTIONS OR SIDE EFFECTS

SYMPTOMS	WHAT TO DO
Life-threatening: None expected.	
Common: Mild nausea.	Continue. Call doctor when convenient.
Infrequent:	
• Mild diarrhea, stomach cramps or vomiting, sore mouth or tongue or have white patches.	Continue. Call doctor when convenient.
• Fever with severe nausea and vomiting, severe stomach pain, unusual tiredness or weakness, yellow eyes or skin, pale stools, skin rash (redness and itching).	Discontinue. Call doctor right away.
Rare: Irregular or slow heartbeat, any hearing loss, fainting.	Discontinue. Call doctor right away.

364

WARNINGS & PRECAUTIONS

Don't take if:
You are allergic to any erythromycin or macrolide antibiotics.

Before you start, consult your doctor if:
* You have had liver disease or impaired liver function or stomach problems.
* You have a hearing loss.
* You have a history of heart rhythm problems.

Over age 60:
You may have increased risk of hearing loss.

Pregnancy:
Decide with your doctor if drug benefits justify risk to unborn child. Risk category B (see page xviii).

Breast-feeding:
Drug passes into milk. Avoid drug or discontinue nursing until you finish medicine. Consult doctor for advice on maintaining milk supply.

Infants & children:
Use only under close medical supervision.

Prolonged use:
* You may become more susceptible to infections caused by germs not responsive to erythromycin.
* Talk to your doctor about the need for follow-up medical examinations or laboratory studies to check liver function.

Skin & sunlight:
No problems expected.

Driving, piloting or hazardous work:
No problems expected.

Discontinuing:
Don't discontinue without doctor's advice until you complete prescribed dose, even though symptoms diminish or disappear.

Others:
* Advise any doctor or dentist whom you consult that you take this medicine.
* If infection symptoms don't start to improve in a few days or they worsen, call your doctor.

POSSIBLE INTERACTION WITH OTHER DRUGS

GENERIC NAME OR DRUG CLASS	COMBINED EFFECT
Benzodiazepines*	Increased effect of benzodiazepine.
Carbamazepine	Increased effect of carbamazepine.
Chloramphenicol	Decreased effect of chloramphenicol.
Cyclosporine	May increase cyclosporin toxicity.
Digoxins*	Increased effect of digoxin.
Enzyme inhibitors*	Increased effect of erythromycin. Avoid.
Hepatotoxics*	Increased risk of liver problems.
HMG-CoA reductase inhibitors	Increased risk of muscle and kidney problems (with lovastatin).
Leukotriene modifiers	Decreased effect of zafirlukast.
Lincomycins*	Decreased lincomycin effect.
Penicillins*	Decreased penicillin effect.
Sibutramine	Increased effect of sibutramine.
Sildenafil	Increased effect of sildenafil.
Xanthines*	Increased effect of xanthine.
Warfarin	Increased risk of bleeding.

POSSIBLE INTERACTION WITH OTHER SUBSTANCES

INTERACTS WITH	COMBINED EFFECT
Alcohol:	Possible liver damage. Avoid.
Beverages: Grapefruit juice.	May increase effect of erythromycin.
Cocaine:	None expected.
Foods: Grapefruit.	May increase effect of erythromycin.
Marijuana:	None expected.
Tobacco:	None expected.

*See Glossary

ESTRAMUSTINE

BRAND NAMES

Emcyt

BASIC INFORMATION

Habit forming? No
Prescription needed? Yes
Available as generic? No
Drug class: Antineoplastic

 USES

Treats prostate cancer.

 DOSAGE & USAGE INFORMATION

How to take:
Capsule—Swallow with liquid. If you can't swallow whole, open capsule and take with liquid or food. Instructions to take on empty stomach mean 1 hour before or 2 hours after eating.

When to take:
According to doctor's instructions. Try to take 1 hour before or 2 hours after eating or drinking any milk products.

If you forget a dose:
If it is almost time for the next dose, wait for the next scheduled dose (don't double this dose).

What drug does:
Suppresses growth of cancer cells.

Time lapse before drug works:
Within 20 hours.

Don't take with:
Any other medicines (including over-the-counter drugs such as cough and cold medicines, laxatives, antacids, diet pills, caffeine, nose drops or vitamins) without consulting your doctor or pharmacist.

 OVERDOSE

SYMPTOMS:
None expected.
WHAT TO DO:
Overdose unlikely to threaten life. If person uses much larger amount than prescribed or if accidentally swallowed, call doctor or poison control center 1-800-222-1222 for help.

 POSSIBLE ADVERSE REACTIONS OR SIDE EFFECTS

SYMPTOMS	WHAT TO DO
Life-threatening: Sudden headaches, chest pain, shortness of breath, leg pain, vision changes, slurred speech.	Seek emergency treatment immediately.
Common: • Skin rash, itching.	Discontinue. Call doctor right away.
• Increased sun sensitivity.	Decrease sun exposure. Call doctor when convenient.
• Diarrhea, dizziness, nausea, vomiting, headache, swelling in hands or feet.	Continue. Call doctor when convenient.
Infrequent: • Joint or muscle pain, difficulty swallowing, sore throat and fever, peeling skin, jaundice.	Discontinue. Call doctor right away.
• Mouth or tongue irritation, breast tenderness or enlargement, decreased interest in sex.	Continue. Call doctor when convenient.
Rare: Bloody urine, hearing loss, back pain, abdominal pain.	Discontinue. Call doctor right away.

WARNINGS & PRECAUTIONS

Don't take if:
* You are allergic to estramustine, estrogens or mechlorethamine. (Estramustine is a combination of an estrogen and mechlorethamine.)
* You have active thromboembolic disorder.

Before you start, consult your doctor if:
* You have jaundice or hepatitis.
* You have history of thrombophlebitis or blood clots.
* You have an ulcer.
* You have asthma.
* You have epilepsy.
* You have bone disease or depressed bone marrow.
* You have kidney or gallbladder disease.
* You have mental depression.
* You suffer from migraine headaches.
* You have or recently had chicken pox.
* You have shingles (herpes zoster).
* You have had a recent heart attack or stroke or have heart or blood vessel disease.

Over age 60:
Adverse reactions and side effects may be more frequent and severe than in younger persons. You may need smaller doses for shorter periods of time.

Pregnancy:
Used in men only. If a male is taking this drug at the time of conception, there may be a risk of birth defects.

Breast-feeding:
Used in men only.

Infants & children:
Not used in this age group.

Prolonged use:
* Talk to your doctor about the need for follow-up medical examinations or laboratory studies to check complete blood counts (white blood cell count, platelet count, red blood cell count, hemoglobin, hematocrit), blood pressure, liver function, serum acid, serum calcium and alkaline phosphatase.
* The drug may cause permanent sterility after it has been taken for a while. Discuss with your doctor any future plans you have for having children.

Skin & sunlight:
No problems expected.

Driving, piloting or hazardous work:
No problems expected.

Discontinuing:
No problems expected.

Others:
* Advise any doctor or dentist whom you consult that you take this medicine.
* May affect results in some medical tests.
* May decrease sperm count in males.
* Do not get any immunizations (vaccinations) while taking this drug unless approved by your doctor.
* Persons in your household should not take an oral polio vaccine while you are taking this drug. They could pass the polio virus on to you. Avoid any persons who have recently taken oral polio vaccine.

POSSIBLE INTERACTION WITH OTHER DRUGS

GENERIC NAME OR DRUG CLASS	COMBINED EFFECT
Adrenocorticoids, systemic	Increased effect of adrenocorticoid.
Calcium supplements*	Decreased absorption of estramustine.
Hepatotoxic medications*	Increased risk of liver toxicity.
Vaccines (killed virus)	Decreased vaccine effect.

POSSIBLE INTERACTION WITH OTHER SUBSTANCES

INTERACTS WITH	COMBINED EFFECT
Alcohol:	Increased "hangover effect" and other gastrointestinal symptoms.
Beverages: Milk and milk products.	Decreased absorption of estramustine. Take drug 1 hour before or 2 hours after milk product.
Cocaine:	None expected.
Foods: Foods high in calcium.	Decreased absorption of estramustine. Take drug 1 hour before or 2 hours after milk product.
Marijuana:	None expected.
Tobacco:	Increased risk of heart attack and blood clots.

*See Glossary

ESTROGENS

GENERIC AND BRAND NAMES

See full list of generic and brand names in *Generic and Brand Name Directory*, page 885.

BASIC INFORMATION

Habit forming? No
Prescription needed? Yes
Available as generic? Yes
Drug class: Female sex hormone (estrogen)

 ## USES

- Treatment for estrogen deficiency.
- Treatment for symptoms of menopause and menstrual cycle irregularity.
- Treatment for estrogen-deficiency osteoporosis (bone softening from calcium loss).
- Treatment for vulvar or vaginal atrophy.
- Treatment for breast or prostate cancer.

 ## DOSAGE & USAGE INFORMATION

How to take:
- Tablet or capsule—Take with or after food to reduce nausea. Swallow with liquid. If you can't swallow whole, crumble tablet or open capsule and take with liquid or food.
- Vaginal cream or suppository—Use as directed on label.
- Gel or emulsion—Apply to skin as directed on product's label.
- Injection—Given by medical professional.
- Transdermal patch or transdermal spray— Follow label instructions.
- Vaginal insert—Follow label instructions.

When to take:
- Oral estrogen—Take at the same time each day.
- Other forms—Follow label instructions for correct dosage schedule.

Continued next column

 ## OVERDOSE

SYMPTOMS:
Nausea, vomiting, fluid retention, breast enlargement and discomfort, abnormal vaginal bleeding, headache, drowsiness.
WHAT TO DO:
Overdose unlikely to threaten life. If person uses much larger amount than prescribed or if accidentally swallowed, call doctor or poison control center 1-800-222-1222 for help.

If you forget a dose:
For oral dosage, take as soon as you remember. If it is almost time for the next dose, wait for the next scheduled dose (don't double this dose). For other forms, follow label instructions.

What drug does:
- Increases estrogen levels in the body.
- Combined with progestins for contraception.

Time lapse before drug works:
10 to 20 days.

Don't take with:
Any other medicine or any dietary supplement without consulting your doctor or pharmacist.

 ## POSSIBLE ADVERSE REACTIONS OR SIDE EFFECTS

SYMPTOMS	WHAT TO DO
Life-threatening: Profuse bleeding.	Seek emergency treatment.
Common:	
• Painful or swollen breasts, swollen feet or ankles, rapid weight gain.	Discontinue. Call doctor right away.
• Appetite loss, nausea, stomach, cramps or bloating, skin irritation in patch or spray users.	Continue. Call doctor when convenient.
Infrequent:	
• Breast lumps or discharge, changes in vaginal bleeding (more, less, spotting, prolonged), migraine headache.	Continue, but call doctor right away.
• Dizziness, contact lens intolerance, vomiting, mild diarrhea, headache, increased or decreased sexual desire, slow weight gain, other unusual symptoms.	Continue. Call doctor when convenient.
Rare:	
• Stomach or side pain, joint or muscle pain, jaundice (yellow skin or eyes).	Discontinue. Call doctor right away.
• Blood clots (severe or sudden headache, severe pain in calf or chest or other body parts, shortness of breath, slurred speech, weakness or numbness, sudden vision changes).	Discontinue. Seek emergency help.

WARNINGS & PRECAUTIONS

Don't take if:
You are allergic to any estrogen-containing drugs.

Before you start, consult your doctor if:
* You have or have had cancer of the breast or reproductive organs, fibrocystic breast disease, fibroid tumors of the uterus or endometriosis, unexplained vaginal bleeding.
* You have migraine headaches, epilepsy or porphyria.
* You have had blood clots, stroke, high blood pressure, congestive heart failure or heart attack.
* You have diabetes, asthma, kidney, liver or gallbladder disease.
* You plan to become pregnant within 3 months.

Over age 60:
Controversial. You and your doctor must decide if risks of drug outweigh benefits.

Pregnancy:
Risk to unborn child outweighs benefits of drug. Don't use. Risk category X (see page xviii).

Breast-feeding:
Drug filters into milk. Consult doctor.

Infants & children:
Not recommended.

Prolonged use:
* Increased growth of fibroid tumors of uterus.
* Talk to your doctor about the need for follow-up medical examinations or laboratory studies to check for drug's effectiveness.

Skin & sunlight:
One or more drugs in this group may cause rash or intensify sunburn in areas exposed to sun or ultraviolet light (photosensitivity reaction). Avoid overexposure. Notify doctor if reaction occurs.

Driving, piloting or hazardous work:
No problems expected.

Discontinuing:
Consult your doctor before discontinuing.

Others:
* For postmenopausal women, the use of hormone replacement therapy (HRT) which combines estrogen and progestin increases slightly the risk for breast cancer, heart attacks and stroke. HRT does not prevent heart disease. HRT is effective for menopause symptoms (used short term), and helps protect against osteoporosis and colon cancer. Other treatments are available for osteoporosis. Discuss with your doctor if HRT is the right treatment for you.
* May interfere with the accuracy of some medical tests.

* Carefully read the paper called "Information for the Patient" that was given to you with your first prescription or a refill. If you lose it, ask your pharmacist for a copy.
* Advise any doctor or dentist whom you consult that you take this medicine.

POSSIBLE INTERACTION WITH OTHER DRUGS

GENERIC NAME OR DRUG CLASS	COMBINED EFFECT
Adrenocorticoids	Increased effect of adrenocorticoid.
Anticoagulants, oral*	Decreased anti-coagulant effect.
Anticonvulsants, hydantoin*	Decreased estrogen effect.
Antidepressants, tricyclic*	Increased toxicity of antidepressants.
Antidiabetics, oral*	Unpredictable increase or decrease in blood sugar.
Antivirals, HIV/AIDS*	Increased risk of pancreatitis.
Bromocriptine	May need to adjust bromocriptine dose.
Cyclosporine	Increased effect of cyclosporine.
Hepatotoxics*	Increased risk of liver problems.
Tamoxifen	Decreased effect of tamoxifen.

POSSIBLE INTERACTION WITH OTHER SUBSTANCES

INTERACTS WITH	COMBINED EFFECT
Alcohol:	None expected.
Beverages: Grapefruit juice.	Possible increased estrogen effect.
Cocaine:	None expected.
Foods:	None expected.
Marijuana:	Possible menstrual irregularities and bleeding between periods.
Tobacco:	Increased risk of blood clots leading to stroke or heart attack.

*See Glossary

ESZOPICLONE

BRAND NAMES

Lunesta

BASIC INFORMATION

Habit forming? Yes
Prescription needed? Yes
Available as generic? No
Drug class: Sedative-hypnotic agent

 ## USES

Treatment for insomnia symptoms such as trouble falling asleep, waking up too often during the night and waking up too early in the morning.

 ## DOSAGE & USAGE INFORMATION

How to take:
Tablet—Swallow whole with liquid.

When to take:
Take immediately before bedtime. For best results do not take with or right after a heavy meal.

If you forget a dose:
Take as soon as you remember. Take drug only when you are able to get 7 hours of sleep before your daily activity begins. Do not exceed prescribed dosage.

What drug does:
The exact mechanism is not known. Acts as a central nervous system depressant which helps decrease sleep problems.

Time lapse before drug works:
Usually within 1 hour. The sleep-inducing affect should last for 6 to 8 hours.

Don't take with:
Any other medicine or any dietary supplement without consulting your doctor or pharmacist.

 ## OVERDOSE

SYMPTOMS:
Drowsiness, weakness, stupor (not able to respond), coma.
WHAT TO DO:
• Dial 911 (emergency) for medical help or call poison control center 1-800-222-1222 for instructions.
• See emergency information on last 3 pages of this book.

 ## POSSIBLE ADVERSE REACTIONS OR SIDE EFFECTS

SYMPTOMS	WHAT TO DO
Life-threatening: Rare allergic reaction—may have hives, rash, itching, swelling, trouble breathing, wheezing, chest pain, dizziness, faintness.	Seek emergency treatment immediately.
Common: Headache, unpleasant taste, drowsiness in the daytime, dizziness.	Continue. Call doctor when convenient.
Infrequent: Indigestion, nausea, nervousness, dry mouth, diarrhea, depression, cold-like symptoms or infection, problems with coordination, lightheadedness, anxiety.	Continue. Call doctor when convenient.
Rare: • Behavioral changes, (agitation, confusion, aggressiveness, suicidal thoughts, other bizarre behaviors), hallucinations, chest pain, swelling of arms or legs, enlarged breasts in men, depression worsens, painful menstruation, sleep-related behaviors.*	Discontinue. Call doctor right away.
• Memory problems (may occur if you wake before the effect of drug is gone), any other symptoms occur that cause concern (they may be due to the drug, an underlying disorder or the effects of lack of sleep).	Continue. Call doctor when convenient.

WARNINGS & PRECAUTIONS

Don't take if:
You are allergic to eszopiclone or zopiclone.

Before you start, consult your doctor if:
- You have respiratory problems.
- You have liver disease.
- You suffer from depression or psychiatric disorder.
- You are an active or recovering alcoholic or drug or substance abuser.

Over age 60:
Side effects may be more frequent and severe than in younger persons. You may need smaller doses for shorter periods of time.

Pregnancy:
Decide with your doctor if drug benefits justify any possible risk to unborn child. Risk category C (see page xviii).

Breast-feeding:
It is unknown if drug passes into milk. Avoid drug or discontinue nursing until you finish medicine. Consult doctor for advice on maintaining milk supply.

Infants & children:
Safety and effectiveness for children under age 18 has not been established.

Prolonged use:
You and your doctor will decide if there is a need to take the drug for prolonged period for chronic insomnia (insomnia at least three nights a week for a period of one month or longer).

Skin & sunlight:
No special problems expected.

Driving, piloting or hazardous work:
Don't drive or pilot aircraft until you learn how medicine affects you. Don't work around dangerous machinery. Don't climb ladders or work in high places. Danger increases if you drink alcohol or take other medicines affecting alertness and reflexes.

Discontinuing:
- Don't discontinue without consulting doctor. Dose may require gradual reduction if you have taken drug for a long time.
- You may have sleeping problems for 1 or 2 nights after stopping drug.
- Withdrawal symptoms may occur after you stop the drug. Consult your doctor if any emotional or physical symptoms do occur.

Others:
- Advise any doctor or dentist whom you consult that you take this medicine.
- Don't take drug if you are traveling on an overnight airplane trip of less than 7 or 8 hours. A temporary memory loss may occur (called traveler's amnesia).

POSSIBLE INTERACTION WITH OTHER DRUGS

GENERIC NAME OR DRUG CLASS	COMBINED EFFECT
Central nervous system (CNS) depressants*	Increased sedative effect.
Enzyme inducers*	Decreased effect of eszopiclone.
Enzyme inhibitors*	Increased effect of eszopiclone.
Ketoconazole	Increased effect of eszopiclone.
Olanzapine	Decreased alertness.

POSSIBLE INTERACTION WITH OTHER SUBSTANCES

INTERACTS WITH	COMBINED EFFECT
Alcohol:	Increased sedation. Avoid.
Beverages:	None expected.
Cocaine:	Unknown. Avoid.
Foods:	Decreased drug effect if taken with a heavy meal.
Marijuana:	Unknown. Avoid.
Tobacco:	None expected.

*See Glossary

ETHIONAMIDE

BRAND NAMES

Trecator

 ## BASIC INFORMATION

Habit forming? No
Prescription needed? Yes
Available as generic? No
Drug class: Antimycobacterial
(antituberculosis)

 ## USES

Treats tuberculosis. Used in combination with other antituberculosis drugs such as isoniazid, streptomycin, rifampin, ethambutol.

 ## DOSAGE & USAGE INFORMATION

How to take:
Tablet—Swallow with liquid or food to lessen stomach irritation. If you can't swallow whole, crumble tablet and take with liquid or food.

When to take:
Usually every 8 to 12 hours, with or after meals.

If you forget a dose:
Take as soon as you remember up to 2 hours late. If more than 2 hours, wait for next scheduled dose. Don't double this dose.

What drug does:
Kills germs that cause tuberculosis.

Time lapse before drug works:
Within 3 hours.

Don't take with:
Any other medicine or any dietary supplement without consulting your doctor or pharmacist.

☠ OVERDOSE

SYMPTOMS:
None expected.
WHAT TO DO:
Overdose unlikely to threaten life. If person uses much larger amount than prescribed or if accidentally swallowed, call doctor or poison control center 1-800-222-1222 for help.

 ## POSSIBLE ADVERSE REACTIONS OR SIDE EFFECTS

SYMPTOMS	WHAT TO DO
Life-threatening: None expected.	
Common:	
• Vomiting.	Discontinue. Call doctor right away.
• Dizziness, sore mouth, nausea, metallic taste.	Continue. Call doctor when convenient.
Infrequent: Jaundice (yellow eyes and skin); numbness, tingling, pain in hands or feet; depression; confusion.	Discontinue. Call doctor right away.
Rare:	
• Hunger, shakiness, rapid heartbeat, blurred vision or other changes in vision, skin rash.	Discontinue. Call doctor right away.
• Gradual swelling in the neck (thyroid gland).	Continue. Call doctor when convenient.
• Enlargement of breasts (male).	No action necessary.

ETHIONAMIDE

WARNINGS & PRECAUTIONS

Don't take if:
You know you are hypersensitive to ethionamide.

Before you start, consult your doctor if:
• You have diabetes.
• You have liver disease.

Over age 60:
No information available.

Pregnancy:
Decide with your doctor if drug benefits justify risk to unborn child. Risk category C (see page xviii).

Breast-feeding:
Effect not documented. Consult your family doctor or pediatrician.

Infants & children:
Effect not documented. Consult your family doctor or pediatrician.

Prolonged use:
No special problems expected.

Skin & sunlight:
No special problems expected.

Driving, piloting or hazardous work:
Don't drive or pilot aircraft until you learn how medicine affects you. Don't work around dangerous machinery. Don't climb ladders or work in high places. Danger increases if you drink alcohol or take medicine affecting alertness and reflexes.

Discontinuing:
Don't discontinue without consulting doctor.

Others:
• Advise any doctor or dentist whom you consult that you take this medicine.
• Request occasional laboratory studies for liver function.
• Request occasional eye examinations.
• Treatment may take months or years.
• You should take pyridoxine (vitamin B-6) supplements while taking ethionamide.

POSSIBLE INTERACTION WITH OTHER DRUGS

GENERIC NAME OR DRUG CLASS	COMBINED EFFECT
Antivirals, HIV/AIDS*	Increased risk of peripheral neuropathy.
Cycloserine	Increased risk of seizures.
Pyridoxine	Increased excretion by kidney. (Should take pyridoxine supplements while on ethionamide to prevent development of neuritis in feet and hands).

POSSIBLE INTERACTION WITH OTHER SUBSTANCES

INTERACTS WITH	COMBINED EFFECT
Alcohol:	Increased incidence of liver diseases.
Beverages: Any alcoholic beverage.	Increased incidence of liver diseases.
Cocaine:	None expected.
Foods:	None expected.
Marijuana:	No interaction expected, but may slow body's recovery.
Tobacco:	No interaction expected, but may slow body's recovery.

*See Glossary

373

ETOPOSIDE

BRAND NAMES

VePesid   **VP-16**

BASIC INFORMATION

Habit forming? No
Prescription needed? Yes
Available as generic? No
Drug class: Antineoplastic

 ## USES

- Treats testicular, lung and bladder cancer.
- Treats Hodgkin's disease and some other forms of cancer.

 ## DOSAGE & USAGE INFORMATION

How to take:
- Capsule—Swallow with liquid. If you can't swallow whole, open capsule and take with liquid or food. Instructions to take on empty stomach mean 1 hour before or 2 hours after eating.
- Injection—Given under doctor's supervision.

When to take:
According to your doctor's instructions.

If you forget a dose:
Skip this dose. Never double dose. Resume regular schedule.

What drug does:
Inhibits DNA in cancer cells.

Time lapse before drug works:
Unpredictable.

Don't take with:
Any other medicines (including over-the-counter drugs such as cough and cold medicines, laxatives, antacids, diet pills, caffeine, nose drops or vitamins) without consulting your doctor or pharmacist.

 ## OVERDOSE

SYMPTOMS:
Rapid pulse, shortness of breath, wheezing, fainting, coma.
WHAT TO DO:
- Dial 911 (emergency) for medical help or call poison control center 1-800-222-1222 for instructions.
- See emergency information on last 3 pages of this book.

 ## POSSIBLE ADVERSE REACTIONS OR SIDE EFFECTS

SYMPTOMS	WHAT TO DO
Life-threatening:	
In case of overdose, see previous column.	
Common:	
• Appetite loss, nausea, vomiting.	Continue. Call doctor when convenient.
• Loss of hair.	No action necessary.
Infrequent:	
Symptoms of low white blood cell count and low platelet count: black, tarry stools; bloody urine; cough; chills or fever; low back pain; bruising.	Discontinue. Call doctor right away.
Rare:	
Mouth sores.	Continue. Call doctor when convenient.

WARNINGS & PRECAUTIONS

Don't take if:
• You have chicken pox.
• You have shingles (herpes zoster).

Before you start, consult your doctor if:
You have liver or kidney disease.

Over age 60:
No special problems expected.

Pregnancy:
Risk to unborn child outweighs drug benefits. Don't use. Risk category D (see page xviii).

Breast-feeding:
Drug passes into milk. Avoid drug or discontinue nursing until you finish medicine. Consult doctor for advice on maintaining milk supply.

Infants & children:
Effect not documented. Consult your doctor.

Prolonged use:
• Talk to your doctor about the need for follow-up medical examinations or laboratory studies to check complete blood counts (white blood cell count, platelet count, red blood cell count, hemoglobin, hematocrit).
• Check mouth frequently for ulcers.

Skin & sunlight:
No problems expected.

Driving, piloting or hazardous work:
Avoid if you feel confused, drowsy or dizzy.

Discontinuing:
May still experience symptoms of bone marrow depression, such as: blood in stools, fever or chills, blood spots under the skin, back pain, hoarseness, bloody urine. If any of these occur, call your doctor right away.

Others:
• Advise any doctor or dentist whom you consult that you take this medicine.
• May affect results in some medical tests.
• Etoposide may be used in combinations with other antineoplastic treatment plans. The incidence and severity of side effects may be different when used in combinations such as doxorubicin, procarbazine and etoposide (APE); etoposide, cyclophosphamide, doxorubicin and vincristine (CAVE, ECHO, CAPO, EVAC or VOCA); cyclophosphamide, doxorubicin and etoposide (CAE or ACE); cisplatin, bleomycin, doxorubicin and etoposide; cisplatin, bleomycin and etoposide; cisplatin and etoposide. For further information regarding these combinations, consult your doctor.

POSSIBLE INTERACTION WITH OTHER DRUGS

GENERIC NAME OR DRUG CLASS	COMBINED EFFECT
Angiotensin-converting enzyme (ACE) inhibitors*	May increase bone marrow depression or make kidney damage more likely.
Antineoplastic (cancer-treating) drugs*	May increase bone marrow depression or make kidney damage more likely.
Clozapine	Toxic effect on bone marrow.
Tiopronin	Increased risk of toxicity to bone marrow.
Vaccines, live or killed virus	Increased likelihood of toxicity or reduced effectiveness of vaccine. Wait 3 months to 1 year after etoposide treatment before getting vaccine.

POSSIBLE INTERACTION WITH OTHER SUBSTANCES

INTERACTS WITH	COMBINED EFFECT
Alcohol:	Increased likelihood of adverse reactions. Avoid.
Beverages: Grapefruit juice.	Decreased effect of etoposide. Avoid.
Cocaine:	Increased likelihood of adverse reactions. Avoid.
Foods:	None expected.
Marijuana:	Increased likelihood of adverse reactions. Avoid.
Tobacco:	None expected.

*See Glossary

EXENATIDE

BRAND NAMES

Byetta

BASIC INFORMATION

Habit forming? No
Prescription needed? Yes
Available as generic? No
Drug class: Antidiabetic; incretin mimetic

 USES

Used in combination with other antidiabetic agents to control blood sugar levels in adults who have type 2 diabetes.

 DOSAGE & USAGE INFORMATION

How to take:
Self injection—Injected under the skin (subcutaneous) of the upper leg (thigh), stomach area (abdomen), or upper arm. The drug comes in a prefilled pen that is used with a small needle. Read and follow the instructions provided with the prescription.

When to take:
Inject it twice a day, at any time within the 60 minutes before the morning and evening meals. Do not inject the drug after eating the meal.

If you forget a dose:
If you forget to inject the dose before you start eating a meal, skip that dose and then inject the next dose as scheduled. Don't double that dose.

Continued next column

 OVERDOSE

SYMPTOMS:
Low blood sugar (hypoglycemia)—See list of symptoms in next column under Infrequent.
WHAT TO DO:
- Eat some type of sugar immediately, such as glucose product, orange juice (add some sugar), nondiet sodas, candy (such as 5 Lifesavers), honey.
- If patient loses consciousness, give glucagon if you have it and know how to use it.
- Dial 911 (emergency) for medical help or call poison control center 1-800-222-1222 for instructions.
- See emergency information on last 3 pages of this book.

What drug does:
- Helps the pancreas produce insulin in response to rising blood sugar levels, inhibits the liver's production of sugar, reduces the rate at which sugar enters the bloodstream by slowing the release of food from the stomach.
- It appears to decrease appetite, which may lead to weight loss.

Time lapse before drug works:
The effects begin right after it is injected.

Don't take with:
Any other medicine or any dietary supplement without consulting your doctor or pharmacist.

 POSSIBLE ADVERSE REACTIONS OR SIDE EFFECTS

SYMPTOMS	WHAT TO DO
Life-threatening:	
Allergic reaction (difficulty breathing, closing of the throat, swelling of the lips or face or tongue, hives).	Seek emergency treatment immediately.
Common:	
Nausea.	Continue. Call doctor if symptom persists.
Infrequent:	
• Stomach symptoms (acid, sour, upset, pain), belching, diarrhea, dizziness, jittery feeling, headache, heartburn, appetite decreased, increased sweating, lack or loss of strength.	Continue. Call doctor when convenient.
• Symptoms of low blood sugar— nervousness, hunger (excessive), cold sweats, rapid pulse, anxiety, cold skin, chills, confusion, drowsiness, loss of concentration, headache, nausea, weakness, shakiness, vision changes.	Seek treatment (eat some form of quick-acting sugar— glucose tablets, sugar, fruit juice, corn syrup, honey).
• Symptoms of high blood sugar— increased urination, unusual thirst, dry mouth, drowsiness, flushed or dry skin, fruit-like breath odor, appetite loss, stomach pain or vomiting, tiredness, trouble breathing, increased blood sugar level.	Check your blood sugar immediately. Call doctor right away.

Rare:

• Abdominal pain (persistent, severe, with or without vomiting).	Discontinue. Call doctor right away.
• Other symptoms that cause concern.	Continue. Call doctor when convenient.

WARNINGS & PRECAUTIONS

Don't take if:
You are allergic to exenatide.

Before you start, consult your doctor if:
• You have type 1 diabetes.
• You require insulin for diabetes treatment.
• You have end-stage renal disease or renal impairment.
• You have severe gastrointestinal disease.

Over age 60:
No special problems expected.

Pregnancy:
Decide with your doctor if drug benefits justify risk to unborn child. Risk category C (see page xviii).

Breast-feeding:
It is unknown if drug passes into milk. Its use is not recommended during breast-feeding. Consult doctor for advice.

Infants & children:
Safety and effectiveness in children has not been established. Consult your child's doctor.

Prolonged use:
Talk to your doctor about the need for follow-up medical examinations and/or laboratory studies to determine continued effectiveness of drug.

Skin & sunlight:
No problems expected.

Driving, piloting or hazardous work:
No problems expected. You do need to be cautious for symptoms of hypoglycemia.

Discontinuing:
Don't discontinue without doctor's advice, even though symptoms diminish or disappear.

Others:
• Notify your doctor if you have a fever, infection, diarrhea, or experience vomiting.
• Advise any doctor or dentist whom you consult that you take this medicine.
• You and your family should educate yourselves about diabetes; learn to recognize the symptoms of hypoglycemia and how to treat it. Hypoglycemia may occur in the treatment of diabetes, as a result of skipped meals, excessive exercise, or alcohol consumption. Carry non-dietetic candy or glucose tablets to treat episodes of low blood sugar.

• Wear or carry medical identification that indicates you have type 2 diabetes and the drugs you take.
• Follow the prescribed diet, medication, and exercise routines closely. Changing any of these things can affect blood sugar levels.
• Store drug in refrigerator. Discard 30 days after first use even if some remains.

POSSIBLE INTERACTION WITH OTHER DRUGS

GENERIC NAME OR DRUG CLASS	COMBINED EFFECT
Drugs taken by mouth that need to pass quickly through the stomach (such as oral contraceptives or antibiotics)	May need to take them 1 hour before injecting exenatide. Consult doctor or pharmacist.

POSSIBLE INTERACTION WITH OTHER SUBSTANCES

INTERACTS WITH	COMBINED EFFECT
Alcohol:	May cause severe low blood sugar. Avoid.
Beverages:	None expected.
Cocaine:	Unknown effect. Avoid.
Foods:	None expected. Do not take drug after a meal. Follow your diabetic diet instructions.
Marijuana:	Possible increase in blood sugar. Avoid.
Tobacco:	None expected. Best to avoid.

*See Glossary

EZETIMIBE

BRAND NAMES

Vytorin   Zetia

BASIC INFORMATION

Habit forming? No
Prescription needed? Yes
Available as generic? No
Drug class: Antihyperlipidemic

 ## USES

Lowers blood cholesterol levels caused by low-density lipoproteins (LDL) in persons who haven't improved by exercising, dieting or using other measures. May be used alone or with other cholesterol lowering drugs (e.g., HMG-CoA reductase inhibitors).

 ## DOSAGE & USAGE INFORMATION

How to take:
Tablet—Swallow with liquid. May be taken on an empty stomach or with food.

When to take:
Once a day at the same time each day.

If you forget a dose:
Take as soon as you remember. If it is almost time for your next dose, skip the missed dose and go back to your regular dosing schedule. Do not double doses.

What drug does:
It lowers the amount of cholesterol your body absorbs from your diet by reducing absorption in the intestines. Other cholesterol lowering drugs alter the production and metabolism of cholesterol in the liver.

Time lapse before drug works:
2 to 4 weeks.

Don't take with:
• A high-fat diet.
• Any other medicine or any dietary supplement without consulting your doctor or pharmacist.

 ## OVERDOSE

SYMPTOMS:
None expected.
WHAT TO DO:
Overdose unlikely to threaten life. If person uses much larger amount than prescribed or if accidentally swallowed, call doctor or poison control center 1-800-222-1222 for help.

 ## POSSIBLE ADVERSE REACTIONS OR SIDE EFFECTS

SYMPTOMS	WHAT TO DO
Life-threatening: None expected.	
Common: None expected.	
Infrequent: Headache, cold or other upper respiratory infection, muscle aches, chest pains, fatigue, dizziness, diarrhea.	Continue. Call doctor when convenient.
Rare: None expected.	

WARNINGS & PRECAUTIONS

Don't take if:
You are allergic to ezetimibe or its components.

Before you start, consult your doctor if:
• You have liver disease.
• You are allergic to any medication, food or other substance.

Over age 60:
No special problems expected.

Pregnancy:
Discuss with your doctor whether drug benefits justify risk to unborn child. Risk category C (see page xviii).

Breast-feeding:
It is unknown if drug passes into breast milk. Avoid drug or discontinue nursing until you finish medicine. Consult doctor for advice on maintaining milk supply.

Infants & children:
Not recommended for children under age 10.

Prolonged use:
Talk to your doctor about the need for follow-up medical examinations or laboratory studies to check liver function and serum cholesterol.

Skin & sunlight:
No problems expected.

Driving, piloting or hazardous work:
No special problems expected.

Discontinuing:
No special problems expected.

Others:
• Advise any doctor or dentist whom you consult that you take this medicine.
• Continue to follow your doctor's instructions about dietary intake, reduced intake of saturated fats, increased fiber intake, weight reduction, and increased physical activity.
• Cholesterol lowering drugs may cause muscle problems or rhabdomyolysis (muscle injury). If you develop persistent muscle aches, pain or weakness or urine turns dark, call the doctor right away.

POSSIBLE INTERACTION WITH OTHER DRUGS

GENERIC NAME OR DRUG CLASS	COMBINED EFFECT
Cholestyramine	Take ezetimibe 2 hours before or 4 hours after.
Colestipol	Take ezetimibe 2 hours before or 4 hours after.
Colesevelam	Take ezetimibe 2 hours before or 4 hours after.
Cyclosporine	Increased effect of ezetimibe.
Fibrates	May require dosage adjustment of either drug.
Gemfibrozil	Increased effect of ezetimibe.

POSSIBLE INTERACTION WITH OTHER SUBSTANCES

INTERACTS WITH	COMBINED EFFECT
Alcohol:	None expected.
Beverages:	None expected.
Cocaine:	None expected.
Foods:	None expected.
Marijuana:	None expected.
Tobacco:	None expected.

FELBAMATE

BRAND NAMES

FBM   **Felbatol**

BASIC INFORMATION

Habit forming? No
Prescription needed? Yes
Available as generic? No
Drug class: Anticonvulsant

 ## USES

- Treatment for partial epileptic seizures.
- Treatment for Lennox-Gastaut syndrome (a severe form of epilepsy in children).

 ## DOSAGE & USAGE INFORMATION

How to take:
- Tablet—Swallow with liquid. May be taken with food to lessen stomach upset unless the doctor has directed taking on an empty stomach.
- Oral suspension—Shake bottle well before measuring. Use specially marked measuring device to measure each dose accurately. Don't measure with a regular household teaspoon.

When to take:
At the same times each day. Your doctor will determine the best schedule. Dosages will gradually be increased over the first 3 weeks.

If you forget a dose:
Take as soon as you remember up to 2 hours late. If more than 2 hours, wait for next scheduled dose (don't double this dose).

What drug does:
- Decreases the frequency of partial seizures that start in a localized part of the brain, including those that progress into more generalized grand mal seizures.
- Decreases seizure activity and improves quality of life in children with Lennox-Gastaut syndrome.

Continued next column

 ## OVERDOSE

SYMPTOMS:
Gastric distress, increased heart rate.
WHAT TO DO:
Overdose unlikely to threaten life. If person uses much larger amount than prescribed or if accidentally swallowed, call doctor or poison control center 1-800-222-1222 for help.

Time lapse before drug works:
May take several weeks for maximum effectiveness.

Don't take with:
Any other medicine or any dietary supplement without consulting your doctor or pharmacist.

 ## POSSIBLE ADVERSE REACTIONS OR SIDE EFFECTS

SYMPTOMS	WHAT TO DO
Life-threatening: None expected.	
Common: • Fever, red or purple spots on skin, walking in unusual manner.	Continue, but call doctor right away.
• Abdominal pain, taste changes, constipation, sleeping difficulty, dizziness, headache, nausea or vomiting, indigestion, appetite loss.	Continue. Call doctor when convenient.
Infrequent: • Mood or mental changes, clumsiness, skin rash, tremor.	Continue, but call doctor right away.
• Vision changes, diarrhea, drowsiness, coughing or sneezing, ear pain or fullness, runny nose, weight loss.	Continue. Call doctor when convenient.
Rare: Black or tarry stools, bloody or dark-colored urine, unusual bruising or bleeding, breathing difficulty, wheezing, pain or tightness in chest, sore throat, mouth or lip sores, swollen face, swollen or painful glands or lymph nodes, yellow skin or eyes, chills, general tired feeling, continuing headache or abdominal pain, hives, itching, muscle cramps, stuffy nose, skin reaction to sunlight.	Continue, but call doctor right away.

WARNINGS & PRECAUTIONS

Don't take if:
You are allergic to felbamate.

Before you start, consult your doctor if:
* You have a sensitivity to other carbamate drugs,* other medications or other substances.
* You have any blood disorder.
* You have a history of bone marrow depression.
* You have or have had any liver disease.

Over age 60:
Adverse reactions and side effects may be more frequent and severe than in younger persons.

Pregnancy:
Decide with your doctor if drug benefits justify risks to unborn child. Risk category B (see page xviii).

Breast-feeding:
Drug passes into milk. Unknown effect. Consult your doctor.

Infants & children:
Give only under close medical supervision.

Prolonged use:
Talk to your doctor about the need for follow-up medical examinations or laboratory studies to check complete blood counts (white blood cell count, platelet count, red blood cell count, hemoglobin, hematocrit), iron concentrations and liver function studies.

Skin & sunlight:
No problems expected.

Driving, piloting or hazardous work:
Don't drive or pilot aircraft until you learn how medicine affects you. Don't work around dangerous machinery. Don't climb ladders or work in high places. Danger increases if you drink alcohol or take other medicines affecting alertness and reflexes such as antihistamines, tranquilizers, sedatives, pain medicine, narcotics and mind-altering drugs.

Discontinuing:
Don't discontinue without doctor's approval due to risk of increased seizure activity.

Others:
* Felbamate may cause serious side effects including blood problems and liver problems (rarely fatal). Decide with your doctor if drug benefits justify risks.
* Advise any doctor or dentist whom you consult that you take this medicine.
* Felbamate may be used alone or combined with other antiepileptic drugs. The dosages of other antiepileptic drugs you currently use will be reduced to minimize side effects and adverse reactions due to interactions.
* Rarely, antiepileptic drugs may lead to suicidal thoughts and behaviors. Call doctor right away if suicidal symptoms or unusual behaviors occur.
* Wear medical identification that indicates the use of this medicine.

POSSIBLE INTERACTION WITH OTHER DRUGS

GENERIC NAME OR DRUG CLASS	COMBINED EFFECT
Carbamazepine	Increased side effects and adverse reactions.
Phenytoin	Increased side effects and adverse reactions.
Valproic acid*	Increased effect of valproic acid.

POSSIBLE INTERACTION WITH OTHER SUBSTANCES

INTERACTS WITH	COMBINED EFFECT
Alcohol:	None expected.
Beverages:	None expected.
Cocaine:	None expected.
Foods:	None expected.
Marijuana:	None expected.
Tobacco:	None expected.

*See Glossary

FIBRATES

GENERIC AND BRAND NAMES

CLOFIBRATE
  Abitrate
  Atromid-S
  Claripex
  Novofibrate
FENOFIBRATE
  Antara
  Fenoglide

FENOFIBRATE (Con't)
  Lipidil
  Lipofen
  Lofibra
  Tricor
  Triglide
FENOFIBRIC ACID
  TriLipix

BASIC INFORMATION

Habit forming? No
Prescription needed? Yes
Available as generic? Yes
Drug class: Antihyperlipidemic

 USES

Used in addition to diet changes to help control levels of blood fats (e.g., lipid disorders such as elevated levels of cholesterol and triglycerides).

 DOSAGE & USAGE INFORMATION

How to take:
• Capsule or tablet—Swallow with liquid. Follow the instructions provided with your prescription about taking the drug with or without food.
• Delayed-release capsule—Swallow with liquid. Do not crush or chew capsule. Take with or without food.

When to take:
At the same time(s) each day. Follow directions on prescription as to when to take each day.

If you forget a dose:
Take as soon as you remember. If it is almost time for the next dose, wait for that dose (don't double this dose) and resume regular schedule.

What drug does:
Helps break down the fats in the blood.

Continued next column

 OVERDOSE

SYMPTOMS:
Diarrhea, headache, muscle pain.
WHAT TO DO:
Overdose unlikely to threaten life. If person uses much larger amount than prescribed or if accidentally swallowed, call doctor or poison control center 1-800-222-1222 for help.

Time lapse before drug works:
3 months or more as measured by laboratory testing.

Don't take with:
Any other medicine or any dietary supplement without consulting your doctor or pharmacist.

 POSSIBLE ADVERSE REACTIONS OR SIDE EFFECTS

SYMPTOMS	WHAT TO DO
Life-threatening: None expected.	
Common: None expected.	
Infrequent:	
• Chest pain, shortness of breath, irregular heartbeat.	Discontinue. Seek emergency treatment.
• Severe symptoms that include nausea, flu-like illness, vomiting.	Discontinue. Call doctor right away.
• Diarrhea, abdominal pain, belching, constipation, muscle aches and pains.	Continue. Call doctor when convenient.
Rare:	
• Cardiac arrhythmias, angina.	Discontinue. Seek emergency treatment.
• Rash, itch; mouth or lip sores; sore throat; swollen feet, legs; blood in urine; painful urination; fever; chills; anemia.	Discontinue. Call doctor right away.
• Dizziness, weakness, drowsiness, muscle cramps, headache, diminished sex drive, hair loss, dry mouth, bloating or stomach pain, chronic indigestion, loss of appetite, unusual bleeding or bruising, unusual tiredness, mild vomiting, yellow eyes or skin.	Continue. Call doctor when convenient.

WARNINGS & PRECAUTIONS

Don't take if:
- You are allergic to any fibrates.
- You have had serious liver disease.

Before you start, consult your doctor if:
- You have had liver or kidney disease.
- You have had peptic ulcer disease.
- You have had gallbladder disease or gallstones.
- You have diabetes.

Over age 60:
Adverse reactions and side effects may be more frequent and severe than in younger persons. May develop flu-like symptoms.

Pregnancy:
Decide with your doctor if drug benefits justify risk to unborn child. Risk category C (see page xviii).

Breast-feeding:
It is unknown if drug passes into milk. Avoid drug or discontinue nursing until you finish medicine. Consult doctor for advice on maintaining milk supply.

Infants & children:
Not recommended.

Prolonged use:
- May cause gallbladder infection.
- Possible cause of stomach cancer.
- Talk to your doctor about the need for follow-up medical examinations or laboratory studies to check cholesterol and triglyceride levels.

Skin & sunlight:
May cause rash or intensify sunburn in areas exposed to sun or ultraviolet light (photosensitivity reaction). Avoid overexposure. Notify doctor if reaction occurs.

Driving, piloting or hazardous work:
Avoid if you feel drowsy or dizzy. Otherwise, no problems expected.

Discontinuing:
Don't discontinue without doctor's advice until you complete prescribed dose, even though symptoms diminish or disappear.

Others:
- Advise any doctor or dentist whom you consult that you take this medicine.
- Periodic blood cell counts and liver-function studies recommended if you take clofibrate for a long time.
- Some medical studies question effectiveness. A number of medical studies warn of toxicity.

POSSIBLE INTERACTION WITH OTHER DRUGS

GENERIC NAME OR DRUG CLASS	COMBINED EFFECT
Anticoagulants, oral*	Increased anticoagulant effect. Dose reduction of anticoagulant necessary.
Antidiabetics, oral*	Increased antidiabetic effect.
Contraceptives, oral*	Decreased fibrate effect.
Cyclosporine	May cause or worsen kidney problems.
Desmopressin	May decrease desmopressin effect.
Dexfenfluramine	Dose may need to be adjusted.
Estrogens*	Decreased fibrate effect.
Furosemide	Possible toxicity of both drugs.
HMG-CoA reductase inhibitors	May cause muscle or kidney problems or make them worse.
Insulin	Increased insulin effect.
Insulin lispro	May need decreased dosage of insulin.
Probenecid	Increased effect and toxicity of fibrate.
Thyroid hormones*	Increased fibrate effect.
Ursodiol	Decreased effect of ursodiol.

POSSIBLE INTERACTION WITH OTHER SUBSTANCES

INTERACTS WITH	COMBINED EFFECT
Alcohol:	None expected.
Beverages:	None expected.
Cocaine:	None expected.
Foods: Fatty foods.	Decreased fibrate effect.
Marijuana:	None expected.
Tobacco:	None expected.

FLAVOXATE

BRAND NAMES

Urispas

BASIC INFORMATION

Habit forming? No
Prescription needed? Yes
Available as generic? Yes
Drug class: Antispasmodic (urinary tract)

 USES

Relieves urinary pain, urgency, nighttime urination, unusual frequency of urination associated with urinary system disorders.

 DOSAGE & USAGE INFORMATION

How to take:
Tablet—Swallow with liquid or food to lessen stomach irritation.

When to take:
30 minutes before meals (unless directed otherwise by doctor).

If you forget a dose:
Take as soon as you remember up to 2 hours late. If more than 2 hours, wait for next scheduled dose (don't double this dose).

What drug does:
Blocks nerve impulses at smooth muscle nerve endings, preventing muscle contractions and gland secretions of organs involved.

Time lapse before drug works:
15 to 30 minutes.

Don't take with:
Any other medicine or any dietary supplement without consulting your doctor or pharmacist.

 OVERDOSE

SYMPTOMS:
Dilated pupils, rapid pulse and breathing, dizziness, fever, hallucinations, confusion, slurred speech, agitation, flushed face, convulsions, coma.
WHAT TO DO:
• **Dial 911 (emergency) for medical help or call poison control center 1-800-222-1222 for instructions.**
• **See emergency information on last 3 pages of this book.**

 POSSIBLE ADVERSE REACTIONS OR SIDE EFFECTS

SYMPTOMS	WHAT TO DO
Life-threatening:	
In case of overdose, see previous column.	
Common:	
• Confusion, delirium, rapid heartbeat.	Discontinue. Call doctor right away.
• Nausea, vomiting, less perspiration, drowsiness.	Continue. Call doctor when convenient.
• Constipation.	Continue. Tell doctor at next visit.
• Dry ears, nose or throat.	No action necessary.
Infrequent:	
• Unusual excitement, irritability, restlessness, clumsiness, hallucinations.	Discontinue. Call doctor right away.
• Headache, increased sensitivity to light, painful or difficult urination.	Continue. Call doctor when convenient.
Rare:	
• Shortness of breath.	Discontinue. Seek emergency treatment.
• Rash or hives, eye pain, blurred vision, sore throat, fever, mouth sores, abdominal pain.	Discontinue. Call doctor right away.
• Dizziness.	Continue. Call doctor when convenient.

WARNINGS & PRECAUTIONS

Don't take if:
- You are allergic to any anticholinergic.
- You have trouble with stomach bloating.
- You have difficulty emptying your bladder completely.
- You have narrow-angle glaucoma.
- You have severe ulcerative colitis.

Before you start, consult your doctor if:
- You have open-angle glaucoma.
- You have angina.
- You have chronic bronchitis or asthma.
- You have liver disease.
- You have hiatal hernia.
- You have enlarged prostate.
- You have myasthenia gravis.
- You have peptic ulcer.
- You will have surgery within 2 months, including dental surgery, requiring general or spinal anesthesia.

Over age 60:
Adverse reactions and side effects, particularly mental confusion, may be more frequent and severe than in younger persons.

Pregnancy:
Consult doctor. Risk category B (see page xviii).

Breast-feeding:
Drug passes into milk. Avoid drug or discontinue nursing until you finish medicine. Consult doctor for advice on maintaining milk supply.

Infants & children:
Use only under medical supervision.

Prolonged use:
Chronic constipation, possible fecal impaction. Consult doctor immediately.

Skin & sunlight:
No problems expected.

Driving, piloting or hazardous work:
Use disqualifies you for piloting aircraft. Don't drive until you learn how medicine affects you. Don't work around dangerous machinery. Don't climb ladders or work in high places. Danger increases if you drink alcohol or take medicine affecting alertness and reflexes, such as antihistamines, tranquilizers, sedatives, pain medicine, narcotics and mind-altering drugs.

Discontinuing:
May be unnecessary to finish medicine. Follow doctor's instructions.

Others:
Advise any doctor or dentist whom you consult that you take this medicine.

 ## POSSIBLE INTERACTION WITH OTHER DRUGS

GENERIC NAME OR DRUG CLASS	COMBINED EFFECT
Antimuscarinics*	Increased effect of flavoxate.
Central nervous system (CNS) depressants, other*	Increased effect of both drugs.
Clozapine	Toxic effect on the central nervous system.
Ethinamate	Dangerous increased effects of ethinamate. Avoid combining.
Fluoxetine	Increased depressant effects of both drugs.
Guanfacine	May increase depressant effects of either drug.
Leucovorin	High alcohol content of leucovorin may cause adverse effects.
Methyprylon	Increased sedative effect, perhaps to dangerous level. Avoid.
Nabilone	Greater depression of central nervous system.
Nizatidine	Increased nizatidine effect.
Sertraline	Increased depressive effects of both drugs.

 ## POSSIBLE INTERACTION WITH OTHER SUBSTANCES

INTERACTS WITH	COMBINED EFFECT
Alcohol:	None expected.
Beverages:	None expected.
Cocaine:	Excessively rapid heartbeat. Avoid.
Foods:	None expected.
Marijuana:	Drowsiness, dry mouth.
Tobacco:	None expected.

*See Glossary

FLECAINIDE ACETATE

BRAND NAMES

Tambocor

BASIC INFORMATION

Habit forming? No
Prescription needed? Yes
Available as generic? Yes
Drug class: Antiarrhythmic

USES

Stabilizes irregular heartbeat.

DOSAGE & USAGE INFORMATION

How to take:
Tablet—Swallow with liquid. If you can't swallow whole, crumble tablet and take with liquid or food.

When to take:
At the same time each day, according to instructions on prescription label. Take tablets approximately 12 hours apart.

If you forget a dose:
Take as soon as you remember up to 4 hours late. If more than 4 hours, wait for next scheduled dose (don't double this dose).

What drug does:
Decreases conduction of abnormal electrical activity in the heart muscle or its regulating systems.

Time lapse before drug works:
1 to 6 hours. May take 3 to 5 days for maximum effect.

Continued next column

OVERDOSE

SYMPTOMS:
Low blood pressure or unconsciousness, irregular or rapid heartbeat, sleepiness, tremor, sweating.
WHAT TO DO:
• **Dial 911 (emergency) for medical help or call poison control center 1-800-222-1222 for instructions.**
• **If person is unconscious, check breathing and pulse. If not breathing, begin mouth-to-mouth rescue breathing. If heart is not beating, begin chest compressions.**
• **See emergency information on last 3 pages of this book.**

Don't take with:
Any other medicine or any dietary supplement without consulting your doctor or pharmacist.

POSSIBLE ADVERSE REACTIONS OR SIDE EFFECTS

SYMPTOMS	WHAT TO DO
Life-threatening:	
In case of overdose, see previous column.	
Common:	
Blurred vision, dizziness.	Continue. Call doctor when convenient.
Infrequent:	
• Chest pain, irregular heartbeat.	Discontinue. Seek emergency treatment.
• Shakiness, rash, nausea, vomiting.	Continue, but call doctor right away.
• Anxiety; depression; weakness; headache; appetite loss; weakness in muscles, bones, joints; swollen feet, ankles or legs; loss of taste; numbness or tingling in hands or feet, abdominal pain.	Continue. Call doctor when convenient.
• Constipation.	Continue. Tell doctor at next visit.
Rare:	
• Shortness of breath.	Discontinue. Seek emergency treatment.
• Sore throat, jaundice, fever.	Continue, but call doctor right away.

WARNINGS & PRECAUTIONS

Don't take if:
You are allergic to flecainide or a local anesthetic such as novocaine, lidocaine or other drug whose generic name ends with "caine."

Before you start, consult your doctor if:
• You have kidney disease.
• You have liver disease.
• You have had a heart attack in past 3 weeks.
• You have a pacemaker.

Over age 60:
Adverse reactions and side effects may be more frequent and severe than in younger persons.

Pregnancy:
Decide with your doctor whether drug benefits justify risk to unborn child. Risk category C (see page xviii).

FLECAINIDE ACETATE

Breast-feeding:
Drug passes into milk. Avoid drug or discontinue nursing until you finish medicine. Consult doctor for advice on maintaining milk supply.

Infants & children:
Not recommended. Safety and dosage have not been established.

Prolonged use:
Talk to your doctor about the need for follow-up medical examinations or laboratory studies to check complete blood counts (white blood cell count, platelet count, red blood cell count, hemoglobin, hematocrit), ECG.*

Skin & sunlight:
No problems expected.

Driving, piloting or hazardous work:
Don't drive or pilot aircraft until you learn how medicine affects you. Don't work around dangerous machinery. Don't climb ladders or work in high places. Danger increases if you drink alcohol or take medicine affecting alertness and reflexes, such as antihistamines, tranquilizers, sedatives, pain medicine, narcotics and mind-altering drugs.

Discontinuing:
Don't discontinue without consulting doctor. Dose may require gradual reduction if you have taken drug for a long time. Doses of other drugs may also require adjustment.

Others:
* Wear identification bracelet or carry an identification card with inscription of medicine you take.
* Advise any doctor or dentist whom you consult that you take this medicine.

 POSSIBLE INTERACTION WITH OTHER DRUGS

GENERIC NAME OR DRUG CLASS	COMBINED EFFECT
Antacids* (high dose)	Possible increased flecainide acetate effect.
Antiarrhythmics, other*	Possible irregular heartbeat.
Beta-adrenergic blocking agents*	Possible decreased efficiency of heart muscle contraction, leading to congestive heart failure.
Bone marrow depressants*	Possible decreased production of blood cells in bone marrow.
Carbonic anhydrase inhibitors*	Possible increased flecainide acetate effect.

Cimetidine	Increased effect of flecainide.
Digitalis preparations*	Possible increased digitalis effect. Possible irregular heartbeat.
Disopyramide	Possible decreased efficiency of heart muscle contraction, leading to congestive heart failure.
Doxepin (topical)	Increased risk of toxicity of both drugs.
Nicardipine	Possible increased effect and toxicity of each drug.
Paroxetine	Increased effect of both drugs.
Propafenone	Increased effect of both drugs and increased risk of toxicity.
Sodium bicarbonate	Possible increased flecainide acetate effect.
Verapamil	Possible decreased efficiency of heart muscle contraction, leading to congestive heart failure.

 POSSIBLE INTERACTION WITH OTHER SUBSTANCES

INTERACTS WITH	COMBINED EFFECT
Alcohol:	May further depress normal heart function.
Beverages: Caffeine-containing beverages.	Possible decreased flecainide effect.
Cocaine:	Possible decreased flecainide effect.
Foods:	None expected.
Marijuana:	Possible decreased flecainide effect.
Tobacco:	Possible decreased flecainide effect.

FLUOROQUINOLONES

GENERIC AND BRAND NAMES

CIPROFLOXACIN
  Cipro
  Cipro XR
  Proquin XR
ENOXACIN
  Penetrex
GEMIFLOXACIN
  Factive
LEVOFLOXACIN
  Levaquin
LOMEFLOXACIN
  Maxaquin

MOXIFLOXACIN
  Avelox
NORFLOXACIN
  Noroxin
OFLOXACIN
  Floxin
SPARFLOXACIN
  Zagam
TROVAFLOXACIN
  Trovan

BASIC INFORMATION

Habit forming? No
Prescription needed? Yes
Available as generic? Yes, for some
Drug class: Antibacterial

USES

- Treats a wide range of bacteria that may cause diarrhea, pneumonia, skin and soft tissue infections, urinary tract infections, conjunctivitis and bone infections.
- Treatment for specific agents that could be used in biologic warfare.

DOSAGE & USAGE INFORMATION

How to take:
- Tablet—Take with full glass of water. Take enoxacin and ofloxacin on an empty stomach. Others may be taken with or without meals.
- Extended release tablet—Swallow whole. Do not crush, break or chew tablet.
- Oral and otic suspension—Take as directed on label.

Continued next column

OVERDOSE

SYMPTOMS:
Confusion and hallucinations, headache, abdominal pain, convulsions.
WHAT TO DO:
- Dial 911 (emergency) for medical help or call poison control center 1-800-222-1222 for instructions.
- See emergency information on last 3 pages of this book.

When to take:
As directed by your doctor.

If you forget a dose:
Take as soon as you remember up to 2 hours late. If more than 2 hours, wait for next scheduled dose (don't double this dose).

What drug does:
Destroys bacteria that is infecting the body.

Time lapse before drug works:
1 to 2 weeks for most infections, but some infections may take 6 weeks or more for cure.

Don't take with:
Any other medicine or any dietary supplement without consulting your doctor or pharmacist.

POSSIBLE ADVERSE REACTIONS OR SIDE EFFECTS

SYMPTOMS	WHAT TO DO
Life-threatening: Hives, rash, intense itching, faintness soon after a dose (anaphylaxis).	Seek emergency treatment immediately.
Common: • Sparfloxacin may cause fainting, slow, irregular heart rate.	Discontinue. Call doctor right away.
• Mild stomach discomfort, nausea, dizziness, drowsiness, nervousness, insomnia, headache, vaginal discharge or pain, lightheadedness, mild diarrhea.	Continue. Call doctor when convenient.
Infrequent: Skin (itching, red, blisters, burning, rash, swelling, peeling).	Discontinue. Call doctor right away.
Rare: • Abdominal pain or cramps or tenderness, agitation, confusion, hallucinations, tremors, shortness of breath, sweating, swelling (neck, face, calves or legs), pale stools, bloody or dark or cloudy urine, joint or calf pain, diarrhea, tired or weak feeling, tendon problems (inflammation, pain, rupture), yellow eyes or skin, seizures, fast or irregular heartbeat, vomiting, fever.	Discontinue. Call doctor right away.

Appetite loss, dreams abnormal, muscle or back pain, skin sensitive to sun, sore mouth or tongue, vision problems, vaginal infection, taste changes, flushing.

Continue. Call doctor when convenient.

WARNINGS & PRECAUTIONS

Don't take if:
You are allergic to fluoroquinolones or quinolone derivatives.

Before you start, consult your doctor if:
* You have any disorder of the central nervous system such as epilepsy or stroke.
* You have had sun sensitivity or tendinitis.
* You have diabetes or liver, kidney or heart disease.

Over age 60:
Risk of tendinitis or tendon rupture (see Others).

Pregnancy:
Decide with your doctor if drug benefits justify risk to unborn child. Risk category C (see page xviii).

Breast-feeding:
Drug passes into milk. Avoid drug or discontinue nursing until you finish medicine. Consult doctor for advice on maintaining milk supply.

Infants & children:
Normally not recommended for ages under 18.

Prolonged use:
Usually not prescribed for long-term use.

Skin & sunlight:
One or more drugs in this group may cause rash or intensify sunburn in areas exposed to sun or ultraviolet light (photosensitivity reaction). Avoid overexposure. Notify doctor if reaction occurs.

Driving, piloting or hazardous work:
Don't drive or pilot aircraft until you learn how medicine affects you. Don't work around dangerous machinery. Don't climb ladders or work in high places. Risk increases if you drink alcohol or take medicine affecting alertness.

Discontinuing:
Don't discontinue without consulting doctor or completing prescribed dosage. Call doctor if symptoms occur after you stop drug (such as stomach cramps, fever, swelling, calf pain, diarrhea that is watery or bloody).

Others:
* Advise any doctor or dentist whom you consult that you take this medicine.
* These drugs increase the risk of tendinitis or tendon rupture in some patients. If tendon pain or inflammation occurs, stop exercising, discontinue drug and call doctor.

*See Glossary

* May affect accuracy of some medical tests.
* Drink plenty of fluids while taking drug.
* Serious liver problems associated with use of trovafloxacin; can lead to liver transplantation and/or death. Consult your doctor about risks.

POSSIBLE INTERACTION WITH OTHER DRUGS

GENERIC NAME OR DRUG CLASS	COMBINED EFFECT
Aminophylline	Increased effect of aminophylline.
Antacids*	Decreased fluoro-quinolone effect.
Antidiabetic agents*	Adverse diabetic reactions.
Anti-inflammatory drugs, nonsteroidal (NSAIDs)*	Increased risk of central nervous system problems.
Caffeine	Increased risk of central nervous system problems.
Calcium supplements	Decreased fluoro-quinolone effect.
Citrates	Decreased trovafloxacin effect.

Continued on page 917

POSSIBLE INTERACTION WITH OTHER SUBSTANCES

INTERACTS WITH	COMBINED EFFECT
Alcohol:	Increased possibility of central nervous system side effects.
Beverages: Caffeine drinks.	Increased effect of caffeine. Don't use with enoxacin.
Cocaine:	Increased possibility of central nervous system side effects.
Foods: Dairy foods.	Decreased effect of fluoroquinolone. Take 2 hours apart.
Marijuana:	Increased possibility of central nervous system side effects.
Tobacco:	Increased possibility of central nervous system side effects.

FLUOROURACIL (Topical)

BRAND NAMES

5-FU   **Fluoroplex**
Efudex

BASIC INFORMATION

Habit forming? No
Prescription needed? Yes
Available as generic? No
Drug class: Antineoplastic (topical)

USES

- Treats precancerous actinic keratoses on skin.
- Treats superficial basal cell carcinomas (skin cancers that don't spread to distant organs and, therefore, do not threaten life).

DOSAGE & USAGE INFORMATION

How to use:
- Apply with cotton-tipped applicator.
- Cream, lotion, ointment—Bathe and dry area before use. Apply small amount and rub gently.
- Wash hands (if fingertips are used to apply) after applying medicine to other parts of body.

When to use:
Once or twice a day or as directed by doctor.

If you forget a dose:
Apply as soon as you remember. Resume basic schedule.

What drug does:
Selectively destroys actively proliferating cells.

Time lapse before drug works:
2 to 3 days.

Don't use with:
Other topical medications unless prescribed by your doctor.

OVERDOSE

SYMPTOMS:
None expected.
WHAT TO DO:
Not for internal use. If child accidentally swallows, dial 911 (emergency) for medical help or call poison control center
1-800-222-1222 for instructions.

POSSIBLE ADVERSE REACTIONS OR SIDE EFFECTS

SYMPTOMS	WHAT TO DO
Life-threatening None expected.	
Common	
• Skin redness or swelling.	Discontinue. Call doctor right away.
• After 1 or 2 weeks of use—Skin itching or oozing; rash, tenderness, soreness.	Continue. Call doctor when convenient.
Infrequent Skin darkening or scaling.	Continue. Call doctor when convenient.
Rare Watery eyes.	Discontinue. Call doctor right away.

WARNINGS & PRECAUTIONS

Don't use if:
You are allergic to fluorouracil.

Before you start, consult your doctor if:
* You have chloasma or acne rosacea.
* You have any other skin problems.

Over age 60:
No problems expected.

Pregnancy:
Consult doctor. Risk category X (see page xviii).

Breast-feeding:
Avoid drug or discontinue nursing until you finish medicine. Consult doctor for advice on maintaining milk supply.

Infants & children:
No problems expected, but check with doctor.

Prolonged use:
No problems expected, but check with doctor.

Skin & sunlight:
May cause rash or intensify sunburn in areas exposed to sun or ultraviolet light (photosensitivity reaction). Avoid overexposure. Notify doctor if reaction occurs.

Driving, piloting or hazardous work:
No problems expected, but check with doctor.

Discontinuing:
Pink, smooth area remains after treatment (usually fades in 1 to 2 months).

Others:
* Skin lesions may need biopsy before treatment.
* Keep medicine out of eyes or mouth.
* Heat and moisture in bathroom medicine cabinet can cause breakdown of medicine. Store someplace else.

POSSIBLE INTERACTION WITH OTHER DRUGS

GENERIC NAME OR DRUG CLASS	COMBINED EFFECT
None significant.	

POSSIBLE INTERACTION WITH OTHER SUBSTANCES

INTERACTS WITH	COMBINED EFFECT
Alcohol:	None expected.
Beverages:	None expected.
Cocaine:	None expected.
Foods:	None expected.
Marijuana:	None expected.
Tobacco:	None expected.

FOLIC ACID (Vitamin B-9)

BRAND NAMES

Apo-Folic   Novo-Folacid
Folvite
Numerous brands of single vitamin and multivitamin combinations may be available.

BASIC INFORMATION

Habit forming? No
Prescription needed?
    High strength: Yes
    Vitamin mixtures: No
Available as generic? Yes
Drug class: Vitamin supplement

 ## USES

- Dietary supplement to promote normal growth, development and good health.
- Dietary supplement during pregnancy to prevent spinal defects.
- Treatment for anemias due to folic acid deficiency occurring from alcoholism, liver disease, hemolytic anemia, sprue, infants on artificial formula, pregnancy, breast feeding and use of oral contraceptives.
- Some studies have found that folic acid supplementation alone or in combination with other vitamins taken before conception and during early pregnancy may reduce the incidence of neural tube defects in infants.

 ## DOSAGE & USAGE INFORMATION

How to take:
Tablet—Swallow with liquid or food to lessen stomach irritation. If you can't swallow whole, crumble tablet and take with liquid or food.

When to take:
At the same time each day.

If you forget a dose:
Take when you remember. Don't double next dose. Resume regular schedule.

Continued next column

 ## OVERDOSE

SYMPTOMS:
None expected.
WHAT TO DO:
Overdose unlikely to threaten life. If child accidentally swallows, dial 911 (emergency) for medical help or call poison control center 1-800-222-1222 for instructions.

What drug does:
Essential to normal red blood cell formation.

Time lapse before drug works:
Not determined.

Don't take with:
Any other medicine or any dietary supplement without consulting your doctor or pharmacist.

 ## POSSIBLE ADVERSE REACTIONS OR SIDE EFFECTS

SYMPTOMS	WHAT TO DO
Life-threatening: None expected.	
Common: Large dose may produce yellow urine.	Continue. Tell doctor at next visit.
Infrequent: None expected.	
Rare: Rash, itching, bronchospasm.	Discontinue. Call doctor right away.

WARNINGS & PRECAUTIONS

Don't take if:
You are allergic to any B vitamin.

Before you start, consult your doctor if:
- You have liver disease.
- You have pernicious anemia. (Folic acid corrects anemia, but nerve damage of pernicious anemia continues.)

Over age 60:
No problems expected.

Pregnancy:
No problems expected. Consult doctor. Risk category A (see page xviii).

Breast-feeding:
No problems expected. Consult doctor.

Infants & children:
No problems expected.

Prolonged use:
No problems expected.

Skin & sunlight:
No problems expected.

Driving, piloting or hazardous work:
No problems expected.

Discontinuing:
Don't discontinue without doctor's advice until you complete prescribed dose, even though symptoms diminish or disappear.

Others:
- Folic acid removed by kidney dialysis. Dialysis patients should increase intake to 300% of RDA or take as directed.
- A balanced diet should provide all the folic acid a healthy person needs and make supplements unnecessary. Best sources are green, leafy vegetables; fruits; liver and kidney.

POSSIBLE INTERACTION WITH OTHER DRUGS

GENERIC NAME OR DRUG CLASS	COMBINED EFFECT
Analgesics*	Decreased effect of folic acid.
Anticonvulsants, hydantoin*	Decreased effect of folic acid. Possible increased seizure frequency.
Chloramphenicol	Possible decreased folic acid effect.
Contraceptives, oral*	Decreased effect of folic acid.
Cortisone drugs*	Decreased effect of folic acid.
Methotrexate	Decreased effect of folic acid.
Para-aminosalicylic acid (PAS)	Decreased effect of folic acid.
Pyrimethamine	Decreased effect of folic acid.
Sulfasalazine	Decreased dietary absorption of folic acid.
Triamterene	Decreased effect of folic acid.
Trimethoprim	Decreased effect of folic acid.
Zinc supplements	Increased need for zinc.

POSSIBLE INTERACTION WITH OTHER SUBSTANCES

INTERACTS WITH	COMBINED EFFECT
Alcohol:	None expected.
Beverages:	None expected.
Cocaine:	None expected.
Foods:	None expected.
Marijuana:	None expected.
Tobacco:	None expected.

*See Glossary

FURAZOLIDONE

BRAND NAMES

Furoxone   **Furoxone Liquid**

BASIC INFORMATION

Habit forming? No
Prescription needed? Yes
Available as generic? No
Drug class: Antiprotozoal, antibacterial
(antibiotic)

USES

- As an adjunct in treating most germs that infect the gastrointestinal tract such as cholera, salmonellosis, E. coli, proteus infections, and other bacterial causes of diarrhea.
- Treats giardiasis.

DOSAGE & USAGE INFORMATION

How to take:
- Liquid—Use a measuring spoon to ensure correct dose.
- Tablet—Swallow with liquid or food to lessen stomach irritation. If you can't swallow whole, crumble tablet and take with liquid or food.

When to take:
At the same time each day, according to instructions on prescription label.

If you forget a dose:
Take as soon as you remember up to 2 hours late. If more than 2 hours, wait for next scheduled dose. Don't double this dose.

What drug does:
Kills microscopic germs.

Time lapse before drug works:
Immediate.

Don't take with:
Any other medicine or any dietary supplement without consulting your doctor or pharmacist.

OVERDOSE

SYMPTOMS:
None expected.
WHAT TO DO:
Overdose unlikely to threaten life. If person uses much larger amount than prescribed or if accidentally swallowed, call doctor or poison control center 1-800-222-1222 for help.

POSSIBLE ADVERSE REACTIONS OR SIDE EFFECTS

SYMPTOMS	WHAT TO DO
Life-threatening:	
None expected except when taken with forbidden foods (see Possible Interaction with Other Substances).	
Common:	
• Nausea, vomiting.	Continue. Call doctor when convenient.
• Dark yellow or brown urine.	No action necessary.
Infrequent:	
• Abdominal pain.	Discontinue. Call doctor right away.
• Headache.	Continue. Call doctor when convenient.
Rare:	
Sore throat, fever, skin rash, itching, joint pain.	Discontinue. Call doctor right away.

WARNINGS & PRECAUTIONS

Don't take if:
- You have G6PD* deficiency.
- You have hypersensitivity to furazolidone, nitrofurantoin (Furadantin), or nitrofurazone (Furacin).

Before you start, consult your doctor if:
You are taking any other prescription or nonprescription medicine.

Over age 60:
No special problems expected.

Pregnancy:
Decide with your doctor if drug benefits justify risk to unborn child. Risk category C (see page xviii).

Breast-feeding:
Drug may pass into milk. Avoid drug or discontinue nursing until you finish medicine. Consult doctor for advice on maintaining milk supply.

Infants & children:
Don't use for infants without specific instructions from your doctor.

Prolonged use:
No special problems expected.

Skin & sunlight:
No special problems expected.

Driving, piloting or hazardous work:
No special problems expected.

Discontinuing:
Food restrictions outlined in Possible Interaction with Other Substances must be continued for at least 2 weeks after furazolidone is discontinued.

Others:
- Should not be taken with foods or drinks high in tyramine (see Possible Interaction with Other Substances).
- Advise any doctor or dentist whom you consult that you take this medicine.

POSSIBLE INTERACTION WITH OTHER DRUGS

GENERIC NAME OR DRUG CLASS	COMBINED EFFECT
Antidepressants, tricyclic*	Sudden, severe increase in blood pressure.
Monoamine oxidase (MAO) inhibitors*	Sudden, severe increase in blood pressure.
Sumatriptan	Adverse effects unknown. Avoid.
Sympathomimetics*	Sudden, severe increase in blood pressure.

POSSIBLE INTERACTION WITH OTHER SUBSTANCES

INTERACTS WITH	COMBINED EFFECT
Alcohol:	Flushed face, shortness of breath, fever, tightness in chest. Avoid.
Beverages: Any alcoholic beverage.	Flushed face, shortness of breath, fever, tightness in chest. Avoid.
Cocaine:	High blood pressure. Avoid.
Foods: Aged cheese; dark beer; red wine (especially Chianti); sherry; liqueurs; caviar; yeast or protein extracts; fava beans; smoked or pickled meat, poultry, fish; pepperoni, salami, summer sausage; over-ripe fruit.	Sudden, severe high blood pressure that may be life-threatening. Avoid.
Marijuana:	High blood pressure. Avoid.
Tobacco:	No special problems expected.

*See Glossary

FUSION INHIBITOR

GENERIC AND BRAND NAMES

ENFUVIRTIDE
Fuzeon

BASIC INFORMATION

Habit forming? No
Prescription needed? Yes
Available as generic? No
Drug class: Fusion inhibitor

 USES

For treatment of HIV and AIDS patients. Used in combination with one or more of the other HIV and AIDS drugs. It is used when other anti-HIV drugs are not effective.

 DOSAGE & USAGE INFORMATION

How to take:
Injection—The drug is injected under the skin using small hypodermic needles. Follow all instructions carefully on the prescription label. Dispose of all needles and syringes as instructed by your doctor.

When to take:
Two shots a day; one taken in the morning and the other 12 hours later at night.

If you forget a dose:
Take as soon as you remember. If it is almost time for your next dose, skip the missed dose and go back to the regular dosing schedule. Do not double doses.

What drug does:
It stops HIV from entering healthy cells. It helps slow the progress of HIV disease, but does not cure it.

Time lapse before drug works:
May require several weeks or months before full benefits are apparent.

Continued next column

 OVERDOSE

SYMPTOMS:
Unknown effects.
WHAT TO DO:
If person takes much larger amount than prescribed, dial 911 (emergency) for medical help or call poison control center 1-800-222-1222 for instructions.

Don't take with:
Any other medicine or any dietary supplement without consulting your doctor or pharmacist. This is very important with antiviral drugs.

 POSSIBLE ADVERSE REACTIONS OR SIDE EFFECTS

SYMPTOMS	WHAT TO DO
Life-threatening:	
Rare allergic reaction— Breathing difficulty; swelling of hands, feet, face, mouth, neck; skin rash.	Discontinue. Seek emergency treatment.
Common:	
• Peripheral neuropathy (burning, tingling, numbness, pain or weakness in arms, hands, feet or legs), pain around cheeks or eyes, fever, chills, runny or stuffy nose, cough, wheezing, tightness in chest.	Continue, but call doctor right away.
• Anxiety, weakness, depression, sores on skin, cold sores, trouble sleeping, weight loss, skin symptoms at site of drug injections, muscle pain, itching.	Continue. Call doctor when convenient.
Infrequent:	
• Eye inflammation (swelling, red and painful), stomach or back pain, dark urine, constipation, appetite loss, nausea or vomiting, indigestion, yellow skin or eyes, skin lump or growth.	Continue, but call doctor right away.
• General ill feeling, diarrhea, headache, joint pain, changes in taste, swollen or painful lymph glands.	Continue. Call doctor when convenient.
Rare:	
Pneumonia symptoms (rapid breathing, short-ness of breath, cough with fever). Any other unusual symptoms that occur (may be due to the illness, this drug or other drugs being taken).	Continue, but call doctor right away.

WARNINGS & PRECAUTIONS

Don't take if:
You are allergic to fusion inhibitors.

Before you start, consult your doctor if:
- You have or have had lung disease.
- You have high viral load or low CD4 cell count.
- You use intravenous (IV) drugs.
- You smoke.

Over age 60:
The drug has not been studied in this age group.

Pregnancy:
Decide with your doctor if drug benefits justify risks to unborn child. Risk category B (see page xviii).

Breast-feeding:
It is unknown if drug passes into milk. It is not recommended that HIV-infected mothers breast-feed. Consult your doctor.

Infants & children:
Safety and efficacy have not been established in children under age 6. Use only under close medical supervision for any children.

Prolonged use:
- Long-term effects have not been established.
- Talk to your doctor about frequent blood counts and liver function studies.

Skin & sunlight:
No problems expected.

Driving, piloting or hazardous work:
Don't drive or pilot aircraft until you learn how medicine affects you. Don't work around dangerous machinery. Don't climb ladders or work in high places. Danger increases if you drink alcohol or take medicine affecting alertness and reflexes.

Discontinuing:
Don't discontinue without doctor's advice. Doses of other drugs may require adjustment.

Others:
- Advise any doctor or dentist whom you consult that you take this medicine.
- Avoid sexual intercourse or use condoms to help prevent the transmission of HIV. Don't share needles or equipment for injections with other persons.
- This drug is combined with others for the best treatment. This increases the risk of side effects or adverse reactions.
- May interfere with results of some blood tests.
- Numerous medical studies are ongoing concerning the use of these and other anti-HIV drugs. Full safety and effectiveness are still being determined.

POSSIBLE INTERACTION WITH OTHER DRUGS

GENERIC NAME OR DRUG CLASS	COMBINED EFFECT
None expected.	

POSSIBLE INTERACTION WITH OTHER SUBSTANCES

INTERACTS WITH	COMBINED EFFECT
Alcohol:	None expected.
Beverages:	None expected.
Cocaine:	Unknown effect. Best to avoid.
Foods:	None expected.
Marijuana:	Unknown effect. Best to avoid.
Tobacco:	None expected.

GABAPENTIN

BRAND NAMES

Neurontin

BASIC INFORMATION

Habit forming? No
Prescription needed? Yes
Available as generic? Yes
Drug class: Anticonvulsant, antiepileptic

 ## USES

- Treatment for partial (focal) epileptic seizures. Used in combination with other antiepileptic drugs.
- Treats postherpetic neuralgia.

 ## DOSAGE & USAGE INFORMATION

How to take:
Capsule—Swallow with liquid. May be taken with or without food.

When to take:
Your doctor will determine the best schedule. Dosages will be increased rapidly over the first 3 days of use. Further increases may be necessary to achieve maximum benefits.

If you forget a dose:
Take as soon as you remember. If it is almost time for the next dose, skip the missed dose and wait for your next scheduled dose (don't double this dose).

What drug does:
The exact mechanism is unknown. The anticonvulsant action may result from an altered transport of brain amino acids. Amino acids play an important part in chemical reactions within the cells.

Time lapse before drug works:
May take several weeks for effectiveness.

Don't take with:
Any other medicine or any dietary supplement without consulting your doctor or pharmacist.

 ## OVERDOSE

SYMPTOMS:
Double vision, slurred speech, drowsiness, tiredness, diarrhea.
WHAT TO DO:
Overdose unlikely to threaten life. If person uses much larger amount than prescribed or if accidentally swallowed, call doctor or poison control center 1-800-222-1222 for help.

 ## POSSIBLE ADVERSE REACTIONS OR SIDE EFFECTS

SYMPTOMS	WHAT TO DO
Life-threatening: None expected.	
Common: Sleepiness, dizziness, fatigue, clumsiness, lack of coordination.	Continue. Call doctor when convenient.
Infrequent: Rapid eye movement (nystagmus), double or blurred vision.	Continue. Call doctor when convenient.
Rare: Rash; nervousness; depression; twitching or swelling in hands, feet or legs; runny nose; dry or sore throat; nausea; vomiting; coughing; dry mouth; constipation; impotence; increased appetite; weight gain; muscle or back ache; forgetfulness; indigestion.	Continue. Call doctor when convenient.

WARNINGS & PRECAUTIONS

Don't take if:
You are allergic to gabapentin.

Before you start, consult your doctor if:
You have kidney disease.

Over age 60:
No special problems expected.

Pregnancy:
Decide with your doctor if drug benefits justify risks to unborn child. Risk category C (see page xviii).

Breast-feeding:
It is unknown if drug passes into milk. Consult your doctor.

Infants & children:
Not recommended for children under age 12.

Prolonged use:
No special problems expected. Follow-up laboratory blood studies may be recommended by your doctor.

Skin & sunlight:
No problems expected.

Driving, piloting or hazardous work:
Don't drive or pilot aircraft until you learn how medicine affects you. Don't work around dangerous machinery. Don't climb ladders or work in high places. Danger increases if you drink alcohol or take other medicines affecting alertness and reflexes such as antihistamines, tranquilizers, sedatives, pain medicine, narcotics and mind-altering drugs.

Discontinuing:
Don't discontinue without doctor's approval due to risk of increased seizure activity.

Others:
* Advise any doctor or dentist whom you consult that you take this medicine.
* Side effects of gabapentin are usually mild to moderate. Because it is normally used with other anticonvulsant drugs, additional side effects may also occur. If they do, discuss them with your doctor.
* Rarely, antiepileptic drugs may lead to suicidal thoughts and behaviors. Call doctor right away if suicidal symptoms or unusual behaviors occur.

POSSIBLE INTERACTION WITH OTHER DRUGS

GENERIC NAME OR DRUG CLASS	COMBINED EFFECT
Antacids*	Allow at least 2 hours between the 2 drugs.

POSSIBLE INTERACTION WITH OTHER SUBSTANCES

INTERACTS WITH	COMBINED EFFECT
Alcohol:	None expected.
Beverages:	None expected.
Cocaine:	None expected.
Foods:	None expected.
Marijuana:	None expected.
Tobacco:	None expected.

GEMFIBROZIL

BRAND NAMES

Lopid

BASIC INFORMATION

Habit forming? No
Prescription needed? Yes
Available as generic? Yes
Drug class: Antihyperlipidemic

 USES

Reduces fatty substances in the blood
(triglycerides) and raises high-density lipoprotein
(HDL) cholesterol levels.

 DOSAGE & USAGE INFORMATION

How to take:
Tablet or capsule—Swallow with liquid or food to
lessen stomach irritation.

When to take:
Take 30 minutes before morning and evening
meals.

If you forget a dose:
Take as soon as you remember up to 2 hours
late. If more than 2 hours, wait for next
scheduled dose (don't double this dose).

What drug does:
Inhibits formation of fatty substances.

Time lapse before drug works:
3 months or more.

Don't take with:
Any other medicine or any dietary supplement
without consulting your doctor or pharmacist.

 OVERDOSE

SYMPTOMS:
Diarrhea, headache, muscle pain.
WHAT TO DO:
Overdose unlikely to threaten life. If person
uses much larger amount than prescribed or
if accidentally swallowed, call doctor or
poison control center 1-800-222-1222 for help.

 POSSIBLE ADVERSE REACTIONS OR SIDE EFFECTS

SYMPTOMS	WHAT TO DO
Life-threatening: None expected.	
Common: Indigestion.	Continue. Call doctor when convenient.
Infrequent: Chest pain, shortness of breath, irregular heartbeat, nausea, vomiting, diarrhea, stomach pain.	Discontinue. Call doctor right away.
Rare: • Rash, itch; sores in mouth, on lips; sore throat; swollen feet, legs; blood in urine; painful urination; fever; chills.	Discontinue. Call doctor right away.
• Dizziness, headache, drowsiness, muscle cramps, dry skin, backache, unusual tiredness, decreased sex drive.	Continue. Call doctor when convenient.

WARNINGS & PRECAUTIONS

Don't take if:
You are allergic to any antihyperlipidemic.

Before you start, consult your doctor if:
- You have had liver or kidney disease.
- You have gallstones or gallbladder disease.
- You have had peptic-ulcer disease.
- You have diabetes.

Over age 60:
Adverse reactions and side effects may be more frequent and severe than in younger persons.

Pregnancy:
Decide with your doctor if drug benefits justify risks to unborn child. Risk category C (see page xviii).

Breast-feeding:
It is not known if drug passes into milk. Avoid drug or discontinue nursing until you finish medicine. Consult doctor for advice on maintaining milk supply.

Infants & children:
Not recommended.

Prolonged use:
Periodic blood cell counts and liver function studies recommended if you take gemfibrozil for a long time.

Skin & sunlight:
No problems expected.

Driving, piloting or hazardous work:
Avoid if you feel drowsy or dizzy. Otherwise, no problems expected.

Discontinuing:
Don't discontinue without doctor's advice until you complete prescribed dose.

Others:
- Some studies question effectiveness. Many studies warn against toxicity.
- May affect results in some medical tests.
- Advise any doctor or dentist whom you consult that you take this medicine.

POSSIBLE INTERACTION WITH OTHER DRUGS

GENERIC NAME OR DRUG CLASS	COMBINED EFFECT
Anticoagulants, oral*	Increased anti-coagulant effect. Dose reduction of anticoagulant necessary.
Antidiabetics, oral*	Increased antidiabetic effect.
Contraceptives, oral*	Decreased gemfibrozil effect.
Dexfenfluramine	May require dosage change as weight loss occurs.
Estrogens*	Decreased gemfibrozil effect.
Furosemide	Possible toxicity of both drugs.
HMG-CoA reductase inhibitors	Increased risk of muscle inflammation and kidney failure.
Insulin	Increased insulin effect.
Lovastatin	Increased risk of kidney problems.
Thyroid hormones*	Increased gemfibrozil effect.

POSSIBLE INTERACTION WITH OTHER SUBSTANCES

INTERACTS WITH	COMBINED EFFECT
Alcohol:	None expected.
Beverages:	None expected.
Cocaine:	Decreased effect of gemfibrozil. Avoid.
Foods: Fatty foods.	Decreased gemfibrozil effect.
Marijuana:	None expected.
Tobacco:	Decreased gemfibrozil absorption. Avoid.

*See Glossary

GLUCAGON

BRAND NAMES

Glucagon for Injection

BASIC INFORMATION

Habit forming? No
Prescription needed? Yes
Available as generic? Yes
Drug class: Antihypoglycemic, diagnostic aid

USES

- Treats low blood sugar (hypoglycemia) in diabetics.
- Used as antidote for overdose of beta-adrenergic blockers, quinidine and tricyclic antidepressants.

DOSAGE & USAGE INFORMATION

How to take:
Injection—As directed by your doctor.

When to take:
When there are signs of low blood sugar (anxiety; chills; cool, pale skin; hunger; nausea; tremors; sweating; weakness; stomach pain; confusion; drowsiness; fast heartbeat; continuing headache; unsteady walk; unusual tiredness or weakness; vision changes; unconsciousness) in diabetics who don't respond to eating some form of sugar.

If you forget a dose:
Single dose only.

What drug does:
Forces liver to make more sugar and release it into the bloodstream.

Time lapse before drug works:
- For hypoglycemic condition—5 to 20 minutes.
- For muscle relaxant—1 to 10 minutes.

Continued next column

OVERDOSE

SYMPTOMS:
Nausea, vomiting, severe weakness, irregular heartbeat, hoarseness, cramps.
WHAT TO DO:
- Dial 911 (emergency) for medical help or call poison control center 1-800-222-1222 for instructions.
- See emergency information on last 3 pages of this book.

Don't take with:
Any other medicines (including over-the-counter drugs such as cough and cold medicines, laxatives, antacids, diet pills, caffeine, nose drops or vitamins) without consulting your doctor or pharmacist.

POSSIBLE ADVERSE REACTIONS OR SIDE EFFECTS

SYMPTOMS	WHAT TO DO
Life-threatening:	
Unconsciousness.	Seek emergency treatment immediately.
Common:	
Nausea.	Continue. Call doctor when convenient.
Infrequent:	
Lightheadedness, breathing difficulty, skin rash.	Discontinue. Call doctor right away.
Rare:	
None expected.	

WARNINGS & PRECAUTIONS

Don't take if:
You can't tolerate glucagon.

Before you start, consult your doctor if:
- You are allergic to beef or pork.
- You have pheochromocytoma.*

Over age 60:
No special problems expected.

Pregnancy:
No proven harm to unborn child, but avoid if possible. Consult doctor. Risk category B (see page xviii).

Breast-feeding:
No special problems expected. Consult doctor.

Infants & children:
No special problems expected.

Prolonged use:
To be used intermittently and not for prolonged periods.

Skin & sunlight:
No problems expected.

Driving, piloting or hazardous work:
Don't drive or pilot aircraft until you learn how medicine affects you. Don't work around dangerous machinery. Don't climb ladders or work in high places. Danger increases if you drink alcohol or take medicine affecting alertness and reflexes.

Discontinuing:
No special problems expected.

Others:
- May affect results in some medical tests.
- Explain to other family members how to inject glucagon.
- Before injecting, try to eat some form of sugar, such as glucose tablets, corn syrup, honey, orange juice, hard candy or sugar cubes.
- Store unmixed glucagon at room temperature. Store mixed glucagon in refrigerator, but don't freeze. Mixed solution is only good for 48 hours.
- Check expiration date regularly and replace drug before it expires.

POSSIBLE INTERACTION WITH OTHER DRUGS

GENERIC NAME OR DRUG CLASS	COMBINED EFFECT
Anticoagulants*	Increased anticoagulant effect.

POSSIBLE INTERACTION WITH OTHER SUBSTANCES

INTERACTS WITH	COMBINED EFFECT
Alcohol:	Decreased glucagon effect.
Beverages:	None expected.
Cocaine:	Increased adverse reactions.
Foods: Sugar, fruit juice, candy.	Enhances glucagon effect.
Marijuana:	Increased adverse reactions.
Tobacco:	None expected.

GLYCOPYRROLATE

BRAND NAMES

Robinul   Robinul Forte

BASIC INFORMATION

Habit forming? No
Prescription needed? Yes
Available as generic? Yes
Drug class: Antispasmodic, anticholinergic

 USES

- Reduces spasms of digestive system.
- Reduces production of saliva during dental procedures.
- Treats peptic ulcer by reducing gastric acid secretion.

 DOSAGE & USAGE INFORMATION

How to take:
Tablet—Swallow with liquid. If you can't swallow whole, crumble tablet and take with small amount of liquid or food.

When to take:
30 minutes before meals (unless directed otherwise by doctor).

If you forget a dose:
Wait for next scheduled dose (don't double this dose).

What drug does:
Blocks nerve impulses at parasympathetic nerve endings, preventing smooth (involuntary) muscle contractions and gland secretions of organs involved.

Time lapse before drug works:
15 to 30 minutes.

Don't take with:
Any other medicine or any dietary supplement without consulting your doctor or pharmacist.

 OVERDOSE

SYMPTOMS:
Dry mouth, blurred vision, low blood pressure, decreased breathing rate, rapid heartbeat, flushed skin, drowsiness.
WHAT TO DO:
- **Dial 911 (emergency) for medical help or call poison control center 1-800-222-1222 for instructions.**
- **See emergency information on last 3 pages of this book.**

 POSSIBLE ADVERSE REACTIONS OR SIDE EFFECTS

SYMPTOMS	WHAT TO DO
Life-threatening: Hives, rash, intense itching, faintness soon after a dose (anaphylaxis).	Seek emergency treatment immediately.
Common: Dry mouth, loss of taste, constipation, difficult urination.	Continue. Call doctor when convenient.
Infrequent:	
• Confusion; dizziness; drowsiness; eye pain; headache; rash; sleep disturbance such as nightmares, frequent waking; nausea; vomiting; rapid heartbeat; lightheadedness.	Discontinue. Call doctor right away.
• Insomnia, blurred vision, diminished sex drive, decreased sweating, nasal congestion, altered taste.	Continue. Call doctor when convenient.
Rare: Rash, hives.	Discontinue. Call doctor right away.

 WARNINGS & PRECAUTIONS

Don't take if:
- You are allergic to any anticholinergic.
- You have trouble with stomach bloating.
- You have difficulty emptying your bladder completely.
- You have narrow-angle glaucoma.
- You have severe ulcerative colitis.

Before you start, consult your doctor if:
- You have open-angle glaucoma.
- You have angina, chronic bronchitis or asthma, liver disease, hiatal hernia, enlarged prostate, myasthenia gravis, peptic ulcer, kidney or thyroid disease.
- You will have surgery within 2 months, including dental surgery, requiring general or spinal anesthesia.

Over age 60:
Adverse reactions and side effects may be more frequent and severe than in younger persons.

Pregnancy:
Consult doctor. Risk category B (see page xviii).

Breast-feeding:
Drug passes into milk and decreases milk flow. Avoid drug or discontinue nursing until you finish medicine. Consult doctor for advice on maintaining milk supply.

Infants & children:
Use only under medical supervision.

Prolonged use:
Chronic constipation, possible fecal impaction. Consult doctor immediately.

Skin & sunlight:
No problems expected.

Driving, piloting or hazardous work:
No problems expected.

Discontinuing:
May be unnecessary to finish medicine. Follow doctor's instructions.

Others:
* Heatstroke more likely if you become overheated during exertion.
* Advise any doctor or dentist whom you consult that you take this medicine.

 POSSIBLE INTERACTION WITH OTHER DRUGS

GENERIC NAME OR DRUG CLASS	COMBINED EFFECT
Adrenocorticoids, systemic	Possible glaucoma.
Antacids*	Decreased glycopyrrolate absorption effect.
Amantadine	Increased glycopyrrolate effect.
Anticholinergics, other*	Increased glycopyrrolate effect.
Antidepressants, tricyclic*	Increased glycopyrrolate effect.
Antidiarrheals*	Decreased glycopyrrolate absorption effect.
Attapulgite	Decreased effect of anticholinergic.
Buclizine	Increased glycopyrrolate effect.
Digitalis	Possible decreased absorption of digitalis.
Haloperidol	Increased internal eye pressure.
Ketoconazole	Decreased ketoconazole effect.

Meperidine	Increased glycopyrrolate effect.
Methylphenidate	Increased anticholinergic effect.
Molindone	Increased nizatidine effect.
Monoamine oxidase (MAO) inhibitors*	Increased glycopyrrolate effect.
Orphenadrine	Increased glycopyrrolate effect.
Phenothiazines	Increased glycopyrrolate effect.
Pilocarpine	Increased glycopyrrolate effect. Loss of pilocarpine effect in glaucoma treatment.
Potassium chloride tabs	Increased side effects of potassium tablets.
Quinidine	Increased glycopyrrolate effect.
Sedatives* or central nervous system (CNS) depressants*	Increased sedative effect of both drugs.
Vitamin C	Increased glycopyrrolate effect. Avoid large vitamin C doses.

 POSSIBLE INTERACTION WITH OTHER SUBSTANCES

INTERACTS WITH	COMBINED EFFECT
Alcohol:	None expected.
Beverages:	None expected.
Cocaine:	Excessively rapid heartbeat.
Foods:	None expected.
Marijuana:	Drowsiness and dry mouth.
Tobacco:	None expected.

*See Glossary

GOLD COMPOUNDS

GENERIC AND BRAND NAMES

AURANOFIN
Ridaura-Oral

**GOLD SODIUM
THIOMALATE**
Myocrisin

BASIC INFORMATION

Habit forming? No
Prescription needed? Yes
Available as generic? No
Drug class: Gold compounds

 USES

Treatment for rheumatoid arthritis and juvenile arthritis.

 DOSAGE & USAGE INFORMATION

How to take:
- Capsule—Swallow with full glass of fluid. Follow prescription directions. Taking too much can cause serious adverse reactions.
- Injection—Under medical supervision.

When to take:
Once or twice daily, morning and night.

If you forget a dose:
Take as soon as you remember up to 6 hours late, then go back to usual schedule.

What drug does:
Modifies disease activity of rheumatoid arthritis by mechanisms not yet understood.

Time lapse before drug works:
3 to 6 months.

Don't take with:
Any other medicine or any dietary supplement without consulting your doctor or pharmacist.

 OVERDOSE

SYMPTOMS:
Confusion, delirium, numbness and tingling in feet and hands.
WHAT TO DO:
- Dial 911 (emergency) for medical help or call poison control center 1-800-222-1222 for instructions.
- See emergency information on last 3 pages of this book.

 POSSIBLE ADVERSE REACTIONS OR SIDE EFFECTS

SYMPTOMS	WHAT TO DO
Life-threatening:	
Hives, rash, intense itching, faintness soon after a dose (anaphylaxis).	Seek emergency treatment immediately.
Common:	
• Itch; hives; sores or white spots in mouth, throat; appetite loss; diarrhea; vomiting; skin rashes; fever.	Discontinue. Call doctor right away.
• Indigestion, constipation.	Continue. Call doctor when convenient.
Infrequent:	
• Excessive fatigue; sore tongue, mouth or gums; metallic or odd taste; unusual bleeding or bruising; blood in urine; vaginal discharge; flushing; fainting; dizziness; sweating after injection.	Discontinue. Call doctor right away.
• Hair loss; pain in muscles, bones and joints (with injections).	Continue. Call doctor when convenient.
Rare:	
• Blood in stool, difficult breathing, coughing, seizures.	Discontinue. Seek emergency treatment.
• Abdominal pain, jaundice, numbness or tingling in hands or feet, muscle weakness.	Discontinue. Call doctor right away.
• "Pink eye."	Continue. Call doctor when convenient.

406

WARNINGS & PRECAUTIONS

Don't take if:
- You have a history of allergy to gold or other metals.
- You have any blood disorder.
- You have kidney disease.

Before you start, consult your doctor if:
- You are pregnant or may become pregnant.
- You have lupus erythematosus.
- You have Sjögren's syndrome.
- You have chronic skin disease.
- You are debilitated.
- You have blood dyscrasias.

Over age 60:
Adverse reactions and side effects may be more frequent and severe than in younger persons.

Pregnancy:
Decide with your doctor if drug benefits justify risks to unborn child. Risk category C (see page xviii).

Breast-feeding:
Drug may filter into milk, causing side effects in infants. Avoid. Consult doctor.

Infants & children:
Not recommended. Safety and dosage have not been established.

Prolonged use:
Request periodic laboratory studies of blood counts, urine and liver function. These should be done before use and at least once a month during treatment.

Skin & sunlight:
- One or more drugs in this group may cause rash or intensify sunburn in areas exposed to sun or ultraviolet light (photosensitivity reaction). Avoid overexposure. Notify doctor if reaction occurs.
- Blue-gray pigmentation in skin exposed to sunlight.

Driving, piloting or hazardous work:
Avoid if you have serious adverse reactions or side effects. Otherwise, no problems expected.

Discontinuing:
Don't discontinue without doctor's advice until you complete prescribed dose.

Others:
- Side effects and adverse reactions may appear during treatment or for many months after discontinuing.
- Gold has been shown to cause kidney tumors and kidney cancer in animals given excessive doses.
- May interfere with the accuracy of some medical tests.

 ## POSSIBLE INTERACTION WITH OTHER DRUGS

GENERIC NAME OR DRUG CLASS	COMBINED EFFECT
Bone marrow depressants*	Increased risk of toxicity of both drugs.
Hepatotoxics*	Increased risk of toxicity of both drugs.
Nephrotoxics*	Increased risk of toxicity of both drugs.
Penicillamine	Increased likelihood of kidney damage.
Phenytoin	Increased phenytoin blood levels. Phenytoin dosage may require adjustment.

 ## POSSIBLE INTERACTION WITH OTHER SUBSTANCES

INTERACTS WITH	COMBINED EFFECT
Alcohol:	None expected.
Beverages:	None expected.
Cocaine:	None expected.
Foods:	None expected.
Marijuana:	None expected.
Tobacco:	None expected.

GRISEOFULVIN

BRAND NAMES

Fulvicin P/G
Fulvicin U/F
Grifulvin V
Grisactin

Grisactin Ultra
Grisovin-FP
Gris-PEG

 BASIC INFORMATION

Habit forming? No
Prescription needed? Yes
Available as generic? Yes
Drug class: Antifungal

 USES

Treatment for fungal infections susceptible to griseofulvin.

 DOSAGE & USAGE INFORMATION

How to take:
• Tablet or capsule—Swallow with liquid or food to lessen stomach irritation. If you can't swallow whole, crumble tablet or open capsule and take with liquid or food.
• Liquid—Follow label instructions.

When to take:
With or immediately after meals.

If you forget a dose:
Take as soon as you remember up to 2 hours late. If more than 2 hours, wait for next scheduled dose (don't double this dose).

What drug does:
Prevents fungi from growing and reproducing.

Time lapse before drug works:
2 to 10 days for skin infections. 2 to 4 weeks for infections of fingernails or toenails. Complete cure of either may require several months.

Don't take with:
Any other medicine or any dietary supplement without consulting your doctor or pharmacist.

 OVERDOSE

SYMPTOMS:
Nausea, vomiting, diarrhea. In sensitive individuals, severe diarrhea may occur without overdosing.
WHAT TO DO:
Overdose unlikely to threaten life. If person uses much larger amount than prescribed or if accidentally swallowed, call doctor or poison control center 1-800-222-1222 for help.

POSSIBLE ADVERSE REACTIONS OR SIDE EFFECTS

SYMPTOMS	WHAT TO DO
Life-threatening: None expected.	
Common: Headache.	Continue. Tell doctor at next visit.
Infrequent: • Confusion; rash, hives, itch; mouth or tongue irritation; soreness; nausea; vomiting; diarrhea; stomach pain.	Discontinue. Call doctor right away.
• Insomnia, tiredness.	Continue. Call doctor when convenient.
Rare: Sore throat, fever, numbness or tingling in hands or feet, cloudy urine, yellow skin or eyes, sensitivity of skin to sunlight (these symptoms are more likely to occur with high doses taken for long periods).	Discontinue. Call doctor right away.

WARNINGS & PRECAUTIONS

Don't take if:
* You are allergic to any antifungal medicine.
* You are allergic to penicillin.
* You have liver disease.
* You have porphyria.
* The infection is minor and will respond to less potent drugs.

Before you start, consult your doctor if:
* You plan to become pregnant within medication period.
* You have lupus.

Over age 60:
Adverse reactions and side effects may be more frequent and severe than in younger persons.

Pregnancy:
Risk to unborn child outweighs drug benefits. Don't use. Risk category X (see page xviii).

Breast-feeding:
No problems expected, but consult your doctor.

Infants & children:
Not recommended for children younger than 2.

Prolonged use:
* You may become susceptible to infections caused by germs not responsive to griseofulvin.
* Talk to your doctor about the need for follow-up medical examinations or laboratory studies to check complete blood counts (white blood cell count, platelet count, red blood cell count, hemoglobin, hematocrit), liver function, kidney function.

Skin & sunlight:
May cause rash or intensify sunburn in areas exposed to sun or ultraviolet light (photosensitivity reaction). Avoid overexposure. Notify doctor if reaction occurs.

Driving, piloting or hazardous work:
Don't drive or pilot aircraft until you learn how medicine affects you. Don't work around dangerous machinery. Don't climb ladders or work in high places. Danger increases if you drink alcohol or take medicine affecting alertness and reflexes.

Discontinuing:
Don't discontinue without doctor's advice until you complete prescribed dose, even though symptoms diminish or disappear.

Others:
* Periodic laboratory blood studies and liver and kidney function tests recommended.
* Advise any doctor or dentist whom you consult that you take this medicine.

POSSIBLE INTERACTION WITH OTHER DRUGS

GENERIC NAME OR DRUG CLASS	COMBINED EFFECT
Anticoagulants, oral*	Decreased anticoagulant effect.
Barbiturates*	Decreased griseofulvin effect.
Contraceptives, oral*	Decreased contraceptive effect.
Photosensitizing medications*	Increased sun hazard.

POSSIBLE INTERACTION WITH OTHER SUBSTANCES

INTERACTS WITH	COMBINED EFFECT
Alcohol:	Increased intoxication. Possible disulfiram reaction.*
Beverages:	None expected.
Cocaine:	None expected.
Foods:	None expected, but foods high in fat will improve drug absorption.
Marijuana:	None expected.
Tobacco:	None expected.

GUAIFENESIN

BRAND NAMES

See full list of brand names in the *Generic and Brand Name Directory*, page 886.

BASIC INFORMATION

Habit forming? No
Prescription needed? No
Available as generic? Yes
Drug class: Expectorant

 ## USES

Loosens mucus in respiratory passages from allergies and infections (hay fever, cough or cold). Guaifenesin may be a single ingredient or it can be combined with other drugs, such as in a cough and cold product.

 ## DOSAGE & USAGE INFORMATION

How to take:
* Tablet or capsule—Swallow with liquid. If you can't swallow whole, crumble tablet or open capsule and take with liquid or food.
* Extended-release tablet or extended-release capsule—Swallow whole with liquid.
* Syrup, oral solution or lozenge—Take as directed on label. Follow with 8 oz. water.
* Soft chew—Take as directed on label.

When to take:
As needed, no more often than every 4 hours for regular forms. The extended-release forms are usually taken every 12 hours.

If you forget a dose:
Take as soon as you remember. If it is almost time for the next dose, skip the missed dose and wait for your next scheduled dose (don't double this dose).

Continued next column

 ## OVERDOSE

SYMPTOMS:
Drowsiness, mild weakness, nausea, vomiting.
WHAT TO DO:
Overdose unlikely to threaten life. If person uses much larger amount than prescribed or if accidentally swallowed, call doctor or poison control center 1-800-222-1222 for help.

What drug does:
Increases production of watery fluids to thin mucus so it can be coughed out or absorbed.

Time lapse before drug works:
15 to 30 minutes. Regular use for 5 to 7 days may be necessary for maximum benefit.

Don't take with:
Any other medicine or any dietary supplement without consulting your doctor or pharmacist.

 ## POSSIBLE ADVERSE REACTIONS OR SIDE EFFECTS

SYMPTOMS	WHAT TO DO
Life-threatening: None expected.	
Common: None expected.	
Infrequent: Drowsiness, rash, stomach pain, diarrhea, nausea, vomiting, dizziness, headache, hives.	Discontinue. Call doctor if symptoms persist.
Rare: None expected.	

**WARNINGS &
PRECAUTIONS**

Don't take if:
You are allergic to any cough or cold preparation containing guaifenesin.

Before you start, consult your doctor if:
You are allergic to any medicine, food or other substance.

Over age 60:
Adverse reactions and side effects may be more frequent and severe than in younger persons. For drug to work, you should drink 8 to 10 glasses of fluid per day.

Pregnancy:
Decide with your doctor if drug benefits justify risks to unborn child. Risk category C (see page xviii).

Breast-feeding:
No proven problems. Consult your doctor.

Infants & children:
Read the label on the product to see if it is approved for your child's age. Always follow the directions on product's label about how to use. If unsure, ask your doctor or pharmacist.

Prolonged use:
No problems expected.

Skin & sunlight:
No problems expected.

Driving, piloting or hazardous work:
Avoid if you feel drowsy. Otherwise, no problems expected.

Discontinuing:
May be unnecessary to finish medicine. Discontinue when symptoms disappear. If symptoms persist more than 1 week, consult doctor.

Others:
* Some guaifenesin syrup products contain alcohol. Read labels for alcohol content if you want to avoid these products.
* Advise any doctor or dentist whom you consult that you take this medicine.

 **POSSIBLE INTERACTION
WITH OTHER DRUGS**

GENERIC NAME OR DRUG CLASS	COMBINED EFFECT
Anticoagulants*	Possible risk of bleeding.

 **POSSIBLE INTERACTION
WITH OTHER SUBSTANCES**

INTERACTS WITH	COMBINED EFFECT
Alcohol:	None expected.
Beverages:	You should drink 8 to 10 glasses of fluid per day for drug to work.
Cocaine:	None expected.
Foods:	None expected.
Marijuana:	None expected.
Tobacco:	None expected.

GUANADREL

BRAND NAMES

Hylorel

BASIC INFORMATION

Habit forming? No
Prescription needed? Yes
Available as generic? No
Drug class: Antihypertensive

 USES

Controls, but doesn't cure, high blood pressure.

 DOSAGE & USAGE INFORMATION

How to take:
Tablet—Swallow with liquid or food to lessen stomach irritation. If you can't swallow whole, crumble tablet and take with liquid or food.

When to take:
At the same time each day.

If you forget a dose:
Take as soon as you remember up to 2 hours late. If more than 2 hours, wait for next scheduled dose (don't double this dose).

What drug does:
Relaxes muscle cells of small arteries.

Time lapse before drug works:
4 to 6 hours. May need to take for lifetime.

Don't take with:
Any other medicine or any dietary supplement without consulting your doctor or pharmacist.

 OVERDOSE

SYMPTOMS:
Severe blood pressure drop; fainting; blurred vision; slow, weak pulse; cold, sweaty skin; loss of consciousness.
WHAT TO DO:
• Dial 911 (emergency) for medical help or call poison control center 1-800-222-1222 for instructions.
• See emergency information on last 3 pages of this book.

 POSSIBLE ADVERSE REACTIONS OR SIDE EFFECTS

SYMPTOMS	WHAT TO DO
Life-threatening:	
In case of overdose, see previous column.	
Common:	
• Diarrhea, more bowel movements, fatigue, weakness.	Continue. Call doctor when convenient.
• Dizziness, lower sex drive, feet and ankle swelling, drowsiness.	Continue. Tell doctor at next visit.
• Stuffy nose, dry mouth.	No action necessary.
Infrequent:	
• Rash, blurred vision, drooping eyelids, chest pain or shortness of breath, muscle pain or tremor.	Discontinue. Call doctor right away.
• Nausea or vomiting, headache.	Continue. Call doctor when convenient.
• Impotence, nighttime urination.	Continue. Tell doctor at next visit
Rare:	
Decreased white blood cells causing sore throat, fever.	Discontinue. Call doctor right away.

 WARNINGS & PRECAUTIONS

Don't take if:
• You are allergic to guanadrel.
• You have taken MAO inhibitors* within 2 weeks.

Before you start, consult your doctor if:
• You have had a stroke or have heart disease.
• You have asthma.
• You have had kidney disease.
• You have peptic ulcer or chronic acid indigestion.
• You will have surgery within 2 months, including dental surgery, requiring general or spinal anesthesia.

Over age 60:
Adverse reactions and side effects may be more frequent and severe than in younger persons. Start with small doses and monitor blood pressure frequently.

Pregnancy:
No proven harm to unborn child. Avoid if possible. Consult doctor. Risk category B (see page xviii).

Breast-feeding:
No proven harm to nursing infant. Avoid if possible. Consult doctor.

Infants & children:
Not recommended.

Prolonged use:
- Due to drug's cumulative effect, dose will require adjustment to prevent wide fluctuations in blood pressure.
- Talk to your doctor about the need for follow-up medical examinations or laboratory studies.

Skin & sunlight:
No problems expected.

Driving, piloting or hazardous work:
Don't drive or pilot aircraft until you learn how medicine affects you. Don't work around dangerous machinery. Don't climb ladders or work in high places. Danger increases if you drink alcohol or take medicine affecting alertness and reflexes, such as antihistamines, tranquilizers, sedatives, pain medicine, narcotics and mind-altering drugs.

Discontinuing:
Don't discontinue without consulting doctor. Dose may require gradual reduction if you have taken drug for a long time. Doses of other drugs may also require adjustment.

Others:
- Hot weather further lowers blood pressure, particularly in patients over 60.
- Advise any doctor or dentist whom you consult that you take this medicine.

POSSIBLE INTERACTION WITH OTHER DRUGS

GENERIC NAME OR DRUG CLASS	COMBINED EFFECT
Angiotensin-converting enzyme (ACE) inhibitors*	Possible excessive potassium in blood.
Antidepressants, tricyclic*	Decreased effect of guanadrel.
Antihypertensives, other*	Increased effect of guanadrel.
Beta-adrenergic blocking agents*	Increased likelihood of dizziness and fainting.
Carteolol	Increased anti-hypertensive effect.
Contraceptives, oral*	Increased side effects of oral contraceptives.
Central nervous system (CNS) depressants* (anticonvulsants,* antihistamines,* muscle relaxants,* narcotics,* sedatives,* tranquilizers*)	Decreased effect of guanadrel.

Diuretics*	Increased likelihood of dizziness and fainting.
Haloperidol	Decreased effect of guanadrel.
Insulin	Increased insulin effect.
Loxapine	Decreased effect of guanadrel.
Monoamine oxidase (MAO) inhibitors*	Severe high blood pressure. Avoid.
Nicardipine	Blood pressure drop. Dosages may require adjustment.
Nimodipine	Dangerous blood pressure drop.
Phenothiazines*	Decreased effect of guanadrel.
Rauwolfia alkaloids*	Increased likelihood of dizziness and fainting.
Sotalol	Increased anti-hypertensive effect.
Sympathomimetics*	Decreased effect of guanadrel.
Terazosin	Decreases effectiveness of terazosin.
Thioxanthenes*	Decreased effect of guanadrel.
Trimeprazine	Decreased effect of guanadrel.

POSSIBLE INTERACTION WITH OTHER SUBSTANCES

INTERACTS WITH	COMBINED EFFECT
Alcohol:	Decreased effect of guanadrel. Avoid.
Beverages: Caffeine.	Decreased effect of guanadrel.
Cocaine:	Increased risk of heart block and high blood pressure.
Foods:	None expected.
Marijuana:	Higher blood pressure. Avoid.
Tobacco:	Higher blood pressure. Avoid.

*See Glossary

HALOPERIDOL

BRAND NAMES

Apo-Haloperidol	Halperon
Haldol	Novo-Peridol
Haldol Decanoate	Peridol
Haldol LA	PMS Haloperidol

BASIC INFORMATION

Habit forming? No
Prescription needed? Yes
Available as generic? Yes
Drug class: Antipsychotic

 ## USES

- Reduces severe anxiety, agitation and psychotic behavior.
- Treatment for Tourette's syndrome.
- Treatment for infantile autism.
- Treatment for Huntington's chorea.

 ## DOSAGE & USAGE INFORMATION

How to take:
- Tablet—Swallow with liquid. If you can't swallow whole, crumble tablet and take with liquid or food.
- Drops—Dilute dose in beverage before swallowing.

When to take:
At the same times each day.

If you forget a dose:
Take as soon as you remember up to 2 hours late. If more than 2 hours, wait for next scheduled dose (don't double this dose).

Continued next column

 ## OVERDOSE

SYMPTOMS:
Weak, rapid pulse; shallow, slow breathing; tremor or muscle weakness; very low blood pressure; convulsions; deep sleep ending in coma.
WHAT TO DO:
- **Dial 911 (emergency) for medical help or call poison control center 1-800-222-1222 for instructions.**
- **If person is unconscious, check breathing and pulse. If not breathing, begin mouth-to-mouth rescue breathing. If heart is not beating, begin chest compressions.**
- **See emergency information on last 3 pages of this book.**

What drug does:
Corrects an imbalance in nerve impulses from brain; blocks effect of dopamine.*

Time lapse before drug works:
Up to 4 weeks.

Don't take with:
Any other medicine or any dietary supplement without consulting your doctor or pharmacist.

 ## POSSIBLE ADVERSE REACTIONS OR SIDE EFFECTS

SYMPTOMS	WHAT TO DO
Life-threatening:	
High fever, rapid pulse, profuse sweating, muscle rigidity, confusion and irritability, seizures.	Discontinue. Seek emergency treatment.
Common:	
• Jerky or involuntary movements, especially of the face, lips, jaw, tongue; slow-frequency tremor of head or limbs, especially while moving; lack of facial expression and slow inflexible movements.	Discontinue. Call doctor right away.
• Pacing or restlessness; intermittent spasms of muscles of face, eyes, tongue, jaw, neck, body or limbs.	Continue. Call doctor when convenient.
Infrequent:	
Dry mouth, blurred vision, constipation, difficulty urinating, sedation, low blood pressure, dizziness.	Continue. Call doctor when convenient.
Rare:	
Other symptoms not listed above.	Continue. Call doctor when convenient.

 ## WARNINGS & PRECAUTIONS

Don't take if:
- You have ever been allergic to haloperidol.
- You are depressed.
- You have Parkinson's disease.
- Patient is younger than 3 years old.

Before you start, consult your doctor if:
- You have a history of mental depression.
- You have had kidney or liver problems.
- You have diabetes, epilepsy, glaucoma, prostate trouble or asthma.
- You have high blood pressure, heart disease or cardiac abnormalities.
- You have QT-prolonging conditions, including electrolyte imbalance (particularly hypokalemia and hypomagnesemia) or familial long QT syndrome.
- You have hyper- or hypothyroidism.
- You drink alcoholic beverages frequently.

Over age 60:
- Adverse reactions and side effects may be more frequent and severe than in younger persons.
- Use of antipsychotic drugs in elderly patients with dementia-related psychosis may increase risk of death. Consult doctor.

Pregnancy:
Decide with your doctor if drug benefits justify risk to unborn child. Risk category C (see page xviii).

Breast-feeding:
Drug passes into milk. Avoid drug or discontinue nursing until you finish medicine. Consult doctor about maintaining milk supply.

Infants & children:
Safety and efficacy have not been established.

Prolonged use:
- May develop tardive dyskinesia (involuntary movements of jaws, lips and tongue).
- Talk to your doctor about the need for follow-up medical examinations or laboratory studies to check blood pressure, liver function.

Skin & sunlight:
- May cause rash or intensify sunburn in areas exposed to sun or ultraviolet light (photosensitivity). Avoid overexposure and use sunscreen. Consult doctor if reaction occurs.
- Avoid getting overheated. The drug affects body temperature and sweating.

Driving, piloting or hazardous work:
Don't drive or pilot aircraft until you learn how medicine affects you. Don't work around dangerous machinery. Don't climb ladders or work in high places. Danger increases if you drink alcohol or take medicine affecting alertness and reflexes.

Discontinuing:
Don't discontinue without consulting doctor. Dose may require gradual reduction if you have taken drug for a long time. Doses of other drugs may also require adjustment.

Others:
- For dry mouth, suck on sugarless hard candy or chew sugarless gum. If dry mouth persists, consult your dentist.

- Higher doses of this drug may increase risk of serious heart rhythm problems (including cases of sudden death). Call doctor right away if heart symptoms occur.
- Advise any doctor or dentist whom you consult that you take this medicine.

 ## POSSIBLE INTERACTION WITH OTHER DRUGS

GENERIC NAME OR DRUG CLASS	COMBINED EFFECT
Anticholinergics*	Increased anticholinergic effect. May cause elevated pressure within the eye.
Anticonvulsants*	Changed seizure pattern.
Antidepressants*	Excessive sedation.
Antihistamines*	Excessive sedation.
Antihypertensives*	May cause severe blood pressure drop.
Barbiturates*	Excessive sedation.
Bupropion	Increased risk of seizures.
Central nervous system (CNS) depressants*	Increased CNS depression; increased blood pressure drop.
Clozapine	Toxic effect on the nervous system.

Continued on page 918

 ## POSSIBLE INTERACTION WITH OTHER SUBSTANCES

INTERACTS WITH	COMBINED EFFECT
Alcohol:	Excessive sedation and depressed brain function. Avoid.
Beverages:	None expected.
Cocaine:	Decreased effect of haloperidol. Avoid.
Foods:	None expected.
Marijuana:	Occasional use—Increased sedation. Frequent use—Possible toxic psychosis.
Tobacco:	None expected.

*See Glossary

HISTAMINE H₂ RECEPTOR ANTAGONISTS

GENERIC AND BRAND NAMES

CIMETIDINE
Apo-Cimetidine
Liquid Tagamet
Novocimetine
Peptol
Tagamet
Tagamet HB
FAMOTIDINE
Fluxid
Mylanta-AR
Pepcid
Pepcid AC
Pepcid Complete
Pepcid RPD
Ulcidine

NIZATIDINE
Axid
RANITIDINE
Apo-Ranitidine
Zantac
Zantac 75
Zantac-C
Zantac Efferdose
Zantac Geldose

BASIC INFORMATION

Habit forming? No
Prescription needed? Yes, for some
Available as generic? Yes, for some
Drug class: Histamine H₂ antagonist

USES

- Treatment for duodenal, gastric and peptic ulcers and other conditions in which stomach produces excess acid.
- Treatment for and prevention of heartburn.
- Maintenance of healing of erosive esophagitis.

DOSAGE & USAGE INFORMATION

How to take:
- Tablet, capsule or liquid—Swallow with liquid.
- Chewable tablet—Chew thoroughly and swallow with water.
- Disintegrating tablet—Let dissolve on tongue.
- Oral suspension or effervescent tablets for oral solution—Follow instructions on prescription.

Continued next column

OVERDOSE

SYMPTOMS:
Confusion, slurred speech, breathing difficulty, rapid heartbeat, delirium.
WHAT TO DO:
Overdose unlikely to threaten life. If person uses much larger amount than prescribed or if accidentally swallowed, call doctor or poison control center 1-800-222-1222 for help.

When to take:
- 1 dose per day—Take at bedtime.
- 2 or more doses per day—Take at the same times each day.

If you forget a dose:
Take as soon as you remember up to 2 hours late. If more than 2 hours, wait for next scheduled dose (don't double this dose).

What drug does:
Blocks histamine release so stomach secretes less acid.

Time lapse before drug works:
- Begins in 30 minutes. May require several days to relieve pain.
- Lower dosages in nonprescription medicines may take 45 minutes to relieve heartburn.

Don't take with:
Any other medicine or any dietary supplement without consulting your doctor or pharmacist.

POSSIBLE ADVERSE REACTIONS OR SIDE EFFECTS

SYMPTOMS	WHAT TO DO
Life-threatening: None expected.	
Common: None expected.	
Infrequent:	
• Dizziness or headache, diarrhea.	Continue. Call doctor when convenient.
• Diminished sex drive, unusual milk flow in females, hair loss.	Continue. Tell doctor at next visit.
Rare:	
• Confusion; rash, hives; sore throat, fever; slow, fast or irregular heartbeat; unusual bleeding or bruising; muscle cramps or pain; fatigue; weakness.	Discontinue. Call doctor right away.
• Constipation.	Continue. Call doctor when convenient.

WARNINGS & PRECAUTIONS

Don't take if:
You are allergic to any histamine H₂ antagonist.

Before you start, consult your doctor if:
- You plan to become pregnant while on medication.
- You take aspirin. Aspirin may irritate stomach.

Over age 60:
Adverse reactions and side effects may be more frequent and severe than in younger persons.

HISTAMINE H₂ RECEPTOR ANTAGONISTS

Pregnancy:
Risk factors vary for drugs in this group. See category list on page xviii and consult doctor.

Breast-feeding:
Drug passes into milk. Avoid drug or discontinue nursing until you finish medicine. Consult doctor about maintaining milk supply.

Infants & children:
Not recommended.

Prolonged use:
- Possible liver damage.
- Talk to your doctor about the need for follow-up medical examinations or laboratory studies.

Skin & sunlight:
No problems expected.

Driving, piloting or hazardous work:
Don't drive or pilot aircraft until you learn how medicine affects you. Don't work around dangerous machinery. Don't climb ladders or work in high places. Danger increases if you drink alcohol or take medicine affecting alertness and reflexes, such as antihistamines, tranquilizers, sedatives, pain medicine, narcotics and mind-altering drugs.

Discontinuing:
Don't discontinue without consulting a doctor. Dose may require gradual reduction if you have taken drug for a long time. Doses of other drugs may also require adjustment.

Others:
- Patients on kidney dialysis—Take at end of dialysis treatment.
- May interfere with the accuracy of some medical tests.
- Advise any doctor or dentist whom you consult that you take this medicine.

POSSIBLE INTERACTION WITH OTHER DRUGS

GENERIC NAME OR DRUG CLASS	COMBINED EFFECT
Alprazolam	Increased effect and toxicity of alprazolam.
Antacids*	Decreased absorption of histamine H₂ receptor antagonist.
Anticoagulants, oral*	Increased anticoagulant effect.
Anticholinergics*	Increased histamine H₂ receptor antagonist effect.
Antivirals, HIV/AIDS*	Increased antiviral effect with cimetidine.
Azelastine	Increased azelastine effect.

Bupropion	Increased bupropion effect.
Carbamazepine	Increased effect and toxicity of carbamazepine.
Carmustine (BCNU)	Severe impairment of red blood cell production; some interference with white blood cell formation.
Chlordiazepoxide	Increased effect and toxicity of chlordiazepoxide.
Cisapride	Decreased histamine H₂ receptor effect.
Citalopram	Increased effect of citalopram.

Continued on page 918

POSSIBLE INTERACTION WITH OTHER SUBSTANCES

INTERACTS WITH	COMBINED EFFECT
Alcohol:	No interactions expected, but alcohol may slow body's recovery. Avoid.
Beverages: Milk.	Enhanced effectiveness. Small amounts useful for taking medication.
Caffeine drinks.	May increase acid secretion and delay healing.
Cocaine:	Decreased effect of histamine H₂ receptor antagonist.
Foods:	Enhanced effectiveness. Protein-rich foods should be eaten in moderation to minimize secretion of stomach acid.
Marijuana:	Increased chance of low sperm count. Marijuana may slow body's recovery. Avoid.
Tobacco:	Reversed effect of histamine H₂ receptor antagonist. Tobacco may slow body's recovery. Avoid.

*See Glossary

417

HMG-CoA REDUCTASE INHIBITORS

GENERIC AND BRAND NAMES

ATORVASTATIN
  Caduet
  Lipitor
FLUVASTATIN
  Lescol
  Lescol XL
LOVASTATIN
  Advicor
  Altocor
  Mevacor
  Mevinolin

PRAVASTATIN
  Eptastatin
  Pravachol
  Pravigard PAC
ROSUVASTATIN
  Crestor
SIMVASTATIN
  Epistatin
  Simcor
  Synvinolin
  Vytorin
  Zocor

BASIC INFORMATION

Habit forming? No
Prescription needed? Yes
Available as generic? Yes, for some
Drug class: Antihyperlipidemic

USES

- Lowers blood cholesterol levels caused by low-density lipoproteins (LDL) in persons who haven't improved by exercising, dieting or using other measures and raises high density lipoproteins (HDL-C).
- Used in combination with a low-fat diet to slow the progression of atherosclerosis in patients with coronary heart disease and high cholesterol levels.
- Reduces risk of heart attacks and strokes in certain patients.
- Lowers triglyceride levels.

DOSAGE & USAGE INFORMATION

How to take:
- Tablet or capsule—Swallow with liquid. If you can't swallow whole, crumble tablet and take with liquid or food.
- Extended release tablet—Swallow with liquid. Do not crumble or chew tablet.

Continued next column

OVERDOSE

SYMPTOMS:
None expected.
WHAT TO DO:
Overdose unlikely to threaten life. If person uses much larger amount than prescribed or if accidentally swallowed, call doctor or poison control center 1-800-222-1222 for help.

When to take:
According to directions on prescription.

If you forget a dose:
Take as soon as you remember up to 2 hours late. If more than 2 hours, wait for next scheduled dose (don't double this dose).

What drug does:
Inhibits an enzyme in the liver.

Time lapse before drug works:
2 to 4 weeks.

Don't take with:
- A high-fat diet.
- Any other medicine or any dietary supplement without consulting your doctor or pharmacist.

POSSIBLE ADVERSE REACTIONS OR SIDE EFFECTS

SYMPTOMS	WHAT TO DO
Life-threatening: None expected.	
Common: None expected.	
Infrequent:	
• Aching muscles, fever, blurred vision.	Discontinue. Call doctor right away.
• Constipation, nausea, dizziness, skin rash, headache, diarrhea, heartburn.	Continue. Call doctor when convenient.
Rare:	
• Muscle or stomach pain, unusual tiredness or weakness.	Discontinue. Call doctor right away.
• Impotence, insomnia.	Continue. Call doctor when convenient.

WARNINGS & PRECAUTIONS

Don't take if:
You are allergic to any HMG-CoA reductase inhibitor.

Before you start, consult your doctor if:
- You take immunosuppressive drugs, particularly following an organ transplant.
- You have low blood pressure.
- You have hormone abnormalities.
- You have an active infection.
- You have active liver disease.
- You have a seizure disorder.
- You have a history of alcohol abuse.
- You have had recent surgery.

Over age 60:
Likely to be more sensitive to drug's side effects.

HMG-CoA REDUCTASE INHIBITORS

Pregnancy:
Consult doctor. Risk category X (see page xviii).

Breast-feeding:
Discontinue nursing until you finish medicine. Consult doctor for advice about milk supply.

Infants & children:
Not recommended for children.

Prolonged use:
Talk to your doctor about the need for follow-up medical examinations or laboratory studies to check liver function, serum cholesterol, eyes.

Skin & sunlight:
No problems expected.

Driving, piloting or hazardous work:
No special problems expected.

Discontinuing:
Don't discontinue without consulting doctor. Dose may require gradual reduction if you have taken drug for a long time. Doses of other drugs may also require adjustment.

Others:
- Request liver function tests and eye examinations before beginning this medicine and repeat every 2 to 6 months.
- Advise any doctor or dentist whom you consult that you take this medicine.
- Cholesterol lowering drugs may cause muscle problems or rhabdomyolysis (muscle injury). If you develop persistent muscle aches, pain or weakness or urine turns dark, call the doctor right away.
- Use an effective form of birth control while taking this drug. Notify your doctor right away if you do become pregnant.

POSSIBLE INTERACTION WITH OTHER DRUGS

GENERIC NAME OR DRUG CLASS	COMBINED EFFECT
Amiodarone	Risk of muscle injury and kidney failure.
Antifungals, azole*	Increased effect of HMG-CoA reductase inhibitor.
Cholestyramine	Decreased effect of HMG-CoA reductase inhibitor if taken at same time.
Colestipol	Decreased effect of HMG-CoA reductase inhibitor if taken at same time.
Cyclosporine	Increased risk of muscle and kidney problems.
Digoxin	Increased digoxin effect.
Diltiazem	Increased effect of HMG-CoA reductase inhibitor.
Erythromycins*	Increased risk of muscle and kidney problems.
Gemfibrozil	Increased risk of muscle and kidney problems and muscle inflammation.
Immunosuppressants*	Increased risk of muscle or kidney problems.
Niacin	Increased risk of muscle and kidney problems.
Orlistat	Increased effect of HMG-CoA reductase inhibitor.
Ranolazine	Increased effect of simvastatin.
Telithromycin	Increased effect of HMG-CoA reductase inhibitor.

POSSIBLE INTERACTION WITH OTHER SUBSTANCES

INTERACTS WITH	COMBINED EFFECT
Alcohol:	Best to avoid alcohol while taking this drug.
Beverages: Grapefruit juice.	May increase effect of HMG-CoA reductase inhibitor.
Cocaine:	None expected.
Foods: Grapefruit.	May increase effect of HMG-CoA reductase inhibitor.
Marijuana:	None expected.
Tobacco:	None expected.

*See Glossary

HYDRALAZINE

BRAND NAMES

Apresoline	Novo-Hylazin
BiDil	

BASIC INFORMATION

Habit forming? No
Prescription needed? Yes
Available as generic? Yes
Drug class: Antihypertensive

 USES

- Treatment for high blood pressure and congestive heart failure.
- The brand name BiDil is approved to treat heart failure specifically in African Americans.

 DOSAGE & USAGE INFORMATION

How to take:
Tablet—Swallow with liquid. If you can't swallow whole, crumble tablet and take with liquid or food.

When to take:
At the same time each day. Should be taken with food.

If you forget a dose:
Take as soon as you remember up to 2 hours late. If more than 2 hours, wait for next scheduled dose (don't double this dose).

What drug does:
Relaxes and expands blood vessel walls, lowering blood pressure.

Time lapse before drug works:
Regular use for several weeks may be necessary to determine drug's effectiveness.

Continued next column

 OVERDOSE

SYMPTOMS:
Rapid and weak heartbeat, fainting, extreme weakness, cold and sweaty skin, flushing.
WHAT TO DO:
- Dial 911 (emergency) for medical help or call poison control center 1-800-222-1222 for instructions.
- If person is unconscious, check breathing and pulse. If not breathing, begin mouth-to-mouth rescue breathing. If heart is not beating, begin chest compressions.
- See emergency information on last 3 pages of this book.

Don't take with:
- Nonprescription drugs containing alcohol without consulting doctor.
- Any other medicine or any dietary supplement without consulting your doctor or pharmacist.

 POSSIBLE ADVERSE REACTIONS OR SIDE EFFECTS

SYMPTOMS	WHAT TO DO
Life-threatening:	
In case of overdose, see previous column.	
Common:	
• Nausea or vomiting, rapid or irregular heartbeat.	Discontinue. Call doctor right away.
• Headache, diarrhea, appetite loss, painful or difficult urination.	Continue. Tell doctor at next visit.
Infrequent:	
• Hives or rash, flushed face, sore throat, fever, chest pain, swelling of lymph glands, skin blisters, swelling in feet or legs.	Discontinue. Call doctor right away.
• Confusion, dizziness, anxiety, depression, joint pain, general discomfort or weakness, muscle pain.	Continue. Call doctor when convenient.
• Watery eyes and irritation, constipation.	Continue. Tell doctor at next visit.
Rare:	
• Weakness and faintness when arising from bed or chair, jaundice.	Discontinue. Call doctor right away.
• Numbness or tingling in hands or feet, nasal congestion, impotence.	Continue. Call doctor when convenient.

 WARNINGS & PRECAUTIONS

Don't take if:
- You are allergic to hydralazine or tartrazine dye.
- You have a history of coronary artery disease or rheumatic heart disease.

HYDRALAZINE

Before you start, consult your doctor if:
- You feel pain in chest, neck or arms on physical exertion.
- You have had lupus.
- You have had a stroke.
- You have had kidney disease or impaired kidney function.
- You will have surgery within 2 months, including dental surgery, requiring general or spinal anesthesia.

Over age 60:
Adverse reactions and side effects may be more frequent and severe than in younger persons.

Pregnancy:
Decide with your doctor if drug benefits justify risk to unborn child. Risk category C (see page xviii).

Breast-feeding:
Drug passes into milk. Avoid drug or discontinue nursing until you finish medicine. Consult doctor about maintaining milk supply.

Infants & children:
Not recommended.

Prolonged use:
- May cause lupus (arthritis-like illness).
- Possible psychosis.
- May cause numbness, tingling in hands or feet.
- Talk to your doctor about the need for follow-up medical examinations or laboratory studies to check blood pressure, complete blood counts (white blood cell count, platelet count, red blood cell count, hemoglobin, hematocrit), ANA titers.*

Skin & sunlight:
No problems expected.

Driving, piloting or hazardous work:
Don't drive or pilot aircraft until you learn how medicine affects you. Don't work around dangerous machinery. Don't climb ladders or work in high places. Danger increases if you drink alcohol or take medicine affecting alertness and reflexes, such as antihistamines, tranquilizers, sedatives, pain medicine, narcotics and mind-altering drugs.

Discontinuing:
Don't discontinue without doctor's advice until you complete prescribed dose, even though symptoms diminish or disappear.

Others:
- Vitamin B-6 diet supplement may be advisable. Consult doctor.
- Some products contain tartrazine dye. Avoid, especially if you are allergic to aspirin.
- May interfere with the accuracy of some medical tests.
- Advise any doctor or dentist whom you consult that you take this medicine.

POSSIBLE INTERACTION WITH OTHER DRUGS

GENERIC NAME OR DRUG CLASS	COMBINED EFFECT
Amphetamines*	Decreased hydralazine effect.
Antihypertensives, other*	Increased antihypertensive effect.
Anti-inflammatory drugs, nonsteroidal (NSAIDs)*	Decreased effect of hydralazine.
Antivirals, HIV/AIDS*	Increased risk of peripheral neuropathy.
Carteolol	Increased antihypertensive effect.
Diazoxide & other anti-hypertensive drugs	Increased antihypertensive effect.
Diuretics, oral*	Increased effects of both drugs. When monitored carefully, combination may be beneficial in controlling hypertension.
Guanfacine	Increased effects of both drugs.

Continued on page 919

POSSIBLE INTERACTION WITH OTHER SUBSTANCES

INTERACTS WITH	COMBINED EFFECT
Alcohol:	May lower blood pressure excessively. Use extreme caution.
Beverages:	None expected.
Cocaine:	Increased risk of heart block and high blood pressure.
Foods:	Increased hydralazine absorption.
Marijuana:	Weakness on standing.
Tobacco:	Possible angina attacks.

*See Glossary

421

HYDRALAZINE & HYDROCHLOROTHIAZIDE

BRAND NAMES

Apresazide

Apresoline-Esidrix

Aprozide

Hydra-Zide

BASIC INFORMATION

Habit forming? No

Prescription needed? Yes

Available as generic? Yes

Drug class: Antihypertensive, diuretic

USES

- Controls, but doesn't cure, high blood pressure.
- Reduces fluid retention (edema).

DOSAGE & USAGE INFORMATION

How to take:

Tablet or capsule—Swallow with liquid. If you can't swallow whole, crumble tablet or open capsule and take with liquid or food.

When to take:

At the same time each day.

If you forget a dose:

Take as soon as you remember up to 2 hours late. If more than 2 hours, wait for next scheduled dose (don't double this dose).

What drug does:

- Forces sodium and water excretion, reducing body fluid.
- Relaxes and expands blood vessel walls, lowering blood pressure.
- Reduced body fluid and relaxed arteries lower blood pressure.

Continued next column

OVERDOSE

SYMPTOMS:

Cramps, drowsiness, weak pulse, rapid and weak heartbeat, fainting, extreme weakness, cold and sweaty skin, coma.

WHAT TO DO:

- **Dial 911 (emergency) for medical help or call poison control center 1-800-222-1222 for instructions.**
- **If person is unconscious, check breathing and pulse. If not breathing, begin mouth-to-mouth rescue breathing. If heart is not beating, begin chest compressions.**
- **See emergency information on last 3 pages of this book.**

Time lapse before drug works:

Regular use for several weeks may be necessary to determine drug's effectiveness.

Don't take with:

- Nonprescription drugs containing alcohol without consulting doctor.
- Any other medicine or any dietary supplement without consulting your doctor or pharmacist.

POSSIBLE ADVERSE REACTIONS OR SIDE EFFECTS

SYMPTOMS	WHAT TO DO
Life-threatening:	
Chest pain, irregular and fast heartbeat, weak pulse.	Discontinue. Seek emergency treatment.
Common:	
• Nausea, vomiting.	Discontinue. Call doctor right away.
• Headache, diarrhea, appetite loss, frequent urination, dry mouth, thirst.	Continue. Call doctor when convenient.
Infrequent:	
• Rash; black, bloody or tarry stool; red or flushed face; sore throat, fever, mouth sores; constipation; lymph glands swelling; blurred vision; skin blisters; swelling in feet or legs.	Discontinue. Call doctor right away.
• Dizziness; confusion; watery eyes; weight gain or loss; joint, muscle or chest pain; depression; anxiety; fever.	Continue. Call doctor when convenient.
Rare:	
• Weakness and faintness when arising from bed or chair, jaundice.	Discontinue. Call doctor right away.
• Numbness or tingling in hands or feet, nasal congestion, impotence.	Continue. Call doctor when convenient.

WARNINGS & PRECAUTIONS

Don't take if:

- You are allergic to hydralazine, any thiazide diuretic drug or tartrazine dye.
- You have history of coronary artery disease or rheumatic heart disease.

HYDRALAZINE & HYDROCHLOROTHIAZIDE

Before you start, consult your doctor if:
- You feel pain in chest, neck or arms on physical exertion.
- You are allergic to any sulfa drug.
- You have had lupus or a stroke.
- You have gout, liver, pancreas or kidney disorder.
- You will have surgery within 2 months, including dental surgery, requiring general or spinal anesthesia.

Over age 60:
Adverse reactions and side effects may be more frequent and severe than in younger persons, especially dizziness and excessive potassium loss.

Pregnancy:
Decide with your doctor if drug benefits justify risk to unborn child. Risk category C (see page xviii).

Breast-feeding:
Drug passes into milk. Avoid drug or discontinue nursing until you finish medicine. Consult doctor for advice on maintaining milk supply.

Infants & children:
Not recommended.

Prolonged use:
- May cause lupus (arthritis-like illness).
- Possible psychosis.
- May cause numbness, tingling in hands or feet.
- Talk to your doctor about the need for follow-up medical examinations or laboratory studies to check blood pressure, complete blood counts (white blood cell count, platelet count, red blood cell count, hemoglobin, hematocrit), ANA titers.*

Skin & sunlight:
One or more drugs in this group may cause rash or intensify sunburn in areas exposed to sun or ultraviolet light (photosensitivity reaction). Avoid overexposure. Notify doctor if reaction occurs.

Driving, piloting or hazardous work:
Don't drive or pilot aircraft until you learn how medicine affects you. Don't work around dangerous machinery. Don't climb ladders or work in high places. Danger increases if you drink alcohol or take medicine affecting alertness and reflexes, such as antihistamines, tranquilizers, sedatives, pain medicine, narcotics and mind-altering drugs.

Discontinuing:
Don't discontinue without consulting doctor's advice until you complete prescribed dose, even though symptoms diminish or disappear.

Others:
- Vitamin B-6 diet supplement may be advisable. Consult doctor.

- Hot weather and fever may cause dehydration and drop in blood pressure. Dose may require temporary adjustment. Weigh daily and report any unexpected weight loss to your doctor.
- May cause rise in uric acid, leading to gout.
- May cause blood sugar rise in diabetics.
- Advise any doctor or dentist whom you consult that you take this medicine.

POSSIBLE INTERACTION WITH OTHER DRUGS

GENERIC NAME OR DRUG CLASS	COMBINED EFFECT
Acebutolol	Decreased anti-hypertensive effect of acebutolol.
Allopurinol	Decreased allopurinol effect.
Amphetamines*	Decreased hydralazine effect.
Antidepressants, tricyclic*	Dangerous drop in blood pressure. Avoid combination unless under medical supervision.
Antihypertensives,* other	Increased anti-hypertensive effect.
Antivirals, HIV/AIDS*	Increased risk of peripheral neuropathy.

Continued on page 919

POSSIBLE INTERACTION WITH OTHER SUBSTANCES

INTERACTS WITH	COMBINED EFFECT
Alcohol:	May lower blood pressure excessively. Use extreme caution.
Beverages:	None expected.
Cocaine:	Dangerous blood pressure rise. Avoid.
Foods: Licorice.	Excessive potassium loss that causes dangerous heart rhythms.
Marijuana:	Weakness on standing. May increase blood pressure.
Tobacco:	Possible angina attacks.

*See Glossary

HYDROCORTISONE (Rectal)

BRAND NAMES

Anamantle HC
  Cream Kit
Anucort
Anusol-H.C.
Cort-Dome High
  Potency
Corticaine

Cortiment-10
Cortiment-40
Dermolate
Hemril-HC
Peranex HC Cream
Proctocort
Rectocort
Xyralid RC

BASIC INFORMATION

Habit forming? No
Prescription needed? Yes
Available as generic? Yes, for some
Drug class: Anti-inflammatory, steroidal
  (rectal); anesthetic (rectal)

 USES

In or around the rectum to relieve swelling,
itching and pain from hemorrhoids (piles) and
other rectal conditions. Frequently used after
hemorrhoid surgery.

 DOSAGE & USAGE INFORMATION

How to use:
- Rectal cream or ointment—Apply to surface of
  rectum with fingers. Insert applicator into
  rectum no farther than halfway and apply
  inside. Wash applicator with warm soapy water
  or discard. Review instructions if unsure.
- Suppository—Remove wrapper and moisten
  with water. Lie on side. Push blunt end of
  suppository into rectum with finger. If
  suppository is too soft, run cold water over it or
  put in refrigerator for 15 to 45 minutes before
  using. Review instructions if unsure.
- Aerosol foam—Read patient instructions.
  Don't insert into rectum. Use the special
  applicator and wash carefully after using.

When to use:
Follow instructions in package or when needed.

Continued next column

 OVERDOSE

SYMPTOMS:
None expected.
WHAT TO DO:
Not intended for internal use. If child
accidentally swallows, dial 911 (emergency)
for medical help or call poison control center
1-800-222-1222 for instructions.

If you forget a dose:
Use as soon as you remember.

What drug does:
- Reduces inflammation.
- Relieves pain and itching.

Time lapse before drug works:
5 to 15 minutes.

Don't use with:
Other rectal medicines without consulting your
doctor or pharmacist.

 POSSIBLE ADVERSE REACTIONS OR SIDE EFFECTS

SYMPTOMS	WHAT TO DO
Life-threatening None expected.	
Common None expected.	
Infrequent • Nervousness, trembling, hives, rash, itch, inflammation or tenderness not present before application, slow heartbeat.	Discontinue. Call doctor right away.
• Dizziness, blurred vision, swollen feet.	Continue. Call doctor when convenient.
Rare • Blood in urine.	Discontinue. Call doctor right away.
• Increased or painful urination.	Continue. Call doctor when convenient.

HYDROCORTISONE (Rectal)

WARNINGS & PRECAUTIONS

Don't use if:
You are allergic to any topical anesthetic.

Before you start, consult your doctor if:
- You have skin infection at site of treatment.
- You have had severe or extensive skin disorders such as eczema or psoriasis.
- You have bleeding hemorrhoids.

Over age 60:
Adverse reactions and side effects may be more frequent and severe than in younger persons.

Pregnancy:
Decide with your doctor if drug benefits justify risk to unborn child. Risk category C (see page xviii).

Breast-feeding:
No problems expected. Consult doctor.

Infants & children:
Don't use without careful medical supervision. Rarely, too much may be absorbed into the blood stream and affect growth.

Prolonged use:
Possible excess absorption. Don't use longer than 3 days for any one problem.

Skin & sunlight:
No problems expected.

Driving, piloting or hazardous work:
No problems expected.

Discontinuing:
May be unnecessary to finish medicine. Follow doctor's instructions.

Others:
- Report any rectal bleeding to your doctor.
- Keep cool, but don't freeze.

POSSIBLE INTERACTION WITH OTHER DRUGS

GENERIC NAME OR DRUG CLASS	COMBINED EFFECT
Sulfa drugs*	Decreased antiinfective effect of sulfa drugs.

POSSIBLE INTERACTION WITH OTHER SUBSTANCES

INTERACTS WITH	COMBINED EFFECT
Alcohol:	None expected.
Beverages:	None expected.
Cocaine:	Possible nervous system toxicity. Avoid.
Foods:	None expected.
Marijuana:	None expected.
Tobacco:	None expected.

*See Glossary

HYDROXYCHLOROQUINE

BRAND NAMES

Plaquenil

BASIC INFORMATION

Habit forming? No
Prescription needed? Yes
Available as generic? No
Drug class: Antiprotozoal, antirheumatic

 ## USES

- Treatment for protozoal infections, such as malaria and amebiasis.
- Treatment for some forms of arthritis and lupus.

 ## DOSAGE & USAGE INFORMATION

How to take:
Tablet—Swallow with food or milk to lessen stomach irritation.

When to take:
- Depends on condition. Is adjusted during treatment.
- Malaria prevention—Begin taking medicine 2 weeks before entering areas where malaria is present and until 8 weeks after return.

If you forget a dose:
- 1 or more doses a day—Take as soon as you remember up to 2 hours late. If more than 2 hours, wait for next scheduled dose (don't double this dose).
- 1 dose weekly—Take as soon as possible, then return to regular dosing schedule.

What drug does:
- Inhibits parasite multiplication.
- Decreases inflammatory response in diseased joint.

Time lapse before drug works:
1 to 2 hours.

Continued next column

 ## OVERDOSE

SYMPTOMS:
Severe breathing difficulty, drowsiness, faintness, headache, seizures.
WHAT TO DO:
- Dial 911 (emergency) for medical help or call poison control center 1-800-222-1222 for instructions.
- See emergency information on last 3 pages of this book.

Don't take with:
Any other medicine or any dietary supplement without consulting your doctor or pharmacist.

 ## POSSIBLE ADVERSE REACTIONS OR SIDE EFFECTS

SYMPTOMS	WHAT TO DO
Life-threatening:	
In case of overdose, see previous column.	
Common:	
Headache, appetite loss, abdominal pain.	Continue. Tell doctor at next visit.
Infrequent:	
• Blurred vision, changes in vision.	Discontinue. Call doctor right away.
• Rash or itch, diarrhea, nausea, vomiting, hair loss, blue-black skin or mouth, dizziness, nervousness.	Continue. Call doctor when convenient.
Rare:	
• Mood or mental changes, seizures, sore throat, fever, unusual bleeding or bruising, muscle weakness, convulsions.	Discontinue. Call doctor right away.
• Ringing or buzzing in ears, hearing loss.	Continue. Call doctor when convenient.

HYDROXYCHLOROQUINE

WARNINGS & PRECAUTIONS

Don't take if:
You are allergic to chloroquine or hydroxychloroquine.

Before you start, consult your doctor if:
- You plan to become pregnant within the medication period.
- You have blood disease.
- You have eye or vision problems.
- You have a G6PD* deficiency.
- You have liver disease.
- You have nerve or brain disease (including seizure disorders).
- You have porphyria.
- You have psoriasis.
- You have stomach or intestinal disease.
- You drink more than 3 oz. of alcohol daily.

Over age 60:
Adverse reactions and side effects may be more frequent and severe than in younger persons.

Pregnancy:
Decide with your doctor if drug benefits justify risk to unborn child. Risk category C (see page xviii).

Breast-feeding:
Drug passes into milk. Avoid drug or discontinue nursing. Consult doctor for advice on maintaining milk supply.

Infants & children:
Not recommended. Dangerous.

Prolonged use:
- Permanent damage to the retina (back part of the eye) or nerve deafness.
- Talk to your doctor about the need for follow-up medical examinations or laboratory studies to check complete blood counts (white blood cell count, platelet count, red blood cell count, hemoglobin, hematocrit), eyes.

Skin & sunlight:
No special problems expected.

Driving, piloting or hazardous work:
Don't drive or pilot aircraft until you learn how medicine affects you. Don't work around dangerous machinery. Don't climb ladders or work in high places. Danger increases if you drink alcohol or take medicine affecting alertness and reflexes.

Discontinuing:
Don't discontinue without doctor's advice until you complete prescribed dose, even though symptoms diminish or disappear.

Others:
- Periodic physical and blood examinations recommended.
- If you are in a malaria area for a long time, you may need to change to another preventive drug every 2 years.

POSSIBLE INTERACTION WITH OTHER DRUGS

GENERIC NAME OR DRUG CLASS	COMBINED EFFECT
Estrogens*	Possible liver toxicity.
Gold compounds*	Risk of severe rash and itch.
Kaolin	Decreased absorption of hydroxychloroquine.
Magnesium trisilicate	Decreased absorption of hydroxychloroquine.
Penicillamine	Possible blood or kidney toxicity.

POSSIBLE INTERACTION WITH OTHER SUBSTANCES

INTERACTS WITH	COMBINED EFFECT
Alcohol:	Possible liver toxicity. Avoid.
Beverages:	None expected.
Cocaine:	None expected.
Foods:	None expected.
Marijuana:	None expected.
Tobacco:	None expected.

*See Glossary

HYDROXYUREA

BRAND NAMES

Droxia   Hydrea

BASIC INFORMATION

Habit forming? No
Prescription needed? Yes
Available as generic? Yes
Drug class: Antineoplastic

USES

- Treats head, neck, ovarian and cervical cancer.
- Treats leukemia, melanoma and polycythemia vera.
- Treats sickle cell disease.

DOSAGE & USAGE INFORMATION

How to take:
Capsule—Swallow with liquid. If you can't swallow whole, open capsule and take with liquid or food. Instructions to take on empty stomach mean 1 hour before or 2 hours after eating.

When to take:
According to doctor's instructions.

If you forget a dose:
Skip this dose. Never double dose. Resume regular schedule.

What drug does:
Probably interferes with synthesis of DNA.

Time lapse before drug works:
2 hours.

Don't take with:
Any other medicines (including over-the-counter drugs such as cough and cold medicines, laxatives, antacids, diet pills, caffeine, nose drops or vitamins) without consulting your doctor or pharmacist.

OVERDOSE

SYMPTOMS:
Black, tarry stools; fainting; seizures.
WHAT TO DO:
- Dial 911 (emergency) for medical help or call poison control center 1-800-222-1222 for instructions.
- See emergency information on last 3 pages of this book.

POSSIBLE ADVERSE REACTIONS OR SIDE EFFECTS

SYMPTOMS	WHAT TO DO
Life-threatening:	
In case of overdose, see previous column.	
Common:	
• Skin rash, fever, chills, cough, back pain.	Discontinue. Call doctor right away.
• Diarrhea, drowsiness, nausea, vomiting.	Continue. Call doctor when convenient.
Infrequent:	
Mouth sores, bruising, constipation, red skin.	Discontinue. Call doctor right away.
Rare:	
Confusion, hallucinations, headache, swollen feet.	Continue. Call doctor when convenient.

WARNINGS & PRECAUTIONS

Don't take if:
You are allergic to hydroxyurea.

Before you start, consult your doctor if:
- You have chicken pox.
- You have shingles (herpes zoster).
- You have anemia or blood disorder.
- You have gout.
- You have an infection.
- You have kidney disease or kidney stones.
- You have taken interferon in the past.

Over age 60:
Adverse reactions and side effects may be more frequent and severe than in younger persons. You may need smaller doses for shorter periods of time.

Pregnancy:
Decide with your doctor if drug benefits justify risk to unborn child. Risk category C (see page xviii).

Breast-feeding:
Drug passes into milk. Avoid drug or discontinue nursing until you finish medicine. Consult doctor for advice on maintaining milk supply.

Infants & children:
Effect not documented. Consult your pediatrician.

Prolonged use:
Talk to your doctor about the need for follow-up medical examinations or laboratory studies to check kidney function, complete blood counts (white blood cell count, platelet count, red blood cell count, hemoglobin, hematocrit) and serum uric acid.

Skin & sunlight:
No problems expected.

Driving, piloting or hazardous work:
Avoid if you feel confused, drowsy or dizzy.

Discontinuing:
May still experience symptoms of bone marrow depression, such as: blood in stools, fever or chills, blood spots under the skin, back pain, hoarseness, bloody urine. If any of these occur, call your doctor right away.

Others:
- Advise any doctor or dentist whom you consult that you take this medicine.
- May affect results in some medical tests.

POSSIBLE INTERACTION WITH OTHER DRUGS

GENERIC NAME OR DRUG CLASS	COMBINED EFFECT
Bone marrow depressants, other*	Dangerous suppression of bone marrow activity.
Clozapine	Toxic effect on bone marrow.
Levamisole	Increased risk of bone marrow depression.
Probenecid	May require increased dosage to treat gout.
Sulfinpyrazone	May require increased dosage to treat gout.
Tiopronin	Increased risk of toxicity to bone marrow.
Vaccines, live or killed virus	Increased risk of side effects.

POSSIBLE INTERACTION WITH OTHER SUBSTANCES

INTERACTS WITH	COMBINED EFFECT
Alcohol:	None expected.
Beverages:	None expected.
Cocaine:	None expected.
Foods:	None expected.
Marijuana:	None expected.
Tobacco:	None expected.

HYDROXYZINE

BRAND NAMES

Ami Rax

Anxanil

Apo-Hydroxyzine

Atarax

Marax

Marax D.F.

Multipax

Novo-Hydroxyzin

Vistaril

BASIC INFORMATION

Habit forming? No

Prescription needed? Yes

Available as generic? Yes

Drug class: Tranquilizer, antihistamine

 USES

* Treatment for anxiety, tension and agitation.
* Relieves itching from allergic reactions.

 DOSAGE & USAGE INFORMATION

How to take:

* Tablet, syrup or capsule—Swallow with liquid. If you can't swallow whole, crumble tablet or open capsule and take with liquid or food.
* Liquid—If desired, dilute dose in beverage before swallowing.

When to take:

At the same times each day.

If you forget a dose:

Take as soon as you remember up to 2 hours late. If more than 2 hours, wait for next scheduled dose (don't double this dose).

What drug does:

Blocks action of histamine after an allergic response triggers histamine release. Histamines cause itching, sneezing, runny nose and eyes and other symptoms.

Time lapse before drug works:

15 to 30 minutes.

Continued next column

 OVERDOSE

SYMPTOMS:

Drowsiness, unsteadiness, agitation, purposeless movements, tremor, convulsions.

WHAT TO DO:

* Dial 911 (emergency) for medical help or call poison control center 1-800-222-1222 for instructions.
* See emergency information on last 3 pages of this book.

Don't take with:

Any other medicine or any dietary supplement without consulting your doctor or pharmacist.

 POSSIBLE ADVERSE REACTIONS OR SIDE EFFECTS

SYMPTOMS	WHAT TO DO
Life-threatening:	
In case of overdose, see previous column.	
Common:	
Drowsiness; dizziness; dryness of mouth, nose or throat; nausea.	Continue. Call doctor when convenient.
Infrequent:	
• Change in vision, clumsiness, rash.	Discontinue. Call doctor right away.
• Less tolerance for contact lenses, painful or difficult urination.	Continue. Call doctor when convenient.
• Appetite loss.	Continue. Tell doctor at next visit.
Rare:	
Nightmares, agitation, irritability, sore throat, fever, rapid heartbeat, unusual bleeding or bruising, fatigue, weakness, confusion, fainting, seizures.	Discontinue. Call doctor right away.

 WARNINGS & PRECAUTIONS

Don't take if:

You are allergic to any antihistamine.

Before you start, consult your doctor if:

* You have asthma or kidney disease.
* You will have surgery within 2 months, including dental surgery, requiring general or spinal anesthesia.

Over age 60:

* Adverse reactions and side effects may be more frequent and severe than in younger persons.
* Drug likely to increase urination difficulty caused by enlarged prostate gland.

Pregnancy:

Decide with your doctor if drug benefits justify risk to unborn child. Risk category C (see page xviii).

Breast-feeding:

Drug passes into milk. Avoid drug or discontinue nursing until you finish medicine. Consult doctor for advice on maintaining milk supply.

Infants & children:
Use only under medical supervision.

Prolonged use:
Tolerance* may develop and reduce effectiveness.

Skin & sunlight:
No problems expected.

Driving, piloting or hazardous work:
Don't drive or pilot aircraft until you learn how medicine affects you. Don't work around dangerous machinery. Don't climb ladders or work in high places. Danger increases if you drink alcohol or take medicine affecting alertness and reflexes, such as antihistamines, tranquilizers, sedatives, pain medicine, narcotics and mind-altering drugs.

Discontinuing:
Don't discontinue without consulting doctor. Dose may require gradual reduction if you have taken drug for a long time. Doses of other drugs may also require adjustment.

Others:
Advise any doctor or dentist whom you consult that you take this medicine.

POSSIBLE INTERACTION WITH OTHER DRUGS

GENERIC NAME OR DRUG CLASS	COMBINED EFFECT
Antidepressants, tricyclic*	Increased effects of both drugs.
Antihistamines*	Increased hydroxyzine effect.
Attapulgite	Decreased hydroxyzine effect.
Carteolol	Decreased antihistamine effect.
Central nervous system (CNS) depressants*	Greater depression of central nervous system.
Clozapine	Toxic effect on the central nervous system.
Fluoxetine	Increased depressant effects of both drugs.
Guanfacine	May increase depressant effects of either drug.
Leucovorin	High alcohol content of leucovorin may cause adverse effects.

Narcotics*	Increased effects of both drugs.
Pain relievers*	Increased effects of both drugs.
Sertraline	Increased depressive effects of both drugs.
Sotalol	Increased antihistamine effect.

POSSIBLE INTERACTION WITH OTHER SUBSTANCES

INTERACTS WITH	COMBINED EFFECT
Alcohol:	Increased sedation and intoxication. Use with caution.
Beverages: Caffeine drinks.	Decreased tranquilizer effect of hydroxyzine.
Cocaine:	Decreased hydroxyzine effect. Avoid.
Foods:	None expected.
Marijuana:	None expected.
Tobacco:	None expected.

*See Glossary

HYOSCYAMINE

BRAND NAMES

Anaspaz	Kinesed
Anaspaz PB	Levbid
Barbidonna	Levsin
Barbidonna 2	Levsin S/L
Belladenal	Levsinex
Cystospaz	Levsinex Timecaps
Cystospaz-M	Neoquess
Gastrosed	Nulev

BASIC INFORMATION

Habit forming? No
Prescription needed?
  Low strength: No
  High strength: Yes
Available as generic? Yes
Drug class: Antispasmodic, anticholinergic

 USES

Reduces spasms of digestive system, bladder and urethra.

 DOSAGE & USAGE INFORMATION

How to take:
- Tablet or liquid—Swallow with liquid or food to lessen stomach irritation. You may chew or crush tablets.
- Extended-release capsule or tablet— Swallow each dose whole.
- Drops—Dilute dose in beverage before swallowing.

When to take:
30 minutes before meals (unless directed otherwise by doctor).

Continued next column

 OVERDOSE

SYMPTOMS:
Dilated pupils, rapid pulse and breathing, dizziness, fever, hallucinations, confusion, slurred speech, agitation, flushed face, convulsions, coma.
WHAT TO DO:
- **Dial 911 (emergency) for medical help or call poison control center 1-800-222-1222 for instructions.**
- **See emergency information on last 3 pages of this book.**

If you forget a dose:
Take as soon as you remember up to 2 hours late. If more than 2 hours, wait for next scheduled dose (don't double this dose).

What drug does:
Blocks nerve impulses at parasympathetic nerve endings, preventing muscle contractions and gland secretions of organs involved.

Time lapse before drug works:
15 to 30 minutes.

Don't take with:
- Antacids* or antidiarrheals* at the same time.
- Any other medicine or any dietary supplement without consulting your doctor or pharmacist.

 POSSIBLE ADVERSE REACTIONS OR SIDE EFFECTS

SYMPTOMS	WHAT TO DO
Life-threatening:	
In case of overdose, see previous column.	
Common:	
• Confusion, delirium, rapid heartbeat.	Discontinue. Call doctor right away.
• Nausea, vomiting, decreased sweating.	Continue. Call doctor when convenient.
• Constipation.	Continue. Tell doctor at next visit.
• Dryness in ears, nose, throat, mouth.	No action necessary.
Infrequent:	
• Headache, painful or difficult urination, nasal congestion, altered taste.	Continue. Call doctor when convenient.
• Lightheadedness.	Discontinue. Call doctor right away.
Rare:	
Rash or hives, eye pain, blurred vision.	Discontinue. Call doctor right away.

 WARNINGS & PRECAUTIONS

Don't take if:
- You are allergic to any anticholinergic.
- You have trouble with stomach bloating.
- You have difficulty emptying your bladder completely.
- You have narrow-angle glaucoma.
- You have severe ulcerative colitis.

Before you start, consult your doctor if:
- You have open-angle glaucoma.
- You have angina.
- You have chronic bronchitis or asthma.
- You have hiatal hernia.
- You have liver, kidney or thyroid disease.
- You have enlarged prostate.
- You have myasthenia gravis.
- You have peptic ulcer.
- You will have surgery within 2 months, including dental surgery, requiring general or spinal anesthesia.

Over age 60:
Adverse reactions and side effects may be more frequent and severe than in younger persons.

Pregnancy:
Decide with your doctor if drug benefits justify risk to unborn child. Risk category C (see page xviii).

Breast-feeding:
Drug passes into milk and decreases milk flow. Avoid drug or discontinue nursing until you finish medicine. Consult doctor for advice on maintaining milk supply.

Infants & children:
Use only under medical supervision.

Prolonged use:
Chronic constipation, possible fecal impaction. Consult doctor immediately.

Skin & sunlight:
No problems expected.

Driving, piloting or hazardous work:
Use disqualifies you for piloting aircraft. Otherwise, no problems expected.

Discontinuing:
May be unnecessary to finish medicine. Follow doctor's instructions.

Others:
Advise any doctor or dentist whom you consult that you take this medicine.

POSSIBLE INTERACTION WITH OTHER DRUGS

GENERIC NAME OR DRUG CLASS	COMBINED EFFECT
Amantadine	Increased hyoscyamine effect.
Anticholinergics, other*	Increased hyoscyamine effect.
Antidepressants, tricyclic*	Increased hyoscyamine effect.
Antihistamines*	Increased hyoscyamine effect.
Cortisone drugs*	Increased internal eye pressure.
Haloperidol	Increased internal eye pressure.
Ketoconazole	Decreased ketoconazole effect.
Meperidine	Increased hyoscyamine effect.
Methylphenidate	Increased hyoscyamine effect.
Molindone	Increased anticholinergic effect.
Monoamine oxidase (MAO) inhibitors*	Increased hyoscyamine effect.
Nizatidine	Increased nizatidine effect.
Orphenadrine	Increased hyoscyamine effect.
Phenothiazines*	Increased hyoscyamine effect.
Pilocarpine	Loss of pilocarpine effect in glaucoma treatment.
Sedatives* or central nervous system (CNS) depressants*	Increased sedative effect of both drugs.
Vitamin C	Decreased hyoscyamine effect. Avoid large doses of vitamin C.

POSSIBLE INTERACTION WITH OTHER SUBSTANCES

INTERACTS WITH	COMBINED EFFECT
Alcohol:	None expected.
Beverages:	None expected.
Cocaine:	Excessively rapid heartbeat. Avoid.
Foods:	None expected.
Marijuana:	Drowsiness and dry mouth.
Tobacco:	None expected.

*See Glossary

IMATINIB

BRAND NAMES

Gleevec

BASIC INFORMATION

Habit forming? No
Prescription needed? Yes
Available as generic? No
Drug class: Antineoplastic

 USES

- Treatment for chronic myeloid leukemia (CML).
- Treatment for gastrointestinal stomal tumors.
- Treatment for certain rare life-threatening disorders with limited treatment options.

 DOSAGE & USAGE INFORMATION

How to take:
Capsule—Swallow with large glass of water to minimize the risk of stomach and gastrointestinal irritation.

When to take:
Usually once a day at mealtime or according to doctor's instructions.

If you forget a dose:
Do not take the missed dose at all. Return to your regular dosing schedule at the prescribed time. Never double a dose to make up for a missed dose. Consult your doctor.

What drug does:
Reduces substantially the level of cancerous cells in the bone marrow and blood of treated patients.

Time lapse before drug works:
Starts working in 2-4 hours, but effectiveness may take 1-3 months.

Don't take with:
Any other medicines (including over-the-counter drugs such as cough and cold medicines, laxatives, antacids, diet pills, caffeine, nose drops or vitamins) without consulting your doctor or pharmacist.

 OVERDOSE

SYMPTOMS:
Unknown effect.
WHAT TO DO:
If person takes much larger amount than prescribed, dial 911 (emergency) for medical help or call poison control center 1-800-222-1222 for instructions.

 POSSIBLE ADVERSE REACTIONS OR SIDE EFFECTS

SYMPTOMS	WHAT TO DO
Life-threatening: Some adverse effects from advanced cancer and/or the medicine can be serious or life threatening.	Seek emergency treatment for any symptoms that appear severe or critical.
Common: Chest pain, shortness of breath, swelling (face, hands, legs. feet), black tarry stools, nausea or vomiting, muscle pain or cramps, blood in urine, decreased or painful urination, fever, chills, pale skin, quick weight gain, stomach cramps, sore throat, sores on body, ulcers or white spots on lips or in mouth, swollen glands, unusual bleeding or tiredness or weakness.	Continue. Call doctor right away.
• Joint or bone pain, diarrhea, skin rash. fatigue.	Continue. Call doctor when convenient.
Infrequent: • Convulsions, irregular heartbeat, wheezing, tightness in chest, numbness or tingling (in hands, feet, or lips), pinpoint red spots on skin.	Continue. Call doctor right away.
• Bloody nose, mood changes, slow weight gain, weight loss, sneezing, joint pain, constipation, loss of appetite, headache, increased thirst, dry mouth.	Continue. Call doctor when convenient.
Rare: Acid indigestion or upset stomach, stuffy nose, itchy skin.	Continue. Call doctor when convenient.

Note: Side effects are often unavoidable with drugs used to treat cancer. Discuss any concerns or questions or other symptoms with your doctor.

WARNINGS & PRECAUTIONS

Don't take if:
You are allergic to imatinib.

Before you start, consult your doctor if:
* You have any infection.
* You have anemia.
* You have leukopenia, neutropenia or thrombocytopenia.
* You have bone marrow depression.
* You have recent chickenpox or herpes zoster.
* You have liver problems.

Over age 60:
Other than a higher incidence of edema, studies to date have not shown problems that would limit the usefulness of imatinib.

Pregnancy:
Not recommended. Consult doctor. Risk category D (see page xviii).

Breast-feeding:
It is unknown if drug passes into milk. Avoid drug or discontinue nursing until you finish medicine. Consult doctor for advice on maintaining milk supply.

Infants & children:
Safety and efficacy have not been established in children under 18 years of age.

Prolonged use:
* Talk to your doctor about the need for follow-up medical examinations or laboratory studies to check your response to the drug, blood studies, weight gain and liver function.
* The long term effects of the drug are not yet known.

Skin & sunlight:
No problems expected.

Driving, piloting or hazardous work:
No problems expected.

Discontinuing:
No special problems expected. Don't discontinue drug without doctor's approval.

Others:
* Advise any doctor or dentist whom you consult that you take this medicine. Consult doctor before having dental work.
* Do not have any immunizations without your doctor's approval. Imatinib may lower your resistance to the infection that you are getting the immunization for.
* Avoid persons who have recently taken the oral polio virus vaccine; they may pass the virus on to you.
* Avoid people with infections, because you have an increased chance of getting the infection. Advise your doctor of any unusual symptoms, infections or injuries.

* Be careful when brushing or flossing teeth, or using a razor or other sharp object to avoid being injured.
* May affect results in some medical tests.
* Avoid contact sports or activities that could cause, injury, bruising or bleeding.

POSSIBLE INTERACTION WITH OTHER DRUGS

GENERIC NAME OR DRUG CLASS	COMBINED EFFECT
Anticoagulants*	Blood clotting problems.
Blood dyscrasia-causing medications*	Increased risk of adverse effects of imatinib.
Bone marrow depressants, other*	Increased bone marrow suppression.
Cyclosporine	Increased effect of cyclosporine.
Enzyme inducers*	Decreased effect of imatinib.
Enzyme inhibitors*	Increased effect of imatinib.
HMG-CoA reductase inhibitors	Increased effect of HMG-CoA reductase inhibitor.
Pimozide	Increased effect of pimozide.
Vaccines (killed)	Decreased effectiveness of vaccine.
Vaccines (live)	Increased risk of getting the disease the vaccine prevents.

POSSIBLE INTERACTION WITH OTHER SUBSTANCES

INTERACTS WITH	COMBINED EFFECT
Alcohol:	None expected.
Beverages:	None expected.
Cocaine:	None expected. Best to avoid.
Foods:	None expected.
Marijuana:	None expected. Best to avoid.
Tobacco:	None expected.

*See Glossary

IMMUNOSUPPRESSIVE AGENTS

GENERIC AND BRAND NAMES

MYCOPHENOLATE
Myfortic
Myfortic Delayed
Release

TACROLIMUS
Prograf

BASIC INFORMATION

Habit forming? No
Prescription needed? Yes
Available as generic? No
Drug class: Immunosuppressant

 USES

Helps to suppress the immune system and prevent rejection in patients who have undergone organ transplants.

 DOSAGE & USAGE INFORMATION

How to take:
- Capsule—Swallow with liquid. Do not open capsule.
- Tablet—Swallow with liquid. Do not crush tablet.
- Delayed-release tablet—Swallow whole with liquid. Do not crush or chew tablet.
- Oral suspension—Take as directed on label.

When to take:
At the same times each day, according to prescription label. Take mycophenolate on an empty stomach (1 hour before or 2 hours after a meal). Tacrolimus may be taken with or without food.

If you forget a dose:
Take as soon as you remember. If it is almost time for the next dose, wait for next scheduled dose (don't double this dose). Consult doctor if you are unsure about dosing schedule.

Continued next column

 OVERDOSE

SYMPTOMS:
Increased severity of adverse reactions, coma, delirium.
WHAT TO DO:
- Dial 911 (emergency) for medical help or call poison control center 1-800-222-1222 for instructions.
- See emergency information on last 3 pages of this book.

What drug does:
Tacrolimus and mycophenolate are 2 different types of immunosuppressive drugs. They suppress immune reactions (to transplanted organs) in certain cells by inhibiting their growth.

Time lapse before drug works:
3 to 3-1/2 hours. May take several weeks to evaluate effectiveness against organ rejection.

Don't take with:
Any other medicine or any dietary supplement without consulting your doctor or pharmacist.

 POSSIBLE ADVERSE REACTIONS OR SIDE EFFECTS

SYMPTOMS	WHAT TO DO
Life-threatening:	
In case of overdose, see previous column.	
Common:	
• Infections (fever, chills, hoarseness, cough, trouble urinating, back or side pain); headache; tingling or numbness of hands or feet; chest pain; blood in urine; trouble sleeping; trembling of hands; shortness of breath.	Continue, but call doctor right away.
• Mild back pain, constipation or diarrhea, stomach pain, heartburn.	Continue. Call doctor when convenient.
Infrequent:	
• Bloody vomit; anxiety; nervousness; white patches on mouth, tongue or throat; weakness; seizures.	Continue, but call doctor right away.
• Hair loss or excess hair growth, nausea, mild vomiting, skin rash or itch, muscle or joint pain, dizziness.	Continue. Call doctor when convenient.
Rare:	
• Bloody, black or tarry stools; small red spots on skin; unusual bleeding or bruising; irregular heartbeat.	Continue, but call doctor right away.
• Mood or mental changes.	Continue. Call doctor when convenient.

 WARNINGS & PRECAUTIONS

Don't take if:
You are allergic to mycophenolate or tacrolimus.

IMMUNOSUPPRESSIVE AGENTS

Before you start, consult your doctor if:
- You have liver or kidney disease.
- You have a digestive system disease.
- You have an infection.
- You have chickenpox (or have recently been exposed) or herpes zoster (shingles).
- You are female and planning pregnancy or are able to bear children.

Over age 60:
No special problems expected.

Pregnancy:
- Mycophenolate is pregnancy risk category D. Avoid use. It increases risk of pregnancy loss and congenital malformations. (see page xviii).
- Tacrolimus is pregnancy risk category C. Decide with your doctor if drug benefits justify risk to unborn child (see page xviii).

Breast-feeding:
Tacrolimus passes into milk; mycophenolate may pass into milk. Avoid drugs or discontinue nursing until you finish medicine. Consult doctor for advice on maintaining milk supply.

Infants & children:
Safety and effectiveness of mycophenolate are not established. Tacrolimus has been used successfully in liver transplants in pediatric patients.

Prolonged use:
- Can cause reduced function of kidneys.
- Can increase risk of developing lymphoma (cancer of lymph glands).
- Talk to your doctor about the need for follow-up medical examinations or laboratory studies to check blood concentration of drug, kidney function, liver function, potassium levels, drug's effectiveness and adverse reactions.

Skin & sunlight:
No special problems expected.

Driving, piloting or hazardous work:
Don't drive or pilot aircraft until you learn how medicine affects you. Don't work around dangerous machinery. Don't climb ladders or work in high places. Danger increases if you drink alcohol or take medicine affecting alertness and reflexes.

Discontinuing:
Don't discontinue without consulting doctor. You will usually require this drug for your lifetime.

Others:
- Advise any doctor or dentist whom you consult that you take this drug. May interfere with results of some medical tests.
- Wear medical identification stating that you have had a transplant and take this drug.
- Check blood pressure routinely at home. Drug may sometimes cause hypertension.
- Avoid any immunizations except those specifically recommended by your doctor.
- Maintain good dental hygiene. Immunosuppression can cause gum problems.

*See Glossary

- Talk to your doctor about forms of birth control before starting treatment with mycophenolate.

POSSIBLE INTERACTION WITH OTHER DRUGS

GENERIC NAME OR DRUG CLASS	COMBINED EFFECT
Acyclovir	Increased effect of mycophenolate.
Antacids*	Decreased effect of mycophenolate.
Cholestyramine	Decreased effect of mycophenolate.
Diuretics, potassium-sparing*	Increased risk of potassium toxicity.
Enzyme inducers*	Decreased effect of tacrolimus.
Enzyme inhibitors*	Increased effect of tacrolimus.
Ganciclovir	Increased effect of mycophenolate.
Immunosuppressants,* other	Increased immunosuppressive effect.
Nephrotoxic medications*	Increased risk of kidney problems.
Nitroimidazoles	Increased tacrolimus effect.
Potassium supplements	Increased risk of potassium toxicity.

Continued on page 920

POSSIBLE INTERACTION WITH OTHER SUBSTANCES

INTERACTS WITH	COMBINED EFFECT
Alcohol:	Increased risk of toxic effects. Avoid.
Beverages: Grapefruit juice.	Increased effect of drug. Avoid.
Cocaine:	Increased risk of toxic effects. Avoid.
Foods: Grapefruit.	Increased effect of drug. Avoid.
Marijuana:	Increased risk of toxic effects. Avoid.
Tobacco:	None expected.

INDAPAMIDE

BRAND NAMES

Lozide   Lozol

BASIC INFORMATION

Habit forming? No
Prescription needed? Yes
Available as generic? Yes
Drug class: Antihypertensive, diuretic

 USES

- Controls, but doesn't cure, high blood pressure.
- Reduces fluid retention (edema) caused by conditions such as heart disorders.

 DOSAGE & USAGE INFORMATION

How to take:
Tablet—Swallow with liquid or food to lessen stomach irritation.

When to take:
At the same times each day, usually at bedtime.

If you forget a dose:
Bedtime dose—If you forget your once-a-day bedtime dose, don't take it more than 3 hours late. Never double dose.

What drug does:
Forces kidney to excrete more sodium and causes excess salt and fluid to be excreted.

Time lapse before drug works:
2 hours for effect to begin. May require 1 to 4 weeks for full effects.

Don't take with:
Any other medicine or any dietary supplement without consulting your doctor or pharmacist.

 OVERDOSE

SYMPTOMS:
Nausea, vomiting, diarrhea, very dry mouth, thirst, weakness, excessive fatigue, very rapid heart rate, weak pulse.
WHAT TO DO:
- **Dial 911 (emergency) for medical help or call poison control center 1-800-222-1222 for instructions.**
- **If person is unconscious, check breathing and pulse. If not breathing, begin mouth-to-mouth rescue breathing. If heart is not beating, begin chest compressions.**
- **See emergency information on last 3 pages of this book.**

 POSSIBLE ADVERSE REACTIONS OR SIDE EFFECTS

SYMPTOMS	WHAT TO DO
Life-threatening:	
In case of overdose, see previous column.	
Common:	
• Excessive tiredness or weakness, muscle cramps.	Discontinue. Call doctor right away.
• Frequent urination.	Continue. Tell doctor at next visit.
Infrequent:	
Insomnia, mood change, dizziness on changing position, headache, excessive thirst, diarrhea, appetite loss, nausea, dry mouth, decreased sex drive.	Continue. Call doctor when convenient.
Rare:	
• Weak pulse.	Discontinue. Seek emergency treatment.
• Itching, rash, hives, irregular heartbeat.	Discontinue. Call doctor right away.

 WARNINGS & PRECAUTIONS

Don't take if:
You are allergic to indapamide or to any sulfa drug or thiazide diuretic.*

Before you start, consult your doctor if:
- You have severe kidney disease.
- You have diabetes.
- You have gout.
- You have liver disease.
- You will have surgery within 2 months, including dental surgery, requiring general or spinal anesthesia.
- You have lupus erythematosus.
- You are pregnant or plan to become pregnant.

Over age 60:
Adverse reactions and side effects may be more frequent and severe than in younger persons.

Pregnancy:
Consult doctor. Risk category B (see page xviii).

Breast-feeding:
Unknown effect on child. Consult doctor.

Infants & children:
Use only under close medical supervision.

Prolonged use:
Request laboratory studies for blood sugar, BUN,* uric acid and serum electrolytes (potassium and sodium).

Skin & sunlight:
May cause rash or intensify sunburn in areas exposed to sun or ultraviolet light (photosensitivity reaction). Avoid overexposure. Notify doctor if reaction occurs.

Driving, piloting or hazardous work:
Don't drive or pilot aircraft until you learn how medicine affects you. Don't work around dangerous machinery. Don't climb ladders or work in high places. Danger increases if you drink alcohol or take medicine affecting alertness and reflexes, such as antihistamines, tranquilizers, sedatives, pain medicine, narcotics and mind-altering drugs.

Discontinuing:
Don't discontinue without consulting doctor. Dose may require gradual reduction if you have taken drug for a long time. Doses of other drugs may also require adjustment.

Others:
Advise any doctor or dentist whom you consult that you take this medicine.

 POSSIBLE INTERACTION WITH OTHER DRUGS

GENERIC NAME OR DRUG CLASS	COMBINED EFFECT
Adrenocorticoids, systemic	Possible excessive potassium loss.
Allopurinol	Decreased allopurinol effect.
Amiodarone	Increased risk of heartbeat irregularity due to low potassium.
Amphotericin B	Increased potassium.
Angiotensin-converting enzyme (ACE) inhibitors*	Decreased blood pressure. Possible excessive potassium in blood.
Antidepressants, tricyclic*	Dangerous drop in blood pressure.
Antidiabetic agents, oral*	Increased blood sugar.
Antihypertensives, other*	Increased anti-hypertensive effect.
Barbiturates*	Increased indapamide effect.
Beta-adrenergic blocking agents*	Increased effect of indapamide.
Calcium supplements*	Increased calcium in blood.

Carteolol	Increased anti-hypertensive effect.
Cholestyramine	Decreased indapamide effect.
Colestipol	Decreased indapamide effect.
Digitalis preparations*	Excessive potassium loss that may cause dangerous heart rhythms.
Diuretics, thiazide*	Increased effect of thiazide diuretics.
Indomethacin	Decreased indapamide effect.
Lithium	High risk of lithium toxicity.
Monoamine oxidase (MAO) inhibitors*	Increased indapamide effect.
Nicardipine	Dangerous blood pressure drop. Dosages may require adjustment.
Nimodipine	Dangerous blood pressure drop.
Opiates*	Weakness and faintness when arising from bed or chair.

Continued on page 920

 POSSIBLE INTERACTION WITH OTHER SUBSTANCES

INTERACTS WITH	COMBINED EFFECT
Alcohol:	Dangerous blood pressure drop. Avoid.
Beverages:	No problems expected.
Cocaine:	Increased risk of heart block and high blood pressure.
Foods: Licorice.	Excessive potassium loss that may cause dangerous heart rhythms.
Marijuana:	Reduced effectiveness of indapamide. Avoid.
Tobacco:	Reduced effectiveness of indapamide. Avoid.

*See Glossary

INSULIN

BRAND NAMES

See full list of brand names in the *Generic and Brand Name Directory*, page 887.

BASIC INFORMATION

Habit forming? No
Prescription needed? No
Available as generic? Yes
Drug class: Antidiabetic

 ## USES

Treats diabetes, a metabolic disorder, in which patients have high levels of sugar in their blood.

 ## DOSAGE & USAGE INFORMATION

How to take:
* Injection—Injected under the skin. Use disposable, sterile needles. Rotate injection sites.
* Inhaled powder—Follow instructions provided.

When to take:
At the same times each day.

If you forget a dose:
Take as soon as you remember. Wait at least 4 hours for next dose. Resume regular schedule.

What drug does:
Facilitates passage of blood sugar through cell membranes so sugar is usable.

Time lapse before drug works:
30 minutes to 8 hours, depending on type of insulin used.

Continued next column

 ## OVERDOSE

SYMPTOMS:
Low blood sugar (hypoglycemia)—Anxiety; chills, cold sweats, pale skin; drowsiness; excessive hunger; headache; nausea; nervousness; fast heartbeat; shakiness; unusual tiredness or weakness.
WHAT TO DO:
* **Eat some type of sugar immediately, such as glucose product, orange juice (add some sugar), nondiet sodas, candy (such as 5 Lifesavers), honey.**
* **If patient loses consciousness, give glucagon if you have it and know how to use it.**
* **Dial 911 (emergency) for medical help or call poison control center 1-800-222-1222 for instructions.**
* **See emergency information on last 3 pages of this book.**

Don't take with:
Any other medicine or any dietary supplement without consulting your doctor or pharmacist.

 ## POSSIBLE ADVERSE REACTIONS OR SIDE EFFECTS

SYMPTOMS	WHAT TO DO
Life-threatening:	
Hives, rash, intense itching, faintness soon after a dose (anaphylaxis).	Seek emergency treatment immediately.
Common:	
None expected.	
Infrequent:	
• Symptoms of low blood sugar—nervousness, hunger (excessive), cold sweats, rapid pulse, anxiety, cold skin, chills, confusion, concentration loss, drowsiness, headache, nausea, weakness, shakiness, vision changes.	Seek treatment (eat some form of quick-acting sugar—glucose tablets, sugar, fruit juice, corn syrup, honey).
• Symptoms of high blood sugar—increased urination, unusual thirst, dry mouth, drowsiness, flushed or dry skin, fruit-like breath odor, appetite loss, stomach pain or vomiting, tiredness, trouble breathing, increased blood sugar level.	Seek emergency treatment immediately.
• Swelling, redness, itch or warmth at injection site.	Continue. Call doctor when convenient.
Rare:	
None expected.	

 ## WARNINGS & PRECAUTIONS

Don't take if:
* Your diagnosis and dose schedule is not established.
* You don't know how to deal with overdose emergencies.
* You are allergic to insulin.

Before you start, consult your doctor if:
* You take MAO inhibitors.
* You have liver or kidney disease or low thyroid function.

Over age 60:
Guard against hypoglycemia. Repeated episodes can cause permanent confusion and abnormal behavior.

Pregnancy:
Adhere rigidly to diabetes treatment program. Risk category B (see page xviii).

Breast-feeding:
No problems expected. Consult doctor.

Infants & children:
Use only under medical supervision.

Prolonged use:
Talk to your doctor about the need for follow-up medical examinations or laboratory studies to check blood sugar, serum potassium, urine.

Skin & sunlight:
No problems expected.

Driving, piloting or hazardous work:
No problems expected after dose is established.

Discontinuing:
Don't discontinue without doctor's advice until you complete prescribed dose, even though symptoms diminish or disappear.

Others:
- Diet and exercise affect how much insulin you need. Work with your doctor to determine accurate dose.
- Notify your doctor if you skip a dose, overeat, have fever or infection.
- Notify doctor if you develop symptoms of high blood sugar: drowsiness, dry skin, orange fruit-like odor to breath, increased urination, appetite loss, unusual thirst.
- Never freeze insulin.
- May interfere with the accuracy of some medical tests.

POSSIBLE INTERACTION WITH OTHER DRUGS

GENERIC NAME OR DRUG CLASS	COMBINED EFFECT
Adrenocorticoids, systemic	Decreased insulin effect.
Anticonvulsants, hydantoin*	Decreased insulin effect.
Antidiabetics, oral*	Increased antidiabetic effect.
Beta-adrenergic blocking agents*	Possible increased difficulty in regulating blood sugar levels.
Bismuth subsalicylate	Increased insulin effect. May require dosage adjustment.

Carteolol	Hypoglycemic effects may be prolonged.
Contraceptives, oral*	Decreased insulin effect.
Dexfenfluramine	May require dosage change as weight loss occurs.
Diuretics, thiazide*	Decreased insulin effect.
Furosemide	Decreased insulin effect.
Insulin analogs	May require dosage adjustment.
Monoamine oxidase (MAO) inhibitors*	Increased insulin effect.
Nicotine	Increased insulin effect.
Oxyphenbutazone	Increased insulin effect.
Phenylbutazone	Increased insulin effect.
Salicylates*	Increased insulin effect.
Smoking deterrents	May require insulin dosage adjustment.
Sulfa drugs*	Increased insulin effect.
Tetracyclines*	Increased insulin effect.
Thyroid hormones*	Decreased insulin effect.

POSSIBLE INTERACTION WITH OTHER SUBSTANCES

INTERACTS WITH	COMBINED EFFECT
Alcohol:	Increased insulin effect. Blood sugar problems. Avoid.
Beverages:	None expected.
Cocaine:	Unknown effect. Avoid.
Foods:	None expected. Follow your diabetic diet instructions.
Marijuana:	Possible increase in blood sugar. Avoid.
Tobacco:	Decreased insulin absorption. Avoid.

*See Glossary

INSULIN ANALOGS

GENERIC AND BRAND NAMES

INSULIN ASPART
Novolog
Novolog FlexPen
Novolog Mix 50/50
INSULIN DETEMIR
Levemir
INSULIN GLARGINE
Lantus
Lantus OptiClik
Lantus Solostar
Pen

INSULIN GLULISINE
Apidra
INSULIN LISPRO
Humalog
Humalog Mix 50/50
Humalog Mix 75/25

BASIC INFORMATION

Habit forming? No
Prescription needed? Yes
Available as generic? No
Drug class: Antidiabetic

 USES

Treats diabetes, a metabolic disorder, in which patients have high levels of sugar in their blood. The drug keeps blood sugar levels from going too high after eating.

 DOSAGE & USAGE INFORMATION

How to take:
Taken by injection under the skin. Use disposable, sterile needles, or disposable pen. Rotate injection sites. Follow instructions provided with product.

Continued next column

 OVERDOSE

SYMPTOMS:
Low blood sugar (hypoglycemia)—Anxiety; chills, cold sweats, pale skin; drowsiness; excessive hunger; headache; nausea; nervousness; fast heartbeat; shakiness; unusual tiredness or weakness.
WHAT TO DO:
• Eat some type of sugar immediately, such as glucose product, orange juice (add some sugar), nondiet sodas, candy (such as 5 Lifesavers), honey.
• If person is unconscious, give glucagon if you have it and know how to use it.
• Dial 911 (emergency) for medical help or call poison control center 1-800-222-1222 for instructions.
• See emergency information on last 3 pages of this book.

When to take:
At the same times each day. If taken at mealtime, use it within a 15 minute period prior to the meal. May need to be taken in combination with a long-acting insulin to prevent hyperglycemia.

If you forget a dose:
Follow your doctor's instructions. If unsure, call your doctor or pharmacist.

What drug does:
These drugs are rapid- or fast-acting and work quickly in the body after injection. They are variations (analogs) of human insulin and more closely mimic the time action of natural insulin that comes from the pancreas.

Time lapse before drug works:
30 minutes to 1 hour, which is faster than regular insulin. Insulin aspart and insulin lispro finish acting in 3-4 hours, insulin glargine in 24 hours.

Don't take with:
Any other medicine or any dietary supplement without consulting your doctor or pharmacist.

 POSSIBLE ADVERSE REACTIONS OR SIDE EFFECTS

SYMPTOMS	WHAT TO DO
Life-threatening: Hives, rash, intense itching, faintness, swelling, breathing difficulty soon after a dose (anaphylaxis).	Seek emergency treatment immediately.
Common: None expected.	
Infrequent: • Symptoms of low blood sugar— nervousness, hunger (excessive), cold sweats, rapid pulse, anxiety, cold skin, chills, confusion, concentration loss, drowsiness, headache, nausea, weakness, shakiness, vision changes.	Seek treatment (eat some form of quick-acting sugar— glucose tablets, sugar, fruit juice, corn syrup, honey).
• Symptoms of high blood sugar— increased urination, unusual thirst, dry mouth, drowsiness, flushed or dry skin, fruit-like breath odor, appetite loss, stomach pain or vomiting, tiredness, trouble breathing, increased blood sugar level.	Seek emergency treatment immediately.

| Swelling, redness, itch or warmth at injection site; other skin changes at injection site (e.g., thinning or thickened skin). | Continue. Call doctor when convenient. |

Rare:

| Dry mouth, excessive thirst, weak or fast pulse, heartbeat irregularities, mental or mood changes, nausea or vomiting, unusual tiredness or weakness, muscle cramps (may be symptoms of hypokalemia). | Continue, but call doctor right away. |

WARNINGS & PRECAUTIONS

Don't take if:
If you are allergic to insulin.

Before you start, consult your doctor if:
- Your diagnosis and dose schedule are not established or you don't know how to deal with overdose emergencies.
- You take MAO inhibitors.*
- You have hypoglycemia, liver or kidney disease or low thyroid function.

Over age 60:
Insulin requirements may change. The family should notify the doctor if abnormal behavior or confusion occurs in an older person.

Pregnancy:
Risk category B for lispro and category C for aspart and glargine. See page xviii and consult doctor.

Breast-feeding:
Unknown if drugs pass into milk. May require dosage adjustment. Consult doctor.

Infants & children:
Use only under medical supervision.

Prolonged use:
Talk to your doctor about the need for follow-up medical examinations or laboratory studies to check effectiveness of drug.

Skin & sunlight:
No problems expected.

Driving, piloting or hazardous work:
No problems expected after dose is established. Need to be cautious for signs of hypoglycemia.

Discontinuing:
Don't discontinue without doctor's advice, even though symptoms diminish or disappear.

Others:
- Diet and exercise affect how much insulin you need. Work with your doctor to determine accurate dose. Monitor your glucose levels as directed.
- Notify your doctor if you have a fever, infection, diarrhea, or experience vomiting.
- Advise any doctor or dentist whom you consult that you take this medicine.
- Never freeze insulin.
- Wear medical identification that indicates you have diabetes and take insulin.
- You and your family should educate yourselves about diabetes; learn to recognize hypoglycemia and treat it with sugar or glucagon.
- May interfere with the accuracy of some medical tests.

POSSIBLE INTERACTION WITH OTHER DRUGS

GENERIC NAME OR DRUG CLASS	COMBINED EFFECT
Antidiabetics, oral*	Increased antidiabetic effect.
Hyperglycemia-causing agents*	May need increased dosage of insulin.
Hypoglycemia-causing agents*	May need decreased dosage of insulin.
Insulin	May need dosage adjustment.
Sympatholytics*	Increased insulin effect.
Smoking deterrents	May require insulin dosage adjustment.

POSSIBLE INTERACTION WITH OTHER SUBSTANCES

INTERACTS WITH	COMBINED EFFECT
Alcohol:	Increased insulin effect. Blood sugar problems. Avoid.
Beverages:	None expected.
Cocaine:	Unknown effect. Avoid.
Foods:	None expected. Follow your diabetic diet instructions.
Marijuana:	Possible increase in blood sugar. Avoid.
Tobacco:	Decreased insulin absorption. Avoid.

*See Glossary

INTEGRASE INHIBITORS

GENERIC AND BRAND NAMES

RALTEGRAVIR
  Isentress

BASIC INFORMATION

Habit forming? No
Prescription needed? Yes
Available as generic? No
Drug class: Antiviral agent

 USES

For treatment of adults infected with human immunodeficiency virus (HIV) who have failed other antiviral drug therapy. The drug is used in combination with other antiviral drugs. HIV is the virus that causes acquired immunodeficiency syndrome (AIDS).

 DOSAGE & USAGE INFORMATION

How to take:
Tablet—Swallow with liquid. May be taken with or without food.

When to take:
Take twice a day at the same times each day.

If you forget a dose:
Take as soon as you remember. If it is almost time for the next dose, wait for next scheduled dose (don't double this dose).

What drug does:
It helps control HIV infection by inhibiting an enzyme that is required for HIV replication. This may reduce the amount of HIV in the blood and may increase immune system cells. The drug does not cure HIV or AIDS.

Time lapse before drug works:
May require several weeks or months before full benefits are apparent.

Don't take with:
Any other medicine or any dietary supplement without consulting your doctor or pharmacist. This is very important with HIV drugs.

 OVERDOSE

SYMPTOMS:
Unknown.
WHAT TO DO:
If person takes much larger amount than prescribed or if accidentally swallowed, call doctor or poison control center
1-800-222-1222 for help.

 POSSIBLE ADVERSE REACTIONS OR SIDE EFFECTS

SYMPTOMS	WHAT TO DO
Life-threatening: Rare allergic reaction (hives, itching, rash, trouble breathing, tightness in chest, swelling of lips or tongue or throat).	Seek emergency treatment immediately.
Common: Diarrhea, nausea, headache, fever.	Continue. Call doctor when convenient.
Infrequent: Lightheadedness or dizziness, mild stomach pain, muscle or joint pain, tiredness, vomiting, dark urine, increased hunger or thirst.	Continue. Call doctor when convenient.
Rare: • Chest pain, fast heartbeat, short-ness of breath.	Discontinue. Call doctor right away.
• Bruising or bleeding, signs of infection, confusion, mood changes, decreased urination, yellow skin or eyes.	Continue, but call doctor right away.
• Body aches, loss of appetite, a feeling of discomfort, body fat increases or fat moves to different areas of body, bloating, weight gain, excessive sweating, swelling, drowsiness, constipation, other unexplained symptoms.	Continue. Call doctor when convenient.

WARNINGS & PRECAUTIONS

Don't take if:
You are allergic to integrase inhibitors.

Before you start, consult your doctor if:
- You are allergic to any medicine, food or other substance, or have a family history of allergies.
- You have a muscle disorder.
- You have kidney or liver disease.

Over age 60:
Use with caution as adverse reactions and side effects may be more frequent and severe than in younger persons.

Pregnancy:
Decide with your doctor if drug benefits justify risk to unborn child. Risk category C (see page xviii). HIV can be passed to the baby if the mother is not properly treated during pregnancy. Talk to your doctor about being included in the Antiretroviral Pregnancy Registry.

Breast-feeding:
It is unknown if drug passes into milk. It is not recommended that HIV-infected mothers breast-feed. Consult your doctor.

Infants & children:
Safety and efficacy have not been established for children under age 16. Consult doctor.

Prolonged use:
- Long-term effects of using this drug have not been established.
- Talk to your doctor about the need for follow up blood tests and liver function studies.

Skin & sunlight:
No problems expected.

Driving, piloting or hazardous work:
No problems expected.

Discontinuing:
Don't discontinue without doctor's advice.

Others:
- Advise any doctor or dentist whom you consult that you take this medicine.
- Taking this drug does not prevent you from passing HIV to another person through sexual contact or sharing needles. Avoid sexual contact or practice safe sex (e.g., using condoms) to help prevent the transmission of HIV. Never share or re-use needles. If you have questions, ask your doctor for advice.
- Consult your doctor right away if you develop a new infection (e.g., fever, chills, sore throat or other symptoms).
- Consult your doctor right away if you develop muscle pain, especially if you take HMG CoA reductase inhibitors or fibrates.
- Take drug daily as prescribed. Do not increase or decrease dosage of drug without doctor's approval.

POSSIBLE INTERACTION WITH OTHER DRUGS

GENERIC NAME OR DRUG CLASS	COMBINED EFFECT
Rifampin	Decreased effect of integrase inhibitor.

POSSIBLE INTERACTION WITH OTHER SUBSTANCES

INTERACTS WITH	COMBINED EFFECT
Alcohol:	None expected.
Beverages:	None expected.
Cocaine:	Unknown effect. Best to avoid.
Foods:	None expected.
Marijuana:	Unknown effect. Best to avoid.
Tobacco:	None expected.

*See Glossary

GENERIC AND BRAND NAMES

CILOSTAZOL
Pletal

BASIC INFORMATION

Habit forming? No
Prescription needed? Yes
Available as generic? No
Drug class: Vasodilator

 ## USES

- Treats intermittent claudication (leg pain caused by poor circulation).
- Improves blood vessel function.
- Treatment for other disorders as determined by your doctor.

 ## DOSAGE & USAGE INFORMATION

How to take:
Tablet—Swallow with liquid. If you can't swallow tablet whole, ask your pharmacist for advice.

When to take:
Twice a day. Take one half hour before or 2 hours after breakfast and dinner.

If you forget a dose:
Take as soon as you remember up to 2 hours late. If more than 2 hours, wait for next scheduled dose (don't double this dose).

What drug does:
Exact way it works is unknown. It increases blood flow by relaxing and expanding blood vessel walls. It keeps blood from clotting.

Time lapse before drug works:
3-4 weeks, but takes 12 weeks for full benefit.

Don't take with:
Any other medicine, herbal remedy or dietary supplements without consulting your doctor or pharmacist.

 ## OVERDOSE

SYMPTOMS:
Severe headache, severe diarrhea, dizziness, change in heartbeat, nausea or vomiting; flushed, hot face.
WHAT TO DO:
Overdose unlikely to threaten life. If person uses much larger amount than prescribed or if accidentally swallowed, call doctor or poison control center 1-800-222-1222 for help.

 ## POSSIBLE ADVERSE REACTIONS OR SIDE EFFECTS

SYMPTOMS	WHAT TO DO
Life-threatening: None expected.	
Common:	
• Fever, rapid or irregular heartbeat.	Discontinue. Call doctor right away.
• Back pain, gas, dizziness, cough, diarrhea, headache, muscle stiffness or pain, runny or stuffy nose, sore throat.	Continue. Call doctor when convenient.
Infrequent: Fainting, stools are bloody or black or tarry, nausea or indigestion or heartburn (severe or ongoing), tongue swelling, stiff neck, nosebleeds, severe stomach pain or cramping, vomiting blood or material like coffee grounds, unusual bleeding or bruising.	Discontinue. Call doctor right away.
Rare: Burning feeling in throat or chest, bone pain, difficulty in swallowing, ringing or buzzing in the ears, hives, joint pain or stiffness, swelling (face, arms, fingers or lower legs).	Continue. Call doctor when convenient.

WARNINGS & PRECAUTIONS

Don't take if:
- You are allergic to cilostazol.
- You have congestive heart failure.

Before you start, consult your doctor if:
- You have heart disease, heart rhythm disorder or a bleeding disorder.
- You have liver or kidney disease.
- You suffer from migraines.
- You are a smoker.

Over age 60:
Adverse reactions and side effects may be more frequent and severe than in younger persons.

Pregnancy:
Decide with your doctor if drug benefits justify risk to unborn child. Risk category C (see page xviii).

Breast-feeding:
Drug passes into milk. Avoid drug or discontinue nursing until you finish medicine. Consult doctor about maintaining milk supply.

Infants & children:
Not recommended. Safety and dosage has not been established.

Prolonged use:
No problems expected.

Skin & sunlight:
No problems expected.

Driving, piloting or hazardous work:
Avoid if you feel dizzy or weak. Otherwise, no problems expected.

Discontinuing:
Don't discontinue without doctor's advice until you complete prescribed dose, even though symptoms diminish or disappear.

Others:
- Response to drug varies. If your symptoms don't improve after 3 weeks of use, consult doctor.
- Avoid smoking while taking this medication, as it may worsen your condition.
- Advise any doctor or dentist whom you consult that you take this medicine.

POSSIBLE INTERACTION WITH OTHER DRUGS

GENERIC NAME OR DRUG CLASS	COMBINED EFFECT
Enzyme inhibitors*	Increased effect of intermittent claudication agent.
Sertraline	Increased effect of intermittent claudication agent

POSSIBLE INTERACTION WITH OTHER SUBSTANCES

INTERACTS WITH	COMBINED EFFECT
Alcohol:	None expected.
Beverages: Grapefruit juice.	Increased effect of intermittent claudication agent.
Cocaine:	Unknown effect. Avoid.
Foods: Grapefruit.	Increased effect of intermittent claudication agent.
Marijuana:	Unknown effect. Avoid.
Tobacco:	Decreased effect of intermittent claudication agent. Also, nicotine narrows your blood vessels. Avoid.

*See Glossary

IODOQUINOL

BRAND NAMES

Diiodohydroxyquin	Yodoquinol
Diodoquin	Yodoxin
Diquinol	

BASIC INFORMATION

Habit forming? No
Prescription needed? Yes
Available as generic? Yes
Drug class: Antiprotozoal, antiparasitic

 ## USES

Treatment for intestinal amebiasis and balantidiasis.

 ## DOSAGE & USAGE INFORMATION

How to take:
Tablet—Mix with applesauce or chocolate syrup if unable to swallow tablets.

When to take:
Three times daily after meals for 20 days. Treatment may be repeated after 2 to 3 weeks.

If you forget a dose:
Take as soon as you remember up to 2 hours late. If more than 2 hours, wait for next scheduled dose (don't double this dose).

What drug does:
Kills amoeba (microscopic parasites) in intestinal tract.

Time lapse before drug works:
May require full course of treatment (20 days) to cure.

Don't take with:
Any other medicine or any dietary supplement without consulting your doctor or pharmacist.

 ## OVERDOSE

SYMPTOMS:
* Prolonged dosing at high level may produce blurred vision, muscle pain, eye pain, numbness and tingling in hands or feet.
* Single overdosage unlikely to threaten life.

WHAT TO DO:
If person takes much larger amount than prescribed, dial 911 (emergency) for medical help or call poison control center 1-800-222-1222 for instructions.

 ## POSSIBLE ADVERSE REACTIONS OR SIDE EFFECTS

SYMPTOMS	WHAT TO DO
Life-threatening: None expected.	
Common: Diarrhea, nausea, vomiting, abdominal pain.	Continue. Call doctor when convenient.
Infrequent:	
• Clumsiness, rash, hives, itching, blurred vision, muscle pain, numbness or tingling in hands or feet, chills, fever, weakness.	Discontinue. Call doctor right away.
• Swelling of neck (thyroid gland).	Continue. Call doctor when convenient.
Rare: Dizziness, headache, rectal itching.	Continue. Call doctor when convenient.

WARNINGS & PRECAUTIONS

Don't take if:
You are allergic to iodoquinol.

Before you start, consult your doctor if:
* You have optic atrophy or thyroid disease.
* You have kidney or liver disease.

Over age 60:
Adverse reactions and side effects may be more frequent and severe than in younger persons.

Pregnancy:
Decide with your doctor if drug benefits justify risk to unborn child. Risk category C (see page xviii).

Breast-feeding:
No proven problems, but avoid if possible. Discontinue nursing until you finish medicine. Consult doctor for advice on maintaining milk supply.

Infants & children:
Not recommended. Safety and dosage has not been established.

Prolonged use:
Not recommended.

Skin & sunlight:
No problems expected.

Driving, piloting or hazardous work:
No problems expected.

Discontinuing:
Don't discontinue without consulting doctor.

Others:
* Thyroid tests may be inaccurate for as long as 6 months after discontinuing iodoquinol treatment.
* May interfere with the accuracy of some medical tests.

POSSIBLE INTERACTION WITH OTHER DRUGS

GENERIC NAME OR DRUG CLASS	COMBINED EFFECT
None expected.	

POSSIBLE INTERACTION WITH OTHER SUBSTANCES

INTERACTS WITH	COMBINED EFFECT
Alcohol:	None expected.
Beverages:	None expected.
Cocaine:	None expected.
Foods:	Taking with food may decrease gastrointestinal side effects.
Marijuana:	None expected.
Tobacco:	None expected.

IPRATROPIUM

BRAND NAMES

Apo-Ipravent

Atrovent

Atrovent Inhalation
Aerosol

Combivent

Duoneb

Kendral-Ipratropium

BASIC INFORMATION

Habit forming? No
Prescription needed? Yes
Available as generic? Yes
Drug class: Bronchodilator, anticholinergic

 USES

- Treats asthma, bronchitis and emphysema.
- Should not be used alone for acute asthma attacks. May be used with inhalation forms of albuterol or fenoterol.
- May be used to treat rhinorrhea (runny nose).

 DOSAGE & USAGE INFORMATION

How to use:
- Inhalation aerosol or solution—Carefully follow the printed instructions provided with the inhaler. Avoid contact with eyes.
- Nasal spray—Prime the nasal spray pump as directed, then spray in each nostril. Avoid contact with eyes.

When to take:
Inhalation form may be started at 2 inhalations, 4 times a day and increased by your doctor as needed. Usual dose of nasal form is 2 sprays in each nostril, 2 to 3 times a day.

If you forget a dose:
Use as soon as you remember. If it is almost time for the next dose, wait for next scheduled dose (don't double this dose).

What drug does:
Dilates (opens or widens) bronchial tubes or nasal passages by direct effect on them.

Continued next column

 OVERDOSE

SYMPTOMS:
None likely.
WHAT TO DO:
Overdose unlikely to threaten life. If person uses much larger amount than prescribed or if accidentally swallowed, call doctor or poison control center 1-800-222-1222 for help.

Time lapse before drug works:
Inhalation form may take 2 to 3 days for full effectiveness. Effect of nasal form may begin right away or take a few days.

Don't take with:
Any other medicines (including over-the-counter drugs such as cough and cold medicines, laxatives, antacids, diet pills, caffeine, nose drops or vitamins) without consulting your doctor or pharmacist.

 POSSIBLE ADVERSE REACTIONS OR SIDE EFFECTS

SYMPTOMS	WHAT TO DO
Life-threatening: Rare allergic reaction— Breathing difficulty; closing of the throat; swelling of hands, feet, face, lips or tongue; hives.	Discontinue. Seek emergency treatment.
Common: Cough, dry mouth, unpleasant taste.	Continue. Call doctor when convenient.
Infrequent: Blurred vision or other vision changes, difficult urination, stuffy nose, sweating, tremors, weakness, dizziness, nervousness, headache,	Continue. Call doctor when convenient.
Rare: Skin rash or hives, ongoing constipation, increased wheezing, chest tightness or difficulty in breathing, pounding heartbeat, stomach pain or bloating, severe eye pain.	Discontinue. Call doctor right away.

WARNINGS & PRECAUTIONS

Don't take if:
You are sensitive to ipratropium, belladonna, atropine or soybeans, soy lecithin or peanuts.

Before you start, consult your doctor if:
* You have prostate trouble.
* You have glaucoma.
* You have difficulty in urinating.

Over age 60:
Adverse reactions and side effects may be more frequent and severe than in younger persons. You may need smaller doses for shorter periods of time.

Pregnancy:
Decide with your doctor if drug benefits justify risk to unborn child. Risk category B (see page xviii).

Breast-feeding:
It is unknown if drug passes into milk. Avoid drug or discontinue nursing until you finish medicine. Consult doctor for advice on maintaining milk supply.

Infants & children:
Inhalation form may be used in children over age 12. Nasal spray may be used in children over age 6.

Prolonged use:
* For inhalation form, see your doctor to verify drug's effectiveness and for dose adjustment if needed and for eye pressure exams.
* Nasal form should not be used for more than 4 days.

Skin & sunlight:
No problems expected.

Driving, piloting or hazardous work:
Avoid if you feel confused, drowsy or dizzy.

Discontinuing:
No special problems expected.

Others:
* Advise any doctor or dentist whom you consult that you take this medicine.
* Do not increase the drug dosage without your doctor's approval.
* Allow 5-minute intervals between ipratropium inhalations and inhalations of cromolyn, cortisone or other inhalant medicines.

POSSIBLE INTERACTION WITH OTHER DRUGS

GENERIC NAME OR DRUG CLASS	COMBINED EFFECT
Anticholinergics*	Increased anticholinergic effect.
Cromolyn (inhalation form)	Wait 5 minutes after using ipratropium before using cromolyn.

POSSIBLE INTERACTION WITH OTHER SUBSTANCES

INTERACTS WITH	COMBINED EFFECT
Alcohol:	None expected.
Beverages:	None expected.
Cocaine:	Unknown effect. Avoid.
Foods:	None expected.
Marijuana:	Unknown effect. Avoid.
Tobacco:	None expected, but smoking should be avoided.

IRON SUPPLEMENTS

GENERIC AND BRAND NAMES

See full list of generic and brand names in the *Generic and Brand Name Directory*, page 887.

BASIC INFORMATION

Habit forming? No
Prescription needed? No
Available as generic? Yes
Drug class: Mineral supplement (iron)

 USES

Treatment for dietary iron deficiency or iron-deficiency anemia from other causes.

 DOSAGE & USAGE INFORMATION

How to take:
• Tablet, capsule or syrup—Swallow with liquid or food to lessen stomach irritation. If you can't swallow whole, crumble tablet or open capsule and take with liquid or food. Place medicine far back on tongue to avoid staining teeth.
• Extended-release capsule—Swallow whole with liquid. Do not crush.
• Chewable tablet—Chew well before swallowing.
• Liquid—Dilute dose in beverage before swallowing and drink through a straw.

When to take:
1 hour before or 2 hours after eating.

If you forget a dose:
Take up to 2 hours late. If more than 2 hours, wait for next dose (don't double this dose).

Continued next column

 OVERDOSE

SYMPTOMS:
• **Moderate overdose—Stomach pain, vomiting, diarrhea, black stools, lethargy.**
• **Serious overdose—Weakness and collapse; pallor, weak and rapid heartbeat; shallow breathing; convulsions and coma.**
WHAT TO DO:
• **Dial 911 (emergency) for medical help or call poison control center 1-800-222-1222 for instructions.**
• **See emergency information on last 3 pages of this book.**

What drug does:
Stimulates bone marrow's production of hemoglobin (red blood cell pigment that carries oxygen to body cells).

Time lapse before drug works:
3 to 7 days. May require 3 weeks for maximum benefit.

Don't take with:
Any other medicine or any dietary supplement without consulting your doctor or pharmacist.

 POSSIBLE ADVERSE REACTIONS OR SIDE EFFECTS

SYMPTOMS	WHAT TO DO
Life-threatening:	
In case of overdose, see previous column.	
Common:	
• Stomach pain that is continuing.	Discontinue. Call doctor right away.
• Dark green or black stool, teeth stained with liquid iron, constipation, diarrhea, mild nausea or vomiting.	Continue. Call doctor when convenient.
Infrequent:	
None expected.	
Rare:	
• Throat pain on swallowing, chest pain, cramps, blood in stool or black stool that has sticky consistency.	Discontinue. Call doctor right away.
• Darkened urine, heartburn.	Continue. Call doctor when convenient.

 WARNINGS & PRECAUTIONS

Don't take if:
• You are allergic to any iron supplement or tartrazine dye.
• You take iron injections.
• You have acute hepatitis, hemosiderosis or hemochromatosis (conditions involving excess iron in body).
• You have hemolytic anemia.

Before you start, consult your doctor if:
• You plan to become pregnant while on medication.
• You have had stomach surgery.
• You have had peptic ulcer, enteritis or colitis.

Over age 60:
May cause hemochromatosis (iron storage disease) with bronze skin, liver damage, diabetes, heart problems and impotence.

Pregnancy:
Take only if your doctor advises. Risk category C (see page xviii).

Breast-feeding:
No problems expected. Take only if your doctor confirms you have a dietary deficiency or an iron-deficiency anemia.

Infants & children:
Use only under medical supervision. Overdose common and dangerous. Keep out of children's reach.

Prolonged use:
- May cause hemochromatosis (iron storage disease) with bronze skin, liver damage, diabetes, heart problems and impotence.
- Talk to your doctor about the need for follow-up medical examinations or laboratory studies to check complete blood counts (white blood cell count, platelet count, red blood cell count, hemoglobin, hematocrit), serum iron, total iron-binding capacity.

Skin & sunlight:
No problems expected.

Driving, piloting or hazardous work:
No problems expected.

Discontinuing:
May be unnecessary to finish medicine. Follow doctor's instructions.

Others:
- Liquid form stains teeth. Mix with water or juice to lessen the effect. Brush with baking soda or hydrogen peroxide to help remove stain.
- Some products contain tartrazine dye. Avoid, especially if you are allergic to aspirin.
- May interfere with the accuracy of some medical tests.
- If using extended-release form or coated tablet and your stools don't turn black, consult doctor. The tablet may not be breaking down, and an underdose may result.

POSSIBLE INTERACTION WITH OTHER DRUGS

GENERIC NAME OR DRUG CLASS	COMBINED EFFECT
Acetohydroxamic acid	Decreased effects of both drugs.
Antacids*	Poor iron absorption.
Chloramphenicol	Decreased effect of iron. Interferes with formation of red blood cells and hemoglobin.
Cholestyramine	Decreased iron effect.
Etidronate	Decreased etidronate effect. Take at least 2 hours after iron supplement.
H₂ antagonists*	Decreased iron effect.
Iron supplements, other*	Possible excess iron storage in liver.
Proton pump inhibitors	May decrease effect of iron supplement.
Tetracyclines*	Decreased tetracycline effect. Take iron 3 hours before or 2 hours after taking tetracycline.
Vitamin E	Decreased iron and vitamin E effect.
Zinc supplements	Increased need for zinc.

POSSIBLE INTERACTION WITH OTHER SUBSTANCES

INTERACTS WITH	COMBINED EFFECT
Alcohol:	Increased iron absorption. May cause organ damage. Avoid or use in moderation.
Beverages: Milk, tea.	Decreased iron effect.
Cocaine:	None expected.
Foods: Dairy foods, eggs, whole-grain bread and cereal.	Decreased iron effect.
Marijuana:	None expected.
Tobacco:	None expected.

ISOMETHEPTENE, DICHLORALPHENAZONE & ACETAMINOPHEN

BRAND NAMES

Amidrine	Migquin
I.D.A.	Migrapap
Iso-Acetazone	Migratine
Isocom	Migrazone
Midchlor	Migrend
Midquin	Migrex
Midrin	Mitride

BASIC INFORMATION

Habit forming? No
Prescription needed? Yes
Available as generic? Yes
Drug class: Analgesic, sedative, vascular headache suppressant

USES

Treatment of vascular (throbbing or migraine type) and tension headaches.

DOSAGE & USAGE INFORMATION

How to take:
Capsule—Take with liquid.

When to take:
At first sign of headache. Usual dose—2 capsules at start, then 1 every hour until fully relieved. Don't exceed 5 capsules in 12 hours.

If you forget a dose:
Use as soon as you remember.

What drug does:
Causes blood vessels in head to constrict or become narrower. Acetaminophen relieves pain by effects on hypothalamus—the part of the brain that helps regulate body heat and receives body's pain messages.

Time lapse before drug works:
30-60 minutes.

Continued next column

OVERDOSE

SYMPTOMS:
Stomach upsets, irritability, sweating, severe diarrhea, convulsions, coma.
WHAT TO DO:
• **Dial 911 (emergency) for medical help or call poison control center 1-800-222-1222 for instructions.**
• **See emergency information on last 3 pages of this book.**

Don't take with:
Any medicine that will decrease mental alertness or reflexes, such as alcohol, other mind-altering drugs, cough/cold medicines, antihistamines, allergy medicine, sedatives, tranquilizers (sleeping pills or "downers") barbiturates, seizure medicine, narcotics, other prescription medicine for pain, muscle relaxants, anesthetics.

POSSIBLE ADVERSE REACTIONS OR SIDE EFFECTS

SYMPTOMS	WHAT TO DO
Life-threatening:	
In case of overdose, see previous column.	
Common:	
Dizziness, drowsiness.	Continue. Call doctor when convenient.
Infrequent:	
Diarrhea, vomiting, nausea, abdominal cramps, upper abdominal pain.	Discontinue. Call doctor right away.
Rare:	
Rash; itchy skin; sore throat, fever, mouth sores; unusual bleeding or bruising; weakness; jaundice.	Discontinue. Call doctor right away.

WARNINGS & PRECAUTIONS

Don't take if:
• You are allergic to acetaminophen or any other component of this combination medicine.
• Your symptoms don't improve after 2 days use. Call your doctor.

Before you start, consult your doctor if:
You have kidney disease, liver damage, glaucoma, heart or blood vessel disorder, hypertension, alcoholism (active).

Over age 60:
Don't exceed recommended dose. You can't eliminate drug as efficiently as younger persons.

Pregnancy:
Decide with your doctor if drug benefits justify risk to unborn child. Risk category C (see page xviii).

Breast-feeding:
Drug passes into milk. Avoid drug or discontinue nursing until you finish medicine. Consult doctor for advice on maintaining milk supply.

Infants & children:
Give under careful medical supervision only.

ISOMETHEPTENE, DICHLORALPHENAZONE & ACETAMINOPHEN

Prolonged use:
- May affect blood system and cause anemia. Limit use to 5 days for children 12 and under, and 10 days for adults.
- Talk to your doctor about the need for follow-up medical examinations or laboratory studies to check complete blood counts (white blood cell count, platelet count, red blood cell count, hemoglobin, hematocrit), liver function.

Skin & sunlight:
No problems expected.

Driving, piloting or hazardous work:
Avoid if you feel drowsy. Otherwise, no restrictions.

Discontinuing:
Discontinue in 2 days if symptoms don't improve.

Others:
Advise any doctor or dentist whom you consult that you take this medicine.

POSSIBLE INTERACTION WITH OTHER DRUGS

GENERIC NAME OR DRUG CLASS	COMBINED EFFECT
Anticoagulants, oral*	May increase anticoagulant effect. If combined frequently, prothrombin time should be monitored.
Anti-inflammatory drugs, nonsteroidal (NSAIDs)*	Long-term combined effect (3 years or longer) increases chance of damage to kidney, including malignancy.
Aspirin or other salicylates*	Long-term combined effect (3 years or longer) increases chance of damage to kidney, including malignancy.
Beta-adrenergic blocking agents*	Narrowed arteries in heart if taken in large doses.
Central nervous system (CNS) depressants*	Increased sedative effect.
Monoamine oxidase (MAO) inhibitors*	Sudden increase in blood pressure.
Phenacetin	Long-term combined effect (3 years or longer) increases chance of damage to kidney, including malignancy.
Phenobarbital	Quicker elimination and decreased effect of acetaminophen.
Tetracyclines* (effervescent granules or tablets)	May slow tetracycline absorption. Space doses 2 hours apart.
Zidovudine (AZT)	Increased toxic effect of zidovudine.

POSSIBLE INTERACTION WITH OTHER SUBSTANCES

INTERACTS WITH	COMBINED EFFECT
Alcohol:	Drowsiness. Toxicity to liver. Avoid.
Beverages:	None expected.
Cocaine:	None expected. However, cocaine may slow body's recovery. Avoid.
Foods:	None expected.
Marijuana:	Increased pain relief. However, marijuana may slow body's recovery. Avoid.
Tobacco:	May decrease effect of drug. Avoid.

*See Glossary

ISONIAZID

BRAND NAMES

INH	PMS Isoniazid
Isotamine	Rifamate
Laniazid	Tubizid
Nydrazid	

BASIC INFORMATION

Habit forming? No
Prescription needed? Yes
Available as generic? Yes
Drug class: Antitubercular

USES

Kills tuberculosis germs.

DOSAGE & USAGE INFORMATION

How to take:
• Tablet—Swallow with liquid to lessen stomach irritation.
• Syrup—Follow label directions.

When to take:
At the same time each day.

If you forget a dose:
Take as soon as you remember up to 12 hours late. If more than 12 hours, wait for next scheduled dose (don't double this dose).

What drug does:
Interferes with TB germ metabolism. Eventually destroys the germ.

Time lapse before drug works:
3 to 6 months. You may need to take drug as long as 2 years.

Don't take with:
Any other medicine or any dietary supplement without consulting your doctor or pharmacist.

OVERDOSE

SYMPTOMS:
Difficult breathing, convulsions, coma.
WHAT TO DO:
• **Dial 911 (emergency) for medical help or call poison control center 1-800-222-1222 for instructions.**
• **If person is unconscious, check breathing and pulse. If not breathing, begin mouth-to-mouth rescue breathing. If heart is not beating, begin chest compressions.**
• **See emergency information on last 3 pages of this book.**

POSSIBLE ADVERSE REACTIONS OR SIDE EFFECTS

SYMPTOMS	WHAT TO DO
Life-threatening:	
In case of overdose, see previous column.	
Common:	
• Muscle pain and pain in joints, tingling or numbness in extremities, jaundice.	Discontinue. Call doctor right away.
• Confusion, unsteady walk.	Continue. Call doctor when convenient.
Infrequent:	
• Swollen glands, nausea, indigestion, diarrhea, vomiting.	Discontinue. Call doctor right away.
• Dizziness, appetite loss.	Continue. Call doctor when convenient.
Rare:	
• Rash, fever, impaired vision, anemia with fatigue, weakness, fever, sore throat, unusual bleeding or bruising.	Discontinue. Call doctor right away.
• Breast enlargement or discomfort.	Continue. Tell doctor at next visit.

WARNINGS & PRECAUTIONS

Don't take if:
You are allergic to isoniazid.

Before you start, consult your doctor if:
• You plan to become pregnant within medication period.
• You are allergic to ethionamide, pyrazinamide or nicotinic acid.
• You drink alcohol.
• You have liver or kidney disease.
• You have epilepsy, diabetes or lupus.

Over age 60:
Adverse reactions and side effects, especially jaundice, may be more frequent and severe than in younger persons. Kidneys may be less efficient.

Pregnancy:
Decide with your doctor if drug benefits justify risk to unborn child. Risk category C (see page xviii).

Breast-feeding:
Drug passes into milk. Avoid drug or discontinue nursing until you finish medicine. Consult doctor for advice on maintaining milk supply.

Infants & children:
Use only under medical supervision.

Prolonged use:
- Numbness and tingling of hands and feet.
- Talk to your doctor about the need for follow-up medical examinations or laboratory studies to check liver function, eyes.

Skin & sunlight:
No problems expected.

Driving, piloting or hazardous work:
Avoid if you feel dizzy. Otherwise, no problems expected.

Discontinuing:
Don't discontinue without doctor's advice until you complete prescribed dose, even though symptoms diminish or disappear.

Others:
- Diabetic patients may have false blood sugar tests.
- Periodic liver function tests and laboratory blood studies recommended.
- Prescription for vitamin B-6 (pyridoxine) recommended to prevent nerve damage.
- Advise any doctor or dentist whom you consult that you take this medicine.

POSSIBLE INTERACTION WITH OTHER DRUGS

GENERIC NAME OR DRUG CLASS	COMBINED EFFECT
Acetaminophen	Increased risk of liver damage.
Adrenocorticoids, systemic	Decreased isoniazid effect.
Alfentanil	Prolonged duration of alfentanil effect (undesirable).
Antacids* (aluminum-containing)	Decreased absorption of isoniazid.
Anticholinergics*	May increase pressure within eyeball.
Anticoagulants, oral*	Increased anticoagulant effect.
Antidiabetics*	Increased antidiabetic effect.
Antihypertensives*	Increased antihypertensive effect.
Antivirals, HIV/AIDS*	Increased risk of peripheral neuropathy.
Carbamazepine	Increased risk of liver damage.

Cycloserine	Increased risk of central nervous system effects.
Disulfiram	Increased effect of disulfiram.
Laxatives*	Decreased absorption and effect of isoniazid.
Hepatotoxics*	Increased risk of liver damage.
Ketoconazole	Increased risk of liver damage.
Narcotics*	Increased narcotic effect.
Phenytoin	Increased phenytoin effect.
Pyridoxine (Vitamin B-6)	Decreased chance of nerve damage in extremities.
Rifampin	Increased isoniazid toxicity to liver.
Sedatives*	Increased sedative effect.
Stimulants*	Increased stimulant effect.

POSSIBLE INTERACTION WITH OTHER SUBSTANCES

INTERACTS WITH	COMBINED EFFECT
Alcohol:	Increased incidence of liver disease and seizures.
Beverages:	None expected.
Cocaine:	None expected.
Foods: Swiss or Cheshire cheese, fish.	Red or itching skin, fast heartbeat. Seek emergency treatment.
Marijuana:	No interactions expected, but marijuana may slow body's recovery.
Tobacco:	No interactions expected, but tobacco may slow body's recovery.

*See Glossary

ISOTRETINOIN

BRAND NAMES

Accutane
Accutane Roche
Amnesteem

Claravis
Sotret

BASIC INFORMATION

Habit forming? No
Prescription needed? Yes
Available as generic? Yes
Drug classification: Antiacne (systemic)

USES

- Decreases cystic acne formation in severe cases.
- Treats certain other skin disorders involving an overabundance of outer skin layer.

DOSAGE & USAGE INFORMATION

How to take:
Capsule—Swallow with liquid or food to lessen stomach irritation. If you can't swallow whole, open capsule and take with liquid or food.

When to take:
Twice a day. Follow prescription directions.

If you forget a dose:
Take as soon as you remember up to 2 hours late. If more than 2 hours, wait for next scheduled dose and double dose.

What drug does:
Reduces sebaceous gland activity and size.

Time lapse before drug works:
May require 15 to 20 weeks to experience full benefit.

Don't take with:
- Vitamin A or supplements containing Vitamin A.
- Any other medicine or any dietary supplement without consulting your doctor or pharmacist.

OVERDOSE

SYMPTOMS:
None reported.
WHAT TO DO:
Overdose unlikely to threaten life. If person uses much larger amount than prescribed or if accidentally swallowed, call doctor or poison control center 1-800-222-1222 for help.

POSSIBLE ADVERSE REACTIONS OR SIDE EFFECTS

SYMPTOMS	WHAT TO DO
Life-threatening: None expected.	
Common:	
• Burning, red, itching eyes; lip scaling; burning pain; nosebleeds.	Discontinue. Call doctor right away.
• Itchy skin.	Continue. Call doctor when convenient.
• Dry mouth.	Continue. Tell doctor at next visit. (Suck ice or chew gum).
Infrequent:	
• Rash, infection, nausea, vomiting.	Discontinue. Call doctor right away.
• Pain in muscles, bones, joints; hair thinning; tiredness.	Continue. Call doctor when convenient.
Rare:	
• Severe stomach pain, bleeding gums, blurred vision, severe diarrhea, continuing headache, vomiting, eye pain, rectal bleeding, yellow skin or eyes, serious depression, psychosis, thoughts of suicide.	Discontinue. Call doctor right away.
• Mild headache, increased sensitivity to light, stomach upset, peeling of skin on palms or soles of feet.	Continue. Call doctor when convenient.

WARNINGS & PRECAUTIONS

Don't take if:
- You are allergic to isotretinoin, etretinate, tretinoin or vitamin A derivatives.
- You are pregnant or plan pregnancy.
- *You are even able to bear children. Read, understand and follow the patient information enclosure with your prescription.*

Before you start, consult your doctor if:
- You have diabetes.
- You or any member of family have high triglyceride levels in blood.
- You or family members have a history of severe depression.

Over age 60:
Adverse reactions and side effects may be more frequent and severe than in younger persons.

Pregnancy:
Causes birth defects in fetus. Don't use. Risk category X (see page xviii).

Breast-feeding:
Effect unknown. Not recommended. Consult doctor.

Infants & children:
Not approved for ages under 12. Use under close medical supervision for ages 13 to 18.

Prolonged use:
* Possible damage to cornea of the eye.
* Talk to your doctor about the need for follow-up medical examinations or laboratory studies to check complete blood counts (white blood cell count, platelet count, red blood cell count, hemoglobin, hematocrit), liver function, blood lipids, blood sugar.

Skin & sunlight:
May cause rash or intensify sunburn in areas exposed to sun or ultraviolet light (photo-sensitivity reaction). Avoid overexposure. Notify doctor if reaction occurs.

Driving, piloting or hazardous work:
Use caution if there is a decrease in your night vision or you are unable to see well. Consult doctor.

Discontinuing:
Single course of treatment is usually all that's needed. If second course required, wait 8 weeks after completing first course.

Others:
* Use only for severe cases of cystic acne that have not responded to less hazardous forms of acne treatment.
* May interfere with the accuracy of some medical tests.
* May cause bone problems (osteoporosis, fractures, delayed healing).
* Don't donate blood for at least 30 days after discontinuing medicine.
* Acne may worsen at the start of treatment.
* Contact lens wearers may experience discomfort during treatment with this drug.
* Contact doctor right away if a person taking this drug develops symptoms of depression, psychosis (severe mental problems) or has any suicide thoughts or suicide behaviors.
* Advise any doctor or dentist whom you consult that you take this medicine.
* **If you are planning pregnancy or at risk of pregnancy, don't take this drug.**

POSSIBLE INTERACTION WITH OTHER DRUGS

GENERIC NAME OR DRUG CLASS	COMBINED EFFECT
Antiacne topical preparations* (other), cosmetics (medicated), skin preparations with alcohol, soaps or cleansers (abrasive)	Severe skin irritation.
Etretinate	Increased chance of toxicity of each drug.
Tetracyclines*	Increased risk of developing pseudo-tumor cerebri.*
Topical drugs or cosmetics	May interact with isotretinoin.
Tretinoin	Increased chance of toxicity.
Vitamin A	Additive toxic effect of each. Avoid.

POSSIBLE INTERACTION WITH OTHER SUBSTANCES

INTERACTS WITH	COMBINED EFFECT
Alcohol:	Increase in trigly-cerides in blood. Avoid.
Beverages:	None expected.
Cocaine:	Increased chance of toxicity of isotretinoin. Avoid.
Foods:	None expected.
Marijuana:	Increased chance of toxicity of isotretinoin. Avoid.
Tobacco:	May decrease absorption of drug. Avoid tobacco during treatment.

ISOXSUPRINE

BRAND NAMES

Vasodilan   Vasoprine

BASIC INFORMATION

Habit forming? No
Prescription needed? Yes
Available as generic? Yes
Drug class: Vasodilator

 USES

- May improve poor blood circulation.
- Management of premature labor.
- Treatment for painful menstruation.

 DOSAGE & USAGE INFORMATION

How to take:
Tablet—Swallow with liquid or food to lessen stomach irritation. If you can't swallow whole, crumble tablet and take with liquid or food.

When to take:
At the same times each day.

If you forget a dose:
Take as soon as you remember up to 2 hours late. If more than 2 hours, wait for next scheduled dose (don't double this dose).

What drug does:
Expands blood vessels, increasing flow and permitting distribution of oxygen and nutrients.

Time lapse before drug works:
1 hour.

Don't take with:
Any other medicine or any dietary supplement without consulting your doctor or pharmacist.

 OVERDOSE

SYMPTOMS:
Headache, dizziness, flush, vomiting, weakness, sweating, fainting, shortness of breath, coma.
WHAT TO DO:
- Dial 911 (emergency) for medical help or call poison control center 1-800-222-1222 for instructions.
- If person is unconscious, check breathing and pulse. If not breathing, begin mouth-to-mouth rescue breathing. If heart is not beating, begin chest compressions.
- See emergency information on last 3 pages of this book.

 POSSIBLE ADVERSE REACTIONS OR SIDE EFFECTS

SYMPTOMS	WHAT TO DO
Life-threatening: In case of overdose, see previous column.	
Common: None expected.	
Infrequent: Nausea, vomiting.	Continue. Call doctor when convenient.
Rare: Rapid or irregular heartbeat, rash, chest pain, shortness of breath.	Discontinue. Call doctor right away.

WARNINGS & PRECAUTIONS

Don't take if:
* You are allergic to any vasodilator.
* You have any bleeding disease.

Before you start, consult your doctor if:
* You have high blood pressure, hardening of the arteries or heart disease.
* You plan to become pregnant within medication period.
* You have glaucoma.

Over age 60:
Adverse reactions and side effects may be more frequent and severe than in younger persons.

Pregnancy:
Decide with your doctor whether drug benefits justify risk to unborn child. Risk category C (see page xviii).

Breast-feeding:
No problems expected, but consult doctor.

Infants & children:
Not recommended.

Prolonged use:
Talk to your doctor about the need for follow-up medical examinations or laboratory studies.

Skin & sunlight:
No problems expected.

Driving, piloting or hazardous work:
Avoid if you feel dizzy or faint. Otherwise, no problems expected.

Discontinuing:
Don't discontinue without doctor's advice until you complete prescribed dose, even though symptoms diminish or disappear.

Others:
* Be cautious when arising from lying or sitting position, when climbing stairs, or if dizziness occurs.
* May interfere with the accuracy of some medical tests.

POSSIBLE INTERACTION WITH OTHER DRUGS

GENERIC NAME OR DRUG CLASS	COMBINED EFFECT
None significant.	

POSSIBLE INTERACTION WITH OTHER SUBSTANCES

INTERACTS WITH	COMBINED EFFECT
Alcohol:	None expected.
Beverages: Milk.	Decreased stomach irritation.
Cocaine:	Decreased blood circulation to extremities. Avoid.
Foods:	None expected.
Marijuana:	Rapid heartbeat.
Tobacco:	Decreased isoxsuprine effect; nicotine constricts blood vessels.

KANAMYCIN

BRAND NAMES

Kantrex

BASIC INFORMATION

Habit forming? No
Prescription needed? Yes
Available as generic? No
Drug class: Bowel preparation

 USES

- To cleanse bowel of bacteria prior to intestinal surgery.
- Treats hepatic coma.

 DOSAGE & USAGE INFORMATION

How to take:
Capsule—Swallow with liquid. If you can't swallow whole, open capsule and take with liquid or food. Instructions to take on empty stomach mean 1 hour before or 2 hours after eating.

When to take:
At the same time each day, according to instructions on prescription label.

If you forget a dose:
Take as soon as you remember up to 2 hours late. If more than 2 hours, wait for next scheduled dose (don't double this dose).

What drug does:
Kills susceptible bacteria in the intestines.

Time lapse before drug works:
15 to 30 minutes.

Don't take with:
Any other medicine or any dietary supplement without consulting your doctor or pharmacist.

 OVERDOSE

SYMPTOMS:
Clumsiness, dizziness, seizures, coma.
WHAT TO DO:
- Dial 911 (emergency) for medical help or call poison control center 1-800-222-1222 for instructions.
- See emergency information on last 3 pages of this book.

 POSSIBLE ADVERSE REACTIONS OR SIDE EFFECTS

SYMPTOMS	WHAT TO DO
Life-threatening: In case of overdose, see previous column.	
Common: Mouth irritation or soreness, nausea.	Continue. Call doctor when convenient.
Infrequent: Vomiting.	Discontinue. Call doctor right away.
Rare: Decreased urine, hearing loss, ringing in ears, clumsiness, unsteadiness, skin rash.	Discontinue. Call doctor right away.

WARNINGS & PRECAUTIONS

Don't take if:
• You are allergic to kanamycin.
• You can't tolerate any aminoglycoside.

Before you start, consult your doctor if:
• You have hearing difficulty.
• You have intestinal obstruction.
• You have severe kidney disease.
• You have ulcerative colitis.

Over age 60:
Adverse reactions and side effects may be more frequent and severe than in younger persons. You may need smaller doses for shorter periods of time.

Pregnancy:
Consult doctor. Risk category D (see page xviii).

Breast-feeding:
No special problems expected. Consult doctor.

Infants & children:
Not recommended for prolonged use.

Prolonged use:
Not recommended for prolonged use.

Skin & sunlight:
No problems expected.

Driving, piloting or hazardous work:
Avoid if you feel confused, drowsy or dizzy.

Discontinuing:
Not recommended for prolonged use.

Others:
No problems expected.

 POSSIBLE INTERACTION WITH OTHER DRUGS

GENERIC NAME OR DRUG CLASS	COMBINED EFFECT
None significant.	

 POSSIBLE INTERACTION WITH OTHER SUBSTANCES

INTERACTS WITH	COMBINED EFFECT
Alcohol:	None expected.
Beverages:	None expected.
Cocaine:	None expected.
Foods:	None expected.
Marijuana:	None expected.
Tobacco:	None expected.

KAOLIN & PECTIN

BRAND NAMES

Donnagel-MB
Kao-Con
Kaotin
Kapectolin
Kapectolin with
  Paregoric

K-C
K-P
K-Pek
Parepectolin

BASIC INFORMATION

Habit forming? No
Prescription needed? No
Available as generic? Yes
Drug class: Antidiarrheal

 ## USES

Treats mild to moderate diarrhea. Used in conjunction with fluids, appropriate diet and rest. Treats symptoms only. Does not cure any disorder that causes diarrhea.

 ## DOSAGE & USAGE INFORMATION

How to take:
Liquid—Swallow prescribed dosage (without diluting) after each loose bowel movement.

When to take:
After each loose bowel movement.

If you forget a dose:
Take when you remember.

What drug does:
Makes loose stools less watery, but may not prevent loss of fluids.

Time lapse before drug works:
15 to 30 minutes.

Don't take with:
Any other medicine or any dietary supplement without consulting your doctor or pharmacist.

 ## OVERDOSE

SYMPTOMS:
Fecal impaction.
WHAT TO DO:
Overdose unlikely to threaten life. If person uses much larger amount than prescribed or if accidentally swallowed, call doctor or poison control center 1-800-222-1222 for help.

 ## POSSIBLE ADVERSE REACTIONS OR SIDE EFFECTS

SYMPTOMS	WHAT TO DO
Life-threatening: None expected.	
Common: None expected.	
Infrequent: None expected.	
Rare: Constipation (mild).	Continue. Call doctor when convenient.

WARNINGS & PRECAUTIONS

Don't take if:
You are allergic to kaolin or pectin.

Before you start, consult your doctor if:
* Patient is child or infant.
* You have any chronic medical problem with heart disease, peptic ulcer, asthma or others.
* You have fever over 101°F.

Over age 60:
Fluid loss caused by diarrhea, especially if taking other medicines, may lead to serious disability. Consult doctor.

Pregnancy:
Consult doctor. Risk category C (see page xviii).

Breast-feeding:
No problems expected.

Infants & children:
Fluid loss caused by diarrhea in infants and children can cause serious dehydration. Consult doctor before giving any medicine for diarrhea.

Prolonged use:
Not recommended.

Skin & sunlight:
No problems expected.

Driving, piloting or hazardous work:
No problems expected.

Discontinuing:
May be unnecessary to finish medicine. Follow doctor's instructions.

Others:
Consult doctor about fluids, diet and rest.

POSSIBLE INTERACTION WITH OTHER DRUGS

GENERIC NAME OR DRUG CLASS	COMBINED EFFECT
Digoxin	Decreases absorption of digoxin. Separate doses by at least 2 hours.
Lincomycins*	Decreases absorption of lincomycin. Separate doses by at least 2 hours.
All other oral medicines	May decrease absorption of other medicines. Separate doses by at least 2 hours.

POSSIBLE INTERACTION WITH OTHER SUBSTANCES

INTERACTS WITH	COMBINED EFFECT
Alcohol:	Increased diarrhea. Prevents action of kaolin and pectin.
Beverages:	None expected.
Cocaine:	Aggravates underlying disease. Avoid.
Foods:	None expected.
Marijuana:	Aggravates underlying disease. Avoid.
Tobacco:	Aggravates underlying disease. Avoid.

*See Glossary

KAOLIN, PECTIN, BELLADONNA & OPIUM

BRAND NAMES

Amogel PG   Kapectolin PG

Donnagel-PG   Quiagel PG

Donnapectolin-PG

BASIC INFORMATION

Habit forming? Yes

Prescription needed? Yes

Available as generic? No

Drug class: Narcotic, antidiarrheal, antispasmodic

 ## USES

Treats mild to moderate diarrhea. Used in conjunction with fluids, appropriate diet and rest. Treats symptoms only. Does not cure any disorder that causes diarrhea.

 ## DOSAGE & USAGE INFORMATION

How to take:

Liquid—Swallow prescribed dosage (without diluting) after each loose bowel movement.

When to take:

As needed for diarrhea, no more often than every 4 hours.

If you forget a dose:

Take when you remember.

Continued next column

 ## OVERDOSE

SYMPTOMS:

Fecal impaction, rapid pulse, dizziness, fever, hallucinations, confusion, slurred speech, agitation, flushed face, convulsions, deep sleep, slow breathing, slow pulse, warm skin, constricted pupils, coma.

WHAT TO DO:

- **Dial 911 (emergency) for medical help or call poison control center 1-800-222-1222 for instructions.**
- **If person is unconscious, check breathing and pulse. If not breathing, begin mouth-to-mouth rescue breathing. If heart is not beating, begin chest compressions.**
- **See emergency information on last 3 pages of this book.**

What drug does:

- Blocks nerve impulses at parasympathetic nerve endings, preventing muscle contractions and gland secretions of organs involved.
- Makes loose stools less watery, but may not prevent loss of fluids.
- Anesthetizes surface membranes of intestines and blocks nerve impulses.

Time lapse before drug works:

15 to 30 minutes.

Don't take with:

Any other medicine or any dietary supplement without consulting your doctor or pharmacist.

 ## POSSIBLE ADVERSE REACTIONS OR SIDE EFFECTS

SYMPTOMS	WHAT TO DO
Life-threatening:	
Unusually rapid heart-beat (over 100), difficult breathing, slow heart-beat (under 50/minute).	Discontinue. Seek emergency treatment.
Common (with large dosage):	
Weakness, increased sweating, red or flushed face, lightheadedness, headache, dry mouth, dry skin, drowsiness, dizziness, frequent urination, decreased sweating, constipation, confusion, tiredness.	Continue. Call doctor when convenient.
Infrequent:	
• Reduced taste sense, nervousness, eyes, sensitive to sunlight, blurred vision.	Discontinue. Call doctor right away.
• Diminished sex drive, memory loss.	Continue. Call doctor when convenient.
Rare:	
Bloating, abdominal cramps and vomiting, eye pain, hallucinations, shortness of breath, rash, itchy skin, slow heartbeat.	Discontinue. Call doctor right away.

 ## WARNINGS & PRECAUTIONS

Don't take if:

- You are allergic to any anticholinergic, narcotic, kaolin or pectin.
- You have trouble with stomach bloating, difficulty emptying your bladder completely, narrow-angle glaucoma, severe ulcerative colitis.

KAOLIN, PECTIN, BELLADONNA & OPIUM

Before you start, consult your doctor if:
- You have open-angle glaucoma, angina, chronic bronchitis or asthma, hiatal hernia, liver disease, enlarged prostate, myasthenia gravis, peptic ulcer, impaired liver or kidney function, fever over 101°F, any chronic medical problem.
- Patient is child or infant.
- You will have surgery within 2 months, including dental surgery, requiring general or spinal anesthesia.

Over age 60:
- Adverse reactions and side effects may be more frequent and severe than in younger persons.
- More likely to be drowsy, dizzy, unsteady or constipated.
- Fluid loss caused by diarrhea, especially if taking other medicines, may lead to serious disability. Consult doctor.

Pregnancy:
Decide with your doctor if drug benefits justify risk to unborn child. Risk category C (see page xviii).

Breast-feeding:
Drug passes into milk. Avoid drug or discontinue nursing until you finish medicine. Consult doctor for advice on maintaining milk supply.

Infants & children:
Fluid loss caused by diarrhea in infants and children can cause serious dehydration. Consult doctor before giving any medicine for diarrhea.

Prolonged use:
- Causes psychological and physical dependence. Not recommended.
- Talk to your doctor about the need for follow-up medical examinations or laboratory studies to check liver function, kidney function.

Skin & sunlight:
No special problems expected.

Driving, piloting or hazardous work:
Don't drive or pilot aircraft until you learn how medicine affects you. Don't work around dangerous machinery. Don't climb ladders or work in high places. Danger increases if you drink alcohol or take medicine affecting alertness and reflexes, such as antihistamines, tranquilizers, sedatives, pain medicine, narcotics and mind-altering drugs.

Discontinuing:
May be unnecessary to finish medicine. Follow doctor's instructions.

Others:
- Great potential for abuse.
- Consult doctor about fluids, diet and rest.
- Advise any doctor or dentist whom you consult that you take this medicine.

POSSIBLE INTERACTION WITH OTHER DRUGS

GENERIC NAME OR DRUG CLASS	COMBINED EFFECT
Amantadine	Increased belladonna effect.
Analgesics*	Increased analgesic effect.
Antidepressants*	Increased sedative effect.
Antihistamines*	Increased sedative effect.
Carteolol	Increased narcotic effect. Dangerous sedation.
Central nervous system (CNS) depressants*	Increased depressant effect of both.
Cortisone drugs*	Increased internal eye pressure.
Digoxin	Decreases absorption of digoxin. Separate doses by at least 2 hours.
Haloperidol	Increased internal eye pressure.

Continued on page 920

POSSIBLE INTERACTION WITH OTHER SUBSTANCES

INTERACTS WITH	COMBINED EFFECT
Alcohol:	Increases alcohol's intoxicating effect, increased diarrhea, prevents action of kaolin and pectin. Avoid.
Beverages:	None expected.
Cocaine:	Aggravates underlying disease. Avoid.
Foods:	None expected.
Marijuana:	Impairs physical and mental performance, aggravates underlying disease. Avoid.
Tobacco:	Aggravates underlying disease. Avoid.

KERATOLYTICS

GENERIC AND BRAND NAMES

See full list of generic and brand names in the *Generic and Brand Name Directory*, page 888.

BASIC INFORMATION

Habit forming? No
Prescription needed? Yes, on some.
Available as generic? Yes
Drug class: Keratolytic, antiacne (topical), antiseborrheic

 ## USES

Treatment for skin disorders such as acne, psoriasis, ichthyosis,keratosis, folliculitis, flat warts, eczema, urticaria, calluses, corns, seborrheic dermatitis, dandruff and others.

 ## DOSAGE & USAGE INFORMATION

How to use:
Cream, gel, lotion, ointment, pads, plaster, shampoo, soap, topical solution, suspension— Always follow instructions on the label or use as directed by your doctor.

When to use:
At the same time each day or as needed.

If you forget an application:
Use as soon as you remember.

What drug does:
Keratolytics are drugs that soften, loosen and remove keratin (the tough outer layer of the skin).

Time lapse before drug works:
2 to 3 weeks. May require 6 weeks for maximum improvement.

Don't use with:
• Benzoyl peroxide. Apply 12 hours apart.
• Any other topical medicine without consulting your doctor or pharmacist.

 ## OVERDOSE

SYMPTOMS:
None expected.
WHAT TO DO:
If person swallows drug, dial 911 (emergency) for medical help or call poison control center 1-800-222-1222 for instructions.

 ## POSSIBLE ADVERSE REACTIONS OR SIDE EFFECTS

SYMPTOMS	WHAT TO DO
Life-threatening: None expected.	
Common:	
• Pigment change in treated area, warmth or stinging, peeling.	Continue. Tell doctor at next visit.
• Sensitivity to wind or cold.	No action necessary.
Infrequent: Blistering, crusting, severe burning, swelling, skin irritation that begins after treatment.	Discontinue. Call doctor right away.
Rare: Symptoms of systemic toxicity (diarrhea, nausea, dizziness, headache, breathing difficulty, tiredness, weakness).	Discontinue. Call doctor right away.

WARNINGS & PRECAUTIONS

Don't take if:
* You are allergic to resorcinol or salicylic acid.
* You are sunburned or windburned or have an open skin wound, skin irritation or infection.

Before you start, consult your doctor if:
* You have eczema.
* You have diabetes.
* You have peripheral vascular disease (blood vessel disease).

Over age 60:
No problems expected.

Pregnancy:
Risk factors vary for drugs in this group. See category list on page xviii and consult doctor.

Breast-feeding:
No problems expected. Consult doctor.

Infants & children:
Not recommended. Increased risk of toxicity.

Prolonged use:
No problems expected.

Skin & sunlight:
No special problems expected.

Driving, piloting or hazardous work:
No problems expected.

Discontinuing:
Follow your doctor's instructions or the directions on the label.

Others:
* Acne may get worse before improvement starts in 2 or 3 weeks. Don't wash face more than 2 or 3 times daily.
* Keep medicine away from mouth or eyes. If it accidentally gets into the eyes, flush immediately with clear water.
* Keep medicine away from heat or flame.

POSSIBLE INTERACTION WITH OTHER DRUGS

GENERIC NAME OR DRUG CLASS	COMBINED EFFECT
Antiacne topical preparations (other)	Severe skin irritation.
Cosmetics (medicated)	Severe skin irritation.
Skin preparations with alcohol	Severe skin irritation.
Soaps or cleansers (abrasive)	Severe skin irritation.

POSSIBLE INTERACTION WITH OTHER SUBSTANCES

INTERACTS WITH	COMBINED EFFECT
Alcohol:	None expected.
Beverages:	None expected.
Cocaine:	None expected.
Foods:	None expected.
Marijuana:	None expected.
Tobacco:	None expected.

LACOSAMIDE

BRAND NAMES

Vimpat

BASIC INFORMATION

Habit forming? Possibly
Prescription needed? Yes
Available as generic? No
Drug class: Anticonvulsant; antiepileptic

 USES

- Treatment of partial-onset seizures in patients with epilepsy. It is used in combination with other antiepileptic drugs.
- Other uses as recommended by your doctor.

 DOSAGE & USAGE INFORMATION

How to take:
- Tablet—Swallow the tablet with a liquid. May be taken with or without food, and on a full or empty stomach.
- Injection—Given by medical professional.

When to take:
Tablet is usually taken twice a day at the same times each day. Your doctor will determine the best schedule. Dosages may be increased weekly to achieve maximum benefits.

If you forget a dose:
Take as soon as you remember. If it is almost time for the next dose, skip the missed dose and wait for your next scheduled dose (don't double this dose).

What drug does:
It helps stabilize electrical activity in the brain, but the exact way it controls seizures is unknown.

Time lapse before drug works:
May take several weeks for full effectiveness.

Don't take with:
Any other medicine or any dietary supplement without consulting your doctor or pharmacist.

 OVERDOSE

SYMPTOMS:
Unknown (may be similar to side effects).
WHAT TO DO:
Overdose unlikely to threaten life. If person uses much larger amount than prescribed or if accidentally swallowed, call doctor or poison control center 1-800-222-1222 for help.

 POSSIBLE ADVERSE REACTIONS OR SIDE EFFECTS

SYMPTOMS	WHAT TO DO
Life-threatening:	
Rare allergic reaction (hives, itching, rash, trouble breathing, tightness in chest, swelling of lips or tongue or face).	Seek emergency treatment immediately.
Common:	
• Dizziness, unsteady walk, shakiness or trembling, unusual drowsiness, lack of coordination.	Continue, but call doctor right away.
• Blurred or double vision, headache, nausea or vomiting.	Continue. Call doctor when convenient.
Infrequent:	
• Mood or mental changes, feeling sad or irritable, forgetfulness, itchy skin, tiredness, trouble sleeping or concentrating, unusual eye movements, depression.	Continue, but call doctor right away.
• Diarrhea, weakness, spinning sensation.	Continue. Call doctor when convenient.
Rare:	
• Tingling or prickling feelings, noises in ears, chills, fever, changes in heartbeat (fast, slow, irregular, pounding), unusual bleeding or bruising, yellow skin or eyes, new or worsening seizures, shortness of breath, fainting, behavior changes, euphoria .	Continue, but call doctor right away.
• Indigestion, heartburn, dry mouth, constipation, muscle spasms.	Continue. Call doctor when convenient.

WARNINGS & PRECAUTIONS

Don't take if:
You are allergic to lacosamide.

Before you start, consult your doctor if:
* You have diabetes or kidney or liver problems.
* You have a history of any heart disorder or blood vessel problem.
* You have a history of mental or mood problems (such as depression) or suicidal thoughts or attempts.
* You are allergic to any medication, food or other substance.

Over age 60:
May be more at risk for side effects or adverse reactions. Use with caution.

Pregnancy:
Decide with your doctor if drug benefits justify risks to unborn child. Risk category C (see page xviii).

Breast-feeding:
It is unknown if drug passes into milk. Avoid drug or discontinue nursing until you finish medicine. Consult doctor for advice on maintaining milk supply.

Infants & children:
Safety and efficacy not established in children younger than age 17.

Prolonged use:
No special problems expected. Follow-up with your doctor on a regular basis to monitor your condition and check for drug side effects.

Skin & sunlight:
No problems expected.

Driving, piloting or hazardous work:
This drug may cause dizziness, coordination problems or blurred or double vision. Don't drive or pilot aircraft until you learn how medicine affects you. Don't work around dangerous machinery. Don't climb ladders or work in high places. The risk of dizziness increases if you drink alcohol.

Discontinuing:
Don't discontinue without doctor's approval due to risk of increased seizure activity. The dosage may need to be gradually decreased before stopping the drug completely.

Others:
* This drug cannot cure epilepsy and will only work to control seizures for as long as you continue to take it.
* Lacosamide is used with other anticonvulsant drugs and additional side effects may occur. If they do, consult your doctor.
* Advise any doctor or dentist whom you consult that you take this medicine.
* Rarely, antiepileptic drugs may lead to suicidal thoughts and behaviors. Call doctor right away if suicidal symptoms or unusual behaviors occur.
* Carry or wear medical identification that lists your seizure disorder and drugs you take.

POSSIBLE INTERACTION WITH OTHER DRUGS

GENERIC NAME OR DRUG CLASS	COMBINED EFFECT
QT interval prolongation-causing drugs*	Increased risk of cardiac (heart) side effects.

POSSIBLE INTERACTION WITH OTHER SUBSTANCES

INTERACTS WITH	COMBINED EFFECT
Alcohol:	Increased risk of dizziness. Avoid.
Beverages:	None expected.
Cocaine:	Unknown effect. Avoid.
Foods:	None expected.
Marijuana:	Unknown effect. Avoid.
Tobacco:	None expected.

---

*See Glossary

LAMOTRIGINE

BRAND NAMES

Lamictal

Lamictal Chewable
Dispersible Tablet

BASIC INFORMATION

Habit forming? No
Prescription needed? Yes
Available as generic? Yes
Drug class: Anticonvulsant, antiepileptic

 USES

- Treatment for partial (focal) epileptic seizures. May be used in combination with other antiepileptic drugs.
- Treatment of primary generalized tonic-clonic (PGTC) seizures, also known as "grand mal" seizures.
- Maintenance therapy for bipolar disorder.

 DOSAGE & USAGE INFORMATION

How to take:
- Tablet—Swallow whole with liquid. May be taken with or without food. Do not crush or chew tablet as it can have a bitter taste.
- Chewable dispersible tablet—Swallow whole or chew. If you chew the tablets, drink a small amount of water or diluted fruit juice to aid in swallowing. To mix it in a liquid, follow directions provided with prescription.

When to take:
Your doctor will determine the best schedule. Dosages may be increased gradually over the first few weeks of use to achieve maximum benefits.

If you forget a dose:
Take as soon as you remember. If it is almost time for the next dose, then skip the missed dose and wait for your next scheduled dose (don't double this dose).

Continued next column

 OVERDOSE

SYMPTOMS:
Severe drowsiness, severe headache, severe dizziness, coma.
WHAT TO DO:
- **Dial 911 (emergency) for medical help or call poison control center 1-800-222-1222 for instructions.**
- **See emergency information on last 3 pages of this book.**

What drug does:
The exact mechanism is unknown. The anticonvulsant action may result from a decrease in the release of stimulatory neurotransmitters (substances that stimulate nerve cells).

Time lapse before drug works:
May take several weeks for effectiveness.

Don't take with:
Any other medicine or any dietary supplement without consulting your doctor or pharmacist.

 POSSIBLE ADVERSE REACTIONS OR SIDE EFFECTS

SYMPTOMS	WHAT TO DO
Life-threatening:	
In case of overdose, see previous column.	
Common:	
• Skin rash, double vision or blurred vision, clumsiness.	Continue, but call doctor right away.
• Dizziness, nausea or vomiting, headache, drowsiness.	Continue. Call doctor when convenient.
Infrequent:	
Anxiety, depression, confusion, irritability, other mood or mental changes, increase in seizure activity, back-and-forth eye movements (nystagmus).	Continue, but call doctor right away.
Rare:	
• Swelling (hands, face, mouth, feet); breathing difficulty; tiredness or weakness; fever; chills; sore throat; unusual bruising or bleeding; skin peeling, blistering or loosening; muscle cramps or pain; sores on mouth or lips; small red or purple dots on skin, slurred speech.	Continue, but call doctor right away.
• Indigestion, runny nose, trembling, trouble sleeping, weakness.	Continue. Call doctor when convenient.

WARNINGS & PRECAUTIONS

Don't take if:
You are allergic to lamotrigine.

Before you start, consult your doctor if:
• You have kidney or liver disease.
• You have any heart disorder.
• You are allergic to any medication, food, or other substance.

Over age 60:
No special problems expected.

Pregnancy:
• Decide with your doctor if drug benefits justify risks to unborn child. Risk category C (see page xviii).
• Use of this drug during the first 3 months of pregnancy may increase chances of baby being born with cleft lip or cleft palate.

Breast-feeding:
Drug passes into milk. Avoid drug or discontinue nursing until you finish medicine. Consult doctor for advice on maintaining milk supply.

Infants & children:
Safety not established for children under age 16. Use only under close medical supervision.

Prolonged use:
Schedule regular visits to your doctor to determine if drug is continuing to be effective in controlling seizures. Follow-up laboratory blood studies may be recommended by your doctor.

Skin & sunlight:
No special problems expected.

Driving, piloting or hazardous work:
Don't drive or pilot aircraft until you learn how medicine affects you. Don't work around dangerous machinery. Don't climb ladders or work in high places. Danger increases if you drink alcohol or take other medicines affecting alertness and reflexes, such as antihistamines, tranquilizers, sedatives, pain medicine, narcotics and mind-altering drugs.

Discontinuing:
Don't discontinue without doctor's approval due to risk of increased seizure activity. Dosage may need to be gradually reduced.

Others:
• Advise any doctor or dentist whom you consult that you take this medicine.
• Use as directed. Don't increase or decrease dosage without doctor's approval.
• A skin rash may indicate a serious, and potentially life-threatening, medical problem. If a skin rash develops, it is usually during the first 4 to 6 weeks after treatment with the drug is started. Call your doctor promptly if you develop any skin rash.

• Rarely, antiepileptic drugs may lead to suicidal thoughts and behaviors. Call doctor right away if suicidal symptoms or unusual behaviors occur.
• Wear or carry medical identification stating that you have a seizure disorder and take this medication.

POSSIBLE INTERACTION WITH OTHER DRUGS

GENERIC NAME OR DRUG CLASS	COMBINED EFFECT
Carbamazepine	Decreased effect of lamotrigine. Increase in risk of side effects.
Central nervous system (CNS) depressants*	Increased sedation.
Folate antagonists,* other	Folic acid deficiency.
Phenobarbital	Decreased effect of lamotrigine.
Phenytoin	Decreased effect of lamotrigine.
Primidone	Decreased effect of lamotrigine.
Valproic acid*	Increased effect of lamotrigine.

POSSIBLE INTERACTION WITH OTHER SUBSTANCES

INTERACTS WITH	COMBINED EFFECT
Alcohol:	Increased sedation. Avoid.
Beverages:	None expected.
Cocaine:	Problems not known. Best to avoid.
Foods:	None expected.
Marijuana:	Problems not known. Best to avoid.
Tobacco:	None expected.

*See Glossary

LAXATIVES, BULK-FORMING

GENERIC AND BRAND NAMES

See full list of generic and brand names in the *Generic and Brand Name Directory*, page 889.

BASIC INFORMATION

Habit forming? No
Prescription needed? No
Available as generic? Yes
Drug class: Laxative, bulk-forming

 ## USES

For short-term relief of simple constipation (bowel movements that are abnormally difficult or infrequent). Normal frequency of bowel movements may vary from 2 to 3 times a day to 2 to 3 times a week. Laxatives treat the symptoms of constipation, not the cause.

 ## DOSAGE & USAGE INFORMATION

How to take:
Powder, oral solution, tablet, capsule, granules, chewable tablet, caramel, effervescent powder, wafer—Follow package instructions. Swallow with full glass of water or fruit juice. Drink 6 to 8 glasses of water each day in addition to one taken with each dose. Mix all powders thoroughly to avoid any risk of unmixed powder causing intestinal blockage.

When to take:
As directed on the label or according to doctor's instructions.

If you forget a dose:
Take as soon as you remember.

What drug does:
Adds dietary fiber that is not digested. Once in the intestine, it helps to increase fecal bulk, lubricate and soften the intestinal contents and facilitate the passage of stools.

Continued next column

 ## OVERDOSE

SYMPTOMS:
Weakness, increased sweating, confusion, irregular heartbeat, muscle cramps.
WHAT TO DO:
Overdose unlikely to threaten life. If person uses much larger amount than prescribed or if accidentally swallowed, call doctor or poison control center 1-800-222-1222 for help.

Time lapse before drug works:
May work in 12 to 24 hours. Sometimes does not work for 2 to 3 days.

Don't take with:
- Any other medicine or any dietary supplement without consulting your doctor or pharmacist.
- Don't take within 2 hours of taking another medicine. Laxative interferes with absorption of medicine.

 ## POSSIBLE ADVERSE REACTIONS OR SIDE EFFECTS

SYMPTOMS	WHAT TO DO
Life-threatening: None expected.	
Common: None expected.	
Infrequent: Mild stomach cramps, throat irritation with liquid form.	Continue. Call doctor when convenient.
Rare: Allergic skin rash or itching, trouble breathing, swallowing difficulty.	Discontinue. Call doctor right away.

WARNINGS & PRECAUTIONS

Don't take if:
- You have symptoms of appendicitis (abdominal pain, cramping, soreness, bloating, nausea and vomiting). Consult doctor.
- You have dysphagia (swallowing difficulty).
- You are allergic to bulk-forming laxatives.
- You have missed a bowel movement for just 1 or 2 days.

Before you start, consult your doctor if:
- You are allergic to any medicine, food, or other substance or have a family history of allergies.
- You have diabetes or heart or kidney disease.
- You have hypertension (high blood pressure) and the laxative contains sodium.
- You have an intestinal obstruction or undiagnosed rectal bleeding.
- You are taking other laxatives.

Over age 60:
No special problems expected.

Pregnancy:
Most bulk-forming laxatives contain sodium or sugars, which may cause fluid retention. Risk factors vary or may not be designated for these laxatives. Read categories on page xviii and consult doctor.

Breast-feeding:
No special problems expected. Consult doctor.

Infants & children:
- Don't give to children under age 6 without doctor's approval. Young children are not able to describe their symptoms accurately, and a proper diagnosis needs to be made before starting any treatment.
- Don't give to a child who refuses to have a bowel movement (toileting refusal). May force a painful bowel movement and cause the child to hold back even more. Consult doctor.
- For children over age 6, follow package instructions or doctor's directions for correct dosage amount.

Prolonged use:
Don't take for more than 1 week unless under doctor's supervision. Bulk-form laxatives are sometimes used for long-term therapy.

Skin & sunlight:
No special problems expected.

Driving, piloting or hazardous work:
No special problems expected.

Discontinuing:
May be unnecessary to finish medicine. Follow doctor's instructions or instructions on label.

Others:
- Don't give to "flush out" the system or as a "tonic."
- Use as directed. Don't increase or decrease dosage without doctor's approval.
- Excessive use of laxatives in a teenager may indicate an eating disorder such as anorexia nervosa or bulimia nervosa. Consult doctor.
- If there is a sudden change in bowel habits or bowel function that lasts longer than 2 weeks, consult doctor.

POSSIBLE INTERACTION WITH OTHER DRUGS

GENERIC NAME OR DRUG CLASS	COMBINED EFFECT
Antacids*	Irritation of stomach or small intestine.
Anticoagulants*	Decreased anti-coagulant effect. Take 2 hours apart.
Digitalis preparations*	Decreased digitalis effect. Take 2 hours apart.
Diuretics, potassium-sparing*	Decreased potassium effect.
Potassium supplements*	Decreased potassium effect.
Salicylates*	Decreased salicylate effect. Take 2 hours apart.
Tetracyclines*	Decreased tetracycline effect. Take 2 hours apart.

POSSIBLE INTERACTION WITH OTHER SUBSTANCES

INTERACTS WITH	COMBINED EFFECT
Alcohol:	None expected.
Beverages:	None expected.
Cocaine:	None expected.
Foods:	None expected.
Marijuana:	None expected.
Tobacco:	None expected.

*See Glossary

LAXATIVES, OSMOTIC

GENERIC AND BRAND NAMES

See full list of generic and brand names in the *Generic and Brand Name Directory*, page 889.

BASIC INFORMATION

Habit forming? No
Prescription needed? No
Available as generic? Yes
Drug class: Laxative, hyperosmotic

 ## USES

For short-term relief of simple constipation (bowel movements that are abnormally difficult or infrequent). Normal frequency of bowel movements may vary from 2 to 3 times a day to 2 to 3 times a week. Laxatives treat the symptoms of constipation, not the cause.

 ## DOSAGE & USAGE INFORMATION

How to take:
- Oral solution, tablet, crystals, effervescent powder, milk of magnesia—Follow package instructions. Swallow with full glass of water or fruit juice. A second glass of liquid is often recommended for best effect. Drink 6 to 8 glasses of water each day, in addition to one taken with each dose.
- Enema or suppository—Read and follow package instructions.

When to take:
Since drug produces stool within 30 minutes to 3 hours following a dose, take it at a time that will not interfere with sleep or other scheduled activities. Don't take late in the day on an empty stomach.

If you forget a dose:
Take as soon as you remember.

Continued next column

 ## OVERDOSE

SYMPTOMS:
Weakness, increased sweating, confusion, irregular heartbeat, muscle cramps.
WHAT TO DO:
Overdose unlikely to threaten life. If person uses much larger amount than prescribed or if accidentally swallowed, call doctor or poison control center 1-800-222-1222 for help.

What drug does:
Draws water into the bowel from surrounding tissue to help loosen and soften the stool and increases bowel action.

Time lapse before drug works:
- Oral forms—30 minutes to 3 hours. May take longer if taken with a meal.
- Rectal forms—2 to 15 minutes.

Don't take with:
- Any other medicine or any dietary supplement without consulting your doctor or pharmacist.
- Don't take within 2 hours of taking another medicine. Laxative interferes with absorption of medicine.

 ## POSSIBLE ADVERSE REACTIONS OR SIDE EFFECTS

SYMPTOMS	WHAT TO DO
Life-threatening: None expected.	
Common: None expected.	
Infrequent:	
• Belching, cramps, nausea, diarrhea, increased thirst.	Continue. Call doctor when convenient.
• Rectal bleeding, burning, itching or pain (with rectal forms).	Discontinue. Call doctor right away.
Rare: When used too often or dose is too high— Confusion, irregular heartbeat, muscle cramps, unusual tiredness or weakness, dehydration.	Discontinue. Call doctor right away.

 ## WARNINGS & PRECAUTIONS

Don't take if:
- You are having symptoms of appendicitis (abdominal pain, cramping, soreness, bloating, nausea and vomiting). Consult doctor.
- You are allergic to osmotic laxatives.
- You have missed a bowel movement for just 1 or 2 days.

Before you start, consult your doctor if:
- You are allergic to any medicine, food or other substance or have a family history of allergies.
- You have hypertension (high blood pressure) and the laxative contains sodium.
- You have an intestinal obstruction, undiagnosed rectal bleeding or a colostomy or ileostomy.
- You have diabetes or heart or kidney disease.
- You are taking other laxatives.

Over age 60:
- Rectal solutions could cause excess fluid in the body. Consult doctor before using.
- No special problems expected with laxatives taken by mouth.

Pregnancy:
Risk factors vary or may not be designated for these laxatives. Read categories on page xviii and consult doctor.

Breast-feeding:
No special problems expected. Consult doctor.

Infants & children:
- Don't give to children under age 6 without doctor's approval. Young children are not able to describe their symptoms accurately, and a proper diagnosis needs to be made before starting any treatment.
- Don't give to a child who refuses to have a bowel movement (toileting refusal). May force a painful bowel movement and cause the child to hold back even more. Consult doctor.
- For children over age 6, follow package instructions or doctor's directions for correct dosage amount.

Prolonged use:
Don't take for more than 1 week unless under doctor's supervision. May cause laxative dependence in which normal bowel function depends on the laxative to produce a bowel movement.

Skin & sunlight:
No special problems expected.

Driving, piloting or hazardous work:
No special problems expected.

Discontinuing:
May be unnecessary to finish medicine. Follow doctor's instructions or instructions on label.

Others:
- Don't give to "flush out" the system or as a "tonic."
- Use as directed. Don't increase or decrease dosage without doctor's approval.
- Excessive use of laxatives in a teenager may indicate an eating disorder such as anorexia nervosa or bulimia nervosa. Consult doctor.
- If there is a sudden change in bowel habits or bowel function that lasts longer than 2 weeks, consult doctor.

 POSSIBLE INTERACTION WITH OTHER DRUGS

GENERIC NAME OR DRUG CLASS	COMBINED EFFECT
Antacids*	Irritation of stomach or small intestine.
Anticoagulants*	Decreased anti-coagulant effect with aluminum- or magnesium-containing laxatives. Avoid.
Ciprofloxacin	Decreased ciprofloxacin effect with magnesium-containing laxatives. Avoid.
Digitalis preparations*	Decreased digitalis effect with aluminum- or magnesium-containing laxatives. Avoid.
Diuretics, potassium-sparing*	Decreased potassium effect.
Etidronate	Decreased etidronate effect if taken with magnesium-containing laxatives. Take 2 hours apart.
Phenothiazines*	Decreased phenothiazine effect with aluminum- or magnesium-containing laxatives. Avoid.
Potassium supplements*	Decreased potassium effect.
Sodium polystyrene	Fluid imbalance in body with magnesium-containing laxatives. Avoid.
Tetracyclines*	Decreased tetracycline effect. Take 2 hours apart.

 POSSIBLE INTERACTION WITH OTHER SUBSTANCES

INTERACTS WITH	COMBINED EFFECT
Alcohol:	None expected.
Beverages:	None expected.
Cocaine:	None expected.
Foods:	None expected.
Marijuana:	None expected.
Tobacco:	None expected.

*See Glossary

LAXATIVES, SOFTENER/LUBRICANT

GENERIC AND BRAND NAMES

See full list of generic and brand names in the *Generic and Brand Name Directory,* page 889.

BASIC INFORMATION

Habit forming? No
Prescription needed? No
Available as generic? Yes
Drug class: Laxative (stool softener-emollient), lubricant

USES

For short-term relief of simple constipation (bowel movements that are abnormally difficult or infrequent). Normal frequency of bowel movements may vary from 2 to 3 times a day to 2 to 3 times a week. Laxatives treat the symptoms of constipation, not the cause.

DOSAGE & USAGE INFORMATION

How to take:
* Tablet, capsule, syrup, chewable tablet, oral solution—Follow package instructions. Swallow with full glass of water, fruit juice or milk. Drink 6 to 8 glasses of water each day in addition to one taken with each dose.
* Enema or suppository—Read and follow package instructions.

When to take:
Produces stool within 30 minutes to 3 hours following a dose. Take drug at a time that will not interfere with sleep or scheduled activities. Don't take late in the day on an empty stomach.

If you forget a dose:
Take as soon as you remember.

Continued next column

OVERDOSE

SYMPTOMS:
Weakness, increased sweating, confusion, irregular heartbeat, muscle cramps.
WHAT TO DO:
Overdose unlikely to threaten life. If person uses much larger amount than prescribed or if accidentally swallowed, call doctor or poison control center 1-800-222-1222 for help.

What drug does:
Softener laxatives help liquids mix into the stool to help prevent hard stool masses. Lubricant laxatives coat the stool surface with a thin film that helps ease the passage of the stool through the intestines.

Time lapse before drug works:
* When taken by mouth, usually works within 1 to 2 days after first dose, but may take 3 to 5 days for full effectiveness.
* Rectal dosage forms work in 2 to 15 minutes.

Don't take with:
* Any other medicine or any dietary supplement without consulting your doctor or pharmacist.
* Other stool softener laxatives or mineral oil.
* Don't take within 2 hours of taking another medicine. Laxative interferes with absorption of medicine.

POSSIBLE ADVERSE REACTIONS OR SIDE EFFECTS

SYMPTOMS	WHAT TO DO
Life-threatening: None expected.	
Common: None expected.	
Infrequent:	
• Mild stomach cramps, throat irritation with liquid forms, diarrhea.	Continue. Call doctor when convenient.
• Rectal bleeding, burning, itching or pain (with rectal forms).	Discontinue. Call doctor right away.
Rare: Skin rash.	Discontinue. Call doctor right away.

WARNINGS & PRECAUTIONS

Don't take if:
* You have symptoms of appendicitis (abdominal pain, cramping, soreness, bloating, nausea and vomiting). Consult doctor.
* You are allergic to a softener-emollient or lubricant laxative.
* You have missed a bowel movement for just 1 or 2 days.

LAXATIVES, SOFTENER/LUBRICANT

Before you start, consult your doctor if:
- You are allergic to any medicine, food or other substance or have a family history of allergies.
- You have hypertension (high blood pressure) and the laxative contains sodium.
- You have an intestinal obstruction, undiagnosed rectal bleeding or a colostomy or ileostomy.
- You are taking other laxatives.
- You have diabetes or heart or kidney disease.
- You have dysphagia (swallowing difficulty) and want to take mineral oil.

Over age 60:
Oral mineral oil is not recommended for bedridden elderly patients; otherwise, no special problems expected.

Pregnancy:
Risk factors vary or may not be designated for these laxatives. Read categories on page xviii and consult doctor.

Breast-feeding:
No special problems expected. Consult doctor.

Infants & children:
- Don't give to children under age 6 without doctor's approval. Young children are not able to describe their symptoms accurately, and a proper diagnosis needs to be made before starting any treatment.
- Don't give to a child who refuses to have a bowel movement (toileting refusal). May force a painful bowel movement and cause the child to hold back even more. Consult doctor.
- For children over age 6, follow package instructions or doctor's directions for correct dosage amount.

Prolonged use:
Don't take for more than 1 week unless under doctor's supervision.

Skin & sunlight:
No special problems expected.

Driving, piloting or hazardous work:
No special problems expected.

Discontinuing:
May be unnecessary to finish medicine. Follow doctor's instructions or instructions on label.

Others:
- Don't give to "flush out" the system or as a "tonic."
- Use as directed. Don't increase or decrease dosage without doctor's approval.
- Excessive use of laxatives in a teenager may indicate an eating disorder such as anorexia nervosa or bulimia nervosa. Consult doctor.
- If there is a sudden change in bowel habits or bowel function that lasts longer than 2 weeks, consult doctor.

POSSIBLE INTERACTION WITH OTHER DRUGS

GENERIC NAME OR DRUG CLASS	COMBINED EFFECT
Antacids*	Irritation of stomach or small intestine.
Anticoagulants*	Decreased anticoagulant effect with mineral oil.
Contraceptives, oral*	Decreased contraceptive effect with mineral oil.
Danthron	Increased danthron effect.
Digitalis preparations*	Decreased digitalis effect with mineral oil.
Diuretics, potassium-sparing*	Decreased potassium effect.
Phenolphthalein	Increased phenophthalein effect.
Potassium supplements*	Decreased potassium effect.
Vitamins A, D, E, K	Decreased vitamin effect with mineral oil.

POSSIBLE INTERACTION WITH OTHER SUBSTANCES

INTERACTS WITH	COMBINED EFFECT
Alcohol:	None expected.
Beverages:	None expected.
Cocaine:	None expected.
Foods:	None expected.
Marijuana:	None expected.
Tobacco:	None expected.

*See Glossary

LAXATIVES, STIMULANT

GENERIC AND BRAND NAMES

See full list of generic and brand names in the *Generic and Brand Name Directory*, page 890.

BASIC INFORMATION

Habit forming? Potentially
Prescription needed? No
Available as generic? Yes
Drug class: Laxative (stimulant)

 USES

For short-term relief of simple constipation (bowel movements that are abnormally difficult or infrequent). Normal frequency of bowel movements may vary from 2 to 3 times a day to 2 to 3 times a week. Laxatives treat the symptoms of constipation, not the cause.

 DOSAGE & USAGE INFORMATION

How to take:
• Tablet, chewable tablet, syrup, chewing gum, oral solution, granules, fluidextract, emulsion, wafer—Follow package instructions. Swallow with full glass of water, fruit juice or milk. Give child 6 to 8 glasses of fluid each day in addition to the one taken with each dose to keep stool soft. Give on an empty stomach. Results may be delayed if given with food.
• Enema—Lubricate rectal area with petroleum jelly before inserting enema applicator. Insert carefully to avoid damage to rectal wall. To mix powder for rectal solution, follow instructions on package.
• Suppository—Remove wrapper and moisten suppository with water. Gently insert tapered end into rectum. Push well into rectum with finger. Retain in rectum 20 to 30 minutes.

Continued next column

 OVERDOSE

SYMPTOMS:
Weakness, increased sweating, confusion, irregular heartbeat, muscle cramps.
WHAT TO DO:
Overdose unlikely to threaten life. If person uses much larger amount than prescribed or if accidentally swallowed, call doctor or poison control center 1-800-222-1222 for help.

When to take:
Usually at bedtime on an empty stomach, unless directed otherwise. Castor oil is usually taken late in the day, as it works within 2 to 6 hours.

If you forget a dose:
Take as soon as you remember.

What drug does:
Acts on smooth muscles of intestinal wall to cause vigorous bowel movement.

Time lapse before drug works:
Oral form within 6 to 10 hours (castor oil 2 to 6 hours). Rectal form within 15 minutes to 1 hour.

Don't take with:
• Any other medicine or any dietary supplement without consulting your doctor or pharmacist.
• Don't take within 2 hours of another medicine. Laxative interferes with absorption of medicine.

 POSSIBLE ADVERSE REACTIONS OR SIDE EFFECTS

SYMPTOMS	WHAT TO DO
Life-threatening: None expected.	
Common: None expected.	
Infrequent:	
• Belching, cramps, nausea, diarrhea, throat irritation.	Continue. Call doctor when convenient.
• Rectal bleeding, burning, itching or pain (with rectal forms).	Discontinue. Call doctor right away.
Rare: Confusion, irregular heartbeat, muscle cramps, unusual tiredness or weakness; pink to red color of urine and stools (with phenolphthalein); pink, red or violet to brown urine color (with cascara, danthron or senna); yellow to brown color of urine (with cascara, phenolphthalein or senna); skin rash (allergy).	Discontinue. Call doctor right away.

WARNINGS & PRECAUTIONS

Don't take if:
- You have symptoms of appendicitis (abdominal pain, cramping, soreness, bloating, nausea and vomiting). Consult doctor.
- You are allergic to a stimulant laxative.
- You have missed a bowel movement for just 1 or 2 days.

Before you start, consult your doctor if:
- You are a allergic to any medicine, food or other substance or have a family history of allergies.
- You have hypertension (high blood pressure) and the laxative contains sodium.
- You have an intestinal obstruction or undiagnosed rectal bleeding.
- You have diabetes or heart or kidney disease.
- You are taking other laxatives.

Over age 60:
Excessive use of stimulant laxatives may cause excess loss of body fluid, resulting in weakness and lack of coordination.

Pregnancy:
Risk factors vary or may not be designated for these laxatives. Read categories on page xviii and consult doctor.

Breast-feeding:
Some of the stimulant laxatives may pass into breast milk. Consult doctor.

Infants & children:
- Don't give to children under age 6 without doctor's approval. Young children are not able to describe their symptoms accurately, and a proper diagnosis needs to be made before starting any treatment.
- Don't give to a child who refuses to have a bowel movement (toileting refusal). May force a painful bowel movement and cause the child to hold back even more. Consult doctor.
- For children over age 6, follow package instructions or doctor's directions for correct dosage amount.

Prolonged use:
Don't take for more than 1 week unless under doctor's supervision.

Skin & sunlight:
No special problems expected.

Driving, piloting or hazardous work:
No special problems expected.

Discontinuing:
May be unnecessary to finish medicine. Follow doctor's instructions or instructions on label.

Others:
- Don't give to "flush out" the system or as a "tonic."
- Use as directed. Don't increase or decrease dosage without doctor's approval.
- Excessive use of laxatives in a teenager may indicate an eating disorder such as anorexia nervosa or bulimia nervosa. Consult doctor.
- If there is a sudden change in bowel habits or bowel function that lasts longer than 2 weeks, consult doctor.

POSSIBLE INTERACTION WITH OTHER DRUGS

GENERIC NAME OR DRUG CLASS	COMBINED EFFECT
Antacids*	Irritation of stomach or small intestine.
Diuretics, potassium-sparing*	Decreased potassium effect.
Histamine H$_2$ receptor antagonists*	Stomach irritation with bisacodyl. Take 1 hour apart.
Potassium supplements*	Decreased potassium effect.

POSSIBLE INTERACTION WITH OTHER SUBSTANCES

INTERACTS WITH	COMBINED EFFECT
Alcohol:	None expected.
Beverages: Milk.	Stomach irritation with bisacodyl. Take 1 hour apart.
Cocaine:	None expected.
Foods:	None expected.
Marijuana:	None expected.
Tobacco:	None expected.

*See Glossary

LEFLUNOMIDE

BRAND NAMES

Arava

BASIC INFORMATION

Habit forming? No
Prescription needed? Yes
Available as generic? Yes
Drug class: Antirheumatic

 USES

Treats symptoms caused by rheumatoid arthritis, such as inflammation, swelling, stiffness and joint pain. Slows deterioration of joint.

 DOSAGE & USAGE INFORMATION

How to take:
Tablet—Take with full glass of water. If you can't swallow whole, crumble tablet and take with liquid or food.

When to take:
At the same time each day.

If you forget a dose:
Take as soon as you remember. However, if it is almost time for your next dose, skip the missed dose and go back to your regular dosing schedule (don't double this dose).

What drug does:
Stops the body from producing too many of the immune cells that are responsible for the swelling and inflammation (immunosuppressive and antiinflammatory).

Time lapse before drug works:
6 to 12 hours.

Don't take with:
Any other medicine or any dietary supplement without consulting your doctor or pharmacist.

 OVERDOSE

SYMPTOMS:
None expected.
WHAT TO DO:
Overdose unlikely to threaten life. If person uses much larger amount than prescribed or if accidentally swallowed, call doctor or poison control center 1-800-222-1222 for help.

 POSSIBLE ADVERSE REACTIONS OR SIDE EFFECTS

SYMPTOMS	WHAT TO DO
Life-threatening: None expected.	
Common:	
• Chest congestion, cough, difficulty in breathing, loss of appetite, nausea, vomiting, yellow eyes or skin, dizziness, fever, sneezing, sore throat, pain or burning while urinating, frequent urge to urinate.	Continue. Call doctor right away.
• Abdominal pain, hair loss, back pain, diarrhea, heartburn, rash, unexplained weight loss.	Continue. Call doctor if symptoms persist.
Infrequent:	
• Unusual tiredness or weakness, shortness of breath, indigestion, pounding heartbeat, burning or tingling sensation in fingers and toes, joint or muscle pain, rapid heartbeat.	Continue. Call doctor right away.
• Acne, loss of appetite, anxiety, red or irritated eyes, constipation, dry mouth, gas, mouth ulcer, pain or burning in throat, itching, runny nose.	Continue. Call doctor when convenient.
Rare: None expected.	

WARNINGS & PRECAUTIONS

Don't take if:
You are allergic to leflunomide.

Before you start, consult your doctor if:
• You are using any other medication.
• You have immune system problems.
• You have severe or uncontrolled infections.
• You have been diagnosed with kidney or liver disease.

Over age 60:
Side effects or problems experienced with this medication appear to be the same in older people as in younger adults.

Pregnancy:
Risk to unborn child outweighs drug benefits. Don't use. Risk category X (see page xviii).

Breast-feeding:
Drug may pass into milk. Avoid drug or discontinue nursing until you finish medicine. Consult doctor for advice on maintaining milk supply.

Infants & children:
Studies on this medicine have been done only in adult patients. Consult doctor before giving this medicine to persons under age 18.

Prolonged use:
Usually not prescribed for long-term use.

Skin & sunlight:
None expected.

Driving, piloting or hazardous work:
None expected.

Discontinuing:
Don't discontinue without consulting doctor or completing prescribed dosage.

Others:
• May affect accuracy of some laboratory test values.
• Women of childbearing age are advised to use reliable contraception before receiving leflunomide. If you become pregnant while taking this drug, notify your doctor immediately.
• Use of leflunomide by men during time of conception may cause birth defects in their children. Therefore, men taking leflunomide should use condoms as a form of birth control.
• Liver injury may occur while taking this drug. Ask your doctor about the need for liver function tests.
• Do not have any immunizations during or after treatment with this drug without your doctor's approval.
• Advise any doctor or dentist whom you consult that you take this medicine.

 POSSIBLE INTERACTION WITH OTHER DRUGS

GENERIC NAME OR DRUG CLASS	COMBINED EFFECT
Charcoal, activated	Decreased leflunomide effect.
Cholestyramine	Decreased leflunomide effect.
Methotrexate	Increased risk of side effects.
Rifampin	May increase risk of leflunomide toxicity.

 POSSIBLE INTERACTION WITH OTHER SUBSTANCES

INTERACTS WITH	COMBINED EFFECT
Alcohol:	Increases the chance of liver problems. Avoid.
Beverages:	None expected.
Cocaine:	Effect unknown. Avoid.
Foods:	None expected.
Marijuana:	Effect unknown. Avoid
Tobacco:	None expected.

*See Glossary

LEUCOVORIN

BRAND NAMES

Citrocovorin Calcium   Folinic Acid
Citrovorum Factor   Wellcovorin

BASIC INFORMATION

Habit forming? No
Prescription needed? Yes
Available as generic? Yes
Drug class: Antianemic

 USES

- Antidote to folic acid antagonists.
- Treats anemia.

 DOSAGE & USAGE INFORMATION

How to take:
Tablet—Swallow with liquid or food to lessen stomach irritation. If you can't swallow whole, crumble tablet and take with liquid or food.

When to take:
At the same time each day, according to instructions on prescription label.

If you forget a dose:
Take as soon as you remember up to 2 hours late. If more than 2 hours, wait for next scheduled dose (don't double this dose).

What drug does:
Favors development of DNA, RNA and protein synthesis.

Time lapse before drug works:
20 to 30 minutes.

Don't take with:
Any other medicine or any dietary supplement without consulting your doctor or pharmacist.

 OVERDOSE

SYMPTOMS:
Unlikely to threaten life. If overdose is suspected, follow instructions below.
WHAT TO DO:
- Dial 911 (emergency) for medical help or call poison control center 1-800-222-1222 for instructions.
- See emergency information on last 3 pages of this book.

 POSSIBLE ADVERSE REACTIONS OR SIDE EFFECTS

SYMPTOMS	WHAT TO DO
Life-threatening:	
Wheezing.	Seek emergency treatment immediately.
Common:	
None expected.	
Infrequent:	
None expected.	
Rare:	
Skin rash, hives.	Discontinue. Call doctor right away.

LEUCOVORIN

 WARNINGS & PRECAUTIONS

Don't take if:
You are allergic to leucovorin.

Before you start, consult your doctor if:
- You have acid urine, ascites, dehydration.
- You have kidney function impairment.
- You have pernicious anemia.
- You have vitamin B-12 deficiency.

Over age 60:
Adverse reactions and side effects may be more frequent and severe than in younger persons. You may need smaller doses for shorter periods of time.

Pregnancy:
Recommended for the treatment of megaloblastic anemia caused by pregnancy. Decide with your doctor if drug benefits justify risk to unborn child. Risk category C (see page xviii).

Breast-feeding:
It is unknown if drug passes into milk. Avoid drug or discontinue nursing until you finish medicine. Consult doctor for advice on maintaining milk supply.

Infants & children:
May increase frequency of seizures. Avoid if possible.

Prolonged use:
No problems expected.

Skin & sunlight:
No problems expected.

Driving, piloting or hazardous work:
Don't drive or pilot aircraft until you learn how medicine affects you. Don't work around dangerous machinery. Don't climb ladders or work in high places. Danger increases if you drink alcohol or take medicine affecting alertness and reflexes.

Discontinuing:
Don't discontinue without consulting doctor. Dose may require gradual reduction if you have taken drug for a long time. Doses of other drugs may also require adjustment.

Others:
- Advise any doctor or dentist whom you consult that you take this medicine.
- No problems expected.

 POSSIBLE INTERACTION WITH OTHER DRUGS

GENERIC NAME OR DRUG CLASS	COMBINED EFFECT
Anticonvulsants, barbiturate and hydantoin*	Large doses of leucovorin may counteract the effects of these medicines.
Central nervous system (CNS) depressants*	High alcohol content of leucovorin may cause adverse effects.
Fluorouracil	Increased levels of fluorouracil.
Primidone	Large doses of leucovorin may counteract the effects of both drugs.

 POSSIBLE INTERACTION WITH OTHER SUBSTANCES

INTERACTS WITH	COMBINED EFFECT
Alcohol:	Increased adverse reactions of both.
Beverages:	None expected.
Cocaine:	Increased adverse reactions of both drugs.
Foods:	None expected.
Marijuana:	Increased adverse reactions of both drugs.
Tobacco:	Increased adverse reactions of both.

*See Glossary

LEUKOTRIENE MODIFIERS

GENERIC AND BRAND NAMES

MONTELUKAST
Singulair
ZAFIRLUKAST
Accolate

ZILEUTON
Zyflo CR

BASIC INFORMATION

Habit forming? No
Prescription needed? Yes
Available as generic? No
Drug class: Antiasthmatic

 USES

- Treatment of mild to moderate asthma. Not used to treat an active asthma attack. May be used with other asthma medications as directed by your doctor. Montelukast is used for prophylaxis (preventive) and chronic treatment of asthma.
- Prevention of exercise-induced broncho-constriction (EIB) in patients age 15 and older.
- Montelukast is used for treatment of seasonal allergies (hay fever) and perennial allergic rhinitis (PAR), also known as indoor allergies.

 DOSAGE & USAGE INFORMATION

How to take:
- Tablet—Swallow with water, with or without food, except for zafirlukast which must be taken on an empty stomach 1 hour before or 2 hours after a meal.
- Chewable tablet—Chew tablet before you swallow it.
- Extended-release tablet—Swallow whole with liquid. Do not cut, chew or crush tablet.
- Oral granules—Take granules directly in the mouth or mix with a spoonful of cold or room temperature soft food.

Continued next column

 OVERDOSE

SYMPTOMS:
It is unknown what symptoms may occur.
WHAT TO DO:
If person uses much larger amount than prescribed, dial 911 (emergency) for medical help or call poison control center 1-800-222-1222 for instructions.

When to take:
- Montelukast—At the same time each day.
- Zafirlukast—Twice a day at the same times.
- Zileuton—Four times a day at the same times. Take extended-release zileuton within one hour after morning and evening meals.

If you forget a dose:
Take as soon as you remember, up to 2 hours late. If more than 2 hours, wait for next scheduled dose. Do not double doses.

What drug does:
Inhibits inflammatory cells associated with asthma. Inhibits reflex reactions to irritants, exercise and cold.

Time lapse before drug works:
30 minutes to 4 hours.

Don't take with:
Any other medicine or any dietary supplement without consulting your doctor or pharmacist.

 POSSIBLE ADVERSE REACTIONS OR SIDE EFFECTS

SYMPTOMS	WHAT TO DO
Life-threatening: None expected.	
Common: Headache, stomach upset, nausea.	Continue. Call doctor when convenient.
Infrequent: Weak feeling, pain in abdomen, headache, unusual tiredness, cough, dental pain, dizziness, heartburn, fever, nasal congestion, skin rash.	Continue. Call doctor when convenient.
Rare: Liver problems (yellow eyes or skin, fatigue, symptoms of flu, itching, pain in upper right abdominal area).	Discontinue. Call doctor right away.

WARNINGS & PRECAUTIONS

Don't take if:
You are allergic to leukotriene modifiers.

Before you start, consult your doctor if:
* You have any other medical problem.
* You have a liver or kidney disease.
* You have a history of alcoholism.

Over age 60:
In some cases older patients taking zafirlukast experienced more infections; otherwise, no problems expected.

Pregnancy:
Decide with your doctor whether drug benefits justify risk to unborn child. Montelukast and zafirlukast—risk category B; zileuton—risk category C (see page xviii).

Breast-feeding:
* Montelukast and zileuton—It is unknown if drug passes into milk. Avoid drug or discontinue nursing until you finish medicine. Consult doctor for advice on maintaining milk supply.
* Zafirlukast—Drug passes into milk. Avoid drug or discontinue nursing until you finish medicine.

Infants & children:
* Montelukast is approved for children 12 months and older.
* Zafirlukast is approved for children over 6 years.
* Zileuton should only be given under close supervision, especially to children under 12 years old.

Prolonged use:
Schedule regular visits with your doctor to determine if the drug continues its effectiveness in controlling asthma symptoms.

Skin & sunlight:
No problems expected.

Driving, piloting or hazardous work:
No problems expected.

Discontinuing:
Don't discontinue without consulting doctor.

Others:
* In a few rare instances, patients taking zafirlukast while having their oral steroid dosage reduced developed Churg-Strauss syndrome (a rare and sometimes fatal condition). It is not known if the problem is caused by zafirlukast. Symptoms of Churg-Strauss syndrome are similar to those caused by flu. Before starting zafirlukast and reducing oral steroids, discuss the benefits and risk factors with your doctor.
* Advise any doctor or dentist you consult that you take this medicine.

* Talk to your doctor if your asthma attacks are not being controlled by the usual dosage of your fast-acting bronchodilator.
* This drug may affect results in some medical tests.
* This drug should be taken every day, even if you are not having asthma symptoms.

POSSIBLE INTERACTION WITH OTHER DRUGS

GENERIC NAME OR DRUG CLASS	COMBINED EFFECT
Beta adrenergic blocking agents	Increased beta blocker effect.
Calcium channel blockers	Increased effect of calcium channel blocker.
Carbamazepine	Increased effect of carbamazepine.
Cisapride	Increased effect of cisapride.
Cyclosporine	Increased effect of cyclosporine.
Dofetilide	Increased dofetilide effect.
Erythromycin	Decreased effect of zafirlukast.
Phenobarbital	Decreased effect of montelukast.
Phenytoin	Increased effect of phenytoin.
Tolbutamide	Increased effect of tolbutamide.
Warfarin	Increased effect of warfarin.

POSSIBLE INTERACTION WITH OTHER SUBSTANCES

INTERACTS WITH	COMBINED EFFECT
Alcohol:	None expected.
Beverages:	None expected.
Cocaine:	Effects unknown. Avoid.
Foods:	None expected.
Marijuana:	Effects unknown. Avoid.
Tobacco:	None expected.

*See Glossary

LEVAMISOLE

BRAND NAMES

Ergamisol

BASIC INFORMATION

Habit forming? No
Prescription needed? Yes
Available as generic? No
Drug class: Anticancer treatment adjunct

 USES

- Treats colorectal cancer when used in combination with fluorouracil.
- Treats malignant melanoma after surgical removal when there is no evidence of spread to organs other than the skin.

 DOSAGE & USAGE INFORMATION

How to take:
Tablet—Swallow with liquid or food to lessen stomach irritation. If you can't swallow whole, crumble tablet and take with liquid or food.

When to take:
At the same time each day, according to instructions on prescription label.

If you forget a dose:
Don't take until you notify your doctor.

What drug does:
Acts to help restore the immune system. May activate T-cell lymphocytes and other white cells. Also elevates mood.

Time lapse before drug works:
1-1/2 to 2 hours.

Don't take with:
Any other medicine or any dietary supplement without consulting your doctor or pharmacist.

 OVERDOSE

SYMPTOMS:
None expected.
WHAT TO DO:
Overdose unlikely to threaten life. If person uses much larger amount than prescribed or if accidentally swallowed, call doctor or poison control center 1-800-222-1222 for help.

 POSSIBLE ADVERSE REACTIONS OR SIDE EFFECTS

SYMPTOMS	WHAT TO DO
Life-threatening: Fever, muscle aches, headache, cough, hoarseness, sore throat, painful or difficult urination, low back or side pain.	Seek emergency treatment.
Common: • Diarrhea, metallic taste, nausea, joint or muscle pain, skin rash, insomnia, mental depression, nightmares, sleepiness or tiredness, increased dental problems.	Continue. Call doctor when convenient.
• Hair loss.	No action necessary.
Infrequent: Mouth, tongue and lip sores.	Call doctor right away.
Rare: Unsteady gait while walking; blurred vision; confusion; tremors; tingling or numbness in hands, feet or face; seizures; smacking and puckering of lips; uncontrolled tongue movements.	Call doctor right away.

WARNINGS & PRECAUTIONS

Don't take if:
You are allergic to levamisole.

Before you start, consult your doctor if:
- You take other drugs for cancer.
- You have an active infection.
- You have a seizure disorder.
- You have allergies to other medications.

Over age 60:
No special problems expected.

Pregnancy:
Adequate studies not yet done. Consult your doctor. Risk category C (see page xviii).

Breast-feeding:
Effect unknown. Consult doctor.

Infants & children:
Effect not documented. Consult your doctor.

Prolonged use:
No special problems expected.

Skin & sunlight:
No special problems expected.

Driving, piloting or hazardous work:
No special problems expected.

Discontinuing:
Don't discontinue without consulting doctor. Dose may require gradual reduction if you have taken drug for a long time. Doses of other drugs may also require adjustment.

Others:
- Advise any doctor or dentist whom you consult that you take this medicine.
- Defer dental treatments until your blood count is normal. Pay particular attention to dental hygiene. You may be subject to additional risk of oral infection, delayed healing and bleeding.
- Avoid aspirin. May increase risk of internal bleeding.
- Avoid constipation. May increase risk of internal bleeding.

POSSIBLE INTERACTION WITH OTHER DRUGS

GENERIC NAME OR DRUG CLASS	COMBINED EFFECT
Anticoagulants*	Increased risk of bleeding.
Aspirin	Increased risk of bleeding.
Bone marrow depressants*	Increased risk of bone marrow depression.

POSSIBLE INTERACTION WITH OTHER SUBSTANCES

INTERACTS WITH	COMBINED EFFECT
Alcohol:	Increased risk of gastritis and internal bleeding.
Beverages:	None expected.
Cocaine:	Increased risk of mental disturbances. Avoid.
Foods:	None expected.
Marijuana:	None expected.
Tobacco:	None expected.

LEVETIRACETAM

BRAND NAMES

Keppra   Keppra XR

BASIC INFORMATION

Habit forming? No
Prescription needed? Yes
Available as generic? Yes
Drug class: Anticonvulsant; antiepileptic

USES

Used to help control some types of seizures in the treatment of epilepsy. This medicine cannot cure epilepsy and will only work to control seizures for as long as you continue to take it.

DOSAGE & USAGE INFORMATION

How to take:
- Tablet or extended-release tablet—Swallow whole with a liquid. Do not crush, chew or break tablet. May be taken with or without food, and on a full or empty stomach.
- Oral solution—Follow instructions on prescription.

When to take:
At the same time(s) each day. Your doctor will determine the schedule. Dose may be increased every two weeks to achieve maximum benefits.

If you forget a dose:
Take as soon as you remember. If it is almost time for the next dose, wait for that dose (don't double this dose) and resume regular schedule.

What drug does:
The exact mechanism of the anticonvulsant activity of levetiracetam is unknown.

Time lapse before drug works:
May take several weeks for effectiveness.

Don't take with:
Any other medicine or any dietary supplement without consulting your doctor or pharmacist.

OVERDOSE

SYMPTOMS:
Possibly drowsiness or other symptoms.
WHAT TO DO:
Overdose unlikely to threaten life. If person uses much larger amount than prescribed or if accidentally swallowed, call doctor or poison control center 1-800-222-1222 for help.

POSSIBLE ADVERSE REACTIONS OR SIDE EFFECTS

SYMPTOMS	WHAT TO DO
Life-threatening: None expected.	
Common: Cough; dizziness; dry or sore throat; hoarseness; loss of strength or energy; muscle pain or weakness; runny nose; sleepiness; tender, swollen glands in neck; trouble in swallowing; unusual tiredness or weakness; voice changes.	Continue. Call doctor when convenient.
Infrequent: • Clumsiness or unsteadiness, crying, depression, double vision, fever or chills, headache, loss of memory or problems with memory, lower back or side pain, mood or mental changes, suicidal thoughts or feelings, nervousness, angry outbursts, pain or tenderness around eyes and cheekbones, painful or difficult urination, paranoia, muscle control problems, overreacting, shortness of breath or trouble breathing, chest tightness, wheezing.	Continue, but call doctor right away. Seek emergency care for severe symptoms.
• Burning, crawling, itching, numbness, prickling, or tingling feelings; feeling of constant movement of self or surroundings; loss of appetite; spinning sensation; weight loss.	Continue. Call doctor when convenient.
Rare: Other symptoms.	Continue. Call doctor when convenient.

WARNINGS & PRECAUTIONS

Don't take if:
You are allergic to levetiracetam.

Before you start, consult your doctor if:
- You have kidney disease.
- You are allergic to any medication, food or other substance.
- You have any other medical problems.

Over age 60:
No special problems expected.

Pregnancy:
Decide with your doctor if drug benefits justify risks to unborn child. Risk category C (see page xviii).

Breast-feeding:
It is unknown if drug passes into milk. Avoid drug or discontinue nursing until you finish medicine. Consult doctor for advice on maintaining milk supply.

Infants & children:
Approved for children four years of age and older. Carefully follow prescription instructions.

Prolonged use:
No special problems expected. Follow-up laboratory blood studies may be recommended by your doctor.

Skin & sunlight:
No problems expected.

Driving, piloting or hazardous work:
Don't drive or pilot aircraft until you learn how medicine affects you. Don't work around dangerous machinery. Don't climb ladders or work in high places. Danger increases if you drink alcohol or take other medicines affecting alertness and reflexes such as antihistamines, tranquilizers, sedatives, pain medicine, narcotics and mind-altering drugs.

Discontinuing:
Don't discontinue without doctor's approval due to risk of increased seizure activity. The dosage may need to be gradually decreased before stopping the drug completely.

Others:
- Advise any doctor or dentist whom you consult that you take this medicine.
- Levetiracetam may be used with other anticonvulsant drugs and additional side effects may also occur. If they do, discuss them with your doctor.
- Rarely, antiepileptic drugs may lead to suicidal thoughts and behaviors. Call doctor right away if suicidal symptoms or unusual behaviors occur.
- Wear or carry medical identification to show your seizure disorder and the drugs you take.

 ## POSSIBLE INTERACTION WITH OTHER DRUGS

GENERIC NAME OR DRUG CLASS	COMBINED EFFECT
Anticonvulsants,* other	May decrease or increase effect of both drugs.
CNS Depressants*	Increased sedative effect.

 ## POSSIBLE INTERACTION WITH OTHER SUBSTANCES

INTERACTS WITH	COMBINED EFFECT
Alcohol:	Increased sedative effect. Avoid.
Beverages:	None expected.
Cocaine:	Unknown effect. Avoid.
Foods:	None expected.
Marijuana:	Unknown effect. Avoid.
Tobacco:	None expected.

*See Glossary

LEVOCARNITINE

BRAND NAMES

Carnitor

Carnitor Sugar-
free Oral Solution

L-Carnitine

VitaCarn

BASIC INFORMATION

Habit forming? No
Prescription needed? Yes
Available as generic? Yes
Drug class: Nutritional supplement

 ## USES

Treats carnitine deficiency, a genetic impairment preventing normal utilization from diet.

 ## DOSAGE & USAGE INFORMATION

How to take:
* Oral solution—Take after meals with liquid to decrease stomach irritation.
* Tablet—Swallow with liquid or food to lessen stomach irritation. If you can't swallow whole, crumble tablet and take with liquid or food.
* Injection—Given by medical professional.

When to take:
Immediately following or during meals to reduce stomach irritation.

If you forget a dose:
Take as soon as you remember up to 2 hours late. If more than 2 hours, wait for next scheduled dose (don't double this dose).

What drug does:
Facilitates normal use of fat to produce energy. Dietary source is meat and milk.

Time lapse before drug works:
Immediate action.

Don't take with:
Any other medicine or any dietary supplement without consulting your doctor or pharmacist.

 ## OVERDOSE

SYMPTOMS:
Severe muscle weakness.
WHAT TO DO:
* Dial 911 (emergency) for medical help or call poison control center 1-800-222-1222 for instructions.
* See emergency information on last 3 pages of this book.

 ## POSSIBLE ADVERSE REACTIONS OR SIDE EFFECTS

SYMPTOMS	WHAT TO DO
Life-threatening: None expected.	
Common: Changed body odor.	Continue. Call doctor when convenient.
Infrequent: Diarrhea, abdominal pain, nausea, vomiting.	Continue, but call doctor right away.
Rare: None expected.	

WARNINGS & PRECAUTIONS

Don't take if:
You are allergic to levocarnitine.

Before you start, consult your doctor if:
• You have seizure disorder.
• You have severe kidney disorder.

Over age 60:
No problems expected.

Pregnancy:
No proven harm to unborn child, but avoid if possible. Consult doctor. Risk category B (see page xviii).

Breast-feeding:
No problems expected. Consult doctor.

Infants & children:
No problems expected. Deficiency can cause impaired growth and development.

Prolonged use:
Talk to your doctor about the need for follow-up medical examinations or laboratory studies to check triglycerides.

Skin & sunlight:
No problems expected.

Driving, piloting or hazardous work:
No problems expected.

Discontinuing:
Don't discontinue without consulting doctor. Dose may require gradual reduction if you have taken drug for a long time. Doses of other drugs may also require adjustment.

Others:
• Advise any doctor or dentist whom you consult that you take this medicine.
• Do not use a product named "vitamin B-T" sold in health food stores. It contains dextro- and levo-carnitine. This product completely negates the effectiveness of levocarnitine (L-carnitine). Only the L-carnitine form is effective in treating carnitine deficiency.

POSSIBLE INTERACTION WITH OTHER DRUGS

GENERIC NAME OR DRUG CLASS	COMBINED EFFECT
None expected.	

POSSIBLE INTERACTION WITH OTHER SUBSTANCES

INTERACTS WITH	COMBINED EFFECT
Alcohol:	None expected.
Beverages:	None expected.
Cocaine:	None expected.
Foods:	None expected.
Marijuana:	None expected.
Tobacco:	None expected.

LEVODOPA

BRAND NAMES

Dopar   Larodopa

BASIC INFORMATION

Habit forming? No
Prescription needed? Yes
Available as generic? Yes
Drug class: Antiparkinsonism

 USES

Controls Parkinson's disease symptoms such as rigidity, tremor and unsteady gait.

 DOSAGE & USAGE INFORMATION

How to take:
Tablet or capsule—Swallow with liquid or food to lessen stomach irritation. If you can't swallow whole, crumble tablet or open capsule and take with liquid or food.

When to take:
At the same times each day.

If you forget a dose:
Take as soon as you remember up to 2 hours late. If more than 2 hours, wait for next scheduled dose (don't double this dose).

What drug does:
Restores chemical balance necessary for normal nerve impulses.

Time lapse before drug works:
2 to 3 weeks to improve; 6 weeks or longer for maximum benefit.

Don't take with:
Any other medicine or any dietary supplement without consulting your doctor or pharmacist.

 OVERDOSE

SYMPTOMS:
Muscle twitch, spastic eyelid closure, nausea, vomiting, diarrhea, irregular and rapid pulse, weakness, fainting, confusion, agitation, hallucination, coma.
WHAT TO DO:
* **Dial 911 (emergency) for medical help or call poison control center 1-800-222-1222 for instructions.**
* **If person is unconscious, check breathing and pulse. If not breathing, begin mouth-to-mouth rescue breathing. If heart is not beating, begin chest compressions.**
* **See emergency information on last 3 pages of this book.**

 POSSIBLE ADVERSE REACTIONS OR SIDE EFFECTS

SYMPTOMS	WHAT TO DO
Life-threatening:	
In case of overdose, see previous column.	
Common:	
• Uncontrollable body movements.	Discontinue. Call doctor right away.
• Mood change, diarrhea, depression, anxiety.	Continue. Call doctor when convenient.
• Dry mouth, body odor.	No action necessary.
Infrequent:	
• Fainting, severe dizziness, headache, insomnia, nightmares, itchy skin, rash, nausea, vomiting, irregular heartbeat, eyelid spasm.	Discontinue. Call doctor right away.
• Flushed face, muscle twitching, discolored or dark urine, difficult urination, blurred vision, appetite loss.	Continue. Call doctor when convenient.
• Constipation, tiredness.	Continue. Tell doctor at next visit.
Rare:	
• High blood pressure.	Discontinue. Call doctor right away.
• Upper abdominal pain, anemia, increased sex drive.	Continue. Call doctor when convenient.

 WARNINGS & PRECAUTIONS

Don't take if:
* You are allergic to levodopa or carbidopa.
* You have taken a monoamine oxidase (MAO) inhibitor* in past 2 weeks.
* You have glaucoma (narrow-angle type).

Before you start, consult your doctor if:
* You have diabetes or epilepsy.
* You have had high blood pressure, heart or lung disease.
* You have had liver or kidney disease.
* You have a peptic ulcer.
* You have malignant melanoma.
* You will have surgery within 2 months, including dental surgery, requiring general or spinal anesthesia.

Over age 60:
Adverse reactions and side effects may be more frequent and severe than in younger persons.

Pregnancy:
Decide with your doctor if drug benefits justify risk to unborn child. Risk category C (see page xviii).

Breast-feeding:
Drug filters into milk. May harm child. Avoid.

Infants & children:
Not recommended.

Prolonged use:
* May lead to uncontrolled movements of head, face, mouth, tongue, arms or legs.
* Talk to your doctor about the need for follow-up medical examinations or laboratory studies to check complete blood counts (white blood cell count, platelet count, red blood cell count, hemoglobin, hematocrit), kidney function, liver function.

Skin & sunlight:
No problems expected.

Driving, piloting or hazardous work:
Don't drive or pilot aircraft until you learn how medicine affects you. Don't work around dangerous machinery. Don't climb ladders or work in high places. Danger increases if you drink alcohol or take medicine affecting alertness and reflexes, such as antihistamines, tranquilizers, sedatives, pain medicine, narcotics and mind-altering drugs.

Discontinuing:
Don't discontinue without doctor's advice until you complete prescribed dose, even though symptoms diminish or disappear.

Others:
* Expect to start with small dose and increase gradually to lessen frequency and severity of adverse reactions.
* Advise any doctor or dentist whom you consult that you take this medicine.

POSSIBLE INTERACTION WITH OTHER DRUGS

GENERIC NAME OR DRUG CLASS	COMBINED EFFECT
Antidepressants, tricyclic (TCA)*	Decreased blood pressure. Weakness and faintness when arising from bed or chair.
Antiparkinsonism drugs, other*	Increased levodopa effect.
Bupropion	Increased levodopa effect.
Haloperidol	Decreased levodopa effect.
Loxapine	Decreased levodopa effect.
MAO inhibitors*	Dangerous rise in blood pressure.
Methyldopa	Decreased levodopa effect.
Molindone	Decreased levodopa effect.
Olanzapine	May decrease levodopa effect.
Papaverine	Decreased levodopa effect.
Phenothiazines*	Decreased levodopa effect.
Phenytoin	Decreased levodopa effect.
Pyridoxine (Vitamin B-6)	Decreased levodopa effect.
Quetiapine	Decreased levodopa effect.
Rauwolfia alkaloids*	Decreased levodopa effect.
Seleginine	May require reduced dosage of levodopa.
Thioxanthenes*	Decreased levodopa effect.
Ziprasidone	Decreased levodopa effect.

POSSIBLE INTERACTION WITH OTHER SUBSTANCES

INTERACTS WITH	COMBINED EFFECT
Alcohol:	None expected.
Beverages:	None expected.
Cocaine:	Increased risk of heartbeat irregularity.
Foods: High-protein diet.	Decreased levodopa effect.
Marijuana:	Increased fatigue, lethargy, fainting.
Tobacco:	None expected.

LINCOMYCIN

BRAND NAMES

Lincocin

BASIC INFORMATION

Habit forming? No
Prescription needed? Yes
Available as generic? Yes
Drug class: Antibacterial

USES

Treatment of bacterial infections that are susceptible to lincomycin.

DOSAGE & USAGE INFORMATION

How to take:
Capsule—Swallow with liquid 1 hour before or 2 hours after eating. Drink 8 ounces of water with each dose.

When to take:
At the same times each day.

If you forget a dose:
Take as soon as you remember up to 2 hours late. If more than 2 hours, wait for next scheduled dose (don't double this dose).

What drug does:
Destroys susceptible bacteria. Does not kill viruses.

Time lapse before drug works:
3 to 5 days.

Don't take with:
Any other medicine or any dietary supplement without consulting your doctor or pharmacist.

OVERDOSE

SYMPTOMS:
Severe nausea, vomiting, diarrhea.
WHAT TO DO:
Overdose unlikely to threaten life. If person uses much larger amount than prescribed or if accidentally swallowed, call doctor or poison control center 1-800-222-1222 for help.

POSSIBLE ADVERSE REACTIONS OR SIDE EFFECTS

SYMPTOMS	WHAT TO DO
Life-threatening:	
Hives, wheezing, faintness, itching, coma.	Seek emergency treatment.
Common:	
Mild diarrhea, mild stomach cramps, nausea.	Continue. Call doctor when convenient.
Infrequent:	
• Unusual thirst; vomiting; stomach cramps; severe and watery diarrhea with blood or mucus; painful, swollen joints; jaundice; fever; tiredness; weakness; weight loss.	Discontinue. Call doctor right away.
• Itch around groin, rectum or armpits; white patches in mouth; vaginal discharge, itching.	Continue. Call doctor when convenient.
Rare:	
Skin rash.	Discontinue. Call doctor right away.

WARNINGS & PRECAUTIONS

Don't take if:
- You are allergic to lincomycins.
- You have had ulcerative colitis.
- Prescribed for infant under 1 month old.

Before you start, consult your doctor if:
- You have had yeast infections of mouth, skin or vagina.
- You will have surgery within 2 months, including dental surgery, requiring general or spinal anesthesia.
- You have kidney or liver disease.
- You have allergies of any kind.

Over age 60:
Adverse reactions and side effects may be more frequent and severe than in younger persons.

Pregnancy:
Decide with your doctor if drug benefits justify risk to unborn child. Risk category C (see page xviii).

Breast-feeding:
Drug passes into milk. Avoid drug or discontinue nursing until you finish medicine. Consult doctor for advice on maintaining milk supply.

Infants & children:
Don't give to infants younger than 1 month. Use for children only under medical supervision.

Prolonged use:
- Severe colitis with diarrhea and bleeding.
- You may become more susceptible to infections caused by germs not responsive to lincomycin.
- Talk to your doctor about the need for follow-up medical examinations or laboratory studies or proctosigmoidoscopy.

Skin & sunlight:
No problems expected.

Driving, piloting or hazardous work:
No problems expected.

Discontinuing:
Don't discontinue without doctor's advice until you complete prescribed dose, even though symptoms diminish or disappear.

Others:
- May interfere with the accuracy of some medical tests.
- Advise any doctor or dentist whom you consult that you take use medicine.

POSSIBLE INTERACTION WITH OTHER DRUGS

GENERIC NAME OR DRUG CLASS	COMBINED EFFECT
Antidiarrheal preparations*	Decreased lincomycin effect.
Attapulgite	May decrease effectiveness of lincomycin.
Chloramphenicol	Decreased lincomycin effect.
Erythromycins*	Decreased lincomycin effect.
Narcotics*	Increased risk of respiratory problems.

POSSIBLE INTERACTION WITH OTHER SUBSTANCES

INTERACTS WITH	COMBINED EFFECT
Alcohol:	None expected.
Beverages:	None expected.
Cocaine:	None expected.
Foods:	None expected.
Marijuana:	None expected.
Tobacco:	None expected.

LINEZOLID

BRAND NAMES

Zyvox

BASIC INFORMATION

Habit forming? No
Prescription needed? Yes
Available as generic? No
Drug class: Antibacterial, antibiotic
  (oxazolidinone)

 ## USES

Treats bacterial infections of the blood, lungs and skin. It may also be used for other conditions as determined by your doctor.

 ## DOSAGE & USAGE INFORMATION

How to take:
* Tablet—Take with full glass of water. If you can't swallow whole, crumble tablet and take with liquid or food.
* Oral suspension—Take as directed on label. The medicine should be gently mixed by inverting the bottle 3 to 5 times before each dose. Do not shake the bottle.

When to take:
As directed by your doctor. Usually every 12 hours.

If you forget a dose:
Take as soon as you remember. However, if it is almost time for your next dose, skip the missed dose and go back to your regular dosing schedule (don't double this dose).

What drug does:
Destroys bacteria in the body, probably by blocking protein production inside bacteria.

Time lapse before drug works:
10 to 14 days for most infections, but some infections may take longer. Continue taking this medicine for the full time of treatment even if you begin to feel better after a few days.

Continued next column

 ## OVERDOSE

SYMPTOMS:
None expected.
WHAT TO DO:
Overdose unlikely to threaten life. If person uses much larger amount than prescribed or if accidentally swallowed, call doctor or poison control center 1-800-222-1222 for help.

Don't take with:
Any other medicine or any dietary supplement without consulting your doctor or pharmacist.

 ## POSSIBLE ADVERSE REACTIONS OR SIDE EFFECTS

SYMPTOMS	WHAT TO DO
Life-threatening: None expected.	
Common:	
• Diarrhea, headache.	Continue. Call doctor when convenient.
• Nausea.	Continue. Call doctor if symptoms persist.
Infrequent:	
• Fever, sore mouth or tongue, rash, black tarry stools, chest pain, chills, cough, painful or difficult urination, unusual bleeding or bruising, unusual tiredness or weakness, vomiting.	Discontinue. Call doctor right away.
• Constipation, change in taste, sleeplessness, vaginal yeast infection.	Continue. Call doctor when convenient.
Rare: None expected.	

WARNINGS & PRECAUTIONS

Don't take if:
You are allergic to linezolid.

Before you start, consult your doctor if:
* You are using any other medication.
* You have a history of bleeding problems, diarrhea, high blood pressure or any other medical problems.

Over age 60:
Side effects or problems experienced with this medication appear to be the same in older people as in younger adults.

Pregnancy:
Decide with your doctor if drug benefits justify risk to unborn child. Risk category C (see page xviii).

Breast-feeding:
It is unknown if drug passes into milk. Avoid drug or discontinue nursing until you finish medicine. Consult doctor for advice on maintaining milk supply.

Infants & children:
Studies on this medicine have been done only in adult patients. Consult doctor before giving this medicine to persons under age 18.

Prolonged use:
Usually not prescribed for long-term use.

Skin & sunlight:
None expected.

Driving, piloting or hazardous work:
None expected.

Discontinuing:
Don't discontinue without consulting doctor or completing prescribed dosage.

Others:
* May affect accuracy of some laboratory test values.
* Do not store in the bathroom, near the kitchen sink or in other damp places. Heat or moisture may cause the medicine to break down.
* Advise any doctor or dentist whom you consult that you take this medicine.

POSSIBLE INTERACTION WITH OTHER DRUGS

GENERIC NAME OR DRUG CLASS	COMBINED EFFECT
Pseudoephedrine	May increase blood pressure.
Serotonergics*	Serotonin syndrome.*

POSSIBLE INTERACTION WITH OTHER SUBSTANCES

INTERACTS WITH	COMBINED EFFECT
Alcohol:	None expected.
Beverages:	None expected.
Cocaine:	Effect unknown. Avoid.
Foods:	None expected.
Marijuana:	Effect unknown. Avoid
Tobacco:	None expected.

LITHIUM

BRAND NAMES

Carbolith	Lithane
Cibalith-S	Lithizine
Duralith	Lithobid
Eskalith	Lithonate
Eskalith CR	Lithotabs

BASIC INFORMATION

Habit forming? No
Prescription needed? Yes
Available as generic? Yes
Drug class: Mood stabilizer

 ## USES

- Normalizes mood and behavior in bipolar (manic-depressive) disorder.
- Treats alcohol toxicity and addiction.
- Treats schizoid personality disorders.

 ## DOSAGE & USAGE INFORMATION

How to take:
- Tablet or capsule—Swallow with liquid or food to lessen stomach irritation. If you can't swallow whole, crumble tablet or open capsule and take with liquid or food. Drink plenty of liquids each day, especially in hot weather.
- Extended-release tablet—Swallow each dose whole. Do not crush.
- Syrup—Take at mealtime. Follow with 8 oz. water.

When to take:
At the same times each day, preferably at mealtime.

If you forget a dose:
Take as soon as you remember up to 2 hours late. If more than 2 hours, wait for next scheduled dose (don't double this dose).

Continued next column

 ## OVERDOSE

SYMPTOMS:
Moderate overdose increases some side effects and may cause diarrhea, nausea. Large overdose may cause vomiting, muscle weakness, convulsions, stupor and coma.
WHAT TO DO:
- Dial 911 (emergency) for medical help or call poison control center 1-800-222-1222 for instructions.
- See emergency information on last 3 pages of this book.

What drug does:
May correct chemical imbalance in brain's transmission of nerve impulses that influence mood and behavior.

Time lapse before drug works:
1 to 3 weeks. May require 3 months before depressive phase of illness improves.

Don't take with:
Any other medicine or any dietary supplement without consulting your doctor or pharmacist.

 ## POSSIBLE ADVERSE REACTIONS OR SIDE EFFECTS

SYMPTOMS	WHAT TO DO
Life-threatening:	
In case of overdose, see previous column.	
Common:	
• Dizziness, diarrhea, nausea, vomiting, shakiness, tremor.	Continue. Call doctor when convenient.
• Dry mouth, thirst, decreased sexual ability, increased urination, anorexia.	Continue. Tell doctor at next visit.
Infrequent:	
• Rash, stomach pain, fainting, heartbeat irregularities, shortness of breath, ear noises, swollen hands or feet, slurred speech.	Discontinue. Call doctor right away.
• Thyroid impairment (coldness; dry, puffy skin). muscle aches. headache. weight gain. fatigue. menstrual irregularities, acnelike breakouts. drowsiness, confusion, weakness.	Continue. Call doctor when convenient.
Rare:	
• Blurred vision, eye pain.	Discontinue. Call doctor right away.
• Jerking of arms and legs, worsening of psoriasis, hair loss.	Continue. Call doctor when convenient.

 ## WARNINGS & PRECAUTIONS

Don't take if:
- You are allergic to lithium or tartrazine dye.
- You have kidney or heart disease.
- Patient is younger than 12.

Before you start, consult your doctor if:
- You plan to become pregnant within medication period.

- You have diabetes, thyroid disorder, epilepsy, brain disease, schizophrenia, difficult urination, heart disease, kidney disorder, Parkinson's or history of leukemia.
- You are on a low-salt diet or drink more than 4 cups of coffee per day.
- You plan surgery within 2 months.

Over age 60:
Adverse reactions and side effects may be more frequent and severe than in younger persons.

Pregnancy:
Some fetal risk, but benefits may outweigh risks. Risk category D (see page xviii).

Breast-feeding:
Drug passes into milk. Avoid drug or discontinue nursing until you finish medicine. Consult doctor for advice on maintaining milk supply.

Infants & children:
Don't give to children younger than 12.

Prolonged use:
- Enlarged thyroid with possible impaired function.
- Talk to your doctor about the need for follow-up medical examinations or laboratory studies to check lithium levels, ECG,* kidney function, thyroid, complete blood counts (white blood cell count, platelet count, red blood cell count, hemoglobin, hematocrit).

Skin & sunlight:
No problems expected.

Driving, piloting or hazardous work:
Don't drive or pilot aircraft until you learn how medicine affects you. Don't work around dangerous machinery. Don't climb ladders or work in high places. Danger increases if you drink alcohol or take medicine affecting alertness and reflexes.

Discontinuing:
Don't discontinue without consulting doctor. Dose may require gradual reduction if you have taken drug for a long time. Doses of other drugs may also require adjustment. Quitting this medication when feeling well creates risk of relapse which may not respond to restarting the medication.

Others:
- Regular checkups, periodic blood tests, and tests of lithium levels and thyroid function recommended.
- Avoid exercise in hot weather and other activities that cause heavy sweating. This contributes to lithium poisoning. It is essential to take adequate fluids during hot weather to avoid toxicity.
- Call your doctor if you have an illness that causes heavy sweating, vomiting, or diarrhea. The loss of too much salt and water from your body could cause lithium toxicity.
- Advise any doctor or dentist whom you consult that you take this medicine.

- Some products contain tartrazine dye. Avoid, especially if allergic to aspirin.

 ## POSSIBLE INTERACTION WITH OTHER DRUGS

GENERIC NAME OR DRUG CLASS	COMBINED EFFECT
Acetazolamide	Decreased lithium effect.
Antihistamines*	Possible excessive sedation.
Anti-inflammatory drugs, nonsteroidal (NSAIDs)*	Increased toxic effect of lithium.
Bupropion	Increased risk of seizures.
Carbamazepine	Increased lithium effect.
Desmopressin	Possible decreased desmopressin effect.
Diazepam	Possible hypothermia.
Diclofenac	Possible increase in effect and toxicity.
Didanosine	Increased risk of peripheral neuropathy.

Continued on page 921

 ## POSSIBLE INTERACTION WITH OTHER SUBSTANCES

INTERACTS WITH	COMBINED EFFECT
Alcohol:	Possible lithium poisoning.
Beverages: Caffeine drinks.	Decreased lithium effect.
Cocaine:	Possible psychosis.
Foods: Salt.	High intake could decrease lithium effect. Low intake could increase lithium effect. *Don't* restrict intake.
Marijuana:	Increased tremor and possible psychosis.
Tobacco:	None expected.

*See Glossary

LOMUSTINE

BRAND NAMES

CCNU   CeeNU

BASIC INFORMATION

Habit forming? No
Prescription needed? Yes
Available as generic? No
Drug class: Antineoplastic

 USES

- Treats brain cancer and Hodgkin's lymphoma.
- Sometimes used to treat breast, lung, skin and gastrointestinal cancer.

 DOSAGE & USAGE INFORMATION

How to take:
Capsule—Swallow with liquid. If you can't swallow whole, open capsule and take with liquid or food. Instructions to take on empty stomach mean 1 hour before or 2 hours after eating. Note: There may be two or more different types of capsules in the container. This is not an error.

When to take:
According to doctor's instructions. Usual course of treatment requires single dosage repeated every 6 weeks.

If you forget a dose:
Take as soon as you remember. Don't ever double doses.

What drug does:
Interferes with growth of cancer cells.

Time lapse before drug works:
None. Works immediately.

Don't take with:
Any other medicine or any dietary supplement without consulting your doctor or pharmacist.

 OVERDOSE

SYMPTOMS:
Decreased urine (kidney failure); high fever, chills (infection); bloody or black stools (bleeding).
WHAT TO DO:
- **Dial 911 (emergency) for medical help or call poison control center 1-800-222-1222 for instructions.**
- **See emergency information on last 3 pages of this book.**

 POSSIBLE ADVERSE REACTIONS OR SIDE EFFECTS

SYMPTOMS	WHAT TO DO
Life-threatening:	
In case of overdose, see previous column.	
Common:	
• Fever, chills, difficult urination, unusual bleeding.	Continue. Call doctor when convenient.
• Appetite loss, nausea, hair loss.	No action necessary.
Infrequent:	
• Anemia, confusion, slurred speech, mouth sores, skin rash.	Continue. Call doctor when convenient.
• Darkened skin.	No action necessary.
Rare:	
• Shortness of breath.	Discontinue. Call doctor right away.
• Jaundice (yellow skin and eyes), cough.	Continue. Call doctor when convenient.

WARNINGS & PRECAUTIONS

Don't take if:
• You have chicken pox.
• You have shingles (herpes zoster).

Before you start, consult your doctor if:
• You have an infection.
• You have kidney or lung disease.
• You have had previous cancer chemotherapy or radiation treatment.

Over age 60:
Adverse reactions and side effects may be more frequent and severe than in younger persons. You may need smaller doses for shorter periods of time.

Pregnancy:
Risk to unborn child outweighs drug benefits. Don't use. Risk category D (see page xviii).

Breast-feeding:
Drug passes into milk. Avoid drug or discontinue nursing until you finish medicine. Consult doctor for advice on maintaining milk supply.

Infants & children:
Effect not documented. Consult your doctor.

Prolonged use:
Talk to your doctor about the need for follow-up medical examinations or laboratory studies to check kidney function, liver function and complete blood counts (white blood cell count, platelet count, red blood cell count, hemoglobin, hematocrit).

Skin & sunlight:
No problems expected.

Driving, piloting or hazardous work:
Don't drive or pilot aircraft until you learn how medicine affects you. Don't work around dangerous machinery. Don't climb ladders or work in high places. Danger increases if you drink alcohol or take medicine affecting alertness and reflexes.

Discontinuing:
Call doctor if any of these occur after discontinuing: black or tarry stools, bloody urine, hoarseness, bleeding or bruising, fever or chills.

Others:
• Advise any doctor or dentist whom you consult that you take this medicine.
• May affect results in some medical tests.
• Most adverse reactions and side effects are unavoidable.
• Avoid immunizations, if possible.
• Avoid persons with infections.
• Check with doctor about brushing or flossing teeth.
• Avoid contact sports.

POSSIBLE INTERACTION WITH OTHER DRUGS

GENERIC NAME OR DRUG CLASS	COMBINED EFFECT
Antineoplastic drugs, other*	Increased chance of drug toxicity.
Blood dyscrasia-causing medicines*	Adverse effect on bone marrow, causing decreased white cells and platelets.
Bone marrow depressants,* other	Increased risk of bone marrow depression.
Clozapine	Toxic effect on bone marrow.
Levamisole	Increased risk of bone marrow depression.
Tiopronin	Increased risk of toxicity to bone marrow.
Vaccines, live or killed virus	Increased chance of toxicity or reduced effectiveness of vaccine. Wait 3 to 12 months after lomustine treatment before getting vaccination.

POSSIBLE INTERACTION WITH OTHER SUBSTANCES

INTERACTS WITH	COMBINED EFFECT
Alcohol:	Increased chance of liver damage.
Beverages:	None expected.
Cocaine:	Increased chance of central nervous system toxicity.
Foods:	None expected.
Marijuana:	None expected.
Tobacco:	None expected.

LOPERAMIDE

BRAND NAMES

Apo-Loperamide
  Caplets
Imodium
Imodium A-D
Imodium Advanced

Imodium Multi
  Symptom Relief
Kaopectate II
  Caplets
Pepto Diarrhea
  Control

BASIC INFORMATION

Habit forming? No, unless taken in high
  doses for long periods.
Prescription needed? Yes, for some
Available as generic? Yes
Drug class: Antidiarrheal

 ## USES

- Treats mild to moderate diarrhea. Used in
  conjunction with fluids, appropriate diet and
  rest. Treats symptoms only. Does not cure any
  disorder that causes diarrhea.
- Treats chronic diarrhea associated with
  inflammatory bowel disease.

 ## DOSAGE & USAGE INFORMATION

How to take:
- Tablet or capsule—Swallow with food to
  lessen stomach irritation.
- Liquid—Follow label instructions and use
  marked dropper.

When to take:
No more often than directed on label.

If you forget a dose:
Take as soon as you remember up to 2 hours
late. If more than 2 hours, wait for next
scheduled dose (don't double this dose).

What drug does:
Blocks digestive tract's nerve supply, which
reduces irritability and contractions in intestinal
tract.

Continued next column

 ## OVERDOSE

SYMPTOMS:
Constipation, lethargy, drowsiness or
unconsciousness.
WHAT TO DO:
Overdose unlikely to threaten life. If person
uses much larger amount than prescribed or
if accidentally swallowed, call doctor or
poison control center 1-800-222-1222 for help.

Time lapse before drug works:
1 to 2 hours.

Don't take with:
Any other medicine or any dietary supplement
without consulting your doctor or pharmacist.

 ## POSSIBLE ADVERSE REACTIONS OR SIDE EFFECTS

SYMPTOMS	WHAT TO DO
Life-threatening: None expected.	
Common: None expected.	
Infrequent: None expected.	
Rare: • Drowsiness, dizziness, dry mouth.	Continue. Call doctor when convenient.
• Nausea, vomiting, bloating, constipation, appetite loss, rash, abdominal pain.	Discontinue. Call doctor right away.

WARNINGS & PRECAUTIONS

Don't take if:
- You have severe colitis.
- You have colitis resulting from antibiotic treatment or infection.
- You are allergic to loperamide.

Before you start, consult your doctor if:
- You are dehydrated from fluid loss caused by diarrhea.
- You have liver disease.

Over age 60:
Adverse reactions and side effects may be more frequent and severe than in younger persons.

Pregnancy:
No proven harm. Avoid if possible. Consult doctor. Risk category B (see page xviii).

Breast-feeding:
No proven problems, but avoid if possible or discontinue nursing until you finish medicine. Consult doctor for advice on maintaining milk supply.

Infants & children:
Don't give to infants or toddlers. Use only under doctor's supervision for children older than 2.

Prolonged use:
Habit forming at high dose.

Skin & sunlight:
No problems expected.

Driving, piloting or hazardous work:
Don't drive or pilot aircraft until you learn how medicine affects you. Don't work around dangerous machinery. Don't climb ladders or work in high places. Danger increases if you drink alcohol or take medicine affecting alertness and reflexes.

Discontinuing:
- May be unnecessary to finish medicine. Follow doctor's instructions.
- After discontinuing, consult doctor if you experience muscle cramps, nausea, vomiting, trembling, stomach cramps or unusual sweating.

Others:
If acute diarrhea lasts longer than 48 hours, discontinue and call doctor. In chronic diarrhea, loperamide is unlikely to be effective if diarrhea doesn't improve in 10 days.

POSSIBLE INTERACTION WITH OTHER DRUGS

GENERIC NAME OR DRUG CLASS	COMBINED EFFECT
Antibiotics*	Increased risk of diarrhea.
Narcotic analgesics	Increased risk of severe constipation.

POSSIBLE INTERACTION WITH OTHER SUBSTANCES

INTERACTS WITH	COMBINED EFFECT
Alcohol:	Depressed brain function. Avoid.
Beverages:	None expected.
Cocaine:	Decreased loperamide effect.
Foods:	None expected.
Marijuana:	None expected.
Tobacco:	None expected.

LOXAPINE

BRAND NAMES

Loxapac
Loxitane

Loxitane C

BASIC INFORMATION

Habit forming? No
Prescription needed? Yes
Available as generic? Yes
Drug class: Tranquilizer, antidepressant

 ## USES

- Treats serious mental illness.
- Treats anxiety and depression.

 ## DOSAGE & USAGE INFORMATION

How to take:
- Oral solution—Take after meals with liquid to decrease stomach irritation.
- Tablet—Swallow with liquid or food to lessen stomach irritation. If you can't swallow whole, crumble tablet and take with liquid or food.
- Capsule—Swallow with liquid or food to lessen stomach irritation. If you can't swallow whole, open capsule and take with liquid or food.

When to take:
At the same times each day, according to instructions on prescription label.

If you forget a dose:
Take as soon as you remember up to 2 hours late. If more than 2 hours, wait for next scheduled dose (don't double this dose).

What drug does:
Blocks the effects of dopamine* in the brain.

Time lapse before drug works:
1/2 to 3 hours.

Don't take with:
Any other medicine or any dietary supplement without consulting your doctor or pharmacist.

 ## OVERDOSE

SYMPTOMS:
Dizziness, drowsiness, severe shortness of breath, muscle spasms, coma.
WHAT TO DO:
- **Dial 911 (emergency) for medical help or call poison control center 1-800-222-1222 for instructions.**
- **See emergency information on last 3 pages of this book.**

 ## POSSIBLE ADVERSE REACTIONS OR SIDE EFFECTS

SYMPTOMS	WHAT TO DO
Life-threatening:	
Severe shortness of breath, skin rash, heartbeat irregularities, profuse sweating, fever, convulsions (rare).	Seek emergency treatment immediately.
Common:	
• Increased dental problems because of dry mouth and less salivation.	Consult your dentist about a prevention program.
• Swallowing difficulty, expressionless face, stiff arms and legs, dizziness.	Discontinue. Call doctor right away.
Infrequent:	
• Chewing movements with lip smacking, loss of balance, shuffling walk, tremor of fingers and hands, uncontrolled tongue movements.	Discontinue. Call doctor right away.
• Constipation, difficult urination, blurred vision, confusion, loss of sex drive, headache, insomnia, menstrual irregularities, weight gain, light sensitivity, nausea.	Continue. Call doctor when convenient.
Rare:	
Rapid heartbeat, fever, sore throat, jaundice, unusual bleeding.	Discontinue. Call doctor right away.

 ## WARNINGS & PRECAUTIONS

Don't take if:
You are allergic to loxapine.

Before you start, consult your doctor if:
- You have a seizure disorder.
- You have an enlarged prostate, glaucoma, Parkinson's disease, heart disease, asthma, emphysema, bronchitis, urinary tract problem, blood pressure problem, blood or blood vessel disorder, kidney or liver disorder or abuse alcohol.

Over age 60:
- Adverse reactions and side effects may be more severe. You may need smaller doses.
- Use of antipsychotic drugs in elderly patients with dementia-related psychosis may increase risk of death. Consult doctor.

Pregnancy:
Decide with your doctor if drug benefits justify risk to unborn child. Risk category C (see page xviii).

Breast-feeding:
Drug may pass into milk. Avoid drug or discontinue nursing until you finish medicine. Consult doctor for advice on maintaining milk supply.

Infants & children:
Not recommended.

Prolonged use:
Talk to your doctor about the need for follow-up medical examinations or laboratory studies.

Skin & sunlight:
May cause rash or intensify sunburn in areas exposed to sun or ultraviolet light (photo-sensitivity reaction). Avoid overexposure and use sunscreen. Notify doctor if reaction occurs.

Driving, piloting or hazardous work:
Don't drive or pilot aircraft until you learn how medicine affects you. Don't work around dangerous machinery. Don't climb ladders or work in high places. Danger increases if you drink alcohol or take medicine affecting alertness and reflexes.

Discontinuing:
* Don't discontinue without consulting doctor. Dose may require gradual reduction if you have taken drug for a long time. Doses of other drugs may also require adjustment.
* These symptoms may occur after medicine has been discontinued: dizziness; nausea; abdominal pain; uncontrolled movements of mouth, tongue and jaw.

Others:
* Use careful oral hygiene.
* Advise any doctor or dentist whom you consult that you take this medicine.

POSSIBLE INTERACTION WITH OTHER DRUGS

GENERIC NAME OR DRUG CLASS	COMBINED EFFECT
Anticonvulsants*	Decreased effect of anticonvulsant.
Antidepressants, tricyclic*	May increase toxic effects of both drugs.
Bupropion	Increased risk of seizures.
Central nervous system (CNS) depressants*	Increased sedative effects of both drugs.
Epinephrine	Rapid heart rate and severe drop in blood pressure.
Extrapyramidal reaction*-causing drugs	Increased risk of side effects.
Fluoxetine	Increased depressant effects of both drugs.
Guanadrel	Decreased effect of guanadrel.
Guanethidine	Decreased effect of guanethidine.
Guanfacine	Increased effects of both drugs.
Haloperidol	May increase toxic effects of both drugs.
Leucovorin	High alcohol content of leucovorin may cause adverse effects.
Methyldopa	May increase toxic effects of both drugs.
Metoclopramide	May increase toxic effects of both drugs.
Molindone	May increase toxic effects of both drugs.
Pemoline	Increased central nervous stimulation.
Pergolide	Decreased pergolide effect.
Phenothiazines*	May increase toxic effects of both drugs.
Pimozide	May increase toxic effects of both drugs.

Continued on page 921

POSSIBLE INTERACTION WITH OTHER SUBSTANCES

INTERACTS WITH	COMBINED EFFECT
Alcohol:	May decrease effect of loxapine. Avoid.
Beverages:	None expected.
Cocaine:	May increase toxicity of both drugs. Avoid.
Foods:	None expected.
Marijuana:	May increase toxicity of both drugs. Avoid.
Tobacco:	May increase toxicity.

*See Glossary

LUBIPROSTONE

BRAND NAMES

Amitiza

BASIC INFORMATION

Habit forming? No
Prescription needed? Yes
Available as generic? No
Drug class: Laxative

 ## USES

- Treatment for chronic idiopathic constipation and its associated symptoms. Idiopathic means the cause of the constipation is unknown or unapparent. The constipation is not caused by a disease or medications.
- Treatment for irritable bowel syndrome with constipation in adult women.
- May be used for treatment of other disorders as determined by your doctor.

 ## DOSAGE & USAGE INFORMATION

How to take:
Capsule—Swallow with liquid and take with food to help reduce any nausea symptoms.

When to take:
At the same time each day, usually twice a day with a meal or snack.

If you forget a dose:
Take as soon as you remember. If it is almost time for the next dose, wait for next scheduled dose (don't double this dose).

What drug does:
It works in the gastrointestinal system to increase fluid secretion. The increased fluid softens the stool and stimulates bowel activity which helps produce bowel movements. The constipation symptoms of bloating, straining and abdominal discomfort are reduced.

Continued next column

 ## OVERDOSE

SYMPTOMS:
Nausea, vomiting, diarrhea, dizziness, loose or watery stools, headache, retching, hot flush or flushing, abdominal pain and possibly other symptoms.
WHAT TO DO:
Overdose unlikely to threaten life. If person uses much larger amount than prescribed or if accidentally swallowed, call doctor or poison control center 1-800-222-1222 for help.

Time lapse before drug works:
Spontaneous bowel movements may occur within 24 hours of taking the first dose. Several spontaneous bowel movements should occur within the first week.

Don't take with:
Any other medicine or any dietary supplement without consulting your doctor or pharmacist.

 ## POSSIBLE ADVERSE REACTIONS OR SIDE EFFECTS

SYMPTOMS	WHAT TO DO
Life-threatening: None expected.	
Common: Nausea, headache, diarrhea, abdominal pain and distension, flatulence.	Continue. Call doctor when convenient.
Infrequent: Severe diarrhea.	Discontinue. Call doctor right away.
Rare: Other symptoms that cause concern (they may or may not be caused by the drug).	Continue. Call doctor when convenient.

WARNINGS & PRECAUTIONS

Don't take if:
You are allergic to lubiprostone.

Before you start, consult your doctor if:
You have a mechanical gastrointestinal obstruction (this can include problems such as adhesions, carcinomas [cancers] or hernias).

Over age 60:
No problems expected.

Pregnancy:
Decide with your doctor whether drug benefits justify risk to unborn child. Risk category C (see page xviii).

Breast-feeding:
It is unknown if drug passes into milk. Avoid drug or discontinue nursing until you finish medicine. Consult doctor for advice on maintaining milk supply.

Infants & children:
It is not approved for use in those under age 18.

Prolonged use:
Talk to your doctor periodically to determine if continued use of the drug is necessary.

Skin & sunlight:
No problems expected.

Driving, piloting or hazardous work:
No problems expected.

Discontinuing:
No problems expected.

Others:
• Advise any doctor or dentist whom you consult that you take this medicine.
• Consult your doctor if severe diarrhea occurs.

POSSIBLE INTERACTION WITH OTHER DRUGS

GENERIC NAME OR DRUG CLASS	COMBINED EFFECT
None expected.	

POSSIBLE INTERACTION WITH OTHER SUBSTANCES

INTERACTS WITH	COMBINED EFFECT
Alcohol:	None expected.
Beverages:	None expected.
Cocaine:	Unknown. Best to avoid.
Foods:	None expected.
Marijuana:	Unknown. Best to avoid.
Tobacco:	None expected.

MACROLIDE ANTIBIOTICS

GENERIC AND BRAND NAMES

AZITHROMYCIN
Zithromax
Zmax

CLARITHROMYCIN
Biaxin
DIRITHROMYCIN
Dynabac

BASIC INFORMATION

Habit forming? No
Prescription needed? Yes
Available as generic? Yes, for some
**Drug class: Antibiotic (macrolide),
antibiotic (erythromycin)**

 USES

Treatment for mild to moderate bacterial
infections responsive to macrolide antibiotics.
These include bronchitis, tonsillitis, some
pneumonias, ear infections, skin infections
(e.g., acne), sinusitis, streptococcal sore throat,
urethritis and others. (Note: Erythromycin is also
a macrolide antibiotic. See its individual chart for
information.)

 **DOSAGE & USAGE
INFORMATION**

How to take:
• Enteric-coated tablet or delayed release
tablet—Swallow with liquid. Do not crush or
chew tablet.
• Tablet or capsule—Swallow with liquid. If you
can't swallow whole, then crumble tablet or
open capsule and take with food or water.
• Oral suspension—Swallow with liquid.

When to take:
At the same time each day. Take azithromycin on
an empty stomach, 1 hour before or 2 hours after
a meal. Clarithromycin may be taken with or
without food. Take dirithromycin with food or
within 1 hour after eating.

Continued next column

 OVERDOSE

SYMPTOMS:
**Possibly diarrhea, nausea, vomiting,
abdominal pain.**
WHAT TO DO:
**Overdose unlikely to threaten life. If person
uses much larger amount than prescribed or
if accidentally swallowed, call doctor or
poison control center 1-800-222-1222 for help.**

If you forget a dose:
Take as soon as you remember. If it is almost
time for the next dose, wait for that dose (don't
double this dose) and resume regular schedule.

What drug does:
Prevents growth and reproduction of susceptible
bacteria.

Time lapse before drug works:
Usually 2 to 5 days. Some infections may take
10 days or longer to resolve.

Don't take with:
Any other medicine or any dietary supplement
without consulting your doctor or pharmacist.

 **POSSIBLE
ADVERSE REACTIONS
OR SIDE EFFECTS**

SYMPTOMS	WHAT TO DO
Life-threatening: Rare allergic reaction— Breathing difficulty; swelling of hands, feet, face, mouth, neck; skin rash; temporary deafness.	Discontinue. Seek emergency treatment.
Common: None expected.	
Infrequent: Nausea, vomiting, abdominal discomfort, diarrhea.	Continue. Call doctor when convenient.
Rare: • Headache, dizziness.	Continue. Call doctor when convenient.
• Allergic reaction (skin rash, itching).	Discontinue. Call right away.

WARNINGS & PRECAUTIONS

Don't take if:
You are allergic to macrolide antibiotics.

Before you start, consult your doctor if:
• You have impaired liver or kidney function.
• You are allergic to any medication, food or other substance.

Over age 60:
No special problems expected.

Pregnancy:
Risk factors vary for drugs in this group. See page xviii and consult doctor.

Breast-feeding:
One or more of these drugs may pass into milk. Avoid drug or discontinue nursing until you finish medicine. Consult doctor for advice on maintaining milk supply.

Infants & children:
Give only under close medical supervision to those under age 12. Young children may not complain or recognize adverse effects of drug. Observe child closely for any reactions.

Prolonged use:
Not recommended. Medicine is discontinued once the infection is cured.

Skin & sunlight:
No special problems expected.

Driving, piloting or hazardous work:
Avoid if you experience dizziness. Otherwise, no problems expected.

Discontinuing:
Don't discontinue without doctor's advice until you complete prescribed dose, even though symptoms diminish or disappear.

Others:
• Advise any doctor or dentist whom you consult that you take this medicine.
• May affect the results of some medical tests.

POSSIBLE INTERACTION WITH OTHER DRUGS

GENERIC NAME OR DRUG CLASS	COMBINED EFFECT
Antacids,* aluminum- or magnesium- containing	Take one hour apart.
Bromocriptine	Increased effect of bromocriptine.
Carbamazepine	Increased effect of carbamazepine.
Cisapride	May increase toxic effects. Avoid.
Cyclosporine	Increased effect of cyclosporine.
Digoxin	Increased effect of digoxin.
Disopyramide	Unknown effect. Use with caution.
Enzyme inhibitors*	Increased effect of enzyme inhibitor (with clarithromycin).
Ergot preparations*	Can cause serious or life-threatening problems with blood circulation. Avoid.
Iron supplements	Decreased effect of dirithromycin. Take 1 hour apart.
Phenytoin	Decreased effect of phenytoin.
Pimozide	May increase toxic effects. Avoid.
Rifabutin	Decreased effect of antibiotic.
Rifampin	Decreased effect of antibiotic.
Tacrolimus	Increased effect of tacrolimus.
Theophylline	Increased effect of theophylline.
Triazolam	Increased risk of triazolam.
Warfarin	Increased risk of bleeding.
Zidovudine	Decreased effect of zidovudine.

POSSIBLE INTERACTION WITH OTHER SUBSTANCES

INTERACTS WITH	COMBINED EFFECT
Alcohol:	None expected.
Beverages:	None expected.
Cocaine:	None expected.
Foods:	None expected
Marijuana:	None expected.
Tobacco:	None expected.

*See Glossary

MAPROTILINE

BRAND NAMES

Ludiomil

BASIC INFORMATION

Habit forming? No
Prescription needed? Yes
Available as generic? Yes
Drug class: Antidepressant

 USES

Treatment for depression or anxiety associated with depression.

 DOSAGE & USAGE INFORMATION

How to take:
Tablet—Swallow with liquid.

When to take:
At the same time each day, usually bedtime.

If you forget a dose:
Bedtime dose—If you forget your once-a-day bedtime dose, don't take it more than 3 hours late. If more than 3 hours, wait for next scheduled dose. Don't double this dose.

What drug does:
Probably affects part of brain that controls messages between nerve cells.

Time lapse before drug works:
Begins in 1 to 2 weeks. May require 4 to 6 weeks for maximum benefit.

Don't take with:
Any other medicine or any dietary supplement without consulting your doctor or pharmacist.

 OVERDOSE

SYMPTOMS:
Respiratory failure, fever, cardiac arrhythmia, muscle stiffness, drowsiness, hallucinations, convulsions, coma.
WHAT TO DO:
* **Dial 911 (emergency) for medical help or call poison control center 1-800-222-1222 for instructions.**
* **If person is unconscious, check breathing and pulse. If not breathing, begin mouth-to-mouth rescue breathing. If heart is not beating, begin chest compressions.**
* **See emergency information on last 3 pages of this book.**

 POSSIBLE ADVERSE REACTIONS OR SIDE EFFECTS

SYMPTOMS	WHAT TO DO
Life-threatening:	
Seizures.	Seek emergency treatment immediately.
Common:	
• Tremor.	Discontinue. Call doctor right away.
• Headache, dry mouth or unpleasant taste, constipation or diarrhea, nausea, indigestion, fatigue, weakness, drowsiness, nervousness, anxiety, excessive sweating.	Continue. Call doctor when convenient.
• Insomnia, craving sweets.	Continue. Tell doctor at next visit.
Infrequent:	
• Hallucinations, shakiness, dizziness, fainting, blurred vision, eye pain, vomiting, irregular heartbeat or slow pulse, inflamed tongue, abdominal pain, jaundice, hair loss, rash, chills, joint pain, palpitations, hiccups, vision changes.	Discontinue. Call doctor right away.
• Painful or difficult urination; fatigue; decreased sex drive; abnormal dreams; nasal congestion; back pain; muscle aches; frequent urination; painful, absent or irregular menstruation.	Continue. Call doctor when convenient.
Rare:	
Itchy skin; sore throat; fever; involuntary movements of jaw, lips and tongue; nightmares; confusion; swollen breasts in men.	Discontinue. Call doctor right away.

WARNINGS & PRECAUTIONS

Don't take if:
* You are allergic to maprotiline.
* You have had a heart attack within 6 weeks.
* You have taken a monoamine oxidase (MAO) inhibitor* within 2 weeks.

Before you start, consult your doctor if:
* You will have surgery within 2 months, including dental surgery, requiring anesthesia.
* You have a history of drug or alcohol abuse.
* You have an enlarged prostate, heart disease or high blood pressure, stomach or intestinal problems, overactive thyroid, asthma, liver disease, schizophrenia, urinary retention, glaucoma, respiratory disorder, seizure disorders, diabetes, or kidney disease.

Over age 60:
More likely to develop urination difficulty and side effects such as hallucinations, shakiness, dizziness, fainting, headache or insomnia.

Pregnancy:
Consult doctor. Risk category B (see page xviii).

Breast-feeding:
Drug passes into milk. Avoid drug or discontinue nursing until you finish medicine. Consult doctor for advice on maintaining milk supply.

Infants & children:
Not approved in ages under 18. If prescribed, carefully read information provided with prescription. Contact doctor right away if symptoms get worse or any there is any talk of suicide or suicide behaviors. Read information under Others.

Prolonged use:
Request blood cell counts, liver function studies; monitor blood pressure closely.

Skin & sunlight:
May cause rash or intensify sunburn in areas exposed to sun or ultraviolet light (photosensitivity reaction). Avoid overexposure and use sunscreen. Notify doctor if reaction occurs.

Driving, piloting or hazardous work:
Don't drive or pilot aircraft until you learn how medicine affects you. Don't work around dangerous machinery. Don't climb ladders or work in high places. Danger increases if you drink alcohol or take medicine affecting alertness and reflexes.

Discontinuing:
Don't discontinue without consulting doctor. Dose may require gradual reduction if you have taken drug for a long time. Doses of other drugs may also require adjustment.

Others:
* Advise any doctor or dentist whom you consult that you take this drug.
* Adults and children taking antidepressants may experience a worsening of the depression symptoms and may display increased suicidal thoughts or behavior. Call doctor right away if these symptoms or behaviors occur.
* For dry mouth, suck sugarless hard candy or chew sugarless gum. If dry mouth persists, consult your dentist.

POSSIBLE INTERACTION WITH OTHER DRUGS

GENERIC NAME OR DRUG CLASS	COMBINED EFFECT
Anticholinergics*	Increased sedation.
Antiglaucoma agents	Heart rhythm problems, high blood pressure.
Antihistamines*	Increased antihistamine effect.
Barbiturates*	Decreased antidepressant effect.
Benzodiazepines*	Increased sedation.
Bupropion	Increased risk of seizures.
Central nervous system (CNS) depressants*	Increased sedation.
Cimetidine	Possible increased antidepressant effect and toxicity.

Continued on page 921

POSSIBLE INTERACTION WITH OTHER SUBSTANCES

INTERACTS WITH	COMBINED EFFECT
Alcohol: Beverages or medicines with alcohol.	Excessive intoxication. Avoid.
Beverages:	None expected.
Cocaine:	Excessive intoxication. Avoid.
Foods:	None expected.
Marijuana:	Excessive drowsiness. Avoid.
Tobacco:	May decrease absorption of maprotiline. Avoid.

*See Glossary

MARAVIROC

BRAND NAMES

Selzentry

BASIC INFORMATION

Habit forming? No
Prescription needed? Yes
Available as generic? No
Drug class: Antiviral agent

USES

Treatment of adults infected with human immunodeficiency virus (HIV) who have failed other antiviral drug therapy. This drug specifically treats patients with CCR5-tropic HIV-1. The drug is used in combination with other antiviral drugs. HIV is the virus that causes acquired immunodeficiency syndrome (AIDS).

DOSAGE & USAGE INFORMATION

How to take:
Tablet—Swallow with liquid. May be taken with or without food.

When to take:
Take twice a day at the same times each day.

If you forget a dose:
Take as soon as you remember. If it is almost time for the next dose, wait for next scheduled dose (don't double this dose).

What drug does:
It helps control HIV infection by blocking the virus from entering your immune system cells. This helps your immune system stay healthy so it can fight the infection. The drug does not cure HIV or AIDS.

Time lapse before drug works:
May require several weeks or months before full benefits are apparent.

Don't take with:
Any other medicine or any dietary supplement without consulting your doctor or pharmacist. This is very important with HIV drugs.

OVERDOSE

SYMPTOMS:
Feeling faint or lightheaded, cold sweats.
WHAT TO DO:
* Call doctor or poison control center 1-800-222-1222 for instructions.
* See emergency information on last 3 pages of this book.

POSSIBLE ADVERSE REACTIONS OR SIDE EFFECTS

SYMPTOMS	WHAT TO DO
Life-threatening: Rare allergic reaction (hives, itching, rash, trouble breathing, tightness in chest, swelling of lips or tongue or throat).	Seek emergency treatment immediately.
Common: Diarrhea, dizziness, fatigue, nausea, cough, fever, other mild cold symptoms, abdominal pain.	Continue. Call doctor when convenient.
Infrequent: Swelling, stomach pain, muscle or joint pain, white patches or sores inside mouth or on lips, constipation, urination problems, changes in body fat, sleeping problems, dizziness when getting up from a sitting or lying down position, cold sores or sores on genital or anal area, itching.	Continue. Call doctor when convenient.
Rare: • Skin rash, liver problem (symptoms may include nausea, stomach pain, loss of appetite, skin rash, dark urine, clay-colored stools, yellow skin or eyes), chest pain, new infection (fever, chills, cough, flu-like symptoms), lightheadedness or near fainting, breathing difficulty.	Discontinue. Call doctor right away.
• Other unexplained symptoms.	Continue. Call doctor when convenient.

MARAVIROC

WARNINGS & PRECAUTIONS

Don't take if:
You are allergic to maraviroc.

Before you start, consult your doctor if:
- You are allergic to any medicine, food or other substance, or have a family history of allergies.
- You have kidney or liver disease (especially hepatitis B or C).
- You have heart disease, low blood pressure, circulation problems or a history of stroke.

Over age 60:
Use with caution as adverse reactions and side effects may be more frequent and severe than in younger persons.

Pregnancy:
Decide with your doctor if drug benefits justify risk to unborn child. Risk category B (see page xviii). HIV can be passed to the baby if the mother is not properly treated during pregnancy. Talk to your doctor about being included in the Antiretroviral Pregnancy Registry.

Breast-feeding:
It is unknown if drug passes into milk. It is not recommended that HIV-infected mothers breast-feed. Consult your doctor.

Infants & children:
Safety and efficacy have not been established for children under age 16. Consult doctor.

Prolonged use:
- Long-term effects of using this drug have not been established.
- Talk to your doctor about the need for follow up blood tests and liver function studies.

Skin & sunlight:
No problems expected.

Driving, piloting or hazardous work:
Don't drive or pilot aircraft until you learn how medicine affects you. Don't work around dangerous machinery. Don't climb ladders or work in high places. Danger increases if you drink alcohol or take medicine affecting alertness and reflexes, such as antihistamines, tranquilizers, sedatives, pain medicine, narcotics and mind-altering drugs.

Discontinuing:
Don't discontinue (even for a short time) without doctor's advice.

Others:
- Advise any doctor or dentist whom you consult that you take this medicine.
- Taking this drug does not prevent you from passing HIV to another person through sexual contact or sharing needles. Avoid sexual contact or practice safe sex (e.g., using condoms) to help prevent the transmission of HIV. Never share or re-use needles. If you have questions, ask your doctor for advice.
- Consult your doctor right away if you develop symptoms of a new infection.
- Take drug daily as prescribed. Do not increase or decrease dosage of drug without doctor's approval.

POSSIBLE INTERACTION WITH OTHER DRUGS

GENERIC NAME OR DRUG CLASS	COMBINED EFFECT
Antihypertensives*	Increased risk of dizziness, Use with caution.
Enzyme inducers*	Decreased effect of maraviroc.
Enzyme inhibitors*	Increased effect of maraviroc.
St. John's wort	Decreased effect of maraviroc. Avoid.

POSSIBLE INTERACTION WITH OTHER SUBSTANCES

INTERACTS WITH	COMBINED EFFECT
Alcohol:	None expected.
Beverages:	None expected.
Cocaine:	Unknown effect. Best to avoid.
Foods:	None expected.
Marijuana:	Unknown effect. Best to avoid.
Tobacco:	None expected.

MASOPROCOL

BRAND NAMES

Actinex

BASIC INFORMATION

Habit forming? No
Prescription needed? Yes
Available as generic? No
Drug class: Antineoplastic (topical)

USES

Treats actinic keratoses (scaly, flat or slightly raised skin lesions).

DOSAGE & USAGE INFORMATION

How to take:
Cream—Wash and dry the skin where lesions are located. Massage cream into affected area. Wash hands immediately after use.

When to take:
Use at the same times each day.

If you forget a dose:
Apply as soon as you remember, then resume regular schedule.

What drug does:
Selectively destroys actively proliferating cells.

Time lapse before drug works:
1 to 2 months.

Don't take with:
Any other medicine or any dietary supplement without consulting your doctor or pharmacist.

OVERDOSE

SYMPTOMS:
None reported.
WHAT TO DO:
Not for internal use. If child accidentally swallows, call poison control center 1-800-222-1222 for help.

POSSIBLE ADVERSE REACTIONS OR SIDE EFFECTS

SYMPTOMS	WHAT TO DO
Life-threatening: None expected.	
Common:	
• Redness and swelling of otherwise normal skin.	Discontinue. Call doctor right away.
• Skin reactions including itching, redness, dryness, flaking where medicine applied.	Continue. Call doctor when convenient.
• Temporary burning sensation right after application.	No action necessary.
Infrequent:	
• Allergic reaction to sulfites—bluish skin, severe dizziness, faintness, wheezing, breathing difficulty.	Discontinue. Seek emergency help.
• Swelling, soreness, persistent burning in treated area.	Continue. Call doctor when convenient.
Rare:	
Bleeding, oozing, blistering skin.	Discontinue. Call doctor right away.

WARNINGS & PRECAUTIONS

Don't take if:
You are allergic to masoprocol.

Before you start, consult your doctor if:
You have a sulfite sensitivity.

Over age 60:
No problems expected.

Pregnancy:
Consult doctor. Risk category B (see page xviii).

Breast-feeding:
Effect not documented. Consult your doctor.

Infants & children:
Not used in this age group.

Prolonged use:
Effects of long-term use unknown. Visit doctor on a regular basis to determine effectiveness of treatment.

Skin & sunlight:
Drug does not cause sensitivity to sunlight. However, keratoses are related to sun exposure, so avoid sunlight when possible.

Driving, piloting or hazardous work:
No problems expected.

Discontinuing:
No problems expected.

Others:
- If you accidentally get masoprocol in your eye, promptly wash the eye with water.
- The cream may stain your clothing.
- Get doctor's approval before using cosmetics or make-up on the skin area you are treating.
- Leave the treated skin areas exposed. Don't cover them with a bandage or a dressing.

POSSIBLE INTERACTION WITH OTHER DRUGS

GENERIC NAME OR DRUG CLASS	COMBINED EFFECT
None significant.	

POSSIBLE INTERACTION WITH OTHER SUBSTANCES

INTERACTS WITH	COMBINED EFFECT
Alcohol:	None expected.
Beverages:	None expected.
Cocaine:	None expected.
Foods:	None expected.
Marijuana:	None expected.
Tobacco:	None expected.

*See Glossary

MECAMYLAMINE

BRAND NAMES

Inversine

BASIC INFORMATION

Habit forming? No
Prescription needed? Yes
Available as generic? No
Drug class: Antihypertensive

 USES

Helps control, but doesn't cure, high blood pressure.

 DOSAGE & USAGE INFORMATION

How to take:
Tablet—Swallow with liquid. If you can't swallow whole, crumble tablet and take with liquid or food. Instructions to take on empty stomach mean 1 hour before or 2 hours after eating.

When to take:
* At the same time each day, according to instructions on prescription label.
* Usually twice a day, every 8 or 12 hours apart. Follow label directions.

If you forget a dose:
Take as soon as you remember up to 2 hours late. If more than 2 hours, wait for next scheduled dose (don't double this dose).

What drug does:
Blocks transmission of electrical impulse where two nerve cells connect. Causes constricted blood vessels to relax.

Time lapse before drug works:
30 minutes to 2 hours.

Don't take with:
Any other medicines (including over-the-counter drugs such as cough and cold medicines, laxatives, antacids, diet pills, caffeine, nose drops or vitamins) without consulting your doctor or pharmacist.

 OVERDOSE

SYMPTOMS:
Confusion, excitement, seizures, coma.
WHAT TO DO:
* Dial 911 (emergency) for medical help or call poison control center 1-800-222-1222 for instructions.
* See emergency information on last 3 pages of this book.

 POSSIBLE ADVERSE REACTIONS OR SIDE EFFECTS

SYMPTOMS	WHAT TO DO
Life-threatening:	
In case of overdose, see previous column.	
Common:	
Dizziness upon arising from chair or bed, blurred vision, decreased sex drive, dry mouth, enlarged pupils, constipation.	Continue. Call doctor when convenient.
Infrequent:	
• Confusion, depression, tremors, shortness of breath.	Discontinue. Call doctor right away.
• Difficult urination, tiredness.	Continue. Tell doctor at next visit.
Rare:	
Appetite loss, nausea and vomiting.	Continue. Tell doctor at next visit.

MECAMYLAMINE

WARNINGS & PRECAUTIONS

Don't take if:
You are allergic to mecamylamine.

Before you start, consult your doctor if:
- You have heart disease.
- You had a recent heart attack.
- You have glaucoma or gout.
- You have kidney disease.

Over age 60:
Adverse reactions and side effects may be more frequent and severe than in younger persons. You may need smaller doses for shorter periods of time.

Pregnancy:
Decide with your doctor if drug benefits justify risk to unborn child. Risk category C (see page xviii).

Breast-feeding:
Effect unknown. Consult doctor.

Infants & children:
Effect not documented. Consult your pediatrician.

Prolonged use:
Talk to your doctor about the need for follow-up medical examinations or laboratory studies to check blood pressure, kidney function and heart function.

Skin & sunlight:
No problems expected.

Driving, piloting or hazardous work:
Avoid if you feel confused, drowsy or dizzy.

Discontinuing:
Don't discontinue without consulting doctor. Dose may require gradual reduction if you have taken drug for a long time. Doses of other drugs may also require adjustment.

Others:
- Advise any doctor or dentist whom you consult that you take this medicine.
- May affect results in some medical tests.
- Get up slowly from chair or bed.
- Dosage may need to be adjusted for hot weather or heavy exercise.

POSSIBLE INTERACTION WITH OTHER DRUGS

GENERIC NAME OR DRUG CLASS	COMBINED EFFECT
Alkalizers, urine*	Prolonged effect of mecamylamine.
Ambenonium	Swallowing difficulty.
Antacids*	Prolonged effect of mecamylamine.
Antibiotics*	Decreased antibiotic effect.
Antiglaucoma, carbonic anhydrase inhibitors	Increased risk of side effects.
Neostigmine	Swallowing difficulty.
Nimodipine	Dangerous blood pressure drop.
Pyridostigmine	Swallowing difficulty.
Sodium bicarbonate	Increased mecamylamine effect.
Sulfa drugs*	Decreased antibiotic effect.

POSSIBLE INTERACTION WITH OTHER SUBSTANCES

INTERACTS WITH	COMBINED EFFECT
Alcohol:	Increased likelihood of fainting.
Beverages:	None expected.
Cocaine:	Increased central nervous system stimulation. Avoid.
Foods: Food with high salt or sodium.	Decreased effectiveness of mecamylamine.
Marijuana:	Increased central nervous system stimulation. Avoid.
Tobacco:	None expected.

MECHLORETHAMINE (Topical)

BRAND NAMES

Mustargen

BASIC INFORMATION

Habit forming? No
Prescription needed? Yes
Available as generic? No
Drug class: Antineoplastic (topical)

 ## USES

- Treats mycosis fungoides.
- Treats other malignancies (by injection).

 ## DOSAGE & USAGE INFORMATION

How to use:
- Solution—It is mixed according to doctor's instructions. Don't inhale vapors or powder. Shower and rinse before treatment. Use rubber gloves to apply over entire body. Avoid contact with eyes, nose and mouth.
- Ointment—Use according to doctor's instructions.

When to use:
Usually once a day.

If you forget a dose:
Apply as soon as you remember. If it is almost time for the next scheduled dose, wait and apply that dose at regular time (don't double this dose).

What drug does:
Destroys cells that produce mycosis fungoides.

Time lapse before drug works:
Starts to work right away, but response to treatment may take 3 to 6 months.

Don't use with:
Any other topical or oral medicines (including over-the-counter drugs such as cough and cold medicines, laxatives, antacids, diet pills, caffeine, nose drops or vitamins) without consulting your doctor or pharmacist.

 ## OVERDOSE

SYMPTOMS:
None expected for topical solutions.
WHAT TO DO:
Not intended for internal use. If child accidentally swallows, call doctor or poison control center 1-800-222-1222 for help.

 ## POSSIBLE ADVERSE REACTIONS OR SIDE EFFECTS

SYMPTOMS	WHAT TO DO
Life-threatening: Immediate hives, shortness of breath.	Seek emergency treatment immediately.
Common: Darkening, dry skin.	Continue. Tell doctor at next visit.
Infrequent: Allergic reaction with rash, itching, hives.	Seek emergency treatment immediately.
Rare: None expected.	

WARNINGS & PRECAUTIONS

Don't use if:
You are allergic to mechlorethamine.

Before you start, consult your doctor if:
• You have chicken pox.
• You have shingles (herpes zoster).
• You have skin infection.

Over age 60:
No special problems expected.

Pregnancy:
Risk to unborn child outweighs drug benefits.
Don't use. Risk category D (see page xviii).

Breast-feeding:
Drug may be absorbed and pass into milk. Avoid drug or discontinue nursing until you finish medicine. Consult doctor for advice on maintaining milk supply.

Infants & children:
Effect unknown. Consult doctor.

Prolonged use:
• Allergic or hypersensitive reactions more likely. The ointment form is less likely to cause a reaction.
• Talk to your doctor about the need for follow-up medical examinations or laboratory studies to check liver function, complete blood counts (white blood cell count, platelet count, red blood cell count, hemoglobin, hematocrit) and hearing tests.

Skin & sunlight:
No problems expected.

Driving, piloting or hazardous work:
Don't drive or pilot aircraft until you learn how medicine affects you. Don't work around dangerous machinery. Don't climb ladders or work in high places. Danger increases if you drink alcohol or take medicine affecting alertness and reflexes.

Discontinuing:
No special problems expected.

Others:
• Advise any doctor or dentist whom you consult that you take this medicine.
• May affect results in some medical tests.
• Don't use if solution is discolored.

POSSIBLE INTERACTION WITH OTHER DRUGS

GENERIC NAME OR DRUG CLASS	COMBINED EFFECT
None significant.	

POSSIBLE INTERACTION WITH OTHER SUBSTANCES

INTERACTS WITH	COMBINED EFFECT
Alcohol:	None expected.
Beverages:	None expected.
Cocaine:	None expected.
Foods:	None expected.
Marijuana:	None expected.
Tobacco:	None expected.

MEGLITINIDES

GENERIC AND BRAND NAMES

NATEGLINIDE
Starlix

REPAGLINIDE
Prandin
PrandiMet

BASIC INFORMATION

Habit forming? No
Prescription needed? Yes
Available as generic? No
Drug class: Antidiabetic

 USES

Helps control, but does not cure type 2 (non-insulin dependent) diabetes. Used alone or in combination with other antidiabetic drugs, along with diet and exercise.

 DOSAGE & USAGE INFORMATION

How to take:
Tablet—Take with water between 15-30 minutes before a meal. If you skip the meal, also skip the dose of medicine. If you have an extra meal, take an extra dose.

When to use:
15-30 minutes before each meal or as directed by doctor.

If you forget a dose:
If it is almost time for your next dose, take only that dose. Do not double doses.

What drug does:
Increases amount of insulin secreted from the pancreas, which helps to control blood sugar.

Continued next column

 OVERDOSE

SYMPTOMS:
Cold sweats, confusion, cool pale skin, difficulty in concentrating, drowsiness, excessive hunger, rapid heartbeat, nausea, nervousness, nightmares, restless sleep, seizures, shakiness, slurred speech, unusual tiredness or weakness, coma.
WHAT TO DO:
- **For mild low blood sugar symptoms, eat or drink something with sugar in it right away.**
- **For more severe symptoms, dial 911 (emergency) for medical help or call poison control center 1-800-222-1222 for instructions.**
- **See emergency information on last 3 pages of this book.**

Time lapse before drug works:
10-30 minutes, peaks in 1 hour.

Don't take with:
Any other medicine or any dietary supplement without consulting your doctor or pharmacist.

 POSSIBLE ADVERSE REACTIONS OR SIDE EFFECTS

SYMPTOMS	WHAT TO DO
Life-threatening: In case of overdose or low blood sugar, see previous column.	
Common: Symptoms of a cold (sore throat, runny or stuffy nose, cough), back pain, diarrhea, joint pain.	Continue. Call doctor when convenient.
Frequent: Low blood sugar symptoms: anxiety, cold sweats, shakiness, rapid heartbeat, blurred vision, pale skin, behavior changes similar to being drunk, confusion or difficulty thinking, drowsiness, excessive hunger, headache, nausea, nightmares, restless sleep, unusual tiredness or weakness.	Treat the low blood sugar. If symptoms are severe, seek emergency treatment.
Infrequent Bloody or cloudy urine, urination problems (burning, painful, difficult, frequent, urge to urinate), wheezing, chills, skin rash or itching or hives, eyes tearing, vomiting.	Discontinue. Call doctor right away.
Rare: • Unusual bleeding or bruising, red spots on skin, black or tarry stools, hoarseness, lower back or side pain, other side effects not listed occur.	Continue, but call doctor right away.
• Indigestion, feeling of warmth or heat or burning, stomach pain, constipation, dizziness.	Continue. Call doctor when convenient.

WARNINGS & PRECAUTIONS

Don't use if:
You are allergic to meglitinides.

Before you start, consult your doctor if:
- You have type 1 diabetes or diabetic ketoacidosis (ketones in the blood).
- You have an infection, fever, an injury or trauma, high stress levels or are planning surgery.
- You have a nervous system disorder.
- You have kidney or liver disease or underactive adrenal or pituitary gland.
- You are weak or undernourished.

Over age 60:
Increased risk of developing low blood sugar.

Pregnancy:
Decide with your doctor if drug benefits justify risk to unborn child. Risk category C (see page xviii).

Breast-feeding:
It is not known if drug passes into milk. Avoid drugs or discontinue nursing until you finish medicine. Consult doctor for advice on maintaining milk supply.

Infants & children:
Not recommended. Safety and dosage have not been established.

Prolonged use:
Talk to your doctor about the need for follow up medical examinations or laboratory studies to check blood glucose levels and glycosylated hemoglobin (HbA1c) values.

Skin & sunlight:
No problems expected.

Driving, piloting or hazardous work:
Don't drive or pilot aircraft until you learn how medicine affects you. Don't work around dangerous machinery. Don't climb ladders or work in high places. Danger increases if you drink alcohol or take medicine affecting alertness and reflexes.

Discontinuing:
Don't discontinue without consulting your doctor even if you feel well. You can have diabetes without feeling any symptoms. Untreated diabetes can cause serious problems.

Others:
- Advise any doctor or dentist whom you consult that you take this medicine. It may interfere with the accuracy of some medical tests.
- Follow any special diet your doctor may prescribe. It can help control diabetes.
- Consult doctor if you become ill with vomiting or diarrhea while taking this drug.
- Use caution when exercising. Ask your doctor about an appropriate exercise program.

- Wear medical identification stating that you have diabetes and take this medication.
- Learn to recognize the symptoms of low and high blood sugar. You and your family need to know what to do if these symptoms occur and when to call the doctor for help.
- Have a glucagon kit and syringe in the event severe low blood sugar occurs.

POSSIBLE INTERACTION WITH OTHER DRUGS

GENERIC NAME OR DRUG CLASS	COMBINED EFFECT
Anti-inflammatory drugs nonsteroidal (NSAIDs)	Increased risk of low blood sugar.
Barbiturates	Blood sugar problems.
Beta adrenergic blocking agents	Blood sugar control problems.
Carbamazepine	Blood sugar problems.
Corticosteroids*	Decreased effect of meglitinide.
Diuretics, thiazide	Decreased effect of repaglinide.
Gemfibrozil	Increased effect of meglitinide.
Hyperglycemia-causing medications*	Increased risk of loss of glycemic control.
Monoamine oxidase (MAO) inhibitors*	Increased risk of low blood sugar.
Salicylates	Increased risk of low blood sugar.
Sympathomimetics*	Decreased effect of meglitinide.
Thyroid hormones	Decreased effect of meglitinide.

POSSIBLE INTERACTION WITH OTHER SUBSTANCES

INTERACTS WITH	COMBINED EFFECT
Alcohol:	Low blood sugar. Avoid.
Beverages:	None expected.
Cocaine:	None expected.
Foods:	None expected.
Marijuana:	None expected.
Tobacco:	None expected.

*See Glossary

MELATONIN

BRAND NAMES

Numerous brand names are available.

BASIC INFORMATION

Habit forming? No
Prescription needed? No
Available as generic? Yes
Drug class: Hormone

 USES

- Melatonin is a hormone produced in the human body by the pineal gland and secreted at night. In most people, the melatonin levels are highest during the normal hours of sleep. The levels increase rapidly in the late evening, peaking after midnight and decreasing toward morning.
- Jet lag: Some research studies have shown that taking melatonin before a flight and continuing for a few days after arrival at the destination helped control jet lag symptoms of fatigue and sleep disturbances. Appears to work best after plane trips that crossed more than six time zones. Timing of doses very important for effectiveness.
- Insomnia and restless leg syndrome: Some research studies have shown that taking melatonin about 2 hours before bedtime decreased the time needed to fall asleep and improved quality of sleep (less wakefulness).
- Other claims that it can slow aging, fight disease, and enhance one's sex life have been less studied and more difficult to prove.

 DOSAGE & USAGE INFORMATION

How to take:
For tablet or capsule—Follow instructions on the label or consult your doctor or pharmacist. Different brands supply different doses. Melatonin, as a product, is marketed as a dietary supplement and is not reviewed by the U.S. Food & Drug Administration (FDA) for effectiveness and

Continued next column

 OVERDOSE

SYMPTOMS:
It is unknown what symptoms may occur.
WHAT TO DO:
If person takes much larger amount than prescribed, dial 911 (emergency) for medical help or call poison control center 1-800-222-1222 for instructions.

safety. The melatonin products being sold are made from animal pineal glands or synthesized. The best dosage amounts are unknown. Use with caution.

When to take:
At the same time each day according to label directions. It is recommended that melatonin be taken at night before bedtime.

If you forget a dose:
Follow label instructions for your particular brand of melatonin. Usually you can take a medication as soon as you remember up to 2 hours late. If more than 2 hours, wait for the next scheduled dose (don't double this dose).

What drug does:
- Glands in the body make chemicals called hormones and release them into the bloodstream. Hormones taken as supplements also end up in the bloodstream. In either case, the blood then carries hormones to different parts of the body. There, hormones influence the way organs and tissues work.
- Hormone supplements may not have the same effects on the body as naturally produced hormones have, because the body processes them differently. Higher doses of supplements may result in higher amounts of hormones in the blood than are healthy.

Time lapse before drug works:
Effectiveness will vary from person to person and will also depend on the reason for taking melatonin.

Don't take with:
Any other medicine or any dietary supplement without consulting your doctor or pharmacist.

 POSSIBLE ADVERSE REACTIONS OR SIDE EFFECTS

SYMPTOMS	WHAT TO DO
Life-threatening: None expected.	
Common: Unknown.	
Infrequent: Drowsiness, confusion, headache or grogginess may occur the following morning.	Reduce dosage or discontinue taking.
Rare: Unknown. If symptoms occur that you are concerned about, talk to your doctor or pharmacist. Further research may uncover other side effects.	

WARNINGS & PRECAUTIONS

Don't use if:
You are allergic to melatonin.

Before you start, consult your doctor if:
- You have any chronic health problem.
- You have high blood pressure (hypertension) or cardiovascular disease. Some studies in animals suggest that melatonin may constrict blood vessels (a condition that could be dangerous for people with these conditions).
- You are allergic to any medication, food or other substance.

Over age 60:
A lower starting dosage is often recommended until a response is determined.

Pregnancy:
Melatonin is not recommended for pregnant women. Decide with your doctor if drug benefits justify risk to unborn child. Risk category is unknown since melatonin is not regulated by the FDA (see page xviii).

Breast-feeding:
It is unknown if drug passes into milk. Avoid drug or discontinue nursing until you finish medicine. Consult doctor for advice on maintaining milk supply.

Infants & children:
Not recommended for children.

Prolonged use:
Effects are unknown. More research is needed to determine long-term effects of melatonin use.

Skin & sunlight:
No problems expected.

Driving, piloting or hazardous work:
Since it causes drowsiness, don't drive or pilot aircraft until you learn how medicine affects you. Don't work around dangerous machinery. Don't climb ladders or work in high places. Danger increases if you drink alcohol or take medicine affecting alertness and reflexes.

Discontinuing:
No problems expected.

Others:
- Advise any doctor or dentist whom you consult that you take melatonin.
- Melatonin is not researched carefully as yet, but there does not appear to be any particular problems. Some studies are promising as to its effect on health.
- Before starting melatonin, talk to your doctor about your sleep problems or try other things that can help sleep, such as avoidance of caffeine, chocolate, and especially, alcohol in any amount.

POSSIBLE INTERACTION WITH OTHER DRUGS

GENERIC NAME OR DRUG CLASS	COMBINED EFFECT
All medications	Effects are unknown. Talk to your doctor or pharmacist.

POSSIBLE INTERACTION WITH OTHER SUBSTANCES

INTERACTS WITH	COMBINED EFFECT
Alcohol:	Disrupts the night-time melatonin effect. Avoid.
Beverages:	None expected.
Cocaine:	Problems not known. Best to avoid.
Foods:	None expected.
Marijuana:	Problems not known. Best to avoid.
Tobacco:	Smoking can disrupt your normal melatonin cycle. Avoid.

MELOXICAM

BRAND NAMES

Mobic

BASIC INFORMATION

Habit forming? No
Prescription needed? Yes
Available as generic? Yes
Drug class: Nonsteroidal anti-inflammatory, antirheumatic

 ## USES

Treatment for joint pain, stiffness, inflammation and swelling of rheumatoid arthritis, osteoarthritis and gout.

 ## DOSAGE & USAGE INFORMATION

How to take:
Tablet—Swallow whole with liquid. May be taken with or without food.

When to take:
At the same time each day.

If you forget a dose:
Take as soon as you remember; however, if it is the next day, skip the missed dose and return to your normal schedule (don't double this dose).

What drug does:
Reduces tissue concentration of prostaglandins (hormones which produce inflammation and pain).

Continued next column

 ## OVERDOSE

SYMPTOMS:
Bloody or black tarry stools; blue lips, fingernails or skin; blurred vision; confusion; changes in urine color or output; difficulty swallowing or breathing; dizziness; fever; chest pain; slow or fast heartbeat; swelling; stomach pain; unusual tiredness or weakness; vomiting of blood or material that looks like coffee grounds; wheezing; yellow eyes or skin.
WHAT TO DO:
* **Dial 911 (emergency) for medical help or call poison control center 1-800-222-1222 for instructions.**
* **See emergency information on last 3 pages of this book.**

Time lapse before drug works:
Begins in 2 to 3 hours. May require 3 weeks of regular use for maximum benefit.

Don't take with:
Any other medicine or any dietary supplement without consulting your doctor or pharmacist.

 ## POSSIBLE ADVERSE REACTIONS OR SIDE EFFECTS

SYMPTOMS	WHAT TO DO
Life-threatening: Hives, rash, intense itching, faintness soon after a dose, breathing difficulties (anaphylaxis).	Seek emergency treatment immediately.
Common: Diarrhea, heartburn, indigestion, gas.	Continue. Call doctor when convenient.
Infrequent: Abdominal pain, anxiety, confusion, constipation, nausea, nervousness, sleepiness.	Continue. Call doctor when convenient.
Rare: Difficulty swallowing, swelling around the face, shortness of breath, tightness in chest, unusual tiredness or weakness, bloody or black tarry stools, vomiting, stomach pain.	Discontinue. Seek emergency treatment.

WARNINGS & PRECAUTIONS

Don't take if:
- You are allergic to aspirin or any other nonsteroidal anti-inflammatory drug (NSAIDs).
- You have nasal polyps.

Before you start, consult your doctor if:
- You have a history of alcohol abuse.
- You have bleeding problems or ulcers.
- You have any condition that causes fluid retention (heart problems or high blood pressure or dehydration).
- You have used tobacco recently.
- You have impaired kidney or liver function.
- You have asthma.

Over age 60:
No problems expected.

Pregnancy:
Decide with your doctor whether drug benefits justify risk to unborn child. Risk category C (see page xviii).

Breast-feeding:
Animal studies show the drug passes into milk. Avoid drug or discontinue nursing until you finish medicine. Consult doctor for advice on maintaining milk supply.

Infants & children:
Not recommended for anyone younger than 18.

Prolonged use:
Talk to your doctor about the need for follow-up medical exams or laboratory studies to check complete blood counts, liver function, stools for blood, and eyes.

Skin & sunlight:
No problems expected.

Driving, piloting or hazardous work:
Don't drive or pilot aircraft until you learn how medicine affects you. Don't work around dangerous machinery. Don't climb ladders or work in high places. Danger increases if you drink alcohol or take medicine affecting alertness and reflexes, such as antihistamines, tranquilizers, sedatives, pain medicine, narcotics and mind-altering drugs.

Discontinuing:
No problems expected. If drug has been taken for a long time, consult doctor before discontinuing.

Others:
- May affect results in some medical tests.
- Advise any doctor or dentist whom you consult that you take this medicine.
- Do not refrigerate.
- Do not store in the bathroom, near the kitchen sink or in other damp places.

POSSIBLE INTERACTION WITH OTHER DRUGS

GENERIC NAME OR DRUG CLASS	COMBINED EFFECT
Angiotensin-converting enzyme (ACE) inhibitors*	May decrease ACE inhibitor effect.
Anti-inflammatory drugs, nonsteroidal (NSAIDs)* other	Increased risk of side effects.
Aspirin	Increased risk of stomach ulcer.
Furosemide	Decreased effect of furosemide.
Lithium	Increased lithium effect.
Warfarin	Increased risk of bleeding problems.

POSSIBLE INTERACTION WITH OTHER SUBSTANCES

INTERACTS WITH	COMBINED EFFECT
Alcohol:	Possible stomach ulcer or bleeding. Avoid.
Beverages:	None expected.
Cocaine:	None expected. Best to avoid.
Foods:	None expected.
Marijuana:	Increased pain relief from NSAIDs.
Tobacco:	Possible stomach ulcer or bleeding.

MELPHALAN

BRAND NAMES

Alkeran

L-PAM

Phenylalanine

Mustard

BASIC INFORMATION

Habit forming? No
Prescription needed? Yes
Available as generic? No
Drug class: Antineoplastic

 ## USES

Treatment for certain types of cancer.

 ## DOSAGE & USAGE INFORMATION

How to take:
* Tablet—Swallow with a full glass of water to help prevent vomiting. Take on an empty stomach, 1 hour before or 2 hours after a meal. If vomiting occurs shortly after taking a dose, consult your doctor for advice.
* IV form—Is given by medical professional.

When to take:
As directed by your doctor. The dosage regimen is individualized. The drug is usually taken for several weeks to start and then followed by a drug rest period for up to 4 weeks.

If you forget a dose:
Skip the missed dose and return to your regular schedule. Don't ever double doses. Consult doctor if you have questions.

What drug does:
It interferes with the growth of cancer cells and causes them to die.

Time lapse before drug works:
May be gradual over weeks or months before your response to the drug can be determined.

Don't take with:
Any other medicine or any dietary supplement without consulting your doctor or pharmacist.

 ## OVERDOSE

SYMPTOMS:
Nausea, vomiting, diarrhea, intestinal bleeding.
WHAT TO DO:
Dial 911 (emergency) for medical help or call poison control center 1-800-222-1222 for instructions.

 ## POSSIBLE ADVERSE REACTIONS OR SIDE EFFECTS

SYMPTOMS	WHAT TO DO
Life-threatening: None expected.	
Common: Nausea and vomiting.	Continue. Call doctor when convenient.
Infrequent: Fever or chills occur with other symptoms (e.g., back or side pain; painful or difficult urination; cough or hoarseness), stools are bloody or tarry or black, bloody urine, fast or irregular heartbeat, small-red spots on skin, shortness of breath, sudden skin rash or itching, troubled breathing, unusual bleeding or bruising, ongoing nausea or vomiting.	Continue, but call doctor right away. Seek emergency care if symptoms are more severe.
Rare: • Mouth or lip sores, difficulty swallowing, joint pain, diarrhea, arms or legs become sore or red, feet or lower legs are swollen, unusual lumps or masses, yellow skin or eyes.	Continue, but call doctor right away.
• Menstrual periods stop, weight loss, other side effects not listed.	Continue. Call doctor when convenient.

WARNINGS & PRECAUTIONS

Don't take if:
* You are allergic to melphalan or prior use of the drug has been ineffective.
* Your doctor has not explained the benefits and risks of taking this medicine.

Before you start, consult your doctor if:
* You have gout.
* You have had kidney stones.
* You have impaired kidney or liver function.
* You have taken other anticancer drugs or had radiation treatment in last 3 weeks.
* You have herpes zoster (shingles) or chicken pox (or been exposed).
* You have heart disease, congestive heart failure or other forms of cancer.
* You have bone marrow depression.
* You have an active infection.

Over age 60:
Adverse reactions and side effects may be more frequent and severe than in younger persons.

Pregnancy:
* Consult doctor. Risk category D (see page xviii).
* This drug may cause birth defects if either the male or female is taking it at the time of conception or if it is taken during pregnancy.

Breast-feeding:
It is unknown if drug passes into milk. Breast-feeding is not recommended while you are taking this drug. Consult doctor.

Infants & children:
Safety and effectiveness in this age group have not been established.

Prolonged use:
* Adverse reactions may be more likely the longer drug is required.
* Talk to your doctor about the need for follow-up medical examinations or laboratory studies to check complete blood counts, kidney function and drug's effectiveness.

Skin & sunlight:
No problems expected.

Driving, piloting or hazardous work:
Use caution until you determine how drug affects you.

Discontinuing:
* Don't discontinue without doctor's advice until you complete prescribed dose.
* Some side effects may follow discontinuing. Report to doctor blurred vision, convulsions, confusion, persistent headache, fever or chills, blood in urine, unusual bleeding or other unexpected symptoms.

Others:
* Can cause sterility which could be permanent.
* Your doctor may advise you to drink extra fluids so that you pass more urine (helps prevent kidney problems).
* The drug increases risk for infections and other malignancies. Consult doctor if you develop new or unexpected symptoms.
* Do not have any immunizations (vaccinations) without doctor's approval. Avoid persons who have taken oral polio vaccine within the last several months.
* Advise any doctor or dentist whom you consult that you take this medicine.

POSSIBLE INTERACTION WITH OTHER DRUGS

GENERIC NAME OR DRUG CLASS	COMBINED EFFECT
None expected	With use of tablet (oral) form of melphalan, but do consult your doctor about any other drugs you take.

POSSIBLE INTERACTION WITH OTHER SUBSTANCES

INTERACTS WITH	COMBINED EFFECT
Alcohol:	None expected.
Beverages:	None expected.
Cocaine:	Unknown. Avoid.
Foods:	None expected.
Marijuana:	Unknown. Avoid.
Tobacco:	Unknown. Avoid.

*See Glossary

MEMANTINE

BRAND NAMES

Namenda   Namenda Oral
                           Solution

BASIC INFORMATION

Habit forming? No
Prescription needed? Yes
Available as generic? No
Drug class: N-methyl-D-aspartate (NMDA)
   receptor antagonist

 ## USES

Treats the symptoms of moderate to severe
Alzheimer's disease. Alzheimer's is a
progressive disease of the brain. Memantine
may be used alone or in combination with other
drugs for Alzheimer's.

 ## DOSAGE & USAGE INFORMATION

How to take:
* Tablet—Swallow with liquid. It may be taken
  with or without food.
* Oral solution—Follow the detailed directions
  provided with the prescription.

When to take:
Once or twice day at the same times each day. A
caregiver should monitor usage.

If you forget a dose:
Take as soon as possible. If it is almost time for
your next dose, skip the missed dose and go
back to the regular dosing schedule. Do not
double doses.

What drug does:
Blocks excess amounts of a brain chemical
called glutamate that can damage or kill nerve
cells. It does not cure Alzheimer's disease or
treat the underlying cause.

Time lapse before drug works:
Improvement may be seen in weeks, but may
take months for maximum benefits. Dosage of
the drug may be increased in one week time
periods for the first few weeks.

Continued next column

 ## OVERDOSE

SYMPTOMS:
Unknown effects.
WHAT TO DO:
If an overdose is suspected, call the doctor
or call poison control center 1-800-222-1222
for help.

Don't take with:
Any other medicine or any dietary supplement
without consulting your doctor or pharmacist.

 ## POSSIBLE ADVERSE REACTIONS OR SIDE EFFECTS

SYMPTOMS	WHAT TO DO
Life-threatening: None expected.	
Common: None expected.	
Infrequent: Dizziness, headache, constipation, confusion.	Continue. Call doctor when convenient.
Rare: Fatigue, back pain, vomiting, sleepiness, high blood pressure. Other symptoms that occur. They may be due to progression of the disease or may be due to the drug.	Continue. Call doctor when convenient.

WARNINGS & PRECAUTIONS

Don't take if:
You are allergic to memantine or its components.

Before you start, consult your doctor if:
• You have kidney, liver or heart problems.
• You have a seizure disorder.
• You are allergic to any medication, food or other substance.

Over age 60:
No special problems expected.

Pregnancy:
Decide with your doctor if drug benefits justify risks to unborn child. Risk category B (see page xviii).

Breast-feeding:
This drug is usually not prescribed for reproductive-age women. It is unknown if drug passes into milk. Consult your doctor.

Infants & children:
Not recommended for this age group.

Prolonged use:
Visit the doctor regularly to determine if the drug is continuing to be effective.

Skin & sunlight:
No special problems expected.

Driving, piloting or hazardous work:
Avoid if you feel dizzy, drowsy or confused.

Discontinuing:
No problems expected. Consult doctor.

Others:
• Advise any doctor or dentist whom the patient consults about the use of this medicine.
• The effects of the drug will differ for different patients. Some patients will improve, others may stay the same, and others continue to deteriorate (get worse).

POSSIBLE INTERACTION WITH OTHER DRUGS

GENERIC NAME OR DRUG CLASS	COMBINED EFFECT
Amantadine	May lead to adverse effects of either drug.
Carbonic anhydrase inhibitors	Increased effect of memantine.
Dextromethorphan	May lead to adverse effects of either drug.
Histamine H$_2$ receptor antagonists	Increased effect of either drug.
Hydrochlorothiazide	Increased effect of both drugs.
Sodium bicarbonate	Increased effect of memantine.
Triamterene	Increased effect of either drug.

POSSIBLE INTERACTION WITH OTHER SUBSTANCES

INTERACTS WITH	COMBINED EFFECT
Alcohol:	None expected. Best to avoid.
Beverages:	None expected.
Cocaine:	Unknown. Best to avoid.
Foods:	None expected.
Marijuana:	Unknown. Best to avoid.
Tobacco:	None expected.

*See Glossary

MEPROBAMATE

BRAND NAMES

See full list of brand names in the *Generic and Brand Name Directory*, page 890.

BASIC INFORMATION

Habit forming? Yes
Prescription needed? Yes
Available as generic? Yes
Drug class: Tranquilizer, antianxiety agent

 ## USES

Reduces mild anxiety, tension and insomnia.

 ## DOSAGE & USAGE INFORMATION

How to take:
• Tablet—Swallow with liquid.
• Extended-release capsule—Swallow each dose whole.

When to take:
At the same times each day.

If you forget a dose:
Take as soon as you remember up to 2 hours late. If more than 2 hours, wait for next scheduled dose (don't double this dose).

What drug does:
Sedates brain centers that control behavior and emotions.

Time lapse before drug works:
1 to 2 hours.

Don't take with:
• Nonprescription drugs containing alcohol or caffeine without consulting doctor.
• Any other medicine or any dietary supplement without consulting your doctor or pharmacist.

 ## OVERDOSE

SYMPTOMS:
Dizziness, slurred speech, stagger, confusion, depressed breathing and heart function, stupor, coma.
WHAT TO DO:
• **Dial 911 (emergency) for medical help or call poison control center 1-800-222-1222 for instructions.**
• **See emergency information on last 3 pages of this book.**

 ## POSSIBLE ADVERSE REACTIONS OR SIDE EFFECTS

SYMPTOMS	WHAT TO DO
Life-threatening:	
Hives, rash, intense itching, faintness soon after a dose, wheezing (anaphylaxis).	Seek emergency treatment immediately.
Common:	
Dizziness, confusion, agitation, drowsiness, unsteadiness, fatigue, weakness.	Continue. Tell doctor at next visit.
Infrequent:	
• Rash, hives, itchy skin; change in vision; diarrhea, nausea or vomiting, slurred speech, blurred vision.	Discontinue. Call doctor right away.
• False sense of well-being, headache.	Continue. Call doctor when convenient.
Rare:	
Sore throat; fever; rapid, pounding, unusually slow or irregular heartbeat; difficult breathing; unusual bleeding or bruising.	Discontinue. Call doctor right away.

WARNINGS & PRECAUTIONS

Don't take if:
You are allergic to meprobamate, tybamate, carbromal or carisoprodol.

Before you start, consult your doctor if:
- You have epilepsy.
- You have impaired liver or kidney function.
- You have tartrazine dye allergy.
- You suffer from drug abuse or alcoholism, active or in remission.
- You have porphyria.

Over age 60:
Adverse reactions and side effects may be more frequent and severe than in younger persons.

Pregnancy:
Risk to unborn child outweighs drug benefits. Don't use. Risk category D (see page xviii).

Breast-feeding:
Drug passes into milk. May cause sedation in child. Avoid drug or discontinue nursing until you finish medicine. Consult doctor for advice on maintaining milk supply.

Infants & children:
Not recommended.

Prolonged use:
- Habit forming.
- May impair blood cell production.

Skin & sunlight:
No problems expected.

Driving, piloting or hazardous work:
Don't drive or pilot aircraft until you learn how medicine affects you. Don't work around dangerous machinery. Don't climb ladders or work in high places. Danger increases if you drink alcohol or take medicine affecting alertness and reflexes, such as antihistamines, tranquilizers, sedatives, pain medicine, narcotics and mind-altering drugs.

Discontinuing:
Don't discontinue without consulting doctor. Dose may require gradual reduction if you have taken drug for a long time. Doses of other drugs may also require adjustment. Report to your doctor any unusual symptom that begins in the first week you discontinue this medicine. These symptoms may include convulsions, confusion, nightmares, insomnia.

Others:
- Advise any doctor or dentist whom you consult that you take this drug.
- For dry mouth, suck sugarless hard candy or chew sugarless gum. If dry mouth persists, consult your dentist.

POSSIBLE INTERACTION WITH OTHER DRUGS

GENERIC NAME OR DRUG CLASS	COMBINED EFFECT
Addictive drugs*	Increased risk of addictive effect.
Antidepressants, tricyclic*	Increased anti-depressant effect.
Antihistamines*	Possible excessive sedation.
Central nervous system (CNS) depressants*	Increased depressive effects of both drugs.
Monoamine oxidase (MAO) inhibitors*	Increased meprobamate effect.
Narcotics*	Increased narcotic effect.
Sertraline	Increased depressive effects of both drugs.

POSSIBLE INTERACTION WITH OTHER SUBSTANCES

INTERACTS WITH	COMBINED EFFECT
Alcohol:	Dangerous increased effect of meprobamate.
Beverages: Caffeine drinks.	Decreased calming effect of meprobamate.
Cocaine:	Decreased meprobamate effect.
Foods:	None expected.
Marijuana:	Increased sedative effect of meprobamate.
Tobacco:	None expected.

MERCAPTOPURINE

BRAND NAMES

6-MP   Purinethol

BASIC INFORMATION

Habit forming? No
Prescription needed? Yes
Available as generic? Yes
Drug class: Antineoplastic,
immunosuppressant

 USES

- Treatment for some kinds of cancer.
- Treatment for regional enteritis and ulcerative colitis and other immune disorders.

 DOSAGE & USAGE INFORMATION

How to take:
Tablet—Swallow with liquid.

When to take:
At the same time each day.

If you forget a dose:
Skip the missed dose. Don't double the next dose.

What drug does:
Inhibits abnormal cell reproduction.

Time lapse before drug works:
May require 6 weeks for maximum effect.

Don't take with:
Any other medicine or any dietary supplement without consulting your doctor or pharmacist.

 OVERDOSE

SYMPTOMS:
Headache, stupor, seizures.
WHAT TO DO:
- **Dial 911 (emergency) for medical help or call poison control center 1-800-222-1222 for instructions.**
- **If person is unconscious, check breathing and pulse. If not breathing, begin mouth-to-mouth rescue breathing. If heart is not beating, begin chest compressions.**
- **See emergency information on last 3 pages of this book.**

 POSSIBLE ADVERSE REACTIONS OR SIDE EFFECTS

SYMPTOMS	WHAT TO DO
Life-threatening:	
In case of overdose, see previous column.	
Common:	
• Black stools or bloody vomit.	Discontinue. Seek emergency treatment.
• Mouth sores, sore throat, unusual bleeding or bruising.	Discontinue. Call doctor right away.
• Abdominal pain, nausea, vomiting, weakness, tiredness.	Continue. Call doctor when convenient.
Infrequent:	
• Seizures.	Discontinue. Seek emergency treatment.
• Diarrhea, headache, confusion, blurred vision, shortness of breath, joint pain, blood in urine, jaundice, back pain, appetite loss, feet and leg swelling.	Discontinue. Call doctor right away.
• Cough.	Continue. Call doctor when convenient.
• Acne, boils, hair loss, itchy skin.	Continue. Tell doctor at next visit.
Rare:	
Fever and chills.	Discontinue. Call doctor right away.

 WARNINGS & PRECAUTIONS

Don't take if:
You are allergic to any antineoplastic.

Before you start, consult your doctor if:
- You are an alcoholic.
- You have blood, liver or kidney disease.
- You have colitis or peptic ulcer.
- You have gout.
- You have an infection.
- You plan to become pregnant within 3 months.

Over age 60:
Adverse reactions and side effects may be more frequent and severe than in younger persons.

Pregnancy:
Risk to unborn child outweighs drug benefits. Don't use. Risk category D (see page xviii).

Breast-feeding:
Avoid drug or discontinue nursing.

Infants & children:
Use only under special medical supervision.

Prolonged use:
* Adverse reactions more likely the longer drug is required.
* Talk to your doctor about the need for follow-up medical examinations or laboratory studies to check complete blood counts (white blood cell count, platelet count, red blood cell count, hemoglobin, hematocrit), liver function, kidney function, uric acid.

Skin & sunlight:
No problems expected.

Driving, piloting or hazardous work:
Avoid if you feel dizzy, drowsy or confused. Otherwise, no problems expected.

Discontinuing:
Don't discontinue without doctor's advice until you complete prescribed dose, even though symptoms diminish or disappear. Some side effects may follow discontinuing. Report to doctor blurred vision, convulsions, confusion, persistent headache, chills or fever, bloody urine or stools, back pain, jaundice.

Others:
* Drink more fluid than usual so you will have more frequent urination.
* Don't give this medicine to anyone else for any purpose. It is a strong drug that requires close medical supervision.
* Advise any doctor or dentist whom you consult that you take this medicine.
* Report for frequent medical follow-up and laboratory studies.

 ## POSSIBLE INTERACTION WITH OTHER DRUGS

GENERIC NAME OR DRUG CLASS	COMBINED EFFECT
Acetaminophen	Increased likelihood of liver toxicity.
Anticoagulants,* oral	May increase or decrease anticoagulant effect.
Antineoplastic drugs,* other	Increased effect of both (may be desirable) or increased toxicity of each.
Chloramphenicol	Increased toxicity of each.
Clozapine	Toxic effect on bone marrow.
Cyclosporine	May increase risk of infection.
Hepatotoxic drugs*	Increased risk of liver toxicity.
Immunosuppressants,* other	Increased risk of infections and neoplasms.*
Isoniazid	Increased risk of liver damage.
Levamisole	Increased risk of bone marrow depression.
Lovastatin	Increased heart and kidney damage.
Probenecid	Increased toxic effect of mercaptopurine.
Sulfinpyrazone	Increased toxic effect of mercaptopurine.
Tiopronin	Increased risk of toxicity to bone marrow.
Vaccines, live or killed	Increased risk of toxicity or reduced effectiveness of vaccine.

 ## POSSIBLE INTERACTION WITH OTHER SUBSTANCES

INTERACTS WITH	COMBINED EFFECT
Alcohol:	May increase chance of intestinal bleeding.
Beverages:	None expected.
Cocaine:	Increased chance of toxicity.
Foods:	Reduced irritation in stomach.
Marijuana:	None expected.
Tobacco:	Increased lung toxicity.

MESALAMINE

BRAND NAMES

5-ASA	Mesalazine
Apriso	Pentasa
Asacol	Rowasa
Canasa	Salofalk
Lialda	

BASIC INFORMATION

Habit forming? No
Prescription needed? Yes
Available as generic? Yes
Drug class: Anti-inflammatory (nonsteroidal)

 USES

- Treats ulcerative colitis.
- Reduces inflammatory conditions of the lower colon and rectum.

 DOSAGE & USAGE INFORMATION

How to use:
- Rectal—Use as an enema. Insert the tip of the pre-packaged medicine container into the rectum. Squeeze container to empty contents. Retain in rectum all night or as long as possible.
- Rectal suppository—Follow instructions on package.
- Delayed-release tablet or extended-release capsule—Swallow with liquid. Do not crush or chew tablet or open capsule. Take Lialda brand with food.

Continued next column

 OVERDOSE

SYMPTOMS:
Confusion, severe diarrhea, lightheadedness or dizziness, severe sleepiness, severe headache, ringing or buzzing in ears, hearing loss, nausea and vomiting, sweating, fast or deep breathing.
WHAT TO DO:
- Dial 911 (emergency) for medical help or call poison control center 1-800-222-1222 for instructions.
- See emergency information on last 3 pages of this book.

When to use:
- Rectal—Each night, preferably after a bowel movement. Continue for 3 to 6 weeks according to your doctor's instructions.
- Rectal suppository—Use 1-3 times a day according to doctor's instructions.
- Oral forms—Follow instructions on label. It may be once-a-day dose or 3 to 4 times a day as directed by doctor.

If you forget a dose:
Take or use as soon as you remember. If it is almost time for the next dose, wait for next scheduled dose (don't double this dose).

What drug does:
It works in the intestinal tract to reduce inflammation and also helps keep the disorder in remission and prevent relapses.

Time lapse before drug works:
3 to 21 days.

Don't take with:
- Oral sulfasalazine concurrently. To do so may increase chances of kidney damage.
- Any other medicine or any dietary supplement without consulting your doctor or pharmacist.

 POSSIBLE ADVERSE REACTIONS OR SIDE EFFECTS

SYMPTOMS	WHAT TO DO
Life-threatening:	
None expected.	
Common:	
None expected.	
Infrequent:	
None expected.	
Rare:	
• Abdominal pain, bloody diarrhea, fever, skin rash, anal irritation, chest pain, shortness of breath.	Discontinue. Call doctor right away.
• Gaseousness, nausea, headache, mild hair loss, diarrhea.	Continue. Call doctor when convenient.

WARNINGS & PRECAUTIONS

Don't take if:
You are allergic to salicylates* or any medication containing sulfasalazine (such as Azulfidine) or mesalamine.

Before you start, consult your doctor if:
- You have had chronic kidney disease.
- You have pancreatitis.
- You have heart inflammation (pericarditis).

Over age 60:
More sensitive to drug. Aggravates symptoms of enlarged prostate. Causes impaired thinking, hallucinations, nightmares. Consult doctor about any of these.

Pregnancy:
Consult doctor. Risk category B (see page xviii).

Breast-feeding:
It is unknown if drug passes into milk. Avoid nursing until you finish medicine. Consult doctor for advice on maintaining milk supply.

Infants & children:
Use for children only under doctor's supervision.

Prolonged use:
Talk to your doctor about the need for follow-up medical examinations or laboratory studies to check urine.

Skin & sunlight:
No problems expected.

Driving, piloting or hazardous work:
Don't drive or pilot aircraft until you learn how medicine affects you. Don't work around dangerous machinery. Don't climb ladders or work in high places. Danger increases if you drink alcohol or take medicine affecting alertness and reflexes.

Discontinuing:
Don't discontinue without consulting doctor. Dose may require gradual reduction if you have taken drug for a long time. Doses of other drugs may also require adjustment.

Others:
- Internal eye pressure should be measured regularly.
- Canasa may stain things it touches.

POSSIBLE INTERACTION WITH OTHER DRUGS

GENERIC NAME OR DRUG CLASS	COMBINED EFFECT
Antacids*	Affects the dosage of brand name Apriso. Avoid.

POSSIBLE INTERACTION WITH OTHER SUBSTANCES

INTERACTS WITH	COMBINED EFFECT
Alcohol:	None expected.
Beverages:	None expected.
Cocaine:	None expected.
Foods:	None expected.
Marijuana:	None expected.
Tobacco:	None expected.

METFORMIN

BRAND NAMES

ACTOplus met	Glumetza
Avandamet	Janumet
Fortamet	Metaglip
Glucophage	PrandiMet
Glucovance	Riomet

BASIC INFORMATION

Habit forming? No
Prescription needed? Yes
Available as generic? Yes
Drug class: Antihyperglycemic, antidiabetic

 ## USES

Treatment for hyperglycemia (excess sugar in the blood) that cannot be controlled by diet alone in patients with diabetes type 2.

 ## DOSAGE & USAGE INFORMATION

How to take:
- Tablet—Swallow with liquid. Take with food.
- Extended release tablet—Swallow whole. Do not break, crush or chew before swallowing. Take with food.
- Oral solution—Follow product instructions.

Continued next column

 ## OVERDOSE

SYMPTOMS:
- **Symptoms of lactic acidosis (acid in the blood)—chills, diarrhea, fatigue, muscle pain, sleepiness, slow heartbeat, breathing difficulty, unusual weakness.**
- **Symptoms of hypoglycemia (low blood sugar)—stomach pain, anxious feeling, cold sweats, chills, confusion, convulsions, cool pale skin, excessive hunger, nausea or vomiting, rapid heartbeat, nervousness, shakiness, unsteady walk, unusual weakness or tiredness, vision changes, unconsciousness.**

WHAT TO DO:
- **For symptoms of lactic acidosis, call doctor immediately.**
- **For mild low blood sugar symptoms, drink or eat something containing sugar right away.**
- **For more severe symptoms, dial 911 (emergency) for medical help or call poison control center 1-800-222-1222 for instructions.**
- **See emergency information on last 3 pages of this book.**

When to take:
Usually 1 to 3 times a day as directed by doctor. Take with meals to lessen stomach irritation. Dosage may be increased on a weekly basis until maximum benefits are achieved.

If you forget a dose:
Take as soon as you remember. If it is almost time for the next dose, skip the missed dose and wait for your next scheduled dose (don't double this dose).

What drug does:
Helps to lower blood sugar when it is too high. Treats the symptoms of diabetes, but does not cure it.

Time lapse before drug works:
May take several weeks for full effectiveness.

Don't take with:
Any other medicine or any dietary supplement without consulting your doctor or pharmacist.

 ## POSSIBLE ADVERSE REACTIONS OR SIDE EFFECTS

SYMPTOMS	WHAT TO DO
Life-threatening: In case of overdose or low blood sugar, see previous column.	
Common:	
• Stomach pain, diarrhea, vomiting.	Continue, but call doctor right away.
• Decreased appetite, changes in taste, gas, headache, weight loss, feeling of fullness or stomach discomfort, nausea.	Continue. Call doctor when convenient.
Infrequent: None expected.	
Rare:	
Lactic acidosis or severe low blood sugar (see symptoms under Overdose).	Discontinue. Call doctor right away or seek emergency help.

 ## WARNINGS & PRECAUTIONS

Don't take if:
You are allergic to metformin.

Before you start, consult your doctor if:
- You have any kidney or liver disease or any heart or blood vessel disorder.
- You have any chronic health problem.
- You have an infection, illness or any condition that can cause low blood sugar.
- You have a history of acid in the blood (metabolic acidosis or ketoacidosis).

METFORMIN

- You are allergic to any medication, food or other substance.

Over age 60:
No special problems expected. A lower starting dosage may be recommended by your doctor.

Pregnancy:
Decide with your doctor if drug benefits justify risks to unborn child. Risk category B (see page xviii).

Breast-feeding:
Drug passes into milk. Avoid drug or discontinue nursing until you finish medicine. Consult doctor for advice on maintaining milk supply.

Infants & children:
Safety and efficacy have not been established. Use only under close medical supervision.

Prolonged use:
- Schedule regular doctor visits to determine if the drug is continuing to be effective in controlling the diabetes and to check for any problems in kidney function.
- You will most likely require an antidiabetic medicine for the rest of your life.
- You will need to test your blood glucose levels several times a day, or for some, once to several times a week.

Skin & sunlight:
No special problems expected.

Driving, piloting or hazardous work:
No special problems expected.

Discontinuing:
Don't discontinue without consulting your doctor, even if you feel well. You can have diabetes without feeling any symptoms. Untreated diabetes can cause serious problems.

Others:
- Advise any doctor or dentist whom you consult that you take this medicine. Drug may interfere with the accuracy of some medical tests.
- Follow any special diet your doctor may prescribe. It can help control diabetes.
- Consult doctor if you become ill with vomiting or diarrhea.
- Use caution when exercising. Ask your doctor about an appropriate exercise program.
- Wear medical identification stating that you have diabetes and take this medication.
- Learn to recognize the symptoms of low blood sugar. You and your family need to know what to do if these symptoms occur.
- Have a glucagon kit and syringe in the event severe low blood sugar occurs. Carry a quick-acting sugar to treat symptoms of mild low blood sugar.
- High blood sugar (hyperglycemia) may occur with diabetes. Ask your doctor about symptoms to watch for and treatment steps to take.

- This drug may be discontinued temporarily prior to x-ray studies or some surgeries.
- Educate yourself about diabetes.

 POSSIBLE INTERACTION WITH OTHER DRUGS

GENERIC NAME OR DRUG CLASS	COMBINED EFFECT
Amiloride	Increased metformin effect.
Calcium channel blockers*	Increased metformin effect.
Cimetidine	Increased metformin effect.
Dexfenfluramine	May require dosage change as weight loss occurs.
Digoxin	Increased metformin effect.
Dofetilide	Increased dofetilide effect.
Furosemide	Increased metformin effect.
Hyperglycemia-causing medications*	Increased risk of hyperglycemia.
Hypoglycemia-causing medications*	Increased risk of hypoglycemia.
Morphine	Increased metformin effect.
Procainamide	Increased metformin effect.
Quinidine	Increased metformin effect.

Continued on page 922

 POSSIBLE INTERACTION WITH OTHER SUBSTANCES

INTERACTS WITH	COMBINED EFFECT
Alcohol:	Increased effect of metformin. Avoid excessive amounts.
Beverages:	None expected.
Cocaine:	None expected.
Foods:	None expected.
Marijuana:	None expected.
Tobacco:	None expected.

*See Glossary

METHENAMINE

BRAND NAMES

Hiprex   **Urex**
Mandelamine

BASIC INFORMATION

Habit forming? No
Prescription needed? Yes
Available as generic? Yes
Drug class: Anti-infective (urinary)

 ## USES

Suppresses chronic urinary tract infections.

 ## DOSAGE & USAGE INFORMATION

How to take:
* Tablet—Swallow with liquid or food to lessen stomach irritation. If you can't swallow whole, crumble tablet and take with liquid or food. If enteric-coated tablet, swallow whole.
* Liquid form—Use a measuring spoon to ensure correct dose.
* Granules—Dissolve dose in 4 oz. of water. Drink all the liquid.

When to take:
At the same times each day.

If you forget a dose:
Take as soon as you remember up to 8 hours late. If more than 8 hours, wait for next scheduled dose (don't double this dose).

What drug does:
A chemical reaction in the urine changes methenamine into formaldehyde, which destroys certain bacteria.

Time lapse before drug works:
Continual use for 3 to 6 months.

Continued next column

 ## OVERDOSE

SYMPTOMS:
Bloody urine, weakness, deep breathing, stupor, coma.
WHAT TO DO:
* **Dial 911 (emergency) for medical help or call poison control center 1-800-222-1222 for instructions.**
* **See emergency information on last 3 pages of this book.**

Don't take with:
Any other medicine or any dietary supplement without consulting your doctor or pharmacist.

 ## POSSIBLE ADVERSE REACTIONS OR SIDE EFFECTS

SYMPTOMS	WHAT TO DO
Life-threatening:	
In case of overdose, see previous column.	
Common:	
• Rash.	Discontinue. Call doctor right away.
• Nausea, difficult urination.	Continue. Call doctor when convenient.
Infrequent:	
• Blood in urine.	Discontinue. Call doctor right away.
• Burning on urination, lower back pain.	Continue. Call doctor when convenient.
Rare:	
None expected.	

WARNINGS & PRECAUTIONS

Don't take if:
- You are allergic to methenamine.
- You have a severe impairment of kidney or liver function.
- Your urine cannot or should not be acidified (check with your doctor).

Before you start, consult your doctor if:
- You have had kidney or liver disease.
- You plan to become pregnant within medication period.
- You have had gout.

Over age 60:
Don't exceed recommended dose.

Pregnancy:
Decide with your doctor if drug benefits justify risk to unborn child. Risk category C (see page xviii).

Breast-feeding:
Drug passes into milk in small amounts. Consult doctor.

Infants & children:
Use only under medical supervision.

Prolonged use:
No problems expected.

Skin & sunlight:
No problems expected.

Driving, piloting or hazardous work:
No problems expected.

Discontinuing:
Don't discontinue without doctor's advice until you complete prescribed dose, even though symptoms diminish or disappear.

Others:
- Requires an acid urine to be effective. Eat more protein foods, cranberries, cranberry juice with vitamin C, plums, prunes.
- Advise any doctor or dentist whom you consult that you take this medicine.

POSSIBLE INTERACTION WITH OTHER DRUGS

GENERIC NAME OR DRUG CLASS	COMBINED EFFECT
Antacids*	Decreased methenamine effect.
Carbonic anhydrase inhibitors*	Decreased methenamine effect.
Citrates*	Decreases effects of methenamine.
Diuretics, thiazide*	Decreased urine acidity.
Sodium bicarbonate	Decreased methenamine effect.
Sulfadoxine and pyrimethamine	Increased risk of kidney toxicity.
Sulfa drugs*	Possible kidney damage.

POSSIBLE INTERACTION WITH OTHER SUBSTANCES

INTERACTS WITH	COMBINED EFFECT
Alcohol:	Possible brain depression. Avoid or use with caution.
Beverages: Milk and other dairy products.	Decreased methenamine effect.
Cocaine:	None expected.
Foods: Citrus, cranberries, plums, prunes.	Increased methenamine effect.
Marijuana:	Drowsiness, muscle weakness or blood pressure drop.
Tobacco:	None expected.

METHOTREXATE

BRAND NAMES

Amethopterin
Folex
Folex PFS
Mexate

Mexate AQ
Rheumatrex
Trexall

BASIC INFORMATION

Habit forming? No
Prescription needed? Yes
Available as generic? Yes
Drug class: Antimetabolite, antipsoriatic

 ## USES

* Treatment for certain types of cancer.
* Treatment for psoriasis in patients with severe problems.
* Treatment for severe rheumatoid arthritis.

 ## DOSAGE & USAGE INFORMATION

How to take:
* Tablet—Swallow with liquid.
* Injectable form—Is sometimes self-injected or used as an oral dose; consult doctor.

When to take:
At the same time each day.

If you forget a dose:
Skip the missed dose. Don't double the next dose.

What drug does:
Inhibits abnormal cell reproduction.

Time lapse before drug works:
May require 6 weeks for maximum effect.

Don't take with:
Any other medicine or any dietary supplement without consulting your doctor or pharmacist.

 ## OVERDOSE

SYMPTOMS:
Headache, stupor, seizures.
WHAT TO DO:
* Dial 911 (emergency) for medical help or call poison control center 1-800-222-1222 for instructions.
* If person is unconscious, check breathing and pulse. If not breathing, begin mouth-to-mouth rescue breathing. If heart is not beating, begin chest compressions.
* See emergency information on last 3 pages of this book.

 ## POSSIBLE ADVERSE REACTIONS OR SIDE EFFECTS

SYMPTOMS	WHAT TO DO
Life-threatening:	
Hives, rash, intense itching, faintness soon after a dose (anaphylaxis).	Seek emergency treatment immediately.
Common:	
• Black stools or bloody vomit.	Discontinue. Seek emergency treatment.
• Sore throat, fever, mouth sores; chills; unusual bleeding or bruising.	Discontinue. Call doctor right away.
• Abdominal pain, nausea, vomiting.	Continue. Call doctor when convenient.
Infrequent:	
• Seizures.	Discontinue. Seek emergency treatment.
• Dizziness when standing after sitting or lying, drowsiness, headache, confusion, blurred vision, shortness of breath, joint pain, blood in urine, jaundice, diarrhea, red skin, back pain.	Discontinue. Call doctor right away.
• Cough, rash, sexual difficulties in males.	Continue. Call doctor when convenient.
• Acne, boils, hair loss, itchy skin.	Continue. Tell doctor at next visit.
Rare:	
Painful urination.	Discontinue. Call doctor right away.

 ## WARNINGS & PRECAUTIONS

Don't take if:
You are allergic to any antimetabolite.

Before you start, consult your doctor if:
* You are an alcoholic.
* You have blood, liver or kidney disease.
* You have colitis or peptic ulcer.
* You have gout.
* You have an infection.
* You plan to become pregnant within 3 months.

Over age 60:
Adverse reactions and side effects may be more frequent and severe than in younger persons.

Pregnancy:
* Psoriasis—Risk to unborn child outweighs drug benefits. Don't use.
* Cancer—Consult doctor.
* Risk category X (see page xviii).

Breast-feeding:
Drug passes into milk. Avoid drug or discontinue nursing.

Infants & children:
Use only under special medical supervision.

Prolonged use:
* Adverse reactions more likely the longer drug is required.
* Talk to your doctor about the need for follow-up medical examinations or laboratory studies to check liver function, kidney function, complete blood counts (white blood cell count, platelet count, red blood cell count, hemoglobin, hematocrit).

Skin & sunlight:
May cause rash or intensify sunburn in areas exposed to sun or ultraviolet light (photosensitivity reaction). Avoid overexposure. Notify doctor if reaction occurs.

Driving, piloting or hazardous work:
Avoid if you feel dizzy, drowsy or confused. Otherwise, no problems expected.

Discontinuing:
Don't discontinue without doctor's advice until you complete prescribed dose, even though symptoms diminish or disappear. Some side effects may follow discontinuing. Report to doctor—blurred vision, convulsions, confusion, persistent headache.

Others:
* Drink more water than usual to cause frequent urination.
* Don't give this medicine to anyone else for any purpose. It is a strong drug that requires close medical supervision.
* Report for frequent medical follow-up and laboratory studies.
* Advise any doctor or dentist whom you consult that you take this medicine.

 POSSIBLE INTERACTION WITH OTHER DRUGS

GENERIC NAME OR DRUG CLASS	COMBINED EFFECT
Anticoagulants,* oral	Increased anticoagulant effect.
Anticonvulsants,* hydantoin	Possible methotrexate toxicity.
Antigout drugs*	Decreased antigout effect. Toxic levels of methotrexate.
Anti-inflammatory drugs, nonsteroidal (NSAIDs)*	Possible increased methotrexate toxicity.
Asparaginase	Decreased methotrexate effect.
Bone marrow depressants,* other	Increased risk of bone marrow depression.
Clozapine	Toxic effect on bone marrow.
Diclofenac	May increase toxicity.
Etretinate	Increased chance of toxicity to liver.
Fluorouracil	Decreased methotrexate effect.
Folic acid	Possible decreased methotrexate effect.
Isoniazid	Increased risk of liver damage.
Leflunomide	Increased risk of side effects.
Leucovorin calcium	Decreased methotrexate toxicity.
Levamisole	Increased risk of bone marrow depression.
Oxyphenbutazone	Possible methotrexate toxicity.
Penicillins*	Increased risk of methotrexate toxicity.
Phenylbutazone	Possible methotrexate toxicity.

Continued on page 922

 POSSIBLE INTERACTION WITH OTHER SUBSTANCES

INTERACTS WITH	COMBINED EFFECT
Alcohol:	Likely liver damage. Avoid.
Beverages:	Extra fluid intake decreases chance of methotrexate toxicity.
Cocaine:	Increased chance of methotrexate adverse reactions. Avoid.
Foods:	None expected.
Marijuana:	None expected.
Tobacco:	None expected.

*See Glossary

METHYLERGONOVINE

BRAND NAMES

Methergine   Methylergometrine

BASIC INFORMATION

Habit forming? No
Prescription needed? Yes
Available as generic? No
Drug class: Ergot preparation (uterine stimulant)

USES

Retards excessive post-delivery bleeding.

DOSAGE & USAGE INFORMATION

How to take:
Tablet—Swallow with liquid or food to lessen stomach irritation.

When to take:
At the same times each day.

If you forget a dose:
Don't take missed dose and don't double next one. Wait for next scheduled dose.

What drug does:
Causes smooth muscle cells of uterine wall to contract and surround bleeding blood vessels of relaxed uterus.

Time lapse before drug works:
20 to 30 minutes.

Don't take with:
Any other medicine or any dietary supplement without consulting your doctor or pharmacist.

OVERDOSE

SYMPTOMS:
Vomiting, diarrhea, weak pulse, low blood pressure, dyspnea, angina, convulsions.
WHAT TO DO:
• Dial 911 (emergency) for medical help or call poison control center 1-800-222-1222 for instructions.
• If person is unconscious, check breathing and pulse. If not breathing, begin mouth-to-mouth rescue breathing. If heart is not beating, begin chest compressions.
• See emergency information on last 3 pages of this book.

POSSIBLE ADVERSE REACTIONS OR SIDE EFFECTS

SYMPTOMS	WHAT TO DO
Life-threatening:	
In case of overdose, see previous column.	
Common:	
Nausea, vomiting, severe lower abdominal menstrual-like cramps.	Discontinue. Call doctor right away.
Infrequent:	
• Confusion, ringing in ears, diarrhea, muscle cramps.	Discontinue. Call doctor right away.
• Unusual sweating.	Continue. Call doctor when convenient.
Rare:	
Sudden, severe headache; shortness of breath; chest pain; numb, cold hands and feet.	Discontinue. Seek emergency treatment.

WARNINGS & PRECAUTIONS

Don't take if:
You are allergic to any ergot preparation.

Before you start, consult your doctor if:
* You have coronary artery or blood vessel disease.
* You have liver or kidney disease.
* You have high blood pressure.
* You have postpartum infection.

Over age 60:
Not recommended.

Pregnancy:
Used only after delivery of baby.

Breast-feeding:
Drug passes into milk. Avoid drug or discontinue nursing until you finish medicine. Consult doctor for advice on maintaining milk supply.

Infants & children:
Not recommended.

Prolonged use:
Talk to your doctor about the need for follow-up medical examinations or laboratory studies to check blood pressure, ECG.*

Skin & sunlight:
No problems expected.

Driving, piloting or hazardous work:
No problems expected.

Discontinuing:
May be unnecessary to finish medicine. Follow doctor's instructions.

Others:
Drug should be used for short time only following childbirth or miscarriage.

POSSIBLE INTERACTION WITH OTHER DRUGS

GENERIC NAME OR DRUG CLASS	COMBINED EFFECT
Antianginals*	Possible vasospasm (peripheral and cardiac).
Ergot preparations,* other	Increased methylergonovine effect.

POSSIBLE INTERACTION WITH OTHER SUBSTANCES

INTERACTS WITH	COMBINED EFFECT
Alcohol:	None expected.
Beverages:	None expected.
Cocaine:	None expected.
Foods:	None expected.
Marijuana:	None expected.
Tobacco:	Decreased methylergonovine effect. Don't smoke.

METHYSERGIDE

BRAND NAMES

Sansert

BASIC INFORMATION

Habit forming? Yes
Prescription needed? Yes
Available as generic? No
Drug class: Vasoconstrictor

 USES

Prevents migraine and other recurring vascular headaches. Not for acute attack.

 DOSAGE & USAGE INFORMATION

How to take:
Tablet—Swallow with liquid or with food to lessen stomach irritation. If you can't swallow whole, crumble tablet and take with liquid or food.

When to take:
At the same times each day.

If you forget a dose:
Don't take missed dose. Wait for next scheduled dose (don't double this dose).

What drug does:
Blocks the action of serotonin, a chemical that constricts blood vessels.

Time lapse before drug works:
About 3 weeks.

Don't take with:
Any other medicine or any dietary supplement without consulting your doctor or pharmacist.

 OVERDOSE

SYMPTOMS:
Nausea, vomiting, abdominal pain, severe diarrhea, lack of coordination, extreme thirst.
WHAT TO DO:
Overdose unlikely to threaten life. If person uses much larger amount than prescribed or if accidentally swallowed, call doctor or poison control center 1-800-222-1222 for help.

 POSSIBLE ADVERSE REACTIONS OR SIDE EFFECTS

SYMPTOMS	WHAT TO DO
Life-threatening: None expected.	
Common: • Itchy skin.	Discontinue. Call doctor right away.
• Nausea, vomiting, diarrhea, numbness or tingling of extremities, leg weakness, abdominal pain.	Continue. Call doctor when convenient.
• Drowsiness, constipation.	Continue. Tell doctor at next visit.
Infrequent: • Anxiety, agitation, hallucinations, unusually fast or slow heartbeat, dizziness.	Discontinue. Call doctor right away.
• Change in vision, nightmares, insomnia.	Continue. Call doctor when convenient.
Rare: • Extreme thirst, chest pain, shortness of breath, fever, pale or swollen extremities, leg cramps, lower back pain, side or groin pain, appetite loss, joint and muscle pain, rash, facial flush, painful or difficult urination.	Discontinue. Call doctor right away.
• Weight change, hair loss.	Continue. Tell doctor at next visit.

WARNINGS & PRECAUTIONS

Don't take if:
You are allergic to any antiserotonin.*

Before you start, consult your doctor if:
- You are allergic to any ergot preparation.
- You have had a peptic ulcer.
- You plan to become pregnant within medication period.
- You have an infection.
- You have a heart or blood vessel disease.
- You have a chronic lung disease or a collagen (connective tissue) disorder.
- You have impaired liver or kidney function.

Over age 60:
Adverse reactions and side effects may be more frequent and severe than in younger persons.

Pregnancy:
Consult doctor. Risk category X (see page xviii).

Breast-feeding:
Drug probably passes into milk. Avoid drug or discontinue nursing until you finish medicine. Consult doctor for advice on maintaining milk supply.

Infants & children:
Not recommended.

Prolonged use:
- May cause fibrosis, a condition in which scar tissue is deposited on heart valves, in lung tissue, blood vessels and internal organs. After 6 months, decrease dose over 2 to 3 weeks. Then discontinue for at least 2 months for re-evaluation.
- Talk to your doctor about the need for follow-up medical examinations or laboratory studies to check retroperitoneal imaging.*

Skin & sunlight:
No problems expected.

Driving, piloting or hazardous work:
Avoid if you feel drowsy or dizzy. Otherwise, no problems expected.

Discontinuing:
- Don't discontinue without consulting doctor. Dose may require gradual reduction if you have taken drug for a long time. Doses of other drugs may also require adjustment.
- Probably should discontinue drug if you don't improve after 3 weeks use.

Others:
- Periodic laboratory tests for liver function and blood counts recommended.
- Advise any doctor or dentist whom you consult that you take this medicine.
- Potential for abuse.
- Some products contain tartrazine dye. Avoid, especially if you are allergic to aspirin.

POSSIBLE INTERACTION WITH OTHER DRUGS

GENERIC NAME OR DRUG CLASS	COMBINED EFFECT
Ergot preparations*	Unpredictable increased or decreased effect of either drug.
Narcotics*	Decreased narcotic effect.

POSSIBLE INTERACTION WITH OTHER SUBSTANCES

INTERACTS WITH	COMBINED EFFECT
Alcohol:	None expected. However, alcohol may trigger a migraine headache.
Beverages: Caffeine drinks.	Decreased methysergide effect.
Cocaine:	May make headache worse.
Foods:	None expected. Avoid foods to which you are allergic.
Marijuana:	No proven problems.
Tobacco:	Blood vessel constriction. Makes headache worse.

*See Glossary

METOCLOPRAMIDE

BRAND NAMES

Apo-Metoclop	Octamide
Clopra	Octamide PFS
Emex	Reclomide
Maxeran	Reglan

BASIC INFORMATION

Habit forming? No
Prescription needed? Yes
Available as generic? Yes
Drug class: Antiemetic, dopaminergic blocker

 USES

* Relieves nausea and vomiting caused by chemotherapy and drug-related postoperative factors.
* Relieves symptoms of esophagitis and stomach swelling in people with diabetes.

 DOSAGE & USAGE INFORMATION

How to take:
Tablet or syrup—Swallow with liquid or food to lessen stomach irritation.

When to take:
30 minutes before symptoms expected, up to 4 times a day.

If you forget a dose:
Take as soon as you remember up to 2 hours late. If more than 2 hours, wait for next scheduled dose (don't double this dose).

What drug does:
* Prevents smooth muscle in stomach from relaxing, thereby helping to empty stomach more quickly.
* Affects vomiting center in brain.

Continued next column

 OVERDOSE

SYMPTOMS:
Severe drowsiness, muscle spasms, mental confusion, trembling, seizure, coma.
WHAT TO DO:
* **Dial 911 (emergency) for medical help or call poison control center 1-800-222-1222 for instructions.**
* **If person is unconscious, check breathing and pulse. If not breathing, begin mouth-to-mouth rescue breathing. If heart is not beating, begin chest compressions.**
* **See emergency information on last 3 pages of this book.**

Time lapse before drug works:
30 to 60 minutes.

Don't take with:
Any other medicine or any dietary supplement without consulting your doctor or pharmacist.

 POSSIBLE ADVERSE REACTIONS OR SIDE EFFECTS

SYMPTOMS	WHAT TO DO
Life-threatening:	
In case of overdose, see previous column.	
Common:	
Drowsiness, restlessness.	Continue. Call doctor when convenient.
Frequent	
Rash.	Continue. Call doctor when convenient.
Infrequent:	
• Wheezing, shortness of breath.	Discontinue. Call doctor right away.
• Dizziness; headache; insomnia; tender, swollen breasts; increased milk flow; menstrual changes; decreased sex drive.	Continue. Call doctor when convenient.
Rare:	
• Abnormal, involuntary movements of jaw, lips and tongue; depression; Parkinson's syndrome.*	Discontinue. Call doctor right away.
• Constipation, nausea, diarrhea, dry mouth.	Continue. Call doctor when convenient.

 WARNINGS & PRECAUTIONS

Don't take if:
You are allergic to procaine, procainamide or metoclopramide.

Before you start, consult your doctor if:
* You have Parkinson's disease.
* You have liver or kidney disease.
* You have epilepsy.
* You have bleeding from gastrointestinal tract or intestinal obstruction.
* You will have surgery within 2 months, including dental surgery, requiring general or spinal anesthesia.

Over age 60:
Adverse reactions and side effects may be more frequent and severe than in younger persons.

Pregnancy:
No proven harm to unborn child. Avoid if possible. Consult doctor. Risk category B (see page xviii).

Breast-feeding:
Unknown effect. Consult doctor.

Infants & children:
Adverse reactions more likely to occur than in adults.

Prolonged use:
Adverse reactions including muscle spasms and trembling hands more likely to occur.

Skin & sunlight:
No problems expected.

Driving, piloting or hazardous work:
Don't drive or pilot aircraft until you learn how medicine affects you. Don't work around dangerous machinery. Don't climb ladders or work in high places. Danger increases if you drink alcohol or take medicine affecting alertness and reflexes, such as antihistamines, tranquilizers, sedatives, pain medicine, narcotics and mind-altering drugs.

Discontinuing:
May be unnecessary to finish medicine. Follow doctor's instructions.

Others:
Advise any doctor or dentist whom you consult that you take this medicine.

 POSSIBLE INTERACTION WITH OTHER DRUGS

GENERIC NAME OR DRUG CLASS	COMBINED EFFECT
Acetaminophen	Increased absorption of acetaminophen.
Anticholinergics*	Decreased metoclopramide effect.
Aspirin	Increased absorption of aspirin.
Bromocriptine	Decreased bromocriptine effect.
Butyrophenone	Increased chance of muscle spasm and trembling.
Central nervous system (CNS) depressants*	Excess sedation.
Clozapine	Toxic effect on the central nervous system.
Digitalis preparations*	Decreased absorption of digitalis.
Ethinamate	Dangerous increased effects of ethinamate. Avoid combining.

Fluoxetine	Increased depressant effects of both drugs.
Guanfacine	May increase depressant effects of either drug.
Insulin	Unpredictable changes in blood glucose. Dosages may require adjustment.
Leucovorin	High alcohol content of leucovorin may cause adverse effects.
Levodopa	Increased absorption of levodopa.
Lithium	Increased absorption of lithium.
Loxapine	May increase toxic effects of both drugs.
Methyprylon	Increased sedative effect, perhaps to dangerous level. Avoid.
Nabilone	Greater depression of central nervous system.
Narcotics*	Decreased metoclopramide effect.
Nizatidine	Decreased nizatidine absorption.
Pergolide	Decreased pergolide effect.

Continued on page 922

 POSSIBLE INTERACTION WITH OTHER SUBSTANCES

INTERACTS WITH	COMBINED EFFECT
Alcohol:	Excess sedation. Avoid.
Beverages: Coffee.	Decreased metoclopramide effect.
Cocaine:	Decreased metoclopramide effect.
Foods:	None expected.
Marijuana:	Decreased metoclopramide effect.
Tobacco:	Decreased metoclopramide effect.

*See Glossary

METYRAPONE

BRAND NAMES

Metopirone

BASIC INFORMATION

Habit forming? No
Prescription needed? Yes
Available as generic? No
Drug class: Antiadrenal

 USES

- To diagnose the function of the pituitary gland.
- Treats Cushing's disease, a disorder characterized by higher than normal concentrations of cortisol (one of the hormones secreted by the adrenal glands) in the blood.

 DOSAGE & USAGE INFORMATION

How to take:

- For medical testing purposes—Take the prescribed number of tablets with milk or food on the day before the scheduled test. On the day of the test, blood and urine studies will show the amount of hormones in your blood. Results of the test will help establish your diagnosis.
- For treatment of Cushing's syndrome— Swallow tablet with liquid. If you can't swallow whole, crumble tablet and take with liquid or food.

When to take:

- For medical testing—Take the prescribed number of tablets on the day before the scheduled test.
- For treatment of Cushing's disease—Take total daily amount in divided doses. Follow prescription directions carefully.

Continued next column

 OVERDOSE

SYMPTOMS:

Nausea (severe), vomiting, diarrhea, abdominal pain, sudden weakness, irregular heartbeat.
WHAT TO DO:

- **Dial 911 (emergency) for medical help or call poison control center 1-800-222-1222 for instructions.**
- **See emergency information on last 3 pages of this book.**

If you forget a dose:

Take as soon as you remember up to 2 hours late. If more than 2 hours, wait for next scheduled dose (don't double this dose).

What drug does:

Prevents one of the chemical reactions in the production of cortisol by the adrenal glands.

Time lapse before drug works:

Approximately 1 hour.

Don't take with:

Cortisone*-like medicines for 48 hours prior to testing. Any other medicine or any dietary supplement without consulting your doctor or pharmacist.

 POSSIBLE ADVERSE REACTIONS OR SIDE EFFECTS

SYMPTOMS	WHAT TO DO?
Life-threatening:	
In case of overdose, see previous column.	
Common:	
Dizziness, headache, nausea.	Continue. Call doctor when convenient.
Infrequent:	
Drowsiness.	Continue. Call doctor when convenient.
Rare:	
Hair loss or excess growth, decreased appetite, confusion, acne (may begin or may worsen if already present).	Continue. Call doctor when convenient.

METYRAPONE

WARNINGS & PRECAUTIONS

Don't take if:
You are allergic to metyrapone.

Before you start, consult your doctor if:
- You have porphyria.
- You have adrenal insufficiency (Addison's disease).
- You have decreased pituitary function.

Over age 60:
No special problems expected.

Pregnancy:
Safety not established. Take only under careful supervision of medical professional. Risk category C (see page xviii).

Breast-feeding:
Drug may pass into milk, although controlled studies in humans have not been performed. Since the possibility exists, avoid nursing until you finish the medicine.

Infants & children:
No special problems expected.

Prolonged use:
No special problems expected.

Skin & sunlight:
No special problems expected.

Driving, piloting or hazardous work:
Don't drive or pilot aircraft until you learn how medicine affects you. Don't work around dangerous machinery. Don't climb ladders or work in high places. Danger increases if you drink alcohol or take medicine affecting alertness and reflexes.

Discontinuing:
No special problems expected.

Others:
Advise any doctor or dentist whom you consult that you take this medicine.

POSSIBLE INTERACTION WITH OTHER DRUGS

GENERIC NAME OR DRUG CLASS	COMBINED EFFECT
Antidiabetics, oral*	Increased risk of adverse reactions.
Contraceptives, oral*	Possible inaccurate test results.
Estrogens*	Possible inaccurate test results.
Insulin	Increased risk of adverse reactions.
Phenytoin	Possible inaccurate test results.

POSSIBLE INTERACTION WITH OTHER SUBSTANCES

INTERACTS WITH	COMBINED EFFECT
Alcohol:	None expected.
Beverages:	None expected.
Cocaine:	None expected.
Foods:	Increased appetite and absorption of nutrients, causing difficulty with weight control.
Marijuana:	None expected.
Tobacco:	None expected.

*See Glossary

MEXILETINE

BRAND NAMES

Mexitil

BASIC INFORMATION

Habit forming? No
Prescription needed? Yes
Available as generic? Yes
Drug class: Antiarrhythmic

 USES

Stabilizes irregular heartbeat.

 DOSAGE & USAGE INFORMATION

How to take:
Capsule—Swallow whole with food, milk or
antacid to lessen stomach irritation.

When to take:
At the same times each day as directed by your
doctor.

If you forget a dose:
Take as soon as you remember up to 4 hours
late. If more than 4 hours, wait for next
scheduled dose (don't double this dose).

What drug does:
Blocks the fast sodium channel in heart tissue.

Time lapse before drug works:
30 minutes to 2 hours.

Don't take with:
Any other medicine or any dietary supplement
without consulting your doctor or pharmacist.

 OVERDOSE

SYMPTOMS:
Nausea, vomiting, seizures, convulsions,
cardiac arrest.
WHAT TO DO:
• **Dial 911 (emergency) for medical help or
call poison control center 1-800-222-1222
for instructions.**
• **See emergency information on last 3 pages
of this book.**

 POSSIBLE ADVERSE REACTIONS OR SIDE EFFECTS

SYMPTOMS	WHAT TO DO
Life-threatening: Chest pain, shortness of breath, irregular or fast heartbeat.	Discontinue. Seek emergency treatment.
Common: Dizziness, anxiety, shakiness, unsteadiness when walking, heartburn, nausea, vomiting.	Discontinue. Call doctor right away.
Infrequent: • Sore throat, fever, mouth sores; blurred vision; confusion; constipation; diarrhea; headache; numbness or tingling in hands or feet; ringing in ears; unexplained bleeding or bruising; rash; slurred speech; insomnia; weakness; difficult swallowing.	Discontinue. Call doctor right away.
• Loss of taste.	Continue. Call doctor when convenient.
Rare: • Seizures.	Discontinue. Seek emergency treatment.
• Hallucinations, psychosis, memory loss, difficult breathing, swollen feet and ankles, hiccups, jaundice.	Discontinue. Call doctor right away.
• Hair loss, impotence.	Continue. Call doctor when convenient.

WARNINGS & PRECAUTIONS

Don't take if:
If you are allergic to mexiletine, lidocaine or tocainide.

Before you start, consult your doctor if:
* You have had liver or kidney disease or impaired kidney function.
* You have had lupus.
* You have a history of seizures.
* You will have surgery within 2 months, including dental surgery, requiring general or spinal anesthesia.
* You have heart disease or low blood pressure.

Over age 60:
Adverse reactions and side effects may be more frequent and severe than in younger persons. Ask doctor about smaller doses.

Pregnancy:
Decide with your doctor if drug benefits justify risk to unborn child. Risk category C (see page xviii).

Breast-feeding:
Drug passes into milk. Avoid drug or discontinue nursing until you finish medicine. Consult doctor for advice on maintaining milk supply.

Infants & children:
Use only under close medical supervision.

Prolonged use:
* May cause lupus*-like illness.
* Talk to your doctor about the need for follow-up medical examinations or laboratory studies to check ECG,* liver function.

Skin & sunlight:
No problems expected.

Driving, piloting or hazardous work:
Use caution if you feel dizzy or weak. Otherwise, no problems expected.

Discontinuing:
Don't discontinue without consulting doctor. Dose may require gradual reduction if you have taken drug for a long time. Doses of other drugs may also require adjustment.

Others:
Advise any doctor or dentist whom you consult that you take this medicine.

POSSIBLE INTERACTION WITH OTHER DRUGS

GENERIC NAME OR DRUG CLASS	COMBINED EFFECT
Cimetidine	Increased mexiletine effect and toxicity.
Encainide	Increased effect of toxicity on the heart muscle.
Nicardipine	Possible increased effect and toxicity of each drug.
Phenobarbital	Decreased mexiletine effect.
Phenytoin	Decreased mexiletine effect.
Propafenone	Increased effect of both drugs and increased risk of toxicity.
Rifampin	Decreased mexiletine effect.
Urinary acidifiers*	May decrease effectiveness of medicine.
Urinary alkalizers*	May slow elimination of mexiletine and cause need to adjust dosage.

POSSIBLE INTERACTION WITH OTHER SUBSTANCES

INTERACTS WITH	COMBINED EFFECT
Alcohol:	Causes irregular effectiveness of mexiletine. Avoid.
Beverages: Caffeine drinks, iced drinks.	Irregular heartbeat.
Cocaine:	Decreased mexiletine effect.
Foods:	None expected.
Marijuana:	Irregular heartbeat. Avoid.
Tobacco:	Dangerous combination. May lead to liver problems and reduce excretion of mexiletine.

*See Glossary

MIFEPRISTONE (RU-486)

BRAND NAMES

Mifeprex

BASIC INFORMATION

Habit forming? No
Prescription needed? Yes
Available as generic? No
Drug class: Abortifacient

 ## USES

Terminates pregnancy in the early stages (up to 7 weeks or 49 days since the beginning of the last menstrual period). Mifepristone is not approved for ending later pregnancies. Requires three trips to your doctor's office: day one for administration, day three for a second medication (if you are still pregnant) and day fourteen for follow-up and determination of the status of your pregnancy.

 ## DOSAGE & USAGE INFORMATION

How to take:
Tablet—Taken on day one under strict compliance in the presence of your doctor. On day three misoprostol is taken in your doctor's office (if you are still pregnant).

When to take:
At your doctors office.

What drug does:
Mifepristone blocks a hormone (progesterone) needed for your pregnancy to continue.

If you forget a dose:
Medication is taken at your doctor's office.

Time lapse before drug works:
A few days to two weeks. If you are still pregnant after two weeks, your doctor will discuss other options you have including a surgical alternative to terminate your pregnancy.

Don't take with:
Any other medicine or any dietary supplement without consulting your doctor or pharmacist.

 ## OVERDOSE

SYMPTOMS:
Symptoms are unknown.
WHAT TO DO:
Overdose unlikely to threaten life. If person uses much larger amount than prescribed or if accidentally swallowed, call doctor or poison control center 1-800-222-1222 for help.

 ## POSSIBLE ADVERSE REACTIONS OR SIDE EFFECTS

SYMPTOMS	WHAT TO DO
Life-threatening: None expected.	
Common: Nausea or vomiting, diarrhea, abdominal pain, back pain, dizziness, unusual tiredness or weakness, headache.	Call doctor if symptoms persist.
Infrequent: • Excessive and heavy vaginal bleeding.	Call doctor right away.
• Pale skin, troubled breathing, unusual bleeding or bruising, anxiety, upset stomach, acid indigestion, fever, insomnia, leg pain, increased clear or white vaginal discharge, shaking, stuffy nose, cough, fainting, genital itching or pain, chills or flu-like symptoms, sinusitis.	Call doctor if symptoms persist.
Rare: None expected.	

MIFEPRISTONE (RU-486)

WARNINGS & PRECAUTIONS

Don't take if:
You are allergic to mifepristone or misoprostol.

Before you start, consult your doctor if:
- You have a history of adrenal failure.
- You have a history of hemorrhagic (bleeding) disorders.
- You have an ectopic pregnancy (a pregnancy outside the uterus).
- You have any other medical problems.
- You have anemia.
- You have an in-place intra-uterine device (IUD).
- You cannot easily get emergency medical help during the two weeks after you take the drug.
- You have a family history of porphyria.

Over age 60:
Not used in this age group.

Pregnancy:
Mifepristone is used to terminate pregnancy.

Breast-feeding:
It is unknown if mifepristone is distributed into breast milk. Avoid drug or discontinue nursing until you finish medicine. Consult doctor for advice on maintaining milk supply.

Infants & children:
Safety and efficacy not established. Not used in this age group.

Prolonged use:
Not intended for prolonged use.

Skin & sunlight:
No problems expected.

Driving, piloting or hazardous work:
No problems expected.

Discontinuing:
Drug is administered in the presence of a licensed medical professional who has registered with the manufacturer.

Others:
- Prior to using this medication, you will be required to sign a statement that you have decided to end your pregnancy.
- Advise any doctor or dentist whom you consult that you take this medicine.
- The follow-up doctor visits are very important. Don't miss them.
- May affect the results in some medical tests.
- An ultrasonographic scan may be scheduled 14 days after mifepristone administration to confirm termination of pregnancy and assess bleeding.
- If you do not want to become pregnant again, start using a birth control method as soon as your pregnancy ends.
- Serious bacterial infection and sepsis (blood infection) may occur without the usual signs of infection, such as fever and pelvic tenderness.
- If you are still pregnant after the two weeks, there may be birth defects if the pregnancy continues. Your doctor will discuss other options to end your pregnancy.

POSSIBLE INTERACTION WITH OTHER DRUGS

GENERIC NAME OR DRUG CLASS	COMBINED EFFECT
Anticoagulants*	Excessive bleeding.
Corticosteroids* (long term use)	Effects unknown. Avoid.
Enzyme inducers*	May decrease effect of mifepristone.
Enzyme inhibitors*	May increase effect of mifepristone.

POSSIBLE INTERACTION WITH OTHER SUBSTANCES

INTERACTS WITH	COMBINED EFFECT
Alcohol:	None expected. Best to avoid.
Beverages: Grapefruit juice	May increase effect of mifepristone.
Cocaine:	Unknown. Avoid.
Foods:	None expected.
Marijuana:	None expected.
Tobacco:	None expected.

*See Glossary

MIGLITOL

BRAND NAMES

Glyset

BASIC INFORMATION

Habit forming? No
Prescription needed? Yes
Available as generic? No
Drug class: Antidiabetic

 USES

Treatment for hyperglycemia (excess sugar in the blood) that cannot be controlled by diet alone in patients with type 2 diabetes. The drug may be used alone or in combination with other antidiabetic drugs.

 DOSAGE & USAGE INFORMATION

How to take:
Tablet—Swallow with liquid. Take at the very beginning of a meal.

When to take:
Usually 3 times a day or as directed by doctor. Dosage may be increased at 4 to 8 week intervals until maximum benefits are achieved.

If you forget a dose:
And your meal is finished, then skip the missed dose and wait for your next meal and next scheduled dose (don't double this dose).

What drug does:
Impedes the digestion and absorption of carbohydrates and their subsequent conversion into glucose. This improves control of blood glucose and may reduce the complications of diabetes. However, miglitol does not cure diabetes.

Continued next column

 OVERDOSE

SYMPTOMS:
An overdose may cause flatulence, diarrhea and abdominal pain. It is unlikely to produce serious side effects. The drug itself will not produce low blood sugar (hypoglycemia).
WHAT TO DO:
Overdose unlikely to threaten life. If person uses much larger amount than prescribed or if accidentally swallowed, call doctor or poison control center 1-800-222-1222 for help.

Time lapse before drug works:
May take several weeks for full effectiveness.

Don't take with:
Any other medicine or any dietary supplement without consulting your doctor or pharmacist.

 POSSIBLE ADVERSE REACTIONS OR SIDE EFFECTS

SYMPTOMS	WHAT TO DO
Life-threatening: None expected from the drug by itself.	
Common: Diarrhea, stomach cramps, gas, bloating feeling.	Continue. Call doctor when convenient.
Infrequent: Skin rash.	Continue. Call doctor when convenient.
Rare: Low blood sugar (hypoglycemia) may occur if you are taking other drugs for diabetes and you do not consume enough calories. Symptoms may include stomach pain, anxious feeling, cold sweats, chills, confusion, convulsions, cool pale skin, excessive hunger, nausea or vomiting, rapid heartbeat, nervousness, shakiness, unsteady walk, unusual weakness or tiredness, vision changes,	For low blood sugar, take glucose or eat honey or drink orange juice. For more severe symptoms, call doctor right away or seek emergency help.

WARNINGS & PRECAUTIONS

Don't take if:
You are allergic to miglitol.

Before you start, consult your doctor if:
- You have any kidney or liver disease or any heart or blood vessel disorder.
- You have any chronic health problem.
- You have an infection, illness or any condition that can cause low blood sugar.
- You have a history of acid in the blood (metabolic acidosis or ketoacidosis).
- You have inflammatory bowel disease or any other intestinal disorder.
- You are allergic to any medication, food or other substance.

Over age 60:
No special problems expected.

Pregnancy:
Decide with your doctor if drug benefits justify risks to unborn child. Risk category B (see page xviii).

Breast-feeding:
Drug passes into milk. It is not recommended for use in nursing mothers.

Infants & children:
Safety and efficacy have not been established. Use only under close medical supervision.

Prolonged use:
- Schedule regular doctor visits to determine if the drug is continuing to be effective in controlling the diabetes and to check for any problems in kidney function.
- You will most likely require an antidiabetic medicine for the rest of your life.
- You will need to test your blood glucose levels several times a day, or for some, once to several times a week.

Skin & sunlight:
No special problems expected.

Driving, piloting or hazardous work:
No special problems expected.

Discontinuing:
Don't discontinue without consulting your doctor even if you feel well. You can have diabetes without feeling any symptoms. Untreated diabetes can cause serious problems.

Others:
- Advise any doctor or dentist whom you consult that you take this medicine.
- It may interfere with the accuracy of some medical tests.
- Follow any special diet your doctor may prescribe. It can help control diabetes.
- Consult doctor if you become ill with vomiting or diarrhea while taking this drug.

- Use caution when exercising. Ask your doctor about an appropriate exercise program.
- Wear medical identification stating that you have diabetes and take this medication.
- Learn to recognize the symptoms of low blood sugar. You and your family need to know what to do if these symptoms occur.
- Have a glucagon kit and syringe in the event severe low blood sugar occurs.
- High blood sugar (hyperglycemia) may occur with diabetes. Ask your doctor about symptoms to watch for and treatment steps to take.
- Educate yourself about diabetes.

POSSIBLE INTERACTION WITH OTHER DRUGS

GENERIC NAME OR DRUG CLASS	COMBINED EFFECT
Amylase (Pancreatic enzyme)	Decreased miglitol effect.
Antidiabetic agents, sulfonylurea	May cause hypoglycemia.
Charcoal, activated	Decreased miglitol effect.
Pancreatin (Pancreatic enzyme)	Decreased miglitol effect.
Pramlintide	Decreased absorption of nutrients.
Propranolol	Decreased effect of propranolol.
Ranitidine	Decreased effect of ranitidine.

POSSIBLE INTERACTION WITH OTHER SUBSTANCES

INTERACTS WITH	COMBINED EFFECT
Alcohol:	May increase effect of miglitol. Avoid excessive amounts.
Beverages:	None expected.
Cocaine:	None expected. Best to avoid.
Foods:	None expected.
Marijuana:	None expected. Best to avoid.
Tobacco:	People with diabetes should not smoke.

*See Glossary

MINOXIDIL

BRAND NAMES

Loniten

BASIC INFORMATION

Habit forming? No
Prescription needed? Yes
Available as generic? Yes
Drug class: Antihypertensive

 USES

- Treatment for high blood pressure in conjunction with other drugs, such as beta-adrenergic blockers and diuretics.
- Treatment for congestive heart failure.
- Can stimulate hair growth.

 DOSAGE & USAGE INFORMATION

How to take:
Tablet—Swallow with liquid. If you can't swallow whole, crumble tablet and take with liquid or food.

When to take:
At the same time each day, according to instructions on prescription label.

If you forget a dose:
Take as soon as you remember up to 2 hours late. If more than 2 hours, wait for next scheduled dose (don't double this dose).

What drug does:
Relaxes small blood vessels (arterioles) so blood can pass through more easily.

Time lapse before drug works:
2 to 3 hours for effect to begin; 3 to 7 days of continuous use may be necessary for maximum blood pressure response.

Don't take with:
Any other medicine or any dietary supplement without consulting your doctor or pharmacist.

 OVERDOSE

SYMPTOMS:
Low blood pressure, fainting, chest pain, shortness of breath, coma.
WHAT TO DO:
- Dial 911 (emergency) for medical help or call poison control center 1-800-222-1222 for instructions.
- See emergency information on last 3 pages of this book.

 POSSIBLE ADVERSE REACTIONS OR SIDE EFFECTS

SYMPTOMS	WHAT TO DO
Life-threatening:	
In case of overdose, see previous column.	
Common:	
• Excessive hair growth, flushed skin or redness.	Continue. Call doctor when convenient.
• Bloating.	Discontinue. Call doctor right away.
Infrequent:	
• Chest pain, irregular or slow heartbeat, shortness of breath, swollen feet or legs, rapid weight gain.	Discontinue. Call doctor right away.
• Numbness of hands, feet or face; headache; tender breasts; darkening of skin.	Continue. Call doctor when convenient.
Rare:	
Rash.	Discontinue. Call doctor right away.

WARNINGS & PRECAUTIONS

Don't take if:
You are allergic to minoxidil.

Before you start, consult your doctor if:
* You have had recent stroke or heart attack or angina pectoris in past 3 weeks.
* You have impaired kidney function.
* You have pheochromocytoma.*

Over age 60:
Adverse reactions and side effects may be more frequent and severe than in younger persons.

Pregnancy:
Decide with your doctor if drug benefits justify risk to unborn child. Risk category C (see page xviii).

Breast-feeding:
Human studies not available. Avoid if possible. Consult doctor.

Infants & children:
Not recommended. Safety and dosage have not been established.

Prolonged use:
Request periodic blood examinations that include potassium levels.

Skin & sunlight:
May cause rash or intensify sunburn in areas exposed to sun or ultraviolet light (photosensitivity reaction). Avoid overexposure. Notify doctor if reaction occurs.

Driving, piloting or hazardous work:
Avoid if you become dizzy or faint. Otherwise, no problems expected.

Discontinuing:
Don't discontinue without consulting doctor. Dose may require gradual reduction if you have taken drug for a long time. Doses of other drugs may also require adjustment.

Others:
* Advise any doctor or dentist whom you consult that you take this medicine.
* Check blood pressure frequently.

POSSIBLE INTERACTION WITH OTHER DRUGS

GENERIC NAME OR DRUG CLASS	COMBINED EFFECT
Anesthesia	Drastic blood pressure drop.
Antihypertensives,* other	Dosage adjustments may be necessary to keep blood pressure at desired level.
Carteolol	Increased anti-hypertensive effect.
Diuretics*	Dosage adjustments may be necessary to keep blood pressure at desired level.
Estrogens*	May increase blood pressure.
Guanadrel	Weakness and faintness when arising from bed or chair.
Guanethidine	Weakness and faintness when arising from bed or chair.
Lisinopril	Increased anti-hypertensive effect. Dosage of each may require adjustment.
Nicardipine	Blood pressure drop. Dosages may require adjustment.
Nimodipine	Dangerous blood pressure drop.
Nitrates*	Drastic blood pressure drop.
Sotalol	Increased anti-hypertensive effect.
Sympathomimetics*	Possible decreased minoxidil effect.
Terazosin	Decreased effectiveness of terazosin.

POSSIBLE INTERACTION WITH OTHER SUBSTANCES

INTERACTS WITH	COMBINED EFFECT
Alcohol:	Possible excessive blood pressure drop.
Beverages:	None expected.
Cocaine:	Increased risk of heart block and high blood pressure.
Foods: Salt substitutes.	Possible excessive potassium levels in blood.
Marijuana:	Increased dizziness.
Tobacco:	May decrease minoxidil effect. Avoid.

MINOXIDIL (Topical)

BRAND NAMES

Dermal   Rogaine for Men
Rogaine   Rogaine for Women
Rogaine Extra
  Strength for Men

BASIC INFORMATION

Habit forming? No
Prescription needed? No
Available as generic? Yes
Drug class: Hair growth stimulant

USES

Treats hair loss on scalp from male and female pattern baldness (alopecia androgenetica).

DOSAGE & USAGE INFORMATION

How to use:
Topical solution
* Apply only to dry hair and scalp. With the provided applicator, apply the amount prescribed to the scalp area being treated. Begin in center of the treated area.
* Wash hands immediately after use.
* Don't use a blow dryer.
* If you are using at bedtime, wait 30 minutes after applying before retiring.

When to use:
Twice a day or as directed.

If you forget a dose:
Use as soon as you remember. No need to ever double the dose.

What drug does:
Stimulates hair growth by possibly dilating small blood capillaries, thereby providing more blood to hair follicles.

Time lapse before drug works:
Varies with individuals.

Don't use with:
Other hair-growth products without consulting your doctor or pharmacist.

OVERDOSE

SYMPTOMS:
None expected.
WHAT TO DO:
Not for internal use. If child accidentally swallows, dial 911 (emergency) for medical help or call poison control center 1-800-222-1222 for instructions.

POSSIBLE ADVERSE REACTIONS OR SIDE EFFECTS

SYMPTOMS	WHAT TO DO
Life-threatening: Fast, irregular heartbeat (rare; represents too much absorbed into body).	Discontinue. Seek emergency treatment.
Common: None expected.	
Infrequent: Itching scalp; flaking, reddened skin.	Continue. Call doctor when convenient.
Rare: Burning scalp, skin rash, swollen face, headache, dizziness or fainting, hands and feet numb or tingling, rapid weight gain.	Discontinue. Call doctor right away.

WARNINGS & PRECAUTIONS

Don't use if:
You are allergic to minoxidil.

Before you start, consult your doctor if:
• You are allergic to anything.
• You have heart disease or high blood pressure.
• You have skin irritation or abrasion or severe sunburn (systemic absorption may be increased).

Over age 60:
No problems expected.

Pregnancy:
Decide with your doctor if drug benefits justify risk to unborn child. Risk category C (see page xviii).

Breast-feeding:
Don't use.

Infants & children:
Don't use.

Prolonged use:
No problems expected.

Skin & sunlight:
No problems expected.

Driving, piloting or hazardous work:
No problems expected.

Discontinuing:
No problems expected.

Others:
• Keep away from eyes, nose and mouth. Flush with plain water if accident occurs.
• New hair will drop out when you stop using minoxidil.
• Keep solution cool, but don't freeze.

POSSIBLE INTERACTION WITH OTHER DRUGS

GENERIC NAME OR DRUG CLASS	COMBINED EFFECT
Adrenocorticoids,* topical	May cause undesirable absorption of minoxidil.
Minoxidil, oral	Increased risk of toxicity.
Petrolatum, topical	May cause undesirable absorption of minoxidil.
Retinoids,* topical	May cause undesirable absorption of minoxidil.

POSSIBLE INTERACTION WITH OTHER SUBSTANCES

INTERACTS WITH	COMBINED EFFECT
Alcohol:	None expected.
Beverages:	None expected.
Cocaine:	None expected.
Foods:	None expected.
Marijuana:	None expected.
Tobacco:	None expected.

*See Glossary

MIRTAZAPINE

BRAND NAMES

Remeron   Remeron SolTab

BASIC INFORMATION

Habit forming? Not expected
Prescription needed? Yes
Available as generic? Yes
Drug class: Antidepressant

 ## USES

Treats symptoms of mental depression.

 ## DOSAGE & USAGE INFORMATION

How to take:
* Tablet—Swallow with liquid. May be taken with or without food.
* Oral disintegrating tablet—Let tablet dissolve in your mouth.

When to take:
At the same time each day, usually in the evening before bedtime.

If you forget a dose:
Take as soon as you remember up to 12 hours late. If more than 12 hours, wait for the next scheduled dose (don't double this dose).

What drug does:
The exact mechanism is unknown. It appears to block certain chemicals in the brain, which in turn helps production of other brain chemicals that play a role in helping to relieve symptoms of depression.

Time lapse before drug works:
Will take up to several weeks to show improvement of the depression symptoms.

Don't take with:
Any other medicine or any dietary supplement without consulting your doctor or pharmacist.

 ## OVERDOSE

SYMPTOMS:
Drowsiness, disorientation, memory impairment, rapid heartbeat.
WHAT TO DO:
* Dial 911 (emergency) for medical help or call poison control center 1-800-222-1222 for instructions.
* See emergency information on last 3 pages of this book.

 ## POSSIBLE ADVERSE REACTIONS OR SIDE EFFECTS

SYMPTOMS	WHAT TO DO
Life-threatening: None expected.	
Common:	
• Sleepiness, increased appetite, weight gain, dizziness, dry mouth, constipation, tiredness, increased thirst.	Continue. Call doctor when convenient.
• Abdominal pain, vomiting, joint pain, increased cough, rash, itching, agitation, anxiety, twitching, apathy.	Discontinue. Call doctor right away.
Infrequent:	
• Slow heartbeat, migraine, dehydration, weight loss, unusual weakness, pain in any part of the body, changes in menstrual periods, changes in vision or hearing, mouth sores, mood or mental changes, breathing difficulty, lack of coordination.	Discontinue. Call doctor right away.
• Forgetfulness, lightheadedness.	Continue. Call doctor when convenient.
Rare:	
• Swelling of hands, feet or legs; infection (fever, chills, aches or pains, sore throat); swollen or discolored tongue; changes in urinary function; hives.	Discontinue. Call doctor right away.
• Muscle aches, strange dreams, headache.	Continue. Call doctor when convenient.

WARNINGS & PRECAUTIONS

Don't take if:
You are allergic to mirtazapine.

Before you start, consult your doctor if:
* You have seizure disorder, heart disease, blood circulation problem or had a stroke.
* You are dehydrated.
* You have a history of drug dependence or drug abuse.
* You have kidney or liver disease.
* You have a history of mood disorders, such as mania, or thoughts of suicide.
* You are allergic to any other medication, food or other substances.

Over age 60:
A lower starting dosage is usually recommended until a response is determined.

Pregnancy:
Decide with your doctor if drug benefits justify risk to unborn child. Risk category C (see page xviii).

Breast-feeding:
It is unknown if drug passes into milk. Avoid drug or discontinue nursing until you finish medicine. Consult doctor for advice on maintaining milk supply.

Infants & children:
Not approved for ages under 18. If prescribed, carefully read information provided with prescription. Contact doctor right away if depression symptoms get worse or there is any talk of suicide or suicide behaviors. Also, read information under Others.

Prolonged use:
Consult with your doctor on a regular basis while taking this drug to check your progress, to discuss any increase or changes in side effects and the need for continued treatment.

Skin & sunlight:
May cause a rash or intensify sunburn in areas exposed to sun or ultraviolet light (photosensitivity reaction). Avoid excessive sun exposure. Consult doctor if reaction occurs.

Driving, piloting or hazardous work:
Don't drive or pilot aircraft until you learn how medicine affects you. Don't work around dangerous machinery. Don't climb ladders or work in high places. Danger increases if you drink alcohol or take medicine affecting alertness and reflexes.

Discontinuing:
Consult doctor before discontinuing this drug.

Others:
* Get up slowly from a sitting or lying position to avoid dizziness, faintness or lightheadedness.
* Advise any doctor or dentist whom you consult that you take this medicine.
* Adults and children taking antidepressants may experience a worsening of the depression symptoms and may display increased suicidal thoughts or behavior. Call doctor right away if these symptoms or behaviors occur.
* Do not increase or reduce dosage without doctor's approval.

POSSIBLE INTERACTION WITH OTHER DRUGS

GENERIC NAME OR DRUG CLASS	COMBINED EFFECT
Benzodiazepines	Increased sedative effect. Avoid.
Monoamine oxidase, (MAO) inhibitors	Potentially life-threatening. Allow 14 days between use of 2 drugs.
Other medications	Complete studies have not been done to evaluate interactions with other drugs, but the potential exists for a variety of possible interactions. Consult doctor or pharmacist.

POSSIBLE INTERACTION WITH OTHER SUBSTANCES

INTERACTS WITH	COMBINED EFFECT
Alcohol:	Increased sedative affect. Avoid.
Beverages:	None expected.
Cocaine:	Unknown effect. Best to avoid.
Foods:	None expected.
Marijuana:	Unknown effect. Best to avoid.
Tobacco:	None expected.

MISOPROSTOL

BRAND NAMES

Arthrotec   Cytotec

BASIC INFORMATION

Habit forming? No
Prescription needed? Yes
Available as generic? No
Drug class: Antiulcer agent

 USES

Prevents development of stomach ulcers in persons taking nonsteroidal anti-inflammatory drugs (NSAIDs), including aspirin.

 DOSAGE & USAGE INFORMATION

How to take:
Tablet—Swallow with liquid. Swallow Arthrotec brand whole. If you can't swallow Cytotec brand whole, crumble tablet and take with liquid or food. Instructions to take on empty stomach mean 1 hour before or 2 hours after eating.

When to take:
Usually 4 times a day while awake, with or after meals and at bedtime.

If you forget a dose:
Take as soon as you remember up to 2 hours late. If more than 2 hours, wait for next scheduled dose (don't double this dose).

What drug does:
- Improves defense against peptic ulcers by strengthening natural defenses of the stomach lining.
- Decreases stomach acid production.

Time lapse before drug works:
10 to 15 minutes.

Don't take with:
Any other medicines (including over-the-counter drugs such as cough and cold medicines, laxatives, antacids, diet pills, caffeine, nose drops or vitamins) without consulting your doctor or pharmacist.

 OVERDOSE

SYMPTOMS:
None expected.
WHAT TO DO:
Overdose unlikely to threaten life. If person uses much larger amount than prescribed or if accidentally swallowed, call doctor or poison control center 1-800-222-1222 for help.

 POSSIBLE ADVERSE REACTIONS OR SIDE EFFECTS

SYMPTOMS	WHAT TO DO
Life-threatening: None expected.	
Common: Abdominal pain, diarrhea.	Discontinue. Call doctor right away.
Infrequent:	
• Nausea or vomiting.	Continue. Call doctor when convenient.
• Constipation, headache.	Continue. Tell doctor at next visit.
Rare:	
• Gaseousness.	Continue. Tell doctor at next visit.
• Vaginal bleeding.	Discontinue. Call doctor right away.

WARNINGS & PRECAUTIONS

Don't take if:
- You are allergic to any prostaglandin.*
- You are pregnant or of child-bearing age.

Before you start, consult your doctor if:
- You have epilepsy.
- You have heart disease.
- You have blood vessel disease of any kind.

Over age 60:
No special problems expected.

Pregnancy:
- Risk to unborn child outweighs drug benefits. Don't use.
- May also lead to serious complications in pregnant women, including excessive bleeding and future infertility.
- Risk category X (see page xviii).

Breast-feeding:
Drug passes into milk. Avoid drug or discontinue nursing until you finish medicine. Consult doctor for advice on maintaining milk supply.

Infants & children:
Not recommended for children under 18.

Prolonged use:
Talk to your doctor about the need for follow-up medical examinations or laboratory studies to check gastric analysis.

Skin & sunlight:
No problems expected.

Driving, piloting or hazardous work:
Avoid if you feel confused, drowsy or dizzy.

Discontinuing:
No special problems expected.

Others:
Advise any doctor or dentist whom you consult that you take this medicine.

POSSIBLE INTERACTION WITH OTHER DRUGS

GENERIC NAME OR DRUG CLASS	COMBINED EFFECT
Antacids,* magnesium-containing	Severe diarrhea.

POSSIBLE INTERACTION WITH OTHER SUBSTANCES

INTERACTS WITH	COMBINED EFFECT
Alcohol:	Decreases misoprostol effect. Avoid.
Beverages: Caffeine-containing.	Decreases misoprostol effect. Avoid.
Cocaine:	Decreases misoprostol effect. Avoid.
Foods:	None expected.
Marijuana:	Decreases misoprostol effect. Avoid.
Tobacco:	Decreases misoprostol effect. Avoid.

MITOTANE

BRAND NAMES

Lysodren   o,p´-DDD

BASIC INFORMATION

Habit forming? No
Prescription needed? Yes
Available as generic? No
Drug class: Antineoplastic, antiadrenal

 USES

- Treatment for some kinds of cancer.
- Treatment of Cushing's disease.

 DOSAGE & USAGE INFORMATION

How to take:
Tablet—Take with liquid after light meal. Don't
drink fluid with meals. Drink extra fluids between
meals. Avoid sweet and fatty foods.

When to take:
At the same time each day.

If you forget a dose:
Take as soon as you remember. Don't ever
double dose.

What drug does:
Suppresses adrenal cortex to prevent
manufacture of excess cortisone.

Time lapse before drug works:
2 to 3 weeks for full effect.

Don't take with:
Any other medicine or any dietary supplement
without consulting your doctor or pharmacist.

 OVERDOSE

SYMPTOMS:
Headache, vomiting blood, stupor, seizure.
WHAT TO DO:
- Dial 911 (emergency) for medical help or
  call poison control center 1-800-222-1222
  for instructions.
- If person is unconscious, check breathing
  and pulse. If not breathing, begin mouth-
  to-mouth rescue breathing. If heart is not
  beating, begin chest compressions.
- See emergency information on last 3 pages
  of this book.

 POSSIBLE ADVERSE REACTIONS OR SIDE EFFECTS

SYMPTOMS	WHAT TO DO
Life-threatening:	
In case of overdose, see previous column.	
Common:	
• Darkened skin, appetite loss, nausea, vomiting.	Continue. Call doctor when convenient.
• Mental depression, drowsiness.	Continue. Tell doctor at next visit.
Infrequent:	
• Fever, chills, sore throat, unusual bleeding or bruising, difficult breathing, blurred vision, seeing double.	Discontinue. Call doctor right away.
• Rash, hair loss, cough, tiredness, weakness, dizziness when standing after sitting or lying down.	Continue. Call doctor when convenient.
Rare:	
Blood in urine.	Continue. Call doctor when convenient.

MITOTANE

 WARNINGS & PRECAUTIONS

Don't take if:
You are allergic to mitotane, corticosteroids* or any antineoplastic drug.

Before you start, consult your doctor if:
• You have liver disease.
• You have infection.

Over age 60:
Adverse reactions and side effects may be more frequent and severe than in younger persons.

Pregnancy:
Decide with your doctor whether drug benefits justify risk to unborn child. Risk category C (see page xviii).

Breast-feeding:
It is unknown if drug passes into milk. Avoid drug or discontinue nursing until you finish medicine. Consult doctor for advice on maintaining milk supply.

Infants & children:
Use only under care of medical supervisors who are experienced in administering anticancer drugs.

Prolonged use:
Adverse reactions more likely the longer drug is required.

Skin & sunlight:
No problems expected.

Driving, piloting or hazardous work:
No problems expected.

Discontinuing:
• Don't discontinue without consulting doctor. Dose may require gradual reduction if you have taken drug for a long time. Doses of other drugs may also require adjustment.
• Some side effects may follow discontinuing. Report any new symptoms.

Others:
Advise any doctor or dentist whom you consult that you take this medicine.

 POSSIBLE INTERACTION WITH OTHER DRUGS

GENERIC NAME OR DRUG CLASS	COMBINED EFFECT
Adrenocorticoids, systemic	Decreased adrenocorticoid effect.
Antidepressants*	Increased central nervous system depression.
Antihistamines*	Increased central nervous system depression.
Central nervous system (CNS) depressants*	Increased sedation.
Phenytoin	Decreased effect of phenytoin.
Spironolactone	Decreased mitotane effect.
Warfarin	Decreased warfarin effect.

 POSSIBLE INTERACTION WITH OTHER SUBSTANCES

INTERACTS WITH	COMBINED EFFECT
Alcohol:	Increased depression. Avoid.
Beverages:	None expected.
Cocaine:	Increased toxicity. Avoid.
Foods:	Reduced irritation in stomach.
Marijuana:	None expected.
Tobacco:	Increased possibility of lung toxicity.

*See Glossary

MOLINDONE

BRAND NAMES

Moban   Moban Concentrate

BASIC INFORMATION

Habit forming? No
Prescription needed? Yes
Available as generic? No
Drug class: Antipsychotic

 ## USES

Treats severe emotional, mental or nervous problems.

 ## DOSAGE & USAGE INFORMATION

How to take:
Tablet or solution—Swallow with liquid or food to lessen stomach irritation. If you can't swallow tablet whole, crumble and take with food or liquid.

When to take:
Follow instructions on prescription label. Doses should be evenly spaced. For example, 4 times a day means every 6 hours.

If you forget a dose:
Take as soon as you remember up to 2 hours late. If more than 2 hours, wait for next scheduled dose (don't double this dose).

What drug does:
Corrects an imbalance in nerve impulses from the brain.

Time lapse before drug works:
Some benefit seen within a week; 4 to 6 weeks for full benefit.

Don't take with:
• Antacid or medicine for diarrhea at same time.
• Any other medicine or any dietary supplement without consulting your doctor or pharmacist.

 ## OVERDOSE

SYMPTOMS:
Stupor, convulsions, coma.
WHAT TO DO:
• **Dial 911 (emergency) for medical help or call poison control center 1-800-222-1222 for instructions.**
• **See emergency information on last 3 pages of this book.**

 ## POSSIBLE ADVERSE REACTIONS OR SIDE EFFECTS

SYMPTOMS	WHAT TO DO
Life-threatening: High fever, rapid pulse, profuse sweating, muscle rigidity, confusion and irritability, seizures.	Discontinue. Seek emergency treatment.
Common: Sedation, low blood pressure and dizziness.	Continue. Call doctor when convenient.
Infrequent: • Jerky or involuntary movements, especially of the face, lips, jaw, tongue; slow-frequency tremor of head or limbs, especially while moving; muscle rigidity, lack of facial expression and slow, inflexible movements.	Discontinue. Call doctor right away.
• Pacing or restlessness, intermittent spasms of muscles (of face, eyes, tongue, jaw, neck, body or limbs), dry mouth, blurred vision, constipation, difficulty urinating.	Continue. Call doctor when convenient.
Rare: Other symptoms not listed above.	Continue. Call doctor when convenient.

 ## WARNINGS & PRECAUTIONS

Don't take if:
• You are allergic to molindone.
• You have a blood or bone marrow disease.

Before you start, consult your doctor if:
• You will have surgery within 2 months, including dental surgery, requiring general or spinal anesthesia.
• You have asthma, emphysema or other lung disorder, glaucoma, prostate trouble, seizure disorders.
• You take nonprescription ulcer medicine, asthma medicine or amphetamines.

Over age 60:
- Adverse reactions and side effects may be more frequent and severe than in younger persons. More likely to develop involuntary movement of jaws, lips, tongue; chewing. Call doctor immediately. Early treatment can help.
- Use of antipsychotic drugs in elderly patients with dementia-related psychosis may increase risk of death. Consult doctor.

Pregnancy:
Decide with your doctor if drug benefits justify risk to unborn child. Risk category C (see page xviii).

Breast-feeding:
Safety not established. Consult doctor.

Infants & children:
Don't give to children younger than 2.

Prolonged use:
- May lead to tardive dyskinesia (involuntary movement of jaws, lips, tongue; chewing).
- Talk to your doctor about the need for follow-up medical examinations or laboratory studies.

Skin & sunlight:
Avoid getting overheated. The drug affects body temperature and sweating.

Driving, piloting or hazardous work:
Don't drive or pilot aircraft until you learn how medicine affects you. Don't work around dangerous machinery. Don't climb ladders or work in high places. Danger increases if you drink alcohol or take medicine affecting alertness and reflexes.

Discontinuing:
- Nervous and mental disorders—Don't discontinue without doctor's advice until you complete prescribed dose, even though symptoms diminish or disappear.
- Notify your doctor if any of the following occurs—Uncontrollable movements of tongue, arms and legs; lip smacking.

Others:
Advise any doctor or dentist whom you consult that you take this medicine.

POSSIBLE INTERACTION WITH OTHER DRUGS

GENERIC NAME OR DRUG CLASS	COMBINED EFFECT
Anticholinergics*	Increased anticholinergic effect.
Antidepressants, tricyclic*	Increased molindone effect.
Antihistamines*	Increased antihistamine effect.
Appetite suppressants*	Decreased appetite suppressant effect.
Beta-adrenergic blocking agents*	Increased tranquilizer effect.
Bupropion	Increased risk of seizures.
Central nervous system (CNS) depressants*	Increased depressive effects of both drugs.
Clozapine	Toxic effect on the central nervous system.
Extrapyramidal reaction-causing medications*	Increased frequency and severity of extrapyramidal effects.
Fluoxetine	Increased depressant effects of both drugs.
Guanethidine	Decreased guanethidine effect.
Guanfacine	May increase depressant effects of either drug.
Leucovorin	High alcohol content of leucovorin may cause adverse effects.
Levodopa	Decreased levodopa effect.
Loxapine	May increase toxic effects of both drugs.
Mind-altering drugs*	Increased effect of mind-altering drugs.
Narcotics*	Increased narcotic effect.
Phenytoin	Increased or decreased phenytoin effect.

Continued on page 922

POSSIBLE INTERACTION WITH OTHER SUBSTANCES

INTERACTS WITH	COMBINED EFFECT
Alcohol:	Dangerous oversedation.
Beverages:	None expected.
Cocaine:	Decreased molindone effect. Avoid.
Foods:	None expected.
Marijuana:	Drowsiness. May increase antinausea effect.
Tobacco:	None expected.

*See Glossary

MONOAMINE OXIDASE (MAO) INHIBITORS

GENERIC AND BRAND NAMES

ISOCARBOXAZID
  Marplan
PHENELZINE
  Nardil

TRANYLCYPROMINE
  Parnate

BASIC INFORMATION

Habit forming? No
Prescription needed? Yes
Available as generic? No
Drug class: MAO (monoamine oxidase) inhibitor, antidepressant

 ## USES

- Treatment for depression and panic disorder.
- Prevention of vascular or tension headaches.

 ## DOSAGE & USAGE INFORMATION

How to take:
Tablet—Swallow with liquid. If you can't swallow whole, crumble tablet and take with liquid or food.

When to take:
At the same times each day.

If you forget a dose:
Take as soon as you remember up to 2 hours late. If more than 2 hours, wait for next scheduled dose (don't double this dose).

What drug does:
Inhibits nerve transmissions in brain that may cause depression.

Time lapse before drug works:
4 to 6 weeks for maximum effect.

Don't take with:
- Foods containing tyramine.* Life-threatening elevation of blood pressure may result.
- Any other medicine or any dietary supplement without consulting your doctor or pharmacist.

 ## OVERDOSE

SYMPTOMS:
Restlessness, agitation, excitement, fever, confusion, dizziness, heartbeat irregularities, hallucinations, sweating, breathing difficulties, insomnia, irritability, convulsions, coma.
WHAT TO DO:
- **Dial 911 (emergency) for medical help or call poison control center 1-800-222-1222 for instructions.**
- **See emergency information on last 3 pages of this book.**

 ## POSSIBLE ADVERSE REACTIONS OR SIDE EFFECTS

SYMPTOMS	WHAT TO DO
Life-threatening:	
In case of overdose, see previous column. Also read information about dangers associated with tyramine.	
Common:	
• Fatigue, weakness.	Continue. Call doctor when convenient.
• Dizziness when changing position, restlessness, tremors, dry mouth, constipation, difficult urination, blurred vision, "sweet tooth."	Continue. Tell doctor at next visit.
Infrequent:	
• Fainting, enlarged pupils, severe headache, chest pain, rapid or pounding heartbeat.	Discontinue. Seek emergency treatment.
• Hallucinations, insomnia, nightmares, diarrhea, swollen feet or legs, joint pain.	Continue. Call doctor when convenient.
• Diminished sex drive.	Continue. Tell doctor at next visit.
Rare:	
Rash, nausea, vomiting, stiff neck, jaundice, fever, increased sweating, dark urine, slurred speech, staggering gait.	Discontinue. Call doctor right away.

 ## WARNINGS & PRECAUTIONS

Don't take if:
- You are allergic to any MAO inhibitor.
- You have heart disease, congestive heart failure, heart rhythm irregularities or high blood pressure.
- You have liver or kidney disease.

Before you start, consult your doctor if:
- You are an alcoholic.
- You have had a stroke.
- You have diabetes, epilepsy, asthma, overactive thyroid, schizophrenia, Parkinson's disease, adrenal gland tumor.
- You will have surgery within 2 months, including dental surgery, requiring anesthesia.

Over age 60:
Adverse effects more likely.

Pregnancy:
Decide with your doctor if drug benefits justify risk to unborn child. Risk category C (see page xviii).

Breast-feeding:
Safety not established. Consult doctor.

Infants & children:
Not approved for ages under 16. If prescribed, carefully read information provided with prescription. Contact doctor right away if depression symptoms get worse or there is any talk of suicide or suicide behaviors. Also, read information under Others.

Prolonged use:
- May be toxic to liver.
- Talk to your doctor about the need for follow-up medical examinations or laboratory studies to check blood pressure, liver function.

Skin & sunlight:
No special problems expected.

Driving, piloting or hazardous work:
Don't drive or pilot aircraft until you learn how medicine affects you. Don't work around dangerous machinery. Don't climb ladders or work in high places. Danger increases if you drink alcohol or take medicine affecting alertness and reflexes.

Discontinuing:
- Don't discontinue without doctor's advice until you complete prescribed dose, even though symptoms diminish or disappear.
- Follow precautions regarding foods, drinks and other medicines for 2 weeks after discontinuing.
- Adverse symptoms caused by this medicine may occur even after discontinuation. If you develop any of the symptoms listed under Overdose, notify your doctor immediately.

Others:
- May affect blood sugar levels in patients with diabetes.
- Advise any doctor or dentist whom you consult about the use of this medicine.
- Adults and children taking antidepressants may experience a worsening of the depression symptoms and may display increased suicidal thoughts or behavior. Call doctor right away if these symptoms or behaviors occur.
- Fever may indicate that MAO inhibitor dose requires adjustment.

 POSSIBLE INTERACTION WITH OTHER DRUGS

GENERIC NAME OR DRUG CLASS	COMBINED EFFECT
Amphetamines*	Blood pressure rise to life-threatening level.
Anticholinergics*	Increased anticholinergic effect.
Anticonvulsants*	Changed seizure pattern.
Antidepressants, tricyclic*	Blood pressure rise to life-threatening level. Possible fever, convulsions, delirium.
Antidiabetic agents, oral* and insulin	Excessively low blood sugar.
Antihypertensives*	Excessively low blood pressure.
Beta-adrenergic blocking agents*	Possible blood pressure rise if MAO inhibitor is discontinued after simultaneous use with acebutolol.
Bupropion	Increased risk of side effects.
Buspirone	Very high blood pressure.
Caffeine	Irregular heartbeat or high blood pressure.
Carbamazepine	Fever, seizures. Avoid.

Continued on page 923

 POSSIBLE INTERACTION WITH OTHER SUBSTANCES

INTERACTS WITH	COMBINED EFFECT
Alcohol:	Increased sedation to dangerous level.
Beverages: Caffeine drinks.	Irregular heartbeat or high blood pressure.
Drinks containing tyramine.*	Blood pressure rise to life-threatening level.
Cocaine:	Overstimulation. Possibly fatal.
Foods: Foods containing tyramine.*	Blood pressure rise to life-threatening level.
Marijuana:	Overstimulation. Avoid.
Tobacco:	None expected.

*See Glossary

MONOAMINE OXIDASE TYPE B (MAO-B) INHIBITORS

GENERIC AND BRAND NAMES

RASAGILINE
  Azilect
SELEGILINE
  Apo-Selegiline
  Atapryl
  Carbex
  Eldepryl
  Emsam

SELEGILINE (con't)
  Gen-Selegiline
  Movergan
  Novo-Selegiline
  Nu-Selegiline
  Selpak
  Zelepar

BASIC INFORMATION

Habit forming? No
Prescription needed? Yes
Available as generic? Yes, for some
Drug class: Antiparkinsonism; antidyskinetic

USES

- Treats symptoms of Parkinson's disease.
- Treats major depressive disorder (MDD).
- Treats other disorders per doctor's advice.

DOSAGE & USAGE INFORMATION

How to take:
- Tablet or capsule—Swallow whole with liquid.
- Oral disintegrating tablet—Let it dissolve on tongue. Do not swallow tablet whole.
- Skin patch—Follow prescription instructions.

When to take:
Take as directed. The oral form is usually taken at breakfast and lunch to help avoid interfering with sleep. Change patch daily at same time.

If you forget a dose:
Take as soon as you remember. If it is almost time for the next dose, wait for that dose (don't double this dose) and resume regular schedule.

Continued next column

OVERDOSE

SYMPTOMS:
Unknown; may cause sweating, dizziness, insomnia, severe headache, hallucinations, excitement, nervousness, irritability, weakness, seizures, high or low blood pressure, muscle spasm, coma.
WHAT TO DO:
- Dial 911 (emergency) for medical help or call poison control center 1-800-222-1222 for instructions.
- See emergency information on last 3 pages of this book.

What drug does:
It helps prevent breakdown of dopamine levels in the brain. Dopamine is a brain chemical having to do with control of movement and coordination.

Time lapse before drug works:
Starts working in 1-2 hours, but may take 4-6 weeks to determine drug's full effectiveness.

Don't take with:
- Foods containing tyramine.* Rarely may cause severe high blood pressure (hypertension).
- Any other medicine or diet supplement without consulting your doctor or pharmacist.

POSSIBLE ADVERSE REACTIONS OR SIDE EFFECTS

SYMPTOMS	WHAT TO DO
Life-threatening:	
Rare hypertensive crisis (chest pain, large pupils, heartbeat fast or slow, severe headache, light sensitivity, fever, cold skin, stiff or sore neck, severe nausea/vomiting). Rare allergic reaction (trouble breathing; closing of throat; hives; swelling of lips, tongue or face).	Discontinue. Seek emergency care.
Common:	
• Mood or mental changes, increase in uncontrolled body movements.	Discontinue. Call doctor right away.
• Stomach pain, dry mouth, dizziness, insomnia, feeling faint, mild nausea or vomiting, patch causes mild skin reaction.	Continue. Call doctor when convenient.
Infrequent:	
Bloody or tarry stools, urination difficult or frequent, trouble with breathing or speaking, dizziness or lightheaded when getting up from sitting or lying down, lip smacking, hallucinations, lack of balance, unusual tongue or chewing movements, stomach pain, restlessness, swollen feet or legs, new or odd movements of arms or legs or other body parts, vomiting blood or coffee-ground-like material, wheezing.	Discontinue. Call doctor right away.

MONOAMINE OXIDASE TYPE B (MAO-B) INHIBITORS

Rare:

Constipation, anxiety, tiredness, eyelid spasm, changes in taste, blurred or double vision, leg pain, ringing in ears, diarrhea, burning of lips or mouth or throat, drowsiness, sensitivity to light, sweating, loss of appetite, memory problems, muscle cramps, nervousness, numbness in fingers or toes, red or raised or itchy skin, taste changes, unusual weight loss, heartburn, jaw clenching or teeth gnashing, excess feeling of well-being.

Continue. Call doctor when convenient.

WARNINGS & PRECAUTIONS

Don't take if:
You are allergic to selegiline or rasagiline.

Before you start, consult your doctor if:
* You have a history of ulcers.
* You have tardive dyskinesia or a tremor.
* Patient has profound dementia or severe psychosis.

Over age 60:
No problems expected.

Pregnancy:
Decide with your doctor if drug benefits justify risk to unborn child. Risk category C (see page xviii).

Breast-feeding:
It is unknown if drug passes into milk. Consult doctor for advice.

Infants & children:
Not recommended.

Prolonged use:
Follow up with your doctor on a regular basis to verify the continued effectiveness of the drug.

Skin & sunlight:
May cause rash or intensify sunburn in areas exposed to sun or ultraviolet light (photosensitivity reaction). Avoid overexposure. Notify doctor if reaction occurs.

Driving, piloting or hazardous work:
Don't drive or pilot aircraft until you learn how medicine affects you. Don't work around dangerous machinery. Don't climb ladders or work in high places. Danger increases if you drink alcohol or take medicine affecting alertness and reflexes.

Discontinuing:
Don't discontinue without your doctor's approval as symptoms may worsen. A gradual reduction in dosage may be required.

Others:
* Avoid sudden rises from lying-down or sitting positions.
* Advise any doctor or dentist whom you consult that you take this medicine.

POSSIBLE INTERACTION WITH OTHER DRUGS

GENERIC NAME OR DRUG CLASS	COMBINED EFFECT
Antidepressants, tricyclic	Serious reactions. Avoid or take at least 14 days apart.
Enzyme inducers*	May decrease effect of rasagiline.
Enzyme inhibitors*	May increase effect of rasagiline.
Levodopa	Increased risk of adverse reactions.
Meperidine	Life-threatening. reactions. Avoid.
Narcotics*	Serious reactions. Avoid.
Serotonergic agents,* other	May cause a serotonin syndrome* type reaction. Avoid.

POSSIBLE INTERACTION WITH OTHER SUBSTANCES

INTERACTS WITH	COMBINED EFFECT
Alcohol:	Increased sedation. Avoid.
Beverages: Caffeine	Increased effect of caffeine. Limit use.
Cocaine:	High blood pressure, rapid heartbeat. Avoid.
Foods: Tyramine-containing*	Severe hypertension. Avoid.
Marijuana:	Excess drowsiness. Avoid.
Tobacco:	None expected.

*See Glossary

MUSCARINIC RECEPTOR ANTAGONISTS

GENERIC AND BRAND NAMES

DARIFENACIN
  Enablex
FESOTERODINE
  Toviaz
OXYBUTYNIN
  Ditropan
  Ditropan XL
  Gelnique
  Oxytrol

SOLIFENACIN
  Vesicare
TOLTERODINE
  Detrol
  Detrol LA
TROSPIUM
  Sanctura
  Sanctura XR

BASIC INFORMATION

Habit forming? No
Prescription needed? Yes
Available as generic? Yes, for some
Drug class: Antispasmodic; anticholinergic

 ## USES

Used to treat an overactive bladder in men and women. Symptoms include urinary frequency, urinary urgency, night-time urination or urge incontinence (inability to control bladder).

 ## DOSAGE & USAGE INFORMATION

How to take:
- Tablet—Swallow whole with liquid. May be taken with or without food. Take trospium 1 hour before eating or on an empty stomach.
- Extended-release capsule or tablet—Swallow whole with liquid. Take with or without food.
- Syrup, skin patch or gel (oxybutynin)—Follow instructions on prescription.

When to take:
Take one or more times (as directed) a day at the same time each day. The patch should be applied twice a week. The gel is applied daily.

Continued next column

 ## OVERDOSE

SYMPTOMS:
Unsteadiness, confusion, dizziness, severe drowsiness, fast heartbeat, fever, red face, hallucinations, difficult breathing, enlarged pupils, unusual nervousness or excitement.
WHAT TO DO:
- Dial 911 (emergency) for medical help or call poison control center 1-800-222-1222 for instructions.
- See emergency information on last 3 pages of this book.

If you forget a dose:
Take as soon as you remember. If it is almost time for the next dose, wait for that dose (don't double this dose) and resume regular schedule.

What drug does:
The drugs increase the amount of urine the bladder can hold and also decrease the pressure involved with the urge to urinate.

Time lapse before drug works:
Symptoms should start to improve in about a week. It may take 4 to 6 weeks for full benefits.

Don't take with:
Any other medicine or any dietary supplement without consulting your doctor or pharmacist.

 ## POSSIBLE ADVERSE REACTIONS OR SIDE EFFECTS

SYMPTOMS	WHAT TO DO
Life-threatening: Rare allergic reaction—Breathing difficulty; closing of the throat; swelling of hands, feet, face, lips or tongue; hives.	Discontinue. Seek emergency treatment.
Common: Constipation, dry mouth, dry eyes or throat, blurred vision, sweating decreased, urinary retention, drowsiness, skin patch causes itching at application site.	Continue. Call doctor if symptoms persist.
Infrequent: Flu-like symptoms, decreased sexual ability, difficulty in urinating, headache, sensitivity to light, nausea, vomiting, abdominal pain, insomnia, dizziness, fatigue, depression, diarrhea, gas.	Continue. Call doctor when convenient.
Rare: • Eye pain, fast heart rate, urinary tract infection, swelling of arms or legs, changes in mental status, confusion, fainting, skin changes (blistering, peeling or loosening), dark color urine, chest pain, high blood pressure.	Discontinue. Call doctor right away.
• Back or muscle pain, dry skin, skin rash.	Continue. Call doctor when convenient.

MUSCARINIC RECEPTOR ANTAGONISTS

WARNINGS & PRECAUTIONS

Don't take if:
You are allergic to muscarinic receptor antagonists or anticholinergic drugs.

Before you start, consult your doctor if:
- You have heart disease, bleeding disorder or high blood pressure.
- You have hiatal hernia; liver, kidney or thyroid disease; enlarged prostate or myasthenia gravis.
- You have any gastrointestinal disorder or intestinal or urinary tract blockage.
- You have a bladder emptying problem.
- You have glaucoma.
- You have severe ulcerative colitis.
- Patient has Alzheimer's or dementia.

Over age 60:
Adverse reactions and side effects may be more frequent and severe than in younger persons.

Pregnancy:
Decide with your doctor if drug benefits justify any possible risk to unborn child. Risk category for oxybutynin is B, others are C (see page xviii).

Breast-feeding:
It is unknown if these drugs pass into milk. Avoid drug or discontinue nursing until you finish medicine. Consult doctor for advice on maintaining milk supply.

Infants & children:
Oxybutynin is approved for use in children over age 5. Safety and effectiveness of other drugs in this group for use in children under age 18 has not been established.

Prolonged use:
No special problems expected.

Skin & sunlight:
No special problems expected.

Driving, piloting or hazardous work:
Don't drive or pilot aircraft until you learn how drug affects you. Don't work around dangerous machinery. Don't climb ladders or work in high places. Danger increases if you drink alcohol or take drugs affecting alertness and reflexes.

Discontinuing:
No special problems expected. Follow doctor's instructions.

Others:
- Advise any doctor or dentist whom you consult that you take this drug.
- Be careful in hot weather, hot tubs or saunas. The drug can increase your risk of heat stroke (due to decreased sweating).
- Chew sugarless gum or suck on ice chips to relieve a dry mouth. Call your doctor or dentist if the dry mouth lasts longer than 2 weeks.

POSSIBLE INTERACTION WITH OTHER DRUGS

GENERIC NAME OR DRUG CLASS	COMBINED EFFECT
Anticholinergics,* other	Increased risk of side effects from either drug.
Antidepressants, tricyclic*	Increased effect of antidepressant.
Cationic drugs*	May increase effect of trospium.
Central nervous system (CNS) depressants*	Increased sedative effect.
Enzyme inducers*	Decreased effect of darifenacin or solifenacin.
Enzyme inhibitors*	Increased effect of darifenacin, solifenacin or tolterodine.
Flecainide	Increased effect of flecainide. Use caution.
Ketoconazole	Increased effect of solifenacin.
QT prolongation-causing drugs*	Increased risk of heart problems.
Thioridazine	Increased effect of thioridazine.

POSSIBLE INTERACTION WITH OTHER SUBSTANCES

INTERACTS WITH	COMBINED EFFECT
Alcohol:	Increased sedative effect. Avoid.
Beverages: Grapefruit juice.	May increase effect. of darifenacin, solifenacin or tolterodine.
Cocaine:	Unknown effect. Avoid.
Foods:	None expected.
Marijuana:	Drowsiness and dry mouth. Avoid.
Tobacco:	None expected.

*See Glossary

575

MUSCLE RELAXANTS, SKELETAL

GENERIC AND BRAND NAMES

CARISOPRODOL
  Rela
  Sodol
  Soma
  Soma Compound
    with Codeine
  Sopridol
  Soridol
CHLORPHENESIN
  Maolate
CHLORZOXAZONE
  Paraflex
  Parafon Forte

METAXALONE
  Skelaxin
METHOCARBAMOL
  Carbacot
  Delaxin
  Marbaxin
  Robamol
  Robaxin
  Robaxisal
  Robomol
  Skelex

BASIC INFORMATION

Habit forming? Possibly
Prescription needed? Yes
Available as generic? Yes, for some.
Drug class: Muscle relaxant

USES

Adjunctive treatment to rest, analgesics and physical therapy for muscle spasms.

DOSAGE & USAGE INFORMATION

How to take:
* Tablet—Swallow with liquid. If you can't swallow whole, crumble tablet and take with liquid or food. Instructions to take on empty stomach mean 1 hour before or 2 hours after eating.
* Extended-release tablet—Swallow whole with liquid. Don't crumble tablet.

When to take:
As needed, no more often than every 4 hours.

Continued next column

OVERDOSE

SYMPTOMS:
Nausea, vomiting, diarrhea, convulsions, headache. May progress to severe weakness, difficult breathing, sensation of paralysis, coma.
WHAT TO DO:
* **Dial 911 (emergency) for medical help or call poison control center 1-800-222-1222 for instructions.**
* **See emergency information on last 3 pages of this book.**

If you forget a dose:
Take as soon as you remember. Wait 4 hours for next dose (don't double this dose).

What drug does:
Blocks body's pain messages to brain. Also causes sedation.

Time lapse before drug works:
30 to 60 minutes.

Don't take with:
Any other medicine or any dietary supplement without consulting your doctor or pharmacist.

POSSIBLE ADVERSE REACTIONS OR SIDE EFFECTS

SYMPTOMS	WHAT TO DO
Life-threatening:	
Hives, rash, intense itching, faintness soon after a dose (anaphylaxis); extreme weakness, transient paralysis, temporary vision loss.	Seek emergency treatment immediately.
Common:	
• Drowsiness, dizziness.	Continue. Call doctor when convenient.
• Orange or red-purple urine.	No action necessary.
Infrequent:	
• Agitation, constipation or diarrhea, nausea, cramps, vomiting, wheezing, shortness of breath, headache, depression, muscle weakness, trembling, insomnia, uncontrolled eye movements, fainting.	Discontinue. Call doctor right away.
• Blurred vision.	Continue. Call Doctor when convenient.
Rare:	
• Black, tarry or bloody stool; convulsions.	Discontinue. Seek emergency treatment.
• Rash, hives, or itch; sore throat; fever; jaundice; tiredness; hiccups.	Discontinue. Call doctor right away.

WARNINGS & PRECAUTIONS

Don't take if:
- You are allergic to any skeletal muscle relaxant.
- You have porphyria.

Before you start, consult your doctor if:
- You have had liver or kidney disease.
- You plan pregnancy within medication period.
- You are allergic to tartrazine dye.
- You suffer from depression.

Over age 60:
Adverse reactions and side effects may be more frequent and severe than in younger persons.

Pregnancy:
Safety not proven. Avoid if possible. Consult doctor. Risk category C (see page xviii).

Breast-feeding:
Drug may pass into milk. Avoid drug or discontinue nursing until you finish medicine. Consult doctor for advice on maintaining milk supply.

Infants & children:
Not recommended.

Prolonged use:
- Talk to your doctor about the need for follow-up medical examinations or laboratory studies to check liver function, kidney function, complete blood counts (white blood cell count, platelet count, red blood cell count, hemoglobin, hematocrit).
- Safety beyond 8 weeks of treatment not established.

Skin & sunlight:
No problems expected.

Driving, piloting or hazardous work:
Don't drive or pilot aircraft until you learn how medicine affects you. Don't work around dangerous machinery. Don't climb ladders or work in high places. Danger increases if you drink alcohol or take medicine affecting alertness and reflexes, such as antihistamines, tranquilizers, sedatives, pain medicine, narcotics and mind-altering drugs.

Discontinuing:
Don't discontinue without doctor's advice until you complete prescribed dose, even though symptoms diminish or disappear.

Others:
- May affect results in some medical tests.
- Advise any doctor or dentist whom you consult that you take this medicine.

POSSIBLE INTERACTION WITH OTHER DRUGS

GENERIC NAME OR DRUG CLASS	COMBINED EFFECT
Antidepressants*	Increased sedation.
Antihistamines*	Increased sedation.
Clozapine	Toxic effect on the central nervous system.
Central nervous system (CNS) depressants*	Increased depressive effects of both drugs.
Dronabinol	Increased effect of dronabinol on central nervous system. Avoid combination.
Mind-altering drugs*	Increased sedation.
Muscle relaxants,* others	Increased sedation.
Narcotics*	Increased sedation.
Sedatives*	Increased sedation.
Sertraline	Increased depressive effects of both drugs.
Sleep inducers*	Increased sedation.
Tranquilizers*	Increased sedation.

POSSIBLE INTERACTION WITH OTHER SUBSTANCES

INTERACTS WITH	COMBINED EFFECT
Alcohol:	Increased sedation.
Beverages:	None expected.
Cocaine:	Lack of coordination, increased sedation.
Foods:	None expected.
Marijuana:	Lack of coordination, drowsiness, fainting.
Tobacco:	None expected.

*See Glossary

NABILONE

BRAND NAMES

Cesamet

BASIC INFORMATION

Habit forming? No
Prescription needed? Yes
Available as generic? No
Drug class: Antiemetic

 ## USES

- Treats nausea and vomiting.
- Prevents nausea and vomiting in patients receiving cancer chemotherapy.

 ## DOSAGE & USAGE INFORMATION

How to take:
Capsule—Swallow with liquid. If you can't swallow whole, open capsule and take with liquid or food.

When to take:
At the same times each day, according to instructions on prescription label.

If you forget a dose:
Take as soon as you remember up to 2 hours late. If more than 2 hours, wait for next scheduled dose (don't double this dose).

What drug does:
Chemically related to marijuana, it probably regulates the vomiting control center in the brain.

Time lapse before drug works:
2 hours.

Continued next column

 ## OVERDOSE

SYMPTOMS:
Mood changes; confusion and delusions; hallucinations; mental depression; nervousness; breathing difficulty; fast, slow or pounding heartbeat; fainting.
WHAT TO DO:
- Dial 911 (emergency) for medical help or call poison control center 1-800-222-1222 for instructions.
- If person is unconscious, check breathing and pulse. If not breathing, begin mouth-to-mouth rescue breathing. If heart is not beating, begin chest compressions.
- See emergency information on last 3 pages of this book.

Don't take with:
- Alcohol or any drug that depresses the central nervous system. See Central Nervous System (CNS) Depressants in the Glossary.
- Any other medicine or any dietary supplement without consulting your doctor or pharmacist.

 ## POSSIBLE ADVERSE REACTIONS OR SIDE EFFECTS

SYMPTOMS	WHAT TO DO
Life-threatening: Mood changes; fainting; hallucinations; fast, slow or pounding heartbeat; confusion and delusions; mental depression; nervousness; breathing difficulty.	Seek emergency treatment.
Common: Dry mouth.	Continue. Call doctor when convenient.
Infrequent: Clumsiness, mental changes, drowsiness, headache, false sense of well-being.	Discontinue. Call doctor right away.
Rare: Blurred vision, dizziness on standing, appetite loss, muscle pain.	Discontinue. Call doctor right away.

WARNINGS & PRECAUTIONS

Don't take if:
- You are allergic to nabilone or marijuana.
- You have schizophrenic, manic or depressive states.

Before you start, consult your doctor if:
- You have abused drugs or are dependent on them, including alcohol.
- You have had high blood pressure or heart disease.
- You have had impaired liver function.

Over age 60:
Adverse reactions and side effects may be more frequent and severe than in younger persons. You may need smaller doses for shorter periods of time.

Pregnancy:
Decide with your doctor whether drug benefits justify risk to unborn child. Risk category C (see page xviii).

Breast-feeding:
Drug passes into milk. Avoid drug or discontinue nursing until you finish medicine. Consult doctor for advice on maintaining milk supply.

Infants & children:
Not recommended for children 18 and younger. Use only under doctor's supervision.

Prolonged use:
- Avoid prolonged use. This medicine is intended to be used only during a cycle of cancer chemotherapy.
- Talk to your doctor about the need for follow-up medical examinations or laboratory studies to check blood pressure, heart function.

Skin & sunlight:
No problems expected.

Driving, piloting or hazardous work:
Don't drive or pilot aircraft until you learn how medicine affects you. Don't work around dangerous machinery. Don't climb ladders or work in high places. Danger increases if you drink alcohol or take medicine affecting alertness and reflexes.

Discontinuing:
No problems expected.

Others:
- Blood pressure should be measured regularly.
- Learn to count and recognize changes in your pulse.
- Get up from bed or chair slowly to avoid fainting.

POSSIBLE INTERACTION WITH OTHER DRUGS

GENERIC NAME OR DRUG CLASS	COMBINED EFFECT
Apomorphine	Decreased effect of apomorphine.
Central nervous system (CNS) depressants,* other	Greater depression of the central nervous system.

POSSIBLE INTERACTION WITH OTHER SUBSTANCES

INTERACTS WITH	COMBINED EFFECT
Alcohol:	Dangerous depression of the central nervous system. Avoid.
Beverages:	None expected.
Cocaine:	Decreased nabilone effect. Avoid.
Foods:	None expected.
Marijuana:	None expected.
Tobacco:	None expected.

*See Glossary

NAFARELIN

BRAND NAMES

Synarel

BASIC INFORMATION

Habit forming? No
Prescription needed? Yes
Available as generic? No
Drug class: Gonadotropin inhibitor

 USES

- Treatment for endometriosis to relieve pain and reduce scattered implants of endometrial tissue.
- Treatment for central precocious puberty.

 DOSAGE & USAGE INFORMATION

How to take:
Nasal spray—Follow instructions on package insert provided with your medicine.

When to take:
As directed by your doctor. Usually two times a day.

If you forget a dose:
Take as soon as you remember. Don't double this dose.

What drug does:
Reduces estrogen production by ovaries.

Time lapse before drug works:
May require 6 months for full effect.

Don't take with:
- Birth control pills.
- Nasal sprays to decongest the membranes in the nose.
- Any other medicine or any dietary supplement without consulting your doctor or pharmacist.

 OVERDOSE

SYMPTOMS:
None expected.
WHAT TO DO:
Overdose unlikely to threaten life. If person uses much larger amount than prescribed or if accidentally swallowed, call doctor or poison control center 1-800-222-1222 for help.

 POSSIBLE ADVERSE REACTIONS OR SIDE EFFECTS

SYMPTOMS	WHAT TO DO
Life-threatening: None expected.	
Common: Hot flashes.	No action necessary.
Infrequent: Decreased sexual desire, vaginal dryness, headache, acne, swelling of hands and feet, reduction of breast size, weight gain, itchy scalp with flaking, muscle ache, nasal irritation.	Continue. Call doctor when convenient.
Rare: Insomnia, depression, weight loss.	Continue. Call doctor when convenient.

NAFARELIN

WARNINGS & PRECAUTIONS

Don't take if:
- You become pregnant.
- You have breast cancer.
- You are allergic to any of the ingredients in nafarelin.
- You have undiagnosed abnormal vaginal bleeding.

Before you start, consult your doctor if:
- You take birth control pills.
- You have diabetes.
- You have heart disease.
- You have epilepsy.
- You have kidney disease.
- You have liver disease.
- You have migraine headaches.
- You need to use topical nasal decongestants.

Over age 60:
Adverse reactions and side effects may be more frequent and severe than in younger persons.

Pregnancy:
Risk to unborn child outweighs drug benefits. Don't use. Stop if you get pregnant. Consult doctor. Risk category X (see page xviii).

Breast-feeding:
Unknown whether medicine filters into milk. Consult doctor.

Infants & children:
Not recommended.

Prolonged use:
- Full effect requires prolonged use. Don't discontinue without consulting doctor.
- Talk to your doctor about the need for mammogram, follow-up medical examinations or laboratory studies to check liver function.

Skin & sunlight:
No special problems expected.

Driving, piloting or hazardous work:
No special problems expected.

Discontinuing:
Don't discontinue without consulting doctor. Menstrual periods may be absent for 2 to 3 months after discontinuation.

Others:
- May alter blood sugar levels in diabetic persons.
- Interferes with accuracy of laboratory tests to study pituitary gonadotropic and gonadal functions.
- Experience with nafarelin has been limited to women 18 years of age and older.
- Bone density decreases during treatment phase, but recovers following treatment.

POSSIBLE INTERACTION WITH OTHER DRUGS

GENERIC NAME OR DRUG CLASS	COMBINED EFFECT
Decongestant nasal sprays*	Decreased absorption of nafarelin.

POSSIBLE INTERACTION WITH OTHER SUBSTANCES

INTERACTS WITH	COMBINED EFFECT
Alcohol:	Excessive nervous system depression. Avoid.
Beverages: Caffeine drinks.	Rapid, irregular heartbeat. Avoid.
Cocaine:	May interfere with expected action of nafarelin. Avoid.
Foods:	None expected.
Marijuana:	May interfere with expected action of nafarelin. Avoid.
Tobacco:	Rapid, irregular heartbeat; increased leg cramps. Avoid.

*See Glossary

NALTREXONE

BRAND NAMES

Barr   Vivitrol
ReVia

BASIC INFORMATION

Habit forming? No
Prescription needed? Yes
Available as generic? Yes
Drug class: Narcotic antagonist

USES

- Treats detoxified former narcotics addicts. It helps maintain a drug-free state.
- May be used to treat alcoholism (along with a counseling program).

DOSAGE & USAGE INFORMATION

How to take:
- *Don't take at all until detoxification has been accomplished.*
- Tablet—Swallow with liquid or food to lessen stomach irritation. If you can't swallow whole, crumble tablet and take with liquid or food.
- Extended-release injectable—Given by a healthcare provider.

When to take:
- Take tablet at the same time every day or every other day as directed.
- Extended-release injectable is given monthly.

If you forget a dose:
Follow detailed instructions from the one who prescribed for you.

What drug does:
It works in the brain to block the pleasurable effects or high feeling you get when you use narcotics or alcohol.

Continued next column

OVERDOSE

SYMPTOMS:
Seizures, nausea, stomach pain, dizziness, coma.
WHAT TO DO:
- **Dial 911 (emergency) for medical help or call poison control center 1-800-222-1222 for instructions.**
- **See emergency information on last 3 pages of this book.**

Time lapse before drug works:
1 hour.

Don't take with:
- Narcotics.
- Any other medicine or any dietary supplement without consulting your doctor or pharmacist.

POSSIBLE ADVERSE REACTIONS OR SIDE EFFECTS

SYMPTOMS	WHAT TO DO
Life-threatening: Hallucinations, very fast heartbeat, fainting, breathing difficulties.	Seek emergency treatment immediately.
Common: Skin rash, chills, constipation, appetite loss, irritability, insomnia, anxiety, headache, nausea, vomiting.	Continue. Call doctor when convenient.
Infrequent: • Nosebleeds, joint pain.	Discontinue. Call doctor right away.
• Abdominal pain, blurred vision, confusion, earache, fever, depression, diarrhea, common cold symptoms, injection site reaction (pain, tender, itching or hard lump).	Continue. Call doctor when convenient.
Rare: • Pain, tenderness or color change in feet.	Discontinue. Call doctor right away.
• Ringing in ears, swollen glands, decreased sex drive.	Continue. Call doctor when convenient.

WARNINGS & PRECAUTIONS

Don't take if:
- You will not have close medical supervision.
- You are currently dependent on drugs.
- You have severe liver disease.

Before you start, consult your doctor if:
You have mild liver disease, kidney disease or bleeding disorder such as hemophilia.

Over age 60:
Adverse reactions and side effects may be more frequent and severe than in younger persons. You may need smaller doses for shorter periods of time.

Pregnancy:
Decide with your doctor whether drug benefits justify risk to unborn child. Risk category C (see page xviii).

Breast-feeding:
Safety not established. Consult doctor.

Infants & children:
Not recommended.

Prolonged use:
- Not recommended.
- Talk to your doctor about the need for follow-up medical examinations or laboratory studies to check kidney function.

Skin & sunlight:
No problems expected.

Driving, piloting or hazardous work:
Don't drive or pilot aircraft until you learn how medicine affects you. Don't work around dangerous machinery. Don't climb ladders or work in high places. Danger increases if you drink alcohol or take medicine affecting alertness and reflexes.

Discontinuing:
Don't discontinue without consulting doctor. Dose may require gradual reduction if you have taken drug for a long time. Doses of other drugs may also require adjustment.

Others:
- Probably not effective in treating people addicted to substances other than opium or morphine derivatives.
- Must be given under close supervision by people experienced in using naltrexone to treat addicts.
- Attempting to use narcotics to overcome effects of naltrexone may lead to coma and death.
- Advise any doctor or dentist whom you consult that you take this medicine.
- Withdraw from medication several days prior to expected surgery.

 POSSIBLE INTERACTION WITH OTHER DRUGS

GENERIC NAME OR DRUG CLASS	COMBINED EFFECT
Narcotic medicines*	1. Precipitates withdrawal symptoms. May lead to cardiac arrest, coma and death (if naltrexone taken while person is dependent on these drugs). 2. If these drugs are taken while person is taking naltrexone, opioid effect (pain relief) will be blocked.
Isoniazid	Increased risk of liver damage.

 POSSIBLE INTERACTION WITH OTHER SUBSTANCES

INTERACTS WITH	COMBINED EFFECT
Alcohol:	Unpredictable effects. Avoid.
Beverages:	None expected.
Cocaine:	Unpredictable effects. Avoid.
Foods:	None expected.
Marijuana:	Unpredictable effects. Avoid.
Tobacco:	None expected.

*See Glossary

NARCOTIC ANALGESICS

GENERIC AND BRAND NAMES

See full list of generic and brand names in the *Generic and Brand Name Directory*, page 891.

BASIC INFORMATION

Habit forming? Yes
Prescription needed? Yes
Available as generic? Yes
Drug class: Narcotic

 ## USES

Relieves pain and diarrhea; suppresses cough.

 ## DOSAGE & USAGE INFORMATION

How to take:
* Tablet, capsule or extended-release tablet— Swallow with liquid. Do not crush, crumble or open extended release forms, especially the Palladone brand (could lead to a fatal dose).
* Liquid form of morphine—Mix with fruit juice just before taking to improve taste.
* Syrup—Mix with one-half glass of water (4 oz.) before swallowing.
* Dispersible tablets—Stir into water or fruit juice just before taking each dose.
* Liquid form—May need to be diluted with water before taking. Follow directions on label.
* Suppositories—Remove wrapper and moisten suppository with water. Gently insert into rectum, small end first.
* Nasal, transmucosal or lozenge form—Follow prescription instructions.
* Transdermal—Follow instructions exactly.
* Buccal tablet—Let tablet dissolve in mouth per instructions. Do not chew or swallow whole.

Continued next column

 ## OVERDOSE

SYMPTOMS:
Deep sleep, slow breathing; slow pulse; respiratory arrest; flushed, warm skin; seizures; constricted pupils.
WHAT TO DO:
* **Dial 911 (emergency) for medical help or call poison control center 1-800-222-1222 for instructions.**
* **If person is unconscious, check breathing and pulse. If not breathing, begin mouth-to-mouth rescue breathing. If heart is not beating, begin chest compressions.**
* **See emergency information on last 3 pages of this book.**

When to take:
When needed. No more often than every 4 hours.

If you forget a dose:
Take as soon as you remember. Wait 4 hours for next dose.

What drug does:
* Blocks pain messages to brain and spinal cord.
* Reduces sensitivity of brain's cough control center.

Time lapse before drug works:
30 minutes.

Don't take with:
Any other medicine or any dietary supplement without consulting your doctor or pharmacist.

 ## POSSIBLE ADVERSE REACTIONS OR SIDE EFFECTS

SYMPTOMS	WHAT TO DO
Life-threatening:	
Irregular or slow heartbeat, difficult breathing, wheezing.	Discontinue. Seek emergency treatment.
Common:	
Dizziness, drowsiness, tiredness, headache, lightheadedness, nausea or vomiting, stomach cramps, overexcitement.	Continue. Call doctor when convenient.
Infrequent:	
• Black, tarry stools; bloody or cloudy urine; painful or frequent urination; fast, slow or pounding heartbeat; hallucinations; breathing problems, wheezing; back or side pain; red dots on skin; red or flushed face; ringing or buzzing in ears; skin rash, hives or itching; sore throat; fever; face swelling; decreased urine; trembling; uncontrolled muscle movements; unusual bleeding or bruising; yellow skin or eyes.	Discontinue. Call doctor right away.
• Feeling depressed, pale stools.	Continue. Call doctor when convenient.
Rare:	
Changes in vision, constipation, dry mouth, loss of appetite, restlessness, nightmares, trouble sleeping.	Discontinue. Call doctor when convenient.

WARNINGS & PRECAUTIONS

Don't take if:
- You are allergic to any narcotic.
- Diarrhea is due to toxic effect of drugs or poisons.

Before you start, consult your doctor if:
- You have asthma or liver or kidney problems.
- You will have surgery within 2 months, including dental surgery, requiring general or spinal anesthesia.

Over age 60:
More likely to be drowsy, dizzy, unsteady or constipated. Use only if absolutely necessary.

Pregnancy:
Risk factors vary for drugs in this group. See category list on page xviii and consult doctor.

Breast-feeding:
Drug passes into milk and may harm child. Avoid drug or discontinue nursing until you finish medicine. Consult doctor for advice on maintaining milk supply.

Infants & children:
Not recommended.

Prolonged use:
- With high doses and long-term use, can cause psychological and physical dependence (addiction).
- May cause chronic constipation.

Skin & sunlight:
No special problems expected.

Driving, piloting or hazardous work:
Don't drive or pilot aircraft until you learn how medicine affects you. Don't work around dangerous machinery. Don't climb ladders or work in high places. Danger increases if you drink alcohol or take medicine affecting alertness and reflexes.

Discontinuing:
- Discontinue in 2 days if symptoms don't improve. Report to the doctor any symptoms that develop after discontinuing, such as gooseflesh, irritability, insomnia, yawning, weakness, large eye pupils.
- If used for several weeks or more, consult doctor before discontinuing.

Others:
- Some products contain tartrazine dye. Avoid, especially if you are allergic to aspirin.
- Advise any doctor or dentist whom you consult that you take this medicine.
- Follow directions exactly for using the fentanyl skin patch to avoid an overdose that could lead to severe side effects (including death).
- Lying down after the first few doses may decrease unwanted effects of nausea, vomiting, lightheadedness or dizziness.

POSSIBLE INTERACTION WITH OTHER DRUGS

GENERIC NAME OR DRUG CLASS	COMBINED EFFECT
Analgesics,* other	Increased analgesic effect.
Anticoagulants,* oral	Possible increased anticoagulant effect.
Anticholinergics*	Increased anticholinergic effect.
Antidepressants*	Increased sedative effect.
Antihistamines*	Increased sedative effect.
Anti-inflammatory drugs, nonsteroidal (NSAIDs)*	Increased narcotic effect.
Butorphanol	Possibly precipitates withdrawal with chronic narcotic use.
Carbamazepine	Increased carbamazepine effect possible with propoxyphene.
Carteolol	Increased narcotic effect. Dangerous sedation.

Continued on page 924

POSSIBLE INTERACTION WITH OTHER SUBSTANCES

INTERACTS WITH	COMBINED EFFECT
Alcohol:	Increased intoxicating effect of alcohol (especially Avinza brand). Do not drink alcohol or take alcohol-containing drugs.
Beverages:	None expected.
Cocaine:	Increased toxic effects of cocaine. Avoid.
Foods:	None expected.
Marijuana:	Impaired physical and mental performance. Avoid.
Tobacco:	None expected.

*See Glossary

NARCOTIC ANALGESICS & ACETAMINOPHEN

GENERIC AND BRAND NAMES

See full list of generic and brand names in the *Generic and Brand Name Directory*, page 892.

BASIC INFORMATION

Habit forming? Yes
Prescription needed? Yes
Available as generic? Yes
Drug class: Narcotic, analgesic, fever reducer

 ## USES

Relieves pain, reduces fever.

 ## DOSAGE & USAGE INFORMATION

How to take:
• Tablet or capsule—Swallow with liquid. If you can't swallow whole, crumble tablet or open capsule and take with liquid or food.
• Syrup—Mix with one-half glass of water (4 oz.) before swallowing.
• Liquid form—May need to be diluted with water before taking. Follow directions on label.

When to take:
When needed. No more often than every 4 hours.

If you forget a dose:
Take as soon as you remember. Wait 4 hours for next dose.

Continued next column

 ## OVERDOSE

SYMPTOMS:
Stomach upset; irritability; sweating, convulsions; deep sleep; slow breathing; slow pulse; flushed, warm skin; constricted pupils; coma.
WHAT TO DO:
• **Dial 911 (emergency) for medical help or call poison control center 1-800-222-1222 for instructions.**
• **If person is unconscious, check breathing and pulse. If not breathing, begin mouth-to-mouth rescue breathing. If heart is not beating, begin chest compressions.**
• **See emergency information on last 3 pages of this book.**

What drug does:
• May affect hypothalamus—the part of the brain that helps regulate body heat and receives body's pain messages.
• Blocks pain messages to brain and spinal cord.
• Reduces sensitivity of brain's cough control center.

Time lapse before drug works:
15 to 30 minutes. May last 4 hours.

Don't take with:
• Other drugs with acetaminophen. Too much acetaminophen can damage liver and kidneys.
• Any other medicine or any dietary supplement without consulting your doctor or pharmacist.

 ## POSSIBLE ADVERSE REACTIONS OR SIDE EFFECTS

SYMPTOMS	WHAT TO DO
Life-threatening:	
Irregular or slow heartbeat, difficult breathing, wheezing.	Discontinue. Seek emergency treatment.
Common:	
Dizziness, drowsiness, tiredness, headache, lightheadedness, nausea or vomiting, stomach cramps, overexcitement.	Continue. Call doctor when convenient.
Infrequent:	
• Black, tarry stools; bloody or cloudy urine; painful or frequent urination; fast, slow or pounding heartbeat; hallucinations; breathing problems, wheezing; back or side pain; red dots on skin; red or flushed face; ringing or buzzing in ears; skin rash, hives or itching; sore throat; fever; face swelling; decreased urine; trembling; uncontrolled muscle movements; unusual bleeding or bruising; yellow skin or eyes.	Discontinue. Call doctor right away.
• Feeling depressed, pale stools.	Continue. Call doctor when convenient.
Rare:	
Changes in vision, constipation, dry mouth, loss of appetite, restlessness, nightmares, trouble sleeping.	Discontinue. Call doctor when convenient.

NARCOTIC ANALGESICS & ACETAMINOPHEN

 WARNINGS & PRECAUTIONS

Don't take if:
- You are allergic to any narcotic or acetaminophen.
- Your symptoms don't improve after 2 days use. Call your doctor.

Before you start, consult your doctor if:
- You have bronchial asthma, kidney disease or liver damage.
- You will have surgery within 2 months, including dental surgery, requiring general or spinal anesthesia.

Over age 60:
More likely to be drowsy, dizzy, unsteady or constipated. Don't exceed recommended dose.

Pregnancy:
Risk factors vary for drugs in this group. See category list on page xviii and consult doctor.

Breast-feeding:
Drug passes into milk and may harm child. Avoid drug or discontinue nursing until you finish medicine. Consult doctor for advice on maintaining milk supply.

Infants & children:
Not recommended.

Prolonged use:
- With high doses and long-term use, can cause psychological and physical dependence (addiction).
- May cause chronic constipation.

Skin & sunlight:
No problems expected.

Driving, piloting or hazardous work:
Don't drive or pilot aircraft until you learn how medicine affects you. Don't work around dangerous machinery. Don't climb ladders or work in high places. Danger increases if you drink alcohol or take medicine affecting alertness and reflexes.

Discontinuing:
- Discontinue in 2 days if symptoms don't improve. Report to your doctor any symptoms that develop after discontinuing, such as gooseflesh, irritability, insomnia, yawning, weakness, large eye pupils.
- If used for several weeks or more, consult doctor before discontinuing.

Others:
- Lying down after the first few doses may decrease unwanted effects of nausea, vomiting, lightheadedness or dizziness.
- Advise any doctor or dentist whom you consult that you take this medicine.

 POSSIBLE INTERACTION WITH OTHER DRUGS

GENERIC NAME OR DRUG CLASS	COMBINED EFFECT
Analgesics,* other	Increased analgesic effect.
Anticoagulants,* other	May increase anticoagulant effect. Prothrombin times should be monitored.
Anticholinergics*	Increased anticholinergic effect.
Antidepressants*	Increased sedative effect.
Antihistamines*	Increased sedative effect.
Carteolol	Increased narcotic effect. Dangerous sedation.
Mind-altering drugs*	Increased sedative effect.
Narcotics,* other	Increased narcotic effect.
Nitrates*	Excessive blood pressure drop.
Phenobarbital and other barbiturates*	Quicker elimination and decreased effect of acetaminophen.

Continued on page 924

 POSSIBLE INTERACTION WITH OTHER SUBSTANCES

INTERACTS WITH	COMBINED EFFECT
Alcohol:	Increased intoxicating effect of alcohol. Do not drink alcohol or take alcohol-containing drugs.
Beverages:	None expected.
Cocaine:	Increased toxic effects of cocaine. Avoid.
Foods:	None expected.
Marijuana:	Impaired physical and mental performance. Avoid.
Tobacco:	None expected.

*See Glossary

NARCOTIC ANALGESICS & ASPIRIN

GENERIC AND BRAND NAMES

See full list of generic and brand names in the *Generic and Brand Name Directory*, page 892.

BASIC INFORMATION

Habit forming? Yes
Prescription needed? Yes
Available as generic? Yes
Drug class: Narcotic, analgesic, anti-inflammatory (nonsteroidal)

 ## USES

Reduces pain, fever, inflammation.

 ## DOSAGE & USAGE INFORMATION

How to take:
Tablet or capsule—Swallow with liquid. If you can't swallow whole, crumble tablet or open capsule and take with liquid or food.

When to take:
When needed. No more often than every 4 hours.

If you forget a dose:
Take as soon as you remember. Wait 4 hours for next dose.

Continued next column

 ## OVERDOSE

SYMPTOMS:
Ringing in ears; nausea; vomiting; dizziness; fever; deep sleep; slow breathing; slow pulse; flushed, warm skin; constricted pupils; hallucinations; convulsions; coma.
WHAT TO DO:
- **Dial 911 (emergency) for medical help or call poison control center 1-800-222-1222 for instructions.**
- **If person is unconscious, check breathing and pulse. If not breathing, begin mouth-to-mouth rescue breathing. If heart is not beating, begin chest compressions.**
- **See emergency information on last 3 pages of this book.**

What drug does:
- Affects hypothalamus, the part of the brain which regulates temperature, by dilating small blood vessels in skin.
- Prevents clumping of platelets (small blood cells) so blood vessels remain open.
- Decreases prostaglandin effect.
- Suppresses body's pain messages.
- Reduces sensitivity of brain's cough control center.

Time lapse before drug works:
30 minutes.

Don't take with:
- Tetracyclines. Space doses 1 hour apart.
- Any other medicine or any dietary supplement without consulting your doctor or pharmacist.

 ## POSSIBLE ADVERSE REACTIONS OR SIDE EFFECTS

SYMPTOMS	WHAT TO DO
Life-threatening:	
Irregular or slow heartbeat, difficult breathing, wheezing.	Discontinue. Seek emergency treatment.
Common:	
Dizziness, drowsiness, tiredness, headache, lightheadedness, nausea or vomiting, stomach cramps, overexcitement.	Continue. Call doctor when convenient.
Infrequent:	
• Black, tarry stools; bloody or cloudy urine; painful or frequent urination; fast, slow or pounding heartbeat; hallucinations; breathing problems, wheezing; back or side pain; red dots on skin; red or flushed face; ringing or buzzing in ears; skin rash, hives or itching; sore throat; fever; face swelling; decreased urine; trembling; uncontrolled muscle movements; unusual bleeding or bruising; yellow skin or eyes.	Discontinue. Call doctor right away.
• Feeling depressed, pale stools.	Continue. Call doctor when convenient.
Rare:	
Changes in vision, constipation, dry mouth, loss of appetite, restlessness, nightmares, trouble sleeping.	Discontinue. Call doctor when convenient.

WARNINGS & PRECAUTIONS

Don't take if:
- You are allergic to any narcotic or subject to any substance abuse.
- You have a peptic ulcer of stomach or duodenum or a bleeding disorder.
- You are allergic to aspirin.

Before you start, consult your doctor if:
- You have impaired liver or kidney function, asthma or nasal polyps.
- You have had stomach or duodenal ulcers, gout.
- You will have surgery within 2 months, including dental surgery, requiring general or spinal anesthesia.

Over age 60:
- More likely to be drowsy, dizzy, unsteady or constipated. Use only if absolutely necessary.
- More likely to cause hidden bleeding in stomach or intestines. Watch for dark stools.

Pregnancy:
Risk factors vary for drugs in this group. See category list on page xviii and consult doctor.

Breast-feeding:
Drug passes into milk and may harm child. Avoid drug or discontinue nursing until you finish medicine. Consult doctor for advice on maintaining milk supply.

Infants & children:
Not recommended.

Prolonged use:
- With high doses and long-term use, can cause psychological and physical dependence (addiction).
- May cause chronic constipation.

Skin & sunlight:
No special problems expected.

Driving, piloting or hazardous work:
Don't drive or pilot aircraft until you learn how medicine affects you. Don't work around danger-ous machinery. Don't climb ladders or work in high places. Danger increases if you drink alcohol or take medicine affecting alertness and reflexes, such as antihistamines, tranquilizers, sedatives, pain medicine, narcotics and mind-altering drugs.

Discontinuing:
- Discontinue in 2 to 3 days if symptoms don't improve. Report to your doctor any symptoms that develop after discontinuing, such as gooseflesh, irritability, insomnia, weakness, large eye pupils.
- If used for several weeks or more, consult doctor before discontinuing.

Others:
- Aspirin can complicate surgery; illness; pregnancy, labor and delivery.
- Urine tests for blood sugar may be inaccurate.

- Advise any doctor or dentist whom you consult that you take this medicine.
- Lying down after the first few doses may decrease unwanted effects of nausea, vomiting, lightheadedness or dizziness.
- Don't use if medicine has a strong vinegar-like odor. This means the aspirin is breaking down.

POSSIBLE INTERACTION WITH OTHER DRUGS

GENERIC NAME OR DRUG CLASS	COMBINED EFFECT
Acebutolol	Decreased anti-hypertensive effect of acebutolol.
Adrenocorticoids, systemic	Increased risk of ulcers. Increased adrenocorticoid effect.
Alendronate	Increased risk of stomach irritation.
Allopurinol	Decreased allopurinol effect.
Angiotensin-converting enzyme (ACE) inhibitors*	Decreased effect of ACE inhibitor.
Antacids*	Decreased aspirin effect.
Anticoagulants,* oral	Increased anticoagulant effect. Abnormal bleeding.
Antidepressants*	Increased sedative effect.

Continued on page 925

POSSIBLE INTERACTION WITH OTHER SUBSTANCES

INTERACTS WITH	COMBINED EFFECT
Alcohol:	Increased intoxicating effect of alcohol. (especially Avinza brand) Do not drink alcohol or take alcohol-containing drugs.
Beverages:	None expected.
Cocaine:	Unknown. Avoid.
Foods:	None expected.
Marijuana:	Impaired physical and mental performance. Avoid.
Tobacco:	None expected.

*See Glossary

NATAMYCIN (Ophthalmic)

BRAND NAMES

Natacyn   Pimaricin

BASIC INFORMATION

Habit forming? No
Prescription needed? Yes
Available as generic? No
Drug class: Antifungal (ophthalmic)

USES

Treats fungus infections of the eye.

DOSAGE & USAGE INFORMATION

How to use:
Eye drops
- Wash hands.
- Apply pressure to inside corner of eye with middle finger.
- Tilt head backward. Pull lower lid away from eye with index finger of the same hand.
- Drop eye drops into pouch and close eye. Don't blink.
- Continue pressure for 1 minute after placing medicine in eye.
- Keep eyes closed for 1 to 2 minutes.
- Don't touch applicator tip to any surface (including the eye). If you accidentally touch tip, clean with warm water and soap.
- Keep container tightly closed.
- Keep drops cool, but don't freeze.
- Wash hands immediately after using.

When to use:
As directed. Usually 1 drop in eye every 1 or 2 hours for 3 or 4 days, then every 3 to 4 hours.

If you forget a dose:
Use as soon as you remember.

What drug does:
Changes cell membrane of fungus causing loss of essential constituents of fungus cell.

Continued next column

OVERDOSE

SYMPTOMS:
None expected.
WHAT TO DO:
Not intended for internal use. If child accidentally swallows, dial 911 (emergency) for medical help or call poison control center 1-800-222-1222 for instructions.

Time lapse before drug works:
Starts to work immediately. May require 2 weeks or more to cure infection.

Don't use with:
Other eye drops without consulting your eye doctor.

POSSIBLE ADVERSE REACTIONS OR SIDE EFFECTS

SYMPTOMS	WHAT TO DO
Life-threatening: None expected.	
Common: None expected.	
Infrequent: Eye irritation not present before using natamycin.	Discontinue. Call doctor right away.
Rare: None expected.	

WARNINGS & PRECAUTIONS

Don't use if:
You are allergic to natamycin or any antifungal medicine.*

Before you start, consult your doctor if:
You have allergies to any substance.

Over age 60:
No problems expected.

Pregnancy:
Decide with your doctor if drug benefits justify risk to unborn child. Risk category C (see page xviii).

Breast-feeding:
No problems expected, but check with doctor.

Infants & children:
No problems expected.

Prolonged use:
May cause eye irritation.

Skin & sunlight:
No problems expected.

Driving, piloting or hazardous work:
No problems expected.

Discontinuing:
Don't discontinue without consulting your eye doctor.

Others:
Notify doctor if condition doesn't improve within 1 week.

 ## POSSIBLE INTERACTION WITH OTHER DRUGS

GENERIC NAME OR DRUG CLASS	COMBINED EFFECT

Clinically significant interactions with oral or injected medicines unlikely.

 ## POSSIBLE INTERACTION WITH OTHER SUBSTANCES

INTERACTS WITH	COMBINED EFFECT
Alcohol:	None expected.
Beverages:	None expected.
Cocaine:	None expected.
Foods:	None expected.
Marijuana:	None expected.
Tobacco:	None expected.

NEFAZODONE

BRAND NAMES

Serzone

BASIC INFORMATION

Habit forming? No
Prescription needed? Yes
Available as generic? Yes
Drug class: Antidepressant
(phenylpiperazine)

 ## USES

Treats symptoms of mental depression.

 ## DOSAGE & USAGE INFORMATION

How to take:
Tablet—Swallow with liquid. May be taken with or without food.

When to take:
At the same times each day. The prescribed dosage may be increased weekly until maximum benefits are achieved.

If you forget a dose:
Take as soon as you remember up to 2 hours late. If more than 2 hours, wait for the next scheduled dose (don't double this dose).

What drug does:
The exact mechanism is unknown. It appears to block reuptake of serotonin and norepinephrine (stimulating chemicals in the brain that play a role in emotions and psychological disturbances).

Time lapse before drug works:
Will take up to several weeks to relieve the depression.

Don't take with:
Any other medicine or any dietary supplement without consulting your doctor or pharmacist.

 ## OVERDOSE

SYMPTOMS:
Drowsiness, nausea, vomiting, low blood pressure (faintness, weakness, dizziness, lightheadedness) or increased severity of adverse reactions.
WHAT TO DO:
- **Dial 911 (emergency) for medical help or call poison control center 1-800-222-1222 for instructions.**
- **See emergency information on last 3 pages of this book.**

 ## POSSIBLE ADVERSE REACTIONS OR SIDE EFFECTS

SYMPTOMS	WHAT TO DO
Life-threatening:	
In case of overdose, see previous column.	
Common:	
• Clumsiness or unsteadiness, blurred vision or other vision changes, fainting, lightheadedness, ringing in the ears, skin rash or itching.	Discontinue. Call doctor right away.
• Strange dreams, constipation or diarrhea, dry mouth, heartburn, fever, chills, flushing or feeling warm, headache, increased appetite, insomnia, coughing, tingling or prickly sensations, sore throat, trembling, drowsiness, confusion or agitation, memory lapses.	Continue. Call doctor when convenient.
Infrequent:	
• Tightness in chest; trouble breathing; wheezing; eye pain; combination of nausea, vomiting, diarrhea and stomach pain.	Discontinue. Call doctor right away.
• Joint pain, breast pain, increased thirst.	Continue. Call doctor when convenient.
Rare:	
• Face swelling, hives, muscle pain or stiffness, chest pain, fast heartbeat, mood or mental changes, difficulty speaking, hallucinations, uncontrolled excited behavior, twitching, ear pain, increased hearing sensitivity, bleeding or bruising, irritated red eyes, eyes sensitive to light, pain in back or side, swollen glands, problems with urination.	Discontinue. Call doctor right away.
• Unusual tiredness or weakness, false sense of well-being, menstrual changes, change in sexual desire or function.	Continue. Call doctor when convenient.

WARNINGS & PRECAUTIONS

Don't use if:
You are allergic to nefazodone or trazodone (phenylpiperazine antidepressants).

Before you start, consult your doctor if:
* You have or have had liver disease.
* You have a seizure disorder, heart disease or blood circulation problem or have had a stroke.
* You are dehydrated.
* You have a history of drug abuse.
* You have a history of mood disorders, such as mania, or thoughts of suicide.
* You are allergic to any medication.

Over age 60:
A lower starting dosage is usually recommended until a response is determined.

Pregnancy:
Decide with your doctor if drug benefits justify risk to unborn child. Risk category C (see page xviii).

Breast-feeding:
It is unknown if drug passes into milk. Avoid drug or discontinue nursing until you finish medicine. Consult doctor for advice on maintaining milk supply.

Infants & children:
Not approved for ages under 18. If prescribed, carefully read information provided with prescription. Contact doctor right away if depression symptoms get worse or there is any talk of suicide or suicide behaviors. Also, read information under Others.

Prolonged use:
Consult with your doctor on a regular basis while taking this drug to check your progress and to discuss any increase or changes in side effects and the need for continued treatment.

Skin & sunlight:
May cause a rash or intensify sunburn in areas exposed to sun or ultraviolet light (photosensitivity reaction). Avoid excess sun exposure and use sunscreen. Call doctor if reaction occurs.

Driving, piloting or hazardous work:
Don't drive or pilot aircraft until you learn how medicine affects you. Don't work around dangerous machinery. Don't climb ladders or work in high places. Danger increases if you drink alcohol or take medicine affecting alertness and reflexes.

Discontinuing:
Don't discontinue this drug without consulting doctor. Dosage may require a gradual reduction before stopping.

Others:
* Get up slowly from a sitting or lying position to avoid dizziness, faintness or lightheadedness.
* Advise any doctor or dentist whom you consult that you take this medicine.
* Take drug only as directed. Do not increase or reduce dosage without doctor's approval.
* Adults and children taking antidepressants may experience a worsening of the depression symptoms and may display increased suicidal thoughts or behavior. Call doctor right away if these symptoms or behaviors occur.
* Use of this drug may result in hepatic (liver) problems that can be life-threatening. Call doctor right away if yellow skin or eyes, stomach problems, appetite loss or fatigue occur.

POSSIBLE INTERACTION WITH OTHER DRUGS

GENERIC NAME OR DRUG CLASS	COMBINED EFFECT
Alprazolam	Increased effect of alprazolam.
Antihypertensives*	Possible too-low blood pressure.
Carbamazepine	Decreased effect of nefazodone. Avoid.
Central nervous system (CNS) depressants*	Increased sedation.
Cisapride	Increased effect of cisapride. Avoid.
Digoxin	Increased digoxin effect.
Fluoxetine	Increased risk of side effects.

Continued on page 925

POSSIBLE INTERACTION WITH OTHER SUBSTANCES

INTERACTS WITH	COMBINED EFFECT
Alcohol:	Increased sedative affect. Avoid.
Beverages:	None expected.
Cocaine:	Unknown. Avoid.
Foods:	None expected.
Marijuana:	Unknown. Best to avoid.
Tobacco:	None expected.

*See Glossary

NEOMYCIN (Oral)

BRAND NAMES

Mycifradin

BASIC INFORMATION

Habit forming? No
Prescription needed? Yes
Available as generic? Yes
Drug class: Antibacterial

USES

- Clears intestinal tract of germs prior to surgery.
- Treats some causes of diarrhea.
- Lowers blood cholesterol.
- Lessens symptoms of hepatic coma.

DOSAGE & USAGE INFORMATION

How to take:
Tablet—Swallow with liquid or food to lessen stomach irritation. If you can't swallow whole, crumble tablet and take with liquid or food.

When to take:
According to directions on prescription.

If you forget a dose:
Take as soon as you remember up to 2 hours late. If more than 2 hours, wait for next scheduled dose (don't double this dose).

What drug does:
Kills germs susceptible to neomycin.

Time lapse before drug works:
2 to 3 days.

Don't take with:
Any other medicine or any dietary supplement without consulting your doctor or pharmacist.

OVERDOSE

SYMPTOMS:
Loss of hearing, difficulty breathing, respiratory paralysis.
WHAT TO DO:
- **Dial 911 (emergency) for medical help or call poison control center 1-800-222-1222 for instructions.**
- **If person is unconscious, check breathing and pulse. If not breathing, begin mouth-to-mouth rescue breathing. If heart is not beating, begin chest compressions.**
- **See emergency information on last 3 pages of this book.**

POSSIBLE ADVERSE REACTIONS OR SIDE EFFECTS

SYMPTOMS	WHAT TO DO
Life-threatening: In case of overdose, see previous column.	
Common: Sore mouth or rectum, nausea, vomiting.	Continue. Call doctor when convenient.
Infrequent: None expected.	
Rare: Clumsiness, dizziness, rash, hearing loss, ringing or noises in ear, frothy stools, gaseousness, decreased frequency of urination, diarrhea.	Discontinue. Call doctor right away.

WARNINGS & PRECAUTIONS

Don't take if:
You are allergic to neomycin or any aminoglycoside.*

Before you start, consult your doctor if:
- You will have surgery within 2 months, including dental surgery, requiring general or spinal anesthesia.
- You have hearing loss or loss of balance secondary to 8th cranial nerve disease.
- You have intestinal obstruction.
- You have myasthenia gravis, Parkinson's disease, kidney disease, ulcers in intestines.

Over age 60:
Adverse reactions and side effects may be more frequent and severe than in younger persons.

Pregnancy:
Risk to unborn child outweighs drug benefits. Don't use. Risk category D (see page xviii).

Breast-feeding:
Avoid if possible. Effect unknown. Consult doctor.

Infants & children:
Give only under close medical supervision.

Prolonged use:
- Adverse effects more likely.
- Talk to your doctor about the need for follow-up medical examinations or laboratory studies to check hearing, kidney function.

Skin & sunlight:
No problems expected.

Driving, piloting or hazardous work:
No problems expected.

Discontinuing:
May be unnecessary to finish medicine. Follow doctor's instructions.

Others:
- No problems expected.
- Advise any doctor or dentist whom you consult that you take this medicine.

POSSIBLE INTERACTION WITH OTHER DRUGS

GENERIC NAME OR DRUG CLASS	COMBINED EFFECT
Aminoglycosides*	Increased chance of toxic effect on hearing, kidneys, muscles.
Beta carotene	Decreased absorption of beta carotene.
Capreomycin	Increased chance of toxic effects on hearing, kidneys.
Cephalothin	Increased chance of toxic effect on kidneys.
Cisplatin	Increased chance of toxic effects on hearing, kidneys.
Ethacrynic acid	Increased chance of toxic effects on hearing, kidneys.
Furosemide	Increased chance of toxic effects on hearing, kidneys.
Mercaptomerin	Increased chance of toxic effects on hearing, kidneys.
Penicillins*	Decreased antibiotic effect.
Tiopronin	Increased risk of toxicity to kidneys.
Vancomycin	Increased chance of toxic effects on hearing, kidneys.

POSSIBLE INTERACTION WITH OTHER SUBSTANCES

INTERACTS WITH	COMBINED EFFECT
Alcohol:	Increased chance of toxicity. Avoid.
Beverages:	None expected.
Cocaine:	Increased chance of toxicity. Avoid.
Foods:	None expected.
Marijuana:	Increased chance of toxicity. Avoid.
Tobacco:	None expected.

*See Glossary

NEOMYCIN (Topical)

BRAND NAMES

Myciguent

BASIC INFORMATION

Habit forming? No
Prescription needed? No
Available as generic? Yes
Drug class: Antibacterial (topical)

USES

Treats skin infections that may accompany burns, superficial boils, insect bites or stings, skin ulcers, minor surgical wounds.

DOSAGE & USAGE INFORMATION

How to take:
Cream, lotion, ointment—Bathe and dry area before use. Apply small amount and rub gently. May cover with gauze or bandage if desired.

When to take:
3 or 4 times daily, or as directed by doctor.

If you forget a dose:
Use as soon as you remember.

What drug does:
Kills susceptible bacteria by interfering with bacterial DNA and RNA.

Time lapse before drug works:
Begins first day. May require treatment for a week or longer to cure infection.

Don't take with:
Any other topical medicine without consulting your doctor or pharmacist.

OVERDOSE

SYMPTOMS:
None expected.
WHAT TO DO:
Dial 911 (emergency) for medical help or call poison control center 1-800-222-1222 for instructions.

POSSIBLE ADVERSE REACTIONS OR SIDE EFFECTS

SYMPTOMS	WHAT TO DO
Life-threatening: None expected.	
Common: None expected.	
Infrequent: Itching, swollen, red skin.	Discontinue. Call doctor right away.
Rare: None expected.	

WARNINGS & PRECAUTIONS

Don't take if:
You are allergic to neomycin or any topical medicine.

Before you start, consult your doctor if:
Any lesions on the skin are open sores.

Over age 60:
No problems expected.

Pregnancy:
Consult doctor. Risk category C (see page xviii).

Breast-feeding:
No problems expected, but check with doctor.

Infants & children:
No problems expected, but check with doctor.

Prolonged use:
No problems expected, but check with doctor.

Skin & sunlight:
No special problems expected.

Driving, piloting or hazardous work:
No problems expected, but check with doctor.

Discontinuing:
No problems expected, but check with doctor.

Others:
* Heat and moisture in bathroom medicine cabinet can cause breakdown of medicine. Store someplace else.
* Keep medicine cool, but don't freeze.

 POSSIBLE INTERACTION WITH OTHER DRUGS

GENERIC NAME OR DRUG CLASS	COMBINED EFFECT
Any other topical medication	Hypersensitivity reactions more likely to occur.

 POSSIBLE INTERACTION WITH OTHER SUBSTANCES

INTERACTS WITH	COMBINED EFFECT
Alcohol:	None expected.
Beverages:	None expected.
Cocaine:	None expected.
Foods:	None expected.
Marijuana:	None expected.
Tobacco:	None expected.

*See Glossary

NIACIN
(Vitamin B-3, Nicotinic Acid, Nicotinamide)

BRAND NAMES

Advicor	Nicotinex
Endur-Acin	Nicotinyl alcohol
Nia-Bid	Papulex
Niac	Roniacol
Niacels	Ronigen
Niacin	Rycotin
Niacor	Simcor
Niaspan	Slo-Niacin
Nico-400	Span-Niacin
Nicobid	Tega-Span
Nicolar	Tri-B3

Numerous brands of single vitamin and multivitamin combinations are available.

BASIC INFORMATION

Habit forming? No
Prescription needed? Yes, for some
Available as generic? Yes
Drug class: Vitamin supplement, vasodilator, antihyperlipidemic

USES

- Replacement for niacin lost due to inadequate diet.
- Treatment for vertigo (dizziness) and ringing in ears.
- Prevention of premenstrual headache.
- Reduction of blood levels of cholesterol and triglycerides.
- Treatment for pellagra.

OVERDOSE

SYMPTOMS:
Body flush, nausea, vomiting, abdominal cramps, diarrhea, weakness, lightheadedness, fainting, sweating.
WHAT TO DO:
Overdose unlikely to threaten life. If person uses much larger amount than prescribed or if accidentally swallowed, call doctor or poison control center 1-800-222-1222 for help.

DOSAGE & USAGE INFORMATION

How to take:
- Tablet, capsule or liquid—Swallow with liquid or food to lessen stomach irritation.
- Extended-release tablets or capsules— Swallow each dose whole.

When to take:
At the same times each day.

If you forget a dose:
Take as soon as you remember. Wait 4 hours for next dose.

What drug does:
- Corrects niacin deficiency.
- Dilates blood vessels.
- In large doses, decreases cholesterol production.

Time lapse before drug works:
15 to 20 minutes.

Don't take with:
Any other medicine or any dietary supplement without consulting your doctor or pharmacist.

POSSIBLE ADVERSE REACTIONS OR SIDE EFFECTS

SYMPTOMS	WHAT TO DO
Life-threatening:	
None expected.	
Common:	
Dry skin.	Continue. Call doctor when convenient.
Infrequent:	
• Upper abdominal pain, diarrhea.	Discontinue. Call doctor right away.
• Headache, dizziness, faintness, temporary numbness and tingling in hands and feet.	Continue. Call doctor when convenient.
• "Hot" feeling, flush.	No action necessary.
Rare:	
Rash, itching, jaundice, double vision, weakness and faintness when arising from bed or chair.	Discontinue. Call doctor right away.

WARNINGS & PRECAUTIONS

Don't take if:
You are allergic to niacin or any niacin-containing vitamin mixtures.

Before you start, consult your doctor if:
- You have sensitivity to tartrazine dye.
- You have diabetes.
- You have gout.
- You have gallbladder or liver disease.
- You have impaired liver function.
- You have active peptic ulcer.

Over age 60:
Response to drug cannot be predicted. Dose must be individualized.

Pregnancy:
Consult doctor. Risk category C (see page xviii).

Breast-feeding:
Studies inconclusive. Consult doctor.

Infants & children:
- Use only under medical supervision.
- Keep vitamin-mineral supplements out of children's reach.

Prolonged use:
- May cause impaired liver function.
- Talk to your doctor about the need for follow-up medical examinations or laboratory studies to check liver function, blood sugar.

Skin & sunlight:
No problems expected.

Driving, piloting or hazardous work:
Avoid if you feel dizzy or faint. Otherwise, no problems expected.

Discontinuing:
May be unnecessary to finish medicine. Follow doctor's instructions.

Others:
- A balanced diet should provide all the niacin a healthy person needs and make supplements unnecessary. Best sources are meat, eggs and dairy products.
- Store in original container in cool, dry, dark place.
- Obesity reduces effectiveness.
- Some nicotinic acid products contain tartrazine dye. Read labels carefully if sensitive to tartrazine.

POSSIBLE INTERACTION WITH OTHER DRUGS

GENERIC NAME OR DRUG CLASS	COMBINED EFFECT
Antidiabetics*	Decreased antidiabetic effect.
Beta-adrenergic blocking agents*	Excessively low blood pressure.
Dexfenfluramine	May require dosage change as weight loss occurs.
HMG-CoA reductase inhibitors*	Increased risk of muscle or kidney problems.
Mecamylamine	Excessively low blood pressure.
Methyldopa	Excessively low blood pressure.
Probenecid	Decreased effect of probenecid.
Sulfinpyrazone	Decreased effect of sulfinpyrazone.

POSSIBLE INTERACTION WITH OTHER SUBSTANCES

INTERACTS WITH	COMBINED EFFECT
Alcohol:	Excessively low blood pressure. Use caution.
Beverages:	None expected.
Cocaine:	Increased flushing.
Foods:	None expected.
Marijuana:	None expected.
Tobacco:	Decreased niacin effect.

*See Glossary

NICOTINE

BRAND NAMES

Commit
Habitrol
Nicoderm
Nicoderm CQ
Nicoderm CQ Thin
  Flex patch
Nicorette

Nicorette DS
Nicorette Fresh Mint
Nicotrol
Nicotrol NS
Prostep
Thrive Gum

BASIC INFORMATION

Habit Forming? Yes
Prescription needed? No
Available as generic? Yes, for some
Drug class: Antismoking agent

 USES

Treatment aid to giving up smoking. Nicotine
replacement is to be used in conjunction with a
medically supervised, behavioral modification
program for smoking cessation.

 DOSAGE & USAGE
INFORMATION

How to use:
* Skin patch—Apply to clean, nonhairy site on
  the trunk or upper outer arm. Fold old patch in
  half (sticky sides together) and dispose of
  where children and pets cannot get to it.
* Chewing gum—Chew gum pieces slowly and
  intermittently (chew several times, then place
  between cheek and gum) for best effect.
* Nasal spray—Spray one or two sprays in each
  nostril.
* Lozenge—Use as directed on package.

Continued next column

 OVERDOSE

SYMPTOMS:
Early symptoms—Nausea, vomiting, severe
diarrhea, increased mouth watering,
abdominal pain, cold sweat, severe
headache, dizziness, confusion, vision
and hearing changes.
Late symptoms—Irregular or fast pulse,
fainting, breathing difficulty, convulsions.
WHAT TO DO:
* Dial 911 (emergency) for medical help or
  call poison control center 1-800-222-1222
  for instructions.
* See emergency information on last 3 pages
  of this book.

When to use:
* Skin patch—Daily. Remove old patch and
  apply new patch to new location on the skin.
* Chewing gum—When there is an urge to
  smoke, chew the gum for about 30 minutes.
  For the brand name Thrive Gum, follow
  instructions on label.
* Nasal spray—Hourly, or as directed. Dosage
  adjustments should be made as needed.
* For all—Always follow product's directions.

If you forget a dose:
* Skin patch—Remove old patch and apply new
  patch as soon as you remember, then return to
  regular schedule.
* Chewing gum or nasal spray—Use as soon as
  you remember (don't double dosages).

What drug does:
Delivers a supply of nicotine to the body for relief
of smoking withdrawal symptoms (irritability,
headache, nervousness, drowsiness, fatigue).
Reduces craving for cigarettes.

Time lapse before drug works:
Minutes to hours depending on type of product.

Don't take with:
Any other medicine or any dietary supplement
without consulting your doctor or pharmacist.

 POSSIBLE
ADVERSE REACTIONS
OR SIDE EFFECTS

SYMPTOMS	WHAT TO DO
Life-threatening:	
In case of overdose, see previous column.	
Common:	
• Skin patch—itching, redness, burning or skin rash at site of patch.	Continue. Call doctor when convenient.
• Chewing gum—dental problems, sore mouth or throat, belching, mouth watering.	Continue. Call doctor when convenient.
• Nasal spray—runny nose, watering eyes, throat irritation, sneezing and cough.	Continue. Call doctor when convenient.
Infrequent:	
Diarrhea, dizziness, indigestion, nervousness, strange dreams, muscle aches, nausea, constipation, increased cough, tiredness, irritability, changes in menstruation, insomnia, headache, increase in sweating.	Continue. Call doctor when convenient.

Rare:
- Allergic reaction (swelling, hives, rash, itching, vomiting, irregular or fast heartbeat); symptoms of overdose occur (high doses of nicotine can cause toxic effects, even in people who are nicotine tolerant). — Discontinue. Call doctor right away.
- Hiccups or hoarseness with chewing gum. — Continue. Call doctor when convenient.

WARNINGS & PRECAUTIONS

Don't take if:
You are allergic to nicotine or any of the components in the skin patch.

Before you start, consult your doctor if:
- You are pregnant.
- You have a skin disorder; mouth, throat, dental or TMJ disorder; long-term nasal disorder (allergy, hay fever, sinusitis, polyps) or asthma.
- You have cardiovascular or peripheral vascular disease or high blood pressure.
- You have liver or kidney disease.
- You have hyperthyroidism, insulin-dependent diabetes, pheochromocytoma, peptic ulcer disease or endocrine disorder.

Over age 60:
Adverse reactions and side effects may be more frequent and severe than in younger persons.

Pregnancy:
Tobacco smoke and nicotine are harmful to the fetus. The specific effects of nicotine from these drugs are unknown. Discuss the risks of both with your doctor. Risk category varies for drugs in this group (see page xviii).

Breast-feeding:
Drug passes into breast milk. Avoid drug or discontinue nursing until you finish medicine. Consult doctor for advice on maintaining milk supply.

Infants & children:
Not recommended.

Prolonged use:
Treatment may take several months. Nicotine replacement therapy is not intended for long-term use.

Skin & sunlight:
No problems expected.

Driving, piloting or hazardous work:
Avoid if you feel dizzy or lightheaded. Otherwise, no problems expected.

Discontinuing:
Adverse reactions and side effects related to nicotine withdrawal may continue for some time after discontinuing.

Others:
- Advise any doctor or dentist whom you consult that you take this medicine.
- May affect results of some medical tests.
- Keep both the used and unused skin patches out of the reach of children and pets. Dispose of old patches according to directions.
- For full benefit from this treatment and to decrease risk of side effects, stop cigarette smoking as soon as you begin treatment.

POSSIBLE INTERACTION WITH OTHER DRUGS

GENERIC NAME OR DRUG CLASS	COMBINED EFFECT
Acetaminophen	Increased effect of acetaminophen.
Beta-adrenergic blocking agents*	Increased effect of beta blocker.
Bronchodilators, xanthine* (except dyphylline)	Increased bronchodilator effect.
Imipramine	Increased effect of imipramine.
Insulin & insulin lispro	May require insulin dosage adjustment.
Isoproterenol	Decreased effect of isoproterenol.
Oxazepam	Increased effect of oxazepam.

Continued on page 926

POSSIBLE INTERACTION WITH OTHER SUBSTANCES

INTERACTS WITH	COMBINED EFFECT
Alcohol:	Increased cardiac irritability. Avoid.
Beverages:	None expected.
Cocaine:	Increased cardiac irritability. Avoid.
Foods:	None expected.
Marijuana:	Increased toxic effects. Avoid.
Tobacco:	Increased adverse effects of nicotine. Must avoid.

*See Glossary

NIMODIPINE

BRAND NAMES

NIMODIPINE

BASIC INFORMATION

Habit Forming? No
Prescription needed? Yes
Available as generic? No
Drug class: Calcium channel blocker

 ## USES

Helps repair the damage caused by a ruptured blood vessel in the head (also called ruptured aneurysm or subarachnoid hemorrhage). Unlike other calcium channel blockers, nimodipine is not used for angina or high blood pressure.

 ## DOSAGE & USAGE INFORMATION

How to take:
Capsule—Swallow it whole. Take with liquid. Do not crush or chew the capsule. If you can't swallow the capsule, ask your doctor for advice. Do not ever inject the drug as it can cause serious and possible fatal adverse effects.

When to take:
Results are best if you begin taking within 96 hours after bleeding into the brain begins. Continue taking for 21 days or as directed by your doctor.

If you forget a dose:
Take as soon as you remember. If it is almost time for the next dose, wait for that dose (don't double this dose) and resume regular schedule.

What drug does:
Relaxes blood vessels and improves blood flow.

Continued next column

 ## OVERDOSE

SYMPTOMS:
Unusually fast or unusually slow heartbeat, loss of consciousness, cardiac arrest.
WHAT TO DO:
- **Dial 911 (emergency) for medical help or call poison control center 1-800-222-1222 for instructions.**
- **If person is unconscious, check breathing and pulse. If not breathing, begin mouth-to-mouth rescue breathing. If heart is not beating, begin chest compressions.**
- **See emergency information on last 3 pages of this book.**

Time lapse before drug works:
1 to 2 hours.

Don't take with:
Any other medicine or any dietary supplement without consulting your doctor or pharmacist.

 ## POSSIBLE ADVERSE REACTIONS OR SIDE EFFECTS

SYMPTOMS	WHAT TO DO
Life-threatening:	
In case of overdose, see previous column.	
Common:	
Tiredness, flushing, swelling of feet, ankles and abdomen.	Continue. Tell doctor at next visit.
Infrequent:	
• Unusually fast or unusually slow heartbeat, wheezing, cough, shortness of breath.	Discontinue. Call doctor right away.
• Dizziness; numbness or tingling in hands or feet; difficult urination.	Continue. Call doctor when convenient.
• Nausea, constipation.	Continue. Tell doctor at next visit.
Rare:	
• Transient blindness, increased angina, chest pain.	Discontinue. Seek emergency treatment.
• Fainting, fever, rash, jaundice, depression, psychosis.	Discontinue. Call doctor right away.
• Pain and swelling in joints, hair loss, vivid dreams.	Continue. Call doctor when convenient.
• Headache.	Continue Tell doctor at next visit.

 ## WARNINGS & PRECAUTIONS

Don't take if:
- You are allergic to any calcium channel blocking drug.*
- You have very low blood pressure.

Before you start, consult your doctor if:
- You have kidney or liver disease.
- You have high blood pressure.
- You have heart disease other than coronary artery disease.

Over age 60:
Adverse reactions and side effects may be more frequent and severe than in younger persons.

Pregnancy:
Decide with your doctor if drug benefits justify risk to unborn child. Risk category C (see page xviii).

Breast-feeding:
Safety not established. Avoid if possible.
Consult doctor.

Infants & children:
Not recommended.

Prolonged use:
Talk to your doctor about the need for follow-up
medical examinations or laboratory studies to
check blood pressure, liver function, kidney
function, ECG.*

Skin & sunlight:
No special problems expected.

Driving, piloting or hazardous work:
Avoid if you feel dizzy. Otherwise, no problems
expected.

Discontinuing:
Don't discontinue without doctor's advice until
you complete prescribed dose, even though
symptoms diminish or disappear.

Others:
- Learn to check your own pulse rate. If it drops
  to 50 beats per minute or lower, don't take
  nimodipine until you consult your doctor.
- Drug may lower blood sugar level if daily dose
  is more than 60 mg.

POSSIBLE INTERACTION WITH OTHER DRUGS

GENERIC NAME OR DRUG CLASS	COMBINED EFFECT
Angiotensin-converting enzyme (ACE) inhibitors*	Possible excessive potassium in blood. Dosages may need adjustment.
Antiarrhythmics*	Increased effect and toxicity of each drug.
Anticoagulants,* oral	Increased anticoagulant effect.
Anticonvulsants, hydantoin*	Increased anti-convulsant effect.
Antihypertensives*	Blood pressure changes. Dosage may need changing.
Beta-adrenergic blocking agents* (oral or ophthalmic)	Irregular heartbeat. May worsen heart failure.
Betaxolol eye drops	Increased effect of nimodipine on heart function.
Calcium (large doses)	Possible decreased nimodipine effect.
Carbamazepine	Increased carbamazepine effect and toxicity.

Cimetidine	Increased effect and toxicity of nimodipine.
Cyclosporine	Increased cyclosporine toxicity.
Disopyramide	May cause dangerously slow, fast or irregular heartbeat.
Diuretics*	Dangerous blood pressure drop.
Levobunolol eye drops	Increased effect of nimodipine on heart function.
Lithium	Decreased lithium effect.
Nicardipine	Increased effect and toxicity of each drug.
Phenytoin	Decreased nimodipine effect.
Quinidine	Increased quinidine effect.
Rifampin	Decreased nimodipine effect.
Theophylline	Increased theophylline effect and toxicity.

Continued on page 926

POSSIBLE INTERACTION WITH OTHER SUBSTANCES

INTERACTS WITH	COMBINED EFFECT
Alcohol:	Dangerously low blood pressure. Avoid.
Beverages:	None expected.
Cocaine:	Possible irregular heartbeat. Avoid.
Foods:	None expected.
Marijuana:	Possible irregular heartbeat. Avoid.
Tobacco:	Possible rapid heartbeat. Avoid.

*See Glossary

NITAZOXANIDE

BRAND NAMES

Alinia

BASIC INFORMATION

Habit forming? No
Prescription needed? Yes
Available as generic? No
Drug class: Antiprotozoal; antidiarrheal

 USES

- Treatment of diarrhea and other symptoms caused by two parasitic infections (*Cryptosporidium parvum* and *Giardia lamblia*). These two types of parasites are common causes of persistent diarrhea in children and adults. Outbreaks have been associated with day care centers, swimming pools, water parks and public water supplies.
- May be used for treatment of other disorders as determined by your doctor.

 DOSAGE & USAGE INFORMATION

How to take:
- Oral suspension—Follow label instructions and take with food.
- Tablet—Swallow with liquid and take with food.

When to take:
Usual dose is twice a day for 3 days.

If you forget a dose:
Take as soon as you remember. If it is almost time for your next dose, skip the missed dose and go back to your regular dosing schedule. Do not double doses.

What drug does:
Prevents enzyme reactions that are needed for the parasites to survive. Thousands of enzymes are present in the body with a range of functions including food digestion and toxin elimination.

Continued next column

 OVERDOSE

SYMPTOMS:
Unknown symptoms.
WHAT TO DO:
Overdose unlikely to threaten life. If person uses much larger amount than prescribed or if accidentally swallowed, call doctor or poison control center 1-800-222-1222 for help.

Time lapse before drug works:
Starts working in a few hours, but takes 3 days for effective treatment.

Don't take with:
Any other medicine or any dietary supplement without consulting your doctor or pharmacist.

 POSSIBLE ADVERSE REACTIONS OR SIDE EFFECTS

SYMPTOMS	WHAT TO DO
Life-threatening: None expected.	
Common: None expected.	
Infrequent: None expected.	
Rare: Abdominal pain, diarrhea, vomiting, headache.	Continue. Call doctor if symptoms persist or are severe.

WARNINGS & PRECAUTIONS

Don't take if:
You are allergic to nitazoxanide.

Before you start, consult your doctor if:
* You have liver or kidney disease.
* You have bile or gallbladder problems.
* You have diabetes (the drug contains sucrose).
* You are immunosuppressed due to illness or drugs.

Over age 60:
No problems expected.

Pregnancy:
Decide with your doctor if drug benefits justify risk to unborn child. Risk category B. (See page xviii).

Breast-feeding:
It is unknown if drug passes into milk. Avoid drug or discontinue nursing until you finish medicine. Consult doctor for advice on maintaining milk supply.

Infants & children:
Approved for children over age one.

Prolonged use:
Not used for more than 3 days.

Skin & sunlight:
No problems expected.

Driving, piloting or hazardous work:
No problems expected.

Discontinuing:
No problems expected.

Others:
* Safety and effectiveness of nitazoxanide for HIV positive patients and immunodeficient patients have not been established.
* Advise any doctor or dentist whom you consult that you take this drug.

POSSIBLE INTERACTION WITH OTHER DRUGS

GENERIC NAME OR DRUG CLASS	COMBINED EFFECT
Protein bound drugs*	May increase effect of nitazoxanide.

Note: Specific studies on interactions of nitazoxanide with other drugs have not been conducted. If you have a concern about an interaction between drugs, consult your doctor or pharmacist.

POSSIBLE INTERACTION WITH OTHER SUBSTANCES

INTERACTS WITH	COMBINED EFFECT
Alcohol:	None expected.
Beverages:	None expected.
Cocaine:	None expected.
Foods:	None expected.
Marijuana:	None expected.
Tobacco:	None expected.

*See Glossary

NITRATES

GENERIC AND BRAND NAMES

See full list of generic and brand names in the *Generic and Brand Name Directory*, page 892.

BASIC INFORMATION

Habit forming? No
Prescription needed? Yes
Available as generic? Yes
Drug class: Antianginal (nitrate)

USES

- Reduces frequency and severity of angina attacks.
- Treats congestive heart failure.
- The brand name BiDil is approved to treat heart failure specifically in African Americans.

DOSAGE & USAGE INFORMATION

How to take:
- Extended-release tablet or capsule— Swallow each dose whole with liquid.
- Chewable tablet—Chew tablet at earliest sign of angina, and hold in mouth for 2 minutes.
- Regular tablet or capsule—Swallow whole with liquid. Don't crush, chew or open.
- Buccal tablet—Allow to dissolve inside of mouth.
- Lingual spray—Spray under tongue according to instructions enclosed with prescription.
- Ointment—Apply as directed.
- Patch—Apply to skin according to package instructions.
- Sublingual tablet—Place under tongue every 3 to 5 minutes at earliest sign of angina. If you don't have complete relief with 3 or 4 tablets, call doctor.

Continued next column

OVERDOSE

SYMPTOMS:
Dizziness; blue fingernails and lips; feeling of pressure in head, fever, fainting; shortness of breath; weak, fast heartbeat; convulsions.
WHAT TO DO:
- **Dial 911 (emergency) for medical help or call poison control center 1-800-222-1222 for instructions.**
- **See emergency information on last 3 pages of this book.**

When to take:
- Swallowed tablet—Take at the same times each day, 1 or 2 hours after meals.
- Sublingual tablet or spray—At onset of angina.
- Ointment—Follow prescription directions.
- Patch—According to physician's instructions.

If you forget a dose:
Take as soon as you remember up to 2 hours late. If more than 2 hours, wait for next scheduled dose (don't double this dose).

What drug does:
Relaxes blood vessels, increasing blood flow to heart muscle.

Time lapse before drug works:
- Sublingual tablets and spray—1 to 3 minutes.
- Other forms—15 to 30 minutes. Will not stop an attack, but may prevent attacks.

Don't take with:
Any other medicine or any dietary supplement without consulting your doctor or pharmacist.

POSSIBLE ADVERSE REACTIONS OR SIDE EFFECTS

SYMPTOMS	WHAT TO DO
Life-threatening:	
In case of overdose, see previous column.	
Common:	
Headache, flushed face and neck, dry mouth, nausea, vomiting.	Continue. Tell doctor at next visit.
Infrequent:	
• Fainting, rapid heartbeat.	Discontinue. Call doctor right away.
• Restlessness, blurred vision, dizziness.	Continue. Call doctor when convenient.
Rare:	
• Rash.	Discontinue. Call doctor right away.
• Severe irritation, peeling skin.	Continue. Call doctor when convenient.

WARNINGS & PRECAUTIONS

Don't take if:
You are allergic to nitrates, including nitroglycerin.

Before you start, consult your doctor if:
* You are taking nonprescription drugs.
* You plan to become pregnant within medication period.
* You have glaucoma.
* You have reacted badly to any vasodilator drug.
* You drink alcoholic beverages or smoke marijuana.

Over age 60:
Adverse reactions and side effects may be more frequent and severe than in younger persons.

Pregnancy:
Decide with your doctor if drug benefits justify risk to unborn child. Risk category C (see page xviii).

Breast-feeding:
Effect unknown. Consult your doctor.

Infants & children:
Not recommended.

Prolonged use:
* Drug may become less effective and require higher doses.
* Talk to your doctor about the need for follow-up medical examinations or laboratory studies to check blood pressure, heart rate.

Skin & sunlight:
No problems expected.

Driving, piloting or hazardous work:
Don't drive or pilot aircraft until you learn how medicine affects you. Don't work around dangerous machinery. Don't climb ladders or work in high places. Danger increases if you drink alcohol or take medicine affecting alertness and reflexes.

Discontinuing:
Except for sublingual tablets, don't discontinue without doctor's advice until you complete prescribed dose, even though symptoms diminish or disappear.

Others:
* If discomfort is not caused by angina, nitrate medication will not bring relief. Call doctor if discomfort persists.
* Periodic urine and laboratory blood studies of white cell counts recommended if you take nitrates.
* Keep sublingual tablets in original container. Always carry them with you, but keep from body heat if possible.

* Sublingual tablets produce a burning, stinging sensation when placed under the tongue. Replace supply if no burning or stinging is noted.
* To avoid development of tolerance, drug-free intervals of 10 hours are sufficient

POSSIBLE INTERACTION WITH OTHER DRUGS

GENERIC NAME OR DRUG CLASS	COMBINED EFFECT
Anticholinergics*	Increased internal eye pressure.
Antihypertensives*	Excessive blood pressure drop.
Beta-adrenergic blocking agents*	Excessive blood pressure drop.
Calcium channel blockers*	Decreased blood pressure.
Carteolol	Possible excessive blood pressure drop.
Guanfacine	Increased effects of both drugs.
Narcotics*	Excessive blood pressure drop.
Phenothiazines*	May decrease blood pressure.
Sildenafil	Increased effect of nitrates.
Sympathomimetics*	Possible reduced effects of both medicines.

POSSIBLE INTERACTION WITH OTHER SUBSTANCES

INTERACTS WITH	COMBINED EFFECT
Alcohol:	Excessive blood pressure drop.
Beverages:	None expected.
Cocaine:	Reduced effectiveness of nitrates.
Foods:	None expected.
Marijuana:	Decreased nitrate effect.
Tobacco:	Decreased nitrate effect.

*See Glossary

NITROFURANTOIN

BRAND NAMES

Apo-Nitrofurantoin
Cyantin
Furadantin
Furalan
Furaloid
Furan
Furanite
Furantoin
Furatine
Furaton
Macrobid
Macrodantin

Nephronex
Nifuran
Nitrex
Nitrofan
Nitrofor
Nitrofuracot
Novofuran
Ro-Antoin
Sarodant
Trantoin
Urotoin

BASIC INFORMATION

Habit forming? No
Prescription needed? Yes
Available as generic? Yes
Drug class: Antimicrobial, antibacterial (antibiotic)

 USES

Treatment for urinary tract infections.

 DOSAGE & USAGE INFORMATION

How to take:
* Tablet or capsule—Swallow with food or milk to lessen stomach irritation. If you can't swallow whole, crumble tablet or open capsule and take with liquid or food.
* Extended-release capsule—Swallow with liquid. Do not open capsule.
* Liquid—Shake well and take with food. Use a measuring spoon to ensure accuracy.

When to take:
At the same times each day.

If you forget a dose:
Take as soon as you remember up to 2 hours late. If more than 2 hours, wait for next scheduled dose (don't double this dose).

Continued next column

 OVERDOSE

SYMPTOMS:
Nausea, vomiting, abdominal pain, diarrhea.
WHAT TO DO:
Overdose unlikely to threaten life. If person uses much larger amount than prescribed or if accidentally swallowed, call doctor or poison control center 1-800-222-1222 for help.

What drug does:
Prevents susceptible bacteria in the urinary tract from growing and multiplying.

Time lapse before drug works:
1 to 2 weeks.

Don't take with:
Any other medicine or any dietary supplement without consulting your doctor or pharmacist.

 POSSIBLE ADVERSE REACTIONS OR SIDE EFFECTS

SYMPTOMS	WHAT TO DO
Life-threatening:	
Hives, rash, intense itching, faintness soon after a dose (anaphylaxis).	Seek emergency treatment immediately.
Common:	
• Diarrhea, appetite loss, nausea, vomiting, chest pain, cough, difficult breathing, chills or unexplained fever, abdominal pain.	Discontinue. Call doctor right away.
• Rusty-colored or brown urine.	No action necessary.
Infrequent:	
• Rash, itchy skin, numbness, tingling or burning of face or mouth, fatigue, weakness.	Discontinue. Call doctor right away.
• Dizziness, headache, drowsiness, paleness (in children), discolored teeth (from liquid form).	Continue. Call doctor when convenient.
Rare:	
Jaundice.	Discontinue. Call doctor right away.

WARNINGS & PRECAUTIONS

Don't take if:
- You are allergic to nitrofurantoin.
- You have impaired kidney function.
- You drink alcohol.

Before you start, consult your doctor if:
- You are prone to allergic reactions.
- You are pregnant and within 2 weeks of delivery.
- You have had kidney disease, lung disease, anemia, nerve damage, or G6PD* deficiency (a metabolic deficiency).
- You have diabetes. Drug may affect urine sugar tests.

Over age 60:
Adverse reactions and side effects may be more frequent and severe than in younger persons.

Pregnancy:
Consult doctor. Risk category B (see page xviii).

Breast-feeding:
Drug passes into milk. Avoid drug or discontinue nursing until you finish medicine. Consult doctor for advice on maintaining milk supply.

Infants & children:
Don't give to infants younger than 1 month. Use only under medical supervision for older children.

Prolonged use:
- Chest pain, cough, shortness of breath.
- Talk to your doctor about the need for follow-up medical examinations or laboratory studies to check liver function, lung function.

Skin & sunlight:
No problems expected.

Driving, piloting or hazardous work:
Avoid if you feel dizzy or drowsy. Otherwise, no problems expected.

Discontinuing:
Don't discontinue without consulting doctor. Dose may require gradual reduction if you have taken drug for a long time. Doses of other drugs may also require adjustment.

Others:
- Periodic blood counts, liver function tests, and chest x-rays recommended.
- Advise any doctor or dentist whom you consult that you take this drug.

POSSIBLE INTERACTION WITH OTHER DRUGS

GENERIC NAME OR DRUG CLASS	COMBINED EFFECT
Antivirals, HIV/AIDS*	Increased risk of pancreatitis and peripheral neuropathy.
Hemolytics,* other	Increased risk of toxicity.
Nalidixic acid	Decreased nitrofurantoin effect.
Neurotoxic medicines*	Increased risk of damage to nerve cells.
Probenecid	Increased nitrofurantoin effect.
Sulfinpyrazone	Possible nitrofurantoin toxicity.

POSSIBLE INTERACTION WITH OTHER SUBSTANCES

INTERACTS WITH	COMBINED EFFECT
Alcohol:	Possible disulfiram reaction.* Avoid.
Beverages:	None expected.
Cocaine:	None expected.
Foods:	None expected.
Marijuana:	None expected.
Tobacco:	None expected.

*See Glossary

NITROIMIDAZOLES

GENERIC AND BRAND NAMES

METRONIDAZOLE
  Apo-Metronidazole
  Flagyl
  Helidac
  Metizol
  Metric 21
  Metro Cream
  MetroGel
  MetroGel-Vaginal
  Neo-Metric
  Noritate

METRONIDAZOLE
  (con't)
  Novonidazol
  PMS Metronidazole
  Protostat
  Pylera
  Satric
  Trikacide
  Vandazole
TINIDAZOLE
  Tindamax

BASIC INFORMATION

Habit forming? No
Prescription needed? Yes
Available as generic? Yes, for some
Drug class: Antiprotozoal; antibacterial

 ## USES

- Treatment for parasitic infections (such as amebiasis, trichomoniasis or giardiasis).
- Treatment for certain bacterial infections.
- Treatment (combined with other drugs) for ulcer caused by *Helicobacter pylori* infection.
- Topical form treats acne rosacea.
- Vaginal forms treats vaginal infections.
- Other uses as determined by your doctor.

 ## DOSAGE & USAGE INFORMATION

How to take:
- Tablet or capsule—Swallow with liquid. Take with food to lessen stomach irritation. The metronidazole tablet may be crushed and taken with food. Ask your pharmacist about crushing tinidazole tablet.
- Extended-release tablet—Swallow with liquid. Take with food to lessen stomach irritation. Do not crush or crumble tablet.
- Cream—Apply to affected area.
- Vaginal form—Follow instructions provided.

Continued next column

 ## OVERDOSE

SYMPTOMS:
Weakness, nausea, vomiting, diarrhea, confusion, dizziness, numbness, seizures.
WHAT TO DO:
Overdose unlikely to threaten life. If person uses much larger amount than prescribed or if accidentally swallowed, call doctor or poison control center 1-800-222-1222 for help.

When to take:
- Oral form—At the same times each day.
- Topical cream—Apply twice a day.
- Vaginal cream, gel or tablet—Use as directed.

If you forget a dose:
Take as soon as you remember. If it is almost time for the next dose, wait for that dose (don't double this dose) and resume regular schedule.

What drug does:
Kills or stops the growth of protozoa or bacteria.

Time lapse before drug works:
Depends on the infection. May take one day or up to 14 days or longer for a complete cure.

Don't take with:
- Drugs (such as some cough remedies) or supplements containing alcohol.
- Any other medicine or any dietary supplement without consulting your doctor or pharmacist.

 ## POSSIBLE ADVERSE REACTIONS OR SIDE EFFECTS

SYMPTOMS	WHAT TO DO
Life-threatening:	
Rare allergic reaction— Breathing difficulty; closing of the throat; swelling of hands, feet, face, lips or tongue; hives.	Discontinue. Seek emergency treatment.
Common:	
Appetite loss, nausea, stomach pain or cramps, diarrhea, vomiting, lightheaded, mild dizziness.	Continue. Call doctor when convenient.
Infrequent:	
• Metallic or bitter taste, dry mouth, headache.	Continue. Call doctor when convenient.
• Numbness, tingling, weakness or pain in hands or feet (peripheral neuropathy).	Discontinue. Call doctor right away.
• Dark urine (will go away after treatment).	No action necessary.
Rare:	
Unsteadiness or clumsiness, mood or mental changes, skin symptoms (rash, hives, redness, itching), sore throat and fever, seizures, severe stomach or back pain, unusual bleeding or bruising, vaginal irritation or dryness or discharge, changes in urination (painful, frequent, unable to control or decreased).	Discontinue. Call doctor right away.

WARNINGS & PRECAUTIONS

Don't take if:
You are allergic to nitroimidazoles or in the first trimester of pregnancy.

Before you start, consult your doctor if:
• You have seizure, nervous system, or brain disorder.
• You have a stomach or intestinal disorder.
• You have a blood disorder,
• You have liver, kidney or heart disease.
• You have a history of alcoholism.

Over age 60:
No special problems expected.

Pregnancy:
Decide with your doctor if drug benefits justify any possible risk to unborn child. The drugs are not recommended during the first trimester of pregnancy. Metronidazole is risk category B and tinidazole is category C (see page xviii).

Breast-feeding:
Drugs pass into milk. Avoid drug or discontinue nursing until you finish medicine. Consult doctor for advice on maintaining milk supply.

Infants & children:
May be used in children, but always under close medical supervision.

Prolonged use:
These drugs are not intended for long-term use.

Skin & sunlight:
No problems expected.

Driving, piloting or hazardous work:
Don't drive or pilot aircraft until you learn how medicine affects you. Don't work around dangerous machinery. Don't climb ladders or work in high places. Danger increases if you drink alcohol or take other medicines affecting alertness and reflexes.

Discontinuing:
Don't discontinue without doctor's advice until you complete prescribed dose, even though symptoms diminish or disappear.

Others:
• Advise any doctor or dentist whom you consult that you take this medicine. May affect results in some medical tests.
• Contact your doctor if symptoms do not improve in 24 to 48 hours.
• If you are being treated for trichomoniasis, your doctor may want your sexual partner treated at the same time (even if the person has no symptoms).
• These drugs may cause a yeast infection (oral or vaginal) to worsen. Contact your doctor if this occurs.

POSSIBLE INTERACTION WITH OTHER DRUGS

GENERIC NAME OR DRUG CLASS	COMBINED EFFECT
Anticoagulants,* oral	Increased anti-coagulant effect. (bleeding or bruising).
Antivirals, HIV/AIDS*	Increased risk of peripheral neuropathy.*
Cholestyramine	Decreased effect of nitroimidazole. Take several hours apart.
Cyclosporine	Increased cyclosporine effect.
Disulfiram	Disulfiram reaction.* Take 2 weeks apart.
Enzyme inducers*	Decreased effect of nitroimidazole.
Enzyme inhibitors*	Increased effect of nitroimidazole.
Fluorouracil	Increased risk of side effects.
Lithium	Increased lithium effect.
Neurotoxic medications*	Increased risk of side effects.
Oxytetracycline	Decreased metronidazole effect.
Phenytoin	Increased phenytoin effect. Decreased nitroimidazole effect.
Tacrolimus	Increased tacrolimus effect.

POSSIBLE INTERACTION WITH OTHER SUBSTANCES

INTERACTS WITH	COMBINED EFFECT
Alcohol:	Possible disulfiram reaction.* Avoid alcohol while taking drug and for 3 days after finishing.
Beverages:	None expected.
Cocaine:	Unknown. Avoid.
Foods:	None expected.
Marijuana:	Unknown. Avoid.
Tobacco:	None expected.

*See Glossary

NON-NUCLEOSIDE REVERSE TRANSCRIPTASE INHIBITORS

GENERIC AND BRAND NAMES

DELAVIRDINE
  Rescriptor
EFAVIRENZ
  Sustiva
  Atripla

ETRAVIRINE
  Intelence
NEVIRAPINE
  Viramune

BASIC INFORMATION

Habit forming? No
Prescription needed? Yes
Available as generic? No
Drug class: Antiviral, HIV and AIDS

 ## USES

For treatment of HIV and AIDS patients. Used in combination with one or more of the other AIDS drugs. May be used to prevent HIV transmission.

 ## DOSAGE & USAGE INFORMATION

How to take:
* Oral suspension—Swallow with liquid.
* Tablet—Swallow with liquid. May be taken with or without food. Efavirenz should not be taken with a high fat meal.

When to take:
At the same time each day. At the start of treatment, one tablet is taken daily for 2 weeks and then increased to 2 tablets daily. This helps to decrease risk of side effects.

If you forget a dose:
* Twice-a-day dose—Take as soon as you remember up to 2 hours late. If more than 2 hours, wait for next scheduled dose (don't double this dose).
* Once-a-day-dose—Take as soon as you remember. If it is almost time for the next dose, wait for the next scheduled dose (don't double this dose).

Continued next column

 ## OVERDOSE

SYMPTOMS:
Swelling, extreme tiredness, fever, insomnia, rash, dizziness, vomiting, feeling of movement.
WHAT TO DO:
Overdose unlikely to threaten life. If person uses much larger amount than prescribed or if accidentally swallowed, call doctor or poison control center 1-800-222-1222 for help.

What drug does:
Interferes with HIV replication. It helps slow the progress of HIV disease, but does not cure it.

Time lapse before drug works:
May require several weeks or months before full benefits are apparent.

Don't take with:
Any other medicine or any dietary supplement without consulting your doctor or pharmacist. This is very important with these antiviral drugs.

 ## POSSIBLE ADVERSE REACTIONS OR SIDE EFFECTS

SYMPTOMS	WHAT TO DO
Life-threatening: Severe skin rash.	Discontinue. Call doctor right away or get emergency help.
Common: Mild to moderate skin rash, chills, fever, sore throat.	Discontinue. Call doctor right away.
Infrequent: • Fever, blistering skin, mouth sores, aching joints or muscles, eye inflammation, unusual tiredness.	Continue, but call doctor right away.
• Headache, nausea, diarrhea burning or tingling feeling, numbness, sleepiness, loss of appetite, constipation, mood or mental changes, intense dreams, anxiety, difficulty concentrating.	Continue. Call doctor when convenient.
Rare: • Yellow skin or eyes, dark urine, heart palpitations, thoughts of suicide.	Discontinue. Call doctor right away.
• Any other unusual symptoms that occur (may be due to the illness, this drug or other drugs being taken).	Continue, but call doctor right away.

WARNINGS & PRECAUTIONS

Don't take if:
You are allergic to non-nucleoside reverse transcriptase inhibitors.

Before you start, consult your doctor if:
* You are allergic to any medicine, food or other substance, or have a family history of allergies.
* You have kidney or liver disease.

Over age 60:
Adverse reactions and side effects may be more frequent and severe than in younger persons.

Pregnancy:
* Decide with your doctor if drug benefits justify risk to unborn child. Risk category C (see page xviii).
* Efavirenz may cause fetal harm when used during the first trimester. Talk to your doctor about this risk.

Breast-feeding:
Drug passes into milk. Avoid drug or discontinue nursing until you finish medicine. Consult doctor for advice on maintaining milk supply.

Infants & children:
Safety and efficacy have not been established. Use only under close medical supervision.

Prolonged use:
* Long-term effects have not been established.
* Talk to your doctor about frequent blood counts and liver function studies.

Skin & sunlight:
No problems expected.

Driving, piloting or hazardous work:
Don't drive or pilot aircraft until you learn how medicine affects you. Don't work around dangerous machinery. Don't climb ladders or work in high places. Danger increases if you drink alcohol or take medicine affecting alertness and reflexes.

Discontinuing:
Don't discontinue without doctor's advice until you complete prescribed dose, even though symptoms diminish or disappear.

Others:
* Advise any doctor or dentist whom you consult that you take this medicine.
* Taking this drug does not prevent you from passing HIV to another person through sexual contact or sharing needles. Avoid sexual contact or practice safe sex (e.g., using condoms) to help prevent the transmission of HIV. Never share or re-use needles. If you have questions, ask your doctor for advice.
* Consult your doctor right away if you develop a new infection (e.g., fever, chills, sore throat or other symptoms).

* Do not increase or decrease dosage of drug without doctor's approval.

POSSIBLE INTERACTION WITH OTHER DRUGS

GENERIC NAME OR DRUG CLASS	COMBINED EFFECT
Amphetamines	May require dosage adjustment of amphetamine.
Antacids	Take 1-2 hours apart.
Benzodiazepines	May require dosage adjustment of benzodiazepine.
Calcium channel blockers	May require dosage adjustment of calcium channel blocker.
Carbamazepine	Decreased antiviral drug effect.
Clarithromycin	Interaction effects vary.
Contraceptives, oral*	Decreased contraceptive effect. Use alternative birth control method.
Didanosine	Take at least 1 hour apart.
Ergot preparations*	May require dosage adjustment of ergot drug.
Fluoxetine	Increased antiviral effect.
Histamine H_2 receptor antagonists	May require dosage adjustment of antiviral drug.

POSSIBLE INTERACTION WITH OTHER SUBSTANCES

INTERACTS WITH	COMBINED EFFECT
Alcohol:	None expected.
Beverages:	None expected.
Cocaine:	Unknown effect. Best to avoid.
Foods:	None expected.
Marijuana:	Unknown effect. Best to avoid.
Tobacco:	None expected.

*See Glossary

NUCLEOSIDE REVERSE TRANSCRIPTASE INHIBITORS

GENERIC AND BRAND NAMES

ABACAVIR
  Epzicom
  Trizivir
  Ziagen
DIDANOSINE
  Videx
  Videx EC
EMTRICITABINE
  Atripla
  Emtriva
LAMIVUDINE
  Combivir
  Epivir
  Epzicom
  Trizivir

STAVUDINE
  d4T
  Zerit
ZIDOVUDINE
  Apo-Zidovudine
  AZT
  Combivir
  Novo-AZT
  Retrovir
  Trizivir

BASIC INFORMATION

Habit forming? No
Prescription needed? Yes
Available as generic? Yes, for some
Drug class: Antiviral

 USES

Treats human immunodeficiency virus (HIV) and acquired immunodeficiency syndrome (AIDS).

 DOSAGE & USAGE INFORMATION

How to take:
* Tablet or capsule—Swallow with water. May be taken with or without food.
* Didanosine tablet—Chew or manually crumble tablet. If crumble tablet, mix with at least 1 oz. of water. Swallow right away. Take 1 hour before or 2 hours after meal.

Continued next column

 OVERDOSE

SYMPTOMS:
Seizures, severe nausea and vomiting, extreme tiredness or weakness, increase in bruising or bleeding, loss of coordination, involuntary eye movements.
WHAT TO DO:
* **Dial 911 (emergency) for medical help or call poison control center 1-800-222-1222 for instructions.**
* **See emergency information on last 3 pages of this book.**

* Syrup—Measure correct dosage with a specially marked measuring device.
* Buffered didanosine for oral solution— Follow instructions on label. Swallow immediately after mixing.

When to take:
At the same time each day, according to instructions on prescription label. Follow directions on label for taking with or without food.

If you forget a dose:
Take as soon as you remember up to 2 hours late. If more than 2 hours, wait for next scheduled dose (don't double this dose).

What drug does:
Suppresses replication of human immuno-deficiency virus.

Time lapse before drug works:
Depends on the progress of the disease.

Don't take with:
Any other medicine or any dietary supplement without consulting your doctor or pharmacist.

 POSSIBLE ADVERSE REACTIONS OR SIDE EFFECTS

SYMPTOMS	WHAT TO DO
Life-threatening:	
In case of overdose, see previous column.	
Common:	
• Tingling, numbness and burning in the feet and ankles (peripheral neuropathy).	Discontinue. Call doctor right away.
• Headache, anxiety, restlessness, digestive disturbances, diarrhea.	Continue. Call doctor when convenient.
Infrequent:	
• Unusual tiredness and weakness, fever, chills, sore throat, unusual bleeding or bruising, yellow skin and eyes, skin rash, pale skin, muscle or joint pain, mouth or throat sores, stomach pain, nausea and vomiting.	Discontinue. Call doctor right away.
• Lack of strength or energy, difficulty sleep-ing, discolored nails.	Continue. Call doctor when convenient.
Rare:	
Seizures, mood or mental changes, confusion.	Discontinue. Call doctor right away.

WARNINGS & PRECAUTIONS

Don't take if:
You are allergic to antivirals for HIV and AIDS.

Before you start, consult your doctor if:
- You have a history of alcoholism.
- You have hypertriglyceridemia, anemia, gout, phenylketonuria or pancreatitis.
- You have a condition that limits sodium intake
- A gene test is needed before starting abacavir.
- You have liver or kidney disease.
- You have peripheral neuropathy.

Over age 60:
No special problems expected.

Pregnancy:
Risk factors vary for drugs in this group. See category list on page xviii and consult doctor.

Breast-feeding:
Unknown effects. Consult doctor.

Infants & children:
May cause depigmentation of the retina. Children should have eye exams every 3 to 6 months to check for vision changes.

Prolonged use:
Talk with your doctor about the need for follow-up medical examination or laboratory studies to check blood serum and uric acid levels.

Skin & sunlight:
No special problems expected.

Driving, piloting or hazardous work:
Don't drive or pilot aircraft until you learn how medicine affects you. Don't work around dangerous machinery. Don't climb ladders or work in high places. Danger increases if you drink alcohol or take medicine affecting alertness and reflexes, such as antihistamines, tranquilizers, sedatives, pain medicines, narcotics and mind-altering drugs.

Discontinuing:
Don't discontinue without consulting doctor. Dose may require gradual reduction if you have taken drug for a long time. Doses of other drugs may require adjustment.

Others:
- Advise any doctor or dentist whom you consult that you take this medicine.
- Taking this drug does not prevent you from passing HIV to another person through sexual contact or sharing needles. Avoid sexual contact or practice safe sex (e.g., using condoms) to help prevent the transmission of HIV. Never share or re-use needles. If you have questions, ask your doctor for advice.
- Consult your doctor right away if you develop a new infection (e.g., fever, chills, sore throat or other symptoms).

- Do not increase or decrease dosage of drug without doctor's approval.

POSSIBLE INTERACTION WITH OTHER DRUGS

GENERIC NAME OR DRUG CLASS	COMBINED EFFECT
Antacids,* aluminum- or magnesium-containing	Decreased effect of zalcitabine.
Bone marrow depressants,* other	Drugs may need dosage changes.
Cimetidine	Increased effect of zalcitabine and zidovudine.
Clarithromycin	Decreased effect of zidovudine.
Dapsone	Increased risk of peripheral neuropathy. Reduced absorption of both drugs.
Fluoroquinolones	Decreased fluoroquinolone effect.
Ganciclovir	Increased toxicity of both drugs. Use with caution.
Itraconazole	Decreased absorption of itraconazole.
Ketoconazole	Decreased effect of ketoconazole.
Pancreatitis-associated drugs*	Increased risk of pancreatitis with didanosine.

Continued on page 926

POSSIBLE INTERACTION WITH OTHER SUBSTANCES

INTERACTS WITH	COMBINED EFFECT
Alcohol:	Risk of adverse effects. Avoid.
Beverages:	None expected.
Cocaine:	None expected.
Foods:	None expected.
Marijuana:	None expected.
Tobacco:	None expected.

*See Glossary

NUCLEOTIDE REVERSE TRANSCRIPTASE INHIBITORS

GENERIC AND BRAND NAMES

TENOFOVIR
Atripla
Truvada
Viread

BASIC INFORMATION

Habit forming? No
Prescription needed? Yes
Available as generic? No
Drug class: Antiviral

 ## USES

- Treats human immunodeficiency virus (HIV) and acquired immunodeficiency syndrome (AIDS). Used in combination with other anti-retroviral agents. Does not cure or prevent HIV or AIDS.
- Treatment of chronic hepatitis B.

 ## DOSAGE & USAGE INFORMATION

How to take:
Tablets —Swallow with water. Take with a meal.

When to take:
At the same time each day, according to instructions on prescription label.

If you forget a dose:
Take as soon as you remember. If it is almost time for the next dose, wait for next scheduled dose (don't double this dose).

What drug does:
Suppresses replication of human immuno-deficiency virus.

Time lapse before drug works:
Depends on the progress of the disease.

Don't take with:
Any other medicine or any dietary supplement without consulting your doctor or pharmacist.

 ## OVERDOSE

SYMPTOMS:
Unknown effects.
WHAT TO DO:
If person takes much larger amount than prescribed, dial 911 (emergency) for medical help or call poison control center 1-800-222-1222 for instructions.

 ## POSSIBLE ADVERSE REACTIONS OR SIDE EFFECTS

SYMPTOMS	WHAT TO DO
Life-threatening: None expected.	
Common: Vomiting, lack or loss of strength.	Continue. Call doctor when convenient.
Infrequent: Gaseousness, weight loss, diarrhea.	Continue. Call doctor when convenient.
Rare: Breathing fast or shallow, shortness of breath, unusual tiredness, sleepiness, stomach discomfort, loss of appetite, muscle cramping or pain, overall feeling of discomfort, any unusual symptoms.	Continue, but call doctor right away.

NUCLEOTIDE REVERSE TRANSCRIPTASE INHIBITORS

WARNINGS & PRECAUTIONS

Don't take if:
You are allergic to tenofovir.

Before you start, consult your doctor if:
You have liver or kidney disease.

Over age 60:
Studies have not been done in this age group.

Pregnancy:
Consult your doctor. Risk category B (see page xviii).

Breast-feeding:
It is unknown if drug passes into milk. It is not recommended that HIV-infected mothers breast-feed if other options are available. Consult your doctor.

Infants & children:
Safety and efficacy have not been established. Use only with close medical supervision.

Prolonged use:
* Talk with your doctor about the need for follow-up medical examination or laboratory studies to check drug's effectiveness.
* Long-term effects of this drug are unknown. Studies are ongoing.

Skin & sunlight:
No special problems expected.

Driving, piloting or hazardous work:
No problems expected.

Discontinuing:
Don't discontinue without consulting doctor.

Others:
* Advise any doctor or dentist whom you consult that you take this medicine.
* Taking this drug does not prevent you from passing HIV to another person through sexual contact or sharing needles. Avoid sexual contact or practice safe sex (e.g., using condoms) to help prevent the transmission of HIV. Never share or re-use needles. If you have questions, ask your doctor for advice.
* Consult your doctor right away if you develop a new infection (e.g., fever, chills, sore throat or other symptoms).
* Do not increase or decrease dosage of drug without doctor's approval.

POSSIBLE INTERACTION WITH OTHER DRUGS

GENERIC NAME OR DRUG CLASS	COMBINED EFFECT
Antivirals for herpes virus	Increased effect of tenofovir.
Didanosine	Increased effect of didanosine. Take tenofovir 2 hours before or 1 hour after didanosine.

POSSIBLE INTERACTION WITH OTHER SUBSTANCES

INTERACTS WITH	COMBINED EFFECT
Alcohol:	None expected.
Beverages:	None expected.
Cocaine:	None expected. Best to avoid.
Foods:	None expected.
Marijuana:	None expected. Best to avoid.
Tobacco:	None expected.

*See Glossary

NYSTATIN

BRAND NAMES

Dermacomb	Mykacet II
Myco II	Mytrex
Mycobiotic II	Nadostine
Mycogen II	Nilstat
Mycolog II	Nystaform
Mycostatin	Nystex
Myco-Triacet II	Tristatin II
Mykacet	

BASIC INFORMATION

Habit forming? No
Prescription needed? Yes
Available as generic? Yes
Drug class: Antifungal

 USES

Treatment of fungus infections of the mouth or vagina that are susceptible to nystatin.

 DOSAGE & USAGE INFORMATION

How to take:
* Tablet—Swallow with liquid. May take with or without food.
* Ointment, cream, lotion or powder—Use as directed by doctor and label.
* Liquid or powder for oral suspension—Take as directed. Instruction varies by preparation.
* Lozenge—Take as directed on label.

When to take:
At the same time each day.

If you forget a dose:
Take as soon as you remember up to 2 hours late. If more than 2 hours, wait for next scheduled dose (don't double this dose).

Continued next column

 OVERDOSE

SYMPTOMS:
Mild overdose may cause nausea, vomiting, diarrhea.
WHAT TO DO:
Overdose unlikely to threaten life. If person uses much larger amount than prescribed or if accidentally swallowed, call doctor or poison control center 1-800-222-1222 for help.

What drug does:
Prevents growth and reproduction of fungus.

Time lapse before drug works:
Begins immediately. May require 3 weeks for maximum benefit, depending on location and severity of infection.

Don't take with:
Any other medicine or any dietary supplement without consulting your doctor or pharmacist.

 POSSIBLE ADVERSE REACTIONS OR SIDE EFFECTS

SYMPTOMS	WHAT TO DO
Life-threatening: None expected.	
Common: (at high doses) Nausea, stomach pain, vomiting, diarrhea.	Discontinue. Call doctor right away.
Infrequent: Mild irritation, itch at application site.	Discontinue. Call doctor right away.
Rare: None expected.	

WARNINGS & PRECAUTIONS

Don't take if:
You are allergic to nystatin.

Before you start, consult your doctor if:
You plan to become pregnant within medication period.

Over age 60:
No problems expected.

Pregnancy:
No proven harm to unborn child. Avoid if possible. Consult doctor. Risk category B (see page xviii).

Breast-feeding:
No proven problems. Consult doctor.

Infants & children:
No problems expected.

Prolonged use:
No problems expected.

Skin & sunlight:
No problems expected.

Driving, piloting or hazardous work:
No problems expected.

Discontinuing:
Don't discontinue without doctor's advice until you complete prescribed dose, even though symptoms diminish or disappear.

Others:
No problems expected.

POSSIBLE INTERACTION WITH OTHER DRUGS

GENERIC NAME OR DRUG CLASS	COMBINED EFFECT
None reported.	

POSSIBLE INTERACTION WITH OTHER SUBSTANCES

INTERACTS WITH	COMBINED EFFECT
Alcohol:	None expected.
Beverages:	None expected.
Cocaine:	None expected.
Foods:	None expected.
Marijuana:	None expected.
Tobacco:	None expected.

OLANZAPINE

BRAND NAMES

Symbyax   Zyprexa Zydis
Zyprexa

BASIC INFORMATION

Habit forming? No
Prescription needed? Yes
Available as generic? No
Drug class: Antipsychotic

 ## USES

- Treatment for symptoms of schizophrenia, acute mania and other psychotic disorders.
- Treatment for bipolar disorder.

 ## DOSAGE & USAGE INFORMATION

How to take:
- Tablet or capsule—Swallow with liquid. May be taken with or without food.
- Oral disintegrating tablet—Let tablet dissolve in mouth.

When to take:
Once a day at the same time each day. The prescribed dosage may be increased over the first few days of use.

If you forget a dose:
Take as soon as you remember. If it is almost time for the next dose, wait for the next scheduled dose (don't double this dose).

What drug does:
The exact mechanism is unknown. It appears to alleviate symptoms by blocking certain nerve impulses between nerve cells.

Time lapse before drug works:
One to 7 days. Further increases in the dosage amount may be necessary to relieve symptoms for some patients.

Don't take with:
Any other medicine or any dietary supplement without consulting your doctor or pharmacist.

 ## OVERDOSE

SYMPTOMS:
Drowsiness and slurred speech; other symptoms may occur that were not observed in medical studies of the drug.
WHAT TO DO:
If person takes much larger amount than prescribed, dial 911 (emergency) for medical help or call poison control center 1-800-222-1222 for instructions.

 ## POSSIBLE ADVERSE REACTIONS OR SIDE EFFECTS

SYMPTOMS	WHAT TO DO
Life-threatening: High fever, rapid pulse, profuse sweating, muscle rigidity, confusion and irritability, seizures (rare neuroleptic malignant syndrome).	Discontinue. Seek emergency treatment.
Common: • Dizziness, difficulty in speaking or swallowing, shaking hands and fingers, trembling, vision problems, weakness, lightheadedness when arising from a sitting or lying position.	Continue. Call doctor right away.
• Drowsiness, constipation, weight gain, agitation, insomnia, headache, nervousness, runny nose, anxiety, dry mouth, arm or leg stiffness.	Continue. Call doctor when convenient.
Infrequent: • Jerky or involuntary movements (in face, lips, jaw, tongue) chest pain, fast heartbeat.	Continue. Call doctor right away.
• Fever, flu-like symptoms, twitching, mood or mental changes, speech unclear, swollen feet or ankles, appetite increased, cough, saliva increased, muscle tightness, muscle spasms (face, neck, back), joint pain, nausea, vomiting, sore throat, incontinence, abdominal pain.	Continue. Call doctor when convenient.
Rare: • Breathing difficulty, high blood sugar (thirstiness, frequent urination, increased hunger, weakness).	Discontinue. Call doctor right away.
• Swollen face, rash, confusion, decreased sex drive, menstrual changes, sluggishness.	Continue. Call doctor when convenient.

WARNINGS & PRECAUTIONS

Don't take if:
You are allergic to olanzapine.

Before you start, consult your doctor if:
- You have liver disease, heart disease, a blood vessel disorder or history of seizures.
- You have a history of breast cancer.
- You have intestinal blockage.
- You are subject to dehydration or low body temperature.
- You have a history of drug abuse/dependence.
- You have a family history of, are at risk for, or have diabetes.
- You have glaucoma or prostate problems.
- Patient has Alzheimer's.
- You are allergic to any medication, food or other substance.

Over age 60:
- Adverse reactions and side effects may be more severe than in younger persons. A lower starting dosage is usually recommended until a response is determined.
- Use of antipsychotic drugs in elderly patients with dementia-related psychosis may increase risk of death. Consult doctor.

Pregnancy:
Decide with your doctor if drug benefits justify any possible risk to unborn child. Risk category C (see page xviii).

Breast-feeding:
It is unknown if drug passes into milk. It is not recommended for nursing mothers.

Infants & children:
Not approved for ages under 18. If prescribed, carefully read information provided with prescription. Contact doctor right away if depression symptoms get worse or there is any talk of suicide or suicide behaviors. Also, read information under Others.

Prolonged use:
Consult with your doctor on a regular basis while taking this drug to check your progress or to discuss any increase or changes in side effects and the need for continued treatment.

Skin & sunlight:
May cause rash or intensify sunburn in areas exposed to sun or ultraviolet light (photosensitivity reaction). Use sunscreen and avoid over-exposure. Notify doctor if reaction occurs.

Driving, piloting or hazardous work:
Don't drive or pilot aircraft until you learn how medicine affects you. Don't work around dangerous machinery. Don't climb ladders or work in high places. Danger increases if you drink alcohol or take drug affecting alertness and reflexes.

Discontinuing:
Don't discontinue this drug without consulting doctor. Dosage may require a gradual reduction before stopping.

Others:
- Get up slowly from a sitting or lying position to avoid any dizziness or lightheadedness.
- Hot temperatures, exercise, and hot baths can increase risk of heatstroke. Drug may affect body's ability to maintain normal temperature.
- Advise any doctor or dentist whom you consult that you take this medicine.
- Take medicine only as directed. Do not increase or reduce dosage without doctor's approval.
- Adults and children taking antidepressants may experience a worsening of the depression symptoms and may display increased suicidal thoughts or behavior. Call doctor right away if these symptoms or behaviors occur.
- Doctor may monitor enzymes in liver to ensure liver functions are not affected by medication.

POSSIBLE INTERACTION WITH OTHER DRUGS

GENERIC NAME OR DRUG CLASS	COMBINED EFFECT
Anticholinergics,* other	Increased risk of side effects.
Antihypertensives*	Increased effect of antihypertensive.
Carbamazepine	Decreased effect of olanzapine.
Enzyme inducers*	May decrease olanzapine effect.
Enzyme inhibitors*	May increase olanzapine effect.

Continued on page 926

POSSIBLE INTERACTION WITH OTHER SUBSTANCES

INTERACTS WITH	COMBINED EFFECT
Alcohol:	Increased sedation and dizziness. Avoid.
Beverages:	None expected.
Cocaine:	Unknown. Avoid.
Foods:	None expected.
Marijuana:	Unknown. Avoid.
Tobacco:	Decreased olanzapine effect. Avoid.

*See Glossary

OLSALAZINE

BRAND NAMES

Dipentum

BASIC INFORMATION

Habit forming? No
Prescription needed? Yes
Available as generic? No
Drug class: Inflammatory bowel disease
  suppressant

 ## USES

- To maintain remission of ulcerative colitis. Generally prescribed when intolerance to sulfasalazine exists.
- Treatment for Crohn's disease.

 ## DOSAGE & USAGE INFORMATION

How to take:
Capsule—Swallow with liquid or food to lessen stomach irritation. If you can't swallow whole, open capsule and take with liquid or food.

When to take:
Usually twice a day, or as directed on prescription label.

If you forget a dose:
- Take as soon as possible.
- Skip if it is almost time for next dose.
- Don't double next dose.
- Notify your doctor if there are questions.

What drug does:
Inhibits prostaglandin production in the colon.

Time lapse before drug works:
1 hour.

Don't take with:
Any other medicine or any dietary supplement without consulting your doctor or pharmacist.

 ## OVERDOSE

SYMPTOMS:
None expected.
WHAT TO DO:
Overdose unlikely to threaten life. If person uses much larger amount than prescribed or if accidentally swallowed, call doctor or poison control center 1-800-222-1222 for help.

 ## POSSIBLE ADVERSE REACTIONS OR SIDE EFFECTS

SYMPTOMS	WHAT TO DO
Life-threatening:	
Fever, sore throat, paleness, unusual bleeding (representing effect on blood, a rare complication).	Seek emergency treatment.
Common:	
Diarrhea, appetite loss, nausea, vomiting.	Continue. Call doctor when convenient.
Infrequent:	
Mood changes, sleeplessness, headache.	Continue. Call doctor when convenient.
Rare:	
Skin eruption (acne-like), muscle aches.	Continue. Call doctor when convenient.

WARNINGS & PRECAUTIONS

Don't take if:
- You are allergic to olsalazine, aspirin or any other salicylate.
- You are allergic to mesalamine.

Before you start, consult your doctor if:
- You have kidney disease.
- You are taking any other prescription or nonprescription medicine.

Over age 60:
No special problems expected.

Pregnancy:
Decide with your doctor if drug benefits justify risk to unborn child. Risk category C (see page xviii).

Breast-feeding:
Unknown effects. Consult doctor.

Infants & children:
Effect not documented. Consult your family doctor or pediatrician.

Prolonged use:
Follow through with full prescribed course of treatment.

Skin & sunlight:
No special problems expected.

Driving, piloting or hazardous work:
Don't drive or pilot aircraft until you learn how medicine affects you. Don't work around dangerous machinery. Don't climb ladders or work in high places. Danger increases if you drink alcohol or take medicine affecting alertness and reflexes.

Discontinuing:
Don't discontinue without consulting doctor. Dose may require gradual reduction if you have taken drug for a long time. Doses of other drugs may also require adjustment.

Others:
Request your doctor to check blood counts and kidney function on a regular basis.

POSSIBLE INTERACTION WITH OTHER DRUGS

GENERIC NAME OR DRUG CLASS	COMBINED EFFECT
None expected since olsalazine is not appreciably absorbed from the gastrointestinal tract into the bloodstream.	

POSSIBLE INTERACTION WITH OTHER SUBSTANCES

INTERACTS WITH	COMBINED EFFECT
Alcohol:	Increased risk of gastrointestinal upset and/or bleeding.
Beverages: Highly spiced beverages.	Will irritate underlying condition that olsalazine treats.
Cocaine:	Avoid.
Foods: Highly spiced foods.	Will irritate underlying condition that olsalazine treats.
Marijuana:	Avoid.
Tobacco:	Will irritate underlying condition that olsalazine treats. Avoid.

OMEGA-3-ACID ETHYL ESTERS

BRAND NAMES

Lovaza

BASIC INFORMATION

Habit forming? No
Prescription needed? Yes
Available as generic? No
Drug class: Antihyperlipidemic

 USES

* Helps to lower very high triglyceride (fat-like substance) levels in the blood. Its use is recommended in combination with an appropriate heart-healthy diet and exercise program.
* May be used for treatment of other disorders as determined by your doctor.

 DOSAGE & USAGE INFORMATION

How to take:
Capsule—Swallow whole with liquid. It is advised that it be taken with food.

When to take:
It may be taken 1 to 2 times a day. Follow the instructions on your prescription.

If you forget a dose:
Take as soon as you remember. If it is almost time for the next dose, wait for next scheduled dose (don't double this dose).

What drug does:
Omega-3-acid ethyl esters are derived from fish oil. They help reduce the production of fatty substances (triglycerides) in the liver. The exact way they work is not completely understood. They may also increase the level of low-density lipoprotein (LDL) cholesterol. LDL is considered the "bad" cholesterol.

Time lapse before drug works:
About two months for measurable results as determined by laboratory testing.

Continued next column

 OVERDOSE

SYMPTOMS:
Exact symptoms are unknown.
WHAT TO DO:
Overdose unlikely to threaten life. If person uses much larger amount than prescribed or if accidentally swallowed, call doctor or poison control center 1-800-222-1222 for help.

Don't take with:
Any other medicine or any dietary supplement without consulting your doctor or pharmacist.

 POSSIBLE ADVERSE REACTIONS OR SIDE EFFECTS

SYMPTOMS	WHAT TO DO
Life-threatening: An allergic reaction is unlikely. Symptoms could include itching, difficulty breathing, chest tightness, closing of the throat, swelling of the lips or face or tongue, hives.	Seek emergency treatment immediately.
Common: Burping, infection, flu-like symptoms, upset stomach, taste changes, back pain.	Continue. Call doctor when convenient
Infrequent: Chest pain.	Discontinue. Call doctor right away.
Rare: None expected.	

WARNINGS & PRECAUTIONS

Don't take if:
You are allergic to any omega-3-acid ethyl esters, fish oil or fish.

Before you start, consult your doctor if:
- You have medical problems that may contribute to high triglycerides (e.g., diabetes or hypothyroidism).
- You take drugs such as beta blockers, estrogens or thiazide diuretics. They can be a risk factor for high triglycerides.
- You have liver disease.
- You are obese.

Over age 60:
No special problems expected.

Pregnancy:
Decide with your doctor if drug benefits justify any possible risk to unborn child. Risk category C (see page xviii).

Breast-feeding:
It is unknown if drug passes into milk. Avoid drug or discontinue nursing until you finish medicine. Consult doctor for advice on maintaining milk supply.

Infants & children:
Safety and effectiveness in children has not been established. Consult your child's doctor.

Prolonged use:
No problems expected. Ask your doctor about routine laboratory studies to verify continued effectiveness of the drug therapy and to check your triglyceride levels.

Skin & sunlight:
No problems expected.

Driving, piloting or hazardous work:
No problems expected.

Discontinuing:
No problems expected.

Others:
- Follow your doctor's advice carefully regarding proper diet and an exercise program. Drugs such as this one are usually prescribed only when more help is needed.
- Consult your doctor about routine monitoring of LDL cholesterol levels to be sure they are not increasing excessively.
- Diabetic patients may experience worsening of blood sugar control.
- Advise any doctor or dentist whom you consult that you take this medicine.
- This drug was previously named Omacor. It was changed to Lovaza.

POSSIBLE INTERACTION WITH OTHER DRUGS

GENERIC NAME OR DRUG CLASS	COMBINED EFFECT
Anticoagulants, oral*	May increase anticoagulant effect. Consult doctor.

POSSIBLE INTERACTION WITH OTHER SUBSTANCES

INTERACTS WITH	COMBINED EFFECT
Alcohol:	None expected. Decreased alcohol intake is often recommended to help reduce triglyceride levels.
Beverages:	None expected.
Cocaine:	None expected. Best to avoid.
Foods:	None expected.
Marijuana:	None expected. Best to avoid.
Tobacco:	None expected. Smoking can contribute to high triglycerides.

ORLISTAT

BRAND NAMES

Alli   Xenical

BASIC INFORMATION

Habit forming? No
Prescription needed? Yes, for Xenical
Available as generic? No
Drug class: Antiobesity; lipase inhibitor

 USES

- Treatment for obesity and weight loss. To be used in conjunction with a reduced-calorie diet. Treatment with this drug is not recommended for cosmetic weight loss.
- Used to delay onset of type 2 diabetes.

 DOSAGE & USAGE INFORMATION

How to take:
Capsule—Swallow with liquid. If you can't swallow whole, open capsule and take with liquid.

When to take:
With or shortly following meals (containing fats) up to three times daily.

If you forget a dose:
Skip the missed dose and return to your regular dosing schedule. Do not double dose.

What drug does:
Blocks some of the normal absorption of fats from the intestines, causing them to be excreted in the feces.

Time lapse before drug works:
Several months or longer for maximum benefit.

Don't take with:
Any other medicine or any dietary supplement without consulting your doctor or pharmacist.

 OVERDOSE

SYMPTOMS:
None expected.
WHAT TO DO:
Overdose unlikely to threaten life. If person uses much larger amount than prescribed or if accidentally swallowed, call doctor or poison control center 1-800-222-1222 for help.

 POSSIBLE ADVERSE REACTIONS OR SIDE EFFECTS

SYMPTOMS	WHAT TO DO
Life-threatening: None expected.	
Common:	
• Flu-like symptoms, runny nose, congestion, sneezing, sore throat, cough, fever.	Continue. Call doctor when convenient.
• Abdominal pain, oily bowel movements, inability to hold bowel movements, immediate need to have bowel movements, gas with leaky bowel movements, oily spotting of underwear, headaches.	Continue. Call doctor if symptoms persist.
Infrequent:	
• Troubled breathing, tightness in chest, wheezing.	Discontinue. Call doctor right away.
• Anxiety, back pain, menstrual irregularities, rectal pain or discomfort, tooth or gum problems.	Continue. Call doctor if symptoms persist.
Rare:	
• Diarrhea, hearing changes, pain in ear, bloody or cloudy urine, difficult or painful urination, frequent urge to urinate.	Discontinue. Call doctor right away.
• Joint pain, dizziness, dry skin, fatigue, insomnia, muscle pain, nausea, skin rash, vomiting.	Continue. Call doctor if symptoms persist.

WARNINGS & PRECAUTIONS

Don't take if:
- You are allergic to orlistat.
- You have been diagnosed with malabsorption.
- You have cholestasis (blocked bile flow).

Before you start, consult your doctor if:
- You are allergic to any foods or dyes.
- You are taking any other medications or dietary supplements for weight loss.
- You have a history of anorexia or bulimia.
- You have kidney stones or gallbladder problems.
- You are pregnant or are planning to become pregnant.

Over age 60:
Adverse reactions and side effects may be more frequent and severe than in younger persons.

Pregnancy:
Not recommended for use during pregnancy. Risk category B (see page xviii).

Breast-feeding:
It is unknown if orlistat passes into milk. Avoid drug or discontinue nursing until you finish medicine. Consult doctor for advice on maintaining milk supply.

Infants & children:
Not recommended for persons under age 12.

Prolonged use:
Talk to your doctor about the need for follow-up medical examinations or laboratory studies.

Skin & sunlight:
No problems expected.

Driving, piloting or hazardous work:
No special problems expected.

Discontinuing:
Don't discontinue without doctor's advice.

Others:
- Expect to start with small doses and increase gradually to lessen frequency and severity of adverse reactions.
- Orlistat may interfere with your body's absorption of certain vitamins; therefore, you should take a multivitamin supplement daily, two hours before or after taking orlistat.
- Drug may affect the results of some medical tests.
- During treatment, you should be on a nutritionally balanced reduced-calorie diet that contains no more than 30 percent of calories from fat.
- Patients with diabetes may require a reduced dosage of oral hypoglycemic medicine or insulin due to weight loss.
- Advise any doctor or dentist whom you consult that you take this medicine.

POSSIBLE INTERACTION WITH OTHER DRUGS

GENERIC NAME OR DRUG CLASS	COMBINED EFFECT
Cyclosporine	Unknown effect. Monitor closely.
Pravastatin	Increased pravastatin effect.
Vitamins A, D, E, K	Decreased vitamin effect.
Warfarin	Increased warfarin effect.

POSSIBLE INTERACTION WITH OTHER SUBSTANCES

INTERACTS WITH	COMBINED EFFECT
Alcohol:	None expected.
Beverages:	None expected.
Cocaine:	Effects unknown. Avoid.
Foods:	None expected.
Marijuana:	Effects unknown. Avoid.
Tobacco:	None expected.

*See Glossary

ORPHENADRINE

BRAND NAMES

Banflex	Myotrol
Blanex	Neocyten
Disipal	Noradex
Flexagin	Norflex
Flexain	O-Flex
Flexoject	Orflagen
Flexon	Orfro
K-Flex	Orphenate
Marflex	Tega-Flex
Myolin	

BASIC INFORMATION

Habit forming? Possibly
Prescription needed?
　U.S.: Yes
　Canada: No
Available as generic? Yes
Drug class: Muscle relaxant, anticholinergic, antihistamine, antiparkinsonism

USES

* Reduces discomfort of muscle strain.
* Relieves symptoms of Parkinson's disease.
* Adjunctive treatment to rest, analgesics and physical therapy for muscle spasms.

DOSAGE & USAGE INFORMATION

How to take:
* Tablet—Swallow with liquid. If you can't swallow whole, crumble tablet and take with liquid or food.
* Extended-release tablet—Swallow whole. Do not crumble.

When to take:
At the same times each day.

Continued next column

OVERDOSE

SYMPTOMS:
Fainting, confusion, blurred vision, difficulty swallowing, difficulty breathing, decreased urination, widely dilated pupils, rapid heartbeat, rapid pulse, paralysis, convulsions, coma.
WHAT TO DO:
* **Dial 911 (emergency) for medical help or call poison control center 1-800-222-1222 for instructions.**
* **See emergency information on last 3 pages of this book.**

If you forget a dose:
Take as soon as you remember up to 6 hours late. If more than 6 hours, wait for next scheduled dose (don't double this dose).

What drug does:
Sedative and analgesic effects reduce spasm and pain in skeletal muscles.

Time lapse before drug works:
1 to 2 hours.

Don't take with:
Any other medicine or any dietary supplement without consulting your doctor or pharmacist.

POSSIBLE ADVERSE REACTIONS OR SIDE EFFECTS

SYMPTOMS	WHAT TO DO
Life-threatening:	
Extreme weakness; transient paralysis; temporary loss of vision; hives, rash, intense itching, faintness soon after a dose (anaphylaxis).	Seek emergency treatment immediately.
Common:	
None expected.	
Infrequent:	
• Weakness, headache, dizziness, agitation, drowsiness, tremor, confusion, rapid or pounding heartbeat, depression, hearing loss.	Discontinue. Call doctor right away.
• Dry mouth, nausea, vomiting, constipation, urinary hesitancy or retention, abdominal pain, muscle weakness.	Continue. Call doctor when convenient.
Rare:	
Rash, itchy skin, blurred vision, hallucinations.	Discontinue. Call doctor right away.

WARNINGS & PRECAUTIONS

Don't take if:
* You are allergic to orphenadrine.
* You are allergic to tartrazine dye.

Before you start, consult your doctor if:
* You have glaucoma.
* You have myasthenia gravis.
* You have difficulty emptying bladder.
* You have had heart disease or heart rhythm disturbance.
* You have had a peptic ulcer.
* You have prostate enlargement.

Over age 60:
Adverse reactions and side effects may be more frequent and severe than in younger persons.

Pregnancy:
Decide with your doctor if drug benefits justify risk to unborn child. Risk category C (see page xviii).

Breast-feeding:
It is unknown if drug passes into milk. Avoid drug or discontinue nursing until you finish medicine. Consult doctor for advice on maintaining milk supply.

Infants & children:
Not recommended for children younger than 12.

Prolonged use:
- Increased internal eye pressure.
- Talk to your doctor about the need for follow-up medical examinations or laboratory studies to check complete blood counts (white blood cell count, platelet count, red blood cell count, hemoglobin, hematocrit), liver function, kidney function.

Skin & sunlight:
No problems expected.

Driving, piloting or hazardous work:
Don't drive or pilot aircraft until you learn how medicine affects you. Don't work around dangerous machinery. Don't climb ladders or work in high places. Danger increases if you drink alcohol or take medicine affecting alertness and reflexes, such as antihistamines, tranquilizers, sedatives, pain medicine, narcotics and mind-altering drugs.

Discontinuing:
May be unnecessary to finish medicine. Follow doctor's instructions.

Others:
Advise any doctor or dentist whom you consult that you take this drug.

POSSIBLE INTERACTION WITH OTHER DRUGS

GENERIC NAME OR DRUG CLASS	COMBINED EFFECT
Anticholinergics*	Increased anticholinergic effect.
Antidepressants, tricyclic*	Increased sedation.
Antihistamines*	Increased sedation.
Attapulgite	Decreased orphenadrine effect.
Carteolol	Decreased antihistamine effect.

Chlorpromazine	Hypoglycemia (low blood sugar).
Cisapride	Decreased orphenadrine effect.
Contraceptives, oral*	Decreased contraceptive effect.
Griseofulvin	Decreased griseofulvin effect.
Levodopa	Increased levodopa effect. (Improves effectiveness in treating Parkinson's disease).
Nabilone	Greater depression of central nervous system.
Nitrates*	Increased internal eye pressure.
Nizatidine	Increased nizatidine effect.
Phenylbutazone	Decreased phenylbutazone effect.
Potassium supplements*	Increased possibility of intestinal ulcers with oral potassium tablets.
Propoxyphene	Possible confusion, nervousness, tremors.

POSSIBLE INTERACTION WITH OTHER SUBSTANCES

INTERACTS WITH	COMBINED EFFECT
Alcohol:	Increased drowsiness. Avoid.
Beverages:	None expected.
Cocaine:	Decreased orphenadrine effect. Avoid.
Foods:	None expected.
Marijuana:	Increased drowsiness, mouth dryness, muscle weakness, fainting.
Tobacco:	None expected.

ORPHENADRINE, ASPIRIN & CAFFEINE

BRAND NAMES

N3 Gesic
N3 Gesic Forte
Norgesic
Norgesic Forte
Norphadrine
Norphadrine Forte
Orphenagesic
Orphenagesic Forte

BASIC INFORMATION

Habit forming? Yes
Prescription needed? Yes
Available as generic? No
Drug class: Stimulant, vasoconstrictor, muscle relaxant, analgesic, anti-inflammatory (nonsteroidal)

 USES

- Reduces discomfort of muscle strain.
- Reduces pain, fever, inflammation.
- Relieves swelling, stiffness, joint pain.
- Treats drowsiness and fatigue.

 DOSAGE & USAGE INFORMATION

How to take:
Tablet—Swallow with liquid. If you can't swallow whole, crumble and take with liquid or food.

When to take:
At the same times each day.

If you forget a dose:
Take as soon as you remember up to 2 hours late. If more than 2 hours, wait for next scheduled dose (don't double this dose).

What drug does:
- Sedative and analgesic effects reduce spasm and pain in skeletal muscles.
- Affects hypothalamus, the part of the brain which regulates temperature by dilating small blood vessels in skin.

Continued next column

 OVERDOSE

SYMPTOMS:
Fainting, confusion, widely dilated pupils, rapid pulse, ringing in ears, nausea, vomiting, dizziness, fever, deep and rapid breathing, excitement, rapid heartbeat, hallucinations, coma.
WHAT TO DO:
- **Dial 911 (emergency) for medical help or call poison control center 1-800-222-1222 for instructions.**
- **See emergency information on last 3 pages of this book.**

- Prevents clumping of platelets (small blood cells) so blood vessels remain open.
- Decreases prostaglandin effect.
- Suppresses body's pain messages.
- Constricts blood vessel walls.
- Stimulates central nervous system.

Time lapse before drug works:
1 hour.

Don't take with:
- Tetracyclines. Space doses 1 hour apart.
- Any other medicine or any dietary supplement without consulting your doctor or pharmacist.

 POSSIBLE ADVERSE REACTIONS OR SIDE EFFECTS

SYMPTOMS	WHAT TO DO
Life-threatening:	
Hives, rash, intense itching, wheezing, faintness soon after a dose (anaphylaxis), convulsions, fever.	Seek emergency treatment immediately.
Common:	
• Nausea, vomiting, abdominal cramps, nervousness, urgent urination, low blood sugar (hunger, anxiety, cold sweats, rapid pulse).	Discontinue. Call doctor right away.
• Ringing in ears, indigestion, heart-burn, insomnia.	Continue. Call doctor when convenient.
Infrequent:	
• Weakness, headache, dizziness, drowsiness, agitation, tremor, confusion, irregular heartbeat, hearing loss, diarrhea, hallucinations.	Discontinue. Call doctor right away.
• Dry mouth, constipation.	Continue. Call doctor when convenient.
Rare:	
• Black or bloody vomit.	Discontinue. Seek emergency treatment.
• Change in vision; blurred vision; black, bloody or tarry stool; bloody urine; dilated pupils; uncontrolled movement of hands; sore throat; fever.	Discontinue. Call doctor right away.

ORPHENADRINE, ASPIRIN & CAFFEINE

WARNINGS & PRECAUTIONS

Don't take if:
- You need to restrict sodium in your diet. Buffered effervescent tablets and sodium salicylate are high in sodium.
- Aspirin has a strong vinegar-like odor, which means it has decomposed.
- You have a peptic ulcer of stomach or duodenum, a bleeding disorder, heart disease.
- You are allergic to any stimulant or orphenadrine.

Before you start, consult your doctor if:
- You have had stomach or duodenal ulcers, gout, heart disease or heart rhythm disturbance, peptic ulcer.
- You have asthma, nasal polyps, irregular heartbeat, hypoglycemia (low blood sugar), epilepsy, glaucoma, myasthenia gravis, difficulty emptying bladder, prostate enlargement.

Over age 60:
- More likely to cause hidden bleeding in stomach or intestines. Watch for dark stools.
- Adverse reactions and side effects may be more frequent and severe than in younger persons.

Pregnancy:
Risk to unborn child outweighs drug benefits. Don't use. Risk category D (see page xviii).

Breast-feeding:
Drug passes into milk. Avoid drug or discontinue nursing until you finish medicine. Consult doctor for advice on maintaining milk supply.

Infants & children:
- Overdose frequent and severe. Keep bottles out of children's reach.
- Consult doctor before giving to persons under age 18 who have fever and discomfort of viral illness, especially chicken pox and influenza. Probably increases risk of Reye's syndrome.
- Not recommended for children under 12.

Prolonged use:
- Kidney damage. Periodic kidney function test recommended.
- Stomach ulcers more likely.
- Increased internal eye pressure.
- Talk to your doctor about the need for follow-up medical examinations or laboratory studies to check liver function, complete blood counts (white blood cell count, platelet count, red blood cell count, hemoglobin, hematocrit).

Skin & sunlight:
No special problems expected.

Driving, piloting or hazardous work:
Don't drive or pilot aircraft until you learn how medicine affects you. Don't work around dangerous machinery. Don't climb ladders or work in high places. Danger increases if you drink alcohol or take medicine affecting alertness and reflexes, such as antihistamines, tranquilizers, sedatives, pain medicine, narcotics and mind-altering drugs.

Discontinuing:
- For chronic illness—Don't discontinue without doctor's advice until you complete prescribed dose, even though symptoms diminish or disappear.
- May be unnecessary to finish medicine if you take it for a short-term illness. Follow doctor's instructions.

Others:
- Aspirin can complicate surgery; illness; pregnancy, labor and delivery.
- For arthritis, don't change dose without consulting doctor.
- Urine tests for blood sugar may be inaccurate.
- May produce or aggravate fibrocystic breast disease in women.

POSSIBLE INTERACTION WITH OTHER DRUGS

GENERIC NAME OR DRUG CLASS	COMBINED EFFECT
Acebutolol	Decreased antihypertensive effect of acebutolol.

Continued on page 926

POSSIBLE INTERACTION WITH OTHER SUBSTANCES

INTERACTS WITH	COMBINED EFFECT
Alcohol:	Possible stomach irritation and bleeding, increased drowsiness. Avoid.
Beverages: Caffeine drinks.	Increased caffeine effect.
Cocaine:	Decreased orphenadrine effect. Overstimulation. Avoid.
Foods:	None expected.
Marijuana:	Increased effect of drugs. May lead to dangerous, rapid heartbeat. Increased dry mouth. Avoid.
Tobacco:	Increased heartbeat. Avoid.

*See Glossary

OXCARBAZEPINE

BRAND NAMES

Trileptal

BASIC INFORMATION

Habit forming? No
Prescription needed? Yes
Available as generic? Yes
Drug class: Anticonvulsant, antiepileptic

 USES

Treatment for partial (focal) epileptic seizures. May be used alone or in combination with other antiepileptic drugs.

 DOSAGE & USAGE INFORMATION

How to take:
Tablet—Swallow with liquid. May be taken with or without food.

When to take:
Your doctor will determine the best schedule. Dosages will be increased rapidly over the first few days of use. Further increases may be necessary to achieve maximum benefits.

If you forget a dose:
Take as soon as you remember. If it is almost time for the next dose, skip the missed dose and wait for your next scheduled dose (don't double this dose).

What drug does:
The exact mechanism is unknown. The anticonvulsant action may result from an altered transport of brain amino acids. Amino acids play an important part in chemical reactions within the cells.

Time lapse before drug works:
May take several weeks for effectiveness.

Don't take with:
Any other medicine or any dietary supplement without consulting your doctor or pharmacist.

 OVERDOSE

SYMPTOMS:
Double vision, slurred speech, drowsiness, tiredness, diarrhea.
WHAT TO DO:
Overdose unlikely to threaten life. If person uses much larger amount than prescribed or if accidentally swallowed, call doctor or poison control center 1-800-222-1222 for help.

 POSSIBLE ADVERSE REACTIONS OR SIDE EFFECTS

SYMPTOMS	WHAT TO DO
Life-threatening: Severe skin reaction.	Seek emergency help.
Common: • Cough with fever and sneezing and sore throat, clumsiness, vision changes, dizziness, crying, depression, false sense of well-being, spinning sensation, uncontrolled eye movement, feeling of constant movement of self or surroundings.	Continue, but call doctor right away.
• Runny or stuffy nose, nausea or vomiting, sleepiness.	Continue. Call doctor when convenient.
Infrequent: • Blurred vision, cloudy or bloody urine, urination changes (decreased or increased, painful, urgent), confusion, falling, bruising, ill feeling, thirstiness, hoarseness, vaginal itching, heartbeat irregularities, facial pain, memory loss, coordination problems, trembling, shortness of breath, unusual tiredness or weakness.	Continue, but call doctor right away.
• Sour stomach, acne, changes in taste, dry mouth, constipation or diarrhea, heartburn, sweating, feeling of warmth in face or chest, back pain, belching, bloody nose.	Continue. Call doctor when convenient.
Rare: Sore or bleeding lips, chills, chest pain, irritability, hives or itching, muscle or joint pain, nervousness, rectal bleeding, peeling or blistering skin, sores in mouth, swollen legs, purple spots on skin, burning feeling in chest or stomach.	Continue, but call, doctor right away.

WARNINGS & PRECAUTIONS

Don't take if:
You are allergic to oxcarbazepine or carbamazepine.

Before you start, consult your doctor if:
- You have a history of kidney disease.
- You have hyponatremia (too little sodium in the body).
- You are allergic to any medication, food or other substance.
- You have any other medical problems.

Over age 60:
No special problems expected.

Pregnancy:
Decide with your doctor if drug benefits justify risks to unborn child. Risk category C (see page xviii).

Breast-feeding:
Drug passes into milk. Avoid drug or discontinue nursing until you finish medicine. Consult doctor for advice on maintaining milk supply.

Infants & children:
No special problems expected for children over age four.

Prolonged use:
No special problems expected. Follow-up laboratory blood studies may be recommended by your doctor.

Skin & sunlight:
No problems expected.

Driving, piloting or hazardous work:
Don't drive or pilot aircraft until you learn how medicine affects you. Don't work around dangerous machinery. Don't climb ladders or work in high places. Danger increases if you drink alcohol or take other medicines affecting alertness and reflexes such as antihistamines, tranquilizers, sedatives, pain medicine, narcotics and mind-altering drugs.

Discontinuing:
Don't discontinue without doctor's approval due to risk of increased seizure activity. The dosage may need to be gradually decreased before stopping the drug completely.

Others:
- Advise any doctor or dentist whom you consult that you take this medicine.
- The effectiveness of oral contraceptives that contain estrogen may be reduced. Talk to your doctor about other forms of birth control.
- Oxcarbazepine may be used with other anticonvulsant drugs and additional side effects may occur. If they do, discuss them with your doctor.
- There is a small risk of life threatening skin reactions while taking this drug. If you develop an allergic reaction or a skin rash, contact your doctor right away.
- This medicine alone may cause drowsiness, dizziness, or lightheadedness, especially when getting up from a sitting or lying position.
- Rarely, antiepileptic drugs may lead to suicidal thoughts and behaviors. Call doctor right away if suicidal symptoms or unusual behaviors occur.
- Wear or carry medical identification to show your seizure disorder and the drugs you take.

POSSIBLE INTERACTION WITH OTHER DRUGS

GENERIC NAME OR DRUG CLASS	COMBINED EFFECT
Anticonvulsants,* other	Increased risk of side effects.
Contraceptives, oral*	Decreased effect of contraceptive.
CNS Depressants*	Increased sedative effect.
Felodipine	Decreased effect of felodipine.
Verapamil	Decreased effect of verapamil.

POSSIBLE INTERACTION WITH OTHER SUBSTANCES

INTERACTS WITH	COMBINED EFFECT
Alcohol:	Increased sedative effect. Avoid.
Beverages:	None expected.
Cocaine:	Unknown effect. Avoid.
Foods:	None expected.
Marijuana:	Unknown effect. Avoid.
Tobacco:	None expected.

*See Glossary

OXYMETAZOLINE (Nasal)

BRAND NAMES

See full list of brand names in the *Generic and Brand Name Directory*, page 893.

BASIC INFORMATION

Habit forming? No
Prescription needed? No
Available as generic? Yes
Drug class: Sympathomimetic

 ## USES

Relieves congestion of nose, sinuses and throat from allergies and infections.

 ## DOSAGE & USAGE INFORMATION

How to take:
Nasal solution, nasal spray—Use as directed on label. Avoid contamination. Don't use same container for more than 1 person.

When to take:
When needed, no more often than every 4 hours.

If you forget a dose:
Take as soon as you remember. Wait 4 hours for next dose.

What drug does:
Constricts walls of small arteries in nose, sinuses and eustachian tubes.

Time lapse before drug works:
5 to 30 minutes. May last 8 to 12 hours.

Continued next column

 ## OVERDOSE

SYMPTOMS:
Headache, sweating, anxiety, agitation, rapid and irregular heartbeat (rare occurrence with systemic absorption).
WHAT TO DO:
• **Dial 911 (emergency) for medical help or call poison control center 1-800-222-1222 for instructions.**
• **If person is unconscious, check breathing and pulse. If not breathing, begin mouth-to-mouth rescue breathing. If heart is not beating, begin chest compressions.**
• **See emergency information on last 3 pages of this book.**

Don't take with:
• Nonprescription drugs for allergy, cough or cold without consulting doctor.
• Any other medicine or any dietary supplement without consulting your doctor or pharmacist.

 ## POSSIBLE ADVERSE REACTIONS OR SIDE EFFECTS

SYMPTOMS	WHAT TO DO
Life-threatening: In case of overdose, see previous column.	
Common: None expected.	
Infrequent: Burning, dry or stinging nasal passages.	Continue. Call doctor when convenient.
Rare: Rebound congestion (increased runny or stuffy nose); headache, insomnia, nervousness (may occur with systemic absorption).	Discontinue. Call doctor right away.

WARNINGS & PRECAUTIONS

Don't take if:
You are allergic to oxymetazoline or other nasal spray.

Before you start, consult your doctor if:
- You have heart disease or high blood pressure.
- You have diabetes.
- You have overactive thyroid.
- You have taken MAO inhibitors in past 2 weeks.
- You have glaucoma.

Over age 60:
Adverse reactions and side effects may be more frequent and severe than in younger persons.

Pregnancy:
Consult doctor. Risk category C (see page xviii).

Breast-feeding:
No proven problems. Consult doctor.

Infants & children:
Don't give to children younger than 2.

Prolonged use:
Drug may lose effectiveness, cause increased congestion (rebound effect*) and irritate nasal membranes.

Skin & sunlight:
No problems expected.

Driving, piloting or hazardous work:
No problems expected.

Discontinuing:
May be unnecessary to finish medicine. Follow doctor's instructions.

Others:
Don't use for more than 3 days in a row.

POSSIBLE INTERACTION WITH OTHER DRUGS

GENERIC NAME OR DRUG CLASS	COMBINED EFFECT
Antidepressants, tricyclic*	Possible rise in blood pressure.
Butorphanol	Delays start of butorphanol effect.
Maprotiline	Possible increased blood pressure.

POSSIBLE INTERACTION WITH OTHER SUBSTANCES

INTERACTS WITH	COMBINED EFFECT
Alcohol:	None expected.
Beverages: Caffeine drinks.	Nervousness or insomnia.
Cocaine:	High risk of heartbeat irregularities and high blood pressure.
Foods:	None expected.
Marijuana:	Overstimulation. Avoid.
Tobacco:	None expected.

PACLITAXEL

BRAND NAMES

Abraxane   Taxol

BASIC INFORMATION

Habit forming? No
Prescription needed? Yes
Available as generic? No
Drug class: Antineoplastic

 USES

Treats ovarian cancer, breast cancer and some lung cancers.

 DOSAGE & USAGE INFORMATION

How to take:
Injection—Administered only by a doctor or under the supervision of a doctor.

When to take:
Your doctor will determine the schedule. Usually the drug is infused over a 24-hour period at 21-day intervals. Other drugs may be given prior to paclitaxel injection to help prevent adverse effects.

If you forget a dose:
Not a concern since drug is administered by a doctor.

What drug does:
Interferes with the growth of cancer cells, which are eventually destroyed.

Time lapse before drug works:
Results may not show for several weeks or months.

Don't take with:
Any other medicine or any dietary supplement without consulting your doctor or pharmacist.

 OVERDOSE

SYMPTOMS:
None expected.
WHAT TO DO:
Overdose is unlikely. You will be monitored by medical personnel during the time of the infusion.

 POSSIBLE ADVERSE REACTIONS OR SIDE EFFECTS

SYMPTOMS	WHAT TO DO
Life-threatening:	
Anaphylactic reaction soon after an injection (hives, rash, intense itching, faintness, breathing difficulty).	Emergency care will be provided.
Common:	
• Paleness, tiredness, flushing of face, skin rash or itching, shortness of breath, fever, chills, cough or hoarseness, back or side pain, difficult or painful urination, unusual bleeding or bruising, black or tarry stools, blood in stool or urine, pinpoint red spots on skin, bleeding gums, delayed wound healing.	Call doctor right away.
• Pain in joints or muscles; diarrhea; nausea and vomiting; numbness, burning or tingling in hands or feet.	Call doctor when convenient.
• Loss of hair (should regrow after treatment completed).	No action necessary.
Infrequent:	
Heart rhythm disturbances, chest pain.	Call doctor right away.
Rare:	
Pain or redness at injection site, mouth or lip sores.	Call doctor right away.

WARNINGS & PRECAUTIONS

Don't take if:
You are allergic to paclitaxel.

Before you start, consult your doctor if:
- You have an infection or any other medical problem.
- You have or recently had chickenpox or herpes zoster (shingles).
- You have heart problems.
- You are pregnant or if you plan to become pregnant.
- You have had radiation therapy or previously taken anticancer drugs.

Over age 60:
No problems expected.

Pregnancy:
Discuss with your doctor whether drug benefits justify risk to unborn child. Risk category D (see page xviii).

Breast-feeding:
Not known if drug passes into milk. Avoid drug or discontinue nursing until you finish medicine. Consult doctor for advice on maintaining milk supply.

Infants & children:
Safety and effectiveness of use in children not established.

Prolonged use:
Not recommended for long-term use.

Skin & sunlight:
No problems expected.

Driving, piloting or hazardous work:
Avoid if you feel side effects such as nausea and vomiting.

Discontinuing:
Your doctor will determine the schedule.

Others:
- Advise any doctor or dentist whom you consult that you take this medicine.
- May affect the results in some medical tests.
- Do not have any immunizations (vaccinations) without doctor's approval. Other household members should not take oral polio vaccine. It could pass the polio virus on to you. Avoid any contact with persons who have taken oral polio vaccine.
- Possible delayed effects (including some types of cancers) may occur months to years after use. Your doctor should discuss with you all risks involving this drug.
- You will have increased risk of infections. Take extra precautions (handwashing), and avoid people with infections. Avoid crowds if possible. Contact your doctor immediately if you develop signs or symptoms of infection.

- Use care in the use of toothbrushes, dental floss and toothpicks. Talk to your medical doctor before you have dental work done.
- Do not touch your eyes or the inside of your nose without carefully washing your hands first.
- Avoid activities (e.g., contact sports) that could cause bruising or injury.
- Avoid cutting yourself when using a safety razor, fingernail or toenail clippers.

POSSIBLE INTERACTION WITH OTHER DRUGS

GENERIC NAME OR DRUG CLASS	COMBINED EFFECT
Blood dyscrasia-causing medicines*	Increased risk of paclitaxel toxicity.
Bone marrow depressants,* (other)	Increased risk of paclitaxel toxicity.

POSSIBLE INTERACTION WITH OTHER SUBSTANCES

INTERACTS WITH	COMBINED EFFECT
Alcohol:	None expected.
Beverages:	None expected.
Cocaine:	None expected.
Foods:	None expected.
Marijuana:	None expected.
Tobacco:	None expected.

PANCRELIPASE

BRAND NAMES

Cotazym
Cotazym E.C.S.
Cotazym-65B
Cotazym-S
Enzymase-16
Ilozyme
Ku-Zyme HP
Lipancreatin
Pancoate

Pancrease MT4
Pancrease MT10
Pancrease MT16
Protilase
Ultrase MT 12
Ultrase MT 20
Ultrase MT 24
Viokase
Zymase

BASIC INFORMATION

Habit forming? No
Prescription needed? Yes
Available as generic? Yes
Drug class: Enzyme (pancreatic)

 USES

- Replaces pancreatic enzymes lost due to surgery or disease.
- Treats fatty stools (steatorrhea).

 DOSAGE & USAGE INFORMATION

How to take:
- Tablet, capsule or delayed-release capsule—Swallow whole. Do not take with milk or milk products.
- Powder—Sprinkle on liquid or soft food.

When to take:
Before meals.

If you forget a dose:
Take as soon as you remember up to 2 hours late. If more than 2 hours, wait for next scheduled dose (don't double this dose).

What drug does:
Enhances digestion of proteins, carbohydrates and fats.

Continued next column

 OVERDOSE

SYMPTOMS:
Shortness of breath, wheezing, diarrhea.
WHAT TO DO:
Overdose unlikely to threaten life. If person uses much larger amount than prescribed or if accidentally swallowed, call doctor or poison control center 1-800-222-1222 for help.

Time lapse before drug works:
30 minutes.

Don't take with:
Any other medicine or any dietary supplement without consulting your doctor or pharmacist.

 POSSIBLE ADVERSE REACTIONS OR SIDE EFFECTS

SYMPTOMS	WHAT TO DO
Life-threatening: None expected.	
Common: None expected.	
Infrequent: Diarrhea, asthma.	Discontinue. Call doctor right away.
Rare:	
• Rash, hives, blood in urine, swollen feet or legs, abdominal cramps.	Discontinue. Call doctor right away.
• Nausea, joint pain.	Continue. Call doctor when convenient.

PANCRELIPASE

WARNINGS & PRECAUTIONS

Don't take if:
You are allergic to pancreatin, pancrelipase, or pork.

Before you start, consult your doctor if:
You take any other medicines.

Over age 60:
Adverse reactions and side effects may be more frequent and severe than in younger persons.

Pregnancy:
Decide with your doctor if drug benefits justify risk to unborn child. Risk category C (see page xviii).

Breast-feeding:
Drug may pass into milk. Avoid drug or discontinue nursing until you finish medicine. Consult doctor for advice on maintaining milk supply.

Infants & children:
Give under close medical supervision only.

Prolonged use:
No additional problems expected.

Skin & sunlight:
No problems expected.

Driving, piloting or hazardous work:
No problems expected.

Discontinuing:
Don't discontinue without consulting doctor. Dose may require gradual reduction if you have taken drug for a long time. Doses of other drugs may also require adjustment.

Others:
* If you take powder form, avoid inhaling.
* Advise any doctor or dentist whom you consult that you take this medicine.

POSSIBLE INTERACTION WITH OTHER DRUGS

GENERIC NAME OR DRUG CLASS	COMBINED EFFECT
Calcium carbonate antacids*	Decreased effect of pancrelipase.
Iron supplements	Decreased iron absorption.
Magnesium hydroxide antacids*	Decreased effect of pancrelipase.

POSSIBLE INTERACTION WITH OTHER SUBSTANCES

INTERACTS WITH	COMBINED EFFECT
Alcohol:	Unknown.
Beverages: Milk.	Decreased effect of pancrelipase.
Cocaine:	Unknown.
Foods: Ice cream, milk products.	Decreased effect of pancrelipase.
Marijuana:	Decreased absorption of pancrelipase.
Tobacco:	Decreased absorption of pancrelipase.

PANTOTHENIC ACID (Vitamin B-5)

GENERIC AND BRAND NAMES

CALCIUM   Dexol T.D.
  PANTOTHENATE
Numerous brands of single vitamin and multivitamin combinations may be available.

BASIC INFORMATION

Habit forming? No
Prescription needed? No
Available as generic? Yes
Drug class: Vitamin supplement

 ## USES

Prevents and treats vitamin B-5 deficiency.

 ## DOSAGE & USAGE INFORMATION

How to take:
Tablet—Swallow with liquid.

When to take:
At the same times each day.

If you forget a dose:
Take as soon as you remember, then resume regular schedule.

What drug does:
Acts as co-enzyme in carbohydrate, protein and fat metabolism.

Time lapse before drug works:
15 to 20 minutes.

Don't take with:
* Levodopa—Small amounts of pantothenic acid will nullify levodopa effect. Carbidopa-levodopa combination not affected by this interaction.
* Any other medicine or any dietary supplement without consulting your doctor or pharmacist.

 ## OVERDOSE

SYMPTOMS:
None expected.
WHAT TO DO:
Overdose unlikely to threaten life. If person uses much larger amount than prescribed or if accidentally swallowed, call doctor or poison control center 1-800-222-1222 for help.

 ## POSSIBLE ADVERSE REACTIONS OR SIDE EFFECTS

SYMPTOMS	WHAT TO DO
Life-threatening: None expected.	
Common: Heartburn.	Discontinue. Call doctor when convenient.
Infrequent: Cramps.	Discontinue. Call doctor when convenient.
Rare: Rash, hives, difficult breathing.	Discontinue. Seek emergency treatment.

PANTOTHENIC ACID (Vitamin B-5)

 WARNINGS &
PRECAUTIONS

Don't take if:
You are allergic to pantothenic acid.

Before you start, consult your doctor if:
You have hemophilia.

Over age 60:
No problems expected.

Pregnancy:
Risk factor not designated. See category list on page xviii and consult doctor.

Breast-feeding:
Don't exceed recommended dose. Consult doctor.

Infants & children:
Don't exceed recommended dose.

Prolonged use:
Large doses for more than 1 month may cause toxicity.

Skin & sunlight:
No problems expected.

Driving, piloting or hazardous work:
No problems expected.

Discontinuing:
No problems expected.

Others:
Regular pantothenic acid supplements are recommended if you take chloramphenicol, cycloserine, ethionamide, hydralazine, immuno-suppressants,* isoniazid or penicillamine. These decrease pantothenic acid absorption and can cause anemia or tingling and numbness in hands and feet.

 POSSIBLE INTERACTION
WITH OTHER DRUGS

GENERIC NAME OR DRUG CLASS	COMBINED EFFECT
None significant.	

 POSSIBLE INTERACTION
WITH OTHER SUBSTANCES

INTERACTS WITH	COMBINED EFFECT
Alcohol:	None expected.
Beverages:	None expected.
Cocaine:	None expected.
Foods:	None expected.
Marijuana:	None expected.
Tobacco:	May decrease pantothenic acid absorption. Decreased pantothenic acid effect.

PAPAVERINE

BRAND NAMES

Cerespan	Pavarine
Genabid	Pavased
Pavabid	Pavatine
Pavabid Plateau Caps	Pavatym
Pavacot	Paverolan
Pavagen	

BASIC INFORMATION

Habit forming? No
Prescription needed? Yes
Available as generic? Yes
Drug class: Vasodilator

 ## USES

- May improve circulation in the extremities or brain.
- Injected into penis to produce erections.

 ## DOSAGE & USAGE INFORMATION

How to take:
- Tablet—Swallow with liquid or food to lessen stomach irritation. If you can't swallow whole, crumble tablet and take with liquid or food.
- Extended-release capsule—Swallow whole with liquid.
- Injections to penis—Follow doctor's instructions.

When to take:
At the same times each day.

If you forget a dose:
Take as soon as you remember up to 2 hours late. If more than 2 hours, wait for next scheduled dose (don't double this dose).

What drug does:
Relaxes and expands blood vessel walls, allowing better distribution of oxygen and nutrients.

Continued next column

 ## OVERDOSE

SYMPTOMS:
Weakness, fainting, flush, sweating, stupor, irregular heartbeat.
WHAT TO DO:
- **Dial 911 (emergency) for medical help or call poison control center 1-800-222-1222 for instructions.**
- **See emergency information on last 3 pages of this book.**

Time lapse before drug works:
30 to 60 minutes.

Don't take with:
Any other medicine or any dietary supplement without consulting your doctor or pharmacist.

 ## POSSIBLE ADVERSE REACTIONS OR SIDE EFFECTS

SYMPTOMS	WHAT TO DO
Life-threatening: None expected.	
Common:	
• Drowsiness, dizziness, headache, flushed face, stomach irritation, indigestion, nausea, mild constipation.	Continue. Call doctor when convenient.
• Dry mouth, throat.	Continue. Tell doctor at next visit.
Infrequent: Rash, itchy skin, blurred or double vision, weakness, fast heartbeat.	Discontinue. Call doctor right away.
Rare: Jaundice.	Discontinue. Call doctor right away.

WARNINGS & PRECAUTIONS

Don't take if:
You are allergic to papaverine.

Before you start, consult your doctor if:
- You plan to become pregnant within medication period.
- You have had a heart attack, heart disease, angina or stroke.
- You have Parkinson's disease.

Over age 60:
Adverse reactions and side effects may be more frequent and severe than in younger persons.

Pregnancy:
Decide with your doctor if drug benefits justify risk to unborn child. Risk category C (see page xviii).

Breast-feeding:
Drug may pass into milk. Avoid drug or discontinue nursing until you finish medicine. Consult doctor for advice on maintaining milk supply.

Infants & children:
Not recommended.

Prolonged use:
No problems expected.

Skin & sunlight:
No problems expected.

Driving, piloting or hazardous work:
Don't drive or pilot aircraft until you learn how medicine affects you. Don't work around dangerous machinery. Don't climb ladders or work in high places. Danger increases if you drink alcohol or take medicine affecting alertness and reflexes, such as antihistamines, tranquilizers, sedatives, pain medicine, narcotics and mind-altering drugs.

Discontinuing:
May be unnecessary to finish medicine. If drug does not help in 1 to 2 weeks, consult doctor about discontinuing.

Others:
- Periodic liver function tests recommended.
- Internal eye pressure measurements recommended if you have glaucoma.
- Advise any doctor or dentist whom you consult that you take this medicine.

POSSIBLE INTERACTION WITH OTHER DRUGS

GENERIC NAME OR DRUG CLASS	COMBINED EFFECT
Levodopa	Decreased levodopa effect.
Narcotics*	Increased sedation.
Pain relievers*	Increased sedation.
Pergolide	Decreased pergolide effect.
Sedatives*	Increased sedation.
Sympathomimetics*	Reversal of the effect of papaverine.
Tranquilizers*	Increased sedation.

POSSIBLE INTERACTION WITH OTHER SUBSTANCES

INTERACTS WITH	COMBINED EFFECT
Alcohol:	None expected.
Beverages:	None expected.
Cocaine:	Decreased papaverine effect.
Foods:	None expected.
Marijuana:	None expected.
Tobacco:	Decrease in papaverine's dilation of blood vessels.

*See Glossary

PAREGORIC

BRAND NAMES

Brown Mixture

Camphorated Opium
  Tincture

Kapectolin with
  Paregoric

Parepectolin

BASIC INFORMATION

Habit forming? Yes
Prescription needed? Yes
Available as generic? Yes
Drug class: Narcotic, antidiarrheal

 USES

Reduces intestinal cramps and diarrhea.

 DOSAGE & USAGE INFORMATION

How to take:
Drops or liquid—Dilute dose in beverage before swallowing.

When to take:
As needed for diarrhea, no more often than every 4 hours.

If you forget a dose:
Take as soon as you remember. Wait 4 hours for next dose.

What drug does:
Anesthetizes surface membranes of intestines and blocks nerve impulses.

Time lapse before drug works:
2 to 6 hours.

Don't take with:
Any other medicine or any dietary supplement without consulting your doctor or pharmacist.

 OVERDOSE

SYMPTOMS:
Deep sleep; slow breathing; slow pulse; flushed, warm skin; constricted pupils.
WHAT TO DO:
* **Dial 911 (emergency) for medical help or call poison control center 1-800-222-1222 for instructions.**
* **If person is unconscious, check breathing and pulse. If not breathing, begin mouth-to-mouth rescue breathing. If heart is not beating, begin chest compressions.**
* **See emergency information on last 3 pages of this book.**

 POSSIBLE ADVERSE REACTIONS OR SIDE EFFECTS

SYMPTOMS	WHAT TO DO
Life-threatening:	
In case of overdose, see previous column.	
Common:	
Dizziness, flushed face, unusual tiredness, difficult urination.	Continue. Call doctor when convenient.
Infrequent:	
Severe constipation, abdominal pain, vomiting.	Discontinue. Call doctor right away.
Rare:	
• Hives, rash, itchy skin, slow heartbeat, irregular breathing.	Discontinue. Call doctor right away.
• Depression.	Continue. Call doctor when convenient.

PAREGORIC

WARNINGS & PRECAUTIONS

Don't take if:
You are allergic to any narcotic.*

Before you start, consult your doctor if:
You have impaired liver or kidney function.

Over age 60:
More likely to be drowsy, dizzy, unsteady or constipated.

Pregnancy:
Risk factor varies with length of pregnancy. See category list on page xviii and consult doctor.

Breast-feeding:
Drug filters into milk. May depress infant. Avoid.

Infants & children:
Use only under medical supervision.

Prolonged use:
Causes psychological and physical dependence.

Skin & sunlight:
No problems expected.

Driving, piloting or hazardous work:
Don't drive or pilot aircraft until you learn how medicine affects you. Don't work around dangerous machinery. Don't climb ladders or work in high places. Danger increases if you drink alcohol or take medicine affecting alertness and reflexes, such as antihistamines, tranquilizers, sedatives, pain medicine, narcotics and mind-altering drugs.

Discontinuing:
May be unnecessary to finish medicine. Follow doctor's instructions.

Others:
Great potential for abuse.

POSSIBLE INTERACTION WITH OTHER DRUGS

GENERIC NAME OR DRUG CLASS	COMBINED EFFECT
Analgesics*	Increased analgesic effect.
Anticholinergics*	Increased risk of constipation.
Antidepressants*	Increased sedation.
Antidiarrheal preparations*	Increased sedative effect. Avoid.
Antihistamines*	Increased sedation.
Central nervous system (CNS) depressants*	Increased central nerve system depression.
Naloxone	Decreased paregoric effect.
Naltrexone	Decreased paregoric effect.
Narcotics,* other	Increased narcotic effect.

POSSIBLE INTERACTION WITH OTHER SUBSTANCES

INTERACTS WITH	COMBINED EFFECT
Alcohol:	Increases alcohol's intoxicating effect. Avoid.
Beverages:	None expected.
Cocaine:	None expected.
Foods:	None expected.
Marijuana:	Impairs physical and mental performance.
Tobacco:	None expected.

*See Glossary

645

PEDICULICIDES (Topical)

GENERIC AND BRAND NAMES

LINDANE
  GBH
  G-Well
  Kwellada
  Kwildane
  PMS Lindane
MALATHION
  Derbac
  Ovide
PERMETHRIN
  Acticin
  Elimite Cream
  Nix Cream Rinse

PYRETHRINS &
  PIPERONYL
  BUTOXIDE
A-200 Gel
A-200 Shampoo
Barc
Blue
Lice-Enz Foam And
  Comb Lice Killing
  Shampoo Kit
Pyrinyl
R&C
TISIT
TISIT Blue
Triple X

BASIC INFORMATION

Habit forming? No
Prescription needed? Yes
Available as generic? Yes, for some
Drug class: Pediculicide, scabicide

USES

- Treats scabies and lice infections of skin or scalp.
- Cream and lotion treats scabies.
- Shampoo treats lice infections.

OVERDOSE

SYMPTOMS:
Rarely (toxic effects from too much absorbed through skin)—Vomiting, muscle cramps, dizziness, seizure, rapid heartbeat.
WHAT TO DO:

- Not for internal use. If child accidentally swallows, call poison center 1-800-222-1222 for instructions.
- Dial 911 (emergency) for medical help or call poison control center 1-800-222-1222 for help.
- See emergency information on last 3 pages of this book.

DOSAGE & USAGE INFORMATION

How to use:
- All household members should be examined for infection and treated if infected.
- Read directions on product for proper application technique and length of time to leave on the body.
- Wear plastic gloves when you apply. Use care not to apply more than directed. Avoid contact with eyes, nose and mouth. Flush eyes with water if product gets in the eyes.
- Bathe before applying. Wash hands after applying.
- Use in well-ventilated room.

When to use:
As directed on package.

If you forget a dose:
Use as soon as you remember.

What drug does:
Absorbed into bodies of lice and scabies organisms, killing them.

Time lapse before drug works:
Cream or lotion requires 8 to 12 hours contact with skin.

Don't use with:
Other medicines for scabies or lice without consulting your doctor or pharmacist.

POSSIBLE ADVERSE REACTIONS OR SIDE EFFECTS

SYMPTOMS	WHAT TO DO
Life-threatening	
None expected.	
Common	
None expected.	
Infrequent	
None expected.	
Rare	
• Skin irritation or rash.	Discontinue. Call doctor right away.
• Skin itch that continues 1 week to several weeks after treatment.	Call doctor when convenient.

WARNINGS & PRECAUTIONS

Don't use if:
You are allergic to any pediculicide.

Before you start, consult your doctor if:
* You are allergic to anything that touches your skin.
* You are using any other medicines, creams, lotions or oils.

Over age 60:
Adverse reactions and side effects may be more frequent and severe than in younger persons. Ask doctor about smaller doses.

Pregnancy:
Risk factors vary for drugs in this group. See category list on page xviii and consult doctor.

Breast-feeding:
Effect unknown. Avoid if possible. Consult doctor.

Infants & children:
* More likely to be toxic. Use only under close medical supervision.
* Lindane is not recommended for use in infants. For other children, follow package instructions. Never use more of the product than instructed.

Prolonged use:
Not recommended. Avoid.

Skin & sunlight:
No problems expected, but check with doctor.

Driving, piloting or hazardous work:
No problems expected, but check with doctor.

Discontinuing:
No problems expected, but check with doctor.

Others:
* Don't use on open sores or wounds.
* Put on freshly dry cleaned or washed clothing after treatment.
* After treatment, boil all bed sheets, covers and towels before using.
* Store items that can't be washed or cleaned in plastic bags for 2 weeks.
* Avoid inhaling or swallowing drug.
* Thoroughly clean house.
* Wash combs and hairbrushes in hot soapy water. Don't share with others.
* Even after successful treatment, itching can continue due to remaining inflammation in the skin. This should not be confused with a reinfection. Consult doctor if you are unsure.

POSSIBLE INTERACTION WITH OTHER DRUGS

GENERIC NAME OR DRUG CLASS	COMBINED EFFECT
Antimyasthenics*	Excessive absorption and chance of toxicity (with malathion only).
Cholinesterase inhibitors*	Excessive absorption and chance of toxicity (with malathion only).

POSSIBLE INTERACTION WITH OTHER SUBSTANCES

INTERACTS WITH	COMBINED EFFECT
Alcohol:	None expected.
Beverages:	None expected.
Cocaine:	None expected.
Foods:	None expected.
Marijuana:	None expected.
Tobacco:	None expected.

PENICILLAMINE

BRAND NAMES

Cuprimine   Depen

BASIC INFORMATION

Habit forming? No
Prescription needed? Yes
Available as generic? No
Drug class: Chelating agent, antirheumatic, antidote (heavy metal)

USES

- Treatment for rheumatoid arthritis.
- Prevention of kidney stones.
- Treatment for heavy metal poisoning.

DOSAGE & USAGE INFORMATION

How to take:
Tablet or capsule—Swallow with liquid on an empty stomach 1 hour before or 2 hours after eating.

When to take:
At the same times each day.

If you forget a dose:
- 1 dose a day—Take as soon as you remember up to 12 hours late. If more than 12 hours, wait for next scheduled dose (don't double this dose).
- More than 1 dose a day—Take as soon as you remember up to 2 hours late. If more than 2 hours, wait for next scheduled dose (don't double this dose).

What drug does:
- Combines with heavy metals so kidney can excrete them.
- Combines with cysteine (amino acid found in many foods) to prevent cysteine kidney stones.
- May improve protective function of some white blood cells against rheumatoid arthritis.

Continued next column

OVERDOSE

SYMPTOMS:
Ulcers, sores, convulsions, coughing up blood, coma.
WHAT TO DO:
- **Dial 911 (emergency) for medical help or call poison control center 1-800-222-1222 for instructions.**
- **See emergency information on last 3 pages of this book.**

Time lapse before drug works:
2 to 3 months.

Don't take with:
Any other medicine or any dietary supplement without consulting your doctor or pharmacist.

POSSIBLE ADVERSE REACTIONS OR SIDE EFFECTS

SYMPTOMS	WHAT TO DO
Life-threatening: In case of overdose, see previous column.	
Common: Rash, itchy skin, swollen lymph glands, appetite loss, nausea, diarrhea, vomiting, decreased taste.	Discontinue. Call doctor right away.
Infrequent: Sore throat, fever, unusual bruising, swollen feet or legs, bloody or cloudy urine, weight gain, fatigue, weakness, joint pain.	Discontinue. Call doctor right away.
Rare: Double or blurred vision; pain; ringing in ears; ulcers, sores, white spots in mouth; difficult breathing; coughing up blood; jaundice; abdominal pain; skin blisters; peeling skin.	Discontinue. Call doctor right away.

WARNINGS & PRECAUTIONS

Don't take if:
- You are allergic to penicillamine.
- You have severe anemia.

Before you start, consult your doctor if:
- You have kidney disease.
- You are allergic to any penicillin antibiotic.

Over age 60:
More likely to damage blood cells and kidneys.

Pregnancy:
Decide with your doctor if drug benefits justify risk to unborn child. Risk category C (see page xviii).

Breast-feeding:
Safety not established. Consult doctor.

Infants & children:
Use only under medical supervision.

Prolonged use:
- May damage blood cells, kidney, liver.
- Talk to your doctor about the need for follow-up medical examinations or laboratory studies to check complete blood counts (white blood cell count, platelet count, red blood cell count, hemoglobin, hematocrit), kidney function, liver function.

Skin & sunlight:
No problems expected.

Driving, piloting or hazardous work:
No problems expected.

Discontinuing:
No problems expected.

Others:
- Request laboratory studies on blood and urine every 2 weeks. Kidney and liver function studies recommended every 6 months.
- Advise any doctor or dentist you consult that you use this medicine.

POSSIBLE INTERACTION WITH OTHER DRUGS

GENERIC NAME OR DRUG CLASS	COMBINED EFFECT
Gold compounds*	Damage to blood cells and kidney.
Immuno-suppressants*	Damage to blood cells and kidney.
Iron supplements*	Decreased effect of penicillamine. Wait 2 hours between doses.
Pyridoxine (vitamin B-6)	Increased need for pyridoxine.

POSSIBLE INTERACTION WITH OTHER SUBSTANCES

INTERACTS WITH	COMBINED EFFECT
Alcohol:	Increased side effects of penicillamine.
Beverages:	None expected.
Cocaine:	Increased side effects of penicillamine.
Foods:	Possible decreased penicillamine effect due to decreased absorption.
Marijuana:	Increased side effects of penicillamine.
Tobacco:	None expected.

PENICILLINS

GENERIC AND BRAND NAMES

See full list of generic and brand names in the *Generic and Brand Name Directory*, page 893.

BASIC INFORMATION

Habit forming? No
Prescription needed? Yes
Available as generic? Yes
Drug class: Antibacterial

 ## USES

Treatment of bacterial infections that are susceptible to penicillin, including lower respiratory tract infections, otitis media, sinusitis, skin and skin structure infections, urinary tract infections, gastrointestinal disorders, ulcers, endocarditis, pharyngitis. Different penicillins treat different kinds of infections.

 ## DOSAGE & USAGE INFORMATION

How to take:
* Tablet or capsule—Swallow with liquid on an empty stomach 1 hour before or 2 hours after eating. You may take amoxicillin, penicillin V, pivampicillin or pivmecillinam on a full stomach.
* Chewable tablet—Chew or crush before swallowing.
* Oral suspension—Measure each dose with an accurate measuring device (not a household teaspoon). Store according to instructions.
* Tablets for oral suspension—Mix one tablet in 2 teaspoonfuls of water. Drink right away.

When to take:
Follow instructions on prescription label, or take as directed by doctor. The number of doses, the time between doses and the length of treatment will depend on the problem being treated.

Continued next column

 ## OVERDOSE

SYMPTOMS:
Severe diarrhea, nausea or vomiting.
WHAT TO DO:
Overdose unlikely to threaten life. If person uses much larger amount than prescribed or if accidentally swallowed, call doctor or poison control center 1-800-222-1222 for help.

If you forget a dose:
Take as soon as you remember, then continue regular schedule. If it is almost time for the next dose, wait for that dose (don't double that dose).

What drug does:
Destroys susceptible bacteria. Does not kill viruses (e.g., colds or influenza), fungi or parasites.

Time lapse before drug works:
May be several days before medicine affects infection.

Don't take with:
Any other medicine or any dietary supplement without consulting your doctor or pharmacist.

 ## POSSIBLE ADVERSE REACTIONS OR SIDE EFFECTS

SYMPTOMS	WHAT TO DO
Life-threatening: Hives, rash, intense itching, shortness of breath, faintness soon after a dose (anaphylaxis).	Seek emergency treatment immediately.
Common: Nausea, vomiting or diarrhea (all mild); sore mouth or tongue; white patches in mouth or on tongue; vaginal itching or discharge; stomach pain.	Continue. Call doctor when convenient.
Infrequent: None expected.	
Rare: Unexplained bleeding or bruising, weakness, sore throat, fever, severe abdominal cramps, diarrhea (watery and severe), convulsions.	Discontinue. Call doctor right away.

WARNINGS & PRECAUTIONS

Don't take if:
You are allergic to penicillins* or cephalosporins.* A life-threatening reaction may occur.

Before you start, consult your doctor if:
- You are allergic to any substance or drug.
- You have mononucleosis.
- You have congestive heart failure.
- You have high blood pressure or any bleeding disorder.
- You have cystic fibrosis.
- You have kidney disease or a stomach or intestinal disorder.

Over age 60:
No special problems expected.

Pregnancy:
Consult doctor. Risk category B (see page xviii).

Breast-feeding:
Drug passes into milk. Child may become sensitive to penicillins and have allergic reactions to penicillin drugs. Discuss risks and benefits with your doctor.

Infants & children:
No special problems expected.

Prolonged use:
- You may become more susceptible to infections caused by germs not responsive to penicillins.
- Talk to your doctor about the need for follow-up medical examinations or laboratory studies.

Skin & sunlight:
No problems expected.

Driving, piloting or hazardous work:
Usually not dangerous. Most hazardous reactions likely to occur a few minutes after taking penicillin.

Discontinuing:
Don't discontinue without doctor's advice until you complete prescribed dose, even though symptoms diminish or disappear.

Others:
- Urine sugar test for diabetes may show false positive result.
- If your symptoms don't improve within a few days (or if they worsen), call your doctor.
- Don't take medicines for diarrhea without your doctor's approval.
- Birth control pills may not be effective. Use additional birth control methods.

POSSIBLE INTERACTION WITH OTHER DRUGS

GENERIC NAME OR DRUG CLASS	COMBINED EFFECT
Chloramphenicol	Decreased effect of both drugs.
Cholestyramine	May decrease penicillin effect.
Colestipol	May decrease penicillin effect.
Contraceptives, oral*	Impaired contraceptive efficiency.
Erythromycins*	Decreased effect of both drugs.
Methotrexate	Increased risk of methotrexate toxicity.
Probenecid	Increased effect of all penicillins.
Sodium benzoate & sodium phenylacetate	May reduce effect of sodium benzoate & sodium phenylacetate.
Sulfonamides*	Decreased penicillin effect.
Tetracyclines*	Decreased effect of both drugs.

POSSIBLE INTERACTION WITH OTHER SUBSTANCES

INTERACTS WITH	COMBINED EFFECT
Alcohol:	Occasional stomach irritation.
Beverages:	None expected.
Cocaine:	None expected.
Foods: Acidic fruits or juices, aged cheese, wines, syrups (if taken with penicillin G).	Decreased antibiotic effect.
Marijuana:	None expected.
Tobacco:	None expected.

---

*See Glossary

PENICILLINS & BETA-LACTAMASE INHIBITORS

GENERIC AND BRAND NAMES

AMOXICILLIN & CLAVULANATE
Augmentin
Augmentin ES-600
Augmentin SR
Clavulin

BASIC INFORMATION

Habit forming? No
Prescription needed? Yes
Available as generic? Yes
Drug class: Antibacterial

USES

Treatment of bacterial infections that are susceptible to penicillin and beta-lactamase inhibitors, including lower respiratory tract infections, otitis media, sinusitis, skin and skin structure infections, and urinary tract infections.

DOSAGE & USAGE INFORMATION

How to take:
- Tablet—Swallow with liquid on a full or empty stomach. Taking with food may lessen any stomach irritation.
- Chewable tablet—Chew or crush before swallowing.
- Oral suspension—Measure each dose with an accurate measuring device (not a household teaspoon).

When to take:
Follow instructions on prescription label, or take as directed by doctor. Normally the drug is taken every 8 hours for 7 to 10 days.

If you forget a dose:
Take as soon as you remember, then continue regular schedule. If it is almost time for the next dose, wait for that dose (don't double it).

Continued next column

OVERDOSE

SYMPTOMS:
Severe diarrhea, nausea or vomiting.
WHAT TO DO:
Overdose unlikely to threaten life. If person uses much larger amount than prescribed or if accidentally swallowed, call doctor or poison control center 1-800-222-1222 for help.

What drug does:
Destroys susceptible bacteria. Does not kill viruses, fungi or parasites. Beta-lactamase inhibitors increase penicillin's effectiveness by inactivating beta-lactamase (a substance in some bacteria which destroys the penicillin).

Time lapse before drug works:
May be several days before medicine affects infection.

Don't take with:
Any other medicine or any dietary supplement without consulting your doctor or pharmacist.

POSSIBLE ADVERSE REACTIONS OR SIDE EFFECTS

SYMPTOMS	WHAT TO DO
Life-threatening: Hives, rash, intense itching, shortness of breath, faintness soon after a dose (anaphylaxis).	Seek emergency treatment immediately.
Common: Nausea, vomiting or diarrhea (all mild); sore mouth or tongue; white patches in mouth or on tongue; vaginal itching or discharge; stomach pain.	Continue. Call doctor when convenient.
Infrequent: None expected.	
Rare: Unexplained bleeding or bruising, weakness, sore throat, fever, severe abdominal cramps, diarrhea (watery and severe), convulsions.	Discontinue. Call doctor right away.

WARNINGS & PRECAUTIONS

Don't take if:
You are allergic to penicillins or cephalosporins. Life-threatening reaction may occur.

Before you start, consult your doctor if:
* You are allergic to any substance or drug.
* You have mononucleosis.
* You have congestive heart failure.
* You have high blood pressure or any bleeding disorder.
* You have cystic fibrosis.
* You have kidney disease or a stomach or intestinal disorder.

Over age 60:
No special problems expected.

Pregnancy:
Consult doctor. Risk category B (see page xviii).

Breast-feeding:
Drug passes into milk. Child may become sensitive to penicillins and have allergic reactions to penicillin drugs. Avoid penicillin or discontinue nursing until you finish medicine. Consult doctor for advice on maintaining milk supply.

Infants & children:
No special problems expected.

Prolonged use:
* You may become more susceptible to infections caused by germs not responsive to penicillins.
* Talk to your doctor about the need for follow-up medical examinations or laboratory studies to check SGPT,* SGOT.*

Skin & sunlight:
No problems expected.

Driving, piloting or hazardous work:
Usually not dangerous. Most hazardous reactions likely to occur a few minutes after taking.

Discontinuing:
Don't discontinue without doctor's advice until you complete prescribed dose, even though symptoms diminish or disappear.

Others:
* Urine sugar test for diabetes may show false positive result.
* If your symptoms don't improve within a few days (or if they worsen), call your doctor.
* Don't take for diarrhea without your doctor's approval.
* Birth control pills may not be effective. Use additional birth control methods.

 ## POSSIBLE INTERACTION WITH OTHER DRUGS

GENERIC NAME OR DRUG CLASS	COMBINED EFFECT
Chloramphenicol	Decreased effect of both drugs.
Cholestyramine	May decrease penicillin effect.
Colestipol	May decrease penicillin effect.
Contraceptives, oral*	Impaired contraceptive efficiency.
Erythromycins*	Decreased effect of both drugs.
Methotrexate	Increased risk of methotrexate toxicity.
Probenecid	Increased effect of all penicillins.
Sodium benzoate & sodium phenylacetate	May reduce effect of sodium benzoate & sodium phenylacetate.
Tetracyclines*	Decreased effect of both drugs.

 ## POSSIBLE INTERACTION WITH OTHER SUBSTANCES

INTERACTS WITH	COMBINED EFFECT
Alcohol:	Occasional stomach irritation.
Beverages:	None expected.
Cocaine:	None expected.
Foods:	None expected.
Marijuana:	None expected.
Tobacco:	None expected.

*See Glossary

PENTAMIDINE

BRAND NAMES

NebuPent   Pneumopent
Pentacarinat

BASIC INFORMATION

Habit forming? No
Prescription needed? Yes
Available as generic? No
Drug class: Antiprotozoal

 ## USES

- Treats pneumocystis pneumonia caused by *Pneumocystis jirovecii.*
- Treats some tropical diseases such as leishmaniasis, African sleeping sickness and others.

 ## DOSAGE & USAGE INFORMATION

How to take:
Inhalation—Follow package instructions.

When to take:
According to doctor's instructions.

If you forget a dose:
Not likely to happen.

What drug does:
Interferes with RNA and DNA of infecting organisms.

Time lapse before drug works:
30 minutes to 1 hour.

Don't take with:
Any other medicines (including over-the-counter drugs such as cough and cold medicines, laxatives, antacids, diet pills, caffeine, nose drops or vitamins) without consulting your doctor or pharmacist.

 ## OVERDOSE

SYMPTOMS:
None expected.
WHAT TO DO:
Overdose unlikely to threaten life. If person uses much larger amount than prescribed or if accidentally swallowed, call doctor or poison control center 1-800-222-1222 for help.

 ## POSSIBLE ADVERSE REACTIONS OR SIDE EFFECTS

SYMPTOMS	WHAT TO DO
Life-threatening:	
Unconsciousness, rapid pulse, cold sweats.	Seek emergency treatment immediately.
Common:	
Chest pain or congestion; wheezing; coughing; difficulty in breathing; skin rash; pain, dryness or sensation of lump in throat.	Discontinue. Call doctor right away.
Infrequent:	
• Abdomen or back pain, nausea, vomiting, anxiety, cold sweats, chills, headache, appetite changes, decreased urination, unusual tiredness.	Discontinue. Call doctor right away.
• Bitter or metallic taste.	No action necessary.
Rare:	
None expected.	

WARNINGS & PRECAUTIONS

Don't take if:
You know you are allergic to pentamidine.

Before you start, consult your doctor if:
You have asthma.

Over age 60:
Adverse reactions and side effects may be more frequent and severe than in younger persons. You may need smaller doses for shorter periods of time.

Pregnancy:
Decide with your doctor if drug benefits justify risk to unborn child. Risk category C (see page xviii).

Breast-feeding:
Unknown effects. Not recommended. Consult doctor.

Infants & children:
Unknown effects. Consult doctor.

Prolonged use:
Talk to your doctor about the need for follow-up medical examinations or laboratory studies to check blood sugar; blood pressure; kidney, liver and heart function; complete blood counts (white blood cell count, platelet count, red blood cell count, hemoglobin, hematocrit); ECG* and serum calcium.

Skin & sunlight:
No problems expected.

Driving, piloting or hazardous work:
Avoid if you feel confused, drowsy or dizzy.

Discontinuing:
No special problems expected.

Others:
* Advise any doctor or dentist whom you consult that you take this medicine.
* May affect results in some medical tests.
* Avoid exposure to people who have infectious diseases.
* To help decrease bitter taste in mouth, dissolve a hard candy after taking medicine.
* Consult your doctor for additional information on the injectable form of this drug.

POSSIBLE INTERACTION WITH OTHER DRUGS

GENERIC NAME OR DRUG CLASS	COMBINED EFFECT
None reported with inhalation form of drug.	

POSSIBLE INTERACTION WITH OTHER SUBSTANCES

INTERACTS WITH	COMBINED EFFECT
Alcohol:	Increased likelihood of adverse reactions. Avoid.
Beverages:	None expected.
Cocaine:	Increased likelihood of adverse reactions. Avoid.
Foods:	None expected.
Marijuana:	Increased likelihood of adverse reactions. Avoid.
Tobacco:	Increased likelihood of adverse reactions. Avoid.

*See Glossary

PENTOXIFYLLINE

BRAND NAMES

Trental

BASIC INFORMATION

Habit forming? No
Prescription needed? Yes
Available as generic? Yes
Drug class: Hemorheologic agent

 USES

- Reduces pain in legs caused by poor blood circulation (usually due to intermittent claudication).
- May be used for other disorders as determined by your doctor.

 DOSAGE & USAGE INFORMATION

How to take:
Extended-release tablet—Swallow whole with liquid. Do not crush or crumble tablet.

When to take:
At mealtimes. Taking with food decreases the likelihood of irritating the stomach to cause nausea. May take with antacids to help prevent stomach irritation.

If you forget a dose:
Take as soon as you remember up to 3 hours late. If more than 3 hours, wait for next scheduled dose (don't double this dose).

What drug does:
- Reduces "stickiness" of red blood cells and improves flexibility of the red cells.
- Improves blood flow through blood vessels.

Time lapse before drug works:
Several weeks for full effect on circulation.

Don't take with:
Any other medicine or any dietary supplement without consulting your doctor or pharmacist.

 OVERDOSE

SYMPTOMS:
Drowsiness, flushed face, fainting, unusual excitement, convulsions.
WHAT TO DO:
- Dial 911 (emergency) for medical help or call poison control center 1-800-222-1222 for instructions.
- See emergency information on last 3 pages of this book.

 POSSIBLE ADVERSE REACTIONS OR SIDE EFFECTS

SYMPTOMS	WHAT TO DO
Life-threatening: None expected.	
Common: None expected.	
Infrequent: Drowsiness, headache, nausea, vomiting, stomach upset.	Continue. Call doctor when convenient.
Rare: Chest pain, irregular heartbeat.	Discontinue. Call doctor right away.

WARNINGS & PRECAUTIONS

Don't take if:
You are allergic to pentoxifylline or other xanthines (caffeine, theophylline, theobromine, aminophylline, dyphylline, or oxtriphylline).

Before you start, consult your doctor if:
- You have coronary artery disease.
- You have active bleeding or any condition where there is a risk of bleeding (e.g., stroke).
- You have cerebrovascular (blood vessels in the brain) disease.
- You have liver or kidney disease.

Over age 60:
Adverse reactions and side effects may be more frequent and severe than in younger persons. Ask doctor about smaller doses.

Pregnancy:
Decide with your doctor if drug benefits justify risk to unborn child. Risk category C (see page xviii).

Breast-feeding:
Drug passes into milk. Avoid drug or discontinue nursing until you finish medicine. Consult doctor for advice on maintaining milk supply.

Infants & children:
Not recommended.

Prolonged use:
No problems expected.

Skin & sunlight:
No problems expected.

Driving, piloting or hazardous work:
Wait to see if drug causes drowsiness. If not, no problems expected.

Discontinuing:
Don't discontinue without doctor's approval.

Others:
- Don't smoke. Nicotine constricts blood vessels and worsens your condition.
- Advise any doctor or dentist you consult that you use this medicine.

POSSIBLE INTERACTION WITH OTHER DRUGS

GENERIC NAME OR DRUG CLASS	COMBINED EFFECT
Anticoagulants,* oral	Possible decreased effect of anticoagulant.
Antihypertensives*	Possible increased effect of hypertensive drug.
Cimetidine	Increased risk of side effects.
Xanthines*	Increased nervous system stimulation.

POSSIBLE INTERACTION WITH OTHER SUBSTANCES

INTERACTS WITH	COMBINED EFFECT
Alcohol:	Unknown. Best to avoid.
Beverages: Coffee, tea or other caffeine-containing beverages.	Increased nervous system stimulation.
Cocaine:	Reduced effect of pentoxifylline. Avoid.
Foods:	None expected.
Marijuana:	Decreased effect of pentoxifylline. Avoid.
Tobacco:	Decreased effect of pentoxifylline. Avoid.

PHENAZOPYRIDINE

BRAND NAMES

Azo-Cheragan
Azo-Gantrisin
Azo-Standard
Baridium
Eridium
Geridium
Phen-Azo
Phenazodine

Pyrazodine
Pyridiate
Pyridium
Pyronium
Urodine
Urogesic
Viridium

BASIC INFORMATION

Habit forming? No
Prescription needed? Yes
Available as generic? Yes
Drug class: Analgesic (urinary)

 ## USES

Relieves pain of lower urinary tract irritation, as in cystitis, urethritis or prostatitis. Relieves symptoms only. Phenazopyridine alone does not cure infections.

 ## DOSAGE & USAGE INFORMATION

How to take:
Tablet—Swallow with liquid or food to lessen stomach irritation.

When to take:
At the same times each day.

If you forget a dose:
Take as soon as you remember up to 2 hours late. If more than 2 hours, wait for next scheduled dose (don't double this dose).

What drug does:
Anesthetizes lower urinary tract. Relieves pain, burning, pressure and urgency to urinate.

Time lapse before drug works:
1 to 2 hours.

Don't take with:
Any other medicine or any dietary supplement without consulting your doctor or pharmacist.

 ## OVERDOSE

SYMPTOMS:
Shortness of breath, weakness.
WHAT TO DO:
Overdose unlikely to threaten life. If person uses much larger amount than prescribed or if accidentally swallowed, call doctor or poison control center 1-800-222-1222 for help.

 ## POSSIBLE ADVERSE REACTIONS OR SIDE EFFECTS

SYMPTOMS	WHAT TO DO
Life-threatening: None expected.	
Common: Red-orange urine.	No action necessary.
Infrequent: Indigestion, fatigue, weakness, dizziness, abdominal pain.	Continue. Call doctor when convenient.
Rare: • Rash, jaundice, bluish skin color.	Discontinue. Call doctor right away.
• Headache.	Continue. Call doctor when convenient.

WARNINGS & PRECAUTIONS

Don't take if:
* You have hepatitis.
* You are allergic to any urinary analgesic.

Before you start, consult your doctor if:
You have kidney or liver disease.

Over age 60:
Adverse reactions and side effects may be more frequent and severe than in younger persons.

Pregnancy:
No proven harm to unborn child. Avoid if possible. Consult doctor. Risk category B (see page xviii).

Breast-feeding:
Effect unknown. Consult doctor.

Infants & children:
Not recommended.

Prolonged use:
* Orange or yellow skin.
* Anemia. Occasional blood studies recommended.

Skin & sunlight:
No problems expected.

Driving, piloting or hazardous work:
No problems expected.

Discontinuing:
May be unnecessary to finish medicine. Follow doctor's instructions.

Others:
Advise any doctor or dentist whom you consult that you take this medicine.

POSSIBLE INTERACTION WITH OTHER DRUGS

GENERIC NAME OR DRUG CLASS	COMBINED EFFECT
None significant.	

POSSIBLE INTERACTION WITH OTHER SUBSTANCES

INTERACTS WITH	COMBINED EFFECT
Alcohol:	None expected.
Beverages:	None expected.
Cocaine:	None expected.
Foods:	None expected.
Marijuana:	None expected.
Tobacco:	None expected.

PHENOTHIAZINES

GENERIC AND BRAND NAMES

See full list of generic and brand names in the *Generic and Brand Name Directory*, page 894.

BASIC INFORMATION

Habit forming? No
Prescription needed? Yes
Available as generic? Yes, for some.
Drug class: Antipsychotic, antiemetic (phenothiazine)

 USES

- Treatment for mental and emotional disorders.
- Treats nausea, vomiting, hiccups.
- May be used for other conditions as determined by your doctor.

 DOSAGE & USAGE INFORMATION

How to take:
- Tablet, sustained release capsule, extended-release capsule—Swallow with liquid or food to lessen stomach irritation.
- Suppository—Remove wrapper and moisten suppository with water. Gently insert into rectum, pointed end first.
- Drops or liquid—Dilute dose in beverage.

When to take:
Times will vary. Take at the same times each day as directed by your doctor.

If you forget a dose:
Take as soon as you remember. If it is almost time for your next dose, skip the missed dose and return to your regular dosing schedule (don't double this dose).

What drug does:
- Suppresses brain centers that control abnormal emotions and behavior.
- Suppresses brain's vomiting center.

Continued next column

 OVERDOSE

SYMPTOMS:
Stupor, convulsions, coma.
WHAT TO DO:
- **Dial 911 (emergency) for medical help or call poison control center 1-800-222-1222 for instructions.**
- **See emergency information on last 3 pages of this book.**

Time lapse before drug works:
Some benefit seen within a week; takes 4 to 6 weeks for full effect.

Don't take with:
- Antacid or medicine for diarrhea at same time.
- Any other medicine or any dietary supplement without consulting your doctor or pharmacist.

 POSSIBLE ADVERSE REACTIONS OR SIDE EFFECTS

SYMPTOMS	WHAT TO DO
Life-threatening: High fever, rapid pulse, profuse sweating, muscle rigidity, confusion and irritability, seizures.	Discontinue. Seek emergency treatment.
Common: Dry mouth, blurred vision, constipation, difficulty urinating; sedation, dizziness, low blood pressure.	Continue. Call doctor when convenient.
Infrequent: Continuous jerky or involuntary movements, especially of the face, lips, jaw, tongue; slow-frequency tremor of head or limbs, especially while moving; muscle rigidity, lack of facial expression and slow, inflexible movements. Pacing or restlessness; intermittent spasms of muscles of face, eyes, tongue, jaw, neck, body or limbs; jaundice (yellow skin or eyes).	Discontinue. Call doctor right away.
Rare: Other symptoms not listed above.	Continue. Call doctor when convenient.

 WARNINGS & PRECAUTIONS

Don't take if:
- You are allergic to any phenothiazine.
- You have a blood or bone marrow disease.

Before you start, consult your doctor if:
- You will have surgery within 2 months, including dental surgery, requiring general or spinal anesthesia.
- You have asthma, emphysema or other lung disorder; glaucoma; or prostate trouble.
- You take nonprescription ulcer medicine, asthma medicine or amphetamines.

Over age 60:
- Adverse reactions and side effects may be more frequent and severe than in younger persons. More likely to develop involuntary movement of jaws, lips, tongue; chewing. Report this to your doctor immediately. Early treatment can help.
- Use of antipsychotic drugs in elderly patients with dementia-related psychosis may increase risk of death. Consult doctor.

Pregnancy:
Risk factors vary for drugs in this group. See category list on page xviii and consult doctor.

Breast-feeding:
Drug passes into milk. Avoid drug or discontinue nursing until you finish medicine. Consult doctor for advice on maintaining milk supply.

Infants & children:
- Don't give to children younger than 2.
- Children more likely than adults to develop adverse reactions from these drugs.

Prolonged use:
May lead to tardive dyskinesia (involuntary movement of jaws, lips, tongue; chewing).

Skin & sunlight:
- One or more drugs in this group may cause rash or intensify sunburn in areas exposed to sun or ultraviolet light (photosensitivity reaction). Use sunscreen and avoid overexposure. Notify doctor if reaction occurs. Sensitivity may remain for 3 months after discontinuing drug.
- Avoid getting overheated or chilled. These drugs affect body temperature and sweating.

Driving, piloting or hazardous work:
Don't drive or pilot aircraft until you learn how medicine affects you. Don't work around dangerous machinery. Don't climb ladders or work in high places. Danger increases if you drink alcohol or take medicine affecting alertness and reflexes.

Discontinuing:
- Nervous and mental disorders—Don't discontinue without doctor's advice until you complete prescribed dose, even though symptoms diminish or disappear.
- Other disorders—Follow doctor's instructions about discontinuing.
- Adverse reactions may occur after drug is discontinued. Consult doctor if new symptoms develop, such as dizziness, nausea, stomach pain, trembling or tardive dyskinesia.*

Others:
- To relieve mouth dryness, chew or suck sugarless gum, candy, or ice.
- Avoid getting the liquid form of the drug on the skin. It may cause a skin rash or irritation.
- Advise any doctor or dentist whom you consult that you take this medicine.

 ## POSSIBLE INTERACTION WITH OTHER DRUGS

GENERIC NAME OR DRUG CLASS	COMBINED EFFECT
Anticholinergics*	Increased phenothiazine effect.
Anticonvulsants*	Increased risk of seizures. May need to increase dosage of anticonvulsant.
Antidepressants, tricyclic*	Increased antidepressant effect.
Antihistamines*	Increased antihistamine effect.
Antihypertensives*	Severe low blood pressure.
Appetite suppressants*	Decreased appetite suppressant effect.
Bupropion	Increased risk of seizures.
Clozapine	Toxic effect on the central nervous system.
Dofetilide	Increased risk of heart problems.

Continued on page 927

 ## POSSIBLE INTERACTION WITH OTHER SUBSTANCES

INTERACTS WITH	COMBINED EFFECT
Alcohol:	Dangerous oversedation. Avoid.
Beverages:	None expected.
Cocaine:	Decreased phenothiazine effect. Avoid.
Foods:	None expected.
Marijuana:	Drowsiness. May increase antinausea effect.
Tobacco:	None expected.

*See Glossary

PHENYLEPHRINE

BRAND NAMES

See full list of brand names in the *Generic and Brand Name Directory*, page 894.

BASIC INFORMATION

Habit forming? No
Prescription needed? No
Available as generic? Yes
Drug class: Sympathomimetic, decongestant

 ## USES

- Temporary relief of congestion of nose and sinuses caused by allergies, colds, hay fever or sinus infection.
- Treats congestion of eustachian tubes caused by middle ear infections.

 ## DOSAGE & USAGE INFORMATION

How to take:

- Nasal drops or spray—Wash hands before use. Blow nose gently, and then use the drops or spray according to instructions on the label.
- Combination drug products—Use according to label directions. Phenylephrine is the decongestant ingredient in many combination cough, cold and hay fever remedies.

When to take:
As needed, no more often than every 4 hours.

If you forget a dose:
Take when you remember. Wait 4 hours or as directed on label for next dose. Never double a dose.

What drug does:
Narrows the blood vessels in the nasal passages or ears which helps relieve the stuffy feeling caused by congestion.

Time lapse before drug works:
5 to 30 minutes.

Continued next column

 ## OVERDOSE

SYMPTOMS:
Sweating, dizziness, extreme tiredness, slow heartbeat, coma.
WHAT TO DO:
- **Dial 911 (emergency) for medical help or call poison control center 1-800-222-1222 for instructions.**
- **See emergency information on last 3 pages of this book.**

Don't take with:
Nonprescription drugs for asthma, cough, cold, allergy, appetite suppressants, sleeping pills or drugs containing caffeine without consulting your doctor or pharmacist.

 ## POSSIBLE ADVERSE REACTIONS OR SIDE EFFECTS

SYMPTOMS	WHAT TO DO
Life-threatening:	
Rare allergic reaction (hives, itching, rash, trouble breathing, tightness in chest, swelling of lips or tongue or face).	Seek emergency treatment immediately.
Common:	
Dizziness, insomnia, nervousness, lightheadedness.	Discontinue. Call doctor if symptoms persist.
Infrequent:	
Nasal product may cause burning, dryness, stinging inside nose.	Discontinue. Call doctor if symptoms persist.
Rare:	
• Unusual behavior, fast or pounding heartbeat, seizure, severe shaking.	Discontinue. Call doctor right away.
• Headache, nausea, vomiting, anxiety, mild shaking, sweating.	Discontinue. Call doctor if symptoms persist.

WARNINGS & PRECAUTIONS

Don't take if:
You are allergic to phenylephrine or any sympathomimetic.*

Before you start, consult your doctor if:
- You have high blood pressure.
- You have heart disease.
- You have diabetes.
- You have overactive thyroid.
- You have prostate problems.
- You have urination problems.
- You have glaucoma.
- You have taken MAO inhibitors in past 2 weeks.

Over age 60:
Adverse reactions and side effects may be more frequent and severe than in younger persons.

Pregnancy:
Decide with your doctor if drug benefits justify risk to unborn child. Risk category C (see page xviii).

Breast-feeding:
It is unknown if drug passes into milk. Avoid drug or discontinue nursing until you finish medicine. Consult doctor for advice on maintaining milk supply.

Infants & children:
Read the label on the product to see if it is approved for your child's age. Always follow the directions on product's label about how to use. If unsure, ask your doctor or pharmacist.

Prolonged use:
Do not use product for longer than advised on label or by doctor. Nasal spray may cause rebound congestion* if used longer than recommended on label.

Skin & sunlight:
No problems expected.

Driving, piloting or hazardous work:
Drug may cause dizziness or lightheadedness. Don't drive or pilot aircraft until you learn how medicine affects you. Don't work around dangerous machinery. Don't climb ladders or work in high places.

Discontinuing:
May be unnecessary to finish medicine. Follow label or doctor's instructions.

Others:
- Call the doctor if symptoms worsen or new symptoms develop with use of this medicine.
- Heed all warnings on the product label.
- Advise any doctor or dentist whom you consult that you take this medicine.

POSSIBLE INTERACTION WITH OTHER DRUGS

GENERIC NAME OR DRUG CLASS	COMBINED EFFECT
Antidepressants, tricyclic*	Increased phenylephrine effect.
Antihypertensives*	Increased risk of high blood pressure.
Monoamine oxidase (MAO) inhibitors*	Serious interaction (possibly fatal). Don't use within 14 days.

POSSIBLE INTERACTION WITH OTHER SUBSTANCES

INTERACTS WITH	COMBINED EFFECT
Alcohol:	Increased dizziness. Avoid.
Beverages:	None expected.
Cocaine:	Unknown effect. Avoid.
Foods:	None expected.
Marijuana:	Unknown effect. Avoid.
Tobacco:	None expected.

*See Glossary

PHENYLEPHRINE (Ophthalmic)

BRAND NAMES

Ak-Dilate	Neofrin
Ak-Nefrin	Ocugestrin
Dilatair	Ocu-Phrin
Dionephrine	Phenoptic
I-Phrine	Prefrin Liquifilm
Isopto Frin	Relief Eye Drops
Minims	for Red Eyes
Phenylephrine	Spersaphrine
Mydfrin	

BASIC INFORMATION

Habit forming? No
Prescription needed? Yes, some strengths
Available as generic? No
Drug class: Mydriatic, decongestant
(ophthalmic)

USES

- High-concentration drops—Dilates pupils.
- Low-concentration drops (available without prescription)—Relieves minor eye irritations caused by colds, hay fever, dust, wind, swimming, sun, smog, hard contact lenses, eye strain, smoke.

DOSAGE & USAGE INFORMATION

How to use:
Eye drops
- Wash hands.
- Apply pressure to inside corner of eye with middle finger.
- Continue pressure for 1 minute after placing medicine in eye.
- Tilt head backward. Pull lower lid away from eye with index finger of the same hand.
- Drop eye drops into pouch and close eye. Don't blink.
- Keep eyes closed for 1 to 2 minutes.
- Don't touch applicator tip to any surface (including the eye). If you accidentally touch tip, clean with warm water and soap.

Continued next column

OVERDOSE

SYMPTOMS:
None expected unless too much is absorbed or drops are accidentally swallowed.
WHAT TO DO:
Call poison control center 1-800-222-1222 or doctor for instructions.

- Keep container tightly closed.
- Keep cool, but don't freeze.
- Wash hands immediately after using.

When to use:
As directed on label.

If you forget a dose:
Use as soon as you remember.

What drug does:
Acts on small blood vessels to make them constrict.

Time lapse before drug works:
15 to 90 minutes.

Don't use with:
- Other eye drops or ointment without consulting your eye doctor.
- Antidepressants,* guanadrel, guanethidine, maprotiline, pargyline, any monoamine oxidase (MAO) inhibitor.*

POSSIBLE ADVERSE REACTIONS OR SIDE EFFECTS

SYMPTOMS	WHAT TO DO
Life-threatening: None expected, unless you use much more than directed.	Discontinue. Call doctor right away.
Common: None expected.	
Infrequent: Burning or stinging eyes, headache, eyes more sensitive to light, watery eyes, eye irritation not present before.	Continue. Call doctor when convenient.
Rare: None expected, unless too much gets absorbed. If so, symptoms will be paleness, dizziness, tremor, increased sweating, irregular or fast heartbeat.	Discontinue. Call doctor right away.

PHENYLEPHRINE (Ophthalmic)

WARNINGS & PRECAUTIONS

Don't use if:
- You are allergic to phenylephrine.
- You have glaucoma.

Before you start, consult your doctor if:
- You have heart disease with irregular heart-beat, high blood pressure, diabetes.
- You take antidepressants,* guanadrel, guanethidine, maprotiline, pargyline, any monoamine oxidase (MAO) inhibitor.*

Over age 60:
Adverse reactions and side effects may be more frequent and severe than in younger persons. Ask doctor about smaller doses.

Pregnancy:
Decide with your doctor if drug benefits justify risk to unborn child. Risk category C (see page xviii).

Breast-feeding:
Safety not established. Consult doctor.

Infants & children:
Use only under close medical supervision.

Prolonged use:
Avoid if possible.

Skin & sunlight:
No special problems expected.

Driving, piloting or hazardous work:
No problems expected.

Discontinuing:
No problems expected.

Others:
Consult doctor if condition doesn't improve in 3 to 4 days.

POSSIBLE INTERACTION WITH OTHER DRUGS

GENERIC NAME OR DRUG CLASS	COMBINED EFFECT
Clinically significant interactions with oral or injected medicines unlikely.	

POSSIBLE INTERACTION WITH OTHER SUBSTANCES

INTERACTS WITH	COMBINED EFFECT
Alcohol:	None expected.
Beverages:	None expected.
Cocaine:	None expected.
Foods:	None expected.
Marijuana:	None expected.
Tobacco:	None expected.

PILOCARPINE (Oral)

BRAND NAMES

Salagen

BASIC INFORMATION

Habit forming? No
Prescription needed? Yes
Available as generic? Yes
Drug class: Cholinergic

 USES

Treatment for dry mouth caused by radiation treatment of patients with cancer (of the head or neck) or patients with Sjogren's syndrome.

 DOSAGE & USAGE INFORMATION

How to take:
Tablet—Follow doctor's directions. May require dosing several times a day.

When to take:
At the same times each day.

If you forget a dose:
Take as soon as you remember. If it is almost time for your next dose, skip the missed dose and return to your regular dosing schedule (don't double this dose).

What drug does:
Stimulates the salivary glands to increase their secretions.

Time lapse before drug works:
20-60 minutes.

Don't take with:
Any other medicine or any dietary supplement without consulting your doctor or pharmacist.

 OVERDOSE

SYMPTOMS:
Stomach cramps or pain, diarrhea, severe nausea or vomiting, rapid heartbeat, chest pain, confusion, fainting, bad headache, severe shortness of breath, unusual trembling or shaking, visual problems.
WHAT TO DO:
* **If person takes much larger amount than prescribed, dial 911 (emergency) for medical help or call poison control center 1-800-222-1222 for instructions.**
* **If symptoms are severe or critical, dial 911 (emergency) for medical help or call poison control center 1-800-222-1222 for help.**

 POSSIBLE ADVERSE REACTIONS OR SIDE EFFECTS

SYMPTOMS	WHAT TO DO
Life-threatening:	
In case of overdose, see previous column.	
Common:	
Runny nose, cough, fever, chills, diarrhea, indigestion, nausea, tiredness or weakness, warm feeling, sweating, skin flushing or red, urinary frequency, joint pain or muscle aches.	Continue. Call doctor when convenient.
Infrequent:	
• Swelling (ankles, feet, face or fingers), rapid heartbeat, visual problems, bloody nose, vomiting.	Discontinue. Call doctor right away.
• Trembling or shaking, trouble with swallowing, voice change, headache.	Continue. Call doctor when convenient.
Rare:	
None expected.	

WARNINGS & PRECAUTIONS

Don't take if:
You are allergic to pilocarpine (ophthalmic or oral) or have uncontrolled asthma.

Before you start, consult your doctor if:
- You have gallbladder problems.
- You have iritis or glaucoma.
- You have had heart or blood vessel disease.
- You have asthma.
- You have any cognitive or psychiatric problem.
- You have or have had kidney disease.
- You have been told you have a tendency for retinal detachment or have retinal disease.
- You have peptic ulcer disease.

Over age 60:
No problems expected.

Pregnancy:
Decide with your doctor if drug benefits justify risk to unborn child. Risk category C (see page xviii).

Breast-feeding:
It is unknown if pilocarpine passes into breast milk. Avoid drug or discontinue nursing until you finish medicine. Consult doctor for advice on maintaining milk supply.

Infants & children:
Safety and efficacy has not been established in children.

Prolonged use:
If no improvement is seen after twelve weeks of using this medicine, consult doctor.

Skin & sunlight:
No problems expected.

Driving, piloting or hazardous work:
May cause visual disturbances, especially at night. Don't drive or pilot aircraft until you learn how medicine affects you. Don't work around dangerous machinery. Don't climb ladders or work in high places. Danger increases if you drink alcohol or take medicine affecting alertness and reflexes.

Discontinuing:
Consult doctor before discontinuing.

Others:
- Advise any doctor or dentist whom you consult that you take this medicine.
- Since this drug causes sweating, be sure to drink plenty of fluids.

POSSIBLE INTERACTION WITH OTHER DRUGS

GENERIC NAME OR DRUG CLASS	COMBINED EFFECT
Anticholinergics*	Decreased effect of both drugs.
Antiglaucoma agents*	Increased antiglaucoma effect.
Antiglaucoma, beta blockers	Increased risk of side effects.
Beta adrenergic blocking agents	Increased risk of side effects.
Bethanechol	Increased risk of side effects.
Cholinergics,* other	Increased effect of both drugs.

POSSIBLE INTERACTION WITH OTHER SUBSTANCES

INTERACTS WITH	COMBINED EFFECT
Alcohol:	None expected.
Beverages:	None expected.
Cocaine:	None expected. Best to avoid.
Foods:	None expected.
Marijuana:	None expected. Best to avoid.
Tobacco:	None expected.

PLATELET INHIBITORS

GENERIC AND BRAND NAMES

CLOPIDOGREL
Plavix

TICLOPIDINE
Ticlid

BASIC INFORMATION

Habit forming? No
Prescription needed? Yes
Available as generic? Yes, for some
Drug class: Antithrombotic; platelet
   aggregation inhibitor

USES

* To reduce the risk of heart attack or stroke. It
is used for patients who have had a heart
attack or stroke or patients who have a blood
circulation problem.
* Used for patients who have had a coronary
stent implanted.

DOSAGE & USAGE INFORMATION

How to take:
Tablet—Swallow with liquid. If you can't
swallow tablet whole, ask your pharmacist for
advice. Take ticlopidine with food. Clopidogrel
may be taken with or without food.

When to take:
Usually twice a day for ticlopidine and once a
day for clopidogrel (or as directed).

If you forget a dose:
Take as soon as you remember up to 2 hours
late. If more than 2 hours, wait for next
scheduled dose (don't double this dose).

What drug does:
Prevents certain blood cells from clumping
together which reduces the risk of blood clots.

Time lapse before drug works:
1-2 hours. It will take several days for full benefit.

Don't take with:
Any other medicine or any dietary supplement
without consulting your doctor or pharmacist.

OVERDOSE

SYMPTOMS:
Bloody vomit or excessive bleeding from
gums, nose or rectum, difficult breathing.
WHAT TO DO:
Dial 911 (emergency) for medical help or call
poison control center 1-800-222-1222 for
instructions.

POSSIBLE ADVERSE REACTIONS OR SIDE EFFECTS

SYMPTOMS	WHAT TO DO
Life-threatening:	
Severe bleeding.	Seek emergency treatment.
Common:	
• Chest pain, general body pain, red or purple spots on skin.	Continue, but call doctor right away.
• Diarrhea, stomach ache, back pain dizziness, heartburn, muscle aches, symptoms of a cold.	Continue. Call doctor when convenient.
Infrequent:	
• Unusual bleeding or bruising, irregular, heart beat, shortness of breath, swelling of feet or legs, vomiting blood or vomit looks like coffee grounds, fainting, heavy or unexpected menstrual bleeding.	Discontinue, but call doctor right away.
• Headache, joint pain, mild weakness.	Continue. Call doctor when convenient.
Rare:	
• Sudden severe headache or weakness, severe stomach. pain, thrombotic thrombocytopenic purpura (mental changes, dark or bloody urine, difficult speaking, pale skin, seizures, yellow eyes or skin, fever, weakness).	Discontinue. Seek emergency. treatment.
• Signs of infection (fever, chills, sore throat, sores in mouth), blistering or flaking or peeling skin, black or tarry stools, nosebleed, blood in urine, painful or frequent urination, problem with coordination.	Continue, but call doctor right away.
• Loss of appetite, gaseousness, nausea, tiredness, feeling anxious or depressed, trouble sleeping, constipation, numbness or tingling.	Continue. Call doctor when convenient.

WARNINGS & PRECAUTIONS

Don't take if:
* You are allergic to clopidogrel or ticlopidine.
* You have reduced white blood cells (neutropenia).

Before you start, consult your doctor if:
* You have liver disease, kidney disease, peptic ulcers or diverticulitis.
* You have had thrombotic thrombocytopenic purpura.
* You have any blood disease or bleeding disorder or any risk of bleeding due to injury or surgery (including dental surgery).

Over age 60:
No special problems expected.

Pregnancy:
Use during pregnancy only if clearly needed. Consult doctor. Risk category B (see page xviii).

Breast-feeding:
It is not known if drug passes into milk. Avoid drug or discontinue nursing until you finish medicine. Consult doctor for advice on maintaining milk supply.

Infants & children:
Not recommended. Safety has not been established.

Prolonged use:
Regular follow up visits to your doctor are important to monitor the effects of the drug.

Skin & sunlight:
No special problems expected.

Driving, piloting or hazardous work:
Don't drive or pilot aircraft until you learn how the medicine affects you. Don't work around dangerous machinery. Don't climb ladders or work in high places.

Discontinuing:
Don't discontinue without medical advice. It could increase your risk for heart attack or stroke.

Others:
* Advise any doctor or dentist whom you consult that you take this medicine. You may be advised to discontinue the drug 1-2 weeks before elective surgery (including dental surgery).
* Wear a medical identification necklace or tag that indicates you are taking this drug.
* May affect results of some medical tests.
* Report any unusual bleeding to your doctor.

POSSIBLE INTERACTION WITH OTHER DRUGS

GENERIC NAME OR DRUG CLASS	COMBINED EFFECT
Antacids*	Decreased ticlopidine effect.
Anticoagulants	Safety not established. Ask doctor.
Aspirin	Increased risk of bleeding.
Anti-inflammatory drugs, nonsteroidal (NSAIDs)*	Increased risk of bleeding.
Enzyme inhibitors*	Increased effect of enzyme inhibitor.
Phenytoin	Increased phenytoin effect.
Proton pump inhibitors	Decreased effect of clopidogrel with some proton pump inhibitors. Consult doctor.
Xanthines*	Increased xanthine effect.

POSSIBLE INTERACTION WITH OTHER SUBSTANCES

INTERACTS WITH	COMBINED EFFECT
Alcohol:	Increased alcohol in blood. Avoid.
Beverages:	None expected.
Cocaine:	Unknown. Avoid.
Foods:	None expected.
Marijuana:	Unknown. Avoid.
Tobacco:	None expected.

*See Glossary

POTASSIUM SUPPLEMENTS

GENERIC AND BRAND NAMES

See full list of generic and brand names in the *Generic and Brand Name Directory*, page 895.

BASIC INFORMATION

Habit forming? No
Prescription needed? Yes
Available as generic? Yes
Drug class: Mineral supplement (potassium), electrolyte replenisher, antihyperthyroid.

 USES

- Treatment for potassium deficiency due to diuretics, cortisone or digitalis medicines.
- Treatment for hypercalcemia due to cancer.
- Treats overactive thyroid disease.
- Treats iodine deficiency.
- Treatment for low potassium associated with some illnesses.

 DOSAGE & USAGE INFORMATION

How to take:
- Tablet or capsule—Take as directed on label.
- Effervescent tablets, granules, powder or liquid—Dilute dose in water.

When to take:
At the same time each day, preferably with food or immediately after meals.

If you forget a dose:
Take as soon as you remember. Don't double next dose.

What drug does:
Preserves or restores normal function of nerve cells, thyroid, heart and skeletal muscle cells and kidneys, as well as stomach juice secretions.

Time lapse before drug works:
30 minutes to 2 hours. Full benefit may require 12 to 24 hours.

Continued next column

 OVERDOSE

SYMPTOMS:
Paralysis of arms and legs, irregular heartbeat, blood pressure drop, convulsions, coma, cardiac arrest.
WHAT TO DO:
- **Dial 911 (emergency) for medical help or call poison control center 1-800-222-1222 for instructions.**
- **See emergency information on last 3 pages of this book.**

Don't take with:
Any other medicine or any dietary supplement without consulting your doctor or pharmacist.

 POSSIBLE ADVERSE REACTIONS OR SIDE EFFECTS

SYMPTOMS	WHAT TO DO
Life-threatening:	
In case of overdose, see previous column.	
Common:	
• Skin rash, swollen salivary glands.	Discontinue. Call doctor right away.
• Diarrhea, nausea abdominal pain.	Continue. Call doctor when convenient.
Infrequent:	
Bone and joint pain, numbness or tingling in hands or feet, vomiting, dizziness.	Discontinue. Call doctor right away.
Rare:	
Confusion; irregular heartbeat; difficult breathing; unusual fatigue; weakness; heaviness of legs; hemorrhage, perforation with enteric-coated tablets (rarely with wax matrix tablets); esophageal ulceration with tablets; bloody stools.	Discontinue. Call doctor right away.

 WARNINGS & PRECAUTIONS

Don't take if:
- You are allergic to any potassium supplement.
- You have acute or chronic kidney disease.

Before you start, consult your doctor if:
- You have Addison's disease or familial periodic paralysis.
- You have heart disease.
- You have intestinal blockage.
- You have a stomach ulcer.
- You use diuretics.
- You have high blood pressure.
- You have kidney disease.
- You have pancreatitis.
- You use heart medicine.
- You use laxatives or have chronic diarrhea.
- You use salt substitutes or low-salt milk.

Over age 60:
Observe dose schedule strictly. Potassium balance is critical. Deviation above or below normal can have serious results.

POTASSIUM SUPPLEMENTS

Pregnancy:
Consult with your doctor before taking potassium supplements, as they may pose a significant risk to your unborn child. Risk category D (see page xviii).

Breast-feeding:
Drug passes into milk. Avoid drug or discontinue nursing until you finish medicine. Consult doctor for advice on maintaining milk supply.

Infants & children:
Use only under doctor's supervision.

Prolonged use:
* Talk to your doctor about the need for follow-up medical examinations or laboratory studies to check serum potassium levels.
* If burning mouth, headache or salivation occur, call doctor.

Skin & sunlight:
No problems expected.

Driving, piloting or hazardous work:
Don't drive or pilot aircraft until you learn how medicine affects you. Don't work around dangerous machinery. Don't climb ladders or work in high places. Danger increases if you drink alcohol or take medicine affecting alertness and reflexes.

Discontinuing:
Don't discontinue without consulting doctor. Dose may require gradual reduction if you have taken drug for a long time. Doses of other drugs may also require adjustment.

Others:
* Overdose or underdose serious. Frequent EKGs and laboratory blood studies to measure serum electrolytes and kidney function recommended.
* Prolonged diarrhea may call for increased dosage of potassium.
* Advise any doctor or dentist you consult that you take this medicine.
* Serious injury may necessitate temporary decrease in potassium.
* Some products contain tartrazine dye. Avoid, especially if you are allergic to aspirin.

 POSSIBLE INTERACTION WITH OTHER DRUGS

GENERIC NAME OR DRUG CLASS	COMBINED EFFECT
Adrenocorticoids, systemic	Decreased potassium effect.
Amiloride	Dangerous rise in blood potassium.
Angiotensin-converting enzyme (ACE) inhibitors*	Possible increased potassium effect.
Antacids*	May decrease potassium absorption.
Anticholinergics, other*	Increased possibility of intestinal ulcers, which sometimes occur with oral potassium tablets.
Anti-inflammatory drugs, nonsteroidal (NSAIDs)*	Increased risk of stomach irritation.
Antithyroid drugs*	Excessive effect of antithyroid drugs.
Beta-adrenergic blocking agents*	Increased potassium levels.
Calcium	Decreased potassium effect.
Cortisone drugs*	Increased fluid retention.
Digitalis preparations*	Possible irregular heartbeat.
Diuretics, thiazide or loop*	Decreased potassium effect.
Laxatives*	Possible decreased potassium effect.
Lithium	Increased chance of producing a thyroid goiter.
Losartan	Increased potassium levels.

Continued on page 928

 POSSIBLE INTERACTION WITH OTHER SUBSTANCES

INTERACTS WITH	COMBINED EFFECT
Alcohol:	None expected.
Beverages:	
• Salty drinks such as tomato juice, commercial thirst quenchers.	Increased fluid retention.
• Low-salt milk or salt substitutes.	Increased potassium levels.
Cocaine:	May cause irregular heartbeat.
Foods: Salty foods.	Increased fluid retention.
Marijuana:	May cause irregular heartbeat.
Tobacco:	None expected.

*See Glossary

PRAMLINTIDE

BRAND NAMES

Symlin   SymlinPen

BASIC INFORMATION

Habit forming? No
Prescription needed? Yes
Available as generic? No
Drug class: Antidiabetic; amylinomimetic

 USES

Treatment for certain patients with type 1 or type 2 diabetes who already use insulin, but still need better blood sugar control.

 DOSAGE & USAGE INFORMATION

How to take:
Self-injection—Injected under the skin (subcutaneous) of the upper leg (thigh) or stomach area (abdomen). Inject pramlintide at a site that is more than 2 inches away from your insulin injection. Read and carefully follow the instructions provided with the prescription. Your doctor will advise you of any necessary changes in your insulin dosages. Never mix insulin and pramlintide. Use different syringes. Rotate injection sites.

When to take:
Inject it just before major meals. A major meal must have at least 250 calories or 30 grams of carbohydrate. Adjust your pre-meal insulin dose and check blood sugar before and after every meal and at bedtime (or as advised by doctor).

If you forget a dose:
If you forget to inject the dose before you start eating a meal, skip that dose and then inject the next dose as scheduled. Don't double that dose.

Continued next column

 OVERDOSE

SYMPTOMS:
Severe nausea, vomiting, diarrhea, dizziness.
WHAT TO DO:
- Overdose unlikely to threaten life. If person uses much larger amount than prescribed or if accidentally swallowed, call doctor or poison control center 1-800-222-1222 for help.
- Be alert to hypoglycemia (low blood sugar) symptoms listed in next column under Infrequent. Pramlintide alone dose not cause hypoglycemia, but it is used with insulin and insulin can induce hypoglycemia.

What drug does:
- Slows down movement of food through the stomach. This affects how fast sugar enters the blood after eating. It reduces blood sugar output by the liver.
- It reduces appetite by creating a feeling of fulness resulting in potential weight loss.

Time lapse before drug works:
Within the 3 hours after a meal.

Don't take with:
Any other medicine or any dietary supplement without consulting your doctor or pharmacist.

 POSSIBLE ADVERSE REACTIONS OR SIDE EFFECTS

SYMPTOMS	WHAT TO DO
Life-threatening: Allergic reaction (difficulty breathing, closing of the throat, swelling of the lips or face or tongue, hives).	Seek emergency treatment immediately.
Common: Nausea.	Continue. Call doctor if symptom persists.
Infrequent: • Indigestion, loss of appetite, vomiting, stomach pain, tiredness, dizziness, injection site reaction (redness, bruising, pain), joint pain, cough, sore throat, headache.	Continue. Call doctor when convenient.
• Symptoms of low blood sugar— nervousness, hunger (excessive), cold sweats, rapid pulse, anxiety, cold skin, chills, confusion, loss of concentration, drowsiness, headache, nausea, weakness, shakiness, vision changes.	Seek treatment (eat some form of quick-acting sugar— glucose tablets, sugar, fruit juice, corn syrup, honey).
• Symptoms of high blood sugar— increased urination, unusual thirst, dry mouth, drowsiness, flushed or dry skin, fruit-like breath odor, appetite loss, stomach pain or vomiting, tiredness, trouble breathing, increased blood sugar level.	Check your blood sugar immediately. Call doctor right away.

Rare:

Other symptoms that cause concern.	Continue. Call doctor when convenient.

WARNINGS & PRECAUTIONS

Don't take if:
You are allergic to pramlintide.

Before you start, consult your doctor if:
- You suffer from gastroparesis (a condition in which the stomach does not empty properly).
- You have difficulty recognizing symptoms of hypoglycemia (low blood sugar).
- You have poor control of your diabetes (A1c is over 9.0%).
- You have difficulty with your insulin regimen or monitoring your blood sugar levels or have recurrent episodes of hypoglycemia.

Over age 60:
No special problems expected.

Pregnancy:
Decide with your doctor if drug benefits justify risk to unborn child. Risk category C (see page xviii).

Breast-feeding:
It is unknown if drug passes into milk. Consult doctor for advice about the risks and benefits.

Infants & children:
Safety and effectiveness in children has not been established. Consult your child's doctor.

Prolonged use:
Talk to your doctor about the need for follow-up medical examinations and/or laboratory studies to check effectiveness of the drug.

Skin & sunlight:
No problems expected.

Driving, piloting or hazardous work:
No problems expected. You do need to be cautious for symptoms of hypoglycemia (especially at the start of drug treatment).

Discontinuing:
Don't discontinue without doctor's advice.

Others:
- Notify your doctor if you have a fever, infection, diarrhea, or experience vomiting.
- Advise any doctor or dentist whom you consult that you take this medicine.
- Wear or carry medical identification that indicates you have type 1 or type 2 diabetes and the drugs you take.
- You and your family should educate yourselves about diabetes; learn to recognize the symptoms of hypoglycemia and how to treat it. Hypoglycemia may occur in the treatment of diabetes as a result of skipped meals, excessive exercise, or alcohol consumption. Carry non-dietetic candy or glucose tablets to treat episodes of low blood sugar.

- Follow your prescribed diet, drug regimen and exercise routines closely. Changing any of these things can affect blood sugar levels.

POSSIBLE INTERACTION WITH OTHER DRUGS

GENERIC NAME OR DRUG CLASS	COMBINED EFFECT
Anticholinergics*	Decreased stomach emptying.
Antidiabetics, oral*	Increased risk of hypoglycemia.
Acarbose	Decreased absorption of nutrients.
Drugs taken by mouth that need to pass quickly through the stomach (such as oral contraceptives or antibiotics)	May need to take them 1 hour before or 2 hours after injecting pramlintide.
Drugs that may increase blood sugar lowering or increase risk of hypoglycemia	Increased risk of hypoglycemia.
Insulin	Possible severe hypoglycemia can occur within 3 hours of pramlintide dose.
Miglitol	Decreased absorption of nutrients.

POSSIBLE INTERACTION WITH OTHER SUBSTANCES

INTERACTS WITH	COMBINED EFFECT
Alcohol:	May cause severe low blood sugar. Avoid.
Beverages:	None expected.
Cocaine:	Unknown effect. Avoid.
Foods:	None expected. Follow your diabetic diet instructions.
Marijuana:	Possible increase in blood sugar. Avoid.
Tobacco:	None expected. Best to avoid.

*See Glossary

PREGABALIN

BRAND NAMES

Lyrica   Lyrica C-V

BASIC INFORMATION

Habit forming? No
Prescription needed? Yes
Available as generic? No
Drug class: Antiepileptic

 ## USES

- Treatment for neuropathic (nerve) pain that is associated with disorders such as diabetic peripheral neuropathy and postherpetic neuralgia (a complication of shingles).
- Treatment for fibromyalgia (a disorder that causes pain, fatigue and sleep problems).
- Used along with other drugs to treat epilepsy.
- Treatment for other disorders as determined by your doctor.

 ## DOSAGE & USAGE INFORMATION

How to take:
Capsule—Swallow with liquid. Take with or without food.

When to take:
2-3 times a day at the same times each day. Dosage may be increased by your doctor after 3-7 days depending on your response.

If you forget a dose:
Take as soon as you remember. If it is almost time for the next dose, wait for that dose (don't double this dose) and resume regular schedule.

What drug does:
The exact mechanism is unclear. It has an affect on certain nerve transmissions in the brain and spinal cord which results in the analgesic (pain relief), anticonvulsant and anti-anxiety activity.

Time lapse before drug works:
Starts working the first day, but may take a week or more to determine full effectiveness.

Continued next column

 ## OVERDOSE

SYMPTOMS:
Unknown (may be similar to side effects).
WHAT TO DO:
Overdose unlikely to threaten life. If person uses much larger amount than prescribed or if accidentally swallowed, call doctor or poison control center 1-800-222-1222 for help.

Don't take with:
Any other medicine or any dietary supplement without consulting your doctor or pharmacist.

 ## POSSIBLE ADVERSE REACTIONS OR SIDE EFFECTS

SYMPTOMS	WHAT TO DO
Life-threatening:	
Rare allergic reaction— Breathing difficulty; closing of the throat; swelling of hands, feet, face, lips or tongue; hives.	Discontinue. Seek emergency treatment.
Common:	
Dizziness, dry mouth, sleepiness, swelling (hands, feet, ankles), blurred or double vision, weight gain, headache, problems with concentration or attention, appetite increased, vomiting, constipation, erectile dysfunction.	Continue. Call doctor when convenient.
Infrequent:	
Emotional changes, diarrhea, unsteady movements (ataxia), euphoric mood, other mood changes, fatigue, sexual function change, hallucinations, unusual dreams, flushing or burning feeling, body symptoms (aches, pain, stiffness, weakness, twitching, tightness), urination changes, dry nose, thirstiness, stomach upset or swollen, eye symptoms (pain, dry, tearing), heartbeat is faster, mild breathing difficulty, rash or hives, insomnia worsens, decreased appetite.	Continue. Call doctor when convenient.
Rare:	
Cold-like symptoms, heartbeat is slower or change in rhythm, changes in blood pressure, menstrual changes, breast pain or discharge, hands or feet feel cold, other new or unexplained symptoms.	Continue. Call doctor when convenient.

WARNINGS & PRECAUTIONS

Don't take if:
- You are allergic to pregabalin.
- You have certain rare hereditary problems (galactose intolerance, the Lapp lactase deficiency or glucose-galactose malabsorption).

Before you start, consult your doctor if:
- You have diabetes.
- You have any kidney disorder.

Over age 60:
If you experience dizziness or sleepiness, take precautions to prevent accidents such as falls.

Pregnancy:
Decide with your doctor if drug benefits justify risk to unborn child. Risk category not determined. (See page xviii).

Breast-feeding:
It is unknown if drug passes into milk. Avoid drug or discontinue nursing until you finish medicine. Consult doctor for advice on maintaining milk supply.

Infants & children:
Safety and effectiveness for children under age 18 has not been established.

Prolonged use:
Talk to your doctor about the need for follow up examinations to determine continued effectiveness of the drug in treating your disorder.

Skin & sunlight:
No special problems expected.

Driving, piloting or hazardous work:
Don't drive or pilot aircraft until you learn how medicine affects you. Don't work around dangerous machinery. Don't climb ladders or work in high places. Danger increases if you drink alcohol or take other medicines affecting alertness and reflexes.

Discontinuing:
Don't discontinue drug without doctor's advice. Dosage may need to be gradually reduced.

Others:
- Don't increase or decrease drug dosage without doctor's approval.
- Advise any doctor or dentist whom you consult that you take this medicine.
- Rarely, antiepileptic drugs may lead to suicidal thoughts and behaviors. Call doctor right away if suicidal symptoms or unusual behaviors occur.
- Wear or carry medical identification to show your seizure disorder and the drugs you take.

POSSIBLE INTERACTION WITH OTHER DRUGS

GENERIC NAME OR DRUG CLASS	COMBINED EFFECT
Central nervous system (CNS) depressants*	May add to any sedative effect.
Lorazepam	Increased effect of lorazepam.
Oxycodone	Increased risk of side effects.

POSSIBLE INTERACTION WITH OTHER SUBSTANCES

INTERACTS WITH	COMBINED EFFECT
Alcohol:	Increased risk of side effects, such as sedation. Avoid.
Beverages:	None expected.
Cocaine:	Effects unknown. Avoid.
Foods:	None expected.
Marijuana:	Effects unknown. Avoid.
Tobacco:	None expected.

---

*See Glossary

PRIMAQUINE

GENERIC NAMES

PRIMAQUINE

BASIC INFORMATION

Habit forming? No
Prescription needed? Yes
Available as generic? Yes
Drug class: Antiprotozoal (antimalarial)

 USES

- Treats some forms of malaria.
- Prevents relapses of some forms of malaria.
- Treats Pneumocystis pneumonia (used in combination with clindamycin).

 DOSAGE & USAGE INFORMATION

How to take:
Tablet—Take with meals or antacids to minimize stomach irritation.

When to take:
At the same time each day, according to instructions on prescription label.

If you forget a dose:
Take as soon as you remember up to 2 hours late. If more than 2 hours, wait for next scheduled dose. Don't double this dose.

What drug does:
Alters the properties of DNA in malaria organisms to prevent them from multiplying.

Time lapse before drug works:
2 to 3 hours.

Don't take with:
Any other medicine or any dietary supplement without consulting your doctor or pharmacist.

 OVERDOSE

SYMPTOMS:
None expected.
WHAT TO DO:
Overdose unlikely to threaten life. If person uses much larger amount than prescribed or if accidentally swallowed, call doctor or poison control center 1-800-222-1222 for help.

 POSSIBLE ADVERSE REACTIONS OR SIDE EFFECTS

SYMPTOMS	WHAT TO DO
Life-threatening: None expected.	
Common: None expected.	
Infrequent: Dark urine; back, leg or stomach pain; appetite loss; pale skin; fever.	Discontinue. Call doctor right away.
Rare: Blue fingernails, lips and skin; dizziness; difficult breathing; extraordinary tiredness; sore throat; fever.	Discontinue. Call doctor right away.

WARNINGS & PRECAUTIONS

Don't take if:
- You have G6PD* deficiency.
- You are hypersensitive to primaquine.

Before you start, consult your doctor if:
You are Black, Oriental, Asian or of Mediterranean origin.

Over age 60:
No special problems expected.

Pregnancy:
Decide with your doctor if drug benefits justify risk to unborn child. Risk category C (see page xviii).

Breast-feeding:
Effect unknown. Consult doctor.

Infants & children:
No special problems expected.

Prolonged use:
No special problems expected.

Skin & sunlight:
No special problems expected.

Driving, piloting or hazardous work:
No special problems expected.

Discontinuing:
No special problems expected.

Others:
- If you are Black, Asian, Oriental or of Mediterranean origin, insist on a test for G6PD* deficiency before taking this medicine.
- Advise any doctor or dentist whom you consult that you take this medicine.

POSSIBLE INTERACTION WITH OTHER DRUGS

GENERIC NAME OR DRUG CLASS	COMBINED EFFECT
Hemolytics,* other	Increased risk of serious side effects affecting the blood.
Quinacrine	Increased toxic effects of primaquine.

POSSIBLE INTERACTION WITH OTHER SUBSTANCES

INTERACTS WITH	COMBINED EFFECT
Alcohol:	Possible liver toxicity. Avoid.
Beverages:	None expected.
Cocaine:	None expected.
Foods:	None expected.
Marijuana:	None expected.
Tobacco:	None expected.

*See Glossary

PRIMIDONE

BRAND NAMES

Apo-Primidone
Myidone
Mysoline

PMS Primidone
Sertan

BASIC INFORMATION

Habit forming? No
Prescription needed? Yes
Available as generic? Yes
Drug class: Anticonvulsant

USES

Prevents some forms of epileptic seizures.

DOSAGE & USAGE INFORMATION

How to take:
- Tablet—Swallow with liquid. If you can't swallow whole, crumble tablet and take with liquid or food.
- Liquid—If desired, dilute dose in beverage before swallowing.

When to take:
Daily in regularly spaced doses, according to doctor's prescription.

If you forget a dose:
Take as soon as you remember up to 2 hours late. If more than 2 hours, wait for next scheduled dose (don't double this dose).

What drug does:
The exact way it works is unknown.It appears to reduce seizures by controlling certain electrical impulses in the brain.

Time lapse before drug works:
2 to 3 weeks for full effectiveness.

Continued next column

OVERDOSE

SYMPTOMS:
Slow, shallow breathing; weak, rapid pulse; confusion, deep sleep, coma.
WHAT TO DO:
- **Dial 911 (emergency) for medical help or call poison control center 1-800-222-1222 for instructions.**
- **If person is unconscious, check breathing and pulse. If not breathing, begin mouth-to-mouth rescue breathing. If heart is not beating, begin chest compressions.**
- **See emergency information on last 3 pages of this book.**

Don't take with:
Any other medicine or any dietary supplement without consulting your doctor or pharmacist.

POSSIBLE ADVERSE REACTIONS OR SIDE EFFECTS

SYMPTOMS	WHAT TO DO
Life-threatening:	
In case of overdose, see previous column.	
Common:	
• Difficult breathing.	Discontinue. Call doctor right away.
• Confusion, change in vision.	Continue. Call doctor when convenient.
• Clumsiness, dizziness, drowsiness.	Continue. Tell doctor at next visit.
Infrequent:	
• Unusual excitement, particularly in children; nausea; vomiting.	Discontinue. Call doctor right away.
• Headache, fatigue, weakness.	Continue. Call doctor when convenient.
Rare:	
• Rash or hives, appetite loss, acute psychosis, hair loss, fever, joint pain.	Discontinue. Call doctor right away.
• Swollen eyelids or legs.	Continue. Call doctor when convenient.
• Decreased sexual ability.	Continue. Tell doctor at next visit.

WARNINGS & PRECAUTIONS

Don't take if:
- You are allergic to primidone.
- You have had porphyria.

Before you start, consult your doctor if:
- You have had liver, kidney or lung disease or asthma.
- You have lupus.

Over age 60:
Adverse reactions and side effects may be more frequent and severe than in younger persons.

Pregnancy:
Consult doctor. Risk category D (see page xviii).

Breast-feeding:
Drug filters into milk. May harm child. Avoid. Consult doctor.

Infants & children:
Use only under medical supervision.

Prolonged use:
- Enlarged lymph and thyroid glands.
- Anemia.
- Rickets in children and osteomalacia (insufficient calcium to bones) in adults.
- Talk to your doctor about the need for follow-up medical examinations or laboratory studies.

Skin & sunlight:
No special problems expected.

Driving, piloting or hazardous work:
Don't drive or pilot aircraft until you learn how medicine affects you. Don't work around dangerous machinery. Don't climb ladders or work in high places. Danger increases if you drink alcohol or take medicine affecting alertness and reflexes.

Discontinuing:
Don't discontinue abruptly or without doctor's advice until you complete prescribed dose, even though symptoms diminish or disappear.

Others:
- Tell doctor if you become ill or injured and must interrupt dose schedule.
- Periodic laboratory blood tests of drug level recommended.
- Rarely, antiepileptic drugs may lead to suicidal thoughts and behaviors. Call doctor right away if suicidal symptoms or unusual behaviors occur.
- Wear or carry medical identification to show your seizure disorder and the drugs you take.

POSSIBLE INTERACTION WITH OTHER DRUGS

GENERIC NAME OR DRUG CLASS	COMBINED EFFECT
Adrenocorticoids, systemic	Decreased adrenocorticoid effect.
Anticoagulants,* oral	Decreased primidone effect.
Anticonvulsants,* other	Changed seizure pattern.
Antidepressants*	Increased antidepressant effect.
Antihistamines*	Increased sedation effect of primidone.
Aspirin	Decreased aspirin effect.
Carbamazepine	Unpredictable increase or decrease of primidone effect.
Carbonic anhydrase inhibitors*	Possible decreased primidone effect.
Central nervous system (CNS) depressants*	Increased CNS depressant effects.
Contraceptives, oral*	Decreased contraceptive effect.
Cyclosporine	Decreased cyclosporine effect.
Digitalis preparations*	Decreased digitalis effect.
Disulfiram	Possible increased primidone effect.
Estrogens*	Decreased estrogen effect.
Griseofulvin	Possible decreased griseofulvin effect.
Isoniazid	Decreased primidone effect.
Lamotrigine	Decreased lamotrigine effect.
Leucovorin (large dose)	May counteract anticonvulsant effect of primidone.
Loxapine	Decreased anticonvulsant effect of primidone.
Metronidazole	Possible decreased metronidazole effect.
Mind-altering drugs*	Increased effect of mind-altering drug.
Monoamine oxidase (MAO) inhibitors*	Increased sedation effect of primidone.
Nabilone	Greater depression of central nervous system.

Continued on page 928

POSSIBLE INTERACTION WITH OTHER SUBSTANCES

INTERACTS WITH	COMBINED EFFECT
Alcohol:	Dangerous sedative effect. Avoid.
Beverages:	None expected.
Cocaine:	Decreased primidone effect.
Foods:	Possible need for more vitamin D.
Marijuana:	Decreased anti-convulsant effect.
Tobacco:	None expected.

*See Glossary

PROBENECID

BRAND NAMES

Benemid   Probalan
Benuryl

BASIC INFORMATION

Habit forming? No
Prescription needed? Yes
Available as generic? Yes
Drug class: Antigout

 ## USES

- Treats chronic gout.
- Increases blood levels of penicillins and cephalosporins.

 ## DOSAGE & USAGE INFORMATION

How to take:
Tablet—Swallow with liquid or food to lessen stomach irritation. If you can't swallow whole, crumble tablet and take with liquid or food.

When to take:
At the same time each day.

If you forget a dose:
Take as soon as you remember up to 12 hours late. If more than 12 hours, wait for next scheduled dose (don't double this dose).

What drug does:
- Forces kidneys to excrete uric acid.
- Reduces amount of penicillin excreted in urine.

Time lapse before drug works:
May require several months of regular use to prevent acute gout.

Don't take with:
- Nonprescription drugs containing aspirin or caffeine.
- Any other medicine or any dietary supplement without consulting your doctor or pharmacist.

 ## OVERDOSE

SYMPTOMS:
Breathing difficulty, severe nervous agitation, vomiting, seizures, convulsions, delirium, coma.
WHAT TO DO:
- **Dial 911 (emergency) for medical help or call poison control center 1-800-222-1222 for instructions.**
- **See emergency information on last 3 pages of this book.**

 ## POSSIBLE ADVERSE REACTIONS OR SIDE EFFECTS

SYMPTOMS	WHAT TO DO
Life-threatening:	
In case of overdose, see previous column.	
Common:	
Headache, appetite loss, nausea, vomiting.	Continue. Call doctor when convenient.
Infrequent:	
• Blood in urine, low back pain, worsening gout.	Discontinue. Call doctor right away.
• Dizziness, flushed face, itchy skin.	Continue. Call doctor when convenient.
• Painful or frequent urination, sore gums.	Continue. Tell doctor at next visit.
Rare:	
Sore throat, fever and chills; difficult breathing; unusual bleeding or bruising; red, painful joint; jaundice; foot, leg or face swelling.	Discontinue. Call doctor right away.

 ## WARNINGS & PRECAUTIONS

Don't take if:
- You are allergic to any uricosuric.*
- You have acute gout.
- Patient is younger than 2.

Before you start, consult your doctor if:
- You have had kidney stones or kidney disease.
- You have a peptic ulcer.
- You have bone marrow or blood cell disease.
- You are undergoing chemotherapy for cancer.

Over age 60:
Adverse reactions and side effects may be more frequent and severe than in younger persons.

Pregnancy:
Consult doctor. Risk category B (see page xviii).

Breast-feeding:
It is unknown if drug passes into milk. Avoid drug or discontinue nursing until you finish medicine. Consult doctor for advice on maintaining milk supply.

Infants & children:
Not recommended.

Prolonged use:
- Possible kidney damage.
- Talk to your doctor about the need for follow-up medical examinations or laboratory studies to check serum uric acid, urine uric acid.

Skin & sunlight:
No problems expected.

Driving, piloting or hazardous work:
Avoid if you feel dizzy. Otherwise, no problems
expected.

Discontinuing:
Don't discontinue without consulting doctor.
Dose may require gradual reduction if you have
taken drug for a long time. Doses of other drugs
may also require adjustment.

Others:
- If signs of gout attack develop while taking
  medicine, consult doctor.
- Advise any doctor or dentist whom you consult
  that you take this medicine.

POSSIBLE INTERACTION WITH OTHER DRUGS

GENERIC NAME OR DRUG CLASS	COMBINED EFFECT
Allopurinol	Increased effect of each drug.
Anticoagulants,* oral	Increased anticoagulant effect.
Anti-inflammatory drugs, nonsteroidal (NSAIDs)*	Increased toxic risk.
Aspirin	Decreased probenecid effect.
Bismuth subsalicylate	Decreased probenecid effect.
Cephalosporins*	Increased cephalosporin effect.
Ciprofloxacin	May cause kidney dysfunction.
Dapsone	Increased dapsone effect. Increased toxicity.
Diclofenac	Increased diclofenac effect.
Diuretics, thiazide*	Decreased probenecid effect.
Hypoglycemics, oral*	Increased hypoglycemic effect.
Indomethacin	Increased adverse effects of indomethacin.
Ketoprofen	Increased risk of ketoprofen toxicity.
Loracarbef	Increased loracarbef effect.

Methotrexate	Increased methotrexate toxicity.
Nitrofurantoin	Increased effect of nitrofurantoin.
Para-aminosalicylic acid	Increased effect of para-aminosalicylic acid.
Penicillins*	Enhanced penicillin effect.
Pyrazinamide	Decreased probenecid effect.
Salicylates*	Decreased probenecid effect.
Sodium benzoate & sodium phenylacetate	May reduce effect of sodium benzoate & sodium phenylacetate.
Sulfa drugs*	Slows elimination. May cause harmful accumulation of sulfa.
Thioguanine	More likelihood of toxicity of both drugs.
Valacyclovir	Increased valacyclovir effect.
Zidovudine	Increased zidovudine toxicity risk.

POSSIBLE INTERACTION WITH OTHER SUBSTANCES

INTERACTS WITH	COMBINED EFFECT
Alcohol:	Decreased probenecid effect.
Beverages: Caffeine drinks.	Loss of probenecid effectiveness.
Cocaine:	None expected.
Foods:	None expected.
Marijuana:	Daily use— Decreased probenecid effect.
Tobacco:	None expected.

PROBENECID & COLCHICINE

BRAND NAMES

Col Benemid   Proben-C
Col-Probenecid

BASIC INFORMATION

Habit forming? No
Prescription needed? Yes
Available as generic? Yes
Drug class: Antigout

 ## USES

- Increases blood levels of penicillins and cephalosporins.
- Relieves joint pain, inflammation, swelling from gout.
- Also used for familial Mediterranean fever, dermatitis herpetiformis.

 ## DOSAGE & USAGE INFORMATION

How to take:
Tablet—Swallow with liquid or food to lessen stomach irritation. If you can't swallow whole, crumble tablet and take with liquid or food.

When to take:
At the same time each day.

If you forget a dose:
Take as soon as you remember up to 12 hours late. If more than 12 hours, wait for next scheduled dose (don't double this dose).

What drug does:
- Forces kidneys to excrete uric acid.
- Reduces amount of penicillin excreted in urine.
- Decreases acidity of joint tissues and prevents deposits of uric acid crystals.

Time lapse before drug works:
12 to 48 hours.

Continued next column

 ## OVERDOSE

SYMPTOMS:
Breathing difficulty, severe nervous agitation, convulsions, bloody urine, diarrhea, vomiting, muscle weakness, fever, stupor, seizures, delirium, coma.
WHAT TO DO:
- **Dial 911 (emergency) for medical help or call poison control center 1-800-222-1222 for instructions.**
- **See emergency information on last 3 pages of this book.**

Don't take with:
- Nonprescription drugs containing aspirin or caffeine.
- Any other medicine or any dietary supplement without consulting your doctor or pharmacist.

 ## POSSIBLE ADVERSE REACTIONS OR SIDE EFFECTS

SYMPTOMS	WHAT TO DO
Life-threatening: Blood in urine; convulsions; severe muscle weakness; difficult breathing; burning feeling of stomach, throat or skin; worsening gout.	Discontinue. Seek emergency treatment.
Common: Diarrhea, headache, abdominal pain.	Discontinue. Call doctor right away.
Infrequent: • Back pain; painful, difficult urination.	Discontinue. Call doctor right away.
• Dizziness, red or flushed face, urgent urination, sore gums, hair loss.	Continue. Call doctor when convenient.
Rare: Sudden decrease in urine output; nausea; vomiting; mood change; fever; chills; jaundice; numbness or tingling in hands or feet; rash; sore throat, fever, mouth sores; swollen face, feet and ankles; unexplained bleeding or bruising; weight gain or loss; low white or red blood cells.	Discontinue. Call doctor right away.

WARNINGS & PRECAUTIONS

Don't take if:
You are allergic to any uricosuric* or colchicine.

Before you start, consult your doctor if:
- You have had kidney stones, kidney disease, heart or liver disease, peptic ulcers or ulcerative colitis.
- You have bone marrow or blood cell disease.
- You will have surgery within 2 months, including dental surgery, requiring general or spinal anesthesia.
- You are undergoing chemotherapy for cancer.

Over age 60:
Adverse reactions and side effects may be more frequent and severe than in younger persons. Colchicine has a narrow margin of safety for people in this age group.

Pregnancy:
Risk factor varies with length of pregnancy. See category list on page xviii and consult doctor.

Breast-feeding:
No problems expected, but consult doctor.

Infants & children:
Not recommended.

Prolonged use:
- Possible kidney damage.
- Permanent hair loss.
- Anemia. Request blood counts.
- Numbness or tingling in hands and feet.
- Talk to your doctor about the need for follow-up medical examinations or laboratory studies to check serum uric acid, urine uric acid.

Skin & sunlight:
No problems expected.

Driving, piloting or hazardous work:
Don't drive or pilot aircraft until you learn how medicine affects you. Don't work around dangerous machinery. Don't climb ladders or work in high places. Danger increases if you drink alcohol or take medicine affecting alertness and reflexes, such as antihistamines, tranquilizers, sedatives, pain medicine, narcotics and mind-altering drugs.

Discontinuing:
- May be unnecessary to finish medicine. Follow doctor's instructions.
- Stop taking if severe digestive upsets occur before symptoms are relieved.

Others:
- If signs of gout attack develop while taking medicine, consult doctor.
- Advise any doctor or dentist whom you consult that you take this medicine

POSSIBLE INTERACTION WITH OTHER DRUGS

GENERIC NAME OR DRUG CLASS	COMBINED EFFECT
Acetohexamide	Increased acetohexamide effect.
Allopurinol	Increased effect of each drug.

Anticoagulants,* oral	Irregular effect on anticoagulation, sometimes increased, sometimes decreased. Follow prothrombin times.
Antidepressants*	Oversedation.
Antihistamines*	Oversedation.
Antihypertensives*	Decreased anti-hypertensive effect.
Anti-inflammatory drugs, nonsteroidal (NSAIDs)*	Increased toxic risk.
Appetite suppressants*	Increased appetite suppressant effect.
Bismuth subsalicylate	Decreased probenecid effect.
Cephalosporins*	Increased cephalosporin effect.
Dapsone	Increased dapsone effect. Increased toxicity.
Diclofenac	Increased diclofenac effect.
Diuretics, thiazide*	Decreased probenecid effect.
Indomethacin	Increased adverse effects of indomethacin.
Ketoprofen	Increased effect of ketoprofen toxicity.

Continued on page 928

POSSIBLE INTERACTION WITH OTHER SUBSTANCES

INTERACTS WITH	COMBINED EFFECT
Alcohol:	Decreased probenecid effect.
Beverages: Caffeine drinks.	Loss of probenecid effectiveness.
Herbal teas.	Increased colchicine effect. Avoid.
Cocaine:	Overstimulation. Avoid.
Foods:	None expected.
Marijuana:	Decreased colchicine and probenecid effect.
Tobacco:	None expected.

*See Glossary

PROCARBAZINE

BRAND NAMES

Matulane   Natulan

BASIC INFORMATION

Habit forming? No
Prescription needed? Yes
Available as generic? No
Drug class: Antineoplastic

 USES

Treatment for some kinds of cancer.

 DOSAGE & USAGE INFORMATION

How to take:
Capsule—Swallow with liquid after light meal. Don't drink fluids with meals. Drink extra fluids between meals. Avoid sweet or fatty foods.

When to take:
At the same time each day.

If you forget a dose:
Take as soon as you remember. Don't double dose ever.

What drug does:
Inhibits abnormal cell reproduction. Procarbazine is an alkylating agent* and an MAO inhibitor.

Time lapse before drug works:
Up to 6 weeks for full effect.

Don't take with:
Any other medicine or any dietary supplement without consulting your doctor or pharmacist.

 OVERDOSE

SYMPTOMS:
Restlessness, agitation, fever, convulsions, bleeding.
WHAT TO DO:
* **Dial 911 (emergency) for medical help or call poison control center 1-800-222-1222 for instructions.**
* **If person is unconscious, check breathing and pulse. If not breathing, begin mouth-to-mouth rescue breathing. If heart is not beating, begin chest compressions.**
* **See emergency information on last 3 pages of this book.**

 POSSIBLE ADVERSE REACTIONS OR SIDE EFFECTS

SYMPTOMS	WHAT TO DO
Life-threatening: In case of overdose, see previous column.	
Common:	
• Nausea, vomiting, decreased urination, numbness or tingling in hands or feet, hair loss, rapid or pounding heartbeat, shortness of breath.	Discontinue. Call doctor right away.
• Fatigue, weakness, confusion.	Continue. Call doctor when convenient.
• Dizziness when changing position, dry mouth, inflamed tongue, constipation, difficult urination.	Continue. Tell doctor at next visit.
Infrequent:	
• Fainting.	Discontinue. Seek emergency treatment.
• Severe headache; abnormal bleeding or bruising; muscle, joint or chest pain, enlarged eye pupils; black, tarry stools; bloody urine.	Discontinue. Call doctor right away.
• Hallucinations, insomnia, nightmares, diarrhea, swollen feet or legs, nervousness, eyes sensitive to light, cough or hoarseness, mouth sores, depression.	Continue, but call doctor right away.
• Diminished sex drive.	Continue. Tell doctor at next visit.
Rare: Rash, stiff neck, jaundice, fever, sore throat, vomiting blood, wheezing.	Discontinue. Call doctor right away.

 WARNINGS & PRECAUTIONS

Don't take if:
You are allergic to any MAO inhibitor.

Before you start, consult your doctor if:
* You are an alcoholic.
* You have asthma.
* You have heart disease, congestive heart failure, heart rhythm irregularities or high blood pressure.
* You have liver or kidney disease.

684

PROCARBAZINE

- You have had a stroke.
- You have diabetes or epilepsy.
- You have overactive thyroid.
- You have schizophrenia.
- You have Parkinson's disease.
- You have adrenal gland tumor.
- You will have surgery within 2 months, including dental surgery, requiring general or spinal anesthesia.

Over age 60:
Adverse reactions and side effects may be more frequent and severe than in younger persons.

Pregnancy:
Consult doctor. Risk category D (see page xviii).

Breast-feeding:
Safety not established. Consult doctor.

Infants & children:
Not recommended.

Prolonged use:
- May be toxic to liver.
- Talk to your doctor about the need for follow-up medical examinations or laboratory studies to check complete blood counts (white blood cell count, platelet count, red blood cell count, hemoglobin, hematocrit), bone marrow, kidney function.

Skin & sunlight:
No special problems expected.

Driving, piloting or hazardous work:
Don't drive or pilot aircraft until you learn how medicine affects you. Don't work around dangerous machinery. Don't climb ladders or work in high places. Danger increases if you drink alcohol or take medicine affecting alertness and reflexes.

Discontinuing:
- Don't discontinue without doctor's advice until you complete prescribed dose, even though symptoms diminish or disappear.
- Follow precautions regarding foods, drinks and other medicines for 2 weeks after discontinuing.

Others:
- May affect blood sugar levels in patients with diabetes.
- Advise any doctor or dentist whom you consult that you take this drug.

POSSIBLE INTERACTION WITH OTHER DRUGS

GENERIC NAME OR DRUG CLASS	COMBINED EFFECT
Amphetamines*	Blood pressure rise to life-threatening level.
Anticonvulsants,* oral	Changed seizure pattern.
Antidepressants, tricyclic*	Blood pressure rise to life-threatening level.
Antidiabetics,* oral and insulin	Excessively low blood sugar.
Antihistamines*	Increased sedation.
Barbiturates*	Increased sedation.
Bone marrow depressants*	Increased toxicity to bone marrow.
Buspirone	Elevated blood pressure.
Caffeine	Irregular heartbeat or high blood pressure.
Carbamazepine	Fever, seizures. Avoid.
Central nervous system (CNS) depressants*	Increased CNS depression.
Clozapine	Toxic effect on bone marrow and central nervous system.
Cyclobenzaprine	Fever, seizures. Avoid.
Dextromethorphan	Fever, hypertension.

Continued on page 929

POSSIBLE INTERACTION WITH OTHER SUBSTANCES

INTERACTS WITH	COMBINED EFFECT
Alcohol:	Increased sedation to dangerous level. Disulfiram-like reaction.*
Beverages: Caffeine drinks.	Irregular heartbeat or high blood pressure.
Drinks containing tyramine.*	Blood pressure rise to life-threatening level.
Cocaine:	Overstimulation. Possibly fatal.
Foods: Foods containing tyramine.*	Blood pressure rise to life-threatening level.
Marijuana:	Overstimulation. Avoid.
Tobacco:	None expected.

*See Glossary

685

PROGESTINS

GENERIC AND BRAND NAMES

See full list of generic and brand names in
Generic and Brand Name Directory, page 896.

BASIC INFORMATION

Habit forming? No
Prescription needed? Yes
Available as generic? Yes, for some.
Drug class: Female sex hormone (progestin)

 USES

- Treatment for menstrual or uterine disorders.
- Contraceptive (used alone or with estrogen).
  May be used for emergency contraception.
- Treatment for symptoms of menopause.
- Treatment for several types of cancer.
- Treatment for female hormone imbalance.
- Megestrol is used for treatment of weight loss
  in AIDS and cancer patients.
- Treatment for female infertility caused by
  progesterone deficiency.
- Treatment for endometrial hyperplasia.

 DOSAGE & USAGE INFORMATION

How to take:
- Capsule—Swallow with liquid. Do not crush,
  chew or break capsule.
- Tablet—Swallow with liquid or food to lessen
  stomach irritation. You may crumble tablet.
- Injection—Given by medical provider.
- Transdermal patch—Follow label instructions.
- Implant—Inserted by a health care provider.
- Oral suspension—Follow label instructions.

When to take:
Daily dose at the same time each day. For other
forms, follow instructions on label.

If you forget a dose:
- Treatment for menstrual disorders—Take up to
  2 hours late. If more than 2 hours, wait for next
  dose (don't double this dose).

Continued next column

 OVERDOSE

SYMPTOMS:
**Nausea, vomiting, fluid retention, breast
discomfort or enlargement, vaginal bleeding.**
WHAT TO DO:
**Overdose unlikely to threaten life. If person
uses much larger amount than prescribed or
if accidentally swallowed, call doctor or
poison control center 1-800-222-1222 for help.**

- Contraceptive—Consult your doctor or label
  instructions. You may need to use another
  birth control method until your next period.

What drug does:
- Progesterone is a female hormone produced
  in the body. Progestins are synthetic
  hormones that have progesterone-like actions.
  They can have multiple effects on the female
  reproductive system.
- The mechanism that produces weight gain or
  helps in cancer treatment is unknown.

Time lapse before drug works:
- Menstrual disorders—24 to 48 hours.
- Contraception—3 weeks.
- Cancer—May require 2 to 3 months regular
  use for maximum benefit.

Don't take with:
Any other medicine or any dietary supplement
without consulting your doctor or pharmacist.

 POSSIBLE ADVERSE REACTIONS OR SIDE EFFECTS

SYMPTOMS	WHAT TO DO
Life-threatening: Anaphylaxis (severe allergic reaction).	Seek emergency treatment immediately.
Common: • Vaginal bleeding changes (heavy, irregular, spotting, stopped).	Continue, but call doctor right away.
• Abdominal cramping, bloating, swollen feet or ankles, tiredness or weakness, mild headache, nausea, mood changes, skin irritation with injection, skin pain with implant.	Continue. Call doctor when convenient.
Infrequent: Depression, acne, tender breasts, changes in facial or body hair, brown spots on skin, loss of sexual desire, insomnia.	Continue. Call doctor when convenient.
Rare: • Rash, changes in breast milk.	Continue, but call doctor right away.
• Blood clot with high doses for noncontraceptive use (sudden headache, pain in calf, vision changes, breathing or speech problems).	Discontinue. Seek emergency help.

WARNINGS & PRECAUTIONS

Don't take if:
You are allergic to any progestin hormone.

Before you start, consult your doctor if:
- You have diabetes, heart or kidney disease.
- You have liver or gallbladder disease.
- You have had thrombophlebitis, embolism or stroke, bleeding disorder or high cholesterol.
- You have unexplained vaginal bleeding.
- You have had breast or uterine cancer.
- You have varicose veins.
- You have a seizure disorder.
- You suffer from migraines or depression.
- You have breast disease (lumps, cysts).

Over age 60:
No special problems expected.

Pregnancy:
Risk factors vary for drugs in this group. See category list on page xviii and consult doctor.

Breast-feeding:
Drug passes into milk in small amounts. The low progestin dose used for contraception has not caused problems. Consult doctor for advice about breast-feeding.

Infants & children:
Use only for female children under medical supervision.

Prolonged use:
No problems expected.

Skin & sunlight:
No problems expected.

Driving, piloting or hazardous work:
No problems expected.

Discontinuing:
Consult doctor. This medicine stays in the body and may cause fetal abnormalities. Wait at least 3 months before becoming pregnant. Side effects may also occur (dizziness, nausea, unusual menstrual bleeding).

Others:
- For postmenopausal women, the use of hormone replacement therapy (HRT) which combines estrogen and progestin increases slightly the risk for breast cancer, heart attacks and stroke. HRT does not prevent heart disease. HRT is effective for menopause symptoms (used short term), and helps protect against osteoporosis and colon cancer. Other treatments are available for osteoporosis. Discuss with your doctor if HRT is the right treatment for you.
- Injection form (Depo-Provera) may result in the loss of bone density. The risk increases, the longer the drug is used. The bone loss may not be reversible.

- Patients with diabetes must be monitored closely. Consult doctor if changes in blood glucose levels occur.
- May affect results in some medical tests.
- Advise any doctor or dentist whom you consult that you take this medicine.
- Carefully read the paper called "Information for the Patient" that was given to you with your first prescription or a refill. If you lose it, ask your pharmacist for a copy.

POSSIBLE INTERACTION WITH OTHER DRUGS

GENERIC NAME OR DRUG CLASS	COMBINED EFFECT
Aminoglutethimide	Decreased progestin effect.
Enzyme inducers*	Decreased progestin effect.

POSSIBLE INTERACTION WITH OTHER SUBSTANCES

INTERACTS WITH	COMBINED EFFECT
Alcohol:	None expected.
Beverages:	None expected.
Cocaine:	Unknown effect. Avoid.
Foods:	None expected.
Marijuana:	Unknown effect. Avoid.
Tobacco: All forms.	Possible blood clots in lung, brain, legs (with high drug doses). Avoid.

*See Glossary

PROGUANIL

BRAND NAMES

Malarone   Paludrine

BASIC INFORMATION

Habit forming? No
Prescription needed? Yes
Available as generic? No
Drug class: Antimalarial

 ## USES

Prevents and treats malaria.

 ## DOSAGE & USAGE INFORMATION

How to take:
Tablet—Swallow whole with liquid after meals.

When to take:
At the same time each day.

If you forget a dose:
Take as soon as you remember; however, if it is almost time for the next dose, skip the missed dose and return to your normal schedule (don't double this dose).

What drug does:
Exact mechanism unknown.

Time lapse before drug works:
1 to 2 weeks.

Don't take with:
Any other medicine or any dietary supplement without consulting your doctor or pharmacist.

 ## OVERDOSE

SYMPTOMS:
Abdominal pain, blood in urine, lower back pain, pain or burning on urination, vomiting.
WHAT TO DO:
If person takes much larger amount than prescribed, dial 911 (emergency) for medical help or call poison control center 1-800-222-1222 for instructions.

 ## POSSIBLE ADVERSE REACTIONS OR SIDE EFFECTS

SYMPTOMS	WHAT TO DO
Life-threatening: None expected.	
Common: Abdominal pain, back pain, coughing, diarrhea, fever, headache, loss of strength, nausea, muscle pain, sore throat, sneezing, vomiting.	Continue. Call doctor if symptoms persist.
Infrequent: Acid or sour stomach, belching, dizziness, flu-like symptoms, heartburn, indigestion, loss of appetite, weight loss, temporary hair loss.	Continue. Call doctor if symptoms persist.
Rare: Skin rash or itching.	Continue. Call doctor when convenient.

WARNINGS & PRECAUTIONS

Don't take if:
You are allergic to proguanil.

Before you start, consult your doctor if:
* You are pregnant or breast-feeding.
* You have kidney problems.

Over age 60:
No problems expected.

Pregnancy:
Decide with your doctor whether drug benefits justify risk to unborn child. Risk category C (see page xviii). Folate supplements should be taken by pregnant women while taking proguanil.

Breast-feeding:
Drug passes into milk. Avoid drug or discontinue nursing until you finish medicine. Consult doctor for advice on maintaining milk supply.

Infants & children:
Not expected to cause different side effects in children than it does in adults.

Prolonged use:
Not intended for long term use.

Skin & sunlight:
No problems expected.

Driving, piloting or hazardous work:
Don't drive or pilot aircraft until you learn how medicine affects you. Don't work around dangerous machinery. Don't climb ladders or work in high places. Danger increases if you drink alcohol or take medicine affecting alertness and reflexes, such as antihistamines, tranquilizers, sedatives, pain medicine, narcotics and mind-altering drugs.

Discontinuing:
Don't discontinue without doctor's advice until you complete the prescribed dosage.

Others:
* Advise any doctor or dentist whom you consult that you take this medicine.
* Persons of Asian or African descent metabolize this drug rapidly, therefore the drug may not reach effective blood levels for protection against malaria.

 POSSIBLE INTERACTION WITH OTHER DRUGS

GENERIC NAME OR DRUG CLASS	COMBINED EFFECT
None expected.	

 POSSIBLE INTERACTION WITH OTHER SUBSTANCES

INTERACTS WITH	COMBINED EFFECT
Alcohol:	None expected.
Beverages:	None expected.
Cocaine:	None expected.
Foods:	None expected.
Marijuana:	None expected.
Tobacco:	None expected.

PROPAFENONE

BRAND NAMES

Rhythmol

BASIC INFORMATION

Habit forming? No
Prescription needed? Yes
Available as generic? Yes
Drug class: Antiarrhythmic

 ## USES

Treats severe heartbeat irregularities (life-threatening ventricular rhythm disturbances).

 ## DOSAGE & USAGE INFORMATION

How to take:
Tablet—Swallow with liquid or food to lessen stomach irritation. If you can't swallow whole, crumble tablet and take with liquid or food.

When to take:
At the same time each day, according to instructions on prescription label.

If you forget a dose:
Take as soon as you remember up to 2 hours late. If more than 2 hours, wait for next scheduled dose. Don't double this dose.

What drug does:
Slows electrical activity in the heart to decrease the excitability of the heart muscle.

Time lapse before drug works:
3-1/2 hours to 1 week for full effect. Begins working almost immediately.

Don't take with:
Any other medicine (including nonprescription drugs such as cough and cold medicines, nose drops, vitamins, laxatives, antacids, diet pills, or caffeine) without consulting your doctor or pharmacist.

 ## OVERDOSE

SYMPTOMS:
Very rapid heart rate that is also irregular.
WHAT TO DO:
Overdose unlikely to threaten life. If person uses much larger amount than prescribed or if accidentally swallowed, call doctor or poison control center 1-800-222-1222 for help.

 ## POSSIBLE ADVERSE REACTIONS OR SIDE EFFECTS

SYMPTOMS	WHAT TO DO
Life-threatening:	
Severe chest pain, severe shortness of breath.	Seek emergency treatment.
Common:	
• Faster or more irregular heartbeat.	Discontinue. Call doctor right away.
• Taste change, dizziness.	Continue. Call doctor when convenient.
Infrequent:	
• Blurred vision, skin rash.	Discontinue. Call doctor right away.
• Constipation, diarrhea.	Continue. Call doctor when convenient.
• Dry mouth, nausea.	Continue. Tell doctor at next visit.
Rare:	
Fever, chills, trembling, joint pain, slow heartbeat.	Discontinue. Call doctor right away.

WARNINGS & PRECAUTIONS

Don't take if:
You are allergic to propafenone.

Before you start, consult your doctor if:
- You have asthma or bronchospasm.
- You have congestive heart failure.
- You have liver disease or kidney disease.
- You have a recent history of heart attack.
- You have a pacemaker.

Over age 60:
More likely to have decreased kidney function and require dosage modification.

Pregnancy:
Decide with your doctor if drug benefits justify risk to unborn child. Risk category C (see page xviii).

Breast-feeding:
No proven problems. Consult doctor.

Infants & children:
Safety and efficacy not established.

Prolonged use:
Don't discontinue without consulting doctor. Dose may require gradual reduction if you have taken drug for a long time. Dosages of other drugs may also require adjustment.

Skin & sunlight:
No special problems expected.

Driving, piloting or hazardous work:
Don't drive or pilot aircraft until you learn how medicine affects you. Don't work around dangerous machinery. Don't climb ladders or work in high places. Danger increases if you drink alcohol or take medicine affecting alertness and reflexes.

Discontinuing:
Don't discontinue without consulting doctor. Dose may require gradual reduction if you have taken drug for a long time. Doses of other drugs may also require adjustment.

Others:
- Advise any doctor or dentist whom you consult that you take this medicine, especially if you are to be anesthetized.
- Report changes in symptoms to your doctor and return for periodic visits to check progress.
- Carry or wear a medical I.D. card or bracelet that indicate your disorder and the drugs you take.

POSSIBLE INTERACTION WITH OTHER DRUGS

GENERIC NAME OR DRUG CLASS	COMBINED EFFECT
Anesthetics, local (e.g., prior to dental procedures)	May increase risk of side effects.
Antiarrhythmics,* other	Increased risk of adverse reactions.
Beta-adrenergic blocking agents*	Increased beta blocker effect.
Digitalis preparations*	Increased digitalis absorption. May require decreased dosage of digitalis preparation.
Doxepin (topical)	Increased risk of toxicity of both drugs.
Warfarin	Increased warfarin effect.

POSSIBLE INTERACTION WITH OTHER SUBSTANCES

INTERACTS WITH	COMBINED EFFECT
Alcohol:	Unpredictable effect on heartbeat. Avoid.
Beverages: Caffeine drinks.	Increased heartbeat irregularity. Avoid.
Cocaine:	Increased heartbeat irregularity. Avoid.
Foods:	None expected.
Marijuana:	Increased heartbeat irregularity. Avoid.
Tobacco:	Increased heartbeat irregularity. Avoid.

*See Glossary

PROPANTHELINE

BRAND NAMES

Pro-Banthine   Propanthel

BASIC INFORMATION

Habit forming? No
Prescription needed?
   High strength: Yes
   Low strength: No
Available as generic? Yes
Drug class: Antispasmodic, anticholinergic

 USES

Reduces spasms of digestive system, bladder and urethra.

 DOSAGE & USAGE INFORMATION

How to take:
Tablet—Swallow with liquid or food to lessen stomach irritation.

When to take:
30 minutes before meals (unless directed otherwise by doctor).

If you forget a dose:
Take as soon as you remember up to 2 hours late. If more than 2 hours, wait for next scheduled dose (don't double this dose).

What drug does:
Blocks nerve impulses at parasympathetic nerve endings, preventing muscle contractions and gland secretions of organs involved.

Time lapse before drug works:
15 to 30 minutes.

Don't take with:
Any other medicine or any dietary supplement without consulting your doctor or pharmacist.

 OVERDOSE

SYMPTOMS:
Dilated pupils, blurred vision, rapid pulse and breathing, dizziness, fever, hallucinations, confusion, slurred speech, agitation, flushed face, convulsions, coma.
WHAT TO DO:
* **Dial 911 (emergency) for medical help or call poison control center 1-800-222-1222 for instructions.**
* **See emergency information on last 3 pages of this book.**

 POSSIBLE ADVERSE REACTIONS OR SIDE EFFECTS

SYMPTOMS	WHAT TO DO
Life-threatening:	
Hives, rash, intense itching, faintness soon after a dose (anaphylaxis).	Seek emergency treatment immediately.
Common:	
• Confusion, delirium, rapid heartbeat.	Discontinue. Call doctor right away.
• Nausea, vomiting, decreased sweating.	Continue. Call doctor when convenient.
• Constipation, loss of taste.	Continue. Tell doctor at next visit.
• Dry ears, nose, throat, mouth.	No action necessary.
Infrequent:	
• Headache, difficult urination, nasal congestion, altered taste, impotence.	Continue. Call doctor when convenient.
• Lightheadedness.	Discontinue. Call doctor right away.
Rare:	
Rash or hives, eye pain, blurred vision.	Discontinue. Call doctor right away.

 WARNINGS & PRECAUTIONS

Don't take if:
* You are allergic to any anticholinergic.
* You have trouble with stomach bloating.
* You have difficulty emptying your bladder completely.
* You have narrow-angle glaucoma.
* You have severe ulcerative colitis.

Before you start, consult your doctor if:
* You have open-angle glaucoma.
* You have angina.
* You have chronic bronchitis or asthma.
* You have hiatal hernia.
* You have liver, kidney or thyroid disease.
* You have enlarged prostate.
* You have myasthenia gravis.
* You have peptic ulcer.
* You will have surgery within 2 months, including dental surgery, requiring general or spinal anesthesia.

Over age 60:
Adverse reactions and side effects may be more frequent and severe than in younger persons.

Pregnancy:
Decide with your doctor whether drug benefits justify risk to unborn child. Risk category C (see page xviii).

Breast-feeding:
Drug passes into milk and decreases milk flow. Avoid drug or discontinue nursing until you finish medicine. Consult doctor for advice on maintaining milk supply.

Infants & children:
Use only under medical supervision.

Prolonged use:
Chronic constipation, possible fecal impaction. Consult doctor immediately.

Skin & sunlight:
No problems expected.

Driving, piloting or hazardous work:
No problems expected.

Discontinuing:
May be unnecessary to finish medicine. Follow doctor's instructions.

Others:
Advise any doctor or dentist whom you consult that you take this medicine.

POSSIBLE INTERACTION WITH OTHER DRUGS

GENERIC NAME OR DRUG CLASS	COMBINED EFFECT
Adrenocorticoids, systemic	Possible glaucoma.
Amantadine	Increased propantheline effect.
Antacids*	Decreased propantheline effect.
Anticholinergics,* other	Increased propantheline effect.
Antidepressants, tricyclic*	Increased propantheline effect. Increased sedation.
Antidiarrhea preparations*	Reduced propantheline effect.
Antihistamines*	Increased propantheline effect.
Attapulgite	Decreased propantheline effect.
Buclizine	Increased propantheline effect.
Digitalis preparations*	Possible decreased absorption of digitalis.
Haloperidol	Increased internal eye pressure.
Ketoconazole	Decreased ketoconazole effect.
Meperidine	Increased propantheline effect.
Methylphenidate	Increased propantheline effect.
Molindone	Increased anticholinergic effect.
Monoamine oxidase (MAO) inhibitors*	Increased propantheline effect.
Nitrates*	Increased internal eye pressure.
Nizatidine	Increased nizatidine effect.
Orphenadrine	Increased propantheline effect.
Phenothiazines*	Increased propantheline effect.
Pilocarpine	Loss of pilocarpine effect in glaucoma treatment.
Potassium supplements*	Increased possibility of intestinal ulcers with oral potassium tablets.
Quinidine	Increased propantheline effect.
Sedatives* or central nervous system (CNS) depressants*	Increased sedative effect of both drugs.
Vitamin C	Decreased propantheline effect. Avoid large doses of vitamin C.

POSSIBLE INTERACTION WITH OTHER SUBSTANCES

INTERACTS WITH	COMBINED EFFECT
Alcohol:	None expected.
Beverages:	None expected.
Cocaine:	Excessively rapid heartbeat. Avoid.
Foods:	None expected.
Marijuana:	Drowsiness and dry mouth.
Tobacco:	None expected.

PROTEASE INHIBITORS

GENERIC AND BRAND NAMES

ATAZANAVIR
  Reyataz
DARUNAVIR
  Prezista
FOSAMPRENAVIR
  Lexiva
INDINAVIR
  Crixivan
LOPINAVIR
  Kaletra

NELFINAVIR
  Viracept
RITONAVIR
  Kaletra
  Norvir
SAQUINAVIR
  Invirase
TIPRANAVIR
  Aptivus

BASIC INFORMATION

Habit forming? No
Prescription needed? Yes
Available as generic? No
Drug class: Protease inhibitor

USES

Used in combination with other drugs as a treatment for HIV infection.

DOSAGE & USAGE INFORMATION

How to take:
* Tablet or capsule—Swallow with liquid. Take with food or meal to enhance drug's absorption. Take tipranavir or darunavir at the same time as ritonavir. Take indinavir 1 hour before or 2 hours after eating. You may take fosamprenavir tablet with or without food. Your doctor may recommend additional methods to help the body absorb the drugs.
* Film-coated tablet (Kaletra)—Can be taken with or without food.
* Liquid ritonavir—Swallow with chocolate milk or liquid nutritional supplement to disguise unpleasant taste.
* Oral solution tipranavir—Take as directed.

When to take:
At the same times each day, according to instructions on prescription label.

Continued next column

OVERDOSE

SYMPTOMS:
Unknown effect.
WHAT TO DO:
Overdose unlikely to threaten life. If person uses much larger amount than prescribed or if accidentally swallowed, call doctor or poison control center 1-800-222-1222 for help.

If you forget a dose:
Take as soon as you remember. If it is almost time for the next dose, wait for next scheduled dose (don't double this dose).

What drug does:
Blocks an enzyme called protease that is vital to the final stages of HIV replication (reproduction). Blocking protease causes HIV to make copies of itself that can't infect new cells.

Time lapse before drug works:
It will take weeks to months of treatment with the drug to determine the benefits of this therapy.

Don't take with:
Any other medicine or any dietary supplement without consulting your doctor or pharmacist.

POSSIBLE ADVERSE REACTIONS OR SIDE EFFECTS

SYMPTOMS	WHAT TO DO
Life-threatening: None expected.	
Common: Diarrhea, abdominal discomfort, nausea, sores in mouth, dizziness, dry mouth, tiredness, appetite loss.	Continue. Call doctor when convenient.
Infrequent: Rash, muscle or joint pain, headache, abdominal pain, weakness, back pain, numbness or tingling in hands or feet, tingling around mouth.	Continue. Call doctor when convenient.
Rare: • Confusion, yellow skin or eyes, severe skin reaction, lack of coordination, seizures, liver problems (fatigue, loss of appetite, nausea, dark urine, yellow skin or eyes, stomach pain). Watch for warning signs of hyperglycemia or diabetes (increased thirst and hunger, unexplained weight loss, increased urination, fatigue and dry itchy skin).	Continue, but call doctor right away.
• Other symptoms not listed. They may be drug-associated or infection-associated.	Continue. Call doctor when convenient.

694

WARNINGS & PRECAUTIONS

Don't take if:
You are allergic to protease inhibitors.

Before you start, consult your doctor if:
- You have any liver or kidney disease.
- You have diabetes or hypertension.
- You have peripheral neuropathy.*

Over age 60:
No special problems expected.

Pregnancy:
Risk factors vary for drugs in this group. See category list on page xviii and consult doctor.

Breast-feeding:
Unknown if drug passes into milk. Breast-feeding not recommended in HIV-infected women.

Infants & children:
Some of these drugs are approved for use in infants and children. Consult your child's doctor.

Prolonged use:
Medical studies have shown that HIV can become resistant to the effects of these drugs.

Skin & sunlight:
No special problems expected.

Driving, piloting or hazardous work:
Don't drive or pilot aircraft until you learn how medicine affects you. Don't work around dangerous machinery. Don't climb ladders or work in high places. Danger increases if you drink alcohol or take medicine affecting alertness and reflexes.

Discontinuing:
Don't discontinue without consulting doctor.

Others:
- Advise any doctor or dentist whom you consult that you take this medicine.
- These drugs do not reduce the risk of transmitting HIV to others through sexual contact. Avoid sexual contact or use condoms to help prevent HIV infection. Don't share needles or equipment for injections with other persons.
- These drugs may cause or aggravate diabetes or hypertension.

POSSIBLE INTERACTION WITH OTHER DRUGS

GENERIC NAME OR DRUG CLASS	COMBINED EFFECT
Alfuzosin	Increased alfuzosin effect with ritonavir.
Antacids*	Take 2 hours apart of protease inhibitor.
Anticonvulsants*	Decreased effect of ritonavir.
Contraceptives, oral	Less contraceptive effect with ritonavir.
Dexamethasone	Decreased effect of ritonavir.
Dofetilide	Increased dofetilide effect.
Enzyme inducers*	Decreased effect of protease inhibitor.
Enzyme inhibitors*	Increased effect of enzyme inhibitor.
Ergot preparations*	Serious or life-threatening problems. Avoid.
Fluticasone	Increased fluticasone effect with ritonavir.
Methadone	Decreased effect of methadone with ritonavir/tipranavir.
Non-nucleoside reverse transcriptase inhibitors	May need dosage adjustment of protease inhibitor.
Proton pump inhibitors	Decreased effect of atazanavir. Avoid.
Rifabutin	Decreased effect of protease inhibitor.
Rifampin	Decreased protease inhibitor effect. Don't use with saquinavir.
Telithromycin	Increased effect of ritonavir.
Trazodone	Increased trazodone effect with ritonavir.

POSSIBLE INTERACTION WITH OTHER SUBSTANCES

INTERACTS WITH	COMBINED EFFECT
Alcohol:	None expected.
Beverages: Grapefruit juice.	May increase effect of protease inhibitor.
Cocaine:	Unknown. Avoid.
Foods: Grapefruit.	May increase effect of protease inhibitor.
Cocaine:	Unknown. Avoid.
Marijuana:	Unknown. Avoid.
Tobacco:	Decreased effect of ritonavir.

*See Glossary

PROTECTANT (Ophthalmic)

GENERIC AND BRAND NAMES

**HYDROXYPROPYL
CELLULOSE**
Lacrisert

**HYDROXYPROPYL
METHYL-
CELLULOSE**
Artificial Tears
Bion Tears
Eye Lube
Gonak
Goniosoft
Goniosol
Isopto Alkaline
Isopto Plain
Isopto Tears
Just Tears
Lacril
Methocel
Moisture Drops
Nature's Tears
Ocutears
Tearisol
Tears Naturale
Tears Naturale Free
Tears Naturale II
Tears Renewed
Ultra Tears

BASIC INFORMATION

Habit forming? No
Prescription needed? Yes
Available as generic? Yes, for some
Drug class: Protectant (ophthalmic), artificial tears

 ## USES

• Relieves eye dryness and irritation caused by inadequate flow of tears.
• Moistens contact lenses and artificial eyes.

 ## OVERDOSE

SYMPTOMS:
None expected.
WHAT TO DO:
Not intended for internal use. If child accidentally swallows, call doctor or poison control center 1-800-222-1222 for help.

 ## DOSAGE & USAGE INFORMATION

How to use:
Eye drops
• Wash hands.
• Apply pressure to inside corner of eye with middle finger.
• Continue pressure for 1 minute after placing medicine in eye.
• Tilt head backward. Pull lower lid away from eye with index finger of the same hand.
• Drop eye drops into pouch and close eye. Don't blink.
• Keep eyes closed for 1 to 2 minutes.
• Don't touch applicator tip to any surface (including the eye). If you accidentally touch tip, clean with warm water and soap.
• Keep container tightly closed.
• Keep cool, but don't freeze.
• Wash hands immediately after using.

When to use:
As directed. Usually every 3 or 4 hours.

If you forget a dose:
Use as soon as you remember.

What drug does:
• Stabilizes and thickens tear film.
• Lubricates and protects eye.

Time lapse before drug works:
2 to 10 minutes.

Don't use with:
Other eye drops without consulting your doctor or pharmacist.

 ## POSSIBLE ADVERSE REACTIONS OR SIDE EFFECTS

SYMPTOMS	WHAT TO DO
Life-threatening None expected.	
Common None expected.	
Infrequent Eye irritation not present before using artificial tears.	Discontinue. Call doctor right away.
Rare None expected.	

PROTECTANT (Ophthalmic)

WARNINGS & PRECAUTIONS

Don't use if:
You are allergic to any artificial tears.

Before you start, consult your doctor if:
You use any other eye drops.

Over age 60:
No problems expected.

Pregnancy:
Risk factor not designated. See category list on page xviii and consult doctor.

Breast-feeding:
No problems expected, but check with doctor.

Infants & children:
Don't use.

Prolonged use:
Don't use for more than 3 or 4 days.

Skin & sunlight:
No problems expected.

Driving, piloting or hazardous work:
No problems expected.

Discontinuing:
May not need all the medicine in container. If symptoms disappear, stop using.

Others:
Check with your doctor if eye irritation continues or becomes worse.

POSSIBLE INTERACTION WITH OTHER DRUGS

GENERIC NAME OR DRUG CLASS	COMBINED EFFECT
Clinically significant interactions with oral or injected medicines unlikely.	

POSSIBLE INTERACTION WITH OTHER SUBSTANCES

INTERACTS WITH	COMBINED EFFECT
Alcohol:	None expected.
Beverages:	None expected.
Cocaine:	None expected.
Foods:	None expected.
Marijuana:	None expected.
Tobacco:	None expected.

PROTON PUMP INHIBITORS

GENERIC AND BRAND NAMES

DEXLANSOPRAZOLE
  Kapidex
ESOMEPRAZOLE
  Nexium Delayed-
    Release Capsules
  Nexium for Delayed-
    Release Oral
    Suspension
LANSOPRAZOLE
  Prevacid
  Prevacid NapraPAC
  Prevacid
    Solutab

OMEPRAZOLE
  Losec
  Prilosec
  Prilosec OTC
  Rapinex Powder
    for Oral
    Suspension
  Zegerid Capsules
  Zegerid Chewable
    Tablets
  Zegerid Powder
PANTOPRAZOLE
  Pantoloc
  Protonix
  Protonix Delayed
    Release Oral
    Suspension
RABEPRAZOLE
  Aciphex

BASIC INFORMATION

Habit forming? No
Prescription needed? Yes, for some
Available as generic? Yes, for some
Drug class: Antiulcer agent; proton pump
  inhibitor

USES

- Treats gastroesophageal reflux disease or GERD (splashing of stomach acid from the stomach up onto the lower end of the esophagus).
- Treats ulcers in the stomach and duodenum.
- Treats any disorder associated with excess production of stomach acid (such as Zollinger-Ellison syndrome).

OVERDOSE

SYMPTOMS:
Severe drowsiness, seizures, breathing
difficulty, decreased body temperature.
WHAT TO DO:
- **Dial 911 (emergency) for medical help or call poison control center 1-800-222-1222 for instructions.**
- **See emergency information on last 3 pages of this book.**

DOSAGE & USAGE INFORMATION

How to take:
- Delayed-release and extended-release capsule—Swallow whole with liquid. Do not crush, chew or open (unless allowed on label).
- Delayed-release oral suspension—Follow instructions on prescription.
- Immediate-release capsule—Swallow whole with water (not other liquids). Do not crush, chew or break open.
- Powder—Follow instructions on prescription.
- Tablet (enteric coated)—Swallow whole with liquid. Do not crush, crumble or chew tablet.

When to take:
Once daily, right before a meal (preferably breakfast), unless otherwise directed by your doctor. Dexlansoprazole can be taken without regard to food. With once-a-day dosing, it is important to take the medicine on schedule.

If you forget a dose:
Take as soon as you remember. If it is almost time for the next dose, wait for next scheduled dose (don't double this dose).

What drug does:
Stops the production of stomach acid.

Time lapse before drug works:
Thirty minutes to 3 hours.

Don't take with:
Any other medicine or any dietary supplement without consulting your doctor or pharmacist.

POSSIBLE ADVERSE REACTIONS OR SIDE EFFECTS

SYMPTOMS	WHAT TO DO
Life-threatening: None expected.	
Common: Diarrhea, stomach pain.	Continue. Call doctor when convenient.
Infrequent: Nausea, loss of appetite, headache, heartburn, muscle pain, skin rash, drowsiness.	Continue. Call doctor when convenient.
Rare: Weakness or unusual tiredness, sore throat and fever, sores in mouth, unusual bleeding or bruising, cloudy or bloody urine, urination changes (difficult, frequent or painful).	Discontinue. Call doctor right away.

WARNINGS & PRECAUTIONS

Don't take if:
You are allergic to proton pump inhibitors (PPIs).

Before you start, consult your doctor if:
* You are allergic to any medicines, foods or other substances.
* You have or have had liver disease.
* You have a stomach infection.

Over age 60:
No special problems expected.

Pregnancy:
Risk factors may vary for drugs in this group. See category list on page xviii and consult doctor.

Breast-feeding:
It is unknown if drug passes into milk. Avoid drug or discontinue nursing until you finish medicine. Consult doctor for advice on maintaining milk supply.

Infants & children:
* Lansoprazole is used in children ages 1 to 17 years.
* Esomeprazole is used in children ages 1 to 17 for the short-term treatment of gastroesophageal reflux disease.
* Rabeprazole is used in children over age 12 to for the short-term treatment of gastroesophageal reflux disease.

Prolonged use:
The length of treatment can run from 4 to 8 weeks or may be indefinite. Though your symptoms may improve in 1 to 2 weeks, your doctor will determine when healing is complete.

Skin & sunlight:
No special problems expected.

Driving, piloting or hazardous work:
No special problems expected.

Discontinuing:
Don't discontinue without consulting doctor until you complete prescribed dose, even though symptoms diminish or disappear.

Others:
* Advise any doctor or dentist whom you consult that you take this medicine.
* If directed by your doctor, it is permissible and sometimes helpful to take with antacids* to relieve upper abdominal pain. Antacids may be used more than once daily if needed.
* The brand name Zegerid contains sodium bicarbonate (a form of salt). If you are on a diet that restricts salt or sodium, consult your doctor before using this drug.
* May affect results of some medical tests.

POSSIBLE INTERACTION WITH OTHER DRUGS

GENERIC NAME OR DRUG CLASS	COMBINED EFFECT
Atazanavir	Decreased effect of atazanavir. Avoid.
Antifungals, azole	Decreased effect of azole antifungal.
Clopidogrel	Decreased effect of clopidogrel with some proton pump inhibitors. Consult doctor.
Diazepam	Increased effect of diazepam.
Digoxin	Increased effect of digoxin.
Iron supplements	Decreased effect of iron supplement.
Phenytoin	Increased effect of phenytoin with omeprazole.
Sucralfate	Decreased effect of some proton pump inhibitors. Take 30 minutes before sucralfate.
Tacrolimus	Increased effect of tacrolimus.
Theophylline	May require dosage adjustment of theophylline with lansoprazole.
Warfarin	May cause abnormal bleeding.

POSSIBLE INTERACTION WITH OTHER SUBSTANCES

INTERACTS WITH	COMBINED EFFECT
Alcohol:	None expected.
Beverages:	None expected.
Cocaine:	None expected.
Foods:	None expected.
Marijuana:	None expected.
Tobacco:	None expected.

*See Glossary

PSEUDOEPHEDRINE

BRAND NAMES

See full list of brand names in the *Generic and Brand Name Directory*, page 896.

BASIC INFORMATION

Habit forming? No
Prescription needed? Yes, for high strength
Available as generic? Yes
Drug class: Sympathomimetic, decongestant

 USES

Reduces congestion of nose, sinuses and ears (eustachian tubes) from infections and allergies.

 DOSAGE & USAGE INFORMATION

How to take:
- Tablet or capsule—Swallow with liquid. You may chew or crush tablet or open capsule.
- Extended-release tablet or capsule—Swallow whole. Do not crush or chew tablet. The capsule may be opened and the contents mixed with jam or jelly and taken with no chewing.
- Syrup—Take as directed on label.
- Drops—Place directly on tongue and swallow.
- Oral solution—Take as directed on label.
- Combination products—Follow instructions on label.

When to take:
- At the same times each day.
- To prevent insomnia, take last dose of day a few hours before bedtime.

If you forget a dose:
Take as soon as you remember. If it is almost time for the next dose, wait for next scheduled dose (don't double this dose).

Continued next column

 OVERDOSE

SYMPTOMS:
Nervousness, restlessness, headache, rapid or irregular heartbeat, sweating, nausea, vomiting, anxiety, confusion, delirium, muscle tremors, convulsions, hallucinations.
WHAT TO DO:
- Dial 911 (emergency) for medical help or call poison control center 1-800-222-1222 for instructions.
- See emergency information on last 3 pages of this book.

What drug does:
Decreases blood volume in nasal tissues, shrinking tissues and enlarging airways.

Time lapse before drug works:
15 to 20 minutes.

Don't take with:
Any other medicine or any dietary supplement without consulting your doctor or pharmacist.

 POSSIBLE ADVERSE REACTIONS OR SIDE EFFECTS

SYMPTOMS	WHAT TO DO
Life-threatening:	
Rare allergic reaction (hives, itching, rash, trouble breathing, tightness in chest, swelling of lips or tongue or throat).	Seek emergency treatment immediately.
Common: None expected.	
Infrequent: Nervousness, restlessness, trouble sleeping.	Discontinue. Call doctor if symptoms persist.
Rare:	
• Hallucinations, seizures, slow or irregular heartbeat, difficult breathing or shortness of breath.	Discontinue. Seek emergency treatment.
• Dizziness or lightheadedness, headache, nausea, vomiting, excess sweating, painful or difficult urination, paleness, weakness, trembling.	Discontinue. Call doctor if symptoms persist.

WARNINGS & PRECAUTIONS

Don't take if:
You are allergic to pseudoephedrine or any sympathomimetic* drug.

Before you start, consult your doctor if:
* You have diabetes or overactive thyroid.
* You have taken any monoamine oxidase (MAO) inhibitor* in past 2 weeks.
* You have high blood pressure or heart or blood vessel disease.
* You have glaucoma.
* You have prostate problems.

Over age 60:
Adverse reactions and side effects may be more frequent and severe than in younger persons.

Pregnancy:
Decide with your doctor if drug benefits justify risk to unborn child. Risk category B (see page xviii).

Breast-feeding:
Drug passes into milk. Avoid drug or discontinue nursing until you finish medicine. Consult doctor for advice on maintaining milk supply.

Infants & children:
Read the label on the product to see if it is approved for your child's age. Always follow the directions on product's label about how to use. If unsure, ask your doctor or pharmacist.

Prolonged use:
Not intended for long-term use. Consult doctor.

Skin & sunlight:
No problems expected.

Driving, piloting or hazardous work:
Avoid if you feel dizzy. Otherwise, no problems expected.

Discontinuing:
May be unnecessary to finish medicine. Follow label directions or doctor's instructions.

Others:
* Call the doctor if symptoms worsen or new symptoms develop with use of this medicine.
* Advise any doctor or dentist whom you consult that you take this medicine.
* Heed all warnings on the product label.
* Most pseudoephedrine-containing products are available without a prescription, but there are restrictions on their sales. This is because pseudoephedrine is a substance often used in the illegal manufacture of methamphetamine or "speed." You will need to ask a pharmacist for the product, show identification, sign a logbook and be limited in the amount you can purchase.

 POSSIBLE INTERACTION WITH OTHER DRUGS

GENERIC NAME OR DRUG CLASS	COMBINED EFFECT
Antihypertensives*	Decreased antihypertensive effect.
Beta-adrenergic blocking agents*	Decreased effect of beta-blocker.
Citrates	Urinary retention. Increased effect of pseudoephedrine.
Digitalis preparations*	Irregular heartbeat.
Methyldopa	Possible increased blood pressure.
Monoamine oxidase (MAO) inhibitors*	Serious reactions (potentially fatal). Take at least 2 weeks apart.
Nitrates*	Possible decreased nitrate effect.
Rauwolfia alkaloids	Decreased effect of pseudoephedrine.
Sympathomimetics,* other	Increased risk of side effects.
Thyroid hormones	Increased effect of either drug.

 POSSIBLE INTERACTION WITH OTHER SUBSTANCES

INTERACTS WITH	COMBINED EFFECT
Alcohol:	None expected.
Beverages: Caffeine drinks.	Nervousness or insomnia.
Cocaine:	High risk of heartbeat irregularities and high blood pressure. Avoid
Foods:	None expected.
Marijuana:	Rapid heartbeat. Avoid.
Tobacco:	None expected.

*See Glossary

PSORALENS

GENERIC AND BRAND NAMES

METHOXSALEN
Oxsoralen
Oxsoralen Topical
Oxsoralen Ultra
UltraMOP

TRIOXSALEN
Trisoralen

BASIC INFORMATION

Habit forming? No
Prescription needed? Yes
Available as generic? No
Drug class: Repigmenting agent (psoralen)

 USES

* Repigmenting skin affected with vitiligo (absence of skin pigment).
* Treatment for psoriasis, when other treatments haven't helped.
* Treatment for mycosis fungoides.

 DOSAGE & USAGE INFORMATION

How to take or apply:
* Tablet or capsule—Swallow with liquid or food to lessen stomach irritation.
* Topical—As directed by doctor.

When to take or apply:
2 to 4 hours before exposure to sunlight or sunlamp.

If you forget a dose:
Take as soon as you remember. Delay sun exposure for at least 2 hours after taking.

What drug does:
Helps pigment cells when used in conjunction with ultraviolet light.

Time lapse before drug works:
* For vitiligo, 6 to 9 months.
* For psoriasis, 10 weeks or longer.
* For tanning, 3 to 4 days.

Don't take with:
Any other medicine that causes skin sensitivity to sun. Ask your pharmacist if you have questions.

 OVERDOSE

SYMPTOMS:
Blistering skin, swelling feet and legs.
WHAT TO DO:
Overdose unlikely to threaten life. If person uses much larger amount than prescribed or if accidentally swallowed, call doctor or poison control center 1-800-222-1222 for help.

POSSIBLE ADVERSE REACTIONS OR SIDE EFFECTS

SYMPTOMS	WHAT TO DO
Life-threatening: None expected.	
Common:	
• Increased skin sensitivity to sun.	Always protect from overexposure.
• Increased eye sensitivity to sunlight.	Always protect with wrap-around sunglasses.
• Nausea.	Continue. Call doctor when convenient.
Infrequent:	
• Skin red and sore.	Discontinue. Call doctor right away.
• Dizziness, headache, depression, leg cramps, insomnia.	Continue. Call doctor when convenient.
Rare:	
Hepatitis with jaundice, blistering and peeling.	Discontinue. Call doctor right away.

WARNINGS & PRECAUTIONS

Don't take if:
* You are allergic to any psoralen.
* You are unwilling or unable to remain under close medical supervision.

Before you start, consult your doctor if:
* You have heart or liver disease.
* You have allergy to sunlight.
* You have cataracts.
* You have albinism.
* You have lupus erythematosus, porphyria, chronic infection, skin cancer or peptic ulcer.
* You will have surgery within 2 months, including dental surgery, requiring general or spinal anesthesia.
* You have skin cancer.

Over age 60:
Adverse reactions and side effects may be more frequent and severe than in younger persons.

Pregnancy:
Risk factors vary for drugs in this group. See category list on page xviii and consult doctor.

Breast-feeding:
Drug may pass into milk. Avoid drug or discontinue nursing until you finish medicine. Consult doctor for advice on maintaining milk supply.

Infants & children:
Not recommended.

Prolonged use:
* Increased chance of toxic effects.
* Talk to your doctor about the need for follow-up medical examinations or laboratory studies to check ANA titers,* complete blood counts (white blood cell count, platelet count, red blood cell count, hemoglobin, hematocrit), liver function, kidney function, eyes.

Skin & sunlight:
* One or more drugs in this group may cause rash or intensify sunburn in areas exposed to sun or ultraviolet light (photosensitivity reaction). Avoid overexposure. Notify doctor if reaction occurs.
* Too much can burn skin. Cover skin for 24 hours before and 8 hours following treatments.

Driving, piloting or hazardous work:
No problems expected. Protect eyes and skin from bright light.

Discontinuing:
Skin may remain sensitive for some time after treatment stops. Use extra protection from sun.

Others:
* Use sunblock on lips.
* Don't use just to make skin tan.
* Don't use hard gelatin capsules interchangeably with soft gelatin capsules.

POSSIBLE INTERACTION WITH OTHER DRUGS

GENERIC NAME OR DRUG CLASS	COMBINED EFFECT
Photosensitizing medications*	Greatly increased likelihood of extreme sensitivity to sunlight.

POSSIBLE INTERACTION WITH OTHER SUBSTANCES

INTERACTS WITH	COMBINED EFFECT
Alcohol:	May increase chance of liver toxicity.
Beverages: Lime drinks.	Avoid—toxic.
Cocaine:	Increased chance of toxicity. Avoid.
Foods: Those containing furocoumarin (limes, parsley, figs, parsnips, carrots, celery, mustard).	May cause toxic reaction to psoralens.
Marijuana:	Increased chance of toxicity. Avoid.
Tobacco:	May cause uneven absorption of medicine. Avoid.

*See Glossary

PYRIDOXINE (Vitamin B-6)

BRAND NAMES

Beesix	Rodex
Hexa-Betalin	Vitabec 6
Pyroxine	

Numerous brands of single vitamin and multivitamin combinations may be available.

BASIC INFORMATION

Habit forming? No
Prescription needed?
   High strength: Yes
   Low strength: No
Available as generic? Yes
Drug class: Vitamin supplement

USES

- Prevention and treatment of pyridoxine deficiency.
- Treatment of some forms of anemia.
- Treatment of INH (isonicotinic acid hydrazide), cycloserine poisoning.

DOSAGE & USAGE INFORMATION

How to take:
- Tablet—Swallow with liquid.
- Extended-release capsule—Swallow each dose whole with liquid.

When to take:
At the same times each day.

If you forget a dose:
Take as soon as you remember, then resume regular schedule.

What drug does:
It is an essential nutrient needed by the body. It acts as co-enzyme in carbohydrate, protein and fat metabolism.

Time lapse before drug works:
15 to 20 minutes.

Don't take with:
Any other medicine or any dietary supplement without consulting your doctor or pharmacist.

OVERDOSE

SYMPTOMS:
None expected.
WHAT TO DO:
Overdose unlikely to threaten life.

POSSIBLE ADVERSE REACTIONS OR SIDE EFFECTS

SYMPTOMS	WHAT TO DO
Life-threatening: None expected.	
Common: None expected.	
Infrequent: Nausea, headache.	Discontinue. Call doctor right away.
Rare: Numbness or tingling in hands or feet (large doses).	Discontinue. Call doctor right away.

PYRIDOXINE (Vitamin B-6)

WARNINGS & PRECAUTIONS

Don't take if:
You are allergic to pyridoxine.

Before you start, consult your doctor if:
You are pregnant or breast-feeding.

Over age 60:
No problems expected.

Pregnancy:
Don't exceed recommended dose. Consult doctor. Risk category A (see page xviii).

Breast-feeding:
Don't exceed recommended dose. Consult doctor.

Infants & children:
Don't exceed recommended dose.

Prolonged use:
Large doses for more than 1 month may cause toxicity.

Skin & sunlight:
No problems expected.

Driving, piloting or hazardous work:
No problems expected.

Discontinuing:
No problems expected.

Others:
- Advise any doctor or dentist whom you consult that you take this medicine.
- Regular pyridoxine supplements recommended if you take chloramphenicol, cycloserine, ethionamide, hydralazine, immuno-suppressants, isoniazid or penicillamine. These decrease pyridoxine absorption and can cause anemia or tingling and numbness in hands and feet.

POSSIBLE INTERACTION WITH OTHER DRUGS

GENERIC NAME OR DRUG CLASS	COMBINED EFFECT
Contraceptives, oral*	Decreased pyridoxine effect.
Cycloserine	Decreased pyridoxine effect.
Estrogens*	Decreased pyridoxine effect.
Ethionamide	Decreased pyridoxine effect.
Hydralazine	Decreased pyridoxine effect.
Hypnotics, barbiturates*	Decreased hypnotic effect.
Immuno-suppressants*	Decreased pyridoxine effect.
Isoniazid	Decreased pyridoxine effect.
Levodopa	Decreased levodopa effect.
Penicillamine	Decreased pyridoxine effect.
Phenobarbital	Possible decreased phenobarbital effect.
Phenytoin	Decreased phenytoin effect.

POSSIBLE INTERACTION WITH OTHER SUBSTANCES

INTERACTS WITH	COMBINED EFFECT
Alcohol:	None expected.
Beverages:	None expected.
Cocaine:	None expected.
Foods:	None expected.
Marijuana:	None expected.
Tobacco:	Decreased pyridoxine effect.

QUETIAPINE

BRAND NAMES

Seroquel

Seroquel XR

BASIC INFORMATION

Habit forming? No
Prescription needed? Yes
Available as generic? No
Drug class: Antipsychotic

 USES

- Treatment for symptoms of schizophrenia.
- Treatment for bipolar disorder (mania and depressive episodes).

 DOSAGE & USAGE INFORMATION

How to take:
- Tablet—Swallow with liquid. May be taken with or without food.
- Extended-release tablet—Swallow each dose whole. Don't crush or chew. Take without food or with a light meal or as advised by doctor.

When to take:
As directed by your doctor—2 to 3 times a day at the same times each day. The dosage may be increased over the first few days of use.

If you forget a dose:
Take as soon as you remember. If it is almost time for the next dose, wait for the next scheduled dose (don't double this dose).

What drug does:
The exact mechanism is unknown. It appears to alleviate symptoms of schizophrenia by blocking certain nerve impulses between nerve cells.

Time lapse before drug works:
One to 7 days. Further increases in the dosage may be needed to relieve symptoms.

Don't take with:
Any other medicine or any dietary supplement without consulting your doctor or pharmacist.

 OVERDOSE

SYMPTOMS:
Drowsiness and slurred speech; other symptoms may occur that were not observed in medical studies of the drug.
WHAT TO DO:
If person takes much larger amount than prescribed, dial 911 (emergency) for medical help or call poison control center 1-800-222-1222 for instructions.

 POSSIBLE ADVERSE REACTIONS OR SIDE EFFECTS

SYMPTOMS	WHAT TO DO
Life-threatening: High fever, rapid pulse, profuse sweating, muscle rigidity, confusion and irritability, seizures (rare neuroleptic malignant syndrome).	Discontinue. Seek emergency treatment.
Common: • Dizziness, difficulty in speaking or swallowing, shaking hands and fingers, trembling, vision problems, weakness, lightheadedness when arising from a sitting or lying position.	Continue. Call doctor right away.
• Drowsiness, constipation, weight gain, agitation, insomnia, headache, nervousness, runny nose, anxiety, dry mouth, arm or leg stiffness.	Continue. Call doctor when convenient.
Infrequent: • Jerky or involuntary movements (in face, lips, jaw, tongue) chest pain, fast heartbeat.	Continue. Call doctor right away.
• Fever, flu-like symptoms, twitching, mood or mental changes, speech unclear, swollen feet or ankles, appetite increased, cough, saliva increased, muscle tightness, muscle spasms (face, neck, back), joint pain, nausea, vomiting, sore throat, incontinence, abdominal pain.	Continue. Call doctor when convenient.
Rare: • Breathing difficulty, high blood sugar (thirstiness, frequent urination, increased hunger, weakness).	Discontinue. Call doctor right away.
• Swollen face, rash, confusion, decreased sex drive, menstrual changes, sluggishness.	Continue. Call doctor when convenient.

QUETIAPINE

WARNINGS & PRECAUTIONS

Don't take if:
You are allergic to quetiapine.

Before you start, consult your doctor if:
- You have a heart problem or disease, high or low blood pressure or blood vessel problem.
- You have Alzheimer's or dementia.
- You have a history of breast cancer.
- You are subject to dehydration or low body temperature.
- You have had suicidal thoughts or behaviors.
- You have a history of alcohol or drug abuse.
- You have diabetes or high blood sugar, thyroid problems, liver or kidney disease or high levels of blood fats.
- You have glaucoma or cataracts.
- You have prostate problems.
- You are allergic to any medication, food or other substance.
- You have a history of seizures.

Over age 60:
- Adverse reactions and side effects may be more severe than in younger persons. A lower starting dosage is usually recommended until a response is determined.
- Use of antipsychotic drugs in elderly patients with dementia-related psychosis may increase risk of death. Consult doctor.

Pregnancy:
Decide with your doctor if drug benefits justify any possible risk to unborn child. Risk category C (see page xviii).

Breast-feeding:
It is unknown if drug passes into milk. It is not recommended for nursing mothers.

Infants & children:
Safety in children under age 18 has not been established. Use only under close medical supervision. Contact doctor right away if depression symptoms get worse or there is any talk of suicide or suicide behaviors.

Prolonged use:
- Consult with your doctor on a regular basis to check your progress or to discuss any increase or changes in side effects and the need for continued treatment.
- Get eyes examined every 6 months.

Skin & sunlight:
May cause rash or intensify sunburn in areas exposed to sun or ultraviolet light (photosensitivity reaction). Use sunscreen and avoid overexposure. Notify doctor if reaction occurs.

Driving, piloting or hazardous work:
Don't drive or pilot aircraft until you learn how medicine affects you. Don't work around dangerous machinery. Don't climb ladders or work in high places. Danger increases if you drink alcohol or take drug affecting alertness.

Discontinuing:
Don't discontinue drug without doctor's advice. Dosage may need to be slowly reduced first.

Others:
- Get up slowly from a sitting or lying position to avoid any dizziness or lightheadedness.
- Advise any doctor or dentist whom you consult that you take this medicine.
- Hot temperatures, exercise, and hot baths can increase risk of heatstroke. Drug may affect body's ability to maintain normal temperature.
- Adults and children taking antidepressants may experience a worsening of the depression symptoms and may display increased suicidal thoughts or behavior. Call doctor right away if these symptoms or behaviors occur.
- Take drug only as directed. Do not increase or reduce dosage without doctor's approval.

POSSIBLE INTERACTION WITH OTHER DRUGS

GENERIC NAME OR DRUG CLASS	COMBINED EFFECT
Antihypertensives*	Increased risk of low blood pressure.
Central nervous system (CNS) depressants,* other	Increased sedative effect.
Enzyme inducers*	May decrease quetiapine effect.
Enzyme inhibitors*	May increase quetiapine effect.

Continued on page 929

POSSIBLE INTERACTION WITH OTHER SUBSTANCES

INTERACTS WITH	COMBINED EFFECT
Alcohol:	Increased sedation and dizziness. Avoid.
Beverages: Grapefruit juice.	Increased effect of drug. Avoid.
Cocaine:	Unknown. Avoid.
Foods:	None expected.
Marijuana:	Unknown. Avoid.
Tobacco:	None expected.

*See Glossary

QUINACRINE

BRAND NAMES

Atabrine

BASIC INFORMATION

Habit forming? No
Prescription needed? Yes
Available as generic? Yes
Drug class: Antiprotozoal

 USES

- Treats disease caused by the intestinal parasite *Giardia lamblia*.
- Treats mild to moderate discoid lupus erythematosus.

 DOSAGE & USAGE INFORMATION

How to take:
Tablet—Swallow with full glass of water, tea or fruit juice. If you can't swallow whole, crumble tablet and mix with jam or chocolate syrup.

When to take:
After meals.

If you forget a dose:
Take as soon as you remember up to 2 hours late. If more than 2 hours, wait for next scheduled dose (don't double this dose).

What drug does:
Destroys *Giardia lamblia* parasites in the gastrointestinal system.

Time lapse before drug works:
1 day.

Continued next column

 OVERDOSE

SYMPTOMS:
Severe abdominal cramps, convulsions, severe diarrhea, fainting, irregular heartbeat, restlessness.
WHAT TO DO:
- Dial 911 (emergency) for medical help or call poison control center 1-800-222-1222 for instructions.
- If person is unconscious, check breathing and pulse. If not breathing, begin mouth-to-mouth rescue breathing. If heart is not beating, begin chest compressions.
- See emergency information on last 3 pages of this book.

Don't take with:
Any other medicine or any dietary supplement without consulting your doctor or pharmacist.

 POSSIBLE ADVERSE REACTIONS OR SIDE EFFECTS

SYMPTOMS	WHAT TO DO
Life-threatening:	
In case of overdose, see previous column.	
Common:	
• Dizziness, nausea, headache.	Discontinue. Call doctor right away.
• Yellow eyes, skin, urine (due to dye-like characteristics of quinacrine).	Report to doctor, but no action necessary.
Infrequent:	
• Mild abdominal cramps; mild diarrhea; appetite loss; skin rash, itching or peeling.	Discontinue. Call doctor right away.
• Mood changes.	Continue. Call doctor when convenient.
Rare:	
Hallucinations, nightmares.	Discontinue. Call doctor right away.

WARNINGS & PRECAUTIONS

Don't take if:
You are allergic to quinacrine.

Before you start, consult your doctor if:
- You have porphyria.
- You have had psoriasis.
- You have a history of severe mental disorders.
- You are on a low-salt, low-sugar or other special diet.

Over age 60:
No special problems.

Pregnancy:
Decide with your doctor whether drug benefits justify risk to unborn child. Treatment best begun after child has been delivered. Risk category C (see page xviii).

Breast-feeding:
Effect unknown. Consult doctor.

Infants & children:
Children tolerate quinacrine poorly. Quinacrine may cause vomiting due to bitter taste. Try crushing tablets in jam, honey or chocolate syrup.

Prolonged use:
- Can cause eye problems, liver disease, aplastic anemia. Don't use for more than 5 days.
- Talk to your doctor about the need for follow-up medical examinations or laboratory studies to check stools for giardiasis.

Skin & sunlight:
No problems expected.

Driving, piloting or hazardous work:
Don't drive or pilot aircraft until you learn how medicine affects you. Don't work around dangerous machinery. Don't climb ladders or work in high places. Danger increases if you drink alcohol or take medicine affecting alertness and reflexes, such as antihistamines, tranquilizers, sedatives, pain medicine, narcotics and mind-altering drugs.

Discontinuing:
Don't discontinue before 5 days without consulting doctor.

Others:
- Advise any doctor or dentist whom you consult that you take this medicine.
- Request 3 stool exams several days apart.

POSSIBLE INTERACTION WITH OTHER DRUGS

GENERIC NAME OR DRUG CLASS	COMBINED EFFECT
Primaquine	Decreased effect of primaquine.

POSSIBLE INTERACTION WITH OTHER SUBSTANCES

INTERACTS WITH	COMBINED EFFECT
Alcohol:	Increased adverse effects of both. Avoid.
Beverages:	None expected.
Cocaine:	None expected.
Foods:	None expected.
Marijuana:	None expected.
Tobacco:	None expected.

QUINIDINE

BRAND NAMES

Apo-Quinidine
Cardioquin
Cin-Quin
Duraquin
Novoquinidin

Quinaglute Dura-
  Tabs
Quinalan
Quinate
Quinidex Extentabs
Quinora

BASIC INFORMATION

Habit forming? No
Prescription needed?
  U.S.: Yes
  Canada: No
Available as generic? Yes
Drug class: Antiarrhythmic

 USES

• Corrects heart rhythm disorders.
• May be used in treatment of malaria.

 DOSAGE & USAGE INFORMATION

How to take:
• Tablet or capsule—Swallow with liquid or food to lessen stomach irritation. If you can't swallow whole, crush tablet or open capsule and take with small amount of food.
• Extended-release tablet—Swallow each dose whole. Don't crush them.

When to take:
At the same times each day.

If you forget a dose:
Take as soon as you remember up to 2 hours late. If more than 2 hours, wait for next scheduled dose (don't double this dose).

Continued next column

 OVERDOSE

SYMPTOMS:
Confusion, severe blood pressure drop, lethargy, breathing difficulty, fainting, seizures, coma.
WHAT TO DO:
• **Dial 911 (emergency) for medical help or call poison control center 1-800-222-1222 for instructions.**
• **If person is unconscious, check breathing and pulse. If not breathing, begin mouth-to-mouth rescue breathing. If heart is not beating, begin chest compressions.**
• **See emergency information on last 3 pages of this book.**

What drug does:
Delays nerve impulses to the heart to regulate heartbeat.

Time lapse before drug works:
2 to 4 hours.

Don't take with:
Any other medicine or any dietary supplement without consulting your doctor or pharmacist.

 POSSIBLE ADVERSE REACTIONS OR SIDE EFFECTS

SYMPTOMS	WHAT TO DO
Life-threatening: Hives, rash, intense itching, faintness soon after a dose (anaphylaxis); wheezing.	Seek emergency treatment immediately.
Common: Bitter taste, diarrhea, nausea, vomiting, appetite loss, abdominal pain.	Discontinue. Call doctor right away.
Infrequent: • Dizziness, light-headedness, fainting, headache, confusion, rash, change in vision, difficult breathing, rapid heartbeat.	Discontinue. Call doctor right away.
• Ringing in ears.	Continue. Call doctor when convenient.
Rare: • Unusual bleeding or bruising, difficulty or pain on swallowing, fever, joint pain, jaundice, hepatitis.	Discontinue. Call doctor right away.
• Weakness.	Continue. Call doctor when convenient.

 WARNINGS & PRECAUTIONS

Don't take if:
• You are allergic to quinidine.
• You have an active infection.

Before you start, consult your doctor if:
• You have an electrolyte disorder.
• You have heart disease or myasthenia gravis.
• You have kidney or liver disease.

Over age 60:
Adverse reactions and side effects may be more frequent and severe than in younger persons.

Pregnancy:
Decide with your doctor if drug benefits justify risk to unborn child. Risk category C (see page xviii).

Breast-feeding:
Drug filters into milk. May harm child. Consult doctor.

Infants & children:
No problems expected.

Prolonged use:
Talk to your doctor about the need for follow-up studies to check complete blood counts (white blood cell count, platelet count, red blood cell count, hemoglobin, hematocrit), liver function, kidney function, serum potassium levels, ECG.*

Skin & sunlight:
May cause rash or intensify sunburn in areas exposed to sun or ultraviolet light (photosensitivity reaction). Avoid overexposure. Notify doctor if reaction occurs.

Driving, piloting or hazardous work:
Don't drive or pilot aircraft until you learn how medicine affects you. Don't work around dangerous machinery. Don't climb ladders or work in high places. Danger increases if you drink alcohol or take medicine affecting alertness and reflexes, such as antihistamines, tranquilizers, sedatives, pain medicine, narcotics and mind-altering drugs.

Discontinuing:
Don't discontinue without doctor's advice until you complete prescribed dose, even though symptoms diminish or disappear.

Others:
Advise any doctor or dentist whom you consult that you take this medicine.

POSSIBLE INTERACTION WITH OTHER DRUGS

GENERIC NAME OR DRUG CLASS	COMBINED EFFECT
Alkalizers, urinary*	Slows quinidine elimination, increasing its effect and toxicity.
Amiodarone	Increased effect of quinidine. Risk of heart rhythm problems.
Antacids	Take at least 2 hours apart.
Anticholinergics	Increased anticholinergic effect.
Anticoagulants,* oral	Possible increased anticoagulant effect.
Antidepressants, tricyclic	Increased risk of heart rhythm problems.

Cimetidine	Increased quinidine effect.
Digitalis preparations	May slow heartbeat. Dose adjustments may be needed.
Diltiazem	Increased quinidine effect.
Enzyme inhibitors*	Increased effect of quinidine.
Erythromycin	Possible irregular heartbeat.
Haloperidol	Possible irregular heartbeat.
Mefloquine	Possible irregular heartbeat. Avoid.
Memantine	Increased effect of either drug.
Metformin	Increased metformin effect.
Nifedipine	Possible decreased quinidine effect.
Phenobarbital	Decreased quinidine effect.
Phenothiazines*	Possible increased quinidine effect.
QT interval prolongation-causing drugs*	Heartbeat irregularities.
Verapamil	Increased quinidine effect.

POSSIBLE INTERACTION WITH OTHER SUBSTANCES

INTERACTS WITH	COMBINED EFFECT
Alcohol:	None expected.
Beverages: Caffeine drinks.	Causes rapid heartbeat. Use with care.
Grapefruit juice.	Toxicity risk. Avoid.
Cocaine:	Irregular heartbeat. Avoid.
Foods:	None expected.
Marijuana:	Can cause fainting.
Tobacco:	Irregular heartbeat. Avoid.

*See Glossary

QUININE

BRAND NAMES

Qualaquin

BASIC INFORMATION

Habit forming? No
Prescription needed? Yes
Available as generic? Yes
Drug class: Antiprotozoal

 ## USES

Treatment or prevention of malaria.

 ## DOSAGE & USAGE INFORMATION

How to take:
Tablet or capsule—Swallow with liquid or food to lessen stomach irritation.

When to take:
* Prevention—At the same time each day, usually at bedtime.
* Treatment—At the same times each day in evenly spaced doses.

If you forget a dose:
* Prevention—Take as soon as you remember up to 12 hours late. If more than 12 hours, wait for next scheduled dose (don't double this dose).
* Treatment—Take as soon as you remember up to 2 hours late. If more than 2 hours, wait for next scheduled dose (don't double this dose).

What drug does:
* Reduces contractions of skeletal muscles.
* Increases blood flow.
* Interferes with genes in malaria micro-organisms.

Time lapse before drug works:
May require several days or weeks for maximum effect.

Continued next column

 ## OVERDOSE

SYMPTOMS:
Severe impairment of vision and hearing; severe nausea, vomiting, diarrhea; shallow breathing, fast heartbeat; apprehension, confusion, delirium.
WHAT TO DO:
Dial 911 (emergency) for medical help or call poison control center 1-800-222-1222 for instructions.

Don't take with:
Any other medicine or any dietary supplement without consulting your doctor or pharmacist.

 ## POSSIBLE ADVERSE REACTIONS OR SIDE EFFECTS

SYMPTOMS	WHAT TO DO
Life-threatening:	
In case of overdose, see previous column.	
Common:	
• Blurred vision or change in vision, eyes sensitive to light.	Discontinue. Call doctor right away.
• Dizziness, headache, abdominal discomfort, mild nausea, vomiting, diarrhea.	Continue. Call doctor when convenient.
• Ringing or buzzing in ears, impaired hearing.	Continue. Tell doctor at next visit.
Infrequent:	
Rash, hives, itchy skin, difficult breathing.	Discontinue. Call doctor right away.
Rare:	
Sore throat, fever, unusual bleeding or bruising, unusual tiredness or weakness, angina.	Discontinue. Call doctor right away.

WARNINGS & PRECAUTIONS

Don't take if:
You are allergic to quinine or quinidine.

Before you start, consult your doctor if:
- You plan to become pregnant within medication period.
- You have asthma.
- You have eye disease, hearing problems or ringing in the ears.
- You have heart disease.
- You have myasthenia gravis.

Over age 60:
Adverse reactions and side effects may be more frequent and severe than in younger persons.

Pregnancy:
Risk to unborn child outweighs drug benefits. Don't use. Risk category X (see page xviii).

Breast-feeding:
Drug filters into milk. May harm child. Consult doctor.

Infants & children:
Use only under medical supervision.

Prolonged use:
May develop headache, blurred vision, nausea, temporary hearing loss, but seldom need to discontinue because of these symptoms.

Skin & sunlight:
May cause rash or intensity sunburn in areas exposed to sun or ultraviolet light (photosensitivity reaction). Avoid overexposure. Notify doctor if reaction occurs.

Driving, piloting or hazardous work:
Avoid if you feel dizzy or have blurred vision. Otherwise, no problems expected.

Discontinuing:
Don't discontinue without doctor's advice until you complete prescribed dose, even though symptoms diminish or disappear.

Others:
- Advise any doctor or dentist whom you consult that you take this medicine.
- Don't confuse with quinidine, a medicine for heart rhythm problems.

POSSIBLE INTERACTION WITH OTHER DRUGS

GENERIC NAME OR DRUG CLASS	COMBINED EFFECT
Alkalizers,* urinary	Possible toxic effects of quinine.
Antacids* (with aluminum hydroxide)	Decreased quinine effect.
Anticoagulants,* oral	Increased anticoagulant effect.
Dapsone	Increased risk of adverse effect on blood cells.
Digitalis	Possible increased digitalis effect.
Digoxin	Possible increased digoxin effect.
Mefloquine	Increased risk of heartbeat irregularities.
Metformin	Increased metformin effect.
Quinidine	Possible toxic effects of quinine.

POSSIBLE INTERACTION WITH OTHER SUBSTANCES

INTERACTS WITH	COMBINED EFFECT
Alcohol:	None expected.
Beverages:	None expected.
Cocaine:	None expected.
Foods:	None expected.
Marijuana:	None expected.
Tobacco:	None expected.

RALOXIFENE

BRAND NAMES

Evista

BASIC INFORMATION

Habit forming? No
Prescription needed? Yes
Available as generic? No
Drug class: Osteoporosis therapy,
  prophylactic

 USES

- Prevents and treats osteoporosis in post-menopausal women. Does not treat hot flashes of menopause.
- Lowers low-density lipoprotein (LDL) cholesterol blood levels.
- Used for reduction of breast cancer risk in postmenopausal women.
- Other uses as determined by your doctor.

 DOSAGE & USAGE INFORMATION

How to take:
Tablet—Swallow with water, with or without food. If you can't swallow whole, crumble tablet and take with liquid or food.

When to take:
At the same time each day.

If you forget a dose:
Take as soon as you remember up to 12 hours late. If more than 12 hours, wait for next scheduled dose (don't double this dose).

What drug does:
It is a selective estrogen receptor modulator or SERM. These drugs can act both like the hormone estrogen (such as in the bones) or block estrogen (such as in the breast tissue).

Time lapse before drug works:
Up to twelve months.

Don't take with:
Any other medicine or any dietary supplement without consulting your doctor or pharmacist.

 OVERDOSE

SYMPTOMS:
None reported.
WHAT TO DO:
Overdose unlikely to threaten life. If person uses much larger amount than prescribed or if accidentally swallowed, call doctor or poison control center 1-800-222-1222 for help.

 POSSIBLE ADVERSE REACTIONS OR SIDE EFFECTS

SYMPTOMS	WHAT TO DO
Life-threatening: Blood clot formation.	Discontinue. Seek emergency treatment immediately.
Common: • Chest pain; bloody or cloudy urine; burning or painful urination; frequent urge to urinate; infection; cold- or flu-like symptoms; leg cramping; skin rash; swelling of hands, ankle or feet; vaginal itching.	Discontinue. Call doctor right away.
• Joint or muscle pain, swollen joints, gas, upset stomach, vomiting, hot flashes, insomnia, white vaginal discharge, depression, sweating, unexplained weight gain.	Continue. Call doctor if symptoms persist.
Infrequent: Abdominal pain, diarrhea, loss of appetite, nausea, weakness, migraine headache, difficulty breathing, fever, congestion.	Discontinue. Call doctor right away.
Rare: Blood clot formation (symptoms include swelling in legs, sharp pain in legs, sudden chest pain, coughing up blood, changes in vision).	Discontinue. Seek emergency treatment immediately.

WARNINGS & PRECAUTIONS

Don't take if:
- You are allergic to raloxifene.
- You are scheduled for surgery within 72 hours.

Before you start, consult your doctor if:
- You plan to become pregnant within the medication period.
- You have or have had a history of blood clot (deep vein thrombosis) formation.
- You have a history of stroke, transient ischemic attacks (TIA) or heart disease.
- You have high triglycerides (a blood fat).
- You have or have had cancer or tumors.
- You have liver disease.

Over age 60:
Adverse reactions and side effects in older adults have been similar to those experienced by women who have just undergone menopause.

Pregnancy:
Use of raloxifene is not recommended during pregnancy. Risk category X (see page xviii).

Breast-feeding:
Unknown whether drug passes into milk and is not recommended during breast-feeding. Presently raloxifene is to be used in post-menopausal women only.

Infants & children:
Not recommended for this age group.

Prolonged use:
No problems expected. Your doctor should periodically evaluate your response to the drug and adjust the dose if necessary.

Skin & sunlight:
No problems expected.

Driving, piloting or hazardous work:
No problems expected.

Discontinuing:
Don't discontinue without consulting doctor.

Others:
- Advise any doctor or dentist whom you consult that you take this medicine.
- This drug is associated with an increased risk of developing blood clots in the veins (deep vein thrombosis) or stroke. Consult doctor.
- In addition to taking the drug, weight-bearing exercise and adequate intake of calcium and vitamin D are essential in preventing bone loss. Periods of prolonged inactivity may worsen your condition. Daily dietary supplements of elemental calcium and vitamin D may be recommended by your doctor.
- May help lower low-density lipoprotein (LDL) cholesterol levels.

POSSIBLE INTERACTION WITH OTHER DRUGS

GENERIC NAME OR DRUG CLASS	COMBINED EFFECT
Cholestyramine	Lessens the effect of raloxifene.
Estrogens	Not recommended for use with raloxifene.
Protein bound drugs*	Caution is recommended; consult doctor before taking any of these in conjunction with raloxifene.
Warfarin	May lessen the effect of warfarin.

POSSIBLE INTERACTION WITH OTHER SUBSTANCES

INTERACTS WITH	COMBINED EFFECT
Alcohol:	Increased risk of adverse effects. Avoid.
Beverages:	None expected.
Cocaine:	Effects unknown. Avoid.
Foods:	None expected.
Marijuana:	Effects unknown. Avoid.
Tobacco:	Increases risk of blood clot. Avoid.

*See Glossary

RAMELTEON

BRAND NAMES

Rozerem

BASIC INFORMATION

Habit forming? No
Prescription needed? Yes
Available as generic? No
Drug class: Melatonin receptor agonist;
nonbenzodiazepine hypnotic

 USES

It is used to help you fall asleep faster when you have trouble falling asleep and experience insomnia.

 DOSAGE & USAGE INFORMATION

How to take:
Tablet—Swallow whole with liquid. Do not crush or chew the tablet. Take it with or without food. Do not take it with, or immediately after, a high fat meal. Doing so can reduce the effectiveness of the drug.

When to take:
Take within 30 minutes of bedtime. Take the drug only when you know that you will get 8 full hours (or more) of sleep after the dose.

If you forget a dose:
Skip the missed dose. Resume dosage schedule the next night if needed to help you sleep. Do not take more than one dose in a 24 hour period.

What drug does:
It stimulates melatonin receptors (chemicals) in the brain that are responsible for the regulation of the body's 24 hour sleep-wake cycle.

Time lapse before drug works:
Usually within 30 to 90 minutes.

Continued next column

 OVERDOSE

SYMPTOMS:
Unknown for sure; may include extreme drowsiness, confusion, dizziness, difficult or slow breathing and unconsciousness.
WHAT TO DO:
* Dial 911 (emergency) for medical help or call poison control center 1-800-222-1222 for instructions.
* See emergency information on last 3 pages of this book.

Don't take with:
Fluvoxamine or any other medicine or any dietary supplement without consulting your doctor or pharmacist.

 POSSIBLE ADVERSE REACTIONS OR SIDE EFFECTS

SYMPTOMS	WHAT TO DO
Life-threatening:	
Allergic reaction (difficulty breathing, closing of the throat, swelling of the lips or face or tongue, hives).	Seek emergency treatment immediately.
Common:	
Dizziness, drowsiness, nausea, headache, fatigue, worsening insomnia.	Discontinue. Call doctor when convenient.
Infrequent:	
Decreased sex drive, menstrual changes, milky discharge from breasts, cold- or flu-like symptoms, muscle or joint or body aches or pain, taste changes, stomach upset.	Discontinue. Call doctor when convenient.
Rare:	
The class of drugs used to treat insomnia are called hypnotics. They can cause a variety of adverse reactions in one's emotions, behavior, cognition (thinking) and mood. Symptoms can include worsening depression, memory problems, confusion, bizarre behaviors, suicidal thoughts, hallucinations, unusual excitement, irritability, aggressiveness, nervousness, sleep-related behaviors,* and possibly others.	Discontinue. Call doctor right away.

WARNINGS & PRECAUTIONS

Don't take if:
- You are allergic to ramelteon.
- You are taking the drug fluvoxamine.

Before you start, consult your doctor if:
- You have or have had liver disease.
- You suffer from depression or a psychiatric disorder or abuse alcohol or drugs.
- You suffer from sleep apnea or emphysema, asthma, bronchitis or other chronic lung disease.

Over age 60:
No special problems expected.

Pregnancy:
Decide with your doctor if drug benefits justify any possible risk to unborn child. Risk category C (see page xviii).

Breast-feeding:
It is unknown if drug passes into milk. It is not recommended during breast-feeding. Consult doctor for advice.

Infants & children:
Safety and effectiveness in children has not been established. Consult your child's doctor.

Prolonged use:
No special problems expected. You and your doctor will decide if there is a need to take the drug for a prolonged period for chronic insomnia (insomnia at least three nights a week for a period of one month or longer).

Skin & sunlight:
No special problems expected.

Driving, piloting or hazardous work:
Don't drive or pilot aircraft until you learn how medicine affects you. Don't work around dangerous machinery. Don't climb ladders or work in high places. Danger increases if you drink alcohol or take other medicines affecting alertness and reflexes.

Discontinuing:
No problems expected. Ramelteon does not appear to produce withdrawal symptoms or lead to physical dependence.

Others:
- Advise any doctor or dentist whom you consult that you take this medicine.
- Consult your doctor if your insomnia symptoms do not improve after taking the drug a few nights.

POSSIBLE INTERACTION WITH OTHER DRUGS

GENERIC NAME OR DRUG CLASS	COMBINED EFFECT
Enzyme inducers*	Decreased effect of ramelteon.
Enzyme inhibitors*	Increased effect of ramelteon. Consult your doctor or pharmacist before using.
Fluvoxamine	Increased effect of ramelteon. Avoid.

POSSIBLE INTERACTION WITH OTHER SUBSTANCES

INTERACTS WITH	COMBINED EFFECT
Alcohol:	Increased sedation. Avoid.
Beverages: Grapefruit juice.	Unknown effect. Consult doctor.
Cocaine:	Unknown. Avoid.
Foods: Grapefruit.	Unknown effect. Consult doctor.
High fat meal	Drug effect is decreased if taken with, or right after, the meal.
Marijuana:	Unknown. Avoid.
Tobacco:	None expected.

RANOLAZINE

BRAND NAMES

Ranexa

BASIC INFORMATION

Habit forming? No
Prescription needed? Yes
Available as generic? No
Drug class: Antianginal

 ## USES

Treatment of chronic angina (chest pain caused by an insufficient supply of oxygen to the heart). It may be used in combination with other drug treatments, such as amlodipine, beta blockers or nitrates.

 ## DOSAGE & USAGE INFORMATION

How to take:
Extended-release tablet—Swallow whole with liquid. It may be taken with or without food. Do not crush, crumble or chew tablet.

When to take:
Usually twice a day at the same times each day. Follow the instructions on your prescription.

If you forget a dose:
Take as soon as you remember. If it is almost time for the next dose, wait for next scheduled dose (don't double this dose).

What drug does:
Exact method of action is unknown. It appears to relax contracted heart muscle and return blood flow to normal levels which relieves the pain.

Time lapse before drug works:
Within a few hours. Dosage may be increased by your doctor as needed for pain relief.

Don't take with:
Any other medicine or any dietary supplement without consulting your doctor or pharmacist.

 ## OVERDOSE

SYMPTOMS:
May include dizziness, "pins and needles" feeling, nausea, vomiting, double vision, confusion and fainting.
WHAT TO DO:
Overdose unlikely to threaten life. If person uses much larger amount than prescribed or if accidentally swallowed, call doctor or poison control center 1-800-222-1222 for help.

 ## POSSIBLE ADVERSE REACTIONS OR SIDE EFFECTS

SYMPTOMS	WHAT TO DO
Life-threatening: None expected.	
Common: Dizziness, headache, constipation, nausea, weakness.	Continue. Call doctor when convenient.
Infrequent: Abdominal pain, tinnitus, vomiting, vertigo, dry mouth, tremor, lightheaded or dizziness when arising from sitting or lying position.	Continue. Call doctor when convenient.
Rare: Palpitations, slow heartbeat, blood in urine, blurred vision, fainting.	Discontinue. Call doctor right away.

WARNINGS & PRECAUTIONS

Don't take if:
You are allergic to ranolazine.

Before you start, consult your doctor if:
- You have pre-existing QT interval prolongation (an abnormality of the heart's electrical system as diagnosed by medical testing).
- You have kidney or liver disease.
- You have uncorrected hypokalemia (low potassium level).
- You have a history of ventricular tachycardia.

Over age 60:
Adverse reactions and side effects may be more frequent and severe than in younger persons. You may need smaller doses at start of therapy.

Pregnancy:
Decide with your doctor if drug benefits justify any possible risk to unborn child. Risk category C (see page xviii).

Breast-feeding:
It is unknown if drug passes into milk. Avoid drug or discontinue nursing until you finish medicine. Consult doctor for advice on maintaining milk supply.

Infants & children:
Safety and effectiveness in children has not been established.

Prolonged use:
No problems expected.

Skin & sunlight:
No problems expected.

Driving, piloting or hazardous work:
Don't drive motor vehicles or pilot aircraft until you learn how medicine affects you. Don't work around dangerous machinery. Don't climb ladders or work in high places.

Discontinuing:
No problems expected. Consult your doctor before stopping the drug.

Others:
- Other antianginal drugs should be tried first due to the risk of QT interval prolongation (abnormality of the heart's electrical system).
- An ECG* should be performed prior to starting the drug and periodically during drug therapy.
- It is important to follow your doctor's advice on diet, exercise, smoking and weight control.
- Advise any doctor or dentist whom you consult that you take this medicine.

POSSIBLE INTERACTION WITH OTHER DRUGS

GENERIC NAME OR DRUG CLASS	COMBINED EFFECT
Antidepressants, tricyclics	Increased effect of tricyclic antidepressant.
Antipsychotics*	Increased effect of antipsychotic.
Digoxin	Increased effect and blood levels of digoxin.
Enzyme inhibitors*	Risk of abnormal heart rhythm. Avoid.
QT interval prolongation-causing drugs,* other	Risk of abnormal heart rhythm. Avoid.
Simvastatin	Increased effect of simvastatin.

POSSIBLE INTERACTION WITH OTHER SUBSTANCES

INTERACTS WITH	COMBINED EFFECT
Alcohol:	None expected.
Beverages: Grapefruit juice.	Risk of abnormal heart rhythm. Avoid.
Cocaine:	Unknown. Best to avoid.
Foods: Grapefruit.	Risk of abnormal heart rhythm. Avoid.
Marijuana:	Unknown. Best to avoid.
Tobacco:	None expected. Persons with angina should not smoke.

RAUWOLFIA ALKALOIDS

GENERIC AND BRAND NAMES

See full list of generic and brand names in the *Generic and Brand Name Directory*, page 897.

BASIC INFORMATION

Habit forming? No
Prescription needed? Yes
Available as generic? Yes
Drug class: Antihypertensive, tranquilizer (rauwolfia alkaloid)

 ## USES

• Treatment for high blood pressure.
• Tranquilizer for mental and emotional disturbances.

 ## DOSAGE & USAGE INFORMATION

How to take:
Tablet—Swallow with liquid or food to lessen stomach irritation. If you can't swallow whole, crumble tablet and take with liquid or food.

When to take:
At the same times each day.

If you forget a dose:
Take as soon as you remember up to 2 hours late. If more than 2 hours, wait for next scheduled dose (don't double this dose).

What drug does:
• Interferes with nerve impulses and relaxes blood vessel muscles, reducing blood pressure.
• Suppresses brain centers that control emotions.

Time lapse before drug works:
3 weeks continual use required to determine effectiveness.

Continued next column

 ## OVERDOSE

SYMPTOMS:
Drowsiness; slow, weak pulse; slow, shallow breathing; diarrhea; coma; flush; low body temperature; pinpoint pupils.
WHAT TO DO:
• **Dial 911 (emergency) for medical help or call poison control center 1-800-222-1222 for instructions.**
• **See emergency information on last 3 pages of this book.**

Don't take with:
Any other medicine or any dietary supplement without consulting your doctor or pharmacist.

 ## POSSIBLE ADVERSE REACTIONS OR SIDE EFFECTS

SYMPTOMS	WHAT TO DO
Life-threatening:	
In case of overdose, see previous column.	
Common:	
• Depression, dizziness.	Continue. Call doctor when convenient.
• Headache, faintness, drowsiness, lethargy, red eyes, stuffy nose, impotence, diminished sex drive, diarrhea, dry mouth.	Continue. Tell doctor at next visit.
Infrequent:	
• Black stool; bloody vomit; chest pain; shortness of breath; irregular or slow heartbeat; stiffness in muscles, bones, joints.	Discontinue. Call doctor right away.
• Trembling hands, foot and leg swelling.	Continue. Call doctor when convenient.
Rare:	
• Rash or itchy skin, sore throat, fever, abdominal pain, nausea, vomiting, unusual bleeding or bruising, jaundice.	Discontinue. Call doctor right away.
• Painful urination, nightmares.	Continue. Call doctor when convenient.

 ## WARNINGS & PRECAUTIONS

Don't take if:
You are allergic to any rauwolfia alkaloid.

Before you start, consult your doctor if:
• You have been depressed.
• You have had peptic ulcer, ulcerative colitis or gallstones.
• You have epilepsy.
• You will have surgery within 2 months, including dental surgery, requiring general or spinal anesthesia.

Over age 60:
Adverse reactions and side effects may be more frequent and severe than in younger persons.

Pregnancy:
Decide with your doctor whether drug benefits justify risk to unborn child. Risk category C (see page xviii).

Breast-feeding:
Drug passes into milk. Avoid drug or discontinue nursing until you finish medicine. Consult doctor for advice on maintaining milk supply.

Infants & children:
Not recommended.

Prolonged use:
* Causes cancer in laboratory animals. Consult your doctor if you have a family or personal history of cancer.
* Talk to your doctor about the need for follow-up medical examinations or laboratory studies.

Skin & sunlight:
No problems expected.

Driving, piloting or hazardous work:
Avoid if you feel drowsy, dizzy or faint. Otherwise, no problems expected.

Discontinuing:
Don't discontinue without consulting doctor. Dose may require gradual reduction if you have taken drug for a long time. Doses of other drugs may also require adjustment.

Others:
* Advise any doctor or dentist whom you consult that you take this medicine.
* Consult your doctor if you do isometric exercises. These raise blood pressure. Drug may intensify blood pressure rise.

 ## POSSIBLE INTERACTION WITH OTHER DRUGS

GENERIC NAME OR DRUG CLASS	COMBINED EFFECT
Anticoagulants,* oral	Unpredictable increased or decreased effect of anticoagulant.
Anticonvulsants*	Serious change in seizure pattern.
Antidepressants*	Increased anti-depressant effect.
Antihistamines*	Increased anti-histamine effect.
Antihypertensives,* other	Increased rauwolfia effect.
Aspirin	Decreased aspirin effect.
Beta-adrenergic blocking agents*	Increased rauwolfia alkaloid effect. Excessive sedation.
Carteolol	Increased anti-hypertensive effect.

Central nervous system (CNS) depressants*	Increased CNS depression.
Clozapine	Toxic effect on the central nervous system.
Digitalis preparations*	Possible irregular heartbeat.
Dronabinol	Increased effects of both drugs. Avoid.
Ethinamate	Dangerous increased effects of ethinamate. Avoid combining.
Fluoxetine	Increased depressant effects of both drugs.
Guanfacine	May increase depressant effects of either medicine.
Leucovorin	High alcohol content of leucovorin may cause adverse effects.
Levodopa	Decreased levodopa effect.

Continued on page 929

 ## POSSIBLE INTERACTION WITH OTHER SUBSTANCES

INTERACTS WITH	COMBINED EFFECT
Alcohol:	Increased intoxication. Use with extreme caution.
Beverages: Carbonated drinks.	Decreased rauwolfia alkaloid effect.
Cocaine:	Increased risk of heart block and high blood pressure.
Foods: Spicy foods.	Possible digestive upset.
Marijuana:	Occasional use—Mild drowsiness. Daily use—Moderate drowsiness, low blood pressure, depression.
Tobacco:	None expected.

RENIN INHIBITORS

GENERIC AND BRAND NAMES

ALISKIREN
Tekturna   Tekturna HCT

BASIC INFORMATION

Habit forming? No
Prescription needed? Yes
Available as generic? No
Drug class: Antihypertensive; renin inhibitor

USES

Treatment for hypertension (high blood pressure). May be used alone or along with other antihypertensive medications.

DOSAGE & USAGE INFORMATION

How to take:
Tablet—Swallow with liquid. May be taken with or without food. Do not remove the special drying agent from the bottle.

When to take:
Once daily at the same time each day, or as directed by your doctor.

If you forget a dose:
Take as soon as you remember. If it is almost time for the next dose, then skip the missed dose and wait for your next scheduled dose (don't double this dose).

What drug does:
It inhibits renin, a kidney enzyme associated with the regulation of blood pressure. This helps the blood vessels to relax and widen so blood pressure is lowered.

Time lapse before drug works:
It starts working within a few hours, but may take several weeks for full effectiveness.

Don't take with:
Any other medicine or any dietary supplement without consulting your doctor or pharmacist.

OVERDOSE

SYMPTOMS:
Unknown. Could cause very low blood pressure (hypotension).
WHAT TO DO:
Overdose unlikely to threaten life. If person uses much larger amount than prescribed or if accidentally swallowed, call doctor or poison control center 1-800-222-1222 for help.

POSSIBLE ADVERSE REACTIONS OR SIDE EFFECTS

SYMPTOMS	WHAT TO DO
Life-threatening: Rare allergic reaction (hives, itching, rash, trouble breathing, tightness in chest, swelling of lips or tongue or throat).	Seek emergency treatment immediately.
Common: Diarrhea, headache.	Continue. Call doctor when convenient.
Infrequent: Cough, rash.	Continue. Call doctor when convenient.
Rare: • Low blood pressure (feeling faint, dizzy or lightheaded), seizure.	Discontinue. Call doctor right away.
• Abdominal pain, bloating, heartburn, nausea, burping, reflux, fatigue, upper respiratory tract infection, back pain, runny or stuffy nose.	Continue. Call doctor when convenient.

WARNINGS & PRECAUTIONS

Don't take if:
- You are allergic to aliskiren.
- You are pregnant.

Before you start, consult your doctor if:
- You have kidney (renal) disease or disorder.
- You have a history of dialysis, nephrotic syndrome, or renovascular hypertension (high blood pressure caused by narrowing of the arteries that carry blood to the kidneys).
- You have hyperkalemia (high level of potassium in the blood).
- You plan to become pregnant.
- You are allergic to any medication, food or other substance.

Over age 60:
No special problems expected.

Pregnancy:
Decide with your doctor if drug benefits justify any possible risk to unborn child. When used in the second and third trimesters, the drug can cause injury and even death to the developing fetus. Risk category C—first trimester and D—second and third trimesters (see page xviii).

Breast-feeding:
It is unknown if drug passes into milk. Avoid drug or discontinue nursing. Consult doctor for advice.

Infants & children:
Not approved for children under age 18.

Prolonged use:
- No special problems expected. Hypertension usually requires life-long treatment.
- Schedule regular doctor visits to determine if drug is continuing to be effective in controlling the hypertension and to check your potassium levels and kidney function.

Skin & sunlight:
No special problems expected.

Driving, piloting or hazardous work:
Use caution if you feel dizzy or are experiencing other side effects.

Discontinuing:
Don't discontinue without consulting your doctor, even if you feel well. You can have hypertension without feeling any symptoms. Untreated high blood pressure can cause serious problems.

Others:
- Advise any doctor or dentist whom you consult that you take this medicine. May interfere with the accuracy of some medical tests.
- Follow any diet or exercise plan your doctor prescribes. It can help control hypertension.
- Get up slowly from a sitting or lying position to avoid any dizziness, faintness or lightheadedness.

POSSIBLE INTERACTION WITH OTHER DRUGS

GENERIC NAME OR DRUG CLASS	COMBINED EFFECT
Antihypertensives, other*	Increased antihypertensive effect.
Furosemide	May decrease furosemide effect.

POSSIBLE INTERACTION WITH OTHER SUBSTANCES

INTERACTS WITH	COMBINED EFFECT
Alcohol:	None expected.
Beverages:	None expected.
Cocaine:	Unknown effect. Avoid.
Foods:	None expected.
Marijuana:	Unknown effect. Avoid.
Tobacco:	None expected. Best to avoid.

*See Glossary

RESERPINE, HYDRALAZINE & HYDROCHLOROTHIAZIDE

BRAND NAMES

Cam-Ap-Es	Serpazide
Cherapas	Tri-Hydroserpine
Ser-A-Gen	Unipres
Seralazide	

BASIC INFORMATION

Habit forming? No
Prescription needed? Yes
Available as generic? Yes
Drug class: Antihypertensive

USES

* Treatment for high blood pressure and congestive heart failure.
* Reduces fluid retention (edema).

DOSAGE & USAGE INFORMATION

How to take:
Tablet—Swallow with liquid. If you can't swallow whole, crumble and take with liquid or food.

When to take:
At the same times each day.

If you forget a dose:
Take as soon as you remember up to 2 hours late. If more than 2 hours, wait for next scheduled dose (don't double this dose).

What drug does:
* Relaxes blood vessels, reducing blood pressure.
* Suppresses brain centers that control emotions.
* Reduces body fluid and relaxes arteries, lowering blood pressure.

Time lapse before drug works:
Regular use for several weeks may be necessary to determine drug's effectiveness.

Continued next column

OVERDOSE

SYMPTOMS:
Drowsiness; slow, shallow breathing; pinpoint pupils; diarrhea; flush; low body temperature; rapid, weak heartbeat; fainting; extreme weakness; cold, sweaty skin; cramps, coma.
WHAT TO DO:
* **Dial 911 (emergency) for medical help or call poison control center 1-800-222-1222 for instructions.**
* **See emergency information on last 3 pages of this book.**

Don't take with:
* Nonprescription drugs containing alcohol without consulting doctor.
* Any other medicine or any dietary supplement without consulting your doctor or pharmacist.

POSSIBLE ADVERSE REACTIONS OR SIDE EFFECTS

SYMPTOMS	WHAT TO DO
Life-threatening:	
Rapid or irregular heartbeat, weak pulse, fainting, black stool, black or bloody vomit, chest pain.	Discontinue. Seek emergency treatment.
Common:	
• Nausea, vomiting.	Discontinue. Call doctor right away.
• Headache, diarrhea, drowsiness, runny nose, appetite loss.	Continue. Call doctor when convenient.
Infrequent:	
• Blurred vision, chest pain, abdominal pain, rash, hives, joint pain.	Discontinue. Call doctor right away.
• Dizziness; mood change; headache; dry mouth; weakness; tiredness; weight gain or loss; eyes red, watery, irritated; confusion; constipation; red or flushed face; joint stiffness; depression; anxiety; foot and leg swelling.	Continue. Call doctor when convenient.
Rare:	
• Jaundice; unexplained bleeding or bruising; sore throat, fever, mouth sores; weakness and faintness when arising from bed or chair.	Discontinue. Call doctor right away.
• Numbness, tingling, burning feeling in feet and hands; nasal congestion; impotence; nightmares.	Continue. Call doctor when convenient.

WARNINGS & PRECAUTIONS

Don't take if:
You are allergic to any rauwolfia alkaloid, hydralazine, any thiazide diuretic drug,* or tartrazine dye.

RESERPINE, HYDRALAZINE & HYDROCHLOROTHIAZIDE

Before you start, consult your doctor if:
- You have been depressed.
- You have had peptic ulcer, ulcerative colitis, gallstones, kidney disease or impaired kidney function, lupus or a stroke.
- You have epilepsy, gout, liver, pancreas or kidney disorder.
- You feel pain in chest, neck or arms on physical exertion.
- You are allergic to any sulfa drug.*
- You will have surgery within 2 months, including dental surgery, requiring general or spinal anesthesia.

Over age 60:
Adverse reactions and side effects may be more frequent and severe than in younger persons, especially dizziness and excessive potassium loss.

Pregnancy:
Decide with your doctor if drug benefits justify risk to unborn child. Risk category C (see page xviii).

Breast-feeding:
Drug passes into milk. Avoid drug or discontinue nursing until you finish medicine. Consult doctor.

Infants & children:
Not recommended.

Prolonged use:
- Causes cancer in laboratory animals. Consult your doctor if you have a family or personal history of cancer.
- Possible psychosis.
- May cause lupus; numbness, tingling in hands or feet.
- Talk to your doctor about the need for follow-up medical examinations or laboratory studies.

Skin & sunlight:
One or more drugs in this group may cause rash or intensify sunburn in areas exposed to sun or ultraviolet light (photosensitivity reaction). Avoid overexposure. Notify doctor if reaction occurs.

Driving, piloting or hazardous work:
Don't drive or pilot aircraft until you learn how medicine affects you. Don't work around dangerous machinery. Don't climb ladders or work in high places. Danger increases if you drink alcohol or take medicine affecting alertness and reflexes.

Discontinuing:
Don't discontinue without consulting doctor. Dose may require gradual reduction if you have taken drug for a long time. Doses of other drugs may also require adjustment.

Others:
- Consult your doctor if you do isometric exercises. These raise blood pressure. Drug may intensify blood pressure rise.

- Vitamin B-6 supplement may be advisable. Consult doctor.
- Hot weather and fever may cause dehydration and drop in blood pressure. Dose may require temporary adjustment. Weigh daily and report any unexpected weight decreases to your doctor.
- Advise any doctor or dentist whom you consult that you take this medicine.
- May cause rise in uric acid, leading to gout.
- May cause blood sugar rise in diabetics.
- Some products contain tartrazine dye. Avoid, especially if you are allergic to aspirin.

 ## POSSIBLE INTERACTION WITH OTHER DRUGS

GENERIC NAME OR DRUG CLASS	COMBINED EFFECT
Acebutolol	Possible increased effects of drugs.
Allopurinol	Decreased allopurinol effect.

Continued on page 930

 ## POSSIBLE INTERACTION WITH OTHER SUBSTANCES

INTERACTS WITH	COMBINED EFFECT
Alcohol:	Increased intoxication. Avoid.
Beverages: Carbonated drinks.	Decreased reserpine effect.
Cocaine:	Dangerous blood pressure rise. Avoid.
Foods: Spicy foods.	Possible digestive upset.
Licorice.	Excessive potassium loss that causes dangerous heart rhythms.
Marijuana:	Weakness on standing. May increase blood pressure. Occasional use— Mild drowsiness. Daily use—Moderate drowsiness, low blood pressure, depression.
Tobacco:	Possible angina attacks.

---

*See Glossary

RETINOIDS (Oral)

GENERIC AND BRAND NAMES

ACITRETIN
Soriatane

BASIC INFORMATION

Habit forming? No
Prescription needed? Yes
Available as generic? No
Drug class: Antipsoriatic

 USES

- Treats psoriasis in patients who don't respond well to standard or usual treatment. It may be combined with phototherapy or other antipsoriatic drugs.
- It may be used to improve arthritis symptoms that accompany psoriasis.
- Treatment for certain other skin disorders.

 DOSAGE & USAGE INFORMATION

How to take:
Capsule—Swallow with liquid and take with food to lessen stomach irritation.

When to take:
At the same times each day, usually twice a day.

If you forget a dose:
One dose a day—Take as soon as you remember, up to 12 hours late. If more than 12 hours, wait for next scheduled dose (don't double this dose).

What drug does:
The exact mechanism of action is unknown. The drug appears to help growth of normal skin cells. It also has anti-inflammatory action.

Time lapse before drug works:
The skin may show improvement in 2 weeks, but full benefit can take 2 to 3 months.

Continued next column

 OVERDOSE

SYMPTOMS:
May include nausea, vomiting, severe headache, drowsiness, loss of balance, itching, irritability.
WHAT TO DO:
Overdose unlikely to threaten life. If person takes much larger amount than prescribed, call doctor, poison control center 1-800-222-1222 or hospital emergency room for help.

Don't take with:
Any other medicine or any dietary supplement without consulting your doctor or pharmacist.

 POSSIBLE ADVERSE REACTIONS OR SIDE EFFECTS

SYMPTOMS	WHAT TO DO
Life-threatening: None expected.	
Common:	
• Severe headache, severe nausea or vomiting.	Discontinue. Call doctor right away.
• Stiffness or pain in bones or joints or muscles, mild headaches, lip symptoms (chapped, redness, sore, cracking, swollen), dryness of nose or eyes, hair loss, skin sensitivity to sunlight, sore mouth, nosebleeds, peeling or scaling (eyelids, palms, fingertips, and soles of feet), runny nose, sore or swollen gums, thirstiness.	Continue. Call doctor when convenient.
Infrequent:	
• Blurred vision, eye pain.	Discontinue. Call doctor right away.
• Fingernails loose or skin around them is sore or red, loss of eyebrows or eye lashes, redness of eye or inside eyelid, eyes watery or sensitive to light, swollen eyelids, problem with contact lens use, psoriasis gets worse in early drug use.	Continue. Call doctor when convenient.
Rare:	
• Double vision, decreased night vision, yellow skin or eyes, stomach pain, dark urine, unusual bruising.	Discontinue. Call doctor right away.
• Skin symptoms (spots, infection, sores, stinging, odd odor, burning, rash), ear pain or itching, flu-like symptoms, stye, cough or hoarseness, trouble in speaking, vaginal discharge or itching or irritation.	Continue. Call doctor when convenient.

WARNINGS & PRECAUTIONS

Don't take if:
- You are female and pregnant or may get pregnant in the next 3 years. Severe birth defects have occurred while using and after discontinuing this drug. Don't start drug until you have 2 negative pregnancy tests. Read all the prescribing information carefully.
- If you are allergic to retinoids or parabens (used as preservative in gelatin capsule).

Before you start, consult your doctor if:
- You have high cholesterol or triglycerides.
- You have diabetes or are an alcoholic.
- You have had problems with too much vitamin A in the body (hypervitaminosis).
- You are a female of reproductive age.
- You have kidney, liver or pancreas disease.

Over age 60:
Adverse reactions and side effects may be more frequent and severe than in younger persons. You may need smaller doses for shorter periods of time.

Pregnancy:
- Risk to unborn child outweighs drug benefits. The drug may cause severe birth defects. Don't use. Risk category X (see page xviii).
- Stop taking the drug and consult your doctor right away if you become pregnant while taking the drug or within 3 years after stopping.

Breast-feeding:
The drug may pass into milk. Avoid drug or discontinue nursing until you finish medicine. Consult doctor for advice on maintaining milk supply.

Infants & children:
It may prevent normal bone growth in children. Use only under close medical supervision.

Prolonged use:
Talk to your doctor about follow-up medical exams or laboratory studies to check blood lipids, liver function, eyes or pregnancy tests.

Skin & sunlight:
May cause rash or intensify sunburn in areas exposed to sun or ultraviolet light (photosensitivity reaction). Use sunscreen with SPF of 15 or higher. Avoid overexposure. Notify doctor if reaction occurs.

Driving, piloting or hazardous work:
Don't drive motor vehicles or pilot aircraft until you learn how medicine affects you. Don't work around dangerous machinery. Don't climb ladders or work in high places.

Discontinuing:
Drug use is discontinued once skin has healed sufficiently. Your psoriasis may recur after stopping the drug. Consult doctor for advice. Don't use leftover drug without doctor's approval.

Others:
- Certain methods of birth control may fail while using this drug, including tubal ligation and progestin (minipill) preparations. Other birth control methods may be affected also. Use two different methods of birth control.
- Don't donate blood during drug treatment or for 3 years thereafter.
- Advise any doctor or dentist whom you consult that you take this medicine.
- May cause liver damage or problems in controlling blood sugar.
- Laboratory blood studies for cholesterol and triglyceride levels should be obtained prior to and during treatment.
- Avoid skin products that cause skin dryness or sensitivity. Consult your doctor for advice.

POSSIBLE INTERACTION WITH OTHER DRUGS

GENERIC NAME OR DRUG CLASS	COMBINED EFFECT
Acne preparations*	Excessive drying effect on skin.
Contraceptives, oral* (progestin-only type)	Decreased effect of oral contraceptive.
Isotretinoin	Increased risk of adverse reactions.
Methotrexate	Risk of hepatitis.
Phenytoin	Increased effect of phenytoin.
Tetracyclines*	Risk of pseudotumor cerebri (pressure in the brain).
Tretinoin	Increased risk of adverse reactions.
Vitamin A	Increased risk of adverse reactions.

POSSIBLE INTERACTION WITH OTHER SUBSTANCES

INTERACTS WITH	COMBINED EFFECT
Alcohol:	Risk of severe side effects during drug use and after stopping. Avoid alcohol.
Beverages:	None expected.
Cocaine:	Unknown. Avoid.
Foods:	None expected.
Marijuana:	Unknown. Avoid.
Tobacco:	None expected.

*See Glossary

RETINOIDS (Topical)

GENERIC AND BRAND NAMES

ADAPALENE
  Differin
  Epiduo
BEXAROTENE
  Targretin
TAZAROTENE
  Avage
  Tazorac
TRETINOIN
  Atralin Gel
  Avita
  Renova
  Retin-A Cream
  Retin-A Cream
    Regimen Kit
  Retin-A Gel
  Retin-A Gel
    Regimen Kit

TRETINOIN (Con't)
  Retin-A Solution
  Retinoic Acid
  Solage
  Stieva-A Cream
  Stieva-A Cream
    Forte
  Stieva-A Ge
  Stieva-A Solution
  Tretin-X
  Tri-Luma
  Vitamin A Acid
    Cream
  Vitamin A Acid Gel
  Ziana Gel

BASIC INFORMATION

Habit forming? No
Prescription needed? Yes
Available as generic? Yes, for some
Drug class: Antiacne (topical), antipsoriatic

USES

* Treatment for acne, psoriasis, ichthyosis, keratosis, folliculitis, flat warts.
* Treatment for sun-damaged skin (wrinkles), mottled skin, rough skin and pigmented skin.
* Bexarotene treats skin cancer (cutaneous T cell lymphoma).
* Tri-Luma is a combination drug—tretinoin and fluocinolone and hydroquinone (not covered in this book).
* Solage is a combination drug—tretinoin plus mequinol (which is not covered in this topic).

OVERDOSE

SYMPTOMS:
None expected.
WHAT TO DO:
* If person accidentally swallows drug, dial 911 (emergency) for medical help or call poison control center 1-800-222-1222 for instructions.
* See emergency information on last 3 pages of this book.

DOSAGE & USAGE INFORMATION

How to use:
Wash skin with nonmedicated soap, pat dry, wait 20 minutes before applying.
* Cream or gel—Apply to affected areas with fingertips and rub in gently.
* Solution—Apply to affected areas with gauze pad or cotton swab. Avoid getting too wet so medicine doesn't drip into eyes or mouth, onto lips or inside nose.
* Follow manufacturer's directions on container.

When to use:
Apply once daily, usually in the evening before going to bed.

If you forget a dose:
Use as soon as you remember if it is still the same day. If more than 12 hours late, wait for the next dose (don't double this dose).

What drug does:
Helps control acne inflammation and prevent new acne outbreaks. Increases skin cell turnover so skin layer peels off more easily.

Time lapse before drug works:
May require 2 to 6 weeks for minimum benefit and 3 to 12 months for full benefit.

Don't use with:
Any other topical medicine without consulting your doctor or pharmacist.

POSSIBLE ADVERSE REACTIONS OR SIDE EFFECTS

SYMPTOMS	WHAT TO DO
Life-threatening: None expected.	
Common: • Mild redness, itching, chapping, dryness of skin during first few weeks of use.	Depending on severity, may reduce frequency of use.
• Worsening of acne or psoriasis during first few weeks of use (due to action of the drug on previous unseen skin breakouts).	Expected effect. No action necessary.
Infrequent: Painful skin irritation, darkening or lightening of skin where treated.	Discontinue. Call doctor when convenient.
Rare: None expected.	

WARNINGS & PRECAUTIONS

Don't take if:
You are allergic to topical retinoids or any of the components of the gel product.

Before you start, consult your doctor if:
- You are using any other prescription or nonprescription medicine for the skin.
- You are using abrasive skin cleansers or medicated cosmetics.

Over age 60:
No problems expected.

Pregnancy:
- Adapalene and tretinoin—Discuss with your doctor if benefits outweigh risks to unborn child. Risk category C (see page xviii).
- Bexarotene and tazarotene—Risk to unborn child outweighs drug's benefits. Don't use. Risk category X (see page xviii).

Breast-feeding:
Effect unknown. Consult doctor.

Infants & children:
Not recommended.

Prolonged use:
No problems expected.

Skin & sunlight:
- May cause rash or intensify sunburn in areas exposed to sun or ultraviolet light. Avoid over-exposure. Notify doctor if reaction occurs.
- If you are normally exposed to considerable sunlight, use extra caution. Use broad spectrum of sunscreen on treated areas and wear protective clothing (e.g., hat).

Driving, piloting or hazardous work:
No problems expected.

Discontinuing:
- May be unnecessary to finish medicine. Discontinue when acne improves. For some patients, this medicine may be used indefinitely to control acne.
- If skin problem doesn't improve after first few weeks of use, consult doctor.

Others:
- Cold or windy weather may further irritate the skin. Avoid if possible.
- Products with a drying effect on the skin may cause irritation when used with retinoids. These include cosmetics, abrasive soaps and cleansers, astringents, and topical products that contain alcohol, spices or lime.
- Advise any doctor or dentist whom you consult that you use this medicine.
- Brand name Solage also contains the drug mequinol.
- Don't apply drug to skin area that has cuts, abrasions, a rash or is sunburned.

POSSIBLE INTERACTION WITH OTHER DRUGS

GENERIC NAME OR DRUG CLASS	COMBINED EFFECT
Antiacne topical* preparations, other	Excessive skin irritation.
Cosmetics (medicated)	Severe skin irritation.
Insect repellents containing DEET	Repellent can be absorbed into skin.
Skin-peeling agents (salicylic acid, sulfur, resorcinol)	Excessive skin irritation.
Skin preparations with alcohol	Severe skin irritation.
Soaps or cleansers (abrasive)	Severe skin irritation.

POSSIBLE INTERACTION WITH OTHER SUBSTANCES

INTERACTS WITH	COMBINED EFFECT
Alcohol:	None expected.
Beverages:	None expected.
Cocaine:	None expected.
Foods:	None expected.
Marijuana:	None expected.
Tobacco:	None expected.

RIBAVIRIN

BRAND NAMES

Tribavirin   Virazole
Virazid

BASIC INFORMATION

Habit forming? No
Prescription needed? Yes
Available as generic? Yes
Drug class: Antiviral

 ## USES

- Treats severe viral pneumonia.
- Treats respiratory syncytial virus (RSV) infections in hospitalized infants or children.
- Treats influenza A and B with some success.
- Does not treat other viruses such as the common cold.
- Brand names Rebetol and Ribasphere are used to treat chronic hepatitis C when combined with another drug. The information in this chart does not include any facts about these two brands. Your doctor will provide you the information and instructions and will follow your therapy carefully.

 ## DOSAGE & USAGE INFORMATION

How to take:
By inhalation of a fine mist through mouth. Requires a special sprayer attached to oxygen mask, face mask for infants or hood.

When to take:
As ordered by your doctor.

If you forget a dose:
Use as soon as you remember.

What drug does:
Kills virus or prevents its growth.

Time lapse before drug works:
Begins working in 1 hour. May require treatment for 12 to 18 hours per day for 3 to 7 days.

Don't take with:
Any other medicine or any dietary supplement without consulting your doctor or pharmacist.

 ## OVERDOSE

SYMPTOMS:
None expected.
WHAT TO DO:
Overdose unlikely to threaten life. If person uses much larger amount than prescribed or if accidentally swallowed, call doctor or poison control center 1-800-222-1222 for help.

 ## POSSIBLE ADVERSE REACTIONS OR SIDE EFFECTS

SYMPTOMS	WHAT TO DO
Life-threatening:	
None expected.	
Common:	
None expected.	
Infrequent:	
• Unusual tiredness or weakness.	Discontinue. Call doctor right away.
• Headache, insomnia, appetite loss, nausea.	Continue. Call doctor when convenient.
Rare:	
Skin irritation or rash.	Continue. Call doctor when convenient.

WARNINGS & PRECAUTIONS

Don't take if:
You are allergic to ribavirin.

Before you start, consult your doctor if:
* You are now on low-salt, low-sugar or other special diet.
* You have severe anemia.

Over age 60:
Adverse reactions and side effects may be more frequent and severe than in younger persons. Ask doctor about smaller doses.

Pregnancy:
Risk to unborn child outweighs drug benefits. Don't use. Risk category X (see page xviii).

Breast-feeding:
Drug may pass into milk. Avoid drug or discontinue nursing until you finish medicine. Consult doctor for advice on maintaining milk supply.

Infants & children:
Use only under close medical supervision.

Prolonged use:
No problems expected.

Skin & sunlight:
No special problems expected.

Driving, piloting or hazardous work:
Don't drive or pilot aircraft until you learn how medicine affects you. Don't work around dangerous machinery. Don't climb ladders or work in high places. Danger increases if you drink alcohol or take medicine affecting alertness and reflexes, such as antihistamines, tranquilizers, sedatives, pain medicine, narcotics and mind-altering drugs.

Discontinuing:
Don't discontinue without consulting doctor. Dose may require gradual reduction if you have taken drug for a long time. Doses of other drugs may also require adjustment.

Others:
* Health care workers exposed to ribavirin may experience headache; eye itching, redness or swelling.
* Female health care workers who are pregnant or may become pregnant should avoid exposure to drug.
* The information in this chart does not cover or include the brand names Rebetol or Ribasphere. Your doctor must provide that information for you.

POSSIBLE INTERACTION WITH OTHER DRUGS

GENERIC NAME OR DRUG CLASS	COMBINED EFFECT
Zidovudine	Decreased effect of ribavirin and zidovudine.

POSSIBLE INTERACTION WITH OTHER SUBSTANCES

INTERACTS WITH	COMBINED EFFECT
Alcohol:	None expected.
Beverages:	None expected.
Cocaine:	None expected.
Foods:	None expected.
Marijuana:	None expected.
Tobacco:	None expected.

RIBOFLAVIN (Vitamin B-2)

BRAND NAMES

Numerous brands of single vitamin and multivitamin combinations are available.

BASIC INFORMATION

Habit forming? No
Prescription needed? No
Available as generic? Yes
Drug class: Vitamin supplement

 ## USES

- Dietary supplement to ensure normal growth and health.
- Dietary supplement to treat symptoms caused by deficiency of B-2: sores in mouth, eyes sensitive to light, itching and peeling skin.

 ## DOSAGE & USAGE INFORMATION

How to take:
Tablet—Swallow with liquid or food to lessen stomach irritation. If you can't swallow whole, crumble tablet and take with liquid or food.

When to take:
At the same times each day.

If you forget a dose:
Take as soon as you remember. Resume regular schedule. Don't double dose.

What drug does:
Promotes normal growth and health.

Time lapse before drug works:
Requires continual intake.

Don't take with:
Any other medicine or any dietary supplement without consulting your doctor or pharmacist.

 ## OVERDOSE

SYMPTOMS:
Dark urine, nausea, vomiting.
WHAT TO DO:
Overdose unlikely to threaten life. If person uses much larger amount than prescribed or if accidentally swallowed, call doctor or poison control center 1-800-222-1222 for help.

 ## POSSIBLE ADVERSE REACTIONS OR SIDE EFFECTS

SYMPTOMS	WHAT TO DO
Life-threatening: None expected.	
Common: Urine yellow in color.	No action necessary.
Infrequent: None expected.	
Rare: None expected.	

WARNINGS & PRECAUTIONS

Don't take if:
- You are allergic to any B vitamin.
- You have chronic kidney failure.

Before you start, consult your doctor if:
You are pregnant or plan pregnancy.

Over age 60:
No problems expected.

Pregnancy:
Take within recommended guidelines. Consult doctor. Risk category A (see page xviii).

Breast-feeding:
Take within recommended guidelines. Consult doctor.

Infants & children:
Consult doctor.

Prolonged use:
No problems expected.

Skin & sunlight:
No problems expected.

Driving, piloting or hazardous work:
No problems expected.

Discontinuing:
No problems expected.

Others:
- Advise any doctor or dentist whom you consult that you take this medicine.
- A balanced diet should provide all the vitamin B-2 a healthy person needs and makes supplements unnecessary during periods of good health. Best sources are milk, meats and green leafy vegetables.

POSSIBLE INTERACTION WITH OTHER DRUGS

GENERIC NAME OR DRUG CLASS	COMBINED EFFECT
Anticholinergics*	Possible increased riboflavin absorption.
Antidepressants, tricyclic*	Decreased riboflavin effect.
Phenothiazines*	Decreased riboflavin effect.
Probenecid	Decreased riboflavin effect.

POSSIBLE INTERACTION WITH OTHER SUBSTANCES

INTERACTS WITH	COMBINED EFFECT
Alcohol:	Prevents uptake and absorption of vitamin B-2.
Beverages:	None expected.
Cocaine:	None expected.
Foods:	None expected.
Marijuana:	None expected.
Tobacco:	Prevents absorption of vitamin B-2 and other vitamins and nutrients.

*See Glossary

RIFAMYCINS

GENERIC AND BRAND NAMES

RIFAMPIN
  Rifadin
  Rifamate
  Rifampicin
  Rimactane

RIFAPENTINE
  Priftin

BASIC INFORMATION

Habit forming? No
Prescription needed? Yes
Available as generic? Yes
Drug class: Antibacterial, antitubercular

 ## USES

Treatment for tuberculosis and other infections. Used in combination with other antitubercular medications.

 ## DOSAGE & USAGE INFORMATION

How to take:
Capsule or tablet—Swallow with liquid or food. If you can't swallow whole, open capsule or crumble tablet and take with liquid or small amount of food. For child, mix with small amount of applesauce or jelly.

When to take:
1 hour before or 2 hours after a meal.

If you forget a dose:
Take as soon as you remember up to 2 hours late. If more than 2 hours, wait for next scheduled dose (don't double this dose).

What drug does:
Prevents multiplication of tuberculosis germs.

Continued next column

 ## OVERDOSE

SYMPTOMS:
Slow, shallow breathing; weak, rapid pulse; cold, sweaty skin; coma.
WHAT TO DO:
* **Dial 911 (emergency) for medical help or call poison control center 1-800-222-1222 for instructions.**
* **If person is unconscious, check breathing and pulse. If not breathing, begin mouth-to-mouth rescue breathing. If heart is not beating, begin chest compressions.**
* **See emergency information on last 3 pages of this book.**

Time lapse before drug works:
Usually 2 weeks. May require 1 to 2 years without missed doses for maximum benefit.

Don't take with:
Any other medicine or any dietary supplement without consulting your doctor or pharmacist.

 ## POSSIBLE ADVERSE REACTIONS OR SIDE EFFECTS

SYMPTOMS	WHAT TO DO
Life-threatening:	
In case of overdose, see previous column.	
Common:	
• Diarrhea; reddish urine, stool, saliva, sweat and tears.	Continue. Call doctor when convenient.
• Blood in urine, joint pain, back or side pain, swelling of feet or legs.	Continue, but call doctor right away.
Infrequent:	
• Rash; flushed, itchy skin of face and scalp; blurred vision; difficulty breathing; nausea, vomiting; abdominal cramps; tiredness; bleeding or bruising.	Continue, but call doctor right away.
• Dizziness, unsteady gait, confusion, muscle or bone pain, heartburn, flatulence, chills, headache, fever, mood or behavior changes.	Continue. Call doctor when convenient.
Rare:	
• Sore throat, mouth or tongue; jaundice.	Discontinue. Call doctor right away.
• Appetite loss, less urination.	Continue. Call doctor when convenient.

 ## WARNINGS & PRECAUTIONS

Don't take if:
* You are allergic to any of the rifamycins.
* You wear soft contact lenses.

Before you start, consult your doctor if:
You are alcoholic or have liver disease.

Over age 60:
Adverse reactions and side effects may be more frequent and severe than in younger persons.

Pregnancy:
Decide with your doctor if drug benefits justify risk to unborn child. Risk category C (see page xviii).

Breast-feeding:
Effect unknown. Consult doctor.

Infants & children:
Use only under medical supervision.

Prolonged use:
* You may become more susceptible to infections caused by germs not responsive to rifamycins.
* Talk to your doctor about the need for follow-up medical examinations or laboratory studies to check liver function.

Skin & sunlight:
No problems expected.

Driving, piloting or hazardous work:
Don't drive or pilot aircraft until you learn how medicine affects you. Don't work around dangerous machinery. Don't climb ladders or work in high places. Danger increases if you drink alcohol or take medicine affecting alertness and reflexes, such as antihistamines, tranquilizers, sedatives, pain medicine, narcotics and mind-altering drugs.

Discontinuing:
Don't discontinue without doctor's advice until you complete prescribed dose, even though symptoms diminish or disappear.

Others:
* Reddish tears may discolor soft contact lenses.
* Advise any doctor or dentist you consult that you are using this medication.

 POSSIBLE INTERACTION WITH OTHER DRUGS

GENERIC NAME OR DRUG CLASS	COMBINED EFFECT
Adrenocorticoids, systemic	Decreased adrenocorticoid effect.
Anticoagulants,* oral	Decreased anticoagulant effect.
Antidepressants,* tricyclic	Decreased antidepressant effect.
Antidiabetics,* oral	Decreased antidiabetic effect.
Antifungals,* azole	Decreased antifungal effect.
Barbiturates*	Decreased barbiturate effect.
Calcium channel* blockers	Decreased channel blocker effect.
Chloramphenicol	Decreased effect of both drugs.
Clarithromycin	Decreased antibiotic effect.
Clofibrate	Decreased clofibrate effect.
Clozapine	Toxic effect on bone marrow.
Contraceptives, oral*	Decreased contraceptive effect.
Cyclosporine	Decreased effect of both drugs.
Dapsone	Decreased dapsone effect.
Diazepam	Decreased diazepam effect.
Digitalis preparations*	Decreased digitoxin effect.
Disopyramide	Decreased disopyramide effect.
Doxycycline	Decreased antibiotic effect.
Estrogens* (including contraceptive pills)	Decreased effect of both drugs.
Haloperidol	Decreased haloperidol effect.
Hepatotoxics*	Increased risk of liver toxicity.
Isoniazid	Possible toxicity to liver.
Leflunomide	Increased risk of leflunomide toxicity.
Levothyroxine	Decreased levothyroxine effect.
Methadone	Decreased methadone effect.
Mexiletine	Decreased mexiletine effect.
Non-nucleoside reverse transcriptase inhibitors	May require dosage adjustment of rifampin.

Continued on page 931

 POSSIBLE INTERACTION WITH OTHER SUBSTANCES

INTERACTS WITH	COMBINED EFFECT
Alcohol:	Possible toxicity to liver.
Beverages:	None expected.
Cocaine:	None expected.
Foods:	None expected.
Marijuana:	None expected.
Tobacco:	None expected.

*See Glossary

RIFAXIMIN

BRAND NAMES

Xifaxan

BASIC INFORMATION

Habit forming? No
Prescription needed? Yes
Available as generic? No
Drug class: Antidiarrheal; antibacterial

 ## USES

Treatment for diarrhea (often called travelers' diarrhea) caused by drinking fluids or eating food contaminated by a bacteria (most often *Escherichia coli*). It may not be effective for diarrhea caused by other bacteria or viruses.

 ## DOSAGE & USAGE INFORMATION

How to take:
Tablet—Swallow with liquid. Take with or without food.

When to take:
Three times a day at the same times each day. It is normally taken for three days.

If you forget a dose:
Take as soon as you remember. If it is almost time for the next dose, wait for that dose (don't double this dose) and resume regular schedule.

What drug does:
It works in the gastrointestinal tract to kill the bacteria causing the diarrhea. It is not absorbed into the bloodstream like most antibiotic drugs.

Time lapse before drug works:
Starts working in a few hours, but takes three days to cure the infection being treated.

Don't take with:
Any other medicine or any dietary supplement without consulting your doctor or pharmacist.

 ## OVERDOSE

SYMPTOMS:
Unknown, but may include: nausea, vomiting, diarrhea and abdominal discomfort.
WHAT TO DO:
Overdose unlikely to threaten life. If person uses much larger amount than prescribed or if accidentally swallowed, call doctor or poison control center 1-800-222-1222 for help.

 ## POSSIBLE ADVERSE REACTIONS OR SIDE EFFECTS

SYMPTOMS	WHAT TO DO
Life-threatening:	
Rare allergic reaction—Breathing difficulty; closing of the throat; swelling of hands, feet, face, lips or tongue; hives.	Discontinue. Seek emergency treatment.
Common:	
Headache.	Continue. Call doctor if symptoms persist.
Infrequent:	
Nausea, vomiting, stomach discomfort, gas, straining with bowel movement, sensitivity reaction including rash.	Continue. Call doctor if symptoms persist.
Rare:	
None expected.	

WARNINGS & PRECAUTIONS

Don't take if:
You are allergic to rifaximin or other antibiotics called rifamycins (including rifampin or rifabutin).

Before you start, consult your doctor if:
* You have a fever.
* You have blood in your stool.
* You have dysentery (a severe form of diarrhea).
* You have pseudomembranous colitis.

Over age 60:
No special problems expected.

Pregnancy:
Decide with your doctor if drug benefits justify risk to unborn child. Risk category C. (See page xviii).

Breast-feeding:
It is unknown if drug passes into milk. Avoid drug or discontinue nursing until you finish medicine. Consult doctor for advice on maintaining milk supply.

Infants & children:
Safety and effectiveness for children under age 12 has not been established.

Prolonged use:
Not recommended. Medicine is discontinued once the infection is cured.

Skin & sunlight:
No special problems expected.

Driving, piloting or hazardous work:
No problems expected.

Discontinuing:
* Don't discontinue without doctor's advice until you complete prescribed dose, even though symptoms diminish or disappear.
* Do discontinue and call your doctor if diarrhea gets worse, you have bloody diarrhea or develop a fever.

Others:
* Be sure to drink plenty of fluids while you have diarrhea symptoms to prevent dehydration.
* Contact your doctor if symptoms do not improve in 24 to 48 hours.
* Advise any doctor or dentist whom you consult that you take this medicine.

POSSIBLE INTERACTION WITH OTHER DRUGS

GENERIC NAME OR DRUG CLASS	COMBINED EFFECT
None expected.	

POSSIBLE INTERACTION WITH OTHER SUBSTANCES

INTERACTS WITH	COMBINED EFFECT
Alcohol:	None expected.
Beverages:	None expected.
Cocaine:	Effects unknown. Avoid.
Foods:	None expected.
Marijuana:	Effects unknown. Avoid.
Tobacco:	None expected.

*See Glossary

RILUZOLE

BRAND NAMES

Rilutek

BASIC INFORMATION

Habit forming? No
Prescription needed? Yes
Available as generic? Yes
Drug class: Amyotrophic lateral sclerosis therapy agent

 USES

Treatment for amyotrophic lateral sclerosis (ALS or Lou Gehrig's disease), a motor neuron disorder that causes weakness and atrophy of the muscles. Riluzole may extend a patient's survival time and delay the need for surgery for complications. It does not cure the disorder.

 DOSAGE & USAGE INFORMATION

How to take:
Tablet—Swallow with liquid. Instructions to take on an empty stomach mean 1 hour before or 2 hours after eating.

When to take:
Usually every 12 hours.

If you forget a dose:
Take as soon as you remember up to 6 hours late. If more than 6 hours, wait for the next dose (don't double this dose).

What drug does:
The cause of ALS is unknown and the exact mechanism of how the drug works is also unknown. It appears to decrease production of certain chemicals in the body and may affect some cellular activity that leads to the progressive weakness caused by the disorder.

Time lapse before drug works:
6 to 18 months for maximum benefits.

Don't take with:
Any other medicine or any dietary supplement without consulting your doctor or pharmacist.

 OVERDOSE

SYMPTOMS:
Unknown.
WHAT TO DO:
If person takes much larger amount than prescribed, dial 911 (emergency) for medical help or call poison control center 1-800-222-1222 for instructions.

 POSSIBLE ADVERSE REACTIONS OR SIDE EFFECTS

SYMPTOMS	WHAT TO DO
Life-threatening: None expected.	
Common:	
• Difficulty breathing, abdominal pain, increased coughing, blood pressure increased.	Discontinue. Call doctor right away.
• Mouth has a burning, or tingling feeling, constipation, nausea, vomiting, dizziness, mild weakness, headache, diarrhea.	Continue. Call doctor when convenient.
Infrequent: Skin symptoms (redness, itching, scaling, bruising, oozing or thickening), fever, sore feet or legs, sores in mouth or on lips, fast heartbeat.	Discontinue. Call doctor right away.
Rare: Changes in vision, tightness in chest, wheezing, memory loss, mood changes, severe drowsiness, hallucinations, mental changes, swelling (face, hands, fingers, feet or legs), nosebleed, blood in urine, unusual bleeding, unusual tiredness or weakness, severe headache, pain in various parts of the body, eyes red or irritated, continued or painful penile erection, noisy breathing, loss of bladder control, hives.	Discontinue. Call doctor right away.

WARNINGS & PRECAUTIONS

Don't take if:
You are sensitive to riluzole.

Before you start, consult your doctor if:
- You are allergic to any medicine, food or other substance, or have a family history of allergies.
- You have liver or kidney disease.

Over age 60:
No problems expected.

Pregnancy:
Decide with your doctor if drug benefits justify risk to unborn child. Risk category C (see page xviii).

Breast-feeding:
Not recommended. Consult doctor.

Infants & children:
Not recommended for this age group.

Prolonged use:
Talk to your doctor about the need for follow-up medical examinations or laboratory studies to check liver function.

Skin & sunlight:
No problems expected.

Driving, piloting or hazardous work:
Don't drive or pilot aircraft until you learn how medicine affects you. Don't work around dangerous machinery. Don't climb ladders or work in high places. Danger increases if you drink alcohol or take other medicines affecting alertness and reflexes.

Discontinuing:
No problems expected.

Others:
- May affect the results of some medical tests.
- Use as directed. Don't increase or decrease dosage without doctor's approval.
- Advise any doctor or dentist whom you consult that you take this medicine.
- Call your doctor if you develop a fever.

POSSIBLE INTERACTION WITH OTHER DRUGS

GENERIC NAME OR DRUG CLASS	COMBINED EFFECT
Hepatotoxics*	Increased risk of adverse effects.
Other medications	Complete studies have not been done to evaluate interactions with other drugs, but the potential exists for a variety of possible interactions. Consult doctor.

POSSIBLE INTERACTION WITH OTHER SUBSTANCES

INTERACTS WITH	COMBINED EFFECT
Alcohol:	Increased risk of adverse effects.
Beverages:	None expected.
Cocaine:	Problems not known. Best to avoid.
Foods:	None expected.
Marijuana:	Problems not known. Best to avoid.
Tobacco:	May decrease riluzole effect.

*See Glossary

RITODRINE

BRAND NAMES

Yutopar

BASIC INFORMATION

Habit forming? No
Prescription needed? Yes
Available as generic? Yes
Drug class: Labor inhibitor, beta-adrenergic stimulator

 ## USES

Halts premature labor in pregnancies of 20 or more weeks.

 ## DOSAGE & USAGE INFORMATION

How to take:
Tablet—Swallow with liquid or food to lessen stomach irritation. If you can't swallow whole, crumble tablet and take with liquid or food.

When to take:
Every 4 to 6 hours until term.

If you forget a dose:
Take as soon as you remember up to 2 hours late. If more than 2 hours, wait for next scheduled dose (don't double this dose).

What drug does:
Inhibits contractions of uterus (womb).

Time lapse before drug works:
30 to 60 minutes (oral form). Faster intravenously.

Don't take with:
Any other medicine or any dietary supplement without consulting your doctor or pharmacist.

 ## OVERDOSE

SYMPTOMS:
Rapid, irregular heartbeat to 120 or more; shortness of breath.
WHAT TO DO:
* **Dial 911 (emergency) for medical help or call poison control center 1-800-222-1222 for instructions.**
* **If person is unconscious, check breathing and pulse. If not breathing, begin mouth-to-mouth rescue breathing. If heart is not beating, begin chest compressions.**
* **See emergency information on last 3 pages of this book.**

 ## POSSIBLE ADVERSE REACTIONS OR SIDE EFFECTS

SYMPTOMS	WHAT TO DO
Life-threatening:	
Hives, rash, intense itching, faintness soon after a dose (anaphylaxis).	Seek emergency treatment immediately.
Common:	
Irregular heartbeat, fast heartbeat.	Discontinue. Call doctor right away.
Infrequent:	
• Shortness of breath.	Discontinue. Call doctor right away.
• Nervousness, trembling, headache, nausea, vomiting.	Continue. Call doctor when convenient.
Rare:	
Rash, angina, jaundice.	Discontinue. Call doctor right away.

WARNINGS & PRECAUTIONS

Don't take if:
- You have heart disease.
- You have eclampsia.
- You have lung congestion.
- You have infection in the uterus.
- You have an overactive thyroid.
- You have a bleeding disorder.

Before you start, consult your doctor if:
- You have asthma.
- You have diabetes.
- You have high blood pressure.
- You have pre-eclampsia.

Over age 60:
Not used.

Pregnancy:
Ritodrine crosses placenta, but animal studies show that it doesn't affect fetuses. Benefits versus risks must be assessed by you and your doctor. Risk category B (see page xviii).

Breast-feeding:
Not applicable.

Infants & children:
Not used.

Prolonged use:
Talk to your doctor about the need for follow-up medical examinations or laboratory studies to check blood sugar, ECG,* fluid and electrolytes.

Skin & sunlight:
No problems expected.

Driving, piloting or hazardous work:
Don't drive or pilot aircraft until you learn how medicine affects you. Don't work around dangerous machinery. Don't climb ladders or work in high places. Danger increases if you drink alcohol or take medicine affecting alertness and reflexes, such as antihistamines, tranquilizers, sedatives, pain medicine, narcotics and mind-altering drugs.

Discontinuing:
Don't discontinue without consulting doctor. Dose may require gradual reduction if you have taken drug for a long time. Doses of other drugs may also require adjustment.

Others:
Advise any doctor or dentist whom you consult that you take this medicine.

POSSIBLE INTERACTION WITH OTHER DRUGS

GENERIC NAME OR DRUG CLASS	COMBINED EFFECT
Adrenal corticosteroids*	Increased chance of fluid in lungs of mother. Avoid.
Anesthetics, general*	Possible cardiac arrhythmias or hypotension.
Beta-adrenergic blocking agents*	Decreased effect of ritodrine.
Diazoxide	Possible cardiac arrhythmias or hypotension.
Magnesium sulfate	Possible cardiac arrhythmias or hypotension.
Meperidine	Possible cardiac arrhythmias or hypotension.
Sympathomimetics*	Increased side effects of both.

POSSIBLE INTERACTION WITH OTHER SUBSTANCES

INTERACTS WITH	COMBINED EFFECT
Alcohol:	Increased adverse effects. Avoid.
Beverages:	None expected.
Cocaine:	Injury to fetus. Avoid.
Foods:	None expected.
Marijuana:	Injury to fetus. Avoid.
Tobacco:	Injury to fetus. Avoid.

*See Glossary

SALICYLATES

GENERIC AND BRAND NAMES

See full list of generic and brand names in the *Generic and Brand Name Directory*, page 897.

BASIC INFORMATION

Habit forming? No
Prescription needed? For some
Available as generic? Yes
Drug class: Analgesic, anti-inflammatory (nonsteroidal)

 ## USES

- Reduces pain, fever, inflammation.
- Relieves swelling, stiffness, joint pain of arthritis or rheumatism.
- Decreases risk of myocardial infarction (aspirin only).

 ## DOSAGE & USAGE INFORMATION

How to take:
- Tablet or capsule—Swallow with liquid.
- Extended-release tablet—Swallow each dose whole.
- Suppository—Remove wrapper and moisten suppository with water. Gently insert into rectum, large end first.

When to take:
Pain, fever, inflammation—As needed, no more often than every 4 hours.

If you forget a dose:
- Pain, fever—Take as soon as you remember. Wait 4 hours for next dose.
- Arthritis—Take as soon as you remember up to 2 hours late. Return to regular schedule.

What drug does:
- Affects hypothalamus, the part of the brain that regulates temperature by dilating small blood vessels in skin.

Continued next column

 ## OVERDOSE

SYMPTOMS:
Ringing in ears; nausea; vomiting; dizziness; fever; deep, rapid breathing; hallucinations; convulsions; coma.
WHAT TO DO
- **Dial 911 (emergency) for medical help or call poison control center 1-800-222-1222 for instructions.**
- **See emergency information on last 3 pages of this book.**

- Prevents clumping of platelets (small blood cells) so blood vessels remain open.
- Decreases prostaglandin effect.
- Suppresses body's pain messages.

Time lapse before drug works:
30 minutes for pain, fever, arthritis.

Don't take with:
- Tetracyclines. Space doses 1 hour apart.
- Any other medicine or any dietary supplement without consulting your doctor or pharmacist.

 ## POSSIBLE ADVERSE REACTIONS OR SIDE EFFECTS

SYMPTOMS	WHAT TO DO
Life-threatening:	
Hives, rash, intense itching, faintness soon after a dose (anaphylaxis); black or bloody vomit; blood in urine.	Seek emergency treatment immediately.
Common:	
• Nausea, vomiting, abdominal pain.	Discontinue. Seek emergency treatment.
• Heartburn, indigestion.	Continue. Call doctor when convenient.
• Ringing in ears.	Continue. Tell doctor at next visit.
Infrequent:	
None expected.	
Rare:	
• Black stools, unexplained fever.	Discontinue. Seek emergency treatment.
• Rash, hives, itchy skin, diminished vision, shortness of breath, wheezing, jaundice.	Discontinue. Call doctor right away.
• Drowsiness, headache.	Continue. Call doctor when convenient.

 ## WARNINGS & PRECAUTIONS

Don't take if:
- You are allergic to salicylates.
- You need to restrict sodium in your diet. Buffered effervescent tablets and sodium salicylate are high in sodium.
- Salicylates have a strong vinegar-like odor, which means they have decomposed.
- You have a bleeding disorder.

Before you start, consult your doctor if:
- You have had stomach or duodenal ulcers.
- You have had gout.
- You have asthma or nasal polyps.

Over age 60:
More likely to cause hidden bleeding in stomach or intestines. Watch for dark stools.

Pregnancy:
Risk factors vary for drugs in this group. See category list on page xviii and consult doctor.

Breast-feeding:
Drug passes into milk. Avoid drug or discontinue nursing until you finish medicine. Consult doctor for advice on maintaining milk supply.

Infants & children:
* Overdose frequent and severe. Keep bottles out of children's reach.
* Do not give to persons under age 18 who have fever and discomfort of viral illness, especially chicken pox and influenza. Probably increases risk of Reye's syndrome.

Prolonged use:
* Kidney damage. Periodic kidney function test recommended.
* Talk to your doctor about the need for follow-up medical examinations or laboratory studies to check liver function.

Skin & sunlight:
No special problems expected.

Driving, piloting or hazardous work:
No restrictions unless you feel drowsy.

Discontinuing:
For chronic illness—Don't discontinue without doctor's advice until you complete prescribed dose, even though symptoms diminish or disappear.

Others:
* Salicylates can complicate surgery, pregnancy, labor and delivery, and illness.
* Advise any doctor or dentist whom you consult that you take this medicine.
* For arthritis—Don't change dose without consulting doctor.
* Urine tests for blood sugar may be inaccurate.

POSSIBLE INTERACTION WITH OTHER DRUGS

GENERIC NAME OR DRUG CLASS	COMBINED EFFECT
Acetaminophen	Increased risk of kidney damage (with high, prolonged dose of each).
Adrenocorticoids, systemic	Decreased salicylate effect.
Allopurinol	Decreased allopurinol effect.
Angiotensin-converting enzyme (ACE) inhibitors*	Decreased ACE inhibitor effect.

Antacids*	Decreased salicylate effect.
Anticoagulants,* oral	Increased anticoagulant effect. Abnormal bleeding.
Antidiabetics,* oral	Low blood sugar.
Anti-inflammatory drugs, nonsteroidal (NSAIDs)*	Risk of stomach bleeding and ulcers.
Aspirin, other	Likely salicylate toxicity.
Beta-adrenergic blocking agents*	Decreased anti-hypertensive effect.
Bismuth subsalicylate	Increased risk of salicylate toxicity.
Bumetanide	Decreased diuretic effect.
Calcium supplements*	Increased salicylate effect.
Carteolol	Decreased antihypertensive effect of carteolol.
Ethacrynic acid	Decreased diuretic effect.
Furosemide	Possible salicylate toxicity.
Gold compounds*	Increased likelihood of kidney damage.
Indomethacin	Risk of stomach bleeding and ulcers.
Insulin	Decreased blood sugar.

Continued on page 931

POSSIBLE INTERACTION WITH OTHER SUBSTANCES

INTERACTS WITH	COMBINED EFFECT
Alcohol:	Possible stomach irritation and bleeding. Avoid.
Beverages:	None expected.
Cocaine:	None expected.
Foods:	None expected.
Marijuana:	Possible increased pain relief, but marijuana may slow body's recovery. Avoid.
Tobacco:	None expected.

*See Glossary

SCOPOLAMINE (Hyoscine)

BRAND NAMES

See full list of brand names in the *Generic and Brand Name Directory*, page 897.

BASIC INFORMATION

Habit forming? No
Prescription needed?
   High strength: Yes
   Low strength: No
Available as generic? Yes
Drug class: Antispasmodic, anticholinergic

USES

- Reduces spasms of digestive system, bladder and urethra.
- Relieves painful menstruation.
- Prevents motion sickness.

DOSAGE & USAGE INFORMATION

How to take:
- Tablet or capsule—Swallow with liquid or food to lessen stomach irritation.
- Drops—Dilute dose in beverage.
- Skin disc—Clean application site. Change application sites with each dose.

When to take:
- Motion sickness—Apply disc 30 minutes before departure.
- Other uses—Take 30 minutes before meals (unless directed otherwise by doctor).

If you forget a dose:
Take up to 2 hours late. If more than 2 hours, wait for next dose (don't double this dose).

What drug does:
Blocks nerve impulses at parasympathetic nerve endings, preventing muscle contractions and gland secretions of organs involved.

Continued next column

OVERDOSE

SYMPTOMS:
Dilated pupils, blurred vision, rapid pulse and breathing, dizziness, fever, hallucinations, confusion, slurred speech, agitation, flushed face, convulsions, coma.
WHAT TO DO:
- **Dial 911 (emergency) for medical help or call poison control center 1-800-222-1222 for instructions.**
- **See emergency information on last 3 pages of this book.**

Time lapse before drug works:
15 to 30 minutes.

Don't take with:
Any other medicine or any dietary supplement without consulting your doctor or pharmacist.

POSSIBLE ADVERSE REACTIONS OR SIDE EFFECTS

SYMPTOMS	WHAT TO DO
Life-threatening:	
Hives, rash, intense itching, faintness soon after a dose (anaphylaxis).	Seek emergency treatment immediately.
Common:	
• Confusion, delirium, rapid heartbeat.	Discontinue. Call doctor right away.
• Nausea, vomiting, decreased sweating.	Continue. Call doctor when convenient.
• Constipation, changes in taste.	Continue. Tell doctor at next visit.
• Dryness in ears, nose, throat, mouth.	No action necessary.
Infrequent:	
Headache, difficult urination, stuffy nose, feeling lightheaded.	Continue. Call doctor when convenient.
Rare:	
Rash or hives, eye pain, blurred vision.	Discontinue. Call doctor right away.

WARNINGS & PRECAUTIONS

Don't take if:
- You are allergic to any anticholinergic.
- You have trouble with stomach bloating.
- You have difficulty emptying your bladder completely.
- You have narrow-angle glaucoma.
- You have severe ulcerative colitis.

Before you start, consult your doctor if:
- You have open-angle glaucoma, angina, chronic bronchitis or asthma, hiatal hernia, liver disease, enlarged prostate, myasthenia gravis, peptic ulcer, kidney or thyroid disease.
- You will have surgery within 2 months, including dental surgery, requiring general or spinal anesthesia.

Over age 60:
Adverse reactions and side effects may be more frequent and severe than in younger persons.

Pregnancy:
Decide with your doctor whether drug benefits justify risk to unborn child. Risk category C (see page xviii).

SCOPOLAMINE (Hyoscine)

Breast-feeding:
Drug passes into milk and decreases milk flow. Avoid drug or discontinue nursing until you finish medicine. Consult doctor for advice on maintaining milk supply.

Infants & children:
Use only under medical supervision.

Prolonged use:
Chronic constipation, possible fecal impaction. Consult doctor immediately.

Skin & sunlight:
No problems expected.

Driving, piloting or hazardous work:
Use disqualifies you for piloting aircraft. Don't drive until you learn how medicine affects you. Don't work around dangerous machinery. Don't climb ladders or work in high places.

Discontinuing:
May be unnecessary to finish medicine. Follow doctor's instructions.

Others:
Advise any doctor or dentist whom you consult that you take this medicine.

POSSIBLE INTERACTION WITH OTHER DRUGS

GENERIC NAME OR DRUG CLASS	COMBINED EFFECT
Adrenocorticoids, systemic	Possible glaucoma.
Amantadine	Increased scopolamine effect.
Antacids*	Decreased scopolamine effect.
Anticholinergics,* other	Increased scopolamine effect.
Antidepressants, tricyclic*	Increased scopolamine effect. Increased sedation.
Antidiarrheals*	Decreased scopolamine effect.
Antihistamines*	Increased scopolamine effect.
Attapulgite	Decreased scopolamine effect.
Buclizine	Increased scopolamine effect.
Clozapine	Toxic effect on the central nervous system.
Digitalis preparations*	Possible decreased absorption of scopolamine.
Encainide	Increased effect of toxicity on heart muscle.
Ethinamate	Dangerous increased effects of ethinamate. Avoid combining.
Fluoxetine	Increased depressant effects of both drugs.
Guanfacine	May increase depressant effects of either medicine.
Haloperidol	Increased internal eye pressure.
Ketoconazole	Decreased ketoconazole effect.
Leucovorin	High alcohol content of leucovorin may cause adverse effects.
Meperidine	Increased scopolamine effect.
Methylphenidate	Increased scopolamine effect.
Methyprylon	May increase sedative effect to dangerous level. Avoid.
Molindone	Increased anticholinergic effect.
Monoamine oxidase (MAO) inhibitors*	Increased scopolamine effect.

Continued on page 932

POSSIBLE INTERACTION WITH OTHER SUBSTANCES

INTERACTS WITH	COMBINED EFFECT
Alcohol:	None expected.
Beverages:	None expected.
Cocaine:	Excessively rapid heartbeat. Avoid.
Foods:	None expected.
Marijuana:	Drowsiness, dry mouth.
Tobacco:	None expected.

*See Glossary

745

SELECTIVE SEROTONIN REUPTAKE INHIBITORS (SSRIs)

GENERIC AND BRAND NAMES

CITALOPRAM
  Celexa
ESCITALOPRAM
  Lexapro
FLUOXETINE
  Prozac
  Prozac Weekly
  Sarafem
  Symbyax

FLUVOXAMINE
  Luvox
  Luvox CR
PAROXETINE
  Paxil
  Paxil CR
SERTRALINE
  Zoloft

BASIC INFORMATION

Habit forming? No
Prescription needed? Yes
Available as generic? Yes, for some
Drug class: Antidepressant, antiobsessional agent, antianxiety agent.

USES

- Treats depression, obsessive compulsive disorder, generalized anxiety disorder, panic disorder, post traumatic stress disorder, social phobia, premenstrual dysphoric disorder and seasonal affective disorder.
- Treats depressive episode of bipolar disorder.

DOSAGE & USAGE INFORMATION

How to take:
- Capsule or tablet—Swallow with water. Take with or without food. If you can't swallow whole, crumble tablet or open capsule and take with liquid or food.
- Oral disintegrating tablet—Dissolve in mouth.
- Oral solution, extended-release capsule or controlled-release tablet—Follow instructions.

When to take:
At the same time each day or weekly, usually in the am. Some dosages may be twice daily.

Continued next column

OVERDOSE

SYMPTOMS:
Dizziness, sweating, nausea, vomiting, tremor, heart rhythm disturbances. In rare cases, amnesia, coma and convulsions.
WHAT TO DO:
- **Dial 911 (emergency) for medical help or call poison control center 1-800-222-1222 for instructions.**
- **See emergency information on last 3 pages of this book.**

If you forget a dose:
Take as soon as you remember. If it is near the time of your next dose, skip the missed dose and resume normal schedule. Don't double this dose.

What drug does:
Affects serotonin, one of the chemicals in the brain called neurotransmitters, that plays a role in emotions and psychological disturbances.

Time lapse before drug works:
1 to 4 weeks.

Don't take with:
Any other medicine or any dietary supplement without consulting your doctor or pharmacist.

POSSIBLE ADVERSE REACTIONS OR SIDE EFFECTS

SYMPTOMS	WHAT TO DO
Life-threatening: Rash, itchy skin, breathing problems, chest pain (allergic reaction).	Seek emergency treatment immediately.
Common: Drowsiness, nausea, cough or hoarseness, lower back or side pain, sores on lips or mouth, constipation or diarrhea, headache, anxiety, changes in sexual desire or function, insomnia, dry mouth, unusual weakness or tiredness.	Continue. Call doctor when convenient.
Infrequent: • Vision changes, confusion, apathy (lack of emotion), breathing difficulty, chills, black or tarry stools, fever, enlarged lymph glands, heart rhythm changes, vomiting, skin rash or itching.	Discontinue. Call doctor right away.
• Abdominal pain, loss of appetite, yawning, tingling, skin burning or prickly feeling, stuffy nose, change in sense of taste, tooth grinding, trembling, increased saliva, gas, heartburn, sweating, urinary changes, hair loss, muscle or joint pain, menstrual changes, weight changes.	Continue. Call doctor when convenient.

SELECTIVE SEROTONIN REUPTAKE INHIBITORS (SSRIs)

Rare:

* Seizures (convulsions). Discontinue. Seek emergency help.

* Abnormal bleeding, breast tenderness or enlargement, red or peeling skin, red or irritated eyes, sore throat, sudden body or facial spasms, dizziness, signs of low blood sugar (anxiety, chills, nervousness, difficulty concentrating), clumsiness. Discontinue. Call doctor right away.

WARNINGS & PRECAUTIONS

Don't take if:

* You are allergic to any SSRIs.
* You currently take (or took in the last two weeks) a monoamine oxidase (MAO) inhibitor.

Before you start, consult your doctor if:

* You have had kidney or liver problems.
* You have a history of seizure disorders.
* You have a history of drug or alcohol abuse.
* You have a history of mood disorders, mania, or thoughts of suicide.

Over age 60:
Adverse reactions and side effects may be more severe and frequent than in younger patients; dosage may need to be adjusted.

Pregnancy:
Decide with your doctor if drug benefits justify risk to unborn child. Risk category C for drugs in this group except paroxetine. Paroxetine (Paxil) is a risk category D. It may cause birth defects. (see page xviii for risk category information).

Breast-feeding:
Drugs pass into milk. Avoid drug or discontinue nursing until you finish medicine. Consult doctor for advice on maintaining milk supply.

Infants & children:
For children under age 18 use only with close medical supervision. Carefully read information provided with prescription. Contact doctor right away if depression symptoms get worse or there is any talk of suicide or suicide behaviors. Read also the information under Others on this page.

Prolonged use:
No problems expected. Your doctor should periodically evaluate your response to the drug and adjust the dose if necessary.

Skin & sunlight:
One or more drugs in this group may cause rash or intensify sunburn in areas exposed to sun or ultraviolet light (photosensitivity reaction). Avoid overexposure. Notify doctor if reaction occurs.

Driving, piloting or hazardous work:
Don't drive or pilot aircraft until you learn how medicine affects you. Don't work around dangerous machinery. Don't climb ladders or work in high places. Danger increases if you drink alcohol or take medicine affecting alertness and reflexes.

Discontinuing:

* Don't discontinue without consulting doctor. You may need to reduce the dose gradually to avoid side effects.
* After discontinuing the drug, call your doctor right away if any new or unusual symptoms develop (emotional or physical).

Others:

* Advise any doctor or dentist whom you consult that you take this medicine.
* Take drug only as directed. Do not increase or reduce dosage without doctor's approval.
* Adults and children taking antidepressants may experience a worsening of the depression symptoms and may display increased suicidal thoughts or behavior. Call doctor right away if these symptoms or behaviors occur.

POSSIBLE INTERACTION WITH OTHER DRUGS

GENERIC NAME OR DRUG CLASS	COMBINED EFFECT
Anticoagulants, oral*	Increased risk of side effects of both drugs.
Antidepressants, tricyclic*	Increased risk of side effects.
Benzodiazepines*	Increased benzodiazepine effect.
Bromocriptine	Increased risk of serotonin syndrome.*

Continued on page 932

POSSIBLE INTERACTION WITH OTHER SUBSTANCES

INTERACTS WITH	COMBINED EFFECT
Alcohol:	Contributes to depression. Avoid.
Beverages: Grapefruit juice.	Toxicity risk. Avoid.
Cocaine:	Unknown. Avoid.
Foods:	None expected.
Marijuana:	Unknown. Avoid.
Tobacco:	None expected.

*See Glossary

SEROTONIN-DOPAMINE ANTAGONISTS

GENERIC AND BRAND NAMES

PALIPERIDONE
Invega

RISPERIDONE
Risperdal
Risperdal Consta
Risperdal M-TAB

BASIC INFORMATION

Habit forming? No
Prescription needed? Yes
Available as generic? Yes, for some
Drug class: Antipsychotic

 USES

- Treatment of schizophrenia.
- Treatment for bipolar disorder.
- Treatment of irritability in children with autism.
- Treats other disorders per doctor's advice.

 DOSAGE & USAGE INFORMATION

How to take:
- Tablet—Swallow with liquid. May be taken with or without food.
- Injection—Patients will go to a medical office once every two weeks for treatment.
- Orally disintegrating tablet—Dissolves in the mouth in seconds. Do not chew.
- Oral solution—Dilute in 3 to 4 ounces of liquid (water, orange juice or low fat milk; don't use cola or tea).
- Extended-release tablet—Swallow whole with liquid.

When to take:
At the same times each day. Take once-a-day dose in morning. Prescribed dosage may be increased gradually over first several days.

If you forget a dose:
Take as soon as you remember. If it is almost time for the next dose, wait for the next scheduled dose (don't double this dose).

Continued next column

 OVERDOSE

SYMPTOMS:
Drowsiness, dizziness, rapid heartbeat, low blood pressure, convulsions, muscle spasms and uncontrolled body movements.
WHAT TO DO:
- **Dial 911 (emergency) for medical help or call poison control center 1-800-222-1222 for instructions.**
- **See emergency information on last 3 pages of this book.**

What drug does:
It appears to act on neurotransmitters (serotonin and dopamine) in the brain to help restore more normal thinking and more normal mood.

Time lapse before drug works:
One to 7 days. A gradual increase in the dosage amount may be necessary to relieve symptoms.

Don't take with:
Any other medicine or diet supplement without consulting your doctor or pharmacist.

 POSSIBLE ADVERSE REACTIONS OR SIDE EFFECTS

SYMPTOMS	WHAT TO DO
Life-threatening:	
Neuroleptic malignant syndrome (high fever, fast heart rate, sweating rigid muscles, unstable blood pressure, confusion, seizures, stupor or coma).	Discontinue. Seek emergency treatment.
Common:	
• Difficulty speaking or swallowing, loss of balance, vision changes, mask-like face, shuffling walk, arms or legs are stiff or weak, trembling or twitching, muscle spasms (face, neck, back), unable to move eyes, body twisting.	Discontinue. Call doctor right away.
• Constipation or diarrhea, drowsiness, dry mouth, headache, heartburn, cough, dreaming more, sore throat, nausea, stuffy or runny nose, unusual tiredness or weakness, weight gain, anxiety or nervousness, mood or mental changes, sexual dysfunction, urination problems, restlessness, insomnia, sweating.	Continue. Call doctor when convenient.
Infrequent:	
• Fast or irregular heartbeat, dizziness, lightheadedness, chest pain, trouble breathing.	Discontinue. Call doctor right away.
• Menstrual changes; skin is dry, darker or oily; rash; excess saliva; joint, back or stomach pain; vomiting; appetite loss; weight loss; unexpected breast milk.	Continue. Call doctor when convenient.

Rare:
- High blood sugar (thirstiness, frequent urination, increased hunger, weakness); lip smacking; uncontrolled movements (arms, legs tongue and chewing); cheek puffing; increased blinking; eyelid spasms; unusual facial or body positions; manic behavior; high or low body temperature; unusual bleeding or bruising.

Discontinue. Call doctor right away.

- Other symptoms that cause concern.

Continue. Call doctor when convenient.

WARNINGS & PRECAUTIONS

Don't take if:
You are allergic to paliperidone or risperidone.

Before you start, consult your doctor if:
- You have or have had liver, kidney or heart disease; stroke; high or low blood pressure; seizures; diabetes or prediabetes; Parkinson's disease; breast cancer; neuroleptic malignant syndrome; phenylketonuria; suicide thoughts; tardive dyskinesia or trouble swallowing.
- Patient is elderly and has dementia.

Over age 60:
- Adverse reactions and side effects may be more severe than in younger persons. A lower starting dosage is usually recommended.
- Use of antipsychotic drugs in elderly patients with dementia-related psychosis may increase risk of death. Consult doctor.

Pregnancy:
Decide with your doctor if drug benefits justify any possible risk to unborn child. Risk category C (see page xviii).

Breast-feeding:
It is unknown if drug passes into milk. Consult your doctor for advice.

Infants & children:
Use only with close medical supervision.

Prolonged use:
Consult with your doctor on a regular basis while taking this drug to check your progress or to discuss any increase or changes in side effects and the need for continued treatment.

Skin & sunlight:
- May cause rash or intensify sunburn in areas exposed to sun or ultraviolet light (photosensitivity reaction). Use sunscreen and avoid overexposure. Notify doctor if reaction occurs.
- Hot temperatures and exercise, hot baths can increase risk of heatstroke. Drug may affect body's ability to maintain normal temperature.

Driving, piloting or hazardous work:
Don't drive or pilot aircraft until you learn how drug affects you. Don't work around dangerous machinery. Don't climb ladders or work in high places. Danger increases if you drink alcohol or take drugs affecting alertness and reflexes.

Discontinuing:
- Don't discontinue this drug without doctor's approval. Dosage may require a gradual reduction before stopping.
- Withdrawal effects may occur after stopping drug. Consult doctor if new symptoms develop that cause you concern.

Others:
- Get up slowly from a sitting or lying position to avoid feeling dizzy, faint or lightheaded.
- Advise any doctor or dentist whom you consult that you take this medicine.
- Take drug only as directed. Do not increase or reduce dosage without doctor's approval.

POSSIBLE INTERACTION WITH OTHER DRUGS

GENERIC NAME OR DRUG CLASS	COMBINED EFFECT
Antihypertensives*	Increased risk of low blood pressure.
Carbamazepine	Decreased effect of risperidone.
Central nervous system (CNS) depressants,* other	Increased sedative effect.
Clozapine	Increased effect of risperidone.
Dopamine agonists*	Decreased dopamine agonist effect.

POSSIBLE INTERACTION WITH OTHER SUBSTANCES

INTERACTS WITH	COMBINED EFFECT
Alcohol:	Increased sedative affect. Avoid.
Beverages:	None expected.
Cocaine:	Effect not known. Best to avoid.
Foods:	None expected.
Marijuana:	Effect not known. Best to avoid.
Tobacco:	None expected.

*See Glossary

SEROTONIN & NOREPINEPHRINE REUPTAKE INHIBITORS (SNRIs)

GENERIC AND BRAND NAMES

DESVENLAFAXINE
  Pristiq
DULOXETINE
  Cymbalta

MILNACIPRAN
  Savella
VENLAFAXINE
  Effexor
  Effexor XR

BASIC INFORMATION

Habit forming? No
Prescription needed? Yes
Available as generic? Yes, for some
Drug class: Antidepressant

 ## USES

- Treatment for major depressive disorder.
- Treatment for diabetic peripheral neuropathy.
- Treatment for generalized anxiety disorder.
- May be used for chronic pain syndrome, social anxiety disorder, fibromyalgia, hot flashes, stress incontinence or other disorders.

 ## DOSAGE & USAGE INFORMATION

How to take:
- Tablet, extended-release capsule or extended-release tablet—Swallow whole with liquid. Take with food if stomach upset occurs. Capsule may be opened and contents sprinkled into a spoonful of applesauce and swallowed.
- Delayed-release capsule—Swallow with liquid. May be taken with or without food. Do not open, crush or chew capsule.

When to take:
At the same times each day (with meals or with a snack for venlafaxine).

Continued next column

 ## OVERDOSE

SYMPTOMS:
Extreme drowsiness or tiredness or weakness, seizure, fast heartbeat, tingling or burning sensation, tremor, nausea, vomiting, agitation, hyperactive, enlarged pupils. In some cases, may have no symptoms.
WHAT TO DO:
- **Dial 911 (emergency) for medical help or call poison control center 1-800-222-1222 for instructions.**
- **See emergency information on last 3 pages of this book.**

If you forget a dose:
Take as soon as you remember. If it is almost time for the next dose, wait for that dose (don't double this dose) and resume regular schedule.

What drug does:
Increases level of two brain chemicals (serotonin and norepinephrine) that affect behavior and mood and play a role in depression.

Time lapse before drug works:
Begins in 1 to 3 weeks, but may take 4 to 6 weeks for maximum benefit.

Don't take with:
Any other medicine or any dietary supplement without consulting your doctor or pharmacist.

 ## POSSIBLE ADVERSE REACTIONS OR SIDE EFFECTS

SYMPTOMS	WHAT TO DO
Life-threatening:	
Rare allergic reaction—Breathing difficulty; closing of the throat; swelling of hands, feet, face, lips or tongue; hives.	Discontinue. Seek emergency treatment.
Common:	
Nausea, dry mouth, increased sweating, appetite loss, insomnia or drowsiness, fatigue, headache, constipation, diarrhea, rash or itching.	Continue. Call doctor when convenient.
Infrequent:	
Mood or behavior or mental changes, dizziness, impotence, less interest in sex or changes in orgasm, skin flushing, stomach upset or pain, vomiting, weight loss, muscle aches or pain, joint pain or swelling, trembling or shaking, vision changes, abnormal dreams, sore throat, stuffy or runny nose, fever, cough, frequent or hesitant urination, nervousness, weakness, lightheadedness.	Continue. Call doctor when convenient.
Rare:	
Seizures, fainting, irregular heartbeat, abnormal behaviors, severe symptoms such as suicide thoughts or behaviors.	Discontinue. Call doctor right away.

SEROTONIN & NOREPINEPHRINE REUPTAKE INHIBITORS (SNRIs)

 WARNINGS & PRECAUTIONS

Don't take if:
You are allergic to serotonin and norepinephrine reuptake inhibitors or take MAO inhibitors.*

Before you start, consult your doctor if:
* You have diabetes; heart, liver, or kidney disease; glaucoma; a blood clotting or bleeding problem or high cholesterol.
* You have high or low blood pressure.
* You have thoughts about suicide.
* You have a brain disorder or brain damage or mental retardation.
* You are losing weight.
* You have bipolar disorder or mania.
* You have a history of seizures or epilepsy.
* You drink excess amounts of alcohol.

Over age 60:
No special problems expected.

Pregnancy:
Decide with your doctor if drug benefits justify any possible risk to unborn child. Risk category C (see page xviii).

Breast-feeding:
Venlafaxine passes into milk. It is unknown if duloxetine passes into milk. Avoid nursing until you finish medicine. Consult doctor for advice on maintaining milk supply.

Infants & children:
Not approved for ages under age 18. If prescribed, carefully read information provided with prescription. Contact doctor right away if depression symptoms get worse or there is any talk of suicide or suicide behaviors. Also, read information under Others.

Prolonged use:
Consult with your doctor on a regular basis while taking this drug to check blood pressure and to determine the need for continued treatment.

Skin & sunlight:
No special problems expected.

Driving, piloting or hazardous work:
Don't drive or pilot aircraft until you learn how medicine affects you. Don't work around dangerous machinery. Don't climb ladders or work in high places. Danger increases if you drink alcohol or take medicine affecting alertness and reflexes.

Discontinuing:
* Don't discontinue without consulting doctor. You may need to reduce the dose gradually.
* If any new or unusual symptoms develop (emotional or physical) after you discontinue the drug, call your doctor right away.

Others:
* Rise slowly from a sitting or lying position to avoid dizziness, faintness or lightheadedness.
* Diabetic patients should consult doctor if blood sugar levels are affected by taking this drug.
* Advise any doctor or dentist whom you consult that you take this drug.
* Adults and children taking antidepressants may experience a worsening of the depression symptoms and may display increased suicidal thoughts or behavior. Call doctor right away if these symptoms or behaviors occur.
* Take drug as directed. Do not increase or reduce dosage without doctor's approval.

 POSSIBLE INTERACTION WITH OTHER DRUGS

GENERIC NAME OR DRUG CLASS	COMBINED EFFECT
Antiarrhythmics*	Increased side effect risk (with duloxetine).
Antidepressants, other	Increased sedative effect.
Antidepressants, tricyclic	Increased side effect risk (with duloxetine).
Central nervous system (CNS) depressants,* other	Increased sedative effect.
Cimetidine	Increased effect of venlafaxine.
Enzyme inhibitors*	Increased effect of either drug.
Monoamine oxidase (MAO) inhibitors*	Severe adverse reactions. Allow 14 days between use.
Phenothiazines	Increased side effect risk (with duloxetine).

Continued on page 933

 POSSIBLE INTERACTION WITH OTHER SUBSTANCES

INTERACTS WITH	COMBINED EFFECT
Alcohol:	Possible severe liver damage. Avoid.
Beverages:	None expected.
Cocaine:	Unknown. Avoid.
Foods:	None expected.
Marijuana:	Unknown. Avoid.
Tobacco:	None expected.

*See Glossary

751

SIBUTRAMINE

BRAND NAMES

Meridia

BASIC INFORMATION

Habit forming? Dependence possible
Prescription needed? Yes
Available as generic? No
Drug class: Appetite suppressant

 USES

Treatment for obesity and maintenance of weight loss. The drug is to be used in conjunction with a reduced calorie diet and weight management program. Treatment with this drug is not recommended for "cosmetic" weight loss—that is when a person's height-to-weight ratio does not provide a medical reason for weight loss. Your doctor will help determine your body mass index (BMI), a method of measuring for obesity.

 DOSAGE & USAGE INFORMATION

How to take:
Capsule—Swallow with liquid. It may be taken with or without food. Read instructions carefully that are provided with the prescription.

When to take:
Once a day usually in the morning.

If you forget a dose:
Take as soon as you remember. If it is almost time for the next dose, then skip the missed dose and wait for your next scheduled dose (don't double this dose).

What drug does:
Allows certain chemicals in the brain to act longer in controlling appetite regulating center.

Time lapse before drug works:
Weight loss should begin within 4 weeks.

Continued next column

 OVERDOSE

SYMPTOMS:
It is unknown what symptoms may occur.
WHAT TO DO:
If person takes much larger amount than prescribed, Dial 911 (emergency) for medical help or call poison control center 1-800-222-1222 for instructions.

Don't take with:
Any other medicine or any dietary supplement without consulting your doctor or pharmacist.

 POSSIBLE ADVERSE REACTIONS OR SIDE EFFECTS

SYMPTOMS	WHAT TO DO
Life-threatening: None known.	
Common: Dry mouth, headache, constipation, insomnia (these symptoms usually go away with continued treatment).	Continue. Call doctor when convenient.
Infrequent: • Increase in blood pressure or heart rate.	Discontinue. Call doctor right away.
• Back pain, flu-like symptoms, stomach pain, increased appetite, nausea, heartburn, muscle aches, dizziness, nervousness, anxiety, depression, sore throat, runny nose.	Continue. Call doctor when convenient.
Rare: Chest pain, fainting, swelling of feet or ankles, allergic reaction including skin rash or hives, seizure, any other symptoms you are concerned about.	Discontinue. Call doctor right away.

WARNINGS & PRECAUTIONS

Don't take if:
- You are allergic to sibutramine.
- You have a history of anorexia nervosa.

Before you start, consult your doctor if:
- You have a history of uncontrolled high blood pressure, any heart disorder, coronary artery disease, stroke (or symptoms of a stroke), seizures, or other medical problem.
- You have any kidney or liver disorder.
- Organic causes of obesity have not been ruled out, such as hypothyroidism.
- You have glaucoma.
- You are allergic to any other medication, food or other substance.

Over age 60:
No special problems expected, but a lower starting dosage may be recommended.

Pregnancy:
Sibutramine is not recommended for pregnant women. Risk category C (see page xviii).

Breast-feeding:
It is unknown if drug passes into milk. Avoid drug or discontinue nursing until you finish medicine. Consult doctor for advice on maintaining milk supply.

Infants & children:
Safety and effectiveness in ages under 16 has not been established.

Prolonged use:
- Schedule regular visits to your doctor to determine if drug is continuing to be effective in controlling weight and to monitor your blood pressure.
- The effectiveness and safety of taking this drug beyond one year have not been established.

Skin & sunlight:
No problems expected.

Driving, piloting or hazardous work:
Don't drive or pilot aircraft until you learn how medicine affects you. Don't work around dangerous machinery. Don't climb ladders or work in high places. Danger increases if you drink alcohol or take other medicines affecting alertness and reflexes.

Discontinuing:
Notify your doctor if any new symptoms occur after the drug is stopped.

Others:
- Advise any doctor or dentist whom you consult that you take this medicine.
- Use as directed. Don't increase or decrease dosage without doctor's approval.
- Notify your doctor if you don't lose at least 4 pounds in the first month of treatment.
- Other weight control agents have been associated with heart valve problems and primary pulmonary hypertension.
- Monitor blood pressure.

POSSIBLE INTERACTION WITH OTHER DRUGS

GENERIC NAME OR DRUG CLASS	COMBINED EFFECT
Appetite suppressants,* other	Unknown effect. Avoid.
Decongestants*	May cause increase in blood pressure or heart rate. Avoid.
Central nervous system (CNS) depressants*	Increased sedation. Avoid.
Erythromycin	Increased effect of sibutramine.
Ketoconazole	Increased effect of sibutramine.
Monoamine oxidase, (MAO) inhibitors	Potentially life-threatening. Allow 14 days between use of 2 drugs.
Serotonergic agents,* other	May cause serotonin syndrome.* Avoid.

POSSIBLE INTERACTION WITH OTHER SUBSTANCES

INTERACTS WITH	COMBINED EFFECT
Alcohol:	Increased sedation. Avoid.
Beverages:	None expected.
Cocaine:	Unknown effect. Best to avoid.
Foods:	None expected.
Marijuana:	Unknown effect. Best to avoid.
Tobacco:	None expected.

*See Glossary

SIMETHICONE

BRAND NAMES

Alka-Seltzer Gas
  Relief
Degas
Di-Gel
Extra Strength Gas-X
Extra Strength
  Maalox Anti-Gas
Extra Strength Maalox
  GRF Gas Relief
  Formula
Flatulex
Gas Aid
Gas Relief
Gas-X
Gas-X Extra Strength
Gas-X Thin Strips
Gas-X with Maalox
Gelusil
Genasyme
Imodium Advanced

Imodium Multi-
  Symptom Relief
Maalox Anti-Gas
Maalox GRF Gas
  Relief Formula
Maximum Strength
  Mylanta Gas Relief
Maximum Strength
  Phazyme
Mygel
Mylanta Gas
Mylicon
Mylicon-80
Mylicon-125
Ovol
Ovol 40
Ovol-80
Phazyme
Phazyme 55
Phazyme 95
Riopan Plus

BASIC INFORMATION

Habit forming? No
Prescription needed? No
Available as generic? Yes, for some
Drug class: Antiflatulent

 ## USES

- Treatment for retention of abdominal gas.
- Used prior to x-ray of abdomen.

 ## DOSAGE & USAGE INFORMATION

How to take:
- Tablet or capsule—Swallow with liquid.
- Liquid—Dissolve in water. Drink all of dose.
- Thin strip—Let it dissolve on your tongue.
- Chewable tablet—Chew completely. Don't swallow whole.

Continued next column

 ## OVERDOSE

SYMPTOMS:
None expected.
WHAT TO DO:
Overdose unlikely to threaten life. If person uses much larger amount than prescribed or if accidentally swallowed, call doctor or poison control center 1-800-222-1222 for help.

When to take:
After meals and at bedtime.

What drug does:
Reduces surface tension of gas bubbles in stomach.

Time lapse before drug works:
10 minutes.

If you forget a dose:
Take when remembered if needed.

Don't take with:
Any other medicine or any dietary supplement without consulting your doctor or pharmacist.

 ## POSSIBLE ADVERSE REACTIONS OR SIDE EFFECTS

SYMPTOMS	WHAT TO DO

Life-threatening:
None expected.

Common:
None expected.

Infrequent:
None expected.

Rare:
None expected.

WARNINGS & PRECAUTIONS

Don't take if:
You are allergic to simethicone.

Before you start, consult your doctor if:
You have allergies to other drugs or substances.

Over age 60:
No problems expected.

Pregnancy:
Consult doctor. Risk category C (see page xviii).

Breast-feeding:
No problems expected. Consult doctor.

Infants & children:
Not recommended.

Prolonged use:
No problems expected.

Skin & sunlight:
No problems expected.

Driving, piloting or hazardous work:
No problems expected.

Discontinuing:
May be unnecessary to finish medicine.
Discontinue when symptoms disappear.

Others:
No problems expected.

POSSIBLE INTERACTION WITH OTHER DRUGS

GENERIC NAME OR DRUG CLASS	COMBINED EFFECT
None significant.	

POSSIBLE INTERACTION WITH OTHER SUBSTANCES

INTERACTS WITH	COMBINED EFFECT
Alcohol:	None expected.
Beverages:	None expected.
Cocaine:	None expected.
Foods:	None expected.
Marijuana:	None expected.
Tobacco:	None expected.

SODIUM BICARBONATE

BRAND NAMES

Alka-Seltzer
  Original
Arm & Hammer Pure
  Baking Soda
Bell/ans
Bromo-Seltzer

Citrocarbonate
  Soda Mint
Zegerid Capsules
Zegerid Chewable
  Tablets
Zegerid Powder

BASIC INFORMATION

Habit forming? No
Prescription needed? No
Available as generic? Yes
Drug class: Alkalizer, antacid

USES

• Treats metabolic acidosis.
• Alkalinizes urine to reduce uric acid kidney stones.
• Treats hyperacidity of the stomach that is present with indigestion, gastroesophageal reflux and peptic ulcer disease.

DOSAGE & USAGE INFORMATION

How to take:
• Tablet—Swallow with liquid. If you can't swallow whole, crumble tablet and take with liquid or food.
• Powder—Mix in a glass of water and drink.
• Effervescent sodium bicarbonate—Mix in a glass of cold water and drink.

When to take:
• For hyperacidity—1 to 3 hours after meals.
• For kidney stones—According to prescription instructions.

If you forget a dose:
Take as soon as you remember up to 2 hours late. If more than 2 hours, wait for next scheduled dose (don't double this dose).

Continued next column

OVERDOSE

SYMPTOMS:
Excessive swelling of feet and lower legs.
WHAT TO DO:
Overdose unlikely to threaten life. If person uses much larger amount than prescribed or if accidentally swallowed, call doctor or poison control center 1-800-222-1222 for help.

What drug does:
• Buffers acid in the stomach.
• Increases excretion of bicarbonate in the urine to help dissolve uric acid stones.

Time lapse before drug works:
Works immediately, but the duration of effect is short.

Don't take with:
Any other medicine or any dietary supplement without consulting your doctor or pharmacist.

POSSIBLE ADVERSE REACTIONS OR SIDE EFFECTS

SYMPTOMS	WHAT TO DO
Life-threatening: None expected.	
Common: None expected.	
Infrequent:	
• Stomach cramps that continue.	Discontinue. Call doctor right away.
• Nausea, headache, appetite loss (with long-term use).	Continue. Call doctor when convenient.
Rare:	
Muscle pain or twitching, nervousness, breathing difficulty, mild swelling of feet or lower legs (with large doses).	Discontinue. Call doctor right away.

WARNINGS & PRECAUTIONS

Don't take if:
You are allergic to sodium bicarbonate.

Before you start, consult your doctor if:
You have heart disease, kidney disease or toxemia of pregnancy.

Over age 60:
Adverse reactions and side effects may be more frequent and severe than in younger persons.

Pregnancy:
May cause weight gain and swelling of feet and ankles. Avoid if you have high blood pressure. Consult doctor. Risk category C (see page xviii).

Breast-feeding:
No problems expected, but consult doctor.

Infants & children:
Not recommended. Safety and dosage have not been established.

Prolonged use:
Don't use for longer than prescribed or recommended. May cause sodium overload.

Skin & sunlight:
No special problems expected.

Driving, piloting or hazardous work:
No special problems expected.

Discontinuing:
May be unnecessary to finish medicine. Follow doctor's instructions.

Others:
* Heat and moisture in bathroom medicine cabinet can cause breakdown of medicine. Store someplace else.
* May interfere with the accuracy of some medical tests (especially acidosis and urinalysis tests).

POSSIBLE INTERACTION WITH OTHER DRUGS

GENERIC NAME OR DRUG CLASS	COMBINED EFFECT
Adrenocorticoids*	Sodium overload.
Cortisone	Sodium overload.
Ketoconazole	Decreased absorption of ketoconazole.
Mecamylamine	Increased mecamylamine effect.
Memantine	Increased effect of memantine.
Methenamine	Decreased methenamine effect.
Tetracyclines*	Greatly reduced absorption of tetracyclines.
Any other medicine	Decreased absorption of other medicine if taken within 1 to 2 hours of taking sodium bicarbonate.

POSSIBLE INTERACTION WITH OTHER SUBSTANCES

INTERACTS WITH	COMBINED EFFECT
Alcohol:	Decreased effectiveness of sodium bicarbonate.
Beverages: Milk and milk products (large amounts).	Increased risk of side effects.
Cocaine:	None expected.
Foods:	None expected.
Marijuana:	None expected.
Tobacco:	Decreased effectiveness of sodium bicarbonate.

SODIUM FLUORIDE

BRAND NAMES

Fluor-A-Day
Fluorident
Fluoritab
Fluorodex
Fluotic
Flura
Karidium

Listermint with
　Fluoride
Luride
Luride-SF
Pediaflor
Pedi-Dent
Solu-Flur

Numerous other multiple vitamin-mineral supplements. Check labels.

BASIC INFORMATION

Habit forming? No
Prescription needed? Yes, for some
Available as generic? Yes
Drug class: Mineral supplement (fluoride)

 USES

* Reduces tooth cavities.
* Treats osteoporosis.

 DOSAGE & USAGE INFORMATION

How to take:
* Tablet—Swallow with liquid or crumble tablet and take with liquid (not milk) or food.
* Liquid—Measure with dropper and take directly or with liquid.
* Chewable tablet—Chew slowly and thoroughly before swallowing.

When to take:
Usually at bedtime after teeth are thoroughly brushed.

If you forget a dose:
Take as soon as you remember. Don't double a forgotten dose. Return to schedule.

Continued next column

 OVERDOSE

SYMPTOMS:
Stomach cramps or pain, nausea, faintness, vomiting (possibly bloody), diarrhea, black stools, shallow breathing, muscle spasms, seizures, arrhythmias.
WHAT TO DO:
* Dial 911 (emergency) for medical help or call poison control center 1-800-222-1222 for instructions.
* See emergency information on last 3 pages of this book.

What drug does:
Provides supplemental fluoride to combat tooth decay.

Time lapse before drug works:
8 weeks to provide maximum effect.

Don't take with:
Any other medicine or any dietary supplement without consulting your doctor or pharmacist.

 POSSIBLE ADVERSE REACTIONS OR SIDE EFFECTS

SYMPTOMS	WHAT TO DO
Life-threatening:	
In case of overdose, see previous column.	
Common:	
Constipation, appetite loss.	Continue. Call doctor when convenient.
Infrequent:	
• Rash.	Discontinue. Call doctor right away.
• Tooth discoloration.	Continue. Call doctor when convenient.
Rare:	
• Severe upsets (digestive) only with overdose.	Discontinue. Seek emergency treatment.
• Mouth and lip sores, aching bones, stiffness.	Discontinue. Call doctor right away.

758

WARNINGS & PRECAUTIONS

Don't take if:
* Your water supply contains 0.7 parts fluoride per million. Too much fluoride stains teeth permanently.
* You are allergic to any fluoride-containing product.
* You have underactive thyroid.

Before you start, consult your doctor if:
* You have kidney disease.
* You have ulcers.
* You have joint pain.

Over age 60:
No problems expected.

Pregnancy:
Consult doctor. Risk category C (see page xviii).

Breast-feeding:
No problems expected. Consult doctor.

Infants & children:
No problems expected except accidental overdose. Keep vitamin-mineral supplements out of children's reach.

Prolonged use:
Excess may cause discolored teeth and decreased calcium in blood.

Skin & sunlight:
No problems expected.

Driving, piloting or hazardous work:
No problems expected.

Discontinuing:
No problems expected.

Others:
* Store in original plastic container. Fluoride decomposes glass.
* Some products contain tartrazine dye. Avoid, especially if you are allergic to aspirin.

POSSIBLE INTERACTION WITH OTHER DRUGS

GENERIC NAME OR DRUG CLASS	COMBINED EFFECT
Calcium supplements*	Decreased effect of calcium and fluoride.

POSSIBLE INTERACTION WITH OTHER SUBSTANCES

INTERACTS WITH	COMBINED EFFECT
Alcohol:	None expected.
Beverages: Milk.	Prevents absorption of fluoride. Space dose 2 hours before or after milk.
Cocaine:	None expected.
Foods:	None expected.
Marijuana:	None expected.
Tobacco:	None expected.

*See Glossary

STIMULANT MEDICATIONS

GENERIC AND BRAND NAMES

DEXMETHYL	METHYLPHENIDATE
PHENIDATE	(con't)
Focalin	Methylin ER
Focalin XR	Methylin Oral
METHYLPHENIDATE	Suspension
Concerta	PMS Methylpheni-
Daytrana	date
Metadate CD	Ritalin
Metadate ER	Ritalin LA
Methylin Chewable	Ritalin SR

BASIC INFORMATION

Habit forming? Yes
Prescription needed? Yes
Available as generic? Yes, for some
Drug class: Central nervous system
    stimulant, sympathomimetic

 ## USES

- Decreases overactivity and lengthens attention span in children and adults with attention-deficit hyperactivity disorder (ADHD). A total treatment plan may also include educational, social and psychological therapies.
- Treatment of depression in adults.
- Treatment for narcolepsy (uncontrollable attacks of sleepiness) and other disorders.

 ## DOSAGE & USAGE INFORMATION

How to take:
- Tablet (short-acting)—Swallow with liquid. Take as directed, usually 30-45 minutes before meals, or with meals if stomach upset occurs. If swallowing is a problem, ask your pharmacist if tablet can be crushed and taken with liquid or small amount of food.

Continued next column

 ## OVERDOSE

SYMPTOMS:
Rapid heartbeat, fever, confusion, vomiting, agitation, hallucinations, convulsions, coma.
WHAT TO DO:
- **Dial 911 (emergency) for medical help or call poison control center 1-800-222-1222 for instructions.**
- **If person is unconscious, check breathing and pulse. If not breathing, begin mouth-to-mouth rescue breathing. If heart is not beating, begin chest compressions.**
- **See emergency information on last 3 pages of this book.**

- Skin patch—Follow instructions on label.
- Extended- or sustained-release tablet and capsule—Swallow whole with liquid, usually before breakfast (or as directed). Do not crush tablet. Do not open capsule (unless your label states that the capsule may be opened and sprinkled over cool applesauce and then swallowed right away).
- Oral solution or chewable tablet—Follow instructions on label.

When to take:
At the same times each day. Regular tablets are often taken at breakfast and lunch (best not to take late in day). Extended-release forms are usually taken in the morning.

If you forget a dose:
Take as soon as you remember. If it is almost time for the next dose, wait for next scheduled dose (don't double this dose).

What drug does:
Stimulates brain to improve alertness, concentration and attention span. Calms the hyperactive child and improves ability to focus.

Time lapse before drug works:
May take 2 or more weeks to see effectiveness. Dosage may be increased or decreased depending on the response and side effects.

Don't take with:
Any other medicine or any dietary supplement without consulting your doctor or pharmacist.

 ## POSSIBLE ADVERSE REACTIONS OR SIDE EFFECTS

SYMPTOMS	WHAT TO DO
Life-threatening:	
In case of overdose, see previous column.	
Common:	
• Fast heartbeat, blood pressure increased.	Discontinue. Call doctor right away.
• Nervousness, appetite loss, trouble sleeping.	Continue. Call doctor when convenient.
Infrequent:	
• Rash or hives, chest or joint pain, unusual bruising or bleeding, unable to control body movements, fever.	Discontinue. Call doctor right away.
• Nausea, dizziness, headache, stomach pain, drowsiness, muscle cramps.	Continue. Call doctor when convenient.
Rare:	
Changed or blurred vision, unusual vocal outbursts, convulsions, abnormal or manic behavior, trouble breathing, fainting, hallucinations, is suspicious.	Discontinue. Call doctor right away.

STIMULANT MEDICATIONS

WARNINGS & PRECAUTIONS

Don't take if:
You are allergic to stimulant medications.

Before you start, consult your doctor if:
- You have epilepsy or have seizures.
- You have high blood pressure, any heart or blood vessel disorder or liver problems.
- You have glaucoma.
- You take MAO inhibitors.*
- You suffer from anxiety, agitation, tension, depressive or psychotic problems or have Tourette's syndrome or motor tics.
- You have a history of drug or alcohol abuse.

Over age 60:
Adverse reactions and side effects may be more frequent and severe than in younger persons.

Pregnancy:
Decide with your doctor if drug benefits justify risk to unborn child. Risk category C (see page xviii).

Breast-feeding:
It is unknown if drug passes into milk. Avoid drug or stop nursing until you finish medicine. Consult doctor for advice on maintaining milk supply.

Infants & children:
Use only under medical supervision for children 6 or older. Regular doctor visits are important to monitor drug's effectiveness and side effects.

Prolonged use:
- Increased risk of weight loss and abnormal behaviors. Rare risk of physical growth retardation in children.
- Talk to your doctor about the need for follow up medical examinations or laboratory studies to check drug's effectiveness and monitor any adverse effects.

Skin & sunlight:
No problems expected.

Driving, piloting or hazardous work:
Don't drive, ride a bicycle or pilot aircraft until you learn how drug affects you. Don't work around dangerous machinery. Don't climb ladders or work in high places. Danger increases if you drink alcohol or take drugs affecting alertness and reflexes.

Discontinuing:
- Don't discontinue without doctor's advice even if symptoms diminish or disappear.
- Withdrawal symptoms may occur after you discontinue the drug. Report to your doctor any new physical or emotional symptoms.

Others:
- Drug may cause serious heart and psychiatric (mental) problems, including sudden death. Read warning information provided with prescription. Call doctor right away if symptoms develop (e.g., chest pain, shortness of breath, fainting, or hallucinations).
- Dose must be carefully adjusted by doctor.
- Advise any doctor or dentist whom you consult about the use of this medicine.

POSSIBLE INTERACTION WITH OTHER DRUGS

GENERIC NAME OR DRUG CLASS	COMBINED EFFECT
Anticholinergics*	Increased anticholinergic effect.
Anticoagulants,* oral	Increased anticoagulant effect.
Anticonvulsants*	Increased anticonvulsant effect, or decreased stimulant effect.
Antidepressants, tricyclic*	Increased antidepressant effect. Decreased stimulant medication effect.
Antihypertensives*	Decreased antihypertensive effect.
Central nervous system (CNS) stimulants*	Overstimulation.
Clonidine	Increased risk of adverse effects.
Dextrothyroxine	Increased stimulant medication effect.
Monoamine oxidase (MAO) inhibitors*	Dangerous rise in blood pressure. Take at least 14 days apart.
Pimozide	May mask the cause of tics.

POSSIBLE INTERACTION WITH OTHER SUBSTANCES

INTERACTS WITH	COMBINED EFFECT
Alcohol:	None expected. Best to avoid.
Beverages:	None expected.
Cocaine:	Unknown. Avoid.
Foods:	None expected.
Marijuana:	Unknown. Avoid.
Tobacco:	None expected.

*See Glossary

STIMULANTS, AMPHETAMINE-RELATED

GENERIC AND BRAND NAMES

ARMODAFINIL
  Nuvigil

MODAFINIL
  Alertec
  Provigil
  Sparlon

BASIC INFORMATION

Habit forming? Possibly
Prescription needed? Yes
Available as generic? Yes, for some
**Drug class: Antinarcoleptic; central nervous
  system stimulant**

USES

- Treatment to help people who have narcolepsy to stay awake during the day. It does not cure narcolepsy.
- Used to improve wakefulness in patients with excessive sleepiness disorders, improve wakefulness for obstructive sleep apnea and shift work sleep disorder.
- Treatment for attention deficit hyperactivity disorder (ADHD).

DOSAGE & USAGE INFORMATION

How to take:
Tablet—Swallow whole with liquid. You may take it with or without food.

When to take:
At the same time each day, usually in the morning. Follow instructions on the label.

If you forget a dose:
Take as soon as you remember, until noon of the same day. If you don't remember until later, skip the missed dose to avoid problems getting to sleep. Return to your regular dosing schedule the next day. Do not double doses.

Continued next column

OVERDOSE

SYMPTOMS:
Symptoms may include agitation, increased blood pressure, increased heart rate and insomnia.
WHAT TO DO:
Overdose unlikely to threaten life. If person uses much larger amount than prescribed or if accidentally swallowed, call doctor or poison control center 1-800-222-1222 for help.

What drug does:
Stimulates the central nervous system. The exact way these drugs work is unknown.

Time lapse before drug works:
2 to 4 hours.

Don't take with:
Any other medicine or any dietary supplement without consulting your doctor or pharmacist.

POSSIBLE ADVERSE REACTIONS OR SIDE EFFECTS

SYMPTOMS	WHAT TO DO
Life-threatening:	
Rare allergic reaction— Breathing difficulty; closing of the throat; swelling of hands, feet, face, lips or tongue; hives, any rash.	Discontinue. Seek emergency treatment.
Common:	
Anxiety, headache, nausea, nervousness, trouble sleeping.	Continue. Call doctor when convenient.
Infrequent:	
Appetite changes, diarrhea, dry mouth, skin symptoms (dryness, flushing or tingling), muscle stiffness, stuffy or runny nose, trembling or shaking, vomiting.	Continue. Call doctor when convenient.
Rare:	
Vision changes, chills or fever, confusion, abnormal heart rate, dizziness, fainting, increased thirst or urination, depression, memory or mood changes, shortness of breath, trouble in urinating, uncontrolled movements (face, mouth and tongue).	Discontinue. Call doctor right away.

WARNINGS & PRECAUTIONS

Don't take if:
You are allergic to armodafinil or modafinil or other central nervous system stimulants.

Before you start, consult your doctor if:
- You have heart disease or have had a heart attack.
- You have or have had high blood pressure.
- You take oral contraceptives.

STIMULANTS, AMPHETAMINE-RELATED

- You have liver or kidney disease.
- You have a history of psychosis, depression, mania, or other severe mental illness.

Over age 60:
No special problems expected.

Pregnancy:
Decide with your doctor if drug benefits justify any possible risk to unborn child. Risk category C (see page xviii).

Breast-feeding:
It is unknown if drugs pass into milk. Avoid drug or discontinue nursing until you finish medicine. Consult doctor for advice on maintaining milk supply.

Infants & children:
Not approved for children. One exception—the brand name Sparlon is approved for treatment of attention deficit hyperactivity disorder in children ages 6-17.

Prolonged use:
May lead to physical or mental dependence. Consult your doctor if any of the following signs of dependence occur:
- A strong desire to continue taking this drug.
- A need to increase the dose to receive the effects of the medicine.
- Withdrawal side effects when you stop taking the medicine.

Skin & sunlight:
No problems expected.

Driving, piloting or hazardous work:
Don't drive or pilot aircraft until you learn how medicine affects you. Don't work around dangerous machinery. Don't climb ladders or work in high places. Danger increases if you drink alcohol or take medicine affecting alertness and reflexes such as antihistamines, tranquilizers or sedatives, pain medicine, narcotics and mind-altering drugs.

Discontinuing:
- Consult your doctor if any new or unusual symptoms occur after discontinuing the drug.
- Dose may require gradual reduction if you have taken drug for a long time.

Others:
- If you are using a birth control method, such as pills or implants, they may not be as effective while taking these drugs and for up to one month after stopping them.
- Stop drug and contact your doctor if you experience any sort of unusual rash or mood changes. Rare cases of serious or life-threatening rash and serious psychiatric adverse experiences (including anxiety, mania, hallucinations and thoughts of suicide) have been reported.
- Advise any doctor or dentist whom you consult that you take this medicine.
- May affect the results in some medical tests.

 POSSIBLE INTERACTION WITH OTHER DRUGS

GENERIC NAME OR DRUG CLASS	COMBINED EFFECT
Antidepressants, tricyclic*	Increased effect of antidepressant.
CNS stimulants*	Increased stimulant effect.
Contraceptives*	Decreased contraceptive effect.
Diazepam	Decreased diazepam effect.
Enzyme inducers*	Decreased stimulant effect.
Enzyme inhibitors*	Increased stimulant effect.
MAO inhibitors*	Unknown effect. Avoid.
Mephenytoin	Mephenytoin dose may need adjustment.
Theophylline	Decreased theophylline effect.
Warfarin	Increased warfarin effect.

 POSSIBLE INTERACTION WITH OTHER SUBSTANCES

INTERACTS WITH	COMBINED EFFECT
Alcohol:	Effects unknown. Avoid.
Beverages: Grapefruit juice.	Unknown effect. Consult doctor.
Cocaine:	Effects unknown. Avoid.
Foods: Grapefruit.	Unknown effect. Consult doctor.
Marijuana:	Effects unknown. Avoid.
Tobacco:	None expected.

*See Glossary

SUCRALFATE

BRAND NAMES

Carafate

Sulcrate

Sulcrate Suspension Plus

BASIC INFORMATION

Habit forming? No
Prescription needed? Yes
Available as generic? Yes
Drug class: Antiulcer agent

 ## USES

- Treatment for duodenal and gastric ulcers.
- Used to relieve side effects of nonsteroidal anti-inflammatory therapy in rheumatoid arthritis.
- Treatment for gastroesophageal reflux disease (GERD).

 ## DOSAGE & USAGE INFORMATION

How to take:
- Tablet—Take as directed on an empty stomach.
- Oral suspension—Follow instructions on package.

When to take:
1 hour before meals and at bedtime. Allow 2 hours to elapse before taking other prescription medicines.

If you forget a dose:
Take as soon as you remember up to 2 hours late. If more than 2 hours, wait for next scheduled dose (don't double this dose).

What drug does:
Covers ulcer site and protects from acid, enzymes and bile salts.

Time lapse before drug works:
Begins in 30 minutes. May require several days to relieve pain.

Don't take with:
Any other medicine or any dietary supplement without consulting your doctor or pharmacist.

 ## OVERDOSE

SYMPTOMS:
None expected.
WHAT TO DO:
Overdose unlikely to threaten life. If person uses much larger amount than prescribed or if accidentally swallowed, call doctor or poison control center 1-800-222-1222 for help.

 ## POSSIBLE ADVERSE REACTIONS OR SIDE EFFECTS

SYMPTOMS	WHAT TO DO
Life-threatening: None expected.	
Common: Constipation.	Continue. Call doctor when convenient.
Infrequent: Dizziness, sleepiness, rash, itchy skin, abdominal pain, indigestion, vomiting, nausea, dry mouth, diarrhea.	Continue. Call doctor when convenient.
Rare: Back pain.	Continue. Call doctor when convenient.

 ## WARNINGS & PRECAUTIONS

Don't take if:
You are allergic to sucralfate.

Before you start, consult your doctor if:
- You will have surgery within 2 months, including dental surgery, requiring general or spinal anesthesia.
- You have gastrointestinal or kidney disease.

Over age 60:
Adverse reactions and side effects may be more frequent and severe than in younger persons.

Pregnancy:
No proven harm to unborn child. Avoid if possible. Consult doctor. Risk category B (see page xviii).

Breast-feeding:
Unknown effects. Consult doctor.

Infants & children:
Safety not established.

Prolonged use:
Request blood counts if medicine needed longer than 8 weeks.

Skin & sunlight:
No problems expected.

Driving, piloting or hazardous work:
Don't drive or pilot aircraft until you learn how medicine affects you. Don't work around dangerous machinery. Don't climb ladders or work in high places. Danger increases if you drink alcohol or take medicine affecting alertness and reflexes, such as antihistamines, tranquilizers, sedatives, pain medicine, narcotics and mind-altering drugs.

Discontinuing:
Don't discontinue without consulting doctor.
Dose may require gradual reduction if you have
taken drug for a long time. Doses of other drugs
may also require adjustment.

Others:
Advise any doctor or dentist whom you consult
that you take this medicine.

POSSIBLE INTERACTION WITH OTHER DRUGS

GENERIC NAME OR DRUG CLASS	COMBINED EFFECT
Anagrelide	May interfere with anagrelide absorption.
Antacids*	Take 1/2 hour before or after sucralfate.
Cimetidine	Possible decreased absorption of cimetidine if taken simultaneously.
Ciprofloxacin	Decreased absorption of ciprofloxacin. Take 2 hours before sucralfate.
Digoxin	Decreased absorption of digoxin. Take 2 hours before sucralfate.
Fluoroquinolones	Decreased fluoroquinolone effect.
Ketoconazole	Decreased ketoconazole effect.
Norfloxacin	Decreased absorption of norfloxacin. Take 2 hours before sucralfate.
Ofloxacin	Decreased absorption of ofloxacin. Take 2 hours before sucralfate.
Phenytoin	Possible decreased absorption of phenytoin if taken simultaneously.
Proton pump inhibitors	May decrease effect of some proton pump inhibitors. Take 30 minutes before sucralfate.
Theophylline	Decreased absorption of theophylline. Take 2 hours before sucralfate.
Vitamins A, D, E, K	Decreased vitamin absorption.

POSSIBLE INTERACTION WITH OTHER SUBSTANCES

INTERACTS WITH	COMBINED EFFECT
Alcohol:	Irritates ulcer. Avoid.
Beverages: Caffeine.	Irritates ulcer. Avoid.
Cocaine:	May make ulcer worse. Avoid.
Foods:	No problems expected.
Marijuana:	May make ulcer worse. Avoid.
Tobacco:	May make ulcer worse. Avoid.

*See Glossary

SULFADOXINE & PYRIMETHAMINE

BRAND NAMES

Fansidar

BASIC INFORMATION

Habit forming? No
Prescription needed? Yes
Available as generic? No
Drug class: Antiprotozoal

 USES

- Treats malaria *(plasmodium falciparum)*.
- Helps prevent malaria when traveling to areas where it exists.
- Also used to prevent isosporiasis in patients with acquired immunodeficiency disease.

 DOSAGE & USAGE INFORMATION

How to take:
Tablet—Swallow with liquid. Instructions to take on empty stomach mean 1 hour before or 2 hours after eating. Drink plenty of fluids while using this drug to help kidneys excrete more urine.

When to take:
Follow doctor's instructions.

If you forget a dose:
Take as soon as you remember. If close to time for next dose, skip this one and wait for next scheduled dose. Don't double dose.

What drug does:
The sulfa component kills bacteria; the pyrimethamine works to kill malaria organisms in red blood cells or human tissue.

Time lapse before drug works:
2 to 6 hours.

Continued next column

 OVERDOSE

SYMPTOMS:
Appetite loss, sore throat and fever, seizure, coma.
WHAT TO DO:
- **Dial 911 (emergency) for medical help or call poison control center 1-800-222-1222 for instructions.**
- **See emergency information on last 3 pages of this book.**

Don't take with:
- Any other medicines (including over-the-counter drugs such as cough and cold medicines, laxatives, antacids, diet pills, caffeine, nose drops or vitamins) without consulting your doctor or pharmacist.
- Mefloquine.

 POSSIBLE ADVERSE REACTIONS OR SIDE EFFECTS

SYMPTOMS	WHAT TO DO
Life-threatening:	
In case of overdose, see previous column.	
Common:	
Loss or change of taste; diarrhea; skin rash; pale skin; sore throat; sore, red tongue; mouth ulcers; fever; excessive bleeding; tiredness; light sensitivity.	Discontinue. Call doctor right away.
Infrequent:	
Aching joints, fever, skin blisters or peeling, jaundice (yellow skin and eyes).	Discontinue. Call doctor right away.
Rare:	
Bloody urine, burning on urination, back pain, swollen neck.	Discontinue. Call doctor right away.

SULFADOXINE & PYRIMETHAMINE

WARNINGS & PRECAUTIONS

Don't take if:
You are allergic to sulfa drugs, furosemide, thiazide diuretics, or carbonic anhydrase inhibitors.

Before you start, consult your doctor if:
- You have AIDS.
- You have anemia, seizures, G6PD* deficiency, liver disease, porphyria, kidney disease.
- You can't tolerate sulfa drugs.

Over age 60:
Adverse reactions and side effects may be more frequent and severe than in younger persons. You may need smaller doses for shorter periods of time.

Pregnancy:
Use birth control so you won't get pregnant while in an endemic malaria area. Should not be taken during pregnancy if it can possibly be avoided. Consult doctor. Risk category C (see page xviii).

Breast-feeding:
Drug passes into milk. Avoid drug or discontinue nursing until you finish medicine. Consult doctor for advice on maintaining milk supply.

Infants & children:
Don't use in infants under 2 months old.

Prolonged use:
Talk to your doctor about the need for follow-up medical examinations or laboratory studies to check complete blood counts (white blood cell count, platelet count, red blood cell count, hemoglobin, hematocrit) and urinalysis.

Skin & sunlight:
May cause rash or intensify sunburn in areas exposed to sun or ultraviolet light (photosensitivity reaction). Avoid overexposure. Notify doctor if reaction occurs.

Driving, piloting or hazardous work:
Avoid if you feel confused, drowsy or dizzy.

Discontinuing:
Don't discontinue for 4 to 6 weeks after you leave endemic malaria areas.

Others:
- Advise any doctor or dentist whom you consult that you take this medicine.
- May affect results in some medical tests.
- Sleep under mosquito netting while in endemic areas. Wear long-sleeved shirts and long pants.
- Report to your doctor if you develop any symptoms of illness while you take this medicine—even if the symptoms seem minor.

POSSIBLE INTERACTION WITH OTHER DRUGS

GENERIC NAME OR DRUG CLASS	COMBINED EFFECT
Anticoagulants*	Increased risk of toxicity.
Anticonvulsants*	Increased risk of toxicity.
Antidiabetics*	Increased risk of toxicity.
Bone marrow depressants*	Increased risk of bleeding or other toxic symptoms.
Clozapine	Toxic effect on the central nervous system.
Contraceptives, oral*	Reduced reliability of the contraceptive.
Hepatotoxic medicines*	Increased risk of liver toxicity.
Methenamine	Increased risk of kidney toxicity.
Methotrexate	Increased risk of toxicity.
Zidovudine	Increased risk of liver toxicity.

POSSIBLE INTERACTION WITH OTHER SUBSTANCES

INTERACTS WITH	COMBINED EFFECT
Alcohol:	Nausea and vomiting. Avoid.
Beverages:	No special problems expected.
Cocaine:	Increased likelihood of adverse reactions or seizures. Avoid.
Foods:	No special problems expected.
Marijuana:	Increased likelihood of adverse reactions. Avoid.
Tobacco:	No special problems expected.

*See Glossary

SULFASALAZINE

BRAND NAMES

Azaline	Salazopyrin
Azulfidine	Salazosulfapyridine
Azulfidine En-Tabs	Salicylazosulfa-
PMS Sulfasalazine	pyridine
PMS Sulfasalazine	S.A.S. Enteric-500
EC	S.A.S.-500

BASIC INFORMATION

Habit forming? No
Prescription needed? Yes
Available as generic? Yes
Drug class: Sulfa (sulfonamide)

 ## USES

* Treatment for ulceration and bleeding from ulcerative colitis and Crohn's disease.
* Treatment for rheumatoid arthritis for patients not responding to other treatments.

 ## DOSAGE & USAGE INFORMATION

How to take:
* Tablet—Swallow with liquid. Instructions to take on empty stomach mean 1 hour before or 2 hours after eating.
* Liquid—Shake carefully before measuring.

When to take:
At the same times each day, evenly spaced.

If you forget a dose:
Take as soon as you remember up to 2 hours late. If more than 2 hours, wait for next scheduled dose (don't double this dose).

What drug does:
Anti-inflammatory action reduces tissue destruction in colon.

Time lapse before drug works:
2 to 5 days.

Don't take with:
Any other medicine or any dietary supplement without consulting your doctor or pharmacist.

 ## OVERDOSE

SYMPTOMS:
Less urine, bloody urine, coma.
WHAT TO DO:
* Dial 911 (emergency) for medical help or call poison control center 1-800-222-1222 for instructions.
* See emergency information on last 3 pages of this book.

 ## POSSIBLE ADVERSE REACTIONS OR SIDE EFFECTS

SYMPTOMS	WHAT TO DO
Life-threatening:	
In case of overdose, see previous column.	
Common:	
• Itchy skin, rash.	Discontinue. Call doctor right away.
• Headache, nausea, vomiting, diarrhea, appetite loss, skin sensitive to sun.	Continue. Call doctor when convenient.
• Orange urine or skin.	Continue. Tell doctor at next visit.
Infrequent:	
• Red, peeling or blistering skin; sore throat; fever; swallowing difficulty; unusual bruising; aching joints or muscles; jaundice.	Discontinue. Call doctor right away.
• Dizziness, tiredness, weakness, impotence.	Continue. Call doctor when convenient.
Rare:	
Painful urination; low back pain; numbness, tingling, burning feeling in feet and hands; bloody urine; neck swelling.	Discontinue. Call doctor right away.

 ## WARNINGS & PRECAUTIONS

Don't take if:
You are allergic to any sulfa drug.*

Before you start, consult your doctor if:
* You are allergic to carbonic anhydrase inhibitors, oral antidiabetics or thiazide or loop diuretics.
* You are allergic by nature.
* You have liver or kidney disease.
* You have porphyria.
* You have developed anemia from use of any drug.

Over age 60:
Adverse reactions and side effects may be more frequent and severe than in younger persons.

Pregnancy:
Consult doctor. Risk category B (see page xviii).

Breast-feeding:
Drug passes into milk. Avoid drug or discontinue nursing until you finish medicine. Consult doctor for advice on maintaining milk supply.

Infants & children:
Don't give to infants younger than 2 years.

Prolonged use:
* May enlarge thyroid gland.
* You may become more susceptible to infections caused by germs not responsive to this drug.
* Request frequent blood counts, liver and kidney function studies.

Skin & sunlight:
May cause rash or intensify sunburn in areas exposed to sun or ultraviolet light (photosensitivity reaction). Avoid overexposure. Notify doctor if reaction occurs.

Driving, piloting or hazardous work:
Avoid if you feel dizzy. Otherwise, no problems expected.

Discontinuing:
Don't discontinue without doctor's advice until you complete prescribed dose, even though symptoms diminish or disappear.

Others:
* Drink 2 quarts of liquid each day to prevent adverse reactions.
* If you require surgery, tell anesthetist you take sulfa.

 POSSIBLE INTERACTION WITH OTHER DRUGS

GENERIC NAME OR DRUG CLASS	COMBINED EFFECT
Aminobenzoates	Possible decreased sulfa effect.
Antibiotics*	Decreased sulfa effect.
Anticoagulants,* oral	Increased anticoagulant effect.
Anticonvulsants, hydantoin*	Toxic effect on brain.
Antidiabetics*	Toxic effect on brain.
Aspirin	Increased sulfa effect.
Calcium supplements*	Decreased sulfa effect.
Clozapine	Toxic effect on the central nervous system.
Digoxin	Decreased digoxin effect.
Hepatotoxic agents*	Increased liver toxicity.
Iron supplements*	Decreased sulfa effect.

Isoniazid	Possible anemia.
Mecamylamine	Decreased antibiotic effect.
Methenamine	Possible kidney blockage.
Methotrexate	Increased methotrexate effect.
Oxyphenbutazone	Increased sulfa effect.
Para-aminosalicylic acid	Decreased sulfa effect.
Penicillins*	Decreased penicillin effect.
Phenylbutazone	Increased sulfa effect.
Probenecid	Increased sulfa effect.
Sulfinpyrazone	Increased sulfa effect.
Sulfonylureas*	May increase hypoglycemic action.
Trimethoprim	Increased sulfa effect.
Vitamin C	Possible kidney damage. Avoid large doses of vitamin C.
Zidovudine	Increased risk of toxic effects of zidovudine.

 POSSIBLE INTERACTION WITH OTHER SUBSTANCES

INTERACTS WITH	COMBINED EFFECT
Alcohol:	Increased alcohol effect.
Beverages: Less than 2 quarts of fluid daily.	Kidney damage.
Cocaine:	None expected.
Foods:	None expected.
Marijuana:	None expected.
Tobacco:	None expected.

*See Glossary

SULFINPYRAZONE

BRAND NAMES

Anturan
Anturane
Apo-Sulfinpyrazone
Novopyrazone

BASIC INFORMATION

Habit forming? No
Prescription needed? Yes
Available as generic? Yes
Drug class: Antigout

USES

- Treatment for chronic gout.
- May be prescribed to reduce the risk of recurrent heart attack.

DOSAGE & USAGE INFORMATION

How to take:
Tablet or capsule—Swallow with liquid or food to lessen stomach irritation. If you can't swallow whole, crumble tablet or open capsule and take with liquid or food.

When to take:
At the same times each day.

If you forget a dose:
Take as soon as you remember up to 2 hours late. If more than 2 hours, wait for next scheduled dose (don't double this dose).

What drug does:
Reduces uric acid level in blood and tissues by increasing amount of uric acid secreted in urine by kidneys.

Time lapse before drug works:
May require 6 months to prevent gout attacks.

Don't take with:
Any other medicine or any dietary supplement without consulting your doctor or pharmacist.

OVERDOSE

SYMPTOMS:
Breathing difficulty, vomiting, imbalance, seizures, convulsions, coma.
WHAT TO DO:
- Dial 911 (emergency) for medical help or call poison control center 1-800-222-1222 for instructions.
- If person is unconscious, check breathing and pulse. If not breathing, begin mouth-to-mouth rescue breathing. If heart is not beating, begin chest compressions.
- See emergency information on last 3 pages of this book.

POSSIBLE ADVERSE REACTIONS OR SIDE EFFECTS

SYMPTOMS	WHAT TO DO
Life-threatening:	
In case of overdose, see previous column.	
Common:	
None expected.	
Infrequent:	
• Painful or difficult urination, worsening gout.	Discontinue. Call doctor right away.
• Rash, nausea, vomiting, abdominal pain, low back pain.	Continue. Call doctor when convenient.
Rare:	
• Black, bloody or tarry stools.	Discontinue. Seek emergency treatment.
• Sore throat; fever; unusual bleeding or bruising; red, painful joints; blood in urine; fatigue or weakness.	Discontinue. Call doctor right away.

WARNINGS & PRECAUTIONS

Don't take if:
- You are allergic to any uricosuric.*
- You have acute gout.
- You have active ulcers (stomach or duodenal), enteritis or ulcerative colitis.
- You have blood cell disorders.
- You are allergic to oxyphenbutazone or phenylbutazone.

Before you start, consult your doctor if:
You have kidney or blood disease.

Over age 60:
Adverse reactions and side effects may be more frequent and severe than in younger persons. You require lower dose because of decreased kidney function.

Pregnancy:
Decide with your doctor whether drug benefits justify risk to unborn child. Risk category C (see page xviii).

Breast-feeding:
Effect unknown. Consult doctor.

Infants & children:
Not recommended.

Prolonged use:
- Possible kidney damage.
- Talk to your doctor about the need for follow-up medical examinations or laboratory studies to check complete blood counts (white blood cell count, platelet count, red blood cell count, hemoglobin, hematocrit), kidney function, serum uric acid and urine uric acid.

Skin & sunlight:
No problems expected.

Driving, piloting or hazardous work:
No problems expected.

Discontinuing:
Don't discontinue without consulting doctor. Dose may require gradual reduction if you have taken drug for a long time. Doses of other drugs may also require adjustment.

Others:
- Drink 10 to 12 glasses of water each day you take this medicine.
- Periodic blood and urine laboratory tests recommended.

 POSSIBLE INTERACTION WITH OTHER DRUGS

GENERIC NAME OR DRUG CLASS	COMBINED EFFECT
Allopurinol	Increased effect of each drug.
Anticoagulants,* oral	Increased anticoagulant effect.
Antidiabetics,* oral	Increased antidiabetic effect.
Aspirin	Bleeding tendency. Decreased sulfinpyrazone effect.
Bismuth subsalicylate	Decreased sulfinpyrazone effect.
Cephalosporins*	Increased risk of bleeding.
Cholestyramine	Decreased sulfinpyrazone effect.
Contraceptives, oral*	Increased bleeding between menstrual periods.
Diuretics*	Decreased sulfinpyrazone effect.
Nitrofurantoin	Increased risk of toxicity.
Penicillins*	Increased penicillin effect.

Salicylates*	Bleeding tendency. Decreased sulfinpyrazone effect.
Sulfa drugs*	Increased effect of sulfa drugs.
Thioguanine	May need increased dosage of sulfinpyrazone.

 POSSIBLE INTERACTION WITH OTHER SUBSTANCES

INTERACTS WITH	COMBINED EFFECT
Alcohol:	Decreased sulfinpyrazone effect.
Beverages: Caffeine drinks.	Decreased sulfinpyrazone effect.
Cocaine:	None expected.
Foods:	None expected.
Marijuana:	Occasional use— None expected. Daily use—May increase blood level of uric acid.
Tobacco:	None expected.

*See Glossary

SULFONAMIDES

GENERIC AND BRAND NAMES

See full list of generic and brand names in the *Generic and Brand Names Directory*, page 898.

BASIC INFORMATION

Habit forming? No
Prescription needed? Yes
Available as generic? Yes, for some
Drug class: Antibacterial (antibiotic), antiprotozoal, sulfa (sulfonamide)

 USES

- Treatment of urinary tract and other infections.
- Sulfamethoxazole in combination with trimethoprim may be used to treat bronchitis, certain types of pneumonia, skin infections, middle ear infections, intestinal tract infections and urinary tract infections.

 DOSAGE & USAGE INFORMATION

How to take:
- Tablet—Swallow with liquid. Instructions to take on empty stomach mean 1 hour before or 2 hours after eating. Drink an extra amount of water daily so that urine output will be adequate.
- Liquid—Shake carefully before measuring.
- Other forms—Follow label instructions.

When to take:
At the same times each day, evenly spaced.

If you forget a dose:
Take as soon as you remember up to 2 hours late. If more than 2 hours, wait for next scheduled dose (don't double this dose).

What drug does:
Interferes with a nutrient (folic acid) necessary for growth and reproduction of bacteria. Will not attack viruses.

Continued next column

 OVERDOSE

SYMPTOMS:
Less urine, bloody urine, stomach pain, light-headedness, headache, drowsiness, coma.
WHAT TO DO:
- **Dial 911 (emergency) for medical help or call poison control center 1-800-222-1222 for instructions.**
- **See emergency information on last 3 pages of this book.**

Time lapse before drug works:
2 to 5 days to affect infection.

Don't take with:
Any other medicine or any dietary supplement without consulting your doctor or pharmacist.

 POSSIBLE ADVERSE REACTIONS OR SIDE EFFECTS

SYMPTOMS	WHAT TO DO
Life-threatening:	
In case of overdose, see previous column.	
Common:	
• Itchy skin, rash.	Discontinue. Call doctor right away.
• Headache, nausea, vomiting, diarrhea, appetite loss, skin sensitive to sun, dizziness.	Continue. Call doctor when convenient.
Infrequent:	
• Red, peeling or blistering skin; sore throat; fever; swallowing difficulty; unusual bruising or bleeding; aching joints or muscles; yellow skin or eyes; pale skin.	Discontinue. Call doctor right away.
• Weakness or tiredness.	Continue. Call doctor when convenient.
Rare:	
Painful urination, low back pain, numbness, stomach pain, bloody diarrhea or urine, neck swelling, mood or behavior changes, increased or decreased urine output, thirst.	Discontinue. Call doctor right away.

 WARNINGS & PRECAUTIONS

Don't take if:
You are allergic to any sulfa drug.

Before you start, consult your doctor if:
- You are allergic to carbonic anhydrase inhibitors, oral antidiabetics or diuretics (thiazide or loop).
- You are allergic by nature.
- You have liver or kidney disease.
- You have glucose 6-phosphate dehydrogenase (G6PD) disease.
- You have porphyria.
- You have anemia or other blood problems.

Over age 60:
Adverse reactions and side effects may be more frequent and severe than in younger persons.

Pregnancy:
Decide with your doctor if drug benefits justify risk to unborn child. Risk category C (see page xviii).

Breast-feeding:
Drug passes into milk. Avoid drug or discontinue nursing until you finish medicine. Consult doctor for advice on maintaining milk supply.

Infants & children:
Don't give to infants younger than 2 months.

Prolonged use:
- You may become more susceptible to infections caused by germs not responsive to this drug.
- Drug may enlarge thyroid gland (rare).
- Talk to your doctor about the need for frequent blood counts, liver and kidney function studies.

Skin & sunlight:
May cause rash or intensify sunburn in areas exposed to sun or ultraviolet light (photosensitivity reaction). Avoid excess exposure. Notify doctor if reaction occurs.

Driving, piloting or hazardous work:
Avoid if you feel dizzy. Otherwise, no problems expected.

Discontinuing:
Don't discontinue without doctor's advice until you complete prescribed dose, even though symptoms diminish or disappear.

Others:
- Drink 2 quarts of liquid each day to prevent side effects or adverse reactions.
- Advise any doctor or dentist whom you consult that you take this medicine.
- If you require surgery, tell anesthetist you take sulfa.

POSSIBLE INTERACTION WITH OTHER DRUGS

GENERIC NAME OR DRUG CLASS	COMBINED EFFECT
Aminobenzoate potassium	Possible decreased sulfonamide effect.
Anticoagulants,* oral	Increased anticoagulant effect.
Anticonvulsants,* hydantoin	Increased anticonvulsant effect.
Antidiabetics,* oral	Increased antidiabetic effect.
Bone marrow depressants*	Increased risk of side effects.
Contraceptives,* oral estrogen	Decreased contraceptive effect.
Cyclosporine	Decreased cyclosporine effect.
Hemolytics,* other	Increased risk of side effects.
Hepatotoxic agents*	Increased liver toxicity.
Mecamylamine	Decreased antibiotic effect.
Methenamine	Possible kidney blockage.
Methotrexate	Increased methotrexate effect.
Penicillins*	Decreased penicillin effect.
Phenylbutazone	Increased sulfonamide effect.
Probenecid	Increased sulfonamide effect.
Sulfinpyrazone	Increased sulfonamide effect.

POSSIBLE INTERACTION WITH OTHER SUBSTANCES

INTERACTS WITH	COMBINED EFFECT
Alcohol:	None expected.
Beverages: Inadequate fluid intake.	Increased risk of side effects.
Cocaine:	None expected.
Foods:	None expected.
Marijuana:	None expected.
Tobacco:	None expected.

*See Glossary

SULFONAMIDES & PHENAZOPYRIDINE

GENERIC AND BRAND NAMES

**SULFAMETHOXA-
ZOLE &
PHENAZOPYRIDINE**
Azo Gantanol
Azo-
  Sulfamethoxazole

**SULFISOXAZOLE &
PHENAZO-
PYRIDINE**
Azo Gantrisin
Azo-Sulfisoxazol
Azo-Truxazole
Sul-Azo

BASIC INFORMATION

Habit forming? No
Prescription needed? Yes
Available as generic? Yes
Drug class: Analgesic (urinary), sulfonamide

USES

- Treats infections responsive to this drug.
- Relieves pain of lower urinary tract irritation, as in cystitis, urethritis or prostatitis.

DOSAGE & USAGE INFORMATION

How to take:
Tablet—Swallow with liquid. Instructions to take on empty stomach mean 1 hour before or 2 hours after eating.

When to take:
At the same times each day, after meals.

If you forget a dose:
Take as soon as you remember up to 2 hours late. If more than 2 hours, wait for next scheduled dose (don't double this dose).

What drug does:
- Interferes with a nutrient (folic acid) necessary for growth and reproduction of bacteria. Will not attack viruses.
- Anesthetizes lower urinary tract. Relieves pain, burning, pressure and urgency to urinate.

Time lapse before drug works:
2 to 5 days to affect infection.

Continued next column

OVERDOSE

SYMPTOMS:
Less urine, bloody urine, shortness of breath, weakness, coma.
WHAT TO DO:
- **Dial 911 (emergency) for medical help or call poison control center 1-800-222-1222 for instructions.**
- **See emergency information on last 3 pages of this book.**

Don't take with:
Any other medicine or any dietary supplement without consulting your doctor or pharmacist.

POSSIBLE ADVERSE REACTIONS OR SIDE EFFECTS

SYMPTOMS	WHAT TO DO
Life-threatening:	
In case of overdose, see previous column.	
Common:	
• Rash, itchy skin.	Discontinue. Call doctor right away.
• Dizziness, diarrhea, headache, appetite loss, nausea, vomiting, skin sensitive to sun.	Continue. Call doctor when convenient.
Infrequent:	
• Joint pain; swallowing difficulty; pale skin; blistering; peeling of skin; sore throat, fever, mouth sores; unexplained bleeding or bruising; jaundice.	Discontinue. Call doctor right away.
• Abdominal pain, indigestion, weakness, tiredness.	Continue. Call doctor when convenient.
Rare:	
Back pain; neck swelling; numbness, tingling, burning feeling in feet and hands; bloody urine; painful urination.	Discontinue. Call doctor right away.

WARNINGS & PRECAUTIONS

Don't take if:
- You are allergic to any sulfa drug or urinary analgesic.
- You have hepatitis.

Before you start, consult your doctor if:
- You are allergic to carbonic anhydrase inhibitors, oral antidiabetics or thiazide or loop diuretics.
- You are allergic by nature.
- You have liver or kidney disease, porphyria.
- You have developed anemia from use of any drug.
- You have G6PD* deficiency.

Over age 60:
Adverse reactions and side effects may be more frequent and severe than in younger persons.

Pregnancy:
Risk factors vary for drugs in this group. See category list on page xviii and consult doctor.

SULFONAMIDES & PHENAZOPYRIDINE

Breast-feeding:
Drug passes into milk. Avoid drug or discontinue nursing until you finish medicine. Consult doctor for advice on maintaining milk supply.

Infants & children:
Don't give to infants younger than 1 month.

Prolonged use:
- May enlarge thyroid gland.
- You may become more susceptible to infections caused by germs not responsive to this drug.
- Request frequent blood counts, liver and kidney function studies.
- Orange or yellow skin.
- Anemia. Occasional blood studies recommended.

Skin & sunlight:
One or more drugs in this group may cause rash or intensify sunburn in areas exposed to sun or ultraviolet light (photosensitivity reaction). Avoid overexposure. Notify doctor if reaction occurs.

Driving, piloting or hazardous work:
Avoid if you feel dizzy. Otherwise, no problems expected.

Discontinuing:
Don't discontinue without doctor's advice until you complete prescribed dose, even though symptoms diminish or disappear.

Others:
- Drink 2 quarts of liquid each day to prevent adverse reactions.
- If you require surgery, tell anesthetist you take sulfa.
- Will probably cause urine to be reddish orange. Requires no action.
- May stain fabrics.

POSSIBLE INTERACTION WITH OTHER DRUGS

GENERIC NAME OR DRUG CLASS	COMBINED EFFECT
Aminobenzoates	Possible decreased sulfa effect.
Anticoagulants,* oral	Increased anticoagulant effect.
Anticonvulsants, hydantoin*	Toxic effect on brain.
Antidiabetics*	Toxic effect on brain.
Aspirin	Increased sulfa effect.
Clozapine	Toxic effect on the central nervous system.
Didanosine	Increased risk of pancreatitis.

Hepatotoxic agents*	Increased liver toxicity.
Isoniazid	Possible anemia.
Mecamylamine	Decreased antibiotic effect.
Methenamine	Possible kidney blockage.
Methotrexate	Increased methotrexate effect.
Oxyphenbutazone	Increased sulfa effect.
Para-aminosalicylic acid	Decreased sulfa effect.
Penicillins*	Decreased penicillin effect.
Phenylbutazone	Increased sulfa effect.
Probenecid	Increased sulfa effect.
Sulfinpyrazone	Increased sulfa effect.
Sulfonylureas*	May increase hypoglycemic action.
Trimethoprim	Increased sulfa effect.
Zidovudine	Increased risk of toxic effects of zidovudine.

POSSIBLE INTERACTION WITH OTHER SUBSTANCES

INTERACTS WITH	COMBINED EFFECT
Alcohol:	Increased alcohol effect.
Beverages: Less than 2 quarts of fluid daily.	Kidney damage.
Cocaine:	None expected.
Foods:	None expected.
Marijuana:	None expected.
Tobacco:	None expected.

*See Glossary

SULFONYLUREAS

GENERIC AND BRAND NAMES

See full list of generic and brand names in the *Generic and Brand Name Directory*, page 898.

BASIC INFORMATION

Habit forming? No
Prescription needed? Yes
Available as generic? Yes, for some.
Drug class: Antidiabetic (oral), sulfonylurea

 ## USES

- Treatment for diabetes in adults who can't control blood sugar by diet, weight loss and exercise.
- Treatment for diabetes insipidus (chlorpropamide).

 ## DOSAGE & USAGE INFORMATION

How to take:
- Tablet—Swallow with liquid or food to lessen stomach irritation. If you can't swallow whole, crumble tablet and take with liquid or food.
- Extended-release tablet—Swallow whole with liquid. Do not crush or chew tablet.

When to take:
At the same times each day.

If you forget a dose:
Take as soon as you remember up to 2 hours late. If more than 2 hours, wait for next scheduled dose (don't double this dose).

What drug does:
Stimulates pancreas to produce more insulin. Insulin in blood forces cells to use sugar in blood.

Time lapse before drug works:
3 to 4 hours. May require 2 weeks for maximum benefit.

Don't take with:
Any other medicine or any dietary supplement without consulting your doctor or pharmacist.

 ## OVERDOSE

SYMPTOMS:
Excessive hunger, nausea, anxiety, cool skin, cold sweats, drowsiness, rapid heartbeat, weakness, unconsciousness, coma.
WHAT TO DO:
- **Dial 911 (emergency) for medical help or call poison control center 1-800-222-1222 for instructions.**
- **See emergency information on last 3 pages of this book.**

 ## POSSIBLE ADVERSE REACTIONS OR SIDE EFFECTS

SYMPTOMS	WHAT TO DO
Life-threatening:	
In case of overdose, see previous column.	
Common:	
• Dizziness.	Discontinue. Call doctor right away.
• Diarrhea, appetite loss, nausea, stomach pain, heartburn, constipation.	Continue. Call doctor when convenient.
Infrequent:	
• Low blood sugar (hunger, anxiety, cold sweats, rapid pulse), shortness of breath.	Discontinue. Seek emergency treatment.
• Headache.	Continue. Call doctor when convenient.
Rare:	
Fatigue, itchy skin or rash, sore throat, fever, ringing in ears, unusual bleeding or bruising, jaundice, edema, weakness, confusion.	Discontinue. Call doctor when convenient.

 ## WARNINGS & PRECAUTIONS

Don't take if:
- You are allergic to any sulfonylurea.
- You have impaired kidney or liver function.

Before you start, consult your doctor if:
- You have a severe infection.
- You have thyroid disease.
- You take insulin.
- You have heart disease.

Over age 60:
Dose usually smaller than for younger adults. Avoid episodes of low blood sugar because repeated ones can damage brain permanently.

Pregnancy:
Discuss any use of these drugs with your doctor. Risk factors vary for drugs in this group. See category list on page xviii and consult doctor.

Breast-feeding:
Drug filters into milk. May lower baby's blood sugar. Avoid.

Infants & children:
Don't give to infants or children.

SULFONYLUREAS

Prolonged use:
- Adverse effects more likely.
- Talk to your doctor about the need for follow-up medical examinations or laboratory studies to check blood sugar, complete blood counts (white blood cell count, platelet count, red blood cell count, hemoglobin, hematocrit), eyes.

Skin and sunlight:
One or more drugs in this group may cause rash or intensify sunburn in areas exposed to sun or ultraviolet light (photosensitivity reaction). Avoid overexposure. Notify doctor if reaction occurs.

Driving, piloting or hazardous work:
No problems expected unless you develop hypoglycemia (low blood sugar). If so, avoid driving or hazardous activity.

Discontinuing:
Don't discontinue without consulting doctor. Dose may require gradual reduction if you have taken drug for a long time. Doses of other drugs may also require adjustment.

Others:
- Don't exceed recommended dose. Hypoglycemia (low blood sugar) may occur, even with proper dose schedule. You must balance medicine, diet and exercise.
- May affect results in some medical tests.
- Advise any doctor or dentist whom you consult that you take this medicine.

 POSSIBLE INTERACTION WITH OTHER DRUGS

GENERIC NAME OR DRUG CLASS	COMBINED EFFECT
Adrenocorticoids, systemic	Decreased antidiabetic effect.
Androgens*	Increased blood sugar lowering.
Anticoagulants*	Unpredictable prothrombin times.
Anticonvulsants, hydantoin*	Decreased blood sugar lowering.
Antifungals, azoles	Increased blood sugar lowering.
Anti-inflammatory nonsteroidal drugs (NSAIDs)*	Increased blood sugar lowering.
Aspirin	Increased blood sugar lowering.
Beta-adrenergic blocking agents*	Increased blood sugar lowering. Possible increased difficulty in regulating blood sugar levels.

Bismuth subsalicylate	Increased insulin effect. May require dosage adjustment.
Chloramphenicol	Increased blood sugar lowering.
Cimetidine	Increased blood sugar lowering.
Clofibrate	Increased blood sugar lowering.
Contraceptives, oral*	Decreased blood sugar lowering.
Dapsone	Increased risk of adverse effect on blood cells.
Desmopressin	May increase desmopressin effect.
Dexfenfluramine	May require dosage change as weight loss occurs.
Dextrothyroxine	Sulfonylurea may require adjustment.
Digoxin	Possible decreased digoxin effect.
Diuretics* (loop, thiazide)	Decreased blood sugar lowering.
Epinephrine	Increased blood sugar lowering.
Estrogens*	Increased blood sugar lowering.
Guanethidine	Unpredictable blood sugar lowering effect.
Hemolytics*	Increased risk of adverse effect on blood cells.

Continued on page 933

 POSSIBLE INTERACTION WITH OTHER SUBSTANCES

INTERACTS WITH	COMBINED EFFECT
Alcohol:	Disulfiram reaction.* Avoid.
Beverages:	None expected.
Cocaine:	None expected.
Foods:	None expected.
Marijuana:	Decreased blood sugar lowering. Avoid.
Tobacco:	None expected.

*See Glossary

TAMOXIFEN

BRAND NAMES

Alpha-Tamoxifen   Soltamox
Med Tamoxifen   Tamofen
Novo-Tamoxifen   Tamone
                   Tamoplex

BASIC INFORMATION

Habit forming? No
Prescription needed? Yes
Available as generic? Yes
Drug class: Antineoplastic

USES

* Treats advanced breast cancer.
* Can help prevent breast cancer in those at risk.

DOSAGE & USAGE INFORMATION

How to take:
* Tablet—Swallow with liquid. If you can't swallow whole, crumble tablet and take with liquid or food. Instructions to take on empty stomach mean 1 hour before or 2 hours after eating.
* Oral solution—Follow the directions provided with the prescription.
* Enteric-coated tablet—Swallow whole. Do not crush or crumble tablet.

When to take:
Follow instructions on prescription.

If you forget a dose:
Skip the missed dose and return to regular schedule. Don't double dose.

What drug does:
Blocks uptake of estradiol and inhibits growth of cancer cells.

Time lapse before drug works:
* 4 to 10 weeks.
* With bone metastases—several months.

Continued next column

OVERDOSE

SYMPTOMS:
None expected.
WHAT TO DO:
Overdose unlikely to threaten life. If person uses much larger amount than prescribed or if accidentally swallowed, call doctor or poison control center 1-800-222-1222 for help.

Don't take with:
Any other medicines (including over-the-counter drugs such as cough and cold medicines, laxatives, antacids, diet pills, caffeine, nose drops or vitamins) without consulting your doctor or pharmacist.

POSSIBLE ADVERSE REACTIONS OR SIDE EFFECTS

SYMPTOMS	WHAT TO DO
Life-threatening:	
Leg pain, shortness of breath.	Seek emergency treatment immediately.
Common:	
Hot flashes, nausea and vomiting, weight gain.	Continue. Call doctor when convenient.
Infrequent:	
Headache, dry skin, menstrual irregularities, vaginal itching, sleepiness.	Continue. Call doctor when convenient.
Rare:	
Blurred vision, confusion.	Discontinue. Call doctor right away.

WARNINGS & PRECAUTIONS

Don't take if:
You are allergic to tamoxifen.

Before you start, consult your doctor if:
- You have cataracts.
- You have blood disorders.
- You have high cholesterol.

Over age 60:
Adverse reactions and side effects may be more frequent and severe than in younger persons. You may need smaller doses for shorter periods of time.

Pregnancy:
Consult doctor. Risk category D (see page xviii).

Breast-feeding:
Effect not documented. Consult your doctor.

Infants & children:
Not intended for use in children.

Prolonged use:
Talk to your doctor about the need for follow-up medical examinations (especially pelvic exams) or laboratory studies to check complete blood counts (white blood cell count, platelet count, red blood cell count, hemoglobin, hematocrit) and serum calcium.

Skin & sunlight:
No problems expected.

Driving, piloting or hazardous work:
Avoid if you feel confused, drowsy or dizzy.

Discontinuing:
No special problems expected.

Others:
- Advise any doctor or dentist whom you consult that you take this medicine.
- May affect results in some medical tests.
- Be sure you and your doctor discuss all aspects of using this drug, and read all instructional materials.
- The Nolvadex brand of tamoxifen has been discontinued in the United States.
- May make you more fertile. Talk to your doctor about using some type of birth control.

POSSIBLE INTERACTION WITH OTHER DRUGS

GENERIC NAME OR DRUG CLASS	COMBINED EFFECT
Antacids*	Decreased tamoxifen effect. Take 1 to 2 hours apart.
Cimetidine	Decreased tamoxifen effect.
Estrogens*	Decreased tamoxifen effect.
Famotidine	Decreased tamoxifen effect.
H_2 antagonist antihistamines*	Decreased tamoxifen effect.
Ranitidine	Decreased tamoxifen effect.

POSSIBLE INTERACTION WITH OTHER SUBSTANCES

INTERACTS WITH	COMBINED EFFECT
Alcohol:	None expected.
Beverages:	None expected.
Cocaine:	None expected.
Foods:	None expected.
Marijuana:	None expected.
Tobacco:	None expected.

TEGASEROD

BRAND NAMES

Zelnorm

BASIC INFORMATION

Habit forming? No
Prescription needed? Yes
Available as generic? No
Drug class: Gastrointestinal serotonin
  receptor agonist

 USES

- Treatment for women with constipation-predominant irritable bowel syndrome (IBS or IBS-C). IBS is a common gastrointestinal disorder affecting women more often than men. Symptoms include abdominal pain and discomfort, bloating, constipation or diarrhea.
- Treatment for chronic constipation.
- May be used for treatment of other disorders as determined by your doctor.

Note: This drug is available in the U.S.
      through a special distribution program.
      Consult your doctor.

 DOSAGE & USAGE
              INFORMATION

How to take:
Tablet—Take with water on an empty stomach.

When to use:
Twice daily just before a meal (usually morning and evening). Follow prescription instructions.

If you forget a dose:
Take the missed dose just before your next meal (don't double this dose). Then resume your regular schedule.

What drug does:
Helps in the movement of stools through the bowels and prevents constipation by activating certain body nerve cells (5-HT4 receptors) located in the stomach and intestines.

Continued next column

 OVERDOSE

SYMPTOMS:
May develop diarrhea, headache and/or
abdominal pain.
WHAT TO DO:
Overdose unlikely to threaten life. If person
uses much larger amount than prescribed or
if accidentally swallowed, call doctor or
poison control center 1-800-222-1222 for help.

Time lapse before drug works:
Symptoms may improve within a day to a week, but may take up to 4 weeks to determine if the drug is effective in controlling the IBS symptoms.

Don't take with:
Any other medicine or any dietary supplement without consulting your doctor or pharmacist.

 POSSIBLE
            ADVERSE REACTIONS
            OR SIDE EFFECTS

SYMPTOMS	WHAT TO DO
Life-threatening: None expected.	
Common: Diarrhea (may stop after one episode), mild abdominal pain, nausea, headache, gaseousness.	Continue. Call doctor when convenient.
Infrequent: Dizziness, flu or cold symptoms, back pain, feeling of fullness.	Continue. Call doctor when convenient.
Rare: Increased severity or worsening of symptoms of abdominal pain or diarrhea (may be bloody), rectal bleeding, dizziness, lightheadedness, fainting.	Discontinue. Call doctor right away.

WARNINGS & PRECAUTIONS

Don't take if:
You are allergic to tegaserod.

Before you start, consult your doctor if:
* You have liver or kidney disease.
* You often have diarrhea.
* You have bowel disease, bowel obstruction, gallbladder disease with symptoms, sphincter disorder, or abdominal adhesions.

Over age 60:
No problems expected.

Pregnancy:
Decide with your doctor if drug benefits justify any possible risk to unborn child. Risk category B (see page xviii).

Breast-feeding:
It is unknown if drug passes into milk. Avoid nursing until you finish medicine. Consult doctor for advice on maintaining milk supply.

Infants & children:
Not approved for children under age 18.

Prolonged use:
The drug is indicated for short term use. Caution is advised for its use longer than 3 months since safety has not been established.

Skin & sunlight:
No problems expected.

Driving, piloting or hazardous work:
No problems expected.

Discontinuing:
No problems expected, but consult your doctor before discontinuing the drug.

Others:
* There has been a small increase in abdominal surgeries in patients taking this drug. It is not known if the drug is involved in the increase. There is some concern that the drug may cause or worsen ovarian cysts. Be sure to discuss any questions with your doctor.
* Advise any doctor or dentist whom you consult that you take this medicine.
* The drug's effectiveness for men with IBS has not been established.
* Follow your doctor's advice and recommendations for any additional treatment steps for IBS. They may involve stress reduction, relaxation techniques, dietary changes and others.
* Take medicine only as directed. Do not increase or reduce dosage without doctor's approval. Have regular medical follow-up while taking this drug.
* Recommended therapy is 4-6 weeks with an additional 4-6 weeks if patient has good response.

POSSIBLE INTERACTION WITH OTHER DRUGS

GENERIC NAME OR DRUG CLASS	COMBINED EFFECT
None expected.	

POSSIBLE INTERACTION WITH OTHER SUBSTANCES

INTERACTS WITH	COMBINED EFFECT
Alcohol:	None expected.
Beverages:	None expected.
Cocaine:	None expected.
Foods:	None expected.
Marijuana:	None expected.
Tobacco:	None expected.

*See Glossary

TELITHROMYCIN

BRAND NAMES

Ketek

BASIC INFORMATION

Habit forming? No
Prescription needed? Yes
Available as generic? No
Drug class: Antibacterial; antibiotic
   (ketolide)

 USES

Treatment for community acquired pneumonia of mild to moderate severity.

 DOSAGE & USAGE INFORMATION

How to take:
Tablet—Swallow with a full glass of water. It may be taken with or without food. Do not crush or chew tablet.

When to take:
Once a day at the same time each day.

If you forget a dose:
Take as soon as you remember. If it is almost time for the next dose, wait for that dose (don't double this dose) and resume regular schedule.

What drug does:
Prevents growth and reproduction of susceptible bacteria.

Time lapse before drug works:
Starts working in a few hours, but takes 5 to 10 days to cure the infection being treated.

Don't take with:
Any other medicine or any dietary supplement without consulting your doctor or pharmacist.

 OVERDOSE

SYMPTOMS:
Unknown effects.
WHAT TO DO:
Overdose unlikely to threaten life. If person uses much larger amount than prescribed or if accidentally swallowed, call doctor or poison control center 1-800-222-1222 for help.

 POSSIBLE ADVERSE REACTIONS OR SIDE EFFECTS

SYMPTOMS	WHAT TO DO
Life-threatening: Rare allergic reaction— Breathing difficulty; closing of the throat; swelling of hands, feet, face, lips or tongue; hives.	Discontinue. Seek emergency treatment.
Common: Diarrhea, nausea.	Continue. Call doctor when convenient.
Infrequent: • Vision changes (blurred or difficulty in focusing or double vision).	Continue, but call doctor right away.
• Abdominal discomfort, belching, heartburn, vomiting, tingling or numbness or prickling sensations, changes in vaginal discharge, headache, dry lips or skin, flushing or red or warm skin, pale urine, urination increased or more frequent, genital itching, appetite loss, changes in sense of smell or taste, facial pain or tenderness or swelling, insomnia, mood changes, confusion, dizziness or feeling lightheaded.	Continue. Call doctor when convenient.
Rare: Stomach or chest, pain, breathing or swallowing difficulty, fainting, fever or chills, heartbeat is irregular or fast or slow, urine is dark or decreased, diarrhea is bloody or watery, yellow skin or eyes, unusual weakness or tiredness, unusual bleeding or bruising, joint or muscle pain, sores or patches on mouth or tongue or throat, skin symptoms (rash, peeling, blistering, itching).	Discontinue. Call doctor right away.

TELITHROMYCIN

WARNINGS & PRECAUTIONS

Don't take if:
You are allergic to ketolide or macrolide antibiotics or take cisapride or pimozide.

Before you start, consult your doctor if:
- You have kidney or liver problems.
- You have hepatitis or jaundice.
- You have heart rhythm problems or a slow heartbeat (bradycardia).
- You have low potassium or low magnesium levels in your blood.
- You have myasthenia gravis.
- You are allergic to any medication, food or other substance.

Over age 60:
No special problems expected.

Pregnancy:
Decide with your doctor whether drug benefits justify risk to unborn child. Risk category C (see page xviii).

Breast-feeding:
Unknown if drug passes into milk. Avoid drug or discontinue nursing until you finish drug. Consult doctor for advice on maintaining milk supply.

Infants & children:
Safety and effectiveness for children under age 18 has not been established.

Prolonged use:
Drug is discontinued once the infection is cured.

Skin & sunlight:
No special problems expected.

Driving, piloting or hazardous work:
Avoid if you experience vision problems or dizziness. Otherwise, no problems expected.

Discontinuing:
Don't discontinue without doctor's advice until you complete prescribed dose, even though symptoms diminish or disappear.

Others:
- Advise any doctor or dentist whom you consult that you take this medicine.
- May affect the results of some medical tests.

POSSIBLE INTERACTION WITH OTHER DRUGS

GENERIC NAME OR DRUG CLASS	COMBINED EFFECT
Antiarrhythmics	Risk of heart rhythm problems.
Antifungals, azoles	Increased effect of telithromycin.
Benzodiazepines*	Increased effect of benzodiazepine.
Cisapride (this drug has limited availability)	Heart problem risk. Avoid.
Digoxin	Increased effect of digoxin.
Enzyme inducers*	Decreased effect of enzyme inducer or telithromycin.
Enzyme inhibitors*	Increased effect of enzyme inhibitor or telithromycin.
Ergot preparations*	Toxicity risk of ergot preparation. Avoid.
HMG-CoA reductase inhibitors	Increased effect of HMG-CoA reductase inhibitor.
Metoprolol	Increased risk of side effects.
Pimozide	Heart problem risk. Avoid.
QT interval prolongation-causing drugs	Effects not clear. Use with caution.
Rifampin	Decreased effect of rifampin. Avoid.
Ritonavir	Increased effect of ritonavir.
Sirolimus	Increased effect of sirolimus.
Sotalol	Decreased effect of sotalol.
Tacrolimus	Increased effect of tacrolimus.
Theophylline	Increased risk of side effects. Take one hour apart.
Warfarin	Risk of side effects—bleeding or bruising.

POSSIBLE INTERACTION WITH OTHER SUBSTANCES

INTERACTS WITH	COMBINED EFFECT
Alcohol:	None expected.
Beverages:	None expected.
Cocaine:	Unknown. Avoid.
Foods:	None expected
Marijuana:	Unknown. Avoid.
Tobacco:	None expected, but you shouldn't smoke.

*See Glossary

TERBINAFINE (Oral)

BRAND NAMES

Lamisil Oral
Granules

Lamisil Tablets

BASIC INFORMATION

Habit forming? No
Prescription needed? Yes
Available as generic? Yes
Drug class: Antifungal

 USES

- Treats fungal infection (called onychomycosis) of the toenails or fingernails.
- May be used for other fungal infections as determined by your doctor.
- Note: Another form of this drug is applied topically to the skin. For information, see the drug chart for Antifungals (Topical).

 DOSAGE & USAGE INFORMATION

How to take:
- Tablet—Swallow with liquid. May be taken with or without food. If you can't swallow whole, crush tablet and take with liquid or food.
- Oral granules—Sprinkle on food. Follow instructions on prescription on what foods to use.

When to take:
- It is usually taken once a day at the same time each day for a period of weeks to months.
- It may be taken daily for one week per month for 2, 3 or 4 months (called pulse therapy).

If you forget a dose:
Take tablet as soon as you remember. If it is almost time for the next dose, wait for the next scheduled dose (don't double this dose).

Continued next column

 OVERDOSE

SYMPTOMS:
May include nausea, vomiting, abdominal pain, dizziness, rash, frequent urination and headache.
WHAT TO DO:
- Dial 911 (emergency) for medical help or call poison control center 1-800-222-1222 for instructions.
- See emergency information on last 3 pages of this book.

What drug does:
During the weeks of treatment, the drug will slowly kill the fungus infecting the nail. In many cases, the nail will then grow out normally.

Time lapse before drug works:
Improvement in symptoms may be seen in days or weeks, but fungus infections can be very slow to clear up. The drug is usually prescribed for 6 weeks for fingernail infections and 12 weeks or longer for toenail infections.

Don't take with:
Any other medicine or diet supplement without consulting your doctor or pharmacist.

 POSSIBLE ADVERSE REACTIONS OR SIDE EFFECTS

SYMPTOMS	WHAT TO DO
Life-threatening:	
Rare allergic reaction (hives, itching, rash, trouble breathing, tightness in chest, swelling of lips or tongue or throat).	Seek emergency treatment immediately.
Common:	
Nausea, vomiting, mild stomach pain, diarrhea, feeling of fullness, mild appetite loss, headache.	Continue. Call doctor when convenient.
Infrequent:	
• Skin rash, itching.	Discontinue. Call doctor right away.
• Taste changes or loss of taste.	Continue. Call doctor when convenient.
Rare:	
• Nausea or vomiting that is persistent, unusual tiredness or weakness, stomach pain or appetite loss that is more severe, yellow eyes or skin, dark urine, pale stools, fever, chills, sore throat, aching muscles, skin symptoms (redness, blistering, peeling, loosening), unusual bleeding or bruising.	Discontinue. Call doctor right away.
• Hair loss.	Continue. Call doctor when convenient.

784

WARNINGS & PRECAUTIONS

Don't take if:
You are allergic to terbinafine.

Before you start, consult your doctor if:
- You have chronic or active liver disease or kidney disease.
- You have lupus erythematosus.
- You are an alcoholic.

Over age 60:
No special problems expected.

Pregnancy:
Decide with your doctor if drug should be taken during pregnancy. Treatment of nail fungal infections can usually be postponed until after delivery. Risk category B (see page xviii).

Breast-feeding:
Drug passes into milk. Avoid drug or discontinue nursing until you finish dosage. Consult doctor for advice on maintaining milk supply.

Infants & children:
The safety and effectiveness in this age group has not been established. Use only with doctor's approval and close medical supervision.

Prolonged use:
Use of the drug is usually limited to weeks or months of treatment.

Skin & sunlight:
No problems expected.

Driving, piloting or hazardous work:
No problems expected.

Discontinuing:
Don't discontinue the drug without doctor's advice until you complete prescribed dose, even though symptoms diminish or disappear.

Others:
- Periodic laboratory blood studies and liver and kidney function tests may be recommended.
- Be patient and persistent in following the treatment regimen for nail care. Consult your doctor if symptoms do not improve within a few weeks (or months for onychomycosis), or if they become worse.
- Taste changes caused by the drug usually improve within several weeks after stopping the drug, but a few cases may last a year or more.
- Very rarely, severe complications may occur with use of this drug. They include serious (and possibly fatal) liver disease, an abnormal blood disorder and Stevens Johnson syndrome (a severe allergic skin reaction).
- Advise any doctor or dentist whom you consult that you take this medicine.

POSSIBLE INTERACTION WITH OTHER DRUGS

GENERIC NAME OR DRUG CLASS	COMBINED EFFECT
Caffeine	Increased effect of caffeine.
Enzyme inducers*	May decrease effect of terbinafine or enzyme inducer.
Enzyme inhibitors*	May increase effect of terbinafine or enzyme inhibitor.
Warfarin	May affect blood clotting ability.

POSSIBLE INTERACTION WITH OTHER SUBSTANCES

INTERACTS WITH	COMBINED EFFECT
Alcohol:	Increased risk of side effects. Avoid.
Beverages:	None expected.
Cocaine:	Unknown. Avoid.
Foods:	None expected.
Marijuana:	Unknown. Avoid.
Tobacco:	None expected.

TETRACYCLINES

GENERIC AND BRAND NAMES

See full list of generic and brand names in the *Generic and Brand Name Directory*, page 898.

BASIC INFORMATION

Habit forming? No
Prescription needed? Yes
Available as generic? Yes
Drug class: Antibacterial, antiacne

USES

- Treatment for bacterial infections susceptible to any tetracycline. Not used for viruses.
- Treatment for acne, ulcers and used as diuretic.
- Treatment for dental bacterial infections.

DOSAGE & USAGE INFORMATION

How to take:
- Tablet or capsule—Take on empty stomach 1 hour before or 2 hours after eating. If you can't swallow whole, crumble tablet or open capsule and take with liquid or food.
- Delayed-release capsule or extended-release tablet—Swallow whole with liquid. Do not open, crush or chew.
- Dental product—Follow package instructions.
- Liquid—Shake well. Take with measuring spoon.

When to take:
At the same times each day, evenly spaced.

If you forget a dose:
Take as soon as you remember up to 2 hours late. If more than 2 hours, wait for next scheduled dose (don't double this dose).

What drug does:
Prevents bacteria growth and reproduction.

Time lapse before drug works:
- Infections—May require 5 days to affect infection.
- Acne—May require 4 weeks to affect acne.

Don't take with:
Any other medicine or any dietary supplement without consulting your doctor or pharmacist.

OVERDOSE

SYMPTOMS:
Severe nausea, vomiting, diarrhea.
WHAT TO DO:
Overdose unlikely to threaten life. If person uses much larger amount than prescribed or if accidentally swallowed, call doctor or poison control center 1-800-222-1222 for help.

POSSIBLE ADVERSE REACTIONS OR SIDE EFFECTS

SYMPTOMS	WHAT TO DO
Life-threatening:	
Hives, rash, intense itching, faintness soon after a dose (anaphylaxis).	Seek emergency treatment immediately.
Common:	
• Mild stomach cramps, diarrhea, nausea or vomiting; dizziness, lightheadedness or unsteadiness (with minocycline).	Continue. Call doctor when convenient.
• Increased sensitivity to sunlight, tooth discoloration (in children age 8 and under).	Discontinue. Call doctor right away.
Infrequent:	
• Frequent or increased urination, excessive thirst, unusual tiredness or weakness (with demeclocycline); darker color or discoloration of skin and mucous membranes (with minocycline).	Discontinue. Call doctor right away.
• Sore mouth or tongue, rectal or genital itch.	Continue. Call doctor when convenient.
• Darkened tongue (will go away when drug is discontinued).	No action necessary.
Rare:	
Changes in vision, yellow skin or eyes, continued vomiting, severe stomach cramps, loss of appetite, ongoing headache, bulging fontanel (soft spot on head of infant).	Discontinue. Call doctor right away.

WARNINGS & PRECAUTIONS

Don't take if:
You are allergic to any tetracycline antibiotic.

Before you start, consult your doctor if:
- You have kidney or liver disease.
- You have lupus.
- You have myasthenia gravis.

Over age 60:
Dosage usually less than in younger adults. More likely to cause itching around rectum. Ask your doctor how to prevent it.

Pregnancy:
Risk to unborn child outweighs drug benefits. Don't use. Risk category D (see page xviii).

Breast-feeding:
Drug passes into milk. Avoid drug or discontinue nursing until you finish medicine. Consult doctor for advice on maintaining milk supply.

Infants & children:
May cause permanent teeth malformation or discoloration in children less than 8 years old. Don't use.

Prolonged use:
- You may become more susceptible to infections caused by germs not responsive to tetracycline.
- May cause rare problems in liver, kidney or bone marrow. Periodic laboratory blood studies, liver and kidney function tests recommended if you use drug a long time.

Skin & sunlight:
May cause rash or intensify sunburn in areas exposed to sun or ultraviolet light (photosensitivity reaction). Avoid overexposure. Notify doctor if reaction occurs.

Driving, piloting or hazardous work:
No problems expected.

Discontinuing:
Don't discontinue without doctor's advice until you complete prescribed dose, even though symptoms diminish or disappear.

Others:
- Avoid using outdated drug.
- May affect results in some medical tests.
- Birth control pills may not be effective. Use additional birth control method.
- Advise any doctor or dentist whom you consult that you take this medicine.

POSSIBLE INTERACTION WITH OTHER DRUGS

GENERIC NAME OR DRUG CLASS	COMBINED EFFECT
Antacids*	Decreased tetracycline effect.
Anticoagulants,* oral	Increased anticoagulant effect.
Antivirals, HIV/AIDS*	Decreased antibiotic effect.
Bismuth subsalicylate	Decreased tetracycline absorption.
Calcium supplements*	Decreased tetracycline effect.
Cefixime	Decreased antibiotic effect of cefixime.
Cholestyramine or colestipol	Decreased tetracycline effect.
Contraceptives, oral*	Decreased contraceptive effect.
Desmopressin	Possible decreased desmopressin effect.
Digitalis preparations*	Increased digitalis effect.
Etretinate	Increased chance of adverse reactions of etretinate.
Lithium	Increased lithium effect.
Mineral supplements* (iron, calcium, magnesium, zinc)	Decreased tetracycline absorption. Separate doses by 1 to 2 hours.
Penicillins*	Decreased penicillin effect.
Sodium bicarbonate	Greatly reduced tetracycline absorption.

Continued on page 934

POSSIBLE INTERACTION WITH OTHER SUBSTANCES

INTERACTS WITH	COMBINED EFFECT
Alcohol:	Possible liver damage. Avoid.
Beverages: Milk.	Decreased tetracycline absorption. Take dose 2 hours after or 1 hour before drinking.
Cocaine:	None expected.
Foods: Dairy products.	Decreased tetracycline absorption. Take dose 2 hours after or 1 hour before eating.
Marijuana:	No interactions expected, but marijuana may slow body's recovery. Avoid.
Tobacco:	None expected.

*See Glossary

THIAMINE (Vitamin B-1)

BRAND NAMES

Betalin S Bewon
Betaxin Biamine

Numerous brands of single vitamin and
multivitamin combinations may be available.

BASIC INFORMATION

Habit forming? No
Prescription needed? No
Available as generic? Yes
Drug class: Vitamin supplement

 USES

* Dietary supplement to promote normal growth,
development and health.
* Treatment for beri-beri (a thiamine-deficiency
disease).
* Dietary supplement for alcoholism, cirrhosis,
overactive thyroid, infection, breast-feeding,
absorption diseases, pregnancy, prolonged
diarrhea, burns.

 **DOSAGE & USAGE
INFORMATION**

How to take:
Tablet or liquid—Swallow with beverage or food
to lessen stomach irritation.

When to take:
At the same time each day.

If you forget a dose:
Take when remembered, then return to regular
schedule.

What drug does:
* Promotes normal growth and development.
* Combines with an enzyme to metabolize
carbohydrates.

Time lapse before drug works:
15 minutes.

Don't take with:
Any other medicine or any dietary supplement
without consulting your doctor or pharmacist.

 OVERDOSE

SYMPTOMS:
Increased severity of adverse reactions and
side effects.
WHAT TO DO:
Overdose unlikely to threaten life. If person
uses much larger amount than prescribed or
if accidentally swallowed, call doctor or
poison center 1-800-222-1222 for help.

 **POSSIBLE
ADVERSE REACTIONS
OR SIDE EFFECTS**

SYMPTOMS	WHAT TO DO
Life-threatening: None expected.	
Common: None expected.	
Infrequent: None expected.	
Rare:	
• Wheezing.	Discontinue. Seek emergency treatment.
• Rash or itchy skin.	Discontinue. Call doctor right away.

WARNINGS & PRECAUTIONS

Don't take if:
You are allergic to any B vitamin.

Before you start, consult your doctor if:
You have liver or kidney disease.

Over age 60:
No problems expected.

Pregnancy:
Consult doctor. Risk category A (see page xviii).

Breast-feeding:
No problems expected in meeting child's normal daily requirements. Consult doctor.

Infants & children:
No problems expected.

Prolonged use:
No problems expected.

Skin & sunlight:
No problems expected.

Driving, piloting or hazardous work:
No problems expected.

Discontinuing:
No problems expected.

Others:
A balanced diet should provide enough thiamine for healthy people to make a supplement unnecessary. Best dietary sources of thiamine are whole-grain cereals and meats.

POSSIBLE INTERACTION WITH OTHER DRUGS

GENERIC NAME OR DRUG CLASS	COMBINED EFFECT
Barbiturates*	Decreased thiamine effect.

POSSIBLE INTERACTION WITH OTHER SUBSTANCES

INTERACTS WITH	COMBINED EFFECT
Alcohol:	None expected.
Beverages: Carbonates, citrates (additives listed on many beverage labels).	Decreased thiamine effect.
Cocaine:	None expected.
Foods: Carbonates, citrates (additives listed on many food labels).	Decreased thiamine effect.
Marijuana:	None expected.
Tobacco:	None expected.

THIAZOLIDINEDIONES

GENERIC AND BRAND NAMES

PIOGLITAZONE
Actos
ACTOplus met
Duetact

ROSIGLITAZONE
Avandamet
Avandaryl
Avandia

BASIC INFORMATION

Habit forming? No
Prescription needed? Yes
Available as generic? Yes, for some
Drug class: Antidiabetic

USES

Treatment for type 2 diabetes. Rosiglitazone or pioglitazone may be used alone, with insulin or with other antidiabetic drugs.

DOSAGE & USAGE INFORMATION

How to take:
Tablet—Swallow with liquid. Take at mealtime. If you can't swallow whole, crumble tablet and take with liquid or food.

When to take:
Once a day or as directed by doctor. Dosage may be increased after several weeks.

If you forget a dose:
Wait for your next meal that same day and take dose then. If you forget until the next day, take that day's regular dose on schedule (don't double this dose).

Continued next column

OVERDOSE

SYMPTOMS:
Symptoms of hypoglycemia—stomach pain, anxious feeling, cold sweats, chills, confusion, convulsions, cool pale skin, excessive hunger, nausea or vomiting, rapid heartbeat, nervousness, shakiness, unsteady walk, unusual weakness or tiredness, vision changes, unconsciousness.
WHAT TO DO:
* **For mild hypoglycemia symptoms, drink or eat something with sugar right away.**
* **For more severe symptoms, dial 911 (emergency) for medical help or call poison control center 1-800-222-1222 for instructions.**
* **See emergency information on last 3 pages of this book.**

What drug does:
Lowers blood glucose by improving target cell response to insulin. These drugs do not cure diabetes.

Time lapse before drug works:
May take several weeks for full effectiveness.

Don't take with:
Any other medicine or any dietary supplement without consulting your doctor or pharmacist.

POSSIBLE ADVERSE REACTIONS OR SIDE EFFECTS

SYMPTOMS	WHAT TO DO
Life-threatening: In case of overdose or low blood sugar, see previous column.	
Common:	
• Pain in back or other body part, infection.	Continue. Call doctor right away.
• Headache, dizziness, nausea, unusual tiredness or weakness.	Continue. Call doctor when convenient.
Infrequent: Sore throat, runny nose, diarrhea.	Continue. Call doctor when convenient.
Rare:	
• Severe low blood sugar (see symptoms under Overdose).	Discontinue. Call doctor right away or seek emergency help.
• Liver problems including jaundice (yellow skin or eyes) and hepatitis that could lead to liver transplantation or death; symptoms of heart failure (excessive, rapid weight gain, shortness of breath and swelling of legs or feet) after starting drug.	Discontinue. Call doctor right away.

WARNINGS & PRECAUTIONS

Don't take if:
You are allergic to any of the thiazolidinediones.

Before you start, consult your doctor if:
* You have liver disease or any heart disorder.
* You have any chronic health problem.
* You have a history of acid in the blood (metabolic acidosis or ketoacidosis).
* You are allergic to any medication, food or other substance.

Over age 60:
No special problems expected.

Pregnancy:
Decide with your doctor if drug benefits justify risks to unborn child. Risk category C for pioglitazone and rosiglitazone (see page xviii).

Breast-feeding:
It is unknown if drug passes into milk. It is not recommended for use in nursing mothers.

Infants & children:
Safety and efficacy have not been established. Use only under close medical supervision.

Prolonged use:
* Schedule regular doctor visits to determine if the drug is continuing to be effective in controlling the diabetes and to check for any liver function problems.
* You will most likely require an antidiabetic medicine for the rest of your life.
* You will need to test your blood glucose levels several times a day, or for some, once to several times a week.

Skin & sunlight:
No special problems expected.

Driving, piloting or hazardous work:
No special problems expected.

Discontinuing:
Don't discontinue without consulting your doctor even if you feel well. You can have diabetes without feeling any symptoms. Untreated diabetes can cause serious problems.

Others:
* Use of these drugs may lead to liver problems. Currently, it is necessary to get liver function studies prior to starting the drug, then every other month for 6 months and periodically thereafter while on the drug.
* Rosiglitazone may increase risk of heart attack and heart-related death in certain patients. Consult doctor.
* Use of these drugs can cause fluid retention which may lead to or worsen chronic heart failure.
* Advise any doctor or dentist whom you consult that you take this medicine. It may interfere with the accuracy of some medical tests.
* May cause ovulation to resume in some women with ovarian disorders. Discuss the need for nonhormonal contraception with your doctor.
* Follow any special diet your doctor may prescribe. It can help control diabetes.
* Consult doctor if you become ill with vomiting or diarrhea while taking this drug.
* Use caution when exercising. Ask your doctor about an appropriate exercise program.
* Wear medical identification stating that you have diabetes and take this medication.

* Learn to recognize the symptoms of low blood sugar. You and your family need to know what to do if these symptoms occur.
* Have a glucagon kit and syringe in the event severe low blood sugar occurs.
* Use of these drugs may raise both HDL and LDL cholesterol levels.
* High blood sugar (hyperglycemia) may occur with diabetes. Ask your doctor about symptoms to watch for and treatment steps to take.
* Educate yourself about diabetes.

 POSSIBLE INTERACTION WITH OTHER DRUGS

GENERIC NAME OR DRUG CLASS	COMBINED EFFECT
Antidiabetic agents, sulfonylurea	May decrease fasting plasma glucose concentrations.
Cholestyramine	Decreased effect of troglitazone. Avoid.
Contraceptives, oral*	Decreased effect of contraceptive.
Cyclosporine	Decreased effect of cyclosporine.
HMG-CoA reductase inhibitors	Decreased effect of HMG-CoA reductase inhibitor.
Tacrolimus	Decreased effect of tacrolimus.

 POSSIBLE INTERACTION WITH OTHER SUBSTANCES

INTERACTS WITH	COMBINED EFFECT
Alcohol:	No special problems. Avoid excessive amounts of alcohol.
Beverages:	None expected.
Cocaine:	No special problems. Best to avoid.
Foods:	None expected.
Marijuana:	No special problems. Best to avoid.
Tobacco:	People with diabetes should not smoke.

*See Glossary

THIOGUANINE

BRAND NAMES

Lanvis

BASIC INFORMATION

Habit forming? No
Prescription needed? Yes
Available as generic? Yes
Drug class: Antineoplastic

 USES

Treats some forms of leukemia.

 DOSAGE & USAGE INFORMATION

How to take:
Tablet—Swallow with liquid. If you can't swallow whole, crumble tablet and take with liquid or food. Instructions to take on empty stomach mean 1 hour before or 2 hours after eating.

When to take:
According to doctor's instructions.

If you forget a dose:
Skip the missed dose and return to regular schedule. Don't double dose.

What drug does:
Interferes with growth of cancer cells.

Time lapse before drug works:
Varies greatly among patients.

Don't take with:
Any other medicines (including over-the-counter drugs such as cough and cold medicines, laxatives, antacids, diet pills, caffeine, nose drops or vitamins) without consulting your doctor or pharmacist.

 OVERDOSE

SYMPTOMS:
None expected.
WHAT TO DO:
Overdose unlikely to threaten life. If person uses much larger amount than prescribed or if accidentally swallowed, call doctor or poison control center 1-800-222-1222 for help.

 POSSIBLE ADVERSE REACTIONS OR SIDE EFFECTS

SYMPTOMS	WHAT TO DO
Life-threatening: None expected.	
Common: • Appetite loss, diarrhea, skin rash.	Continue. Call doctor when convenient.
• Nausea.	No action necessary.
Infrequent: Bloody urine; hoarseness or cough; fever or chills; lower back or side pain; painful or difficult urination; red spots on skin; unusual bleeding or bruising; joint pain; swollen feet and legs; unsteady gait; black, tarry stools.	Discontinue. Call doctor right away.
Rare: Mouth and lip sores; jaundice (yellow skin and eyes).	Discontinue. Call doctor right away.

WARNINGS & PRECAUTIONS

Don't take if:
- You are allergic to thioguanine.
- You have chicken pox or shingles.

Before you start, consult your doctor if:
- You have gout.
- You have an infection.
- You have kidney or liver disease.
- You have had radiation or cancer chemotherapy within 6 weeks.

Over age 60:
Adverse reactions and side effects may be more frequent and severe than in younger persons. You may need smaller doses for shorter periods of time.

Pregnancy:
Risk to unborn child outweighs drug benefits. Don't use. Risk category D (see page xviii).

Breast-feeding:
Drug may pass into milk. Avoid drug or discontinue nursing until you finish medicine. Consult doctor for advice on maintaining milk supply.

Infants & children:
No special problems expected.

Prolonged use:
- Increased likelihood of side effects.
- Talk to your doctor about the need for follow-up medical examinations or laboratory studies to check kidney and liver function, serum uric acid, and complete blood counts (white blood cell count, platelet count, red blood cell count, hemoglobin, hematocrit).

Skin & sunlight:
No problems expected.

Driving, piloting or hazardous work:
No problems expected.

Discontinuing:
Report to your doctor any of these symptoms that occur after discontinuing: black, tarry stools; bloody urine; hoarseness or cough; fever or chills; lower back or side pain; painful or difficult urination; red spots on skin; unusual bleeding or bruising.

Others:
- Advise any doctor or dentist whom you consult that you take this medicine.
- May affect results in some medical tests.
- Don't use birth control pills for contraception.

POSSIBLE INTERACTION WITH OTHER DRUGS

GENERIC NAME OR DRUG CLASS	COMBINED EFFECT
Antigout drugs*	May need increased antigout dosage.
Bone marrow depressants,* other	Increased risk of bone marrow depression.
Vaccines, live or killed	Increased risk of toxicity or reduced effectiveness of vaccine.
Zidovudine	More likelihood of toxicity of both drugs.

POSSIBLE INTERACTION WITH OTHER SUBSTANCES

INTERACTS WITH	COMBINED EFFECT
Alcohol:	Increased side effects.
Beverages:	None expected.
Cocaine:	Increased side effects.
Foods:	None expected.
Marijuana:	None expected.
Tobacco:	None expected.

THIOTHIXENE

BRAND NAMES

Navane

Thiothixene HCl
Intensol

BASIC INFORMATION

Habit forming? No
Prescription needed? Yes
Available as generic? Yes
Drug class: Antipsychotic (thioxanthene)

 ## USES

Reduces anxiety, agitation, psychosis.

 ## DOSAGE & USAGE INFORMATION

How to take:
• Capsule—Swallow with liquid. If you can't swallow whole, open capsule and take with liquid or food.
• Syrup—Dilute dose in beverage before swallowing.

When to take:
At the same times each day.

If you forget a dose:
Take as soon as you remember up to 2 hours late. If more than 2 hours, wait for next scheduled dose (don't double this dose).

What drug does:
Corrects imbalance of nerve impulses.

Time lapse before drug works:
3 weeks.

Continued next column

 ## OVERDOSE

SYMPTOMS:
Drowsiness, dizziness, weakness, muscle rigidity, twitching, tremors, confusion, dry mouth, blurred vision, rapid pulse, shallow breathing, low blood pressure, convulsions, coma.
WHAT TO DO:
• **Dial 911 (emergency) for medical help or call poison control center 1-800-222-1222 for instructions.**
• **If person is unconscious, check breathing and pulse. If not breathing, begin mouth-to-mouth rescue breathing. If heart is not beating, begin chest compressions.**
• **See emergency information on last 3 pages of this book.**

Don't take with:
Any other medicine or any dietary supplement without consulting your doctor or pharmacist.

 ## POSSIBLE ADVERSE REACTIONS OR SIDE EFFECTS

SYMPTOMS	WHAT TO DO
Life-threatening:	
High fever, rapid pulse, profuse sweating, muscle rigidity, confusion and irritability, seizures.	Discontinue. Seek emergency treatment.
Common:	
• Jerky or involuntary movements, especially of the face, lips, jaw, tongue; slow-frequency tremor of head or limbs, especially while moving; muscle rigidity, lack of facial expression and slow, inflexible movements.	Discontinue. Call doctor right away.
• Pacing or restlessness; intermittent spasms of muscles of face, eyes, tongue, jaw, neck, body or limbs; dry mouth; blurred vision; constipation, difficulty urinating.	Continue. Call doctor when convenient.
Infrequent:	
• Sedation, low blood pressure and dizziness.	Continue. Call doctor when convenient.
• Other symptoms not listed above.	Continue. Call doctor when convenient.

 ## WARNINGS & PRECAUTIONS

Don't take if:
• You are allergic to any thioxanthene or phenothiazine tranquilizer.
• You have serious blood disorder.
• You have Parkinson's disease.
• Patient is younger than 12.

Before you start, consult your doctor if:
- You have had liver or kidney disease.
- You have epilepsy, glaucoma, prostate trouble.
- You have high blood pressure or heart disease (especially angina).
- You use alcohol daily.
- You will have surgery within 2 months, including dental surgery, requiring general or spinal anesthesia.

Over age 60:
- Adverse reactions and side effects may be more frequent and severe than in younger persons.
- Use of antipsychotic drugs in elderly patients with dementia-related psychosis may increase risk of death. Consult doctor.

Pregnancy:
Decide with your doctor if drug benefits justify risk to unborn child. Risk category C (see page xviii).

Breast-feeding:
Studies inconclusive. Consult your doctor.

Infants & children:
Not recommended.

Prolonged use:
- Pigment deposits in lens and retina of eye.
- Involuntary movements of jaws, lips, tongue (tardive dyskinesia).
- Talk to your doctor about the need for follow-up medical examinations or laboratory studies to check complete blood counts (white blood cell count, platelet count, red blood cell count, hemoglobin, hematocrit), liver function, eyes.

Skin & sunlight:
- May cause rash or intensify sunburn in areas exposed to sun or ultraviolet light (photosensitivity reaction). Use sunscreen and avoid overexposure. Notify doctor if reaction occurs.
- Hot temperatures and exercise, hot baths can increase risk of heatstroke. Drug may affect body's ability to maintain normal temperature.

Driving, piloting or hazardous work:
Don't drive or pilot aircraft until you learn how medicine affects you. Don't work around dangerous machinery. Don't climb ladders or work in high places. Danger increases if you drink alcohol or take medicine affecting alertness and reflexes.

Discontinuing:
Don't discontinue without consulting doctor. Dose may require gradual reduction if you have taken drug for a long time. Doses of other drugs may also require adjustment.

Others:
- Advise any doctor or dentist whom you consult that you take this medicine.
- For dry mouth, suck sugarless hard candy or chew sugarless gum. If dry mouth persists, consult your dentist.

POSSIBLE INTERACTION WITH OTHER DRUGS

GENERIC NAME OR DRUG CLASS	COMBINED EFFECT
Anticonvulsants*	Change in seizure pattern.
Antidepressants, tricyclic*	Increased thiothixene effect. Excessive sedation.
Antihistamines*	Increased thiothixene effect. Excessive sedation.
Antihypertensives*	Excessively low blood pressure.
Barbiturates*	Increased thiothixene effect. Excessive sedation.
Bupropion	Increased risk of seizures.
Epinephrine	Excessively low blood pressure.
Guanethidine	Decreased guanethidine effect.
Levodopa	Decreased levodopa effect.
Mind-altering drugs*	Increased thiothixene effect. Excessive sedation.
Monoamine oxidase (MAO) inhibitors*	Excessive sedation.
Narcotics*	Increased thiothixene effect. Excessive sedation.

Continued on page 934

POSSIBLE INTERACTION WITH OTHER SUBSTANCES

INTERACTS WITH	COMBINED EFFECT
Alcohol:	Excessive brain depression. Avoid.
Beverages:	None expected.
Cocaine:	Decreased thiothixene effect. Avoid.
Foods:	None expected.
Marijuana:	Daily use—Fainting likely, possible psychosis.
Tobacco:	None expected.

*See Glossary

THYROID HORMONES

GENERIC AND BRAND NAMES

LEVOTHYROXINE
  Eltroxin
  Levo-T
  Levothroid
  Novothyrox
LIOTHYRONINE
  Cytomel
LIOTRIX
  Euthroid
  Thyrolar

THYROGLOBULIN
  Levoxyl
  L-Thyroxine
  Proloid
  Synthroid
THYROID
  Armour Thyroid
  Thyrar
  Thyroid Strong
  Westhroid

BASIC INFORMATION

Habit forming? No
Prescription needed? Yes
Available as generic? Yes, for some
Drug class: Thyroid hormone

 USES

Replacement for thyroid hormones lost due to deficiency.

 DOSAGE & USAGE INFORMATION

How to take:
Tablet—Swallow with liquid. Levothyroxine tablet should be taken with full glass of water.

When to take:
At the same time each day before a meal or on awakening.

If you forget a dose:
Take as soon as you remember up to 12 hours late. If more than 12 hours, wait for next scheduled dose (don't double this dose).

What drug does:
Increases cell metabolism rate.

Continued next column

 OVERDOSE

SYMPTOMS:
"Hot" feeling, heart palpitations, nervousness, sweating, hand tremors, insomnia, rapid and irregular pulse, headache, irritability, diarrhea, weight loss, muscle cramps, angina, congestive heart failure possible.
WHAT TO DO:
Overdose unlikely to threaten life. If person uses much larger amount than prescribed or if accidentally swallowed, call doctor or poison control center 1-800-222-1222 for help.

Time lapse before drug works:
48 hours.

Don't take with:
Any other medicine or any dietary supplement without consulting your doctor or pharmacist.

 POSSIBLE ADVERSE REACTIONS OR SIDE EFFECTS

SYMPTOMS	WHAT TO DO
Life-threatening: In case of overdose, see previous column.	
Common: Tremor, headache, irritability, insomnia, appetite change, diarrhea, leg cramps, menstrual irregularities, fever, heat sensitivity, unusual sweating, weight loss, nervousness.	Continue. Call doctor when convenient.
Infrequent: Hives, rash, vomiting, chest pain, rapid and irregular heartbeat, shortness of breath.	Discontinue. Call doctor right away.
Rare: None expected.	

 WARNINGS & PRECAUTIONS

Don't take if:
* You have had a heart attack within the past 6 weeks.
* You have no thyroid deficiency, but want to use this to lose weight.

Before you start, consult your doctor if:
* You have heart disease or high blood pressure.
* You have diabetes.
* You have Addison's disease, have had adrenal gland deficiency or use epinephrine, ephedrine or isoproterenol for asthma.

Over age 60:
More sensitive to thyroid hormone. May need smaller doses.

Pregnancy:
Considered safe if for thyroid deficiency only. Consult doctor. Risk category A (see page xviii).

Breast-feeding:
Present in milk. Consult doctor.

Infants & children:
Use only under medical supervision.

Prolonged use:
- No problems expected if dose is correct.
- Talk to your doctor about the need for follow-up medical examinations or laboratory studies to check thyroid, heart.

Skin & sunlight:
No problems expected.

Driving, piloting or hazardous work:
No problems expected.

Discontinuing:
Don't discontinue without consulting doctor. Dose may require gradual reduction if you have taken drug for a long time. Doses of other drugs may also require adjustment.

Others:
- Digestive upsets, tremors, cramps, nervousness, insomnia or diarrhea may indicate need for dose adjustment.
- Different brands can cause different results. Do not change brands without consulting doctor.
- Advise any doctor or dentist whom you consult that you take this medicine.

POSSIBLE INTERACTION WITH OTHER DRUGS

GENERIC NAME OR DRUG CLASS	COMBINED EFFECT
Adrenocorticoids, systemic	May require thyroid hormone dosage change.
Amphetamines*	Increased amphetamine effect.
Anticoagulants,* oral	Increased anti-coagulant effect.
Antidepressants, tricyclic*	Increased anti-depressant effect. Irregular heartbeat.
Antidiabetics,* oral or insulin	Antidiabetic may require adjustment.
Aspirin (large doses, continuous use)	Increased effect of thyroid hormone.
Barbiturates*	Decreased barbiturate effect.
Beta-adrenergic blocking agents*	Possible decreased effect of beta blocker.
Cholestyramine	Decreased effect of thyroid hormone.
Colestipol	Decreased effect of thyroid hormone.
Contraceptives, oral*	Decreased effect of thyroid hormone.

Digitalis preparations*	Decreased digitalis effect.
Ephedrine	Increased ephedrine effect.
Epinephrine	Increased epinephrine effect.
Estrogens*	Decreased effect of thyroid hormone.
Meglitinides	Increased blood sugar levels.
Methylphenidate	Increased methylphenidate effect.
Phenytoin	Possible decreased effect of thyroid hormone.
Sympathomimetics*	Increased risk of rapid or irregular heartbeat.

POSSIBLE INTERACTION WITH OTHER SUBSTANCES

INTERACTS WITH	COMBINED EFFECT
Alcohol:	None expected.
Beverages:	None expected.
Cocaine:	Excess stimulation. Avoid.
Foods:	None expected.
Marijuana:	None expected.
Tobacco:	None expected.

*See Glossary

TIAGABINE

BRAND NAMES

Gabitril

BASIC INFORMATION

Habit forming? No
Prescription needed? Yes
Available as generic? No
Drug class: Anticonvulsant; antiepileptic

 USES

Treatment of partial seizures in patients with epilepsy. It is used in combination with other antiepileptic drugs.

 DOSAGE & USAGE INFORMATION

How to take:
Tablet—Swallow whole with a liquid. Take with food or on a full stomach.

When to take:
Usually once a day to start, then taken 2 to 4 times a day at the same times each day. Your doctor will determine the schedule. Dosage may be increased slowly to achieve best results.

If you forget a dose:
Take as soon as you remember. If it is almost time for the next dose, skip the missed dose and wait for your next scheduled dose (don't double this dose).

What drug does:
It is not known exactly how the drug works. It increases the amount of a brain chemical (called GABA) that helps prevent seizure activity.

Continued next column

 OVERDOSE

SYMPTOMS:
Seizures including status epilepticus, lack of coordination, confusion, drowsiness, muscle spasms, hostility, impaired speech, agitation, lethargy, stupor, tremors, disorientation, vomiting, temporary paralysis, coma.
WHAT TO DO:
* **Dial 911 (emergency) for medical help or call poison control center 1-800-222-1222 for instructions.**
* **If person is unconscious, check breathing and pulse. If not breathing, begin mouth-to-mouth rescue breathing. If heart is not beating, begin chest compressions.**
* **See emergency information on last 3 pages of this book.**

Time lapse before drug works:
May take several weeks for full effectiveness.

Don't take with:
Any other medicine or any dietary supplement without consulting your doctor or pharmacist.

 POSSIBLE ADVERSE REACTIONS OR SIDE EFFECTS

SYMPTOMS	WHAT TO DO
Life-threatening: Rare allergic reaction (hives, itching, rash, trouble breathing, tightness in chest, swelling of lips or tongue or face); rare Stevens Johnson syndrome (mucous membranes and skin have redness, blisters, peeling, looseness).	Seek emergency treatment immediately.
Common: Dizziness, weakness, tremor, drowsiness, concentration problems, infection (chills, fever, headache, sore throat), nervousness.	Continue. Call doctor when convenient.
Infrequent: • Numbness or burning or tingling sensations, speech problems, agitation, confusion, hostility, memory problems, vision changes, clumsiness.	Continue, but call doctor right away.
• Stomach pain, increased cough, muscle aches or pain or weakness, nausea, sleeping problems, pain, unusual tiredness vomiting, diarrhea.	Continue. Call doctor when convenient.
Rare: • Status epilepticus (ongoing seizures), severe weakness, suicidal thoughts.	Seek emergency treatment immediately.
• New or increased, seizures, severe rash, depression, unusual behaviors.	Continue, but call doctor right away.
• Itching, flushing, mild rash, appetite increased, mouth sores, emotional upsets.	Continue. Call doctor when convenient.

WARNINGS & PRECAUTIONS

Don't take if:
You are allergic to tiagabine.

Before you start, consult your doctor if:
* You do not have seizures or epilepsy.
* You have any type of liver disorder.
* You have a history of mental or mood problems (such as depression) or suicidal thoughts or attempts.
* You are allergic to any medication, food or other substance.

Over age 60:
No problems expected.

Pregnancy:
Decide with your doctor if drug benefits justify risks to unborn child. Risk category C (see page xviii).

Breast-feeding:
It is unknown if drug passes into milk. Avoid drug or discontinue nursing until you finish medicine. Consult doctor for advice on maintaining milk supply.

Infants & children:
Safety and efficacy not established in children younger than age 12.

Prolonged use:
No special problems expected. Follow-up with your doctor on a regular basis to monitor your condition and check for drug side effects.

Skin & sunlight:
No problems expected.

Driving, piloting or hazardous work:
This drug may cause dizziness and drowsiness. Don't drive or pilot aircraft until you learn how medicine affects you. Don't work around dangerous machinery. Don't climb ladders or work in high places. The risk of dizziness increases if you drink alcohol.

Discontinuing:
Don't discontinue without doctor's approval due to risk of increased seizure activity. The dosage may need to be gradually decreased before stopping the drug completely.

Others:
* This drug cannot cure epilepsy and will only work to control seizures for as long as you continue to take it.
* Tiagabine is used with other anticonvulsant drugs and additional side effects may occur. If they do, consult your doctor.
* Advise any doctor or dentist whom you consult that you take this medicine.
* Rarely, antiepileptic drugs may lead to suicidal thoughts and behaviors. Call doctor right away if suicidal symptoms or unusual behaviors occur.
* Carry or wear medical identification that lists your seizure disorder and drugs you take.
* Use of this drug in patients without epilepsy may lead to new onset seizures and status epilepticus. Nonepileptic patients who develop seizures should discontinue the drug. Consult doctor to see if you have a seizure disorder.

POSSIBLE INTERACTION WITH OTHER DRUGS

GENERIC NAME OR DRUG CLASS	COMBINED EFFECT
Enzyme inducing, antiepileptic drugs*	Decreased effect of tiagabine.
Other drugs	Unknown. Consult doctor or pharmacist.
Protein bound drugs*	Increased effect of both drugs.
Seizure threshold lowering drugs*	Increased risk of seizures.
Valproate	May alter affect of either drug. Consult doctor.

POSSIBLE INTERACTION WITH OTHER SUBSTANCES

INTERACTS WITH	COMBINED EFFECT
Alcohol:	Increased risk of dizziness. Avoid.
Beverages:	Ask your doctor about drinking grapefruit juice.
Cocaine:	Unknown effect. Avoid.
Foods:	None expected.
Marijuana:	Unknown effect. Avoid.
Tobacco:	None expected.

*See Glossary

TIOPRONIN

BRAND NAMES

Capen

Captimer

Epatiol

Mucolysin

Sutilan

Thiola

Thiosol

Tioglis

Vincol

BASIC INFORMATION

Habit forming? No

Prescription needed? Yes

Available as generic? No

Drug class: Antiurolithic

 USES

Prevents the formation of kidney stones when there is too much cystine in the urine.

 DOSAGE & USAGE INFORMATION

How to take:

Tablet—Swallow with liquid. If you can't swallow whole, crumble tablet and take with liquid or food. Instructions to take on empty stomach mean 1 hour before or 2 hours after eating.

When to take:

3 times daily (once approximately every 8 hours).

If you forget a dose:

Take as soon as you remember up to 2 hours late. If more than 2 hours, wait for next scheduled dose (don't double this dose).

What drug does:

Removes high levels of cystine from the body.

Time lapse before drug works:

It starts working right away, but full benefit may take weeks to months. Laboratory studies are used to measure the cystine in the urine.

Continued next column

 OVERDOSE

SYMPTOMS:

None expected. If massive overdose is suspected, follow instructions below.

WHAT TO DO:

• Dial 911 (emergency) for medical help or call poison control center 1-800-222-1222 for instructions.

• See emergency information on last 3 pages of this book.

Don't take with:

• Medicines that are known to cause kidney damage or depress bone marrow.

• Any other medicine or any dietary supplement without consulting your doctor or pharmacist.

 POSSIBLE ADVERSE REACTIONS OR SIDE EFFECTS

SYMPTOMS	WHAT TO DO
Life-threatening:	
In case of overdose, see previous column.	
Common:	
• Skin rash, itching skin, mouth sores, mouth ulcers.	Discontinue. Call doctor right away.
• Abdominal pain, gaseousness, diarrhea, nausea or vomiting.	Continue. Call doctor when convenient.
Infrequent:	
• Cloudy urine, chills, breathing difficulty, joint pain.	Discontinue. Call doctor right away.
• Impaired smell or taste.	Continue. Call doctor when convenient.
Rare:	
Coughing up blood, fever, unusual tiredness or weakness, double vision, muscle weakness.	Discontinue. Call doctor right away.

TIOPRONIN

WARNINGS & PRECAUTIONS

Don't take if:
You are allergic to tiopronin or penicillamine.

Before you start, consult your doctor if:
You have had any of the following in the past:
* Agranulocytosis.
* Aplastic anemia.
* Thrombocytopenia.
* Impaired kidney function.

Over age 60:
May require dosage adjustment if kidney function is impaired.

Pregnancy:
Decide with your doctor if drug benefits justify risk to unborn child. Risk category C (see page xviii).

Breast-feeding:
Drug passes into milk. Avoid or discontinue nursing until you finish medicine. Consult doctor for advice on maintaining milk supply.

Infants & children:
Safety not established. Consult doctor.

Prolonged use:
No special problems expected.

Skin & sunlight:
No special problems expected.

Driving, piloting or hazardous work:
Don't drive or pilot aircraft until you learn how medicine affects you. Don't work around dangerous machinery. Don't climb ladders or work in high places. Danger increases if you drink alcohol or take medicine affecting alertness and reflexes.

Discontinuing:
No special problems expected.

Others:
* Advise any doctor or dentist whom you consult that you take this medicine.
* May affect results of some medical tests.

POSSIBLE INTERACTION WITH OTHER DRUGS

GENERIC NAME OR DRUG CLASS	COMBINED EFFECT
Bone marrow depressants*	May increase possibility of toxic effects of tiopronin.
Medications toxic to kidneys (nephrotoxins*)	May increase possibility of toxic effects of tiopronin.

POSSIBLE INTERACTION WITH OTHER SUBSTANCES

INTERACTS WITH	COMBINED EFFECT
Alcohol:	None expected.
Beverages: Water.	Enhances effects of tiopronin. Drink 8 to 10 glasses daily.
Cocaine:	None expected.
Foods:	None expected.
Marijuana:	None expected.
Tobacco:	None expected.

*See Glossary

801

TIOTROPIUM

BRAND NAMES

Spiriva

BASIC INFORMATION

Habit forming? No
Prescription needed? Yes
Available as generic? No
Drug class: Antimuscarinic bronchodilator;
  anticholinergic

 ## USES

Maintenance treatment for bronchospasms that occur with chronic obstructive pulmonary disease (COPD), including chronic bronchitis and emphysema. It is not used to relieve an attack of breathing difficulty.

 ## DOSAGE & USAGE INFORMATION

How to take:
Inhalation powder—Use the capsule only in the HandiHaler device. Do not swallow the capsule. Use care to not get the powder in the eyes. Follow instructions provided with the product. Review them often. Don't depend on memory.

When to take:
Once a day at the same time each day.

If you forget a dose:
Take as soon as you remember. If it is almost time for your next dose, skip the missed dose and go back to the regular dosing schedule. Do not double doses.

What drug does:
Relaxes the muscles around narrowed airways in the lungs and helps to keep them open and make breathing easier.

Continued next column

 ## OVERDOSE

SYMPTOMS:
Inhaled overdose is unlikely. Dry mouth and conjunctivitis may occur. Swallowed capsule is unlikely to cause symptoms as capsule is not well-absorbed by the gastrointestinal tract.
WHAT TO DO:
If person inhales much larger amount than prescribed or someone accidentally swallows a capsule, dial 911 (emergency) for medical help or call poison control center 1-800-222-1222 for instructions.

Time lapse before drug works:
Begins working right away, but will take abut 2-3 weeks for full maintenance benefits.

Don't take with:
Any other medicine or any dietary supplement without consulting your doctor or pharmacist.

 ## POSSIBLE ADVERSE REACTIONS OR SIDE EFFECTS

SYMPTOMS	WHAT TO DO
Life-threatening: None expected.	
Common: Dry mouth.	Continue. Tell doctor at next visit.
Infrequent: Constipation, painful or frequent urination, urinary retention, upset stomach, sore throat, sinus or cold symptoms.	Continue. Call doctor when convenient.
Rare: • Increased heart, rate, chest pain, bloody nose, induced bronchospasm (wheezing), allergic reaction.	Discontinue. Call doctor right away.
• Heartburn, rash, vomiting, muscle or bone aches.	Continue. Call doctor when convenient.

WARNINGS & PRECAUTIONS

Don't take if:
You are allergic to atropine or similar medicines or tiotropium.

Before you start, consult your doctor if:
- You have kidney disorder.
- You have blockage of the drainage passage of the bladder (bladder neck obstruction).
- You have enlarged prostate gland (prostatic hypertrophy).
- You have narrow angle glaucoma.
- You are allergic to any medications.

Over age 60:
No special problems expected.

Pregnancy:
Decide with your doctor if drug benefits justify risk to unborn child. Risk category C (see page xviii).

Breast-feeding:
It is not known if drug passes into milk. Avoid drug or discontinue nursing until you finish medicine. Consult doctor for advice on maintaining milk supply.

Infants & children:
Not recommended for this age group. COPD does not normally occur in children.

Prolonged use:
No problems expected.

Skin & sunlight:
No problems expected.

Driving, piloting or hazardous work:
No problems expected.

Discontinuing:
No problems expected. Consult your doctor before discontinuing.

Others:
- Advise any doctor or dentist whom you consult that you take this medicine.
- For dry mouth, suck sugarless hard candy or chew sugarless gum. If dry mouth continues, consult your dentist.

POSSIBLE INTERACTION WITH OTHER DRUGS

GENERIC NAME OR DRUG CLASS	COMBINED EFFECT
Anticholinergics,* other	Unknown effect. Avoid or ask doctor.

POSSIBLE INTERACTION WITH OTHER SUBSTANCES

INTERACTS WITH	COMBINED EFFECT
Alcohol:	None expected.
Beverages:	None expected.
Cocaine:	Unknown effect. Best to avoid.
Foods:	None expected.
Marijuana:	Unknown effect. Best to avoid.
Tobacco:	May decrease effect of drug. People with COPD should not smoke.

TIZANIDINE

BRAND NAMES

Zanaflex

BASIC INFORMATION

Habit forming? No
Prescription needed? Yes
Available as generic? Yes
Drug class: Antispastic, muscle relaxant

USES

- Relieves muscle spasticity caused by diseases such as multiple sclerosis. It does not appear to improve muscle weakness.
- Relieves muscle spasticity caused by injury to spinal cord.

DOSAGE & USAGE INFORMATION

How to take:
Tablet or capsule—Swallow with liquid. Follow instructions on your prescription about whether to take with food or not. Food can change the amount of the drug absorbed by your body.

When to take:
Up to three times a day or as directed by your doctor.

If you forget a dose:
Take as soon as you remember up to 1 hour late. If more than 1 hour, wait for next scheduled dose (don't double this dose).

What drug does:
Slows nerve impulses that stimulate skeletal muscles, decreasing cramping.

Time lapse before drug works:
Within hours. Dosage may be increased over a several week period to achieve maximum effectiveness.

Don't take with:
Any other medicine or any dietary supplement without consulting your doctor or pharmacist.

OVERDOSE

SYMPTOMS:
Breathing difficulties, heartbeat irregularities; other symptoms may occur that were not observed in medical studies of the drug.
WHAT TO DO:
If person takes much larger amount than prescribed, dial 911 (emergency) for medical help or call poison control center 1-800-222-1222 for instructions.

POSSIBLE ADVERSE REACTIONS OR SIDE EFFECTS

SYMPTOMS	WHAT TO DO
Life-threatening:	
In case of overdose, see previous column.	
Common:	
• Nervousness, sensation changes (tingling, burning, prickling), skin sores, anxiety, tiredness or weakness, constipation, back pain, dizziness, dry mouth, depression, drowsiness, heartburn, lightheadedness when getting up from a sitting or lying position, increase in muscle spasm, muscle weakness, sore throat, runny nose, increased sweating.	Continue. Call doctor when convenient.
• Fever, liver problems, (weight loss, nausea, vomiting, yellow skin or eyes), pain or burning when urinating, involuntary movements, diarrhea, vomiting, stomach pain, speech problems.	Discontinue. Call doctor when convenient.
Infrequent:	
• Heartbeat irregularity, black or tarry stools, seizures, bloody vomit, fever and chills, fainting.	Discontinue. Call doctor right away
• Mental changes, mood changes, dry skin, swelling of hands or feet or other areas of the body, difficulty swallowing, migraine, neck pain, trembling or shaking, weight loss, joint or muscle pain, skin rash, feeling of coldness, puffy skin, weight gain, cough, white patches on tongue or in mouth, visual changes or eye pain.	Continue. Call doctor when convenient.
Rare:	
Other symptoms not mentioned above.	Continue. Call doctor when convenient.

WARNINGS & PRECAUTIONS

Don't take if:
You are allergic to tizanidine.

Before you start, consult your doctor if:
- You have liver disease.
- You have kidney disease.
- You are allergic to any medication, food or other substance.
- You are taking an alpha-adrenergic blood pressure medicine.

Over age 60:
Adverse reactions and side effects may be more frequent and severe than in younger persons. Lower dosage may be recommended to start.

Pregnancy:
Decide with your doctor if drug benefits justify risk to unborn child. Risk category C (see page xviii).

Breast-feeding:
It is unknown if drug passes into milk. Avoid nursing or discontinue until you finish drug. Consult doctor.

Infants & children:
Safety and dosage have not been established.

Prolonged use:
Talk to your doctor about the need for liver function studies while using this drug.

Skin & sunlight:
No special problems expected.

Driving, piloting or hazardous work:
Don't drive or pilot aircraft until you learn how medicine affects you. Don't work around dangerous machinery. Don't climb ladders or work in high places. Danger increases if you drink alcohol or take medicine affecting alertness and reflexes, such as antihistamines, tranquilizers, sedatives, pain medicine, narcotics and mind-altering drugs.

Discontinuing:
Don't discontinue without consulting doctor.

Others:
- May interfere with the results in some medical tests.
- Get up slowly from a sitting or lying position to avoid any dizziness, faintness or lightheadedness.
- Advise any doctor or dentist whom you consult that you take this medicine.
- The brand name Zanaflex is available as a tablet and a capsule. The two formulations are not interchangeable. Switching from the capsule to the tablet may increase risk of side effects.
- Take medicine only as directed. Do not increase or reduce dosage without doctor's approval.

POSSIBLE INTERACTION WITH OTHER DRUGS

GENERIC NAME OR DRUG CLASS	COMBINED EFFECT
Central nervous system (CNS) depressants *	Increased sedation.
Ciprofloxacin	Dangerous increased tizanidine effect. Avoid.
Contraceptives, oral	Increased effect of tizanidine.
Enzyme Inhibitors*	Increased effect of tizanidine.
Fluvoxamine	Dangerous increased tizanidine effect. Avoid.
Hypotension-causing drugs,* other	Increased effect of hypotension.

POSSIBLE INTERACTION WITH OTHER SUBSTANCES

INTERACTS WITH	COMBINED EFFECT
Alcohol:	Increased sedation, low blood pressure. Avoid.
Beverages:	None expected.
Cocaine:	Increased spasticity. Avoid.
Foods:	None expected.
Marijuana:	Increased spasticity or sedation. Avoid.
Tobacco:	May interfere with absorption of medicine.

*See Glossary

TOLCAPONE

BRAND NAMES

Tasmar

BASIC INFORMATION

Habit forming? No
Prescription needed? Yes
Available as generic? No
Drug class: Antidyskinetic,
antiparkinsonism

 ## USES

Used in combination with levodopa and carbidopa for the treatment of the symptoms of Parkinson's disease.

 ## DOSAGE & USAGE INFORMATION

How to take:
Tablet—Swallow whole with a full glass of water. Do not crush or chew tablet before swallowing. May be taken with or without food.

When to take:
At the same times each day as directed by your doctor.

If you forget a dose:
Take as soon as possible. If it is almost time for your next dose, skip the missed dose and go back to your regular dosing schedule. Do not double doses.

What drug does:
Increases the blood levels of levodopa and carbidopa to restore the chemical balance necessary for normal nerve impulses.

Time lapse before drug works:
Up to two hours.

Don't take with:
Any other medicine or any dietary supplement without consulting your doctor or pharmacist.

 ## OVERDOSE

SYMPTOMS:
Nausea, vomiting and dizziness.
WHAT TO DO:
Overdose unlikely to threaten life. If person uses much larger amount than prescribed or if accidentally swallowed, call doctor or poison control center 1-800-222-1222 for help.

 ## POSSIBLE ADVERSE REACTIONS OR SIDE EFFECTS

SYMPTOMS	WHAT TO DO
Life-threatening: None expected.	
Common:	
• Abdominal pain, loss of appetite, diarrhea, dizziness, twitching or unusual body movements, hallucinations, headache, fainting, sleeplessness, nausea, drowsiness, fainting; cough, fever, congestion, runny nose, sneezing, sore throat, vomiting.	Discontinue. Call doctor right away.
• Constipation, excessive dreaming, increased sweating, dry mouth.	Continue. Call doctor if symptoms persist.
• Change in urine color to bright yellow.	No action necessary.
Infrequent:	
• Chest pain, confusion, difficulty breathing, fatigue, falling, blood in urine, hyperactivity, flu-like symptoms, loss of balance control.	Discontinue. Call doctor right away.
• Heartburn, gas.	Continue. Call doctor if symptoms persist.
Rare: Agitation; joint pain; redness or swelling; burning feet; chest discomfort; low blood pressure; difficulty thinking or concentrating; muscle cramps; neck pain; burning, prickling or tingling sensations; sinus congestion; stiffness; bloody or cloudy urine; difficult or painful urination; frequent urge to urinate.	Discontinue. Call doctor right away.

WARNINGS & PRECAUTIONS

Don't take if:
* You have been diagnosed with liver problems.
* You are allergic to tolcapone or any other substances such as food preservatives or dyes.

Before you start, consult your doctor if:
* You have any other medical problem.
* You suffer from hallucinations.
* You have ever been diagnosed with kidney problems.
* You have low blood pressure or are dizzy when getting up suddenly from a sitting or lying position.

Over age 60:
The risk of hallucinations (seeing, hearing or feeling things that are not there) may be increased in patients older than 75 years of age.

Pregnancy:
Decide with your doctor whether drug benefits justify risk to unborn child. Risk category C (see page xviii).

Breast-feeding:
It is not known if drug passes into milk. Avoid drugs or discontinue nursing until you finish medicine. Consult doctor for advice on maintaining milk supply.

Infants & children:
There is no identified potential use of tolcapone in children.

Prolonged use:
No problems expected.

Skin & sunlight:
No problems expected.

Driving, piloting or hazardous work:
Don't drive or pilot aircraft until you learn how medicine affects you. Don't work around dangerous machinery. Don't climb ladders or work in high places. Danger increases if you drink alcohol or take medicine affecting alertness and reflexes.

Discontinuing:
Because of the risk of liver failure, this drug should be stopped if no improvement in 3 weeks.

Others:
* Tolcapone has been indicated in several life-threatening cases of liver failure. This medication should not be used as a first-line treatment for Parkinson's disease.
* You will need frequent liver-function blood tests while you take this medicine.
* Advise any doctor or dentist whom you consult that you take this medicine.

POSSIBLE INTERACTION WITH OTHER DRUGS

GENERIC NAME OR DRUG CLASS	COMBINED EFFECT
Apomorphine	May require adjustment in dosage of apomorphine.
Desipramine	May increase incidence of adverse effects of tolcapone.
Dobutamine	May require adjustment in dosage of dobutamine.
Isoproterenol	May require adjustment in dosage of isoproterenol.
Methyldopa	May require adjustment in dosage of methyldopa.
Monoamine oxidase (MAO) inhibitor*	May reduce the effectiveness of the MAO inhibitor.
Warfarin	May require adjustment in dosage of warfarin.

POSSIBLE INTERACTION WITH OTHER SUBSTANCES

INTERACTS WITH	COMBINED EFFECT
Alcohol:	May increase incidence of hallucinations. Do not use.
Beverages:	None expected.
Cocaine:	May increase incidence of hallucinations. Do not use.
Foods:	None expected.
Marijuana:	May increase incidence of hallucinations. Do not use.
Tobacco:	None expected.

*See Glossary

TOPIRAMATE

BRAND NAMES

Topamax   Topamax Sprinkle
            Capsules

BASIC INFORMATION

Habit forming? No
Prescription needed? Yes
Available as generic? Yes
Drug class: Anticonvulsant, antiepileptic

 ## USES

- Treatment for partial (focal) epileptic seizures. May be used alone or in combination with other antiepileptic drugs.
- Prophylaxis (prevention) of migraine headaches in adults.

 ## DOSAGE & USAGE INFORMATION

How to take:
- Tablet—Swallow the tablets whole with a drink of water; do not crush or chew (the tablet has a bitter taste). May be taken with or without food and on a full or empty stomach.
- Sprinkle capsules—Can be swallowed whole or opened carefully and the contents sprinkled on a small amount of soft food, such as applesauce, pudding, ice cream, oatmeal, or yogurt. Swallow this mixture immediately. Do not chew or store for later use.

When to take:
Your doctor will determine the best schedule. Dosages will be increased rapidly over the first weeks of use. Further increases may be necessary to achieve maximum benefits.

Continued next column

 ## OVERDOSE

SYMPTOMS:
Slow or irregular heartbeat, confusion, dizziness, faintness, unusual tiredness or weakness, blue skin or fingernails, breathing difficulty, coma.
WHAT TO DO:
- **Dial 911 (emergency) for medical help or call poison control center 1-800-222-1222 for instructions.**
- **See emergency information on last 3 pages of this book.**

If you forget a dose:
Take as soon as you remember. If it is almost time for the next dose, skip the missed dose and wait for your next scheduled dose (don't double this dose).

What drug does:
The exact mechanism of the anticonvulsant effect is unknown. It appears to block the spread of seizures rather than raise the seizure threshold like other anticonvulsants. Topiramate's anticonvulsant actions involve several mechanisms.

Time lapse before drug works:
May take several weeks for effectiveness.

Don't take with:
Any other medicine or any dietary supplement without consulting your doctor or pharmacist.

 ## POSSIBLE ADVERSE REACTIONS OR SIDE EFFECTS

SYMPTOMS	WHAT TO DO
Life-threatening:	
In case of overdose, see previous column.	
Common:	
• Burning, prickling, or tingling sensations; clumsiness or unsteadiness; confusion; continuous, uncontrolled back-and-forth or rolling eye movements; dizziness; double vision or other vision problems; drowsiness; generalized slowing of mental and physical activity; memory problems; menstrual changes; menstrual pain; nervousness; speech or language problems; trouble in concentrating or paying attention; unusual tiredness or weakness.	Continue, but call doctor right away.
• Breast pain in women, nausea, tremor.	Continue. Call doctor when convenient.
Infrequent:	
• Abdominal pain, fever, chills, sore throat, lessening of sensations or perception; loss of appetite; mood or mental changes (such as aggression, agitation, apathy, irritability, and depression) red, irritated, or bleeding gums; weight loss.	Continue, but call doctor right away.

• Back pain, chest pain, constipation, heartburn, hot flushes, increased sweating, leg pain.

Continue. Call doctor when convenient.

Rare:

Eye pain, frequent or difficult urination, bloody urine, hearing loss, itching, unsteadiness, loss of bladder control, lower back or side pain, nosebleeds, pale skin, red or irritated eyes, ringing or buzzing in ears, skin rash, swelling, troubled breathing.

Continue, but call doctor right away.

WARNINGS & PRECAUTIONS

Don't take if:
You are allergic to topiramate.

Before you start, consult your doctor if:
• You have a history of liver disease.
• You have kidney disease or kidney stones (nephrolithiasis).
• You are allergic to any medication, food or other substance.
• You have any other medical problems.

Over age 60:
No special problems expected.

Pregnancy:
Decide with your doctor if drug benefits justify risks to unborn child. Risk category C (see page xviii).

Breast-feeding:
It is unknown if drug passes into milk. Avoid drug or discontinue nursing until you finish medicine. Consult doctor for advice on maintaining milk supply.

Infants & children:
This medicine is approved for use from age 2 on. Dose is according to body weight. This medicine is not expected to cause different side effects or problems in children than it does in adults.

Prolonged use:
No special problems expected. Follow-up laboratory blood studies may be recommended by your doctor.

Skin & sunlight:
No problems expected.

Driving, piloting or hazardous work:
Don't drive or pilot aircraft until you learn how medicine affects you. Don't work around dangerous machinery. Don't climb ladders or work in high places. Danger increases if you drink alcohol or take other medicines affecting alertness and reflexes.

Discontinuing:
Don't discontinue without doctor's approval due to risk of increased seizure activity. The dosage may need to be gradually decreased before stopping the drug completely.

Others:
• Advise any doctor or dentist whom you consult that you take this medicine.
• Drink plenty of fluids while taking topiramate. If you have had kidney stones in the past, this will help to reduce your chances of forming kidney stones.
• Topiramate may be used with other anticonvulsant drugs and additional side effects may also occur. If they do, discuss them with your doctor.
• Rarely, antiepileptic drugs may lead to suicidal thoughts and behaviors. Call doctor right away if suicidal symptoms or unusual behaviors occur.
• Wear or carry medical identification to show your seizure disorder and the drugs you take.

POSSIBLE INTERACTION WITH OTHER DRUGS

GENERIC NAME OR DRUG CLASS	COMBINED EFFECT
Anticonvulsants,* other	May decrease or increase effect of both drugs.
Carbonic anhydrase inhibitors*	Increased risk of kidney stones.
Contraceptives, oral*	Decreased effect of contraceptive.
Central nervous system (CNS) depressants*	Increased sedative effect.
Digoxin	May decrease effect of digoxin.

POSSIBLE INTERACTION WITH OTHER SUBSTANCES

INTERACTS WITH	COMBINED EFFECT
Alcohol:	Increased sedative effect. Avoid.
Beverages:	None expected.
Cocaine:	Unknown effect. Avoid.
Foods:	None expected.
Marijuana:	Unknown effect. Avoid.
Tobacco:	None expected.

*See Glossary

TOREMIFENE

BRAND NAMES

Fareston

BASIC INFORMATION

Habit forming? No
Prescription needed? Yes
Available as generic? No
Drug class: Antineoplastic

 ## USES

Used to treat breast cancer in postmenopausal women.

 ## DOSAGE & USAGE INFORMATION

How to take:
Tablet—Swallow with water and take with or without food. If you can't swallow whole, crumble tablet and take with liquid or food.

When to take:
At the same time each day.

If you forget a dose:
Take as soon as possible. If it is almost time for your next dose, skip the missed dose and go back to your regular dosing schedule. Do not double doses.

What drug does:
Exact mechanism unknown. Appears to block growth-stimulating effects of estrogen in the tumor.

Time lapse before drug works:
4 to 6 weeks to determine effectiveness.

Don't take with:
Any other medicine or any dietary supplement without consulting your doctor or pharmacist.

 ## OVERDOSE

SYMPTOMS:
Dizziness, headache, nausea and vomiting.
WHAT TO DO:
Overdose unlikely to threaten life. If person uses much larger amount than prescribed or if accidentally swallowed, call doctor or poison control center 1-800-222-1222 for help.

 ## POSSIBLE ADVERSE REACTIONS OR SIDE EFFECTS

SYMPTOMS	WHAT TO DO
Life-threatening:	
Pain or swelling of feet or lower legs, chest pain, shortness of breath.	Seek emergency treatment immediately.
Common:	
Hot flashes, nausea.	Continue. Call doctor if symptoms persist.
Infrequent:	
• Change in vaginal discharge, pain or feeling of pressure in pelvis, vaginal bleeding, confusion, increased urination, loss of appetite, unusual tiredness, changes in vision.	Continue. Call doctor right away.
• Dizziness, dry eyes, bone pain, vomiting.	Continue. Call doctor if symptoms persist.
Rare:	
None expected.	

WARNINGS & PRECAUTIONS

Don't take if:
- You are allergic to toremifene.
- You have a history of blood clots or have been diagnosed with thromboembolic disease.

Before you start, consult your doctor if:
- You have any other medical problem.
- You have any blood or bleeding disorder.
- You have ever been diagnosed with endometrial hyperplasia (unusual growth of the lining of the uterus).
- You have a tumor that has spread to your bone.

Over age 60:
No problems expected.

Pregnancy:
Consult doctor. Risk category D (see page xviii).

Breast-feeding:
Drug may pass into milk. Avoid drug or discontinue nursing until you finish medicine. Consult doctor about maintaining milk supply.

Infants & children:
There is no identified potential use of toremifene in children.

Prolonged use:
Talk to your doctor about the need for follow-up laboratory studies to check complete blood count, blood calcium concentrations and liver function.

Skin & sunlight:
Avoid prolonged or extended exposure to direct sunlight and/or artificial sunlight while using this medication.

Driving, piloting or hazardous work:
No problems expected.

Discontinuing:
Don't discontinue without consulting doctor.

Others:
- Advise any doctor or dentist you consult that you are taking this medication.
- May interfere with the accuracy of some medical tests.

POSSIBLE INTERACTION WITH OTHER DRUGS

GENERIC NAME OR DRUG CLASS	COMBINED EFFECT
Anticoagulants	May increase time it takes blood to clot.
Diuretics, thiazide	Possible increased calcium.
Enzyme inducers*	May lessen the effect of toremifene.
Enzyme inhibitors*	May increase the effect of toremifene.

POSSIBLE INTERACTION WITH OTHER SUBSTANCES

INTERACTS WITH	COMBINED EFFECT
Alcohol:	None expected.
Beverages:	None expected.
Cocaine:	Effects unknown. Avoid.
Foods:	None expected.
Marijuana:	Effects unknown. Avoid.
Tobacco:	None expected.

TRAMADOL

BRAND NAMES

Ryzolt	Ultram ER
Ultracet	Ultram ODT
Ultram	

BASIC INFORMATION

Habit forming? Yes
Prescription needed? Yes
Available as generic? Yes
Drug class: Analgesic

USES

Treatment for moderate to moderately severe pain (used more for chronic than acute pain).

DOSAGE & USAGE INFORMATION

How to take:
• Tablet or extended-release tablet—Swallow whole with liquid. May be taken with or without food. Do not crush, chew or split tablet. It is for oral use only. Read prescription instructions.
• Disintegrating tablet—Let tablet dissolve in mouth. Do not crush, chew or split tablet. It is for oral use only. Read prescription instructions.

When to take:
Every 4 to 6 hours as needed for pain. Extended release form is taken once a day.

If you forget a dose:
Take as soon as you remember. If it is almost time for the next dose, wait for next scheduled dose (don't double this dose).

What drug does:
Exact mechanism unknown. It appears to block pain messages to the brain and spinal cord.

Continued next column

OVERDOSE

SYMPTOMS:
Breathing difficulty, sleepiness, seizures, cold/clammy skin, slow heartbeat, low blood pressure, stupor, coma. Deaths due to overdose have been reported with abuse and misuse of tramadol, by ingesting, inhaling, or injecting the crushed tablets.
WHAT TO DO:
• **Dial 911 (emergency) for medical help or call poison control center 1-800-222-1222 for instructions.**
• **See emergency information on last 3 pages of this book.**

Time lapse before drug works:
Within 60 minutes.

Don't take with:
Any other medicine or any dietary supplement without consulting your doctor or pharmacist.

POSSIBLE ADVERSE REACTIONS OR SIDE EFFECTS

SYMPTOMS	WHAT TO DO
Life-threatening: Rare allergic reaction (hives, itching, rash, trouble breathing, tightness in chest, swelling of lips or tongue or face).	Seek emergency treatment immediately.
Common: Constipation, nausea, headache, drowsiness, clumsiness, dizziness, itching, flushing or redness of skin, trouble sleeping.	Continue. Call doctor when convenient.
Infrequent: • Constant urge to urinate or inability to urinate, blurred vision.	Discontinue. Call doctor right away.
• Loss of appetite, stomach pain, dry mouth, weakness, confusion, sweating, diarrhea, gas, hot flashes, nervousness, heartburn, tiredness.	Continue. Call doctor when convenient.
Rare: Seizures, balancing difficulty, skin reaction (itching, redness and swelling), memory problems, shortness of breath, difficulty performing tasks, hallucinations, light-headedness when getting up from a sitting or lying position, sensations in hands and feet (burning, tingling, pain, weakness, trembling or shaking), faintness, fast heartbeat.	Discontinue. Call doctor right away.

WARNINGS & PRECAUTIONS

Don't take if:
You are allergic to tramadol or narcotic drugs or you are sensitive to any ingredients in the drug.

Before you start, consult your doctor if:
- You have kidney or liver disease, seizure disorder, stomach disorder or prior head injury.
- You have a history of depression, mental illness or suicidal thoughts or behaviors.
- You have a history of drug abuse or substance abuse, including alcohol abuse.
- You have respiratory problems.

Over age 60:
Increased risk of side effects. Patients over age 75 usually require a dosage adjustment.

Pregnancy:
Decide with your doctor if drug benefits justify risk to unborn child. Risk category C (see page xviii).

Breast-feeding:
Drug passes into milk. Avoid drug or discontinue nursing until you finish medicine. Consult doctor for advice on maintaining milk supply.

Infants & children:
Safety in children under age 18 has not been established.

Prolonged use:
- Consult with your doctor on a regular basis while using this drug.
- Can cause drug dependence, addiction and withdrawal symptoms.

Skin & sunlight:
No special problems expected.

Driving, piloting or hazardous work:
Don't drive or pilot aircraft until you learn how medicine affects you. Don't work around dangerous machinery. Don't climb ladders or work in high places. Danger increases if you drink alcohol or take medicine affecting alertness and reflexes.

Discontinuing:
If you have taken this drug for a long time, consult with your doctor before discontinuing. Withdrawal symptoms may occur if drug is discontinued abruptly. Symptoms include: anxiety, sweating, insomnia, pain, nausea, tremors, diarrhea, breathing problems and hallucinations. Call doctor if symptoms occur.

Others:
- Don't increase dosage or frequency of use without your doctor's approval. Development of a potentially life-threatening serotonin syndrome* or overdose (which can be fatal) may occur with the use of tramadol.
- Advise any doctor or dentist whom you consult that you take this medicine.

POSSIBLE INTERACTION WITH OTHER DRUGS

GENERIC NAME OR DRUG CLASS	COMBINED EFFECT
Carbamazepine	Decreased effect of tramadol.
Central nervous system (CNS) depressants*	Serious adverse events including breathing difficulty.
Clozapine	May increase risk of seizures.
Cyclobenzaprine	May increase risk of seizures.
Digoxin	May increase risk of digoxin toxicity.
Enzyme inducers*	May decrease effect of tramadol.
Enzyme inhibitors*	May increase effect of tramadol.
Monoamine oxidase (MAO) inhibitors*	Serious adverse events including seizures and serotonin syndrome.*
Narcotics*	Increased risk of side effects and seizures.
Phenothiazines*	Increased risk of side effects.
Quinidine	Unknown effect. May need to adjust dose.
Serotonergics*	Increased risk of seizures and serotonin syndrome.*
Tranquilizers*	Increased risk of side effects.
Warfarin	May increase risk of bleeding.

POSSIBLE INTERACTION WITH OTHER SUBSTANCES

INTERACTS WITH	COMBINED EFFECT
Alcohol:	Serious side effects. Avoid.
Beverages:	None expected.
Cocaine:	Unknown. Avoid.
Foods:	None expected.
Marijuana:	Unknown. Avoid.
Tobacco:	None expected.

*See Glossary

TRAZODONE

BRAND NAMES

Trazon   Trialodine

BASIC INFORMATION

Habit forming? No
Prescription needed? Yes
Available as generic? Yes
Drug class: Antidepressant (nontricyclic)

 USES

- Treats mental depression.
- Treats anxiety.
- Helps promote sleep.
- Treats some types of chronic pain.

 DOSAGE & USAGE INFORMATION

How to take:
Tablet—Swallow with liquid or food to lessen stomach irritation. If you can't swallow whole, crumble tablet and take with liquid or food.

When to take:
According to prescription directions. Bedtime dose usually higher than other doses.

If you forget a dose:
Take as soon as you remember up to 2 hours late. If more than 2 hours, wait for next scheduled dose (don't double this dose).

What drug does:
Inhibits serotonin* uptake in brain cells.

Time lapse before drug works:
2 to 4 weeks for full effect.

Don't take with:
Any other medicine or any dietary supplement without consulting your doctor or pharmacist.

 OVERDOSE

SYMPTOMS:
Fainting, irregular heartbeat, respiratory arrest, chest pain, seizures, coma.
WHAT TO DO:
- **Dial 911 (emergency) for medical help or call poison control center 1-800-222-1222 for instructions.**
- **If person is unconscious, check breathing and pulse. If not breathing, begin mouth-to-mouth rescue breathing. If heart is not beating, begin chest compressions.**
- **See emergency information on last 3 pages of this book.**

 POSSIBLE ADVERSE REACTIONS OR SIDE EFFECTS

SYMPTOMS	WHAT TO DO
Life-threatening:	
In case of overdose, see previous column.	
Common:	
Drowsiness.	Continue. Call doctor when convenient.
Infrequent:	
• Prolonged penile erections that may be very painful (priapism).	Seek emergency treatment immediately.
• Tremor, fainting, incoordination, blood pressure rise or drop, rapid heartbeat, shortness of breath.	Discontinue. Call doctor right away.
• Disorientation, confusion, fatigue, dizziness on standing, headache, nervousness, rash, itchy skin, blurred vision, ringing in ears, dry mouth, bad taste, diarrhea, nausea, vomiting, constipation, aching, menstrual changes, diminished sex drive, nightmares, vivid dreams.	Continue. Call doctor when convenient.
Rare:	
Unusual excitement.	Discontinue. Call doctor right away.

 WARNINGS & PRECAUTIONS

Don't take if:
- You are allergic to trazodone.
- You are thinking about suicide.

Before you start, consult your doctor if:
- You have heart rhythm problem.
- You have any heart disease.
- You will have surgery within 2 months, including dental surgery, requiring general or spinal anesthesia.
- You have bipolar (manic-depressive) disorder.
- You have liver or kidney disease.

Over age 60:
Adverse reactions and side effects may be more frequent and severe than in younger persons.

Pregnancy:
Decide with your doctor if drug benefits justify risk to unborn child. Risk category C (see page xviii).

Breast-feeding:
Drug passes into milk. Avoid drug or discontinue nursing until you finish medicine. Consult doctor for advice on maintaining milk supply.

Infants & children:
Not approved for ages under 18. If prescribed, carefully read information provided with prescription. Contact doctor right away if depression symptoms get worse or there is any talk of suicide or suicide behaviors. Also, read information under Others.

Prolonged use:
See your doctor for occasional blood counts, especially if you have fever and sore throat.

Skin & sunlight:
May cause rash or intensify sunburn in areas exposed to sun or ultraviolet light (photosensitivity reaction). Use sunscreen and avoid overexposure. Notify doctor if reaction occurs.

Driving, piloting or hazardous work:
Don't drive or pilot aircraft until you learn how medicine affects you. Don't work around dangerous machinery. Don't climb ladders or work in high places. Danger increases if you drink alcohol or take medicine affecting alertness and reflexes, such as antihistamines, tranquilizers, sedatives, pain medicine, narcotics and mind-altering drugs.

Discontinuing:
Don't discontinue without consulting doctor. Dose may require gradual reduction if you have taken drug for a long time. Doses of other drugs may also require adjustment.

Others:
- Advise any doctor or dentist whom you consult that you take this medicine.
- Adults and children taking antidepressants may experience a worsening of the depression symptoms and may display increased suicidal thoughts or behavior. Call doctor right away if these symptoms or behaviors occur.
- For dry mouth, suck on sugarless hard candy or chew sugarless gum.
- Electroconvulsive therapy* should be avoided. Combined effect is unknown.

 ## POSSIBLE INTERACTION WITH OTHER DRUGS

GENERIC NAME OR DRUG CLASS	COMBINED EFFECT
Antidepressants,* other	Excess drowsiness.
Antihistamines*	Excess drowsiness.
Antihypertensives*	Possible too-low blood pressure. Avoid.
Barbiturates*	Too-low blood pressure and drowsiness. Avoid.
Bupropion	Increased risk of seizures.
Central nervous system (CNS) depressants*	Increased sedation.
Digoxin	Possible increased digitalis effect.
Enzyme Inhibitors*	Increased effect of trazodone.
Guanabenz	Increased effects of both medicines.
Monoamine oxidase (MAO) inhibitors*	May add to toxic effect of each.
Narcotics*	Excess drowsiness.
Phenytoin	Possible increased phenytoin effect.
Ritonavir	Possible increased effect of trazodone.

 ## POSSIBLE INTERACTION WITH OTHER SUBSTANCES

INTERACTS WITH	COMBINED EFFECT
Alcohol:	Excess sedation. Avoid.
Beverages: Caffeine.	May add to heartbeat irregularity. Avoid.
Cocaine:	May add to heartbeat irregularity. Avoid.
Foods:	None expected.
Marijuana:	May add to heartbeat irregularity. Avoid.
Tobacco:	May add to heartbeat irregularity. Avoid.

*See Glossary

TRIAZOLAM

BRAND NAMES

Apo-Triazo   Novo-Triolam
Halcion   Nu-Triazo

BASIC INFORMATION

Habit forming? Yes
Prescription needed? Yes
Available as generic? Yes
Drug class: Sedative-hypnotic agent

 USES

- Treatment for insomnia (short term).
- Prevention or treatment of transient insomnia associated with sudden sleep schedule changes, such as travel across several time zones.

 DOSAGE & USAGE INFORMATION

How to take:
Tablet—Swallow with liquid. If you can't swallow whole, crumble tablet and take with liquid or food.

When to take:
At the same time each day, according to instructions on prescription label. You should be in bed when you take your dose.

If you forget a dose:
Take as soon as you remember up to 2 hours late. If more than 2 hours, wait for next scheduled dose (don't double this dose).

What drug does:
Affects limbic system of brain, the part that controls emotions.

Time lapse before drug works:
Within 30 minutes.

Continued next column

 OVERDOSE

SYMPTOMS:
Drowsiness, weakness, tremor, stupor, coma.
WHAT TO DO:
- **Dial 911 (emergency) for medical help or call poison control center 1-800-222-1222 for instructions.**
- **If person is unconscious, check breathing and pulse. If not breathing, begin mouth-to-mouth rescue breathing. If heart is not beating, begin chest compressions.**
- **See emergency information on last 3 pages of this book.**

Don't take with:
Any other medicine or any dietary supplement without consulting your doctor or pharmacist.

 POSSIBLE ADVERSE REACTIONS OR SIDE EFFECTS

SYMPTOMS	WHAT TO DO
Life-threatening:	
Rare allergic reaction (hives, itching, rash, wheezing, tightness in chest, swelling of lips or tongue or throat).	Seek emergency treatment immediately.
Common:	
Clumsiness, drowsiness, dizziness.	Continue. Call doctor when convenient.
Infrequent:	
• Amnesia, hallucinations, confusion, depression, irritability, rash, itch, vision changes, sore throat, fever, chills, dry mouth.	Discontinue. Call doctor right away.
• Constipation or diarrhea, nausea, vomiting, difficult urination, vivid dreams, behavior changes, abdominal pain, headache.	Continue. Call doctor when convenient.
Rare:	
• Slow heartbeat, breathing difficulty.	Discontinue. Seek emergency treatment.
• Mouth, throat ulcers; jaundice. sleep-related behaviors.*	Discontinue. Call doctor right away.
• Decreased sex drive.	Continue. Call doctor when convenient.

 WARNINGS & PRECAUTIONS

Don't take if:
- You are allergic to any benzodiazepine.
- You have myasthenia gravis.
- You are an active or recovering alcoholic.
- Patient is younger than 6 months.

Before you start, consult your doctor if:
- You have liver, kidney or lung disease.
- You have diabetes, epilepsy or porphyria.
- You have glaucoma.

Over age 60:
Adverse reactions and side effects may be more frequent and severe than in younger persons. You may need smaller doses for shorter periods.

Pregnancy:
Risk to unborn child outweighs drug benefits.
Don't use. Risk category X (see page xviii).

Breast-feeding:
Drug may pass into milk. Avoid drug or
discontinue nursing until you finish medicine.
Consult doctor for advice on maintaining milk
supply.

Infants & children:
Not recommended.

Prolonged use:
May impair liver function.

Skin & sunlight:
No problems expected.

Driving, piloting or hazardous work:
Don't drive or pilot aircraft until you learn how
medicine affects you. Don't work around
dangerous machinery. Don't climb ladders or
work in high places. Danger increases if you
drink alcohol or take medicine affecting alertness
and reflexes.

Discontinuing:
Don't discontinue without consulting doctor.
Dose may require gradual reduction if you have
taken drug for a long time. Doses of other drugs
may also require adjustment.

Others:
* Hot weather, heavy exercise and profuse
  sweating may reduce excretion and cause
  overdose.
* Blood sugar may rise in diabetics, requiring
  insulin adjustment.
* Don't use for insomnia more than 4-7 days.
* Advise any doctor or dentist whom you consult
  that you take this medicine.
* Triazolam has a very short duration of action
  in the body.

POSSIBLE INTERACTION WITH OTHER DRUGS

GENERIC NAME OR DRUG CLASS	COMBINED EFFECT
Anticonvulsants*	Change in seizure frequency or severity.
Antidepressants*	Increased sedative effects of both drugs.
Antihistamines*	Increased sedative effects of both drugs.
Antihypertensives*	Excessively low blood pressure.
Central nervous system (CNS) depressants,* other	Increased central nervous system depression.

Cimetidine	Increased triazolam effect. May be dangerous.
Clozapine	Toxic effect on the central nervous system.
Contraceptives, oral*	Increased triazolam effect and toxicity.
Disulfiram	Increased triazolam effect and toxicity.
Erythromycins*	Increased triazolam effect and toxicity.
Isoniazid	Increased triazolam effect and toxicity.
Ketoconazole	Increased triazolam effect and toxicity.
Levodopa	Possible decreased levodopa effect.
Molindone	Increased tranquilizer effect.
Monoamine oxidase (MAO) inhibitors*	Convulsions, deep sedation, rage.
Narcotics*	Increased sedative effects of both drugs.
Nefazodone	Increased effects of both drugs.
Omeprazole	Delayed excretion of triazolam causing increased amount of triazolam in blood.
Probenecid	Increased triazolam effect.
Zidovudine	Increased toxicity of zidovudine.

POSSIBLE INTERACTION WITH OTHER SUBSTANCES

INTERACTS WITH	COMBINED EFFECT
Alcohol:	Heavy sedation or amnesia. Avoid.
Beverages: Grapefruit juice	Increased triazolam effect.
Cocaine:	Decreased triazolam effect.
Foods:	None expected.
Marijuana:	Heavy sedation. Avoid.
Tobacco:	Decreased triazolam effect.

*See Glossary

TRILOSTANE

BRAND NAMES

Modrastane

BASIC INFORMATION

Habit forming? No
Prescription needed? Yes
Available as generic? No
Drug class: Antiadrenal

 ## USES

Temporary treatment of Cushing's syndrome until surgery on adrenals or radiation to pituitary gland can be performed.

 ## DOSAGE & USAGE INFORMATION

How to take:
Capsule—Swallow with liquid. If you can't swallow whole, open capsule and take with liquid or food. Instructions to take on empty stomach mean 1 hour before or 2 hours after eating.

When to take:
Follow doctor's instructions.

If you forget a dose:
Take as soon as you remember up to 2 hours late. If more than 2 hours, wait for next scheduled dose (don't double this dose).

What drug does:
Decreases function of the adrenal cortex.

Time lapse before drug works:
8 hours.

Don't take with:
Any other medicines (including over-the-counter drugs such as cough and cold medicines, laxatives, antacids, diet pills, caffeine, nose drops or vitamins) without consulting your doctor or pharmacist.

 ## OVERDOSE

SYMPTOMS:
None expected.
WHAT TO DO:
Overdose unlikely to threaten life. If person uses much larger amount than prescribed or if accidentally swallowed, call doctor or poison control center 1-800-222-1222 for help.

 ## POSSIBLE ADVERSE REACTIONS OR SIDE EFFECTS

SYMPTOMS	WHAT TO DO
Life-threatening: None expected.	
Common: Diarrhea, abdominal pain.	Discontinue. Call doctor right away.
Infrequent: Muscle ache, bloating, watery eyes, nausea, increased salivation, flushing, burning mouth or nose.	Continue. Call doctor when convenient.
Rare: Darkening skin, tiredness, appetite loss, depression, skin rash, vomiting.	Continue. Call doctor when convenient.

WARNINGS & PRECAUTIONS

Don't take if:
You know you are allergic to trilostane.

Before you start, consult your doctor if:
- You have an infection.
- You will have surgery while taking.
- You have a head injury.
- You have kidney disease.

Over age 60:
Adverse reactions and side effects may be more frequent and severe than in younger persons. You may need smaller doses for shorter periods of time.

Pregnancy:
Risk to unborn child outweighs drug benefits. Don't use. Risk category X (see page xviii).

Breast-feeding:
Safety not established. Consult doctor.

Infants & children:
Effect not documented. Consult your pediatrician.

Prolonged use:
- Not intended for prolonged use.
- Talk to your doctor about the need for follow-up medical examinations or laboratory studies.

Skin & sunlight:
No problems expected.

Driving, piloting or hazardous work:
Avoid if you feel confused, drowsy or dizzy.

Discontinuing:
No special problems expected.

Others:
- Advise any doctor or dentist whom you consult that you take this medicine.
- May affect results in some medical tests.

POSSIBLE INTERACTION WITH OTHER DRUGS

GENERIC NAME OR DRUG CLASS	COMBINED EFFECT
Aminoglutethimide	Too much decrease in adrenal function.
Mitotane	Too much decrease in adrenal function.

POSSIBLE INTERACTION WITH OTHER SUBSTANCES

INTERACTS WITH	COMBINED EFFECT
Alcohol:	None expected.
Beverages:	None expected.
Cocaine:	None expected.
Foods:	None expected.
Marijuana:	None expected.
Tobacco:	None expected.

TRIMETHOBENZAMIDE

BRAND NAMES

Tigan

BASIC INFORMATION

Habit forming? No
Prescription needed? Yes
Available as generic? Yes
Drug class: Antiemetic

 USES

Reduces nausea and vomiting.

 DOSAGE & USAGE INFORMATION

How to take:
Capsule—Swallow with liquid. If you can't swallow whole, open capsule and take with liquid or food.

When to take:
When needed, no more often than label directs.

If you forget a dose:
Take when you remember. Wait as long as label directs for next dose.

What drug does:
Exact mechanism unknown. Possibly blocks nerve impulses to brain's vomiting centers.

Time lapse before drug works:
20 to 40 minutes.

Don't take with:
Any other medicine or any dietary supplement without consulting your doctor or pharmacist.

 OVERDOSE

SYMPTOMS:
Confusion, convulsions, coma.
WHAT TO DO:
* Dial 911 (emergency) for medical help or call poison control center 1-800-222-1222 for instructions.
* If person is unconscious, check breathing and pulse. If not breathing, begin mouth-to-mouth rescue breathing. If heart is not beating, begin chest compressions.
* See emergency information on last 3 pages of this book.

 POSSIBLE ADVERSE REACTIONS OR SIDE EFFECTS

SYMPTOMS	WHAT TO DO
Life-threatening:	
In case of overdose, see previous column.	
Common:	
Drowsiness.	Continue. Call doctor when convenient.
Infrequent:	
Rash, blurred vision, diarrhea, dizziness, headache, muscle cramps, unusual tiredness.	Discontinue. Call doctor right away.
Rare:	
Seizures, tremor, depression, sore throat, fever, repeated vomiting, back pain, yellow skin or eyes, body spasm (head and heels bent backward and body bowed forward).	Discontinue. Call doctor right away.

 WARNINGS & PRECAUTIONS

Don't take if:
You are allergic to trimethobenzamide.

Before you start, consult your doctor if:
You have reacted badly to antihistamines.

Over age 60:
More susceptible to low blood pressure and sedative effects of this drug.

Pregnancy:
Decide with your doctor if drug benefits justify risk to unborn child. Risk category C (see page xviii).

Breast-feeding:
Effect unknown. Avoid if possible. Consult doctor.

Infants & children:
Avoid during viral infections. Drug may contribute to Reye's syndrome.

Prolonged use:
- Damages blood cell production of bone marrow.
- Causes Parkinson's-like symptoms of tremors, rigidity.

Skin & sunlight:
No special problems expected.

Driving, piloting or hazardous work:
Don't drive until you learn how medicine affects you. Don't work around dangerous machinery. Don't climb ladders or work in high places. Danger increases if you drink alcohol or take medicine affecting alertness and reflexes, such as antihistamines, tranquilizers, sedatives, pain medicine, narcotics and mind-altering drugs.

Discontinuing:
May be unnecessary to finish medicine. Follow doctor's instructions.

Others:
No problems expected.

 POSSIBLE INTERACTION WITH OTHER DRUGS

GENERIC NAME OR DRUG CLASS	COMBINED EFFECT
Antidepressants*	Increased sedative effect.
Antihistamines*	Increased sedative effect.
Barbiturates*	Increased effect of both drugs.
Belladonna	Increased effect of both drugs.
Cholinergics*	Increased effect of both drugs.
Clozapine	Toxic effect on the central nervous system.
Ethinamate	Dangerous increased effects of ethinamate. Avoid combining.
Fluoxetine	Increased depressant effects of both drugs.
Guanfacine	May increase depressant effects of either medicine.
Leucovorin	High alcohol content of leucovorin may cause adverse effects.
Methyprylon	May increase sedative effect to dangerous level. Avoid.
Mind-altering drugs*	Increased effect of mind-altering drug.
Nabilone	Greater depression of central nervous system.
Narcotics*	Increased sedative effect.
Ototoxic medications*	May mask the symptoms of ototoxicity.
Phenothiazines*	Increased effect of both drugs.
Sedatives*	Increased sedative effect.
Sertraline	Increased depressive effects of both drugs.
Sleep inducers*	Increased effect of sleep inducer.
Tranquilizers*	Increased sedative effect.

 POSSIBLE INTERACTION WITH OTHER SUBSTANCES

INTERACTS WITH	COMBINED EFFECT
Alcohol:	Oversedation. Avoid.
Beverages:	None expected.
Cocaine:	None expected.
Foods:	None expected.
Marijuana:	Increased antinausea effect.
Tobacco:	None expected.

TRIMETHOPRIM

BRAND NAMES

Apo-Sulfatrim	SMZ-TMP
Apo-Sulfatrim DS	Sulfamethoprim
Bactrim	Sulfamethoprim DS
Bactrim DS	Sulfaprim
Bethaprim	Sulfaprim DS
Cotrim	Sulfatrim
Cotrim DS	Sulfatrim DS
Co-trimaxizole	Sulfoxaprim
Novotrimel	Sulfoxaprim DS
Novotrimel DS	Sulmeprim
Nu-Cotrimox	Triazole
Nu-Cotrimox DS	Triazole DS
Proloprim	Trimeth-Sulfa
Protrin	Trimpex
Roubac	Trisulfam
Septra	Uroplus DS
Septra DS	Uroplus SS

BASIC INFORMATION

Habit forming? No
Prescription needed? Yes
Available as generic? Yes
Drug class: Antimicrobial (antibacterial)

 USES

- Treats urinary tract infections susceptible to trimethoprim.
- Helps prevent recurrent urinary tract infections if taken once a day.
- Treats Pneumocystis pneumonia.

 DOSAGE & USAGE INFORMATION

How to take:
- Tablet—Swallow with liquid or food to lessen stomach irritation. If can't swallow whole, crush or crumble tablet and take with food or liquid.
- Oral suspension (in combination with sulfamethoxazole)—Follow directions on label.

Continued next column

 OVERDOSE

SYMPTOMS:
Nausea, vomiting, diarrhea.
WHAT TO DO:
Overdose unlikely to threaten life. If person uses much larger amount than prescribed or if accidentally swallowed, call doctor or poison control center 1-800-222-1222 for help.

When to take:
Space doses evenly in 24 hours to keep constant amount in urine.

If you forget a dose:
Take as soon as possible. Wait 5 to 6 hours before next dose. Then return to regular schedule.

What drug does:
Stops harmful bacterial germs from multiplying. Will not kill viruses.

Time lapse before drug works:
2 to 5 days.

Don't take with:
Any other medicine or any dietary supplement without consulting your doctor or pharmacist.

 POSSIBLE ADVERSE REACTIONS OR SIDE EFFECTS

SYMPTOMS	WHAT TO DO
Life-threatening: None expected.	
Common: None expected.	
Infrequent: Diarrhea, nausea, vomiting, stomach cramps, headache.	Continue. Call doctor when convenient.
Rare: Blue fingernails, lips and skin; difficult breathing; sore throat; fever; anemia; jaundice; unusual bleeding or bruising; unusual tiredness or weakness; skin changes (rash, itch, redness, blisters, peeling or loosening); aching joints or muscles.	Discontinue. Call doctor right away.

WARNINGS & PRECAUTIONS

Don't take if:
- You are allergic to trimethoprim or any sulfa drug.*
- You are anemic due to folic acid deficiency.

Before you start, consult your doctor if:
You have had liver or kidney disease.

Over age 60:
- Reduced liver and kidney function may require reduced dose.
- More likely to have severe anal and genital itch.
- Increased susceptibility to anemia.

Pregnancy:
Decide with your doctor whether drug benefits justify risk to unborn child. Risk category C (see page xviii).

Breast-feeding:
No proven harm to unborn child. Avoid if possible. Consult doctor.

Infants & children:
Use under medical supervision only.

Prolonged use:
- Anemia.
- Talk to your doctor about the need for follow-up medical examinations or laboratory studies to check complete blood counts (white blood cell count, platelet count, red blood cell count, hemoglobin, hematocrit).

Skin & sunlight:
May cause rash or intensify sunburn in areas exposed to sun or ultraviolet light (photosensitivity reaction). Avoid overexposure. Notify doctor if reaction occurs.

Driving, piloting or hazardous work:
No problems expected.

Discontinuing:
Don't discontinue without doctor's advice until you complete prescribed dose, even though symptoms diminish or disappear.

Others:
Advise any doctor or dentist whom you consult that you take this medicine.

POSSIBLE INTERACTION WITH OTHER DRUGS

GENERIC NAME OR DRUG CLASS	COMBINED EFFECT
Anticonvulsants*	Increased risk of anemia.
Bone marrow depressants*	Increased possibility of bone marrow suppression.
Folate antagonists,* other	Increased risk of anemia.
Metformin	Increased metformin effect.
Phenytoin	Increased phenytoin effect.

POSSIBLE INTERACTION WITH OTHER SUBSTANCES

INTERACTS WITH	COMBINED EFFECT
Alcohol:	Increased alcohol effect with Bactrim or Septra.
Beverages:	None expected.
Cocaine:	None expected.
Foods:	None expected.
Marijuana:	None expected.
Tobacco:	None expected.

TRIPTANS

GENERIC AND BRAND NAMES

ALMOTRIPTAN
Axert
ELETRIPTAN
Relpax
FROVATRIPTAN
Frova
NARATRIPTAN
Amerge
RIZATRIPTAN
Maxalt
Maxalt-MLT

SUMATRIPTAN
Imitrex
Imitrex Nasal Spray
Treximet
ZOLMITRIPTAN
Zomig
Zomig-Nasal Spray
Zomig-ZMT

BASIC INFORMATION

Habit forming? No
Prescription needed? Yes
Available as generic? Yes, for sumatriptan
Drug class: Antimigraine

 ## USES

- Treatment for acute migraine headaches not relieved by other medications (e.g., aspirin or acetaminophen). Does not prevent migraines.
- Treatment for cluster headaches.

 ## DOSAGE & USAGE INFORMATION

How to take:
- Injection (sumatriptan is self-administered)— Inject under the skin (subcutaneous) of the outer thigh or outer upper arm. Follow doctor's instructions for proper injection technique and method for disposal of the cartridges.
- Tablet—Swallow whole with liquid. Do not crush, break or chew tablet.
- Orally disintegrating tablet—Place on tongue, let it dissolve and swallow with saliva.
- Wafers (rizatriptan)—Place on tongue to dissolve and be swallowed with saliva.
- Nasal spray—One spray into one nostril as a single dose or as instructed by doctor.

Continued next column

 ## OVERDOSE

SYMPTOMS:
Dizziness, sleepiness, vomiting, slow heart-beat, chest pain, tremor, warm feeling, large pupil, irregular breathing, uncoordination.
WHAT TO DO:
- Dial 911 (emergency) for medical help or call poison control center 1-800-222-1222 for instructions.
- See emergency information on last 3 pages of this book.

When to take:
- At the first sign of a migraine (aura or pain). After using drug, lie down in a quiet, dark room to increase effectiveness of treatment.
- An additional dose may be helpful if the migraine returns. Do not exceed the prescribed quantity or frequency. Do not use additional dose if first dose does not bring substantial relief.
- For treatment of cluster headaches, follow your doctor's instructions.

If you forget a dose:
Triptans are not taken on a routine schedule. They are taken when migraines occur.

What drug does:
Enlarged (dilated) blood vessels in the brain cause migraines. Triptans work by narrowing (constricting) these blood vessels.

Time lapse before drug works:
Relief usually begins within 30 minutes for oral dosage (tablets/wafers), 10 minutes for injection and 15 minutes for nasal spray.

Don't take with:
- Ergotamine-containing drugs. Delay 24 hours.
- Any other medicine or any dietary supplement without consulting your doctor or pharmacist.

 ## POSSIBLE ADVERSE REACTIONS OR SIDE EFFECTS

SYMPTOMS	WHAT TO DO
Life-threatening: Rare allergic reaction (hives, itching, rash, wheezing, tightness in chest, swelling of lips or tongue or throat).	Seek emergency treatment immediately.
Common: Nausea and\or vomiting (may be from migraine or from drug), drowsiness or dizziness, migraine recurs.	Continue. Call doctor when convenient.
Infrequent: Sensation of burning, warmth, numbness, cold or tingling; light-headedness; flushing; discomfort of jaw, mouth, throat, nose or sinuses; anxiety; tiredness; vision changes; just feeling ill; muscle weakness, aches, cramps or stiffness; burning, pain, or redness at injection site.	Continue. Call doctor when convenient.

Rare:

Pain, pressure or tightness in the chest; difficulty swallowing; irregular heartbeat, shortness of breath, severe stomach pain	Discontinue. Call doctor right away or seek emergency help for severe symptoms.

WARNINGS & PRECAUTIONS

Don't take if:
- You are allergic to any triptans.
- You have angina pectoris, a history of myocardial infarction or myocardial ischemia, Prinzmetal's angina, stroke or uncontrolled hypertension (high blood pressure).

Before you start, consult your doctor if:
- You have heart rhythm problems or coronary artery disease.
- You have liver or kidney disease.

Over age 60:
Adverse reactions and side effects may be more frequent and severe than in younger persons. Consult doctor.

Pregnancy:
Decide with your doctor whether drug benefits justify risk to unborn child. Risk category C (see page xviii).

Breast-feeding:
Unknown effects. Decide with your doctor whether drug benefits justify possible risk.

Infants & children:
Not recommended for patients under age 18.

Prolonged use:
No problems expected.

Skin & sunlight:
No problems expected.

Driving, piloting or hazardous work:
Avoid if you feel drowsy or dizzy. Otherwise no problems expected.

Discontinuing:
No problems expected. Talk to your doctor if you have plans to discontinue use of drug.

Others:
- Advise any doctor or dentist whom you consult that you take this medicine.
- Rarely, the drug may affect results in some medical tests.
- Follow your doctor's recommendations for any additional treatments for prevention of migraines.
- Sensitivity to light is a symptom of migraine and is not drug-related.

POSSIBLE INTERACTION WITH OTHER DRUGS

GENERIC NAME OR DRUG CLASS	COMBINED EFFECT
Dihydroergotamine	Increased vasoconstriction. Delay 24 hours between drugs.
Enzyme inhibitors*	Increased effect of eletriptan.
Ergotamine	Increased vasoconstriction. Delay 24 hours between drugs.
Monoamine oxidase (MAO) inhibitors*	Adverse effects unknown. Avoid.
Propranolol	Increased effect of rizatriptan.
Selective serotonin reuptake inhibitors (SSRIs)	Risk of serotonin syndrome.*
Serotonergics*	Risk of serotonin syndrome.*
Serotonin & norepinephrine reuptake inhibitors (SNRIs)	Risk of serotonin syndrome.*
Triptans, other	Increased vasoconstriction. Delay 24 hours between drugs.

POSSIBLE INTERACTION WITH OTHER SUBSTANCES

INTERACTS WITH	COMBINED EFFECT
Alcohol:	No interaction known, but alcohol aggravates migraines. Avoid.
Beverages:	Grapefruit juice may increase the effect of eletriptan.
Cocaine:	Unknown. Avoid.
Foods:	Grapefruit may increase the effect of eletriptan.
Marijuana:	Unknown. avoid.
Tobacco:	None expected.

*See Glossary

TUMOR NECROSIS FACTOR BLOCKERS

GENERIC AND BRAND NAMES

ADALIMUMAB	**ETANERCEPT**
Humira	Enbrel
CERTOLIZUMAB	**INFLIXIMAB**
Cimzia	Remicade

BASIC INFORMATION

Habit forming? No
Prescription needed? Yes
Available as generic? No
Drug class: Antirheumatic; biological response modifier

 USES

- Treatment of moderately to severely active rheumatoid arthritis. Used for patients who have not responded to one or more disease modifying antirheumatic drugs (DMARDs). May be used alone or in combination with certain other arthritis drugs (e.g., methotrexate).
- Treats Crohn's disease, ulcerative colitis, moderate to severe ankylosing spondylitis, psoriatic arthritis, and moderate to severe plaque psoriasis.
- May be used for other disorders as determined by your doctor.

 DOSAGE & USAGE INFORMATION

How to take:
- Self injection—The drug may be self-injected under the skin (subcutaneously). Follow your doctor's instructions and the directions provided with the prescription on how and where to inject. Do not use the medication unless you are sure about the proper method for injection. Store medication in the refrigerator (do not freeze) until you plan to use it. After each use, throw away the syringe and any medicine left in it (ask your pharmacist about disposal methods). Never reuse the needles or syringes.

Continued next column

 OVERDOSE

SYMPTOMS:
None expected.
WHAT TO DO:
If an overdose is suspected, dial 911 (emergency) for medical help or call poison control center 1-800-222-1222 for instructions.

- Infliximab—The drug is given by injection in a medical office. With training, some patients may be able to self-inject the drug.

When to take:
Usually etanercept is used once or twice a week, adalimumab is used every other week, and infliximab is given several times a year. Read prescription labels for specific instructions.

If you forget a dose:
Inject as soon as possible. If it is almost time for your next dose, skip the missed dose and go back to your regular dosing schedule. Do not double doses.

What drug does:
Blocks the damage done to healthy cells by the tumor necrosis factor (TNF), a protein in the body. The drug helps prevent the progressive joint destruction of rheumatoid arthritis.

Time lapse before drug works:
It will take several weeks before full benefits of the drug are noticeable.

Don't use with:
Any other medicine or any dietary supplement without consulting your doctor or pharmacist.

 POSSIBLE ADVERSE REACTIONS OR SIDE EFFECTS

SYMPTOMS	WHAT TO DO
Life-threatening: None expected.	
Common: Chills, fever, chest pain or tightness, hives or itching, flushed face, breathing difficulty, stuffy or runny nose, headache, sneezing, wheezing, sore throat, unusual tiredness or weakness, vomiting, rash (on face, scalp or stomach), reaction at injection site.	Call doctor right away.
Infrequent: Painful or frequent or difficult urination, bloody or colored urine, fast heartbeat, faintness, pain or stiffness in muscles and joints, pain (stomach, back, face, shoulder, rectum), dizziness, diarrhea, sores on mouth or tongue, vaginal itching or burning, sore fingernails or toenails.	Call doctor right away.

Rare:

Allergic reaction (itching, rash hives, swelling of face or lips, wheezing), black or tarry stools, vision problems, constipation, feeling of fullness, yellow skin or eyes, swollen glands, fungal infection (fever, cough, tiredness, weight loss, sweats, shortness of breath).

Call doctor right away.

WARNINGS & PRECAUTIONS

Don't take if:
You are allergic to tumor necrosis factor blockers or their components.

Before you start, consult your doctor if:
- You have congestive heart failure (CHF).
- You have or have had tuberculosis.
- You have a central nervous system disorder or a blood disorder or diabetes.
- You are scheduled for surgery.
- You are allergic to rubber or latex (it is used in the drug product's needle covering).
- You have an active infection.
- You have a chronic disorder or infection, a malignancy, or are immunosuppressed.

Over age 60:
Used with caution in elderly patients, since infections are more common in this age group.

Pregnancy:
Risk factors vary for drugs in this group. See category list on page xviii and consult doctor.

Breast-feeding:
It is unknown if drug passes into milk. Consult doctor for advice on breast-feeding if you use this medication.

Infants & children:
Use only with close medical supervision. Infliximab is used in children 6 and older with active Crohn's disease. Etanercept is used in children ages 4 and older who have juvenile rheumatoid arthritis (JRA).

Prolonged use:
- No specific problems expected.
- Talk to your doctor about the need for follow-up medical examinations or laboratory studies to check effectiveness of the drug and to monitor for infections or adverse effects.

Skin & sunlight:
No problems expected.

Driving, piloting or hazardous work:
No problems expected.

Discontinuing:
No problems expected. Consult doctor first.

Others:
- Serious infections (such as tuberculosis and fungal infections) and death have been reported in patients using these drugs. Consult your doctor if any signs or symptoms of infection occur.
- Infliximab use may lead to liver toxicity and liver failure with symptoms of yellow skin or eyes, vomiting, and abdominal pain. It may also cause blood abnormalities or blood vessel inflammation with symptoms of vision changes, weakness, numbness or tingling, paleness, fever, or easy bruising or bleeding. Call doctor right away if symptoms occur.
- Slight increased risk of cancer and lupus-like syndromes. Ask your doctor about your risks.
- Advise any doctor or dentist whom you consult that you take this medicine.
- See your doctor for regular visits while using this drug.
- Avoid immunizations unless doctor approved.

POSSIBLE INTERACTION WITH OTHER DRUGS

GENERIC NAME OR DRUG CLASS	COMBINED EFFECT
Anakinra	Risk of serious infection. Avoid.
Immunosuppressants*	May increase risk of infection.
Live vaccines	May decrease vaccine effect.

Note: Consult your doctor or pharmacist about other possible interactions.

POSSIBLE INTERACTION WITH OTHER SUBSTANCES

INTERACTS WITH	COMBINED EFFECT
Alcohol:	None expected.
Beverages:	None expected.
Cocaine:	None expected. However, cocaine may slow body's recovery. Avoid.
Foods:	None expected.
Marijuana:	None expected. However, marijuana may slow body's recovery. Avoid.
Tobacco:	None expected.

*See Glossary

URSODIOL

BRAND NAMES

Actigall   Ursofalk
Urso

BASIC INFORMATION

Habit forming? No
Prescription needed? Yes
Available as generic? Yes
Drug class: Anticholelithic

 ## USES

- Dissolves cholesterol gallstones in selected patients who either can't tolerate surgery or don't require surgery for other reasons. Not used when surgery is clearly indicated.
- Prevention of gallstone formation during rapid weight loss.
- Treatment for primary biliary cirrhosis.

 ## DOSAGE & USAGE INFORMATION

How to take:
Capsule or tablet—Swallow with a full glass of water. You may take with food to lessen stomach irritation. If you can't swallow whole, open capsule and take with liquid or food. Ask pharmacist for information about crushing tablet form.

When to take:
With meals, 2 or 3 times a day according to your doctor's instructions.

If you forget a dose:
Take as soon as you remember up to 2 hours late. If more than 2 hours, wait for next scheduled time. Don't double this dose.

Continued next column

 ## OVERDOSE

SYMPTOMS:
Severe diarrhea.
WHAT TO DO:
Overdose unlikely to threaten life. If person uses much larger amount than prescribed or if accidentally swallowed, call doctor or poison control center 1-800-222-1222 for help.

What drug does:
Decreases secretion of cholesterol into bile by suppressing production and secretion of cholesterol by the liver. Ursodiol will not help gallstone problems unless the gallstones are made of cholesterol. It works best when the stones are small.

Time lapse before drug works:
Unpredictable. Varies among patients. If taken for gallstones, the drug may need to be taken for a long time.

Don't take with:
Any other medicine or any dietary supplement without consulting your doctor or pharmacist.

 ## POSSIBLE ADVERSE REACTIONS OR SIDE EFFECTS

SYMPTOMS	WHAT TO DO
Life-threatening: Rare allergic reaction— Breathing difficulty; closing of the throat; swelling of hands, feet, face, lips or tongue; hives.	Discontinue. Seek emergency treatment.
Common: None expected.	
Infrequent: Diarrhea, nausea, upset stomach, headache.	Continue. Call doctor when convenient.
Rare: Any unusual symptoms occur.	Continue. Call doctor when convenient.

WARNINGS & PRECAUTIONS

Don't take if:
You are allergic to any bile acids.

Before you start, consult your doctor if:
* You have complications of gallstones, such as infection, cholecystitis or obstruction of the bile ducts.
* You have had pancreatitis.
* You have heart, liver or kidney disease.

Over age 60:
No special problems expected.

Pregnancy:
Decide with your doctor whether drug benefits justify risk to unborn child. Pregnancy risk category B (see page xviii).

Breast-feeding:
It is unknown if drug passes into milk; however, similar substances appear in breast milk. Consult doctor for advice on breast-feeding if you use this medication.

Infants & children:
Not recommended. Adequate studies have not been performed.

Prolonged use:
* No special problems expected.
* Talk to your doctor about the need for follow-up medical examinations or laboratory studies to check kidney function.

Skin & sunlight:
No problems expected.

Driving, piloting or hazardous work:
Don't pilot aircraft until you learn how medicine affects you. Don't work around dangerous machinery. Don't climb ladders or work in high places. Danger increases if you drink alcohol or take medicine affecting alertness and reflexes, such as antihistamines, tranquilizers, sedatives, pain medicine, narcotics and mind-altering drugs.

Discontinuing:
Don't discontinue without consulting doctor.

Others:
* Plan regular visits to your doctor while you take ursodiol. Have ultrasound and liver function studies done at appropriate intervals. Liver damage is unlikely, but theoretically could happen.
* Advise any doctor or dentist whom you consult that you take this medicine.

POSSIBLE INTERACTION WITH OTHER DRUGS

GENERIC NAME OR DRUG CLASS	COMBINED EFFECT
Antacids* (aluminum-containing)	Decreased absorption of ursodiol.
Cholestyramine	Decreased absorption of ursodiol.
Clofibrate	Decreased effect of ursodiol.
Colestipol	Decreased absorption of ursodiol.
Estrogens*	Decreased effect of ursodiol.
Progestins	Decreased effect of ursodiol.

POSSIBLE INTERACTION WITH OTHER SUBSTANCES

INTERACTS WITH	COMBINED EFFECT
Alcohol:	None expected, unless you have impaired liver function from alcohol abuse.
Beverages:	None expected.
Cocaine:	None expected.
Foods:	None expected.
Marijuana:	None expected.
Tobacco:	None reported. However, tobacco may possibly impair absorption from the intestinal tract. Better to avoid.

*See Glossary

VALPROIC ACID

BRAND NAMES

Depakene   Stavzor

BASIC INFORMATION

Habit forming? No
Prescription needed? Yes
Available as generic? Yes
Drug class: Anticonvulsant

USES

• Treatment of various types of epilepsy.
• Treatment for bipolar (manic-depressive) disorder.
• Prevention of migraine headaches.

DOSAGE & USAGE INFORMATION

How to take:
• Capsule or syrup—Swallow with liquid or food to lessen stomach irritation. Do not crush or chew capsule.
• Delayed-release capsule—Swallow whole with a glass of water. Do not crush or chew.

When to take:
One to three times a day as directed by doctor.

If you forget a dose:
Take as soon as you remember. If it is almost time for the next dose, wait for the next scheduled dose (don't double this dose).

What drug does:
It helps stabilize electrical and chemical activity in the brain.

Time lapse before drug works:
1 to 4 hours, but full effect may take weeks.

Don't take with:
Any other medicine or any dietary supplement without consulting your doctor or pharmacist.

OVERDOSE

SYMPTOMS:
Extreme drowsiness, heart problems, loss of consciousness.
WHAT TO DO:
• Dial 911 (emergency) for medical help or call poison control center 1-800-222-1222 for instructions.
• See emergency information on last 3 pages of this book.

POSSIBLE ADVERSE REACTIONS OR SIDE EFFECTS

SYMPTOMS	WHAT TO DO
Life-threatening: Rare allergic reaction (hives, itching, rash, wheezing, tightness in chest, swelling (lips, tongue or throat).	Seek emergency treatment immediately.
Common: Mild appetite loss, indigestion, nausea, vomiting, abdominal cramps, diarrhea, tremor, weight gain or loss, menstrual changes in girls, headache.	Continue. Call doctor when convenient.
Infrequent: Clumsiness or unsteadiness, constipation, skin rash, dizziness, drowsiness, irritable or excited, hair loss.	Continue. Call doctor when convenient.
Rare: Mood or behavior changes; continued nausea, vomiting and appetite loss; increase in seizures; swelling (face, feet, legs); clay-color stools; confusion, yellow skin or eyes; tiredness or weakness; back-and-forth eye movements; seeing spots/seeing double; unusual bleeding or bruising; dark urine; low fever; severe stomach cramps.	Continue, but call doctor right away or seek emergency care for severe symptoms.

WARNINGS & PRECAUTIONS

Don't take if:
You are allergic to valproic acid.

Before you start, consult your doctor if:
• You have liver, kidney, blood or brain disorder or pancreatitis or urea cycle disorder.
• Drug is to be used for a young child.
• You have a history of depression or suicide thoughts or suicidal behavior.
• You are a woman of childbearing age.

Over age 60:
Adverse reactions and side effects may be more frequent and severe than in younger persons.

Pregnancy:
Risk of birth defects to unborn child exists. Use only if benefits of drug greatly exceed fetal risk. Risk category D (see page xviii).

Breast-feeding:
Drug passes into milk. Avoid drug or discontinue nursing until you finish medicine. Consult doctor for advice on maintaining milk supply.

Infants & children:
Increased risk for side effects and adverse reactions. Use under close medical supervision only.

Prolonged use:
Request periodic blood tests, liver and kidney function tests. These tests are necessary for safe and effective use.

Skin & sunlight:
No problems expected.

Driving, piloting or hazardous work:
Don't drive or pilot aircraft until you learn how medicine affects you. Don't work around dangerous machinery. Don't climb ladders or work in high places. Danger increases if you drink alcohol or take medicine affecting alertness and reflexes.

Discontinuing:
Don't discontinue without consulting doctor. Dose may require gradual reduction if you have taken drug for a long time. Doses of other drugs may also require adjustment.

Others:
- Read the insert provided with the drug. Follow all instructions and heed all warnings.
- Advise any doctor or dentist whom you consult that you take this drug.
- In rare cases, the drug can cause life-threatening liver failure (especially in children under age 2) or life-threatening pancreatitis (inflammation of the pancreas). Consult your doctor about your risks.
- Rarely, antiepileptic (anticonvulsant) drugs may lead to suicidal thoughts and behaviors. Call doctor right away if suicidal symptoms or unusual behaviors occur.
- Wear or carry medical identification to show your seizure disorder and the drugs you take.

POSSIBLE INTERACTION WITH OTHER DRUGS

GENERIC NAME OR DRUG CLASS	COMBINED EFFECT
Anticoagulants,* oral	Increased risk of bleeding problems.
Anticonvulsants,* other	Each drug may need dosage adjusted.
Anti-inflammatory drugs, nonsteroidal* (NSAIDs)	Increased risk of bleeding problems.
Aspirin	Increased effect of valproic acid.
Carbamazepine	Decreased effect of valproic acid.
Central nervous system (CNS) depressants*	Increased sedative effect.
Clonazepam	May prolong seizure.
Diazepam	Increased effect of diazepam.
Enzyme inducers*	May Increase effect of some enzyme inducers and decrease effect of valproic acid.
Felbamate	Increased effect of valproic acid.
Hepatotoxics*	Increased risk of liver problems.
Lamotrigine	Increased effect of lamotrigine and risk of life-threatening rash.
Phenobarbital	Increased effect of phenobarbital and decreased effect of valproic acid.
Phenytoin	Increased phenytoin effect; decreased valproic acid effect.
Primidone	Increased effect of primidone.
Rifampin	Decreased effect of valproic acid.

Continued on page 934

POSSIBLE INTERACTION WITH OTHER SUBSTANCES

INTERACTS WITH	COMBINED EFFECT
Alcohol:	Excess sedation. Avoid.
Beverages:	None expected.
Cocaine:	Unknown. Avoid.
Foods:	None expected.
Marijuana:	Unknown. Avoid.
Tobacco:	None expected.

*See Glossary

VANCOMYCIN

BRAND NAMES

Vancocin

BASIC INFORMATION

Habit forming? No
Prescription needed? Yes
Available as generic? Yes
Drug class: Antibacterial

 USES

- Treats colitis when caused by *Clostridium* infections.
- Treats some forms of severe diarrhea and other disorders as determined by your doctor.

 DOSAGE & USAGE INFORMATION

How to take:
- Capsule—Swallow with liquid. If you can't swallow whole, open capsule and take with liquid or food. Instructions to take on empty stomach mean 1 hour before or 2 hours after eating.
- Oral solution—Use the calibrated measuring device. Swallow with other liquid to prevent nausea.
- There is also an injectable form. This information applies to the oral form only.

When to take:
According to doctor's instructions. Usually every 6 hours.

If you forget a dose:
Take as soon as you remember up to 2 hours late. If more than 2 hours, wait for next scheduled dose (don't double this dose).

What drug does:
Kills bacterial cells.

Time lapse before drug works:
None. Works right away. This medicine is not absorbed to a great extent through the intestinal tract.

Continued next column

 OVERDOSE

SYMPTOMS:
None expected.
WHAT TO DO:
Overdose unlikely to threaten life. If person uses much larger amount than prescribed or if accidentally swallowed, call doctor or poison control center 1-800-222-1222 for help.

Don't take with:
Any other medicines (including over-the-counter drugs such as cough and cold medicines, laxatives, antacids, diet pills, caffeine, nose drops or vitamins) without consulting your doctor or pharmacist.

 POSSIBLE ADVERSE REACTIONS OR SIDE EFFECTS

SYMPTOMS	WHAT TO DO
Life-threatening: None expected.	
Common: Bitter taste.	Continue. Tell doctor at next visit.
Infrequent: Nausea or vomiting.	Continue. Call doctor when convenient.
Rare: Hearing loss, ears ringing or buzzing.	Discontinue. Call doctor right away.

WARNINGS & PRECAUTIONS

Don't take if:
You are allergic to vancomycin.

Before you start, consult your doctor if:
• You have hearing problems.
• You have severe kidney disease.
• You have intestinal obstruction.

Over age 60:
Adverse reactions and side effects may be more frequent and severe than in younger persons. You may need smaller doses for shorter periods of time.

Pregnancy:
Consult doctor. Risk category B (see page xviii).

Breast-feeding:
No special problems expected. Consult doctor.

Infants & children:
No special problems expected.

Prolonged use:
Talk to your doctor about the need for follow-up medical examinations or laboratory studies to check hearing acuity, kidney function, vancomycin serum concentration and urinalysis.

Skin & sunlight:
No problems expected.

Driving, piloting or hazardous work:
No problems expected.

Discontinuing:
No special problems expected.

Others:
• Advise any doctor or dentist whom you consult that you take this medicine.
• May affect results in some medical tests.

POSSIBLE INTERACTION WITH OTHER DRUGS

GENERIC NAME OR DRUG CLASS*	COMBINED EFFECT
Cholestyramine	Decreased therapeutic effect of vancomycin.
Colestipol	Decreased therapeutic effect of vancomycin.
Metformin	Increased metformin effect.
Nephrotoxics*	Increased risk of liver toxicity.

POSSIBLE INTERACTION WITH OTHER SUBSTANCES

INTERACTS WITH	COMBINED EFFECT
Alcohol:	None expected.
Beverages:	None expected.
Cocaine:	None expected.
Foods:	None expected.
Marijuana:	None expected.
Tobacco:	None expected.

*See Glossary

VARENICLINE

BRAND NAMES

Chantix

BASIC INFORMATION

Habit Forming? No
Prescription needed? Yes
Available as generic? No
Drug class: Antismoking agent

 USES

Helps adults quit smoking. It is recommended that patients combine use of this drug with a stop-smoking program (such as counseling, support groups and/or patient education).

 DOSAGE & USAGE INFORMATION

How to take:
Tablet—Swallow whole with a full glass (8 ounces) of water.

When to use:
• The tablet is taken twice a day after eating.
• The first step in treatment is to set a date to quit smoking. Then start taking the drug one week before that date. A lower dose is taken at the start of treatment and increased over the first few days. In most cases, treatment time is 12 weeks. It may be continued for another 12 weeks to improve long-term success in quitting smoking.

If you forget a dose:
Take tablet as soon as you remember. If it is almost time for the next dose, wait for the next scheduled dose (don't double this dose).

Continued next column

 OVERDOSE

SYMPTOMS:
Symptoms of an overdose are unknown.
WHAT TO DO:
• Dial 911 (emergency) for medical help or call poison control center 1-800-222-1222 for instructions.
• See emergency information on last 3 pages of this book.

What drug does:
It is a nicotine-free drug that acts on the brain to reduce cravings for cigarettes (and other tobacco products). It also blocks the pleasurable effects of smoking. This helps to decrease the desire to smoke and reduces the unpleasant smoking withdrawal symptoms.

Time lapse before drug works:
It may take several days to see the effects. Full benefit may take 12 weeks of treatment.

Don't take with:
Any other medicine or diet supplement without consulting your doctor or pharmacist.

 POSSIBLE ADVERSE REACTIONS OR SIDE EFFECTS

SYMPTOMS	WHAT TO DO
Life-threatening:	
Rare allergic reaction (hives, itching, rash, trouble breathing, tightness in chest, swelling of lips or tongue or throat).	Seek emergency treatment immediately.
Common:	
Nausea (may go on for several months), insomnia, headache.	Continue. Call doctor when convenient.
Infrequent:	
Strange dreams, gas, abdominal pain, upset stomach, taste changes, constipation, weak or tired feeling, vomiting.	Continue. Call doctor when convenient.
Rare:	
Chest pain, fast or slow or irregular heartbeat, memory loss, seizures, severe or persistent nausea, suicidal thoughts, unusual mental or mood changes, vision changes, drowsiness, other unusual symptoms.	Discontinue. Call doctor right away.

WARNINGS & PRECAUTIONS

Don't take if:
You are allergic to varenicline.

Before you start, consult your doctor if:
* You have kidney disease.
* You have or have had depression or a psychiatric illness.
* You have any chronic medical or health problem.

Over age 60:
Adverse reactions and side effects may be more frequent and severe than in younger persons.

Pregnancy:
Decide with your doctor if drug benefits justify risk to unborn child. Risk category C (see page xviii). (Tobacco smoke and nicotine are known to be harmful to a fetus.)

Breast-feeding:
It is unknown if drug passes into milk. Avoid drug or discontinue nursing until you finish dosage. Consult doctor for advice on maintaining milk supply.

Infants & children:
Safety and effectiveness in children under age 18 has not been established. Consult doctor.

Prolonged use:
It is not intended for long-term use. Usually prescribed for one or two 12-week periods of time.

Skin & sunlight:
No problems expected.

Driving, piloting or hazardous work:
Drug may cause drowsiness. Don't drive or pilot aircraft until you learn how medicine affects you. Don't work around dangerous machinery. Don't climb ladders or work in high places.

Discontinuing:
* Don't discontinue abruptly without doctor's advice. It could increase risk of feeling irritable and cause sleep disturbance.
* Nicotine withdrawal symptoms may occur during and after treatment. These include increased appetite, weight gain, tension, irritability, insomnia, headache and others. Consult doctor if withdrawal symptoms persist.

Others:
* Advise any doctor or dentist whom you consult that you take this medicine.
* For full benefit from a stop-smoking program, follow your doctor's advice.
* Even if you smoke after your quit date, continue to try to quit. Advise your doctor if you do continue to smoke after a few weeks of treatment.

* Patients who are attempting to quit smoking with this drug should be observed for serious mood or behavior changes. Symptoms may include depressed mood, agitation, agressiveness, other emotional changes and thoughts about suicide or possible suicide attempts. Consult your doctor about your risks or call doctor right away if any symptoms occur.

POSSIBLE INTERACTION WITH OTHER DRUGS

GENERIC NAME OR DRUG CLASS	COMBINED EFFECT
Cimetidine	May increase effect of varenicline.
Insulin	No interaction, but dosage may need adjustment once you quit smoking.
Nicotine replacement	May increase risk of side effects.
Theophylline	No interaction, but dosage may need adjustment once you quit smoking.
Warfarin	No interaction, but dosage may need adjustment once you quit smoking.

POSSIBLE INTERACTION WITH OTHER SUBSTANCES

INTERACTS WITH	COMBINED EFFECT
Alcohol:	None expected.
Beverages:	None expected.
Cocaine:	Unknown. Avoid.
Foods:	None expected.
Marijuana:	Unknown. Avoid.
Tobacco:	As intended, varenicline blocks the pleasurable effect of nicotine.

*See Glossary

VITAMIN A

BRAND NAMES

Acon
Afaxin
Alphalin

Aquasol A
Dispatabs
Sust-A

Numerous brands of single vitamin and multivitamin combinations are available.

BASIC INFORMATION

Habit forming? No
Prescription needed? No
Available as generic? Yes
Drug class: Vitamin supplement

 ## USES

- Dietary supplement to ensure normal growth and health, especially of eyes and skin.
- Beta carotene form decreases severity of sun exposure in patients with porphyria.

 ## DOSAGE & USAGE INFORMATION

How to take:
- Drops or capsule—Swallow with liquid. If you can't swallow whole, open capsule and take with liquid or food.
- Oral solution—Swallow with liquid.
- Tablet—Swallow with liquid.

When to take:
At the same time each day.

If you forget a dose:
Take as soon as you remember, then resume regular schedule.

What drug does:
Promotes normal growth and health.

Continued next column

 ## OVERDOSE

SYMPTOMS:
Increased adverse reactions and side effects. Jaundice (rare, but may occur with large doses), malaise, vomiting, irritability, bleeding gums, seizures, double vision, peeling skin.
WHAT TO DO:
If person takes much larger amount than prescribed, dial 911 (emergency) for medical help or call poison control center 1-800-222-1222 for instructions.

Time lapse before drug works:
Requires continual intake.

Don't take with:
Any other medicine or any dietary supplement without consulting your doctor or pharmacist.

 ## POSSIBLE ADVERSE REACTIONS OR SIDE EFFECTS

SYMPTOMS	WHAT TO DO
Life-threatening: In case of overdose, see previous column.	
Common: None expected.	
Infrequent: Confusion; dizziness; drowsiness; headache; irritability; dry, cracked lips; peeling skin; hair loss; sensitivity to light.	Continue. Call doctor when convenient.
Rare: • Bulging soft spot on baby's head, double vision, bone or joint pain, abdominal pain, frequent urination, vomiting.	Discontinue. Call doctor right away.
• Diarrhea, appetite loss, nausea.	Continue. Call doctor when convenient.

WARNINGS & PRECAUTIONS

Don't take if:
You have chronic kidney failure.

Before you start, consult your doctor if:
You have any kidney disorder.

Over age 60:
No problems expected.

Pregnancy:
Risk factor determined by length of pregnancy and dosage amount. See category list on page xviii and consult doctor.

Breast-feeding:
No problems expected. Consult doctor.

Infants & children:
• Avoid large doses.
• Keep vitamin-mineral supplements out of children's reach.

Prolonged use:
No problems expected.

Skin & sunlight:
No special problems expected.

Driving, piloting or hazardous work:
No problems expected.

Discontinuing:
Don't discontinue without doctor's advice until you complete prescribed dose, even though symptoms diminish or disappear.

Others:
• Don't exceed recommended dosage. Too much over a long time may be harmful.
• A balanced diet will help provide vitamin A. Best sources are liver; yellow-orange fruits and vegetables; dark-green, leafy vegetables; milk; butter and margarine.

POSSIBLE INTERACTION WITH OTHER DRUGS

GENERIC NAME OR DRUG CLASS	COMBINED EFFECT
Anticoagulants*	Increased anticoagulant effect with large doses (over 10,000 I.U.) of vitamin A.
Calcium supplements*	Decreased vitamin effect.
Cholestyramine	Decreased vitamin A absorption.
Colestipol	Decreased vitamin absorption.
Contraceptives, oral*	Increased vitamin A levels.
Etretinate	Increased risk of toxic effects.
Isotretinoin	Increased risk of toxic effect of each.
Mineral oil (long-term)	Decreased vitamin A absorption.
Neomycin	Decreased vitamin absorption.
Vitamin A derivatives, other	Increased toxicity risk.
Vitamin E (excess dose)	Vitamin A depletion.

POSSIBLE INTERACTION WITH OTHER SUBSTANCES

INTERACTS WITH	COMBINED EFFECT
Alcohol:	None expected.
Beverages:	None expected.
Cocaine:	None expected.
Foods:	None expected.
Marijuana:	None expected.
Tobacco:	None expected.

*See Glossary

VITAMIN B-12 (Cyanocobalamin)

GENERIC AND BRAND NAMES

CYANOCOBALAMIN
- Anocobin
- Bedoz
- Berubigen
- Betalin 12
- CaloMist
- Cyanabin
- Kaybovite
- Kaybovite-1000
- Nascobal
- Redisol
- Rubion
- Rubramin
- Rubramin-PC

HYDROXOCOBAL-AMIN
- Acti-B-12
- Alpha Redisol
- Alphamin
- Codroxomin
- Droxomin

Numerous brands of single vitamin and multivitamin combinations may be available.

BASIC INFORMATION

Habit forming? No
Prescription needed? Yes, for some
Available as generic? Yes
Drug class: Vitamin supplement

USES

- Dietary supplement for normal growth, development and health.
- Treatment for nerve damage.
- Treatment for pernicious anemia.
- Treatment and prevention of vitamin B-12 deficiencies in people who have had stomach or intestines surgically removed.
- Prevention of vitamin B-12 deficiency in strict vegetarians and persons with absorption diseases.

OVERDOSE

SYMPTOMS:
Increased adverse reactions and side effects.
WHAT TO DO:
Overdose unlikely to threaten life. If person uses much larger amount than prescribed or if accidentally swallowed, call doctor or poison control center 1-800-222-1222 for help.

DOSAGE & USAGE INFORMATION

How to take:
- Tablet—Swallow with liquid.
- Extended-release tablet— Swallow whole with liquid. Do not crush or chew.
- Injection—Follow doctor's directions.
- Nasal gel or nasal spray—Follow instructions on product. Use nasal spray 1 hour before or 1 hour after eating hot foods or drinking hot liquids.

When to take:
- Oral—At the same time each day.
- Injection—Follow doctor's directions.
- Nasal gel or spray—Use weekly or as directed on prescription.

If you forget a dose:
Take when remembered. Don't double next dose. Resume regular schedule.

What drug does:
Acts as enzyme to promote normal fat and carbohydrate metabolism and protein synthesis.

Time lapse before drug works:
15 minutes.

Don't take with:
Any other medicine or any dietary supplement without consulting your doctor or pharmacist.

POSSIBLE ADVERSE REACTIONS OR SIDE EFFECTS

SYMPTOMS	WHAT TO DO
Life-threatening:	
Hives, rash, intense itching, faintness soon after a dose (anaphylaxis).	Seek emergency treatment immediately.
Common:	
None expected.	
Infrequent:	
None expected.	
Rare:	
• Itchy skin, wheezing.	Discontinue. Call doctor right away.
• Diarrhea.	Continue. Call doctor when convenient.

VITAMIN B-12 (Cyanocobalamin)

WARNINGS & PRECAUTIONS

Don't take if:
- You are allergic to any B vitamin.
- You have Leber's disease (optic nerve atrophy).

Before you start, consult your doctor if:
- You have gout.
- You have heart disease.

Over age 60:
Don't take more than recommended amount per day unless prescribed by your doctor.

Pregnancy:
Risk factor determined by length of pregnancy and dosage amount. See category list on page xviii and consult doctor.

Breast-feeding:
Effect unknown. Consult doctor.

Infants & children:
No problems expected.

Prolonged use:
No problems expected.

Skin & sunlight:
No problems expected.

Driving, piloting or hazardous work:
No problems expected.

Discontinuing:
Don't discontinue without doctor's advice until you complete prescribed dose, even though symptoms diminish or disappear.

Others:
- A balanced diet should provide all the vitamin B-12 a healthy person needs and make supplements unnecessary. Best sources are meat, fish, egg yolk and cheese.
- Tablets should be used only for diet supplements. All other uses of vitamin B-12 require injections.
- Don't take large doses of vitamin C (1,000 mg or more per day) unless prescribed by your doctor.

POSSIBLE INTERACTION WITH OTHER DRUGS

GENERIC NAME OR DRUG CLASS	COMBINED EFFECT
Anticonvulsants*	Decreased absorption of vitamin B-12.
Chloramphenicol	Decreased vitamin B-12 effect.
Cholestyramine	Decreased absorption of vitamin B-12.
Cimetidine	Decreased absorption of vitamin B-12.
Colchicine	Decreased absorption of vitamin B-12.
Famotidine	Decreased absorption of vitamin B-12.
H₂ antagonists*	Decreased absorption of vitamin B-12.
Neomycin	Decreased absorption of vitamin B-12.
Para-aminosalicylic acid	Decreased effects of para-aminosalicylic acid.
Potassium (extended-release forms)	Decreased absorption of vitamin B-12.
Ranitidine	Decreased absorption of vitamin B-12.
Vitamin C (ascorbic acid)	Destroys vitamin B-12 if taken at same time. Take 2 hours apart.

POSSIBLE INTERACTION WITH OTHER SUBSTANCES

INTERACTS WITH	COMBINED EFFECT
Alcohol:	Decreased absorption of vitamin B-12.
Beverages:	None expected.
Cocaine:	None expected.
Foods:	None expected.
Marijuana:	None expected.
Tobacco:	None expected.

*See Glossary

VITAMIN C (Ascorbic Acid)

BRAND NAMES

Ascorbicap	Ce-Vi-Sol
Cecon	Cevita
Cemill	C-Span
Cenolate	Flavorcee
Cetane	Redoxon
Cevalin	Sunkist
Cevi-Bid	

Numerous brands of single vitamin and multivitamin combinations are available.

BASIC INFORMATION

Habit forming? No
Prescription needed? No
Available as generic? Yes
Drug class: Vitamin supplement

 ## USES

- Prevention and treatment of scurvy and other vitamin C deficiencies.
- Treatment of anemia.
- Maintenance of acid urine.

 ## DOSAGE & USAGE INFORMATION

How to take:
- Tablet or capsule—Swallow with liquid.
- Extended-release tablet or extended-release capsule—Swallow whole with liquid. Do not crush or chew.
- Chewable tablet—Chew well, then swallow.
- Effervescent tablet—Follow label instructions. Let tablet dissolve in water and drink entire mixture.
- Suspension, solution or drops—Use a dropper or dose-measuring spoon to measure doses.
- Syrup—Follow label instructions. Use a dose-measuring spoon to measure dosage and then swallow.
- Lozenge—Let dissolve completely in mouth.
- Powder or crystal—Measure and mix as directed. Drink all the mixture right away.

Continued next column

 ## OVERDOSE

SYMPTOMS:
Diarrhea, vomiting, dizziness.
WHAT TO DO:
Overdose unlikely to threaten life. If person uses much larger amount than prescribed or if accidentally swallowed, call doctor or poison control center 1-800-222-1222 for help.

When to take:
1, 2 or 3 times per day, as prescribed on label.

If you forget a dose:
Take as soon as you remember, then return to regular schedule.

What drug does:
- May help form collagen.
- Increases iron absorption from intestine.
- Contributes to hemoglobin and red blood cell production in bone marrow.

Time lapse before drug works:
1 week.

Don't take with:
Any other medicine or any dietary supplement without consulting your doctor or pharmacist.

 ## POSSIBLE ADVERSE REACTIONS OR SIDE EFFECTS

SYMPTOMS	WHAT TO DO
Life-threatening: None expected.	
Common: None expected.	
Infrequent:	
• Mild diarrhea, nausea, vomiting.	Discontinue. Call doctor right away.
• Flushed face.	Continue. Call doctor when convenient.
Rare:	
• Kidney stones with high doses, anemia, abdominal pain.	Discontinue. Call doctor right away.
• Headache.	Continue. Tell doctor at next visit.

VITAMIN C (Ascorbic Acid)

WARNINGS & PRECAUTIONS

Don't take if:
You are allergic to vitamin C.

Before you start, consult your doctor if:
- You have sickle-cell or other anemia.
- You have had kidney stones.
- You have gout.

Over age 60:
Don't take more than recommended amount per day unless prescribed by your doctor.

Pregnancy:
Risk factor determined by length of pregnancy and dosage amount. See category list on page xviii and consult doctor.

Breast-feeding:
Avoid large doses. Consult doctor.

Infants & children:
- Avoid large doses. Follow instructions on label.
- Keep vitamin-mineral supplements out of children's reach.

Prolonged use:
Large doses for longer than 2 months may cause kidney stones.

Skin & sunlight:
No problems expected.

Driving, piloting or hazardous work:
No problems expected.

Discontinuing:
No problems expected.

Others:
- Store in cool, dry place.
- May cause inaccurate tests for sugar in urine or blood in stool.
- May cause crisis in patients with sickle-cell anemia.
- A balanced diet should provide all the vitamin C a healthy person needs and make supplements unnecessary. Best sources are citrus, strawberries, cantaloupe and raw peppers.
- Don't take large doses of vitamin C (1,000 mg or more per day) unless prescribed by your doctor.
- Some products contain tartrazine dye. Avoid, if allergic (especially aspirin hypersensitivity).

POSSIBLE INTERACTION WITH OTHER DRUGS

GENERIC NAME OR DRUG CLASS	COMBINED EFFECT
Amphetamines*	Possible decreased amphetamine effect.
Anticholinergics*	Possible decreased anticholinergic effect.
Anticoagulants,* oral	Possible decreased anticoagulant effect.
Antidepressants, tricyclic (TCA)*	Possible decreased antidepressant effect.
Aspirin	Decreased vitamin C effect and salicylate excretion.
Barbiturates*	Decreased vitamin C effect. Increased barbiturate effect.
Cellulose sodium phosphate	Decreased vitamin C effect.
Contraceptives, oral*	Decreased vitamin C effect.
Estrogens*	Increased likelihood of adverse effects from estrogen with 1 g or more of vitamin C per day.
Iron supplements*	Increased iron absorption.
Mexiletine	Possible decreased effectiveness of mexiletine.
Quinidine	Possible decreased quinidine effect.
Salicylates*	Decreased vitamin C effect and salicylate excretion. May lead to salicylate toxicity.
Tranquilizers* (phenothiazine)	May decrease phenothiazine effect if no vitamin C deficiency exists.

POSSIBLE INTERACTION WITH OTHER SUBSTANCES

INTERACTS WITH	COMBINED EFFECT
Alcohol:	None expected.
Beverages:	None expected.
Cocaine:	None expected.
Foods:	None expected.
Marijuana:	None expected.
Tobacco:	Increased requirement for vitamin C.

*See Glossary

VITAMIN D

GENERIC AND BRAND NAMES

ALFACALCIDOL
One-Alpha
CALCIFEDIOL
Calderol
CALCITRIOL
Rocaltrol
CHOLECALCIFEROL
Fosamax Plus D
Fosavance

(Many other name
brands are available)

**DIHYDROTACHY
STEROL**
DHT
DHT Intensol
Hytakerol
DOXERCALCIFEROL
Hectorol
ERGOCALCIFEROL
Calciferol
Drisdol
Osto Forte
Radiostol
Radiostol Forte

BASIC INFORMATION

Habit forming? No
Prescription needed? Only for high strength
Available as generic? Yes
Drug class: Vitamin supplement

USES

- Dietary supplement.
- Prevention of rickets (bone disease).
- Treatment for hypocalcemia (low blood calcium) in kidney disease.
- Supplement in those who use sunscreen daily.

DOSAGE & USAGE INFORMATION

How to take:
- Tablet or capsule—Swallow with liquid.
- Extended-release tablet or extended-release capsule—Swallow whole with liquid. Do not crush or chew.
- Chewable tablet—Chew well, then swallow.
- Effervescent tablet—Follow label instructions. Dissolve tablet in water. Drink entire mixture.

Continued next column

OVERDOSE

SYMPTOMS:
Severe stomach pain, nausea, vomiting, weight loss; bone and muscle pain; increased urination, cloudy urine; mood or mental changes (possible psychosis); high blood pressure, irregular heartbeat; eye irritation or light sensitivity; itchy skin.
WHAT TO DO:
Overdose unlikely to threaten life. If person uses much larger amount than prescribed or if accidentally swallowed, call doctor or poison control center 1-800-222-1222 for help.

- Suspension, solution or drops—Use a dropper or dose-measuring spoon to measure doses.
- Syrup—Follow label instructions. Use a dose-measuring spoon to measure dosage and then swallow.
- Lozenge—Let dissolve completely in mouth.
- Powder or crystal—Measure and mix as directed. Drink all the mixture right away.

When to take:
As directed, usually once a day at the same time each day. Some are taken once a week/month.

If you forget a dose:
Take up to 12 hours late. If more than 12 hours, wait for next dose (don't double this dose).

What drug does:
- Maintains growth and health.
- Prevents rickets.
- Essential so body can use calcium and phosphate.

Time lapse before drug works:
2 hours. May require 2 to 3 weeks of continual use for maximum effect.

Don't take with:
Any other medicine or any dietary supplement without consulting your doctor or pharmacist.

POSSIBLE ADVERSE REACTIONS OR SIDE EFFECTS

SYMPTOMS	WHAT TO DO
Life-threatening:	
In case of overdose, see previous column.	
Common:	
None expected.	
Infrequent:	
Headache, metallic taste in mouth, thirst, dry mouth, constipation, appetite loss, nausea, vomiting, weakness, cloudy urine, sensitivity to light.	Continue. Call doctor when convenient.
Rare:	
• Increased urination, pink eye, psychosis, severe abdominal pain, fever.	Discontinue. Call doctor right away.
• Muscle pain, bone pain, diarrhea.	Continue. Tell doctor when convenient.

WARNINGS & PRECAUTIONS

Don't take if:
You are allergic to medicine containing vitamin D.

Before you start, consult your doctor if:
- You plan to become pregnant while taking vitamin D.
- You have epilepsy.
- You have heart or blood-vessel disease.
- You have kidney disease.

Over age 60:
Adverse reactions and side effects may be more frequent and severe than in younger persons.

Pregnancy:
Risk factor determined by length of pregnancy and dosage amount. See category list on page xviii and consult doctor.

Breast-feeding:
No problems expected, but consult doctor.

Infants & children:
- Avoid large doses.
- Keep vitamins out of children's reach.

Prolonged use:
- No problems expected.
- Talk to your doctor about the need for follow-up medical examinations or laboratory studies to check kidney function, liver function, serum calcium.

Skin & sunlight:
No special problems expected.

Driving, piloting or hazardous work:
No problems expected.

Discontinuing:
Don't discontinue without doctor's advice until you complete prescribed dose, even though symptoms diminish or disappear.

Others:
- Don't exceed dose. Too much over a long time may be harmful.
- A balanced diet should provide all the vitamin D a healthy person needs and make supplements unnecessary. Best sources are fish and vitamin D-fortified milk and bread.
- Some products contain tartrazine dye. Avoid, if allergic (especially aspirin hypersensitivity).
- Sunscreen prevents the body from manufacturing vitamin D from sunshine. Consider supplementary vitamin D if you use sunscreen daily. Ask doctor for advice.

 ## POSSIBLE INTERACTION WITH OTHER DRUGS

GENERIC NAME OR DRUG CLASS	COMBINED EFFECT
Antacids* (magnesium-containing)	Possible excess magnesium.
Anticonvulsants, hydantoin*	Decreased vitamin D effect.
Calcium (high doses)	Excess calcium in blood.
Calcium channel blockers*	Possible decreased effect of calcium channel blockers.
Calcium supplements*	Excessive absorption of vitamin D.
Cholestyramine	Decreased vitamin D effect.
Colestipol	Decreased vitamin D absorption.
Cortisone	Decreased vitamin D effect.
Digitalis preparations*	Heartbeat irregularities.
Diuretics, thiazide*	Possible increased calcium.
Mineral oil	Decreased vitamin D effect.
Neomycin	Decreased vitamin D absorption.
Nicardipine	Decreased nicardipine effect.
Phenobarbital	Decreased vitamin D effect.
Phosphorus preparations*	Accumulation of excess phosphorus.
Rifampin	Possible decreased vitamin D effect.
Vitamin D, other	Possible toxicity.

 ## POSSIBLE INTERACTION WITH OTHER SUBSTANCES

INTERACTS WITH	COMBINED EFFECT
Alcohol:	None expected.
Beverages:	None expected.
Cocaine:	None expected.
Foods:	None expected.
Marijuana:	None expected.
Tobacco:	None expected.

*See Glossary

VITAMIN D (Topical)

GENERIC AND BRAND NAMES

CALCIPOTRIENE
Dovonex
Taclonex

CALCITRIOL
(topical)
Vectical

BASIC INFORMATION

Habit forming? No
Prescription needed? Yes
Available as generic? Yes, for some
Drug class: Antipsoriatic

 ## USES

Treats discoid or "plaque" psoriasis, the most common form of the disorder.

 ## DOSAGE & USAGE INFORMATION

How to use:
Cream, ointment or topical solution—Apply a thin layer to the affected skin or scalp as per instructions. Rub in gently and completely. Avoid your face and eyes. Wash hands after use.

When to use:
Twice a day or as advised by your doctor.

If you forget a dose:
Apply as soon as you remember, then return to regular schedule.

What drug does:
It helps slow the growth of abnormal skin cells.

Time lapse before drug works:
2 weeks. May take up to 8 weeks for maximum benefits that can include marked improvement in symptoms for most patients or complete clearing for others.

Don't use with:
Other topical or oral drugs without consulting with your doctor or pharmacist.

 ## OVERDOSE

SYMPTOMS:
May be absorbed into the body through excess topical application and increase the levels of calcium and cause nausea, vomiting, loss of appetite, increased thirst and urination, unusual tiredness or weakness.
WHAT TO DO:
Overdose unlikely to threaten life. If person uses much larger amount than prescribed or if accidentally swallowed, call doctor or poison control center 1-800-222-1222 for help.

 ## POSSIBLE ADVERSE REACTIONS OR SIDE EFFECTS

SYMPTOMS	WHAT TO DO
Life-threatening: None expected.	
Common: Irritation, burning, itching of the skin.	Discontinue. Call doctor when convenient.
Infrequent: Redness, dryness, peeling, rash, worsening of psoriasis.	Discontinue. Call doctor when convenient.
Rare: Darkening of treated areas of skin, pus in hair follicles: very rare symptoms may occur if drug absorbed into body (nausea, vomiting, loss of appetite, increased thirst and urination, unusual tiredness or weakness).	Discontinue. Call doctor when convenient.

WARNINGS & PRECAUTIONS

Don't use if:
- You are allergic to topical vitamin D.
- You have hypercalcemia (excess of calcium in the body).

Before you start, consult your doctor if:
- You have had allergic reaction to other topical drugs, oral drugs, food or other substances.
- You are taking calcium supplements, oral vitamin D or thiazide diuretics.

Over age 60:
Adverse reactions and side effects may be more frequent and severe than in younger persons.

Pregnancy:
Decide with your doctor if drug benefits justify any possible risk to unborn child. Risk category C (see page xviii).

Breast-feeding:
It is unknown if drugs pass into milk. Avoid drug or discontinue nursing until you finish medicine. Consult doctor for advice on maintaining milk supply.

Infants & children:
Approved for use in age 18 and older. Safety in children has not been established. Use only under close medical supervision. Adverse reactions and side effects may be more frequent and severe.

Prolonged use:
Talk to your doctor about the need for follow-up laboratory studies to check calcium levels in your blood or urine.

Skin & sunlight:
Your skin may be more sensitive to sunlight when using this drug. Sunlight exposure (even brief periods) may cause a skin rash, itching, redness, other skin discoloration or a severe sunburn. When you begin using this drug, try to stay out of direct sunlight, especially between the hours of 10:00 a.m. and 3:00 p.m. Apply a sunblock product that has a skin protection factor (SPF). Wear protective clothing, including a hat and sunglasses. Do not use a sun lamp or tanning bed or booth. Consult your doctor if you have any concerns.

Driving, piloting or hazardous work:
No special problems expected.

Discontinuing:
No special problems expected.

Others:
- Wash hands after applying the drug.
- Advise any doctor or dentist whom you consult that you use this medicine.
- One or more of these products is flammable. Read label. Do not use near an open flame.

POSSIBLE INTERACTION WITH OTHER DRUGS

GENERIC NAME OR DRUG CLASS	COMBINED EFFECT
Calcium supplements	Increased calcium in the blood.
Diuretics, thiazide	Increased calcium in the blood.
Vitamin D (oral)	Increased calcium in the blood.

POSSIBLE INTERACTION WITH OTHER SUBSTANCES

INTERACTS WITH	COMBINED EFFECT
Alcohol:	None expected.
Beverages:	None expected.
Cocaine:	None expected.
Foods:	None expected.
Marijuana:	None expected.
Tobacco:	None expected.

VITAMIN E

BRAND NAMES

Aquasol E   Epsilan-M
Chew-E   Pheryl-E
Eprolin   Viterra E

Numerous brands of single vitamin and multivitamin combinations are available.

BASIC INFORMATION

Habit forming? No
Prescription needed? No
Available as generic? Yes
Drug class: Vitamin supplement

 ## USES

- Dietary supplement to promote normal growth, development and health.
- Treatment and prevention of vitamin E deficiency, especially in premature or low-birth-weight infants.
- Treatment for fibrocystic disease of the breast.
- Treatment for circulatory problems to the lower extremities.
- Treatment for sickle-cell anemia.
- Treatment for lung toxicity from air pollution.

 ## DOSAGE & USAGE INFORMATION

How to take:
- Tablet or capsule—Swallow with liquid.
- Extended-release tablet or extended-release capsule—Swallow whole with liquid. Do not crush or chew.
- Chewable tablet—Chew well, then swallow.
- Effervescent tablet—Follow label instructions. Let tablet dissolve in water and drink entire mixture.
- Suspension, solution or drops—Use a dropper or dose-measuring spoon to measure doses.
- Syrup—Follow label instructions. Use a dose-measuring spoon to measure dosage and then swallow.
- Lozenge—Let dissolve completely in mouth.
- Powder or crystal—Measure and mix as directed. Drink all the mixture right away.

Continued next column

 ## OVERDOSE

SYMPTOMS:
Nausea, vomiting, fatigue.
WHAT TO DO:
Overdose unlikely to threaten life. If person uses much larger amount than prescribed or if accidentally swallowed, call doctor or poison control center 1-800-222-1222 for help.

When to take:
At the same times each day.

If you forget a dose:
Take when you remember. Don't double next dose.

What drug does:
- Promotes normal growth and development.
- Prevents oxidation in body.

Time lapse before drug works:
Will vary depending on the disorder being treated.

Don't take with:
Any other medicine or any dietary supplement without consulting your doctor or pharmacist.

 ## POSSIBLE ADVERSE REACTIONS OR SIDE EFFECTS

SYMPTOMS	WHAT TO DO
Life-threatening: None expected.	
Common: Breast enlargement, dizziness, headache.	Continue. Call doctor when convenient.
Infrequent: Nausea, abdominal pain, muscle aches, pain in lower legs, fever, tiredness, weakness.	Continue. Call doctor when convenient.
Rare: Blurred vision, diarrhea.	Discontinue. Call doctor right away.

WARNINGS & PRECAUTIONS

Don't take if:
You are allergic to vitamin E.

Before you start, consult your doctor if:
- You have had blood clots in leg veins (thrombophlebitis).
- You have liver disease.

Over age 60:
No problems expected. Avoid excessive doses.

Pregnancy:
No problems expected with normal daily requirements. Don't exceed prescribed dose. Consult doctor.

Breast-feeding:
No problems expected. Consult doctor.

Infants & children:
Use only under medical supervision.

Prolonged use:
Toxic accumulation of vitamin E. Don't exceed recommended dose.

Skin & sunlight:
No problems expected.

Driving, piloting or hazardous work:
No problems expected.

Discontinuing:
No problems expected.

Others:
A balanced diet should provide all the vitamin E a healthy person needs and make supplements unnecessary. Best sources are vegetable oils, whole-grain cereals, liver.

POSSIBLE INTERACTION WITH OTHER DRUGS

GENERIC NAME OR DRUG CLASS	COMBINED EFFECT
Anticoagulants,* oral	Increased anticoagulant effect.
Cholestyramine	Decreased vitamin E absorption.
Colestipol	Decreased vitamin E absorption.
Iron supplements*	Possible decreased effect of iron supplement in patients with iron-deficiency anemia. Decreased vitamin E effect in healthy persons.
Mineral oil	Decreased vitamin E effect.
Neomycin	Decreased vitamin E absorption.
Vitamin A	Recommended dose of vitamin E— Increased benefit and decreased toxicity of vitamin A. Excess dose of vitamin E—Vitamin A depletion.

POSSIBLE INTERACTION WITH OTHER SUBSTANCES

INTERACTS WITH	COMBINED EFFECT
Alcohol:	None expected.
Beverages:	None expected.
Cocaine:	None expected.
Foods:	None expected.
Marijuana:	None expected.
Tobacco:	None expected.

*See Glossary

VITAMIN K

GENERIC AND BRAND NAMES

MENADIOL
Synkayvite

PHYTONADIONE
Mephyton

Numerous brands of single vitamin and multivitamin combinations may be available.

BASIC INFORMATION

Habit forming? No
Prescription needed? No
Available as generic? Yes
Drug class: Vitamin supplement

 USES

- Dietary supplement.
- Treatment for bleeding disorders and malabsorption diseases due to vitamin K deficiency.
- Treatment for hemorrhagic disease of the newborn.
- Treatment for bleeding due to overdose of oral anticoagulants.

 DOSAGE & USAGE INFORMATION

How to take:
- May be given by injection in hospital or doctor's office.
- Tablet or capsule—Swallow with liquid.
- Extended-release tablet or extended-release capsule—Swallow whole with liquid. Do not crush or chew.
- Chewable tablet—Chew well, then swallow.
- Effervescent tablet—Follow label instructions. Let tablet dissolve in water and drink entire mixture.
- Suspension, solution or drops—Use a dropper or dose-measuring spoon to measure doses.
- Syrup—Follow label instructions. Use a dose-measuring spoon to measure dosage and then swallow.
- Lozenge—Let dissolve completely in mouth.
- Powder or crystal—Measure and mix as directed. Drink all the mixture right away.

Continued next column

 OVERDOSE

SYMPTOMS:
Nausea, vomiting.
WHAT TO DO:
Overdose unlikely to threaten life. If person uses much larger amount than prescribed or if accidentally swallowed, call doctor or poison control center 1-800-222-1222 for help.

When to take:
At the same time each day.

If you forget a dose:
Take as soon as you remember up to 12 hours late. If more than 12 hours, wait for next scheduled dose (don't double this dose).

What drug does:
- Promotes growth, development and good health.
- Supplies a necessary ingredient for blood clotting.

Time lapse before drug works:
15 to 30 minutes to support blood clotting. For some problems, it may take weeks or months.

Don't take with:
Any other medicine or any dietary supplement without consulting your doctor or pharmacist.

 POSSIBLE ADVERSE REACTIONS OR SIDE EFFECTS

SYMPTOMS	WHAT TO DO
Life-threatening: None expected.	
Common: None expected.	
Infrequent: Unusual taste, face flushing.	Continue. Call doctor when convenient.
Rare: Rash, hives.	Discontinue. Call doctor right away.

WARNINGS & PRECAUTIONS

Don't take if:
- You are allergic to vitamin K.
- You have G6PD* deficiency.
- You have liver disease.

Before you start, consult your doctor if:
You are pregnant.

Over age 60:
No problems expected.

Pregnancy:
Risk factor determined by length of pregnancy and dosage amount. See category list on page xviii and consult doctor.

Breast-feeding:
No problems expected. Consult doctor.

Infants & children:
Phytonadione is the preferred form for hemorrhagic disease of the newborn.

Prolonged use:
Talk to your doctor about the need for follow-up medical examinations or laboratory studies to check prothrombin time.

Skin & sunlight:
No problems expected.

Driving, piloting or hazardous work:
No problems expected.

Discontinuing:
No problems expected.

Others:
- Tell all doctors and dentists you consult that you take this medicine.
- Don't exceed dose. Too much over a long time may be harmful.
- A balanced diet should provide all the vitamin K a healthy person needs and make supplements unnecessary. Best sources are green, leafy vegetables, meat or dairy products.

POSSIBLE INTERACTION WITH OTHER DRUGS

GENERIC NAME OR DRUG CLASS	COMBINED EFFECT
Anticoagulants,* oral	Decreased anticoagulant effect.
Cholestyramine	Decreased vitamin K effect.
Colestipol	Decreased vitamin K absorption.
Dapsone	Increased risk of adverse effect on blood cells.
Mineral oil (long-term)	Vitamin K deficiency.
Neomycin	Decreased vitamin K absorption.
Sulfa drugs*	Vitamin K deficiency.

POSSIBLE INTERACTION WITH OTHER SUBSTANCES

INTERACTS WITH	COMBINED EFFECT
Alcohol:	None expected.
Beverages:	None expected.
Cocaine:	None expected.
Foods:	None expected.
Marijuana:	None expected.
Tobacco:	None expected.

*See Glossary

VITAMINS & FLUORIDE

GENERIC AND BRAND NAMES

Adeflor
Cari-Tab
Mulvidren-F
Poly-Vi-Flor

Tri-Vi-Flor
Vi-Daylin/F
Vi-Penta F

Also brands are available in the forms of multiple vitamins & fluoride; vitamins A, D & C & fluoride.

BASIC INFORMATION

Habit forming? No
Prescription needed? Yes
Available as generic? No
Drug class: Vitamins, minerals

 USES

- Reduces incidence of tooth cavities (fluoride). Children who need supplements should take until age 16.
- Prevents deficiencies of vitamin included in formula (some contain multiple vitamins whose content varies among products; others contain only vitamins A, D and C).

 DOSAGE & USAGE INFORMATION

How to take:
- Chewable tablet—Chew or crush before swallowing.
- Oral liquid—Measure with specially marked dropper. May mix with food, fruit juice, cereal.

When to take:
- Bedtime or with or just after meals.
- If at bedtime, brush teeth first.

If you forget a dose:
Take as soon as you remember up to 2 hours late. If more than 2 hours, wait for next scheduled dose (don't double this dose).

Continued next column

 OVERDOSE

SYMPTOMS:
Minor overdose—Black, brown or white spots on teeth.
Massive overdose—Shallow breathing, black or tarry stools, bloody vomit.
WHAT TO DO:
- **Dial 911 (emergency) for medical help or call poison control center 1-800-222-1222 for instructions.**
- **See emergency information on last 3 pages of this book.**

What drug does:
Provides supplemental fluoride to combat tooth decay.

Time lapse before drug works:
8 weeks to provide maximum benefit.

Don't take with:
- Other medicine at the same time.
- Any other medicine or any dietary supplement without consulting your doctor or pharmacist.

 POSSIBLE ADVERSE REACTIONS OR SIDE EFFECTS

SYMPTOMS	WHAT TO DO
Life-threatening: Fainting, bloody vomit, bloody or black stool, breathing difficulty.	Discontinue. Seek emergency treatment.
Common: White, black or brown spots on teeth; nausea; vomiting.	Discontinue. Call doctor right away.
Infrequent: • Drowsiness; abdominal pain; increased salivation; watery eyes; weight loss; sore throat, fever, mouth sores; constipation; bone pain; rash; muscle stiffness; weakness; tremor; agitation.	Discontinue. Call doctor right away.
• Diarrhea.	Continue. Call doctor when convenient.
Rare: None expected.	

850

WARNINGS & PRECAUTIONS

Don't take if:
* Your water supply contains 0.7 parts fluoride per million. Too much fluoride stains teeth permanently.
* You are allergic to any fluoride-containing product.
* You have underactive thyroid.

Before you start, consult your doctor or dentist:
For proper dosage.

Over age 60:
No problems expected.

Pregnancy:
Risk factor determined by length of pregnancy and dosage amount. See category list on page xviii and consult doctor.

Breast-feeding:
No problems expected. Consult doctor.

Infants & children:
No problems expected in children over 3 years of age except in case of accidental overdose. Keep vitamin-mineral supplements out of children's reach.

Prolonged use:
Excess may cause discolored teeth and decreased calcium in blood.

Skin & sunlight:
No problems expected.

Driving, piloting or hazardous work:
No problems expected.

Discontinuing:
No problems expected.

Others:
* Store in original plastic container. Fluoride decomposes glass.
* Check with dentist once or twice a year to keep cavities at a minimum. Topical applications of fluoride may also be helpful.
* Fluoride probably not necessary if water contains about 1 part per million of fluoride or more. Check with health department.
* Don't freeze.
* Don't keep outdated medicine.

POSSIBLE INTERACTION WITH OTHER DRUGS

GENERIC NAME OR DRUG CLASS	COMBINED EFFECT
Anticoagulants*	Decreased effect of anticoagulant.
Iron supplements*	Decreased effect of any vitamin if iron is present in multivitamin product.
Vitamin A	May lead to vitamin A toxicity if vitamin A is in combination.
Vitamin D	May lead to vitamin D toxicity if vitamin D is in combination.

POSSIBLE INTERACTION WITH OTHER SUBSTANCES

INTERACTS WITH	COMBINED EFFECT
Alcohol:	None expected.
Beverages: Milk.	Prevents absorption of fluoride. Space dose 2 hours before or after milk.
Cocaine:	None expected.
Foods:	None expected.
Marijuana:	None expected.
Tobacco:	None expected.

XYLOMETAZOLINE

BRAND NAMES

Chlorohist-LA
Inspire
Neo-Synephrine II
  Long Acting Nasal
  Spray Adult Strength
Neo-Synephrine II
  Long Acting Nose
  Drops Adult Strength
Otrivin Decongestant
  Nose Drops

Otrivin Nasal Drops
Otrivin Nasal Spray
Otrivin Pediatric
  Decongestant
  Nose Drops
Otrivin Pediatric
  Nasal Drops
Otrivin Pediatric
  Nasal Spray
Otrivin with M-D
  Pump
Triaminic Deconges
  tant Spray Nasal &
  Sinus Congestion

BASIC INFORMATION

Habit forming? No
Prescription needed? No
Available as generic? Yes
Drug class: Sympathomimetic

 USES

Relieves congestion of nose, sinuses and throat from allergies and infections.

 DOSAGE & USAGE INFORMATION

How to take:
Nasal solution, nasal spray—Use as directed on label. Avoid contamination. Don't use same container for more than 1 person.

Continued next column

 OVERDOSE

SYMPTOMS:
Headache, sweating, anxiety, agitation, rapid and irregular heartbeat (rare occurrence with systemic absorption).
WHAT TO DO:
• Dial 911 (emergency) for medical help or call poison control center 1-800-222-1222 for instructions.
• If person is unconscious, check breathing and pulse. If not breathing, begin mouth-to-mouth rescue breathing. If heart is not beating, begin chest compressions.
• See emergency information on last 3 pages of this book.

When to take:
When needed, no more often than every 4 hours.

If you forget a dose:
Take as soon as you remember. Wait 4 hours for next dose.

What drug does:
Constricts walls of small arteries in nose, sinuses and eustachian tubes.

Time lapse before drug works:
5 to 30 minutes.

Don't take with:
• Nonprescription drugs for allergy, cough or cold without consulting doctor.
• Any other medicine or any dietary supplement without consulting your doctor or pharmacist.

 POSSIBLE ADVERSE REACTIONS OR SIDE EFFECTS

SYMPTOMS	WHAT TO DO
Life-threatening:	
In case of overdose, see previous column.	
Common:	
None expected.	
Infrequent:	
Burning, dry or stinging nasal passages.	Continue. Call doctor when convenient.
Rare:	
Rebound congestion (increased runny or stuffy nose), headache, insomnia, nervousness (may occur with systemic absorption).	Discontinue. Call doctor when convenient.

WARNINGS & PRECAUTIONS

Don't take if:
You are allergic to any sympathomimetic nasal spray.

Before you start, consult your doctor if:
- You have heart disease or high blood pressure.
- You have diabetes.
- You have overactive thyroid.
- You have taken a monoamine oxidase (MAO) inhibitor* in past 2 weeks.
- You have glaucoma.

Over age 60:
Adverse reactions and side effects may be more frequent and severe than in younger persons.

Pregnancy:
Decide with your doctor if drug benefits justify risk to unborn child. Risk category C (see page xviii).

Breast-feeding:
No proven problems. Consult doctor.

Infants & children:
Don't give to children younger than 2.

Prolonged use:
Drug may lose effectiveness, cause increased congestion (rebound effect*) and irritate nasal membranes.

Skin & sunlight:
No problems expected.

Driving, piloting or hazardous work:
No problems expected.

Discontinuing:
May be unnecessary to finish medicine. Follow doctor's instructions.

Others:
No problems expected.

POSSIBLE INTERACTION WITH OTHER DRUGS

GENERIC NAME OR DRUG CLASS	COMBINED EFFECT
Antidepressants, tricyclic*	Possible increased blood pressure.
Maprotiline	Possible increased blood pressure.
Monoamine oxidase (MAO) inhibitors*	Possible increased blood pressure.

POSSIBLE INTERACTION WITH OTHER SUBSTANCES

INTERACTS WITH	COMBINED EFFECT
Alcohol:	None expected.
Beverages: Caffeine drinks.	Nervousness or insomnia.
Cocaine:	High risk of heartbeat irregularities and high blood pressure.
Foods:	None expected.
Marijuana:	Overstimulation. Avoid.
Tobacco:	None expected.

ZALEPLON

BRAND NAMES

Sonata

BASIC INFORMATION

Habit forming? Yes
Prescription needed? Yes
Available as generic? Yes
Drug class: Anti-insomnia, hypnotic,
  sedative

 USES

Short-term treatment for insomnia (trouble sleeping).

 DOSAGE & USAGE INFORMATION

How to take:
Capsule—Swallow with liquid. If you can't swallow whole, open capsule and take with liquid or food.

When to take:
Take immediately before bedtime. Ensure that you can get at least 4 hours of rest after taking your medication. Zaleplon may be taken with or without food; however, if taken after a heavy or fatty meal, it may not work as fast as it should.

If you forget a dose:
Skip the missed dose and return to your regular dosing schedule. Do not double dose.

What drug does:
Acts as a central nervous system depressant, decreasing sleep problems such as trouble falling asleep, waking up too often during the night and waking up too early in the morning.

Continued next column

 OVERDOSE

SYMPTOMS:
Clumsiness, unsteadiness, stupor, severe dizziness or fainting, troubled breathing and sluggishness.
WHAT TO DO:
* **Dial 911 (emergency) for medical help or call poison control center 1-800-222-1222 for instructions.**
* **If person is unconscious, check breathing and pulse. If not breathing, begin mouth-to-mouth rescue breathing. If heart is not beating, begin chest compressions.**
* **See emergency information on last 3 pages of this book.**

Time lapse before drug works:
Within 2 hours.

Don't take with:
Any other medicine or any dietary supplement without consulting your doctor or pharmacist.

 POSSIBLE ADVERSE REACTIONS OR SIDE EFFECTS

SYMPTOMS	WHAT TO DO
Life-threatening: Rare allergic reaction (hives, itching, rash, wheezing, tightness in chest, swelling of lips or tongue or throat).	Seek emergency treatment immediately.
Common: Dizziness, headache, muscle pain, nausea.	Continue. Call doctor when convenient.
Infrequent: • Anxiety, vision problems, not feeling like oneself.	Discontinue. Call doctor right away.
• Abdominal pain, burning or prickling or tingling, constipation, cough, dry mouth, eye pain, fever, indigestion, arthritis, amnesia, skin rash, menstrual pain, nervousness, sensitive hearing, tightness in chest, trembling or shaking, unusual weakness, depression or tiredness, wheezing.	Continue. Call doctor if symptoms persist.
Rare: • Nosebleed, hallucinations, sleep-induced behaviors.*	Discontinue. Call doctor right away.
• Loss of appetite, back pain, chest pain, ear pain, general feeling of discomfort, sense of smell difficulty, swelling, rapid weight gain, sensitivity of skin and eyes to sunlight, redness, burning, sunburn.	Continue. Call doctor if symptoms persist.

WARNINGS & PRECAUTIONS

Don't take if:
You have had an allergic reaction to zaleplon.

Before you start, consult your doctor if:
- You have a history of alcohol or drug abuse.
- You have impaired kidney or liver function.
- You are pregnant or nursing.
- You have been diagnosed with clinical depression.

Over age 60:
Adverse reactions and side effects may be more frequent and severe than in younger persons.

Pregnancy:
Decide with your doctor whether drug benefits justify risk to unborn child. Risk category C (see page xviii).

Breast-feeding:
Drug passes into milk. Avoid drug or discontinue nursing until you finish medicine. Consult doctor for advice on maintaining milk supply.

Infants & children:
Not recommended.

Prolonged use:
Not intended for long term use.

Skin & sunlight:
No problems expected.

Driving, piloting or hazardous work:
Don't drive or pilot aircraft, work around dangerous machinery, climb ladders or work in high places for at least 4 hours after taking this medication. Danger increases if you drink alcohol or take medicine affecting alertness and reflexes, such as antihistamines, tranquilizers, sedatives, pain medicine, narcotics and mind-altering drugs.

Discontinuing:
Dose may require gradual reduction. If drug has been taken for a long time, consult doctor before discontinuing. You may have trouble sleeping for the first few nights after you stop taking zaleplon.

Others:
Advise any doctor or dentist whom you consult that you take this medicine.

POSSIBLE INTERACTION WITH OTHER DRUGS

GENERIC NAME OR DRUG CLASS	COMBINED EFFECT
Antidepressants, tricyclic*	Increased effect of either drug. Avoid.
Central nervous system (CNS) depressants*	May increase effect of depressant.
Enzyme inducers*	Decreased zaleplon effect.
Enzyme inhibitors*	Increased zaleplon effect.

POSSIBLE INTERACTION WITH OTHER SUBSTANCES

INTERACTS WITH	COMBINED EFFECT
Alcohol:	Increased sedation. Avoid.
Beverages:	None expected.
Cocaine:	None expected.
Foods:	None expected.
Marijuana:	Increased sedation. Avoid.
Tobacco:	None expected.

ZINC SUPPLEMENTS

GENERIC AND BRAND NAMES

ZINC ACETATE
 Galzin
ZINC GLUCONATE
 Orazinc

ZINC SULFATE
 Egozinc
 PMS Egozinc
 Verazinc
 Zinc-220
 Zincate

Many other multivitamins/mineral products.

BASIC INFORMATION

Habit forming? No
Prescription needed? No
Available as generic? Yes
Drug class: Nutritional supplement (mineral)

USES

- Treats zinc deficiency that may lead to growth retardation, appetite loss, changes in taste or smell, skin eruptions, slow wound healing, decreased immune function, diarrhea or impaired night vision.
- In absence of a deficiency, is used to treat burns, eating disorders, liver disorders, prematurity in infants, intestinal diseases, parasitism, kidney disorders, skin disorders and stress.
- May be useful as a supplement for those who are breast-feeding or pregnant (under a doctor's supervision).
- Zinc acetate is used for treatment of Wilson's disease.

DOSAGE INFORMATION

How to take:
Tablet or capsule—Swallow with liquid. If you can't swallow whole, crumble tablet or open capsule and take with liquid or food.

When to take:
At the same time each day, according to a doctor's instructions or the package label.

Continued next column

OVERDOSE

SYMPTOMS:
Dizziness, yellow eyes and skin, shortness of breath, chest pain, vomiting.
WHAT TO DO:
- **Have patient drink lots of water.**
- **Dial 911 (emergency) for medical help or call poison control center 1-800-222-1222 for instructions.**

If you forget a dose:
Take as soon as you remember up to 2 hours late. If more than 2 hours, wait for next scheduled dose (don't double this dose).

What drug does:
Required by the body for the utilization of many enzymes, nucleic acids and proteins and for cell growth.

Time lapse before drug works:
2 hours.

Don't take with:
Any other medicine or any dietary supplement without consulting your doctor or pharmacist.

POSSIBLE ADVERSE REACTIONS OR SIDE EFFECTS

SYMPTOMS	WHAT TO DO
Life-threatening: None expected.	
Common: None expected.	
Infrequent: None expected.	
Rare:	
• Indigestion, heartburn, nausea and vomiting (only with large doses).	Continue. Call doctor when convenient.
• Fever, chills, sore throat, ulcers in throat or mouth, unusual tiredness or weakness (only with large doses).	Discontinue. Call doctor right away.

WARNINGS & PRECAUTIONS

Don't take if:
You are allergic to zinc.

Before you start, consult your doctor if:
You are pregnant or breast-feeding.

Over age 60:
No special problems expected. Nutritional supplements may be helpful if the diet is restricted in any way.

Pregnancy:
Adequate zinc intake is important. Risk factor not designated. See category list on page xviii and consult doctor.

Breast-feeding:
Adequate zinc intake important. Consult a doctor.

Infants & children:
Normal daily requirements vary with age. Consult a doctor.

Prolonged use:
No special problems expected.

Skin & sunlight:
No special problems expected.

Driving, piloting or hazardous work:
No special problems expected.

Discontinuing:
No special problems expected.

Others:
The best natural sources of zinc are red meats, oysters, herring, peas and beans.

POSSIBLE INTERACTION WITH OTHER DRUGS

GENERIC NAME OR DRUG CLASS	COMBINED EFFECT
Copper supplements	Inhibited absorption of copper.
Diuretics, thiazide*	Increased need for zinc.
Folic acid	Increased need for zinc.
Iron supplements*	Increased need for zinc.
Tetracyclines*	Decreased absorption of tetracycline if taken within 2 hours of each other.

POSSIBLE INTERACTION WITH OTHER SUBSTANCES

INTERACTS WITH	COMBINED EFFECT
Alcohol:	May increase need for zinc.
Beverages:	None expected.
Cocaine:	None expected.
Foods: High-fiber.	May decrease zinc absorption.
Marijuana:	None expected.
Tobacco:	May increase need for zinc.

*See Glossary

ZIPRASIDONE

BRAND NAMES

Geodon

BASIC INFORMATION

Habit forming? No
Prescription needed? Yes
Available as generic? No
Drug class: Antipsychotic

 ## USES

* Treatment for schizophrenia.
* Treatment for acute bipolar mania.

 ## DOSAGE & USAGE INFORMATION

How to take:
Capsule—Swallow with liquid. Should be taken with food. Do not chew capsule.

When to take:
At the same times each day. The prescribed dosage may gradually be increased over the first few days or weeks of use.

If you forget a dose:
Take as soon as you remember. If it is almost time for the next dose, wait for the next scheduled dose (don't double this dose).

What drug does:
The exact mechanism is unknown. It appears to block certain nerve impulses between nerve cells.

Time lapse before drug works:
One to 7 days. A further increase in the dosage amount may be necessary to relieve symptoms for some patients.

Don't take with:
Any other medicine or any dietary supplement without consulting your doctor or pharmacist.

 ## OVERDOSE

SYMPTOMS:
Extreme drowsiness, sleepiness, slurring of speech, high blood pressure.
WHAT TO DO:
* **If symptoms appear serious or severe, dial 911 (emergency) for medical help or call poison control center 1-800-222-1222 for instructions.**
* **See emergency information on last 3 pages of this book.**

 ## POSSIBLE ADVERSE REACTIONS OR SIDE EFFECTS

SYMPTOMS	WHAT TO DO
Life-threatening:	
Rare allergic reaction (hives, itching, rash, wheezing, tightness in chest, swelling of lips or tongue or throat).	Seek emergency treatment immediately.
Common:	
Constipation or diarrhea, indigestion or heartburn, weight gain, rash, belching, stomach pain, nausea, drowsiness, dizziness, restlessness, feeling weak or a loss of strength, lack of muscle and balance control, coordination problems, trouble in speaking, drooling, twisting body movements (of face, neck and back), arms and legs or muscles feel stiff, muscles tremble, shuffling walk.	Continue. Call doctor when convenient.
Infrequent:	
Appetite loss and weight loss, runny or stuffy nose, dry mouth, sneezing, vision changes, red and itchy skin, dystonia (unable to move eyes, eyelid twitching, eyes blinking more, tongue wants to stick out, trouble in breathing or speaking or swallowing), muscles feel tight or ache, feel faint upon standing after sitting or lying.	Continue, but call doctor right away.
Rare:	
Faintness, persistent and painful erection, heartbeat irregular or fast or pounding, palpitations, convulsions, high blood sugar (thirstiness, frequent urination, increased hunger, weakness).	Discontinue. Call doctor right away.

WARNINGS & PRECAUTIONS

Don't take if:
You are allergic to ziprasidone.

Before you start, consult your doctor if:
- You have liver or kidney disease, heart disease, heart rhythm problems, QT prolongation, heart failure or recent heart attack.
- You have a history of seizures.
- The patient has Alzheimer's.
- You have a family history of, or have diabetes.
- You have tardive dyskinesia.
- You have hypokalemia (low potassium) or hypomagnesemia (low magnesium).
- You have neuroleptic malignant syndrome (serious or fatal problems may occur).

Over age 60:
- Adverse reactions and side effects may be more severe than in younger persons. A lower starting dosage is usually recommended until a response is determined.
- Use of antipsychotic drugs in elderly patients with dementia-related psychosis may increase risk of death. Consult doctor

Pregnancy:
Decide with your doctor if drug benefits justify any possible risk to unborn child. Risk category C (see page xviii).

Breast-feeding:
It is unknown if drug passes into milk. Avoid nursing until you finish medicine. Consult doctor for advice on maintaining milk supply.

Infants & children:
Safety and efficacy has not been established. Use only under close medical supervision.

Prolonged use:
Consult with your doctor on a regular basis while taking this drug to check your progress or to discuss any increase or changes in side effects and the need for continued treatment. Also to check blood levels of potassium and magnesium and to monitor you for any heart problems.

Skin & sunlight:
Hot temperatures and exercise, hot baths can increase risk of heatstroke. Drug may affect body's ability to maintain normal temperature.

Driving, piloting or hazardous work:
Don't drive or pilot aircraft until you learn how medicine affects you. Don't work around dangerous machinery. Don't climb ladders or work in high places. Danger increases if you drink alcohol or take medicine affecting alertness and reflexes.

Discontinuing:
Don't discontinue this drug without consulting doctor. Dosage may require a gradual reduction before stopping.

Others:
- Get up slowly from a sitting or lying position to avoid dizziness, faintness or lightheadedness.
- Advise any doctor or dentist whom you consult that you take this medicine.
- Take medicine only as directed. Do not increase or reduce dosage without doctor's approval.

POSSIBLE INTERACTION WITH OTHER DRUGS

GENERIC NAME OR DRUG CLASS	COMBINED EFFECT
Antihypertensives*	Increased antihypertensive effect.
Carbamazepine	Decreased effect of ziprasidone.
Central nervous system (CNS) depressants*	Increased sedative effect. Increased effect of ziprasidone.
Central nervous system (CNS) stimulants	Unknown effect. Avoid.
Dopamine agonists*	Decreased effect of dopamine agonist.
Enzyme inhibitors*	Increased effect of ziprasidone.
Levodopa	May decrease levodopa effect.
QT interval prolongation-causing drugs*	Heart rhythm problems. Avoid.

POSSIBLE INTERACTION WITH OTHER SUBSTANCES

INTERACTS WITH	COMBINED EFFECT
Alcohol:	Increased sedative affect. Avoid.
Beverages: Grapefruit juice	May increase the effect of ziprasidone.
Cocaine:	Effect not known. Best to avoid.
Foods:	None expected.
Marijuana:	Effect not known. Best to avoid.
Tobacco:	None expected.

*See Glossary

ZOLPIDEM

BRAND NAMES

Ambien   ZolpiMist
Ambien CR

BASIC INFORMATION

Habit forming? Yes
Prescription needed? Yes
Available as generic? Yes
Drug class: Sedative-hypnotic agent

 USES

- Short-term treatment for insomnia.
- May be used for other disorders as determined by your doctor.

 DOSAGE & USAGE INFORMATION

How to take:
- Tablet—Swallow with liquid.
- Controlled-release tablet—Swallow tablet whole. Do not crumble, crush or chew tablet.
- Oral spray—Follow instructions provided with prescription.

When to take:
Take immediately before bedtime. For best results, do not take with a meal or immediately after eating a meal.

If you forget a dose:
Take as soon as you remember. Take drug only when you are able to get 7 to 8 hours of sleep before your daily activity begins. Do not exceed prescribed dosage.

What drug does:
Acts as a central nervous system depressant, decreasing sleep problems such as trouble falling asleep, waking up too often during the night and waking up too early in the morning.

Continued next column

 OVERDOSE

SYMPTOMS:
Drowsiness, weakness, stupor, coma.
WHAT TO DO:
- Dial 911 (emergency) for medical help or call poison control center 1-800-222-1222 for instructions.
- If person is unconscious, check breathing and pulse. If not breathing, begin mouth-to-mouth rescue breathing. If heart is not beating, begin chest compressions.
- See emergency information on last 3 pages of this book.

Time lapse before drug works:
Within 1 to 2 hours.

Don't take with:
Any other medicine or any dietary supplement without consulting your doctor or pharmacist.

 POSSIBLE ADVERSE REACTIONS OR SIDE EFFECTS

SYMPTOMS	WHAT TO DO
Life-threatening:	
Rare allergic reaction (hives, itching, rash, wheezing, tightness in chest, swelling of lips or tongue or throat).	Seek emergency treatment immediately.
Common:	
Daytime drowsiness, lightheadedness, dizziness, clumsiness, headache, diarrhea, nausea.	Continue. Call doctor when convenient.
Infrequent:	
Dry mouth, muscle aches or pain, tiredness, indigestion, joint pain, memory problems.	Continue. Call doctor when convenient.
Rare:	
Behavioral changes, agitation, confusion, hallucinations, worsening of depression, bloody or cloudy urine, painful or difficult urination, increased urge to urinate, skin rash or hives, itching, sleep-induced behaviors.*	Discontinue. Call doctor right away.

WARNINGS & PRECAUTIONS

Don't take if:
You are allergic to zolpidem.

Before you start, consult your doctor if:
- You have respiratory problems.
- You have kidney or liver disease.
- You suffer from depression.
- You are an active or recovering alcoholic or substance abuser.

Over age 60:
Adverse reactions and side effects may be more frequent and severe than in younger persons. You may need smaller doses for shorter periods of time.

Pregnancy:
Consult doctor. Risk category B (see page xviii).

Breast-feeding:
Drug passes into milk. Avoid drug or discontinue nursing until you finish medicine. Consult doctor for advice on maintaining milk supply.

Infants & children:
Not recommended for patients under age 18.

Prolonged use:
Not recommended for long-term usage. Don't take for longer than 1 to 2 weeks unless under doctor's supervision.

Skin & sunlight:
No special problems expected.

Driving, piloting or hazardous work:
Don't drive or pilot aircraft until you learn how medicine affects you. Don't work around dangerous machinery. Don't climb ladders or work in high places. Danger increases if you drink alcohol or take other medicines affecting alertness and reflexes.

Discontinuing:
- Don't discontinue without consulting doctor. Dose may require gradual reduction if you have taken drug for a long time.
- You may have sleeping problems for 1 or 2 nights after stopping drug.

Others:
- Advise any doctor or dentist whom you consult that you take this medicine.
- Don't take drug if you are traveling on an overnight airplane trip of less than 7 or 8 hours. A temporary memory loss may occur (traveler's amnesia).

POSSIBLE INTERACTION WITH OTHER DRUGS

GENERIC NAME OR DRUG CLASS	COMBINED EFFECT
Central nervous system (CNS) depressants*	Increased sedative effect. Avoid.
Chlorpromazine	Increased sedative effect. Avoid.
Imipramine	Increased sedative effect. Avoid.

POSSIBLE INTERACTION WITH OTHER SUBSTANCES

INTERACTS WITH	COMBINED EFFECT
Alcohol:	Increased sedation. Avoid.
Beverages:	None expected.
Cocaine:	None expected.
Foods:	Decreased sedative effect if taken with a meal or right after a meal.
Marijuana:	None expected.
Tobacco:	None expected.

*See Glossary

ZONISAMIDE

BRAND NAMES

Zonegran

BASIC INFORMATION

Habit forming? No
Prescription needed? Yes
Available as generic? Yes
Drug class: Anticonvulsant, antiepileptic

 ## USES

Treatment for partial (focal) epileptic seizures.
May be used alone or in combination with other
antiepileptic drugs.

 ## DOSAGE & USAGE INFORMATION

How to take:
Capsule—Swallow with liquid. Do not break or
chew capsule. May be taken with or without food
and on a full or empty stomach.

When to take:
Your doctor will determine the best schedule.
Dosages will be increased rapidly over the first
weeks of use. Further increases may be
necessary to achieve maximum benefits.

If you forget a dose:
Take as soon as you remember. If it is almost
time for the next dose, skip the missed dose and
wait for your next scheduled dose (don't double
this dose).

What drug does:
The exact mechanism is unknown. Studies have
suggested different ways in which the drug
provides anticonvulsant activity.

Time lapse before drug works:
May take several weeks for full effectiveness.

Don't take with:
Any other medicine or any dietary supplement
without consulting your doctor or pharmacist.

 ## OVERDOSE

SYMPTOMS:
**Slow or irregular heartbeat, confusion,
dizziness, faintness, unusual tiredness or
weakness, blue skin or fingernails, breathing
difficulty, coma.**
WHAT TO DO:
* **Dial 911 (emergency) for medical help or
call poison control center 1-800-222-1222
for instructions.**
* **See emergency information on last 3 pages
of this book.**

 ## POSSIBLE ADVERSE REACTIONS OR SIDE EFFECTS

SYMPTOMS	WHAT TO DO
Life-threatening: In case of overdose, see previous column.	
Common:	
• Unsteady walk, shakiness.	Continue, but call doctor right away.
• Sleepiness, dizziness, anxiety, restlessness, loss of appetite.	Continue. Call doctor when convenient.
Infrequent:	
• Agitation, delusions, hallucinations, bruising of the skin, depression, unusual mood or mental changes, double vision.	Continue, but call doctor right away.
• Constipation or diarrhea, heartburn, dry mouth, flu-like symptoms (chills, fever, headache, aching muscles and joints), problems with speech, difficulty in concentrating, sour stomach, belching, back and forth eye movement, nausea, runny or stuffy nose, tingling or burning sensations.	Continue. Call doctor when convenient.
Rare: Other symptoms.	Continue. Call doctor when convenient.

ZONISAMIDE

WARNINGS & PRECAUTIONS

Don't take if:
You are allergic to zonisamide or any other sulfonamides.*

Before you start, consult your doctor if:
- You have a history of liver disease.
- You have renal failure (inability of the kidneys to function properly).
- You are allergic to any medication, food or other substance.
- You have any other medical problems.

Over age 60:
No special problems expected.

Pregnancy:
Decide with your doctor if drug benefits justify risks to unborn child. Risk category C (see page xviii).

Breast-feeding:
Drug passes into milk. Avoid drug or discontinue nursing until you finish medicine. Consult doctor for advice on maintaining milk supply.

Infants & children:
Zonisamide has not been studied in children under age 16. Use only under medical supervision.

Prolonged use:
No special problems expected. Follow-up laboratory blood studies may be recommended by your doctor.

Skin & sunlight:
No problems expected.

Driving, piloting or hazardous work:
Don't drive or pilot aircraft until you learn how medicine affects you. Don't work around dangerous machinery. Don't climb ladders or work in high places. Danger increases if you drink alcohol or take other medicines affecting alertness and reflexes such as antihistamines, tranquilizers, sedatives, pain medicine, narcotics and mind-altering drugs.

Discontinuing:
Don't discontinue without doctor's approval due to risk of increased seizure activity. The dosage may need to be gradually decreased before stopping the drug completely.

Others:
- Advise any doctor or dentist whom you consult that you take this medicine.
- Zonisamide may be used with other anticonvulsant drugs and additional side effects may also occur. If they do, discuss them with your doctor.
- May alter some laboratory tests.
- Rarely, antiepileptic drugs may lead to suicidal thoughts and behaviors. Call doctor right away if suicidal symptoms or unusual behaviors occur.
- Wear or carry medical identification to show your seizure disorder and the drugs you take.

POSSIBLE INTERACTION WITH OTHER DRUGS

GENERIC NAME OR DRUG CLASS	COMBINED EFFECT
Anticonvulsants,* other	Decreased effect of zonisamide.
Central nervous system (CNS) depressants*	Increased sedative effect.

POSSIBLE INTERACTION WITH OTHER SUBSTANCES

INTERACTS WITH	COMBINED EFFECT
Alcohol:	Increased sedative effect. Decreased effect of zonisamide. Avoid.
Beverages:	None expected.
Cocaine:	Unknown effect. Avoid.
Foods:	None expected.
Marijuana:	Unknown effect. Avoid.
Tobacco:	None expected.

Generic and Brand Name Directory

How to Read the Lists Below

On some of the drug charts in this book you are referred to this directory to see a listing of the generic and brand names of the drugs. There are just too many names to fit on the chart page itself, so they are listed here for your reference. It is almost impossible to list all brand names available. Those not listed should be considered as effective as those that are listed.

First, look up the drug chart name (printed in large capital letters). ACETAMINOPHEN is the first name listed in this directory. Under that name, you will find the brand names of drugs (in alphabetical order) that contain the generic drug acetaminophen.

The titles on some drug charts are *drug class* names, such as ADRENOCORTICOIDS (Systemic). In this directory, this *drug class* name is followed first by a numbered list of *generic drug names* in that class. Following that list is the *brand name* list. Each *brand name* has a small number at the end that can be used to match up to the number on the *generic name* list.

For example, under ADRENOCORTICOIDS (Systemic), you will find the brand-name drug **Aristocort**[9]. The number [9] means it contains the generic drug 9. TRIAMCINOLONE.

ACETAMINOPHEN

Abenol
Acephen
Aceta
AcetaDrink
Acetaminophen Uniserts
Aclophen
Actamin
Actamin Extra
Actamin Super
Actimol
Advanced Formula Dristan Caplets
Alba-Temp 300
Alka-Seltzer Plus Cold & Cough Effervescent
Alka-Seltzer Plus Cold & Sinus Liquid-Gels
Alka-Seltzer Plus Night-Time Effervescent
Alka-Seltzer Plus Night-Time Liquid-Gels
Alka-Seltzer Plus Original Effervescent
Alka-Seltzer PM
Allerest No-Drowsiness
All-Nite Cold Formula
Amaphen
Aminofen
Aminofen Max
Anacin-3
Anacin-3 Extra Strength
Anolor 300
Anoquan
Anuphen
Apacet Capsules
Apacet Elixir
Apacet Extra Strength Caplets
Apacet Extra Strength Tablets
Apacet Oral Solution
Apacet Regular Strength Tablets

APAP
Apo-Acetaminophen
Arcet
Aspirin Free Anacin Maximum Strength Caplets
Aspirin Free Anacin Maximum Strength Tablets
Aspirin Free Bayer Select Maximum Strength Headache Plus Caplets
Aspirin-Free Excedrin Caplets
Atasol Caplets
Atasol Drops
Atasol Forte
Atasol Forte Caplets
Atasol Forte Tablets
Atasol Oral Solution
Atasol Tablets
Bancap
Banesin
Bayer Select Maximum Strength Pain Relief Formula
Benadryl Allergy/Sinus Headache Caplets
Benylin All-In-One Cold & Flu Caplets
Benylin All-In-One Cold & Flu Night Caplets
Benylin All-In-One Cold & Flu Nightime Syrup
Benylin All-In-One Cold & Flu Syrup
Benylin All-In-One Day & Night Caplets
Benylin Cold & Sinus
Benylin Cold & Sinus Plus
Benylin Cold & Flu With Codeine Narcotic
Benylin DM 12 Hour Nightime Cough Syrup
Bromo-Seltzer
Bucet
Buffets

Campain
Children's Panadol
Coldrine
Colrex Compound
Comtrex Deep Chest Cold
Conacetol
Conar-A
Congespirin
Congespirin for Children Cold Tablets
Congespirin for Children Liquid Cold Medicine
Congestant D
Contac Allergy/Sinus Day Caplets
Contac Allergy/Sinus Night Caplets
Contac Maximum Strength Sinus Caplets
Contac Night Caplets
Contac Non-Drowsy Formula Sinus Caplets
Contac Severe Cold Formula
Contac Severe Cold Formula Night Strength
Coricidin HBP
Dapa
Datril Extra Strength
Diabetic Tussin Cold & Flu
Diabetic Tussin Night Time Formula
Dolanex
Dolmar
Dristan AF
Dristan AF Plus
Dristan Cold and Flu
Dristan Cold Caplets
Dristan Cold Maximum Strength Caplets
Dristan Cold Multi-Symptom Formula
Dristan Juice Mix-in Cold, Flu, and Cough

Drixoral Cold and Flu
Drixoral Plus
Drixoral Sinus
Duoprin
Duradyne
Endolor
Esgic
Esgic Plus
Excedrin Caplets
Excedrin Extra Strength
   Caplets
Excedrin Back & Body
Excedrin Extra Strength
   Tablets
Excedrin Migraine
Excedrin Tension Headache
Exdol
Exdol Strong
Ezol
Febridyne
Femcet
Fendol
Feverall Children's
Feverall Infants'
Feverall Junior Strength
Feverall Sprinkle Caps
Fioricet
Gelpirin
Gemnisyn
Genapap
Genapap Children's Elixir
Genapap Children's Tablets
Genapap Extra Strength
Genapap Infants'
Genapap Regular Strength
   Tablets
Gendecon
Gen-D-phen
Genebs
Genebs Extra Strength
Genebs Regular Strength
   Tablets
Genex
Goody's Extra Strength
   Tablets
Goody's Headache Powders
Halenol
Halenol Extra Strength
Histagesic Modified
Histosal
Hycomine Compound
Improved Sino-Tuss
Infants' Anacin-3
Infants' Apacet
Infants' Genapap
Infants' Panadol
Infants' Tylenol
Infants' Tylenol Suspension
   Drops
Isopap
Kolephrin
Kolephrin/DM Caplets
Liquiprin Children's Elixir

Liquiprin Infants' Drops
Maximum Strength Tylenol
   Allergy Sinus Caplets
Maximum Strength Tylenol Flu
   Gelcaps
Meda Cap
Meda Tab
Medigesic
Myapap Elixir
ND-Gesic
Neocitrin Colds and Flu Calorie
   Reduced
NeoCitrin Extra Strength Colds
   and Flu
NeoCitrin Extra Strength Sinus
Neopap
Nighttime Pamprin
NyQuil Liquicaps
Nytcold Medicine
Omnicol
Oraphen-PD
Ornex Maximum Strength
   Caplets
Ornex No Drowsiness Caplets
Pacaps
Panadol
Panadol Extra Strength
Panadol Junior Strength
   Caplets
Panadol Maximum Strength
   Caplets
Panadol Maximum Strength
   Tablets
Panex
Panex 500
Paracetamol
Parafon Forte
Pedric
Pertussin All Night PM
Phenapap Sinus Headache &
   Congestion
Phenaphen
Phrenilin
Phrenilin Forte
Presalin
Redutemp
Refenesen Chest Congestion
   & Pain Relief PE
Remcol-C
Repan
Rhinogesic
Rid-A-Pain Compound
Robigesic
Robitussin Honey Flu
Robitussin Night Relief
Robitussin Night Relief Colds
   Formula Liquid
Rounox
S-A-C
Salphenyl
Sedapap
Semcet
Sinubid

Sinus Relief
Slo-Phyllin GG
Snaplets-FR
St. Joseph Aspirin Free Fever
   Reducer for Children
Sudafed Multi-Symptom Cold
   & Cough
Summit
Supac
Suppap
Tapanol
Tapanol Extra Strength
Tapar
Tavist Allergy/Sinus/Headache
Tempra
Tempra Caplets
Tempra Chewable Tablets
Tempra Double Strength
Tempra Drops
Tempra D.S.
Tempra Infants
Tempra Syrup
Tencet
Tenol
Tenol Plus
Theracof Plus Multi-Symptom
   Cough and Cold Reliever
Theraflu Cold & Sore Throat
   Hot Liquid
Theraflu Daytime Severe Cold
   Caplets
Theraflu Flu & Chest
   Congestion Hot Liquid
Theraflu Flu & Sore Throat
   Hot Liquid
Theraflu Nighttime Severe
   Cold Caplets
Theraflu Nighttime Severe
   Cold Hot Liquid
Theraflu Warming Relief
   Daytime
Theraflu Warming Relief
   Nighttime
Triad
Triaminic Cough & Sore
   Throat
Triaminic Flu, Cough & Fever
Triaminic Softchews Cough &
   Sore Throat
Triaprin
Trigesic
Tri-Pain
Two-Dyne
Tylenol
Tylenol 8 Hour
Tylenol Allergy Multi-Symptom
Tylenol Allergy Multi-Symptom
   Nighttime
Tylenol Arthritis Pain
Tylenol Chest Congestion
Tylenol Cold Head Congestion
   Daytime

Tylenol Cold Head Congestion
  Nighttime
Tylenol Cold Head Congestion
  Severe
Tylenol Concentrated Infants'
  Drops
Tylenol Cough & Severe
  Congestion Daytime
Tylenol Cough & Sore Throat
  Daytime
Tylenol Cough & Sore Throat
  Nighttime
Tylenol Extra Strength
Tylenol Extra Strength Rapid
  Release Gels
Tylenol Junior Strength
Tylenol PM
Tylenol Severe Allergy
Tylenol Sinus Congestion &
  Pain Daytime
Tylenol Sinus Congestion &
  Pain Nighttime
Tylenol Sinus Congestion &
  Pain Severe
Tylenol Sinus Severe
  Congestion Daytime
Tylenol Sore Throat Daytime
Tylenol Sore Throat Nighttime
Ty-Pap
Ultracet
Valadol
Valadol Liquid
Valorin
Valorin Extra
Vanquis
Vicks DayQuil Cold/Flu Relief
Vicks DayQuil Cold & Flu
  Symptom Relief Plus
  Vitamin C
Vicks DayQuil Sinus
  LiquiCaps
Vicks Formula 44 Custom
  Care Body Aches
Vicks Formula 44 Custom
  Care Cough & Cold PM
Vicks NyQuil Cold & Flu Relief
Vicks NyQuil Cold & Flu
  Symptom Relief Plus
  Vitamin C
Vicks NyQuil D
Vicks NyQuil Sinus LiquiCaps
Women's Tylenol Menstrual
  Relief Caplets

ADRENOCORTICOIDS
  (Systemic)

GENERIC NAMES
1. BETAMETHASONE
2. BUDESONIDE
3. CORTISONE
4. DEXAMETHASONE

5. HYDROCORTISONE
   (Cortisol)
6. METHYLPREDNISOLONE
7. PREDNISOLONE
8. PREDNISONE
9. TRIAMCINOLONE

BRAND NAMES
Apo-Prednisone[8]
Aristocort[9]
Betnelan[1]
Betnesol[1]
Celestone[1]
Cortef[5]
Cortenema[5]
Cortifoam[5]
Cortone[3]
Cortone Acetate[3]
Decadron[4]
Delta-Cortef[7]
Deltasone[8]
Deronil[4]
Dexasone[4]
Dexone 0.5[4]
Dexone 0.75[4]
Dexone 1.5[4]
Dexone 4[4]
Entocort EC[2]
Flo-Pred[7]
Hexadrol[4]
Hydeltrasol[7]
Hydrocortone[5]
Kenacort[9]
Kenacort Diacetate[9]
Medrol[6]
Meprolone[6]
Meticorten[8]
Mymethasone[4]
Nor-Pred-TBA[7]
Oradexon[4]
Orapred[7]
Orapred ODT[7]
Orasone 1[8]
Orasone 5[8]
Orasone 10[8]
Orasone 20[8]
Orasone 50[8]
Pediapred[7]
Prednisone Intensol[8]
Prednicen-M[8]
Prelone[7]
Sterapred DS[8]
Solurex[4]
Solurex LA[4]
Winpred[8]

ADRENOCORTICOIDS
  (Topical)

GENERIC NAMES
1. ALCLOMETASONE (Topical)
2. AMCINONIDE (Topical)
3. BECLOMETHASONE
   (Topical)

4. BETAMETHASONE (Topical)
5. CLOBETASOL (Topical)
6. CLOBETASONE (Topical)
7. CLOCORTOLONE (Topical)
8. CORTISOL
9. DESONIDE (Topical)
10. DESOXIMETASONE
    (Topical)
11. DEXAMETHASONE
    (Topical)
12. DIFLORASONE (Topical)
13. DIFLUCORTOLONE
    (Topical)
14. FLUMETHASONE (Topical)
15. FLUOCINOLONE (Topical)
16. FLUOCINONIDE (Topical)
17. FLURANDRENOLIDE
    (Topical)
18. FLUTICASONE (Topical)
19. HALCINONIDE (Topical)
20. HALOBETASOL
21. HYDROCORTISONE
    (Dental)
22. HYDROCORTISONE
    (Topical)
23. MOMETASONE (Topical)
24. PREDNICARBATE
25. TRIAMCINOLONE (Topical)

BRAND NAMES
9-1-1[22]
Aclovate[1]
Acticort-100[22]
Adcortyl[25]
Aeroseb-Dex[11]
Aeroseb-HC[22]
Ala-Cort[22]
Ala-Scalp HP[22]
Allercort[22]
Alphaderm[22]
Alphatrex[4]
Anucort-HC[22]
Anusol-HC[22]
Anusol-HC 2.5%[22]
Aristocort[25]
Aristocort A[25]
Aristocort C[25]
Aristocort D[25]
Aristocort R[25]
Bactine[22]
Barriere-HC[22]
Beben[4]
Beta HC[22]
Betacort Scalp Lotion[4]
Betaderm[4]
Betaderm Scalp Lotion[4]
Betamethacot[4]
Betatrex[4]
Beta-Val[4]
Betnovate[4]
Betnovate 1/2[4]
Bio-Syn[15]
CaldeCORT Anti-Itch[22]
CaldeCORT-Light[22]

Carmol-HC[22]
Celestoderm-V[4]
Celestoderm-V/2[4]
Cetacort[22]
Cipro HC[22]
Clobex[5]
Cloderm[7]
Cloderm Pump[7]
Coraz Lotion[22]
Cordran[17]
Cordran SP[17]
Cormax[5]
Cortacet[22]
Cortaid[22]
Cortaid FastStick[22]
Cortate[22]
Cort-Dome[22]
Cort-Dome High Potency[22]
Cortef[22]
Cortef Feminine Itch[22]
Corticaine[22]
Corticreme[22]
Cortifair[22]
Cortiment-10[22]
Cortiment-40[22]
Cortoderm[22]
Cortril[22]
Cultivate[18]
Cyclocort[2]
Decaderm[11]
Decadron[11]
Decaspray[11]
Delacort[22]
Delta-Tritex[25]
Demarest DriCort[22]
Dermabet[4]
Dermacomb[25]
Dermacort[22]
Dermalleve[22]
DermAtop[24]
DermiCort[22]
Dermovate[5]
Dermovate Scalp Application[5]
Dermtex HC[22]
Desonate[9]
DesOwen[9]
Diprolene[4]
Diprolene AF[4]
Diprosone[4]
Drenison[17]
Drenison-1/4[17]
Ectosone[4]
Ectosone Regular[4]
Ectosone Scalp Lotion[4]
Efcortelan[22]
Elocon[23]
Emo-Cort[22]
Emo-Cort Scalp Solution[22]
Epifoam[8]
Eumovate[6]
Fludroxycortide[17]
Fluocet[15]
Fluocin[16]

Fluoderm[15]
Fluolar[15]
Fluonid[15]
Fluonide[15]
Flurosyn[15]
Flutex[25]
Foille Cort[22]
Gly-Cort[22]
Gynecort[22]
Gynecort 10[22]
Halciderm[19]
Halog[19]
Halog E[19]
Hi-Cor 1.0[22]
Hi-Cor 2.5[22]
Hyderm[22]
Hydro-Tex[22]
Hytone[22]
Kenac[25]
Kenalog[25]
Kenalog in Orabase[25]
Kenalog-H[25]
Kenonel[25]
Lacticare-HC[22]
Lanacort[22]
Lanacort 10[22]
Lemoderm[22]
Licon[16]
LidaMantle HC[22]
Lidemol[16]
Lidex[16]
Lidex-E[16]
Locacorten[14]
Locoid[22]
Lotrisone[4]
Lyderm[16]
Maxiflor[12]
Maximum Strength Cortaid[22]
Maxivate[4]
Metaderm Mild[4]
Metaderm Regular[4]
Metosyn[16]
Metosyn FAPG[16]
Myco II[25]
Mycogen II[25]
Mycolog II[25]
My Cort[22]
Myco-Triacet II[25]
Mytrex[25]
Nerisone[13]
Nerisone Oily[13]
Novobetamet[4]
Novohydrocort[22]
Nutracort[22]
Olux[5]
Olux-E[5]
Orabase HCA[22]
Oracort[25]
Oralone[25]
Pandel[22]
Penecort[22]
Pentacort[22]
Pharma-Cort[22]

Prevex B[4]
Prevex HC[4]
Propaderm[3]
Psorcon[12]
Rederm[22]
Rhulicort[22]
Sarna HC[22]
Sential[22]
S-T Cort[22]
Synacort[22]
Synalar[15]
Synalar HP[15]
Synamol[15]
Synemol[15]
Taclonex[4]
Teladar[4]
Temovate[5]
Temovate E[5]
Temovate Emollient[5]
Temovate Gel[5]
Temovate Scalp Application[5]
Texacort[22]
Topicort[10]
Topicort LP[10]
Topicort Mild[10]
Topilene[4]
Topisone[4]
Topsyn[16]
Triacet[25]
Triaderm[25]
Trianide Mild[25]
Trianide Regular[25]
Tristatin II[25]
Triderm[25]
Tridesilon[9]
Tri-Luma[15]
Trymex[25]
Ultravate[20]
Unicort[22]
Uticort[4]
Valisone[4]
Valisone Reduced Strength[4]
Valisone Scalp Lotion[4]
Valnac[4]
Vanos[16]
Verdeso Foam[9]
Vioform-Hydrocortisone
  Lotion[22]
Westcort[22]
Xyralid Cream[22]
Xyralid LP Lotion[22]
Zytopic Cream[25]

ANDROGENS

GENERIC NAMES
1. ETHYLESTRENOL
2. FLUOXYMESTERONE
3. METHYLTESTOSTERONE
4. NANDROLONE
5. OXANDROLONE
6. OXYMETHOLONE
7. STANOZOLOL
8. TESTOSTERONE

BRAND NAMES
Anabolin[4]
Anabolin LA 100[4]
Anadrol-50[6]
Anapolon 50[6]
Andro 100[8]
Andro-Cyp 100[8]
Andro-Cyp 200[8]
Androderm[8]
Androgel[8]
Android-10[3]
Android-25[3]
Android-T[8]
Andro-LA 200[8]
Androlone[4]
Andronaq-50[8]
Andronaq-LA[8]
Andronate 100[8]
Andronate 200[8]
Andropository 100[8]
Andryl 200[8]
Deca-Durabolin[4]
Delatest[8]
Delatestryl[8]
Dep Andro 100[8]
Dep Andro 200[8]
Depotest[8]
Depo-Testosterone[8]
Durabolin[4]
Durabolin-50[4]
Duratest 100[8]
Duratest-200[8]
Durathate 200[8]
Everone[8]
Halotestin[2]
Histerone-50[8]
Histerone-100[8]
Hybolin Decanoate[4]
Dep-Androgyn[5]
Depo-Testadiol[5]
Depotestogen[5]
Duo-Cyp[5]
Duo-Gen L.A.[5]
Duogex L.A.[5]
Dura-Dumone 90/4[5]
Duratestin[5]
Estratest[3]
Estratest H.S.[3]
Halodrin[4]
Menoject L.A.[5]
Neo-Pause[5]
OB[5]
Premarin with
   Methyltestosterone[1]
Striant[8]
Teev[5]
Tes Est Cyp[5]
Test-Estro Cypionate[5]
Testim[8]
Tylosterone[2]
Valertest No. 1[5]
Valertest No. 2[5]

ANESTHETICS (Topical)
GENERIC NAMES
1. BENZOCAINE
2. BENZOCAINE & MENTHOL
3. BUTAMBEN
4. DIBUCAINE
5. LIDOCAINE
6. LIDOCAINE & PRILOCAINE
7. PRAMOXINE
8. TETRACAINE
9. TETRACAINE & MENTHOL
10. TETRACAINE &
    LIDOCAINE

BRAND NAMES
Americaine[1]
Amercaine Topical Anesthetic
   First Aid Ointment[1]
Amercaine Topical Anesthetic
   Spray[1]
Anestafoam[5]
Benzocol[2]
Butesin Picrate[3]
Butyl Aminobenzoate[2]
Cinchocaine[4]
Dermoplast[2]
Emla[6]
Endocaine[1]
Ethyl Aminobenzoate[1]
Lagol[1]
LidaMantle[5]
Lidoderm[5]
Lignocaine[5]
Nupercainal Cream[4]
Nupercainal Ointment[4]
Pontocaine Cream[8]
Pontocaine Ointment[9]
Pramegel[7]
Prax[7]
Synera[10]
Tronothane[7]
Unguentine[1]
Unguentine Plus[1]
Unguentine Spray[1]
Xylocaine[5]
Xyralid Cream[5]
Xyralid LP Lotion[5]
Zostrix Neuropathy Cream[5]

ANGIOTENSIN-CONVERTING ENZYME (ACE) INHIBITORS
GENERIC NAMES
1. BENAZEPRIL
2. CAPTOPRIL
3. ENALAPRIL
4. FOSINOPRIL
5. LISINOPRIL
6. MOEXIPRIL
7. PERINDOPRIL
8. QUINAPRIL
9. RAMIPRIL

10. TRANDOLAPRIL
BRAND NAMES
Accupril[8]
Aceon[7]
Altace[9]
Apo-Capto[2]
Capoten[2]
Lotensin[1]
Lotrel[1]
Mavik[10]
Monopril[4]
Novo-Captoril[2]
Prinivil[5]
Syn-Captopril[2]
Tarka[10]
Teczem[3]
Uniretic[6]
Univasc[6]
Vasotec[3]
Zestril[5]

ANGIOTENSIN-CONVERTING ENZYME (ACE) INHIBITORS & HYDROCHLORO-THIAZIDE
GENERIC NAMES
1. CAPTOPRIL &
   HYDROCHLOROTHIAZIDE
2. ENALAPRIL &
   HYDROCHLOROTHIAZIDE
3. LISINOPRIL &
   HYDROCHLOROTHIAZIDE
4. QUINAPRIL &
   HYDROCHLOROTHIAZIDE

BRAND NAMES
Accuretic[4]
Capozide[1]
Prinzide[3]
Vaseretic[2]
Zestoretic[3]

ANTACIDS
GENERIC NAMES
1. ALUMINA & MAGNESIA
2. ALUMINA & MAGNESIUM
   CARBONATE
3. ALUMINA & MAGNESIUM
   TRISILICATE
4. ALUMINA, MAGNESIA, &
   CALCIUM CARBONATE
5. ALUMINA, MAGNESIA, &
   SIMETHICONE
6. ALUMINA, MAGNESIUM,
   CALCIUM CARBONATE &
   SIMETHICONE
7. ALUMINA, MAGNESIUM
   TRISILICATE, & SODIUM
   BICARBONATE
8. ALUMINUM CARBONATE,
   BASIC

9. ALUMINUM HYDROXIDE
10. CALCIUM & MAGNESIUM
    CARBONATES
11. CALCIUM CARBONATE
12. CALCIUM CARBONATE &
    MAGNESIA
13. CALCIUM CARBONATE &
    MAGNESIUM HYDROXIDE
14. CALCIUM CARBONATE &
    SIMETHICONE
15. CALCIUM CARBONATE,
    MAGNESIA, & SIMETHICONE
16. MAGALDRATE
17. MAGALDRATE &
    SIMETHICONE
18. MAGNESIUM HYDROXIDE
19. MAGNESIUM OXIDE

BRAND NAMES
Acid + All[14]
Advanced Formula Di-Gel[15]
Alamag[1]
Algenic Alka[2]
Algenic Alka Improved[2]
Algicon[9]
Alka-Mints[11]
Alkets[11]
Alkets Extra Strength[11]
Almacone[5]
Almacone II[5]
Alma-Mag #4 Improved[5]
Alma-Mag Improved[5]
AlternaGEL[9]
Alu-Cap[9]
Aludrox[5]
Alu-Tab[9]
Amitone[12]
Amphojel[9]
Amphojel 500[1]
Amphojel Plus[4]
AntaGel[5]
AntaGel-II[5]
Basaljel[9]
Calglycine[11]
Camalox[4]
Chooz[11]
Dialume[9]
Di-Gel[5]
Diovol Ex[1]
Diovol Plus[5]
Duracid[9]
Equilet[11]
Foamicon[3]
Gas-X with Maalox[14]
Gaviscon[2]
Gaviscon Extra Strength Relief
    Formula[9]
Gaviscon-2[7]
Gelusil[5]
Gelusil Extra-Strength[1]
Genalac[11]
Genaton[2]
Genaton Extra Strength[2]

Glycate[11]
Kudrox Double Strength[5]
Losopan[16]
Losopan Plus[17]
Lowsium[16]
Lowsium Plus[17]
Maalox[1]
Maalox HRF[2]
Maalox Plus[5]
Maalox Plus, Extra Strength[5]
Maalox Quick Dissolving
    Chews[11]
Maalox TC[1]
Magnalox[5]
Magnalox Plus[5]
Mag-Ox 400[19]
Mallamint[11]
Maox[19]
Marblen[10]
Mi-Acid[5]
Mi-Acid Double Strength[5]
Mintox[1]
Mintox Extra Strength[5]
Mygel[5]
Mygel II[5]
Mylagen[5]
Mylagen II[5]
Mylanta[5]
Mylanta Calci Tabs[12]
Mylanta Double Strength[5]
Mylanta Double Strength
    Plain[5]
Mylanta Gelcaps[10]
Mylanta Maximum Strength[13]
Mylanta Night Time Strength[9]
Mylanta Regular Strength[5]
Mylanta Plain[5]
Mylanta-II[5]
Nephrox[9]
Neutralca-S[1]
Pepcid Complete[13]
Phillips' Milk of Magnesia[18]
Riopan[16]
Riopan Extra Strength[16]
Riopan Plus[17]
Riopan Plus Double Strength[17]
Riopan Plus Extra Strength[17]
Rolaids[12]
Rolaids Antacid Cool[12]
Rolaids Calcium Rich[11]
Rolaids Chewable[11]
Rolaids Extra Strength[12]
Rolaids Sodium Free[11]
Rulox[1]
Rulox No. 1[1]
Rulox No. 2[1]
Rulox Plus[5]
Simaal 2 Gel[5]
Simaal Gel[5]
Tempo[6]
Titralac[11]
Titralac Plus[11]
Triconsil[7]

Tums[11]
Tums E-X[11]
Tums Extra Strength[11]
Tums Kids[11]
Tums Lasting Effects[11]
Tums Liquid Extra Strength[11]
Tums Liquid Extra Strength
    with Simethicone[14]
Tums QuikPak[11]
Tums Smooth Dissolve[11]
Univol[1]
Uro-Mag[19]
Zygerid Chewable Tablets[18]

ANTIBACTERIALS
(Ophthalmic)
GENERIC NAMES
1. AZITHROMYCIN
    (Ophthalmic)
2. CHLORAMPHENICOL
    (Ophthalmic)
3. CIPROFLOXACIN
    (Ophthalmic)
4. ERYTHROMYCIN
    (Ophthalmic)
5. GATIFLOXACIN
    (Ophthalmic)
6. GENTAMICIN (Ophthalmic)
7. LEVOFLOXACIN
    (Ophthalmic)
8. MOXIFLOXACIN
    (Ophthalmic)
9. NEOMYCIN & POLYMYXIN B
10. NEOMYCIN, POLYMYXIN B
    & BACITRACIN
11. NEOMYCIN, POLYMYXIN B
    & GRAMICIDIN
12. NORFLOXACIN
    (Ophthalmic)
13. OFLOXACIN (Ophthalmic)
14. SULFACETAMIDE
    (Ophthalmic)
15. SULFISOXAZOLE
    (Ophthalmic)
16. TOBRAMYCIN
    (Ophthalmic)

BRAND NAMES
Ak-Chlor Ophthalmic Ointment[2]
Ak-Chlor Ophthalmic Solution[2]
Ak-Spore[9]
Ak-Spore H.C.[11]
Ak-Sulf[14]
Aktob[16]
Alcomicin[7]
AzaSite[1]
Bleph-10[14]
Cetamide[14]
Chibroxin[12]
Chloracol Ophthalmic Solution
    (Ophthalmic)[2]
Chlorofair Ophthalmic
    Ointment[2]

Chlorofair Ophthalmic
Solution[2]
Chloromycetin Ophthalmic
Ointment[2]
Chloromycetin Ophthalmic
Solution[2]
Chloroptic Ophthalmic
Solution[2]
Chloroptic S.O.P.[2]
Ciloxan[3]
Econochlor Ophthalmic
Ointment[2]
Econochlor Ophthalmic
Solution[2]
Fenicol Ophthalmic Ointment[1]
Gantrisin[15]
Garamycin[7]
Genoptic[6]
Gentacidin[7]
Gentafair[7]
Gentak[6]
Gentasol[7]
Gentrasul[6]
I-Chlor Ophthalmic Solution[2]
Ilotycin[4]
Iquix[7]
I-Sulfacet[14]
Mycitracin[10]
Neociden Ophthalmic
Ointment[10]
Neociden Ophthalmic
Solution[11]
Neosporin Ophthalmic
Ointment[10]
Neosporin Ophthalmic
Solution[11]
Neotal[10]
Neotricin HC[9]
Ocu-Chlor Ophthalmic
Ointment[2]
Ocu-Chlor Ophthalmic
Solution[2]
Ocuflox[13]
Ocu-Mycin[6]
Ocu-Spor-B[10]
Ocu-Spor-G[11]
Ocusporin[10]
Ocu-Sul-10[14]
Ocu-Sul-15[14]
Ocu-Sul-30[14]
Ocusulf-10[14]
Ocutricin Ophthalmic
Ointment[10]
Ocutricin Ophthalmic
Solution[11]
Ophthacet[14]
Ophthochlor Ophthalmic
Solution[2]
Ophtho-Chloram Ophthalmic
Solution[2]
Pentamycetin[2]
Pentamycetin Ophthalmic
Ointment[12]

Pentamycetin Ophthalmic
Solution[2]
P.N. Ophthalmic[11]
Quixin[7]
Sodium Sulamyd[14]
Sopamycetin Ophthalmic
Ointment[2]
Sopamycetin Ophthalmic
Solution[2]
Spectro-Chlor Ophthalmic
Ointment[2]
Spectro-Chlor Ophthalmic
Solution[2]
Spectro-Genta[6]
Spectro-Sporin[10]
Spectro-Sulf[14]
Steri-Units Sulfacetamide[14]
Sulamyd[14]
Sulf-10[14]
Sulfair[14]
Sulfair 10[14]
Sulfair 15[14]
Sulfair Forte[14]
Sulfamide[14]
Sulfex[14]
Sulten-10[14]
Tobradex[16]
Tobrex[16]
Tribiotic[11]
Tri-Ophthalmic[11]
Vigamox[8]
Zylet[16]
Zymar[5]

ANTICHOLINERGICS

GENERIC NAMES
1. ANISOTROPINE
2. ATROPINE
3. HOMATROPINE
4. ISOPROPAMIDE
5. MEPENZOLATE
6. METHANTHELINE
7. METHSCOPOLAMINE
8. OXYPHENCYCLIMINE
9. PIRENZEPINE
10. TRIDIHEXETHYL

BRAND NAMES
AH-Chew[7]
AlleRx D[7]
AlleRx Dose Pack DF[7]
AlleRx Dose Pack PE[7]
Amdry-D[7]
Banthine[6]
Cantil[5]
Codan[3]
D.A. Chewable[7]
Dallergy[3]
Dallergy Caplets[3]
Darbid[4]
Daricon[8]
Durahist[7]
Dura-Vent/DA[7]

Extendryl[7]
Extendryl JR[7]
Extendryl SR[7]
Gastrozepin[9]
Hista-Vent PSE[7]
Homapin[3]
Hycodan[3]
Hydromet[3]
Hydropane[6]
OMNIhist L.A.[7]
Pamine[7]
Pamine Forte[7]
Pathilon[10]
Prehist D[7]
Tussigon[3]
Valpin 50[1]

ANTIDEPRESSANTS, TRICYCLIC

GENERIC NAMES
1. AMITRYPTILINE
2. AMOXAPINE
3. CLOMIPRAMINE
4. DESIPRAMINE
5. DOXEPIN
6. IMIPRAMINE
7. NORTRIPTYLINE
8. PROTRIPTYLINE
9. TRIMIPRAMINE

BRAND NAMES
Adapin[5]
Anafranil[3]
Apo-Amitriptyline[1]
Apo-Imipramine[6]
Apo-Trimip[9]
Asendin[2]
Aventyl[7]
Endep[1]
Etrafon[1]
Etrafon-A[1]
Etrafon-D[1]
Etrafon-F[1]
Etrafon-Forte[1]
Impril[6]
Levate[1]
Norfranil[6]
Norpramin[4]
Novo-Doxepin[5]
Novopramine [6]
Novo-Tripramine[9]
Novotriptyn[1]
Pamelor[7]
PMS Amitriptyline[1]
PMS Impramine[6]
PMS Levazine[8]
Rhotrimine[9]
Sinequan[5]
Surmontil[9]
Tipramine[9]
Tofranil[6]
Tofranil-PM[6]
Triadapin[5]

Triavil[8]
Triptil[8]
Vivactil[8]

ANTIDYSKINETICS

GENERIC NAMES
1. BENZTROPINE
2. BIPERIDEN
3. ENTACAPONE
4. ETHOPROPAZINE
5. PIMOZIDE
6. PRAMIPEXOLE
7. PROCYCLIDINE
8. ROPINIROLE
9. TRIHEXYPHENIDYL

BRAND NAMES
Akineton[2]
Apo-Benztropine[1]
Apo-Trihex[4]
Artane[9]
Artane Sequels[9]
Cogentin[1]
Comtan[3]
Mirapex[6]
Orap[5]
Parsidol[4]
Parsitan[4]
PMS Benztropine[1]
PMS Procyclidine[7]
PMS Trihexyphenidyl[9]
Procyclid[7]
Requip[8]
Requip XL[8]
Stalevo[3]
Trihexane[9]
Trihexy[9]

ANTIFUNGALS (Topical)

GENERIC NAMES
1. AMPHOTERICIN B
2. BUTENAFINE
3. CICLOPIROX
4. CLOTRIMAZOLE
5. ECONAZOLE
6. FLUCONAZOLE
7. HALOPROGIN
8. KETOCONAZOLE (Topical)
9. MICONAZOLE
10. NAFTIFINE
11. NYSTATIN
12. OXICONAZOLE (Topical)
13. SERTACONAZOLE
14. SULCONAZOLE
15. TERBINAFINE
16. TOLNAFTATE
17. UNDECYLENIC ACID

BRAND NAMES
Aftate for Athlete's Foot
   Aerosol Spray Liquid[16]
Aftate for Athlete's Foot
   Aerosol Spray Powder[16]
Aftate for Athlete's Foot Gel[16]
Aftate for Athlete's Foot
   Sprinkle Powder[16]
Aftate for Jock Itch Aerosol
   Spray Powder[16]
Aftate for Jock Itch Gel[16]
Aftate for Jock Itch Sprinkle
   Powder[16]
Caldesene Medicated Powder[17]
Canesten Cream[4]
Canesten Solution[4]
Cruex Aerosol Powder[17]
Cruex Antifungal Cream[17]
Cruex Antifungal Powder[17]
Cruex Antifungal Spray
   Powder[17]
Cruex Cream[17]
Cruex Powder[17]
Decylenes[17]
Decylenes Powder[17]
Desenex Aerosol Powder[17]
Desenex Antifungal Cream[17]
Desenex Antifungal Liquid[17]
Desenex Antifungal
   Ointment[17]
Desenex Antifungal
   Penetrating Foam[17]
Desenex Antifungal Powder[17]
Desenex Antifungal Spray
   Powder[17]
Desenex Max Cream[17]
Desenex Ointment[17]
Desenex Powder[17]
Desenex Solution[17]
Ecostatin[5]
Ertazo[13]
Exelderm[14]
Extina[8]
Extina Foam[8]
Fungizone[1]
Genaspore Cream[16]
Gordochom Solution[17]
Halotex[7]
Lamisil[15]
Lamisil Solution 1%[15]
Loprox[3]
Lotriderm[4]
Lotrimin AF[4]
Lotrimin Cream[4]
Lotrimin Lotion[4]
Lotrimin Ointment[4]
Lotrimin Ultra[2]
Lotrisone[4]
Mentax[2]
Mentax TC[2]
Micatin[9]
Monistat-Derm[9]
Mycelex Cream[4]
Mycelex Solution[4]
Myclo Cream[4]
Myclo Solution[4]
Myclo Spray[4]
Mycostatin[11]

Nadostine[11]
Naftin[10]
Nilstat[11]
Nizoral A-D[8]
Nizoral Shampoo[8]
NP-27 Cream[16]
NP-27 Powder[16]
NP-27 Solution[16]
NP-27 Spray Powder[16]
Nyaderm[11]
Nystex[11]
Nystop[11]
Oxistat[12]
Penlac[3]
Pitrex Cream[16]
Spectazole[5]
Tinactin Aerosol Liquid[16]
Tinactin Aerosol Powder[16]
Tinactin Antifungal
   Deodorant
   Powder Aerosol[16]
Tinactin Cream[16]
Tinactin Jock Itch Aerosol
   Powder[16]
Tinactin Jock Itch Cream[16]
Tinactin Jock Itch Spray
   Powder[16]
Tinactin Plus Powder[16]
Tinactin Powder[16]
Tinactin Solution[16]
Ting Antifungal Cream[16]
Ting Antifungal Powder[16]
Ting Antifungal Spray Liquid[16]
Ting Antifungal Spray
   Powder[16]
Vusion[9]
Xolegel Gel[8]
Zeasorb-AF Powder[9]

ANTIFUNGALS (Vaginal)

GENERIC NAMES
1. BUTOCONAZOLE
2. CLOTRIMAZOLE
3. ECONAZOLE
4. GENTIAN VIOLET
5. MICONAZOLE
6. NYSTATIN
7. TERCONAZOLE
8. TIOCONAZOLE

BRAND NAMES
Canesten[2]
Canesten 1[2]
Canesten 3[2]
Canesten 10%[2]
Ecostatin[3]
FemCare[2]
Femizole Prefil[2]
Femizole-7[2]
Genapax[4]
Gyne-Lotrimin[2]
Gyne-Lotrimin 3[2]
Gyno-Trosyd[8]

Monistat[5]
Monistat 1[8]
Monistat 3[5]
Monistat 5[5]
Monistat 7[5]
Mycelex-7[2]
Mycelex-G[2]
Myclo[2]
Mycostatin[6]
Nadostine[6]
Nilstat[6]
Nyaderm[6]
Terazol 3[7]
Terazol 7[7]
Three Day Cream[2]
Vagistat[8]
Vagistat-1[8]

ANTIHISTAMINES

GENERIC NAMES
1. ACRIVASTINE
2. AZATADINE
3. BROMODIPHENHYDRAMINE
4. BROMPHENIRAMINE
5. CARBINOXAMINE
6. CHLORPHENIRAMINE
7. CLEMASTINE FUMARATE
8. CYPROHEPTADINE
9. DEXBROMPHENIRAMINE
10. DEXCHLORPHENIRAMINE
11. DIMENHYDRINATE
12. DIPHENHYDRAMINE
13. DIPHENYLPYRALINE
14. DOXYLAMINE
15. PHENINDAMINE
16. PHENIRAMINE
17. PHENYLTOLOXAMINE
18. PYRILAMINE
19. TRIPELENNAMINE
20. TRIPROLIDINE

BRAND NAMES
Aclophen[6]
Actacin[20]
Actagen[20]
Actagen-C Cough[20]
Actidil[18]
Advil Multi-Symptom Cold[6]
AH-Chew[6]
Alersule[6]
Alka-Seltzer Plus Cold & Cough Liquid Gels[6]
Alka-Seltzer PM[12]
Allent[5]
Alleract[18]
Aller-Chlor[6]
Allercon[20]
Allerdryl[12]
Allerest Maximum Strength[6]
Allerfrim[20]
AllerMax Caplets[12]
Aller-med[12]
Allerphed[20]

Allert[6]
AlleRx Dose Pack DF[6]
AlleRx Dose Pack PE[6]
AlleRx Suspension[6]
All-Nite Cold Formula[14]
Ambay Cough[3]
Ambenyl Cough[3]
Ambophen Expectorant[3]
Anamine[6]
Anamine HD[6]
Anamine T. D.[6]
Apo-Dimenhydrinate[11]
Atrohist Pediatric[6]
Atrohist Pediatric Suspension Dye Free[618]
Atrohist Sprinkle[6]
Banophen[12]
Banophen Caplets[12]
Beldin[12]
Belix[12]
Bena-D 10[12]
Bena-D 50[12]
Benadryl Allergy and Sinus Fastmelt[12]
Benadryl Allergy/Sinus Headache Caplets[12]
Benahist 10[12]
Benahist 50[12]
Ben-Allergin 50[12]
Benaphen[12]
Benoject-10[12]
Benoject-50[12]
Benylin All-In-One Cold & Flu Night Caplets[12]
Benylin All-In-One Cold & Flu Nightime Syrup[6]
Benylin Cold & Sinus Plus[6]
Brexin-L.A[6]
Brofed[5]
Bromanyl[3]
Bromatane DX Cough[5]
Bromfed[5]
Bromfed-DM[5]
Bromfed-PD[5]
Bydramine Cough[12]
Calm X[11]
Calmylin with Codeine[10]
Carbodec[5]
Carbodec DM Drops[5]
Carbodec TR[5]
Cenafed Plus[20]
Cerose-DM[6]
Children's Benadryl Allergy & Cold Fastmelt[12]
Children's Benadryl Perfect Measure[12]
Children's Dramamine[11]
Children's Triaminic Thin Strips Night Time Cold & Cough[12]
Chlo-Amine[6]
Chlor-100[6]
Chlorate[6]

Chlorgest-HD[6]
Chlor-Niramine[6]
Chlorphed[3]
Chlorphedrine SR[3]
Chlor-Pro[6]
Chlor-Pro 10[6]
Chlorspan-12[6]
Chlortab-4[6]
Chlortab-8[6]
Chlor-Trimeton 4 Hour Relief[6]
Chlor-Trimeton 12 Hour Relief[6]
Chlor-Tripolon[6]
Citra Forte[6]
CoActifed Expectorant[20]
Codehist DH[6]
Codeprex[6]
Codimal DH[18]
Codimal DM[6]
Codimal PH[18]
Codimal-A[5]
Codimal-L.A.[6]
Codimal-L.A. Half[6]
Colfed-A[6]
Colrex Compound[6]
Colrex Cough[6]
Coltab Children's[6]
Comhist[6]
Comhist LA[6]
Compoz[12]
Congestant D[6]
Conjec-B[5]
Contac 12-Hour[6]
Contac 12-Hour Allergy[7]
Contac Allergy/Sinus Night Caplets[7]
Contac Night Caplets[12]
Contac Severe Cold Formula[6]
Contac Severe Cold Formula Night Strength[6]
Coricidin HBP[6]
Cotridin[20]
D.A. Chewable[6]
Dallergy[6]
Dallergy Jr[5]
Decohistine DH[6]
Deconamine[6]
Deconamine SR[6]
Dexaphen SA[9]
Dexchlor[10]
Dexophed[9]
Diabetic Tussin Allergy Relief[6]
Diabetic Tussin Cold & Flu[6]
Diabetic Tussin Night Time Formula[12]
Diamine T.D.[5]
Dihistine[6]
Dihistine DH[6]
Dimetabs[11]
Dimetane[5]
Dimetapp Plus Caplets[5]
Dimetapp with Codeine[5]
Dimetapp-A[5]
Dimetapp-A Pediatric[5]

Dimetapp-DM[5]
Dimetapp-DM Cough and Cold[5]
Dimetapp-DM Elixir[5]
Dinate[11]
Diphen Cough[12]
Diphenacen-10[12]
Diphenacen-50[12]
Diphenadryl[12]
Disobrom[9]
Disophrol[9]
Disophrol Chronotabs[9]
Dommanate[11]
Donatussin[6]
Donatussin Drops[6]
Dondril[6]
Dormarex 2[12]
Dormin[12]
Dramamine[11]
Dramamine Chewable[11]
Dramamine Liquid[11]
Dramanate[11]
Dramocen[11]
Dramoject[11]
Dristan AF[6]
Dristan Cold and Flu[6]
Dristan Cold Maximum Strength
   Caplets[5]
Dristan Cold Multi-Symptom
   Formula[6]
Dristan Formula P[18]
Drixoral[9]
Drixoral Cold and Allergy[9]
Drixoral Cold and Flu[9]
Drixoral Plus[9]
Drixoral Sinus[9]
Drixtab[9]
Durahist[6]
Dura-Vent/DA[6]
Dymenate[11]
Ed A-Hist[6]
Endagen-HD[6]
Endal HD[6]
Endal-HD Plus[6]
Extendryl[6]
Extendryl JR[6]
Extendryl SR[6]
Father John's Medicine Plus[6]
Fedahist[6]
Fedahist Decongestant[6]
Fedahist Gyrocaps[6]
Fedahist Timecaps[6]
Fenylhist[12]
Fynex[12]
Genahist[12]
GenAllerate[6]
Gendecon[6]
Gen-D-phen[12]
Gravol[11]
Gravol L/A[11]
Hayfebrol[6]
Histagesic Modified[6]
Histaject Modified[5]

Histalet[6]
Histalet-DM[6]
Histatab Plus[6]
Histatan[6]
Hista-Vent PSE[6]
Histex i/E[5]
Histor-D[6]
Histor-D Timecelles[6]
Hycomine Compound[6]
Hycomine-S Pediatric[6]
Hydramine[12]
Hydramine Cough[12]
Hydramyn[12]
Hydrate[11]
Hydril[12]
Hyrexin-50[12]
Improved Sino-Tuss[6]
Insomnal[12]
Klerist-D[6]
Kolephrin[6]
Kolephrin/DM Caplets[6]
Kronofed-A[6]
Kronofed-A Jr.[6]
Lodrane LD[4]
Lodrane 12Hour ER[4]
Lodrane 24D[4]
Marmine[11]
Maximum Strength Tylenol
   Allergy Sinus Caplets[6]
Meda Syrup Forte[6]
Motion-Aid[12]
Myidil[20]
Nasahist B[5]
Nauseatol[11]
ND Clear T.D.[6]
ND Stat Revised[5]
ND-Gesic[6]
Neocitran A[16]
Neocitran Colds and Flu
   Calorie Reduced[16]
NeoCitran DM Coughs & Cold[16]
NeoCitran Extra Strength
   Colds and Flu[16]
Nervine Night-time Sleep-Aid[12]
Nico-Vert[11]
Nidryl[12]
Nisaval[17]
Nolahist[18]
Noradryl[12]
Norafed[18]
Nordryl[10]
Nordryl Cough[10]
Novodimenate[11]
Novopheniram[6]
NyQuil Cough[14]
Nytol Maximum Strength[12]
Nytol with DPH[12]
Omnicol[6]
OMNIhist L.A.[6]
Optimine[2]
Oraminic II[5]
Palgic[5]
PBZ[19]

PBZ-SR[19]
Pediacof Cough[6]
Pelamine[19]
Periactin[8]
Pertussin All Night PM[14]
Pfeiffer's Allergy[6]
Phenapap Sinus Headache &
   Congestion[6]
Phendry[12]
Phendry Children's Allergy
   Medicine[12]
Phenetron[6]
Phenetron Lanacaps[6]
PMS-Dimenhydrinate[11]
Poladex T.D.[10]
Prehist[6]
Prehist Cough Mixture 4[6]
Prehist D[6]
Pseudo-Chlor[6]
P-V-Tussin[6]
Pyribenzamine[19]
Pyrilamine Maleate Tablets[18]
Remcol-C[6]
Rescon-JR[6]
Rhinatate[6]
Rhinogesic[6]
Rhinosyn[6]
Rhinosyn-DM[6]
Rhinosyn-PD[6]
Robitussin Children's Cough
   & Cold Long-Acting[6]
Robitussin Cough & Cold
   Long-Acting[6]
Robitussin Cough & Cold
   Nighttime[12]
Robitussin with Codeine[16]
Rolatuss Expectorant[6]
Rolatuss Plain[6]
Rondec[5]
Rondec Drops[5]
Rondec-DM[5]
Rondec-DM Drops[5]
Rondec-TR[5]
R-Tannamine[6]
R-Tannamine Pediatric[6]
R-Tannate[6]
R-Tannate Pediatric[6]
Ryna[6]
Ryna-C Liquid[6]
Rynatan[6]
Rynatan Pediatric[6]
Rynatan-S Pediatric[6]
Rynatuss[6]
Rynatuss Pediatric[6]
Salphenyl[6]
Scot-Tussin DM[6]
Scot-Tussin Original 5-Action
   Cold Medicine[14]
Semprex-D[1]
Siladryl[12]
Silphen[12]
Simply Sleep[12]
Sleep-Eze 3[12]

Sominex Formula 2[12]
Sudafed PE Cold & Cough Caplets[12]
Tanoral[6]
Tavist[7]
Tavist-1[7]
Tavist Allergy/Sinus/Headache[7]
Tega-Vert[11]
Telachlor[6]
Teldrin[6]
Theraflu Cold & Cough Hot Liquid[16]
Theraflu Flu & Sore Throat Hot Liquid[16]
Theraflu Nighttime Severe Cold & Cough[12]
Theraflu Nighttime Severe Cold Hot Liquid[12]
Theraflu Thin Strips Multi Symptom[12]
Theraflu Thin Strips Nighttime Severe Cold & Cough[12]
Theraflu Thin Strips Nighttime Severe Cold & Sore Throat[12]
Theraflu Warming Relief Nighttime Severe Cold & Cough[12]
Touro A&H[5]
Travamine[11]
Triafed[20]
Triafed with Codeine[20]
Triaminic-D Multi-Symptom Cold[6]
Triaminic Flu, Cough & Fever[6]
Triaminic Night Time Cough & Cold[6]
Triaminic Softchews Cough & Runny Nose[6]
Triaminic Thin Strips Cough & Runny Nose[12]
Triaminic Thin Strips Night Time Cold & Cough[12]
Tricodene Sugar Free[6]
Trimedine Liquid[6]
Tri-Nefrin Extra Strength[6]
Triotann[6]
Triotann Pediatric[6]
Trip-Tone[11]
Tritann Pediatric[6]
Tri-Tannate[6]
Tri-Tannate Plus Pediatric[6]
Trymegen[6]
Tussanil Plain[6]
Tussar DM[6]
TussiCaps[6]
Tussi-12[18]
Tussionex[6]
Tussirex with Codeine Liquid[16]
Tusstat[12]
Twilite[12]
Tylenol Allergy Multi-Symptom[6]

Tylenol Allergy Multi-Symptom Nighttime[12]
Tylenol Cold Head Congestion Nighttime[6]
Tylenol Cold Multi-Symptom Nighttime[14]
Tylenol Cough & Sore Throat Nighttime[14]
Tylenol Severe Allergy[12]
Tylenol Sinus Congestion & Pain Nighttime[6]
Uni-Bent Cough[12]
Unisom Nighttime Sleep Aid[14]
Unisom SleepGels Maximum Strength[12]
Vanex Forte R[6]
Vanex-HD[6]
Veltane[5]
Vertab[11]
Vicks Children's NyQuil[6]
Vicks Formula 44 Custom Care Cough & Cold PM[6]
Vicks NyQuil Cold & Flu Relief[14]
Vicks NyQuil Cold & Flu Symptom Relief Plus Vitamin C[14]
Vicks NyQuil Cough[14]
Vicks NyQuil D[14]
Vicks Pediatric Formula 44m Cough & Cold Relief[6]
Viravan DM[18]
Wehamine[11]
Wehdryl[12]
Wehdryl-10[12]
Wehdryl-50[12]

ANTIHISTAMINES, PHENOTHIAZINE-DERIVATIVE

GENERIC NAMES
1. PROMETHAZINE
2. TRIMEPRAZINE

BRAND NAMES
Anergan 25[1]
Anergan 50[1]
Antinaus 50[1]
Histantil[1]
Mallergan-VC with Codeine[1]
Panectyl[2]
Penazine VC with Cough[1]
Pentazine[1]
Phenameth DM[1]
Phenameth VC with Codeine[1]
Phenazine 25[1]
Phenazine 50[1]
Phencen-50[1]
Phenergan[1]
Phenergan Fortis[1]
Phenergan Plain[1]
Phenergan VC[1]
Phenergan VC with Codeine[1]

Phenergan with Codeine[1]
Phenergan with Dextromethorphan[1]
Phenoject-50[1]
Pherazine DM[1]
Pherazine VC[1]
Pherazine VC with Codeine[1]
Pherazine with Codeine[1]
PMS Promethazine[1]
Pro-Med 50[1]
Promehist with Codeine[1]
Promerhegan[1]
Promet[1]
Prometh VC with Codeine[1]
Prometh VC Plain[1]
Prometh with Dextromethorphan[1]
Prometh-25[1]
Prometh-50[1]
Promethazine DM[1]
Promethazine VC[1]
Prorex-25[1]
Prorex-50[1]
Prothazine[1]
Prothazine Plain[1]
Shogan[1]
TV-Gan-25[1]
V-Gan-50[1]

ANTI-INFLAMMATORY DRUGS, NON-STEROIDAL (NSAIDs)

GENERIC NAMES
1. DICLOFENAC
2. DIFLUNISAL
3. ETODOLAC
4. FENOPROFEN
5. FLOCTAFENINE
6. FLURBIPROFEN
7. IBUPROFEN
8. INDOMETHACIN
9. KETOPROFEN
10. KETOROLAC
11. MECLOFENAMATE
12. MEFENAMIC ACID
13. NABUMETONE
14. NAPROXEN
15. OXAPROZIN
16. PHENYLBUTAZONE
17. PIROXICAM
18. SULINDAC
19. TENOXICAM
20. TIAPROFENIC ACID
21. TOLMETIN

BRAND NAMES
Aches-N-Pain[7]
Advil[7]
Advil Caplets[7]
Advil Chewable Tablets[7]
Advil Cold and Sinus Caplets[7]
Advil Cold and Sinus LiquiGels[7]
Advil First[7]

Advil Flu & Body Ache[7]
Advil Liqui-Gel[9]
Advil Migraine[7]
Albert Tiafen[20]
Aleve[14]
Aleve Liquid Gels[14]
Aleve-D Sinus & Cold[14]
Alka-Butazolidin[16]
Alkabutazone[16]
Alka-Phenylbutazone[16]
Alrheumat[9]
Amersol[7]
Anaprox[14]
Anaprox DS[14]
Ansaid[6]
Apo-Diclo[1]
Apo-Diflunisal[2]
Apo-Flurbiprofen[6]
Apo-Ibuprofen[7]
Apo-Indomethacin[8]
Apo-Keto[9]
Apo-Keto-E[9]
Apo-Naproxen[14]
Apo-Phenylbutazone[16]
Apo-Piroxicam[17]
Apsifen[7]
Apsifen-F[7]
Arthrotec[1]
Bayer Select Ibuprofen Caplets[7]
Bayer Select Pain Relief
  Formula Caplets[7]
Brufen[7]
Butacote[16]
Butazone[16]
Cataflam[1]
Children's Advil[7]
Children's Advil Cold[7]
Children's Motrin[7]
Clinoril[18]
CoAdvil Caplets[7]
Combunox[7]
Cotybutazone[16]
Cramp End[7]
Daypro[15]
Dimetapp Sinus Caplets[7]
Dolgesic[7]
Dolobid[2]
Dristan Sinus Caplets[7]
EC-Naprosyn[14]
Excedrin-IB Caplets[7]
Excedrin-IB Tablets[7]
Feldene[17]
Feldene Melt[17]
Fenopron[4]
Froben[6]
Froben SR[6]
Genpril[7]
Genpril Caplets[7]
Haltran[7]
Ibifon-600 Caplets[7]
Ibren[7]
Ibu[7]
Ibu-4[7]

Ibu-6[7]
Ibu-8[7]
Ibu-200[7]
Ibudone[7]
Ibumed[7]
Ibuprin[7]
Ibupro-600[7]
Ibu-Tab[7]
Ibutex[7]
Idarac[5]
Ifen[7]
Imbrilon[3]
Indameth[8]
Indocid[8]
Indocid SR[8]
Indocin SR[8]
Lodine[2]
Lodine XL[2]
Meclofen[11]
Meclomen[11]
Medipren[7]
Medipren Caplets[7]
Midol 200[7]
Midol-IB[7]
Mobiflex[19]
Motrin[7]
Motrin, Children's[7]
Motrin Cold and Flu[7]
Motrin, Infants[7]
Motrin-IB[7]
Motrin-IB Caplets[7]
Motrin-IB Cold & Sinus[7]
Motrin Migraine[7]
Nalfon[4]
Nalfon 200[4]
Naprelan[14]
Naprosyn[14]
Naprosyn-E[14]
Naprosyn-SR[14]
Naxen[14]
Novobutazone[16]
Novo-Keto-EC[9]
Novomethacin[8]
Novonaprox[14]
Novopirocam[17]
Novoprofen[7]
Novo-Sundac[18]
Nu-Indo[8]
Nu-Pirox[17]
Nuprin[7]
Nuprin Caplets[7]
Orudis[9]
Orudis-E[9]
Orudis-KT[9]
Orudis-SR[9]
Oruvail[9]
Pamprin-IB[7]
Paxofen[7]
Pedia[7]
Phenylone Plus[16]
Ponstan[12]
Ponstel[12]
Prevacid NapraPac[14]

Progesic[4]
Reprexain[7]
Rhodis[9]
Rhodis-EC[9]
Ro-Profen[7]
Rufen[7]
Saleto-200[7]
Saleto-400[7]
Saleto-600[7]
Saleto-800[7]
Sine-Aid IB[7]
Surgam[20]
Surgam SR[20]
Synflex[14]
Synflex DS[14]
Telectin DS[21]
Toradol[10]
Trendar[7]
Treximet[14]
Vicoprofen[6]
Voltaren[1]
Voltaren Rapide[1]
Voltaren SR[1]
Voltaren XR[1]
Voltarol[1]
Voltarol Retard[1]

ANTI-INFLAMMATORY DRUGS, STEROIDAL (Ophthalmic)

GENERIC NAMES
1. BETAMETHASONE
   (Ophthalmic)
2. DEXAMETHASONE
   (Ophthalmic)
3. FLUOROMETHOLONE
4. HYDROCORTISONE
   (Ophthalmic)
5. LOTEPREDNOL
6. MEDRYSONE
7. PREDNISOLONE
   (Ophthalmic)
8. RIMEXOLONE

BRAND NAMES
Ak-Pred[7]
AK-Spore H.C.[4]
AK-Tate[7]
Alrex[5]
Baldex[2]
Betnesol[1]
Cortamed[4]
Decadron[2]
Dexair[2]
Dexotic[2]
Dexsone[2]
Diodex[2]
Econopred[7]
Econopred Plus[7]
Eflone[3]
Flarex[3]
Fluor-Op[3]
FML Forte[3]

875

FML Liquifilm[3]
FML S.O.P.[3]
HMS Liquifilm[6]
Inflamase Forte[7]
Inflamase-Mild[7]
Lite-Pred[7]
Lotemax[5]
Maxidex[2]
Neotricin[4]
Ocu-Dex[2]
Ocu-Pred[7]
Ocu-Pred Forte[7]
Ocu-Pred-A[7]
PMS-Dexamethasone Sodium
   Phosphate[2]
Pred Forte[7]
Pred Mild[7]
Predair[7]
Predair Forte[7]
Predair-A[7]
Spersadex[2]
Storz-Dexa[2]
Tobradex[2]
Ultra Pred[7]
Vexol[8]
Zylet[5]

ANTISEBORRHEICS
(Topical)

GENERIC NAMES
1. CHLOROXINE
2. PYRITHIONE
3. SALICYLIC ACID, SULFUR
   & COAL TAR
4. SELENIUM SULFIDE

BRAND NAMES
Capitrol[1]
Dan-Gard[2]
DHS Zinc Dandruff Shampoo[2]
Exsel[4]
Glo-Sel[4]
Head & Shoulders[2]
Head & Shoulders Antidandruff
   Cream Shampoo Normal to
   Dry Formula[2]
Head & Shoulders Antidandruff
   Cream Shampoo Normal to
   Oily Formula[2]
Head & Shoulders Antidandruff
   Lotion Shampoo 2 in 1
   Formula[2]
Head & Shoulders Antidandruff
   Lotion Shampoo Normal to
   Dry Formula[2]
Head & Shoulders Antidandruff
   Lotion Shampoo Normal to
   Oily Formula[2]
Head & Shoulders Dry Scalp
   2 in 1 Formula Lotion
   Shampoo[2]

Head & Shoulders Dry Scalp
   Conditioning Formula Lotion
   Shampoo[2]
Head & Shoulders Dry Scalp
   Regular Formula Lotion
   Shampoo[2]
Head & Shoulders Intensive
   Treatment 2 in 1 Formula
   Dandruff Lotion Shampoo[4]
Head & Shoulders Intensive
   Treatment Conditioning
   Formula Dandruff Lotion
   Shampoo[4]
Head & Shoulders Intensive
   Treatment Regular Formula
   Dandruff Lotion Shampoo[4]
Meted Maximum Strength
   Anti-Dandruff Shampoo with
   Conditioners[3]
Sebex-T Tar Shampoo[2]
Sebulex Conditioning
   Suspension Shampoo[3]
Sebulex Lotion Shampoo[3]
Sebulon[2]
Sebutone[3]
Selsun[4]
Selsun Blue[4]
Selsun Blue Dry Formula[4]
Selsun Blue Extra
   Conditioning Formula[4]
Selsun Blue Extra Medicated
   Formula[4]
Selsun Blue Oily Formula[4]
Selsun Blue Regular Formula[4]
Tersi Foam[4]
Theraplex Z[2]
Vanseb Cream Dandruff
   Shampoo[3]
Vanseb Lotion Dandruff
   Shampoo[3]
Vanseb-T[3]
Zincon[2]
ZNP[2]

APPETITE
SUPPRESSANTS

GENERIC NAMES
1. BENZPHETAMINE
2. DIETHYLPROPION
3. MAZINDOL
4. PHENDIMETRAZINE
5. PHENTERMINE

BRAND NAMES
Adipex-P[5]
Adipost[4]
Adphen[4]
Anorex SR[4]
Anoxine-AM[5]
Appecon[4]
Bontril PDM[4]
Bontril Slow Release[4]
Dapex-37.5[5]

Didrex[1]
Dital[4]
Dyrexan-OD[4]
Fastin[5]
Ionamin[5]
Mazanor[3]
Melfiat-105 Unicelles[4]
Metra[4]
M-Orexic[2]
Obalan[4]
Obe-Del[4]
Obe-Mar[5]
Obe-Nix[5]
Obephen[5]
Obermine[5]
Obestin-30[5]
Obezine[4]
Oby-Trim[5]
Panrexin M[4]
Panrexin MTP[4]
Panshape[5]
Parzine[4]
Phendiet[4]
Phendimet[4]
Phentercot[5]
Phentra[5]
Phentride[5]
Phentrol[5]
Phenzine[4]
Plegine[4]
Prelu-2[4]
Preludin-Endurets[4]
PT 105[4]
Rexigen[4]
Rexigen Forte[4]
Sanorex[3]
Slynn-LL[4]
Statobex[4]
T-Diet[5]
Tega-Nil[4]
Tenuate[2]
Tenuate Dospan[2]
Tepanil[2]
Tepanil Ten-Tab[2]
Teramin[5]
Trimstat[4]
Trimtabs[4]
Wehless[4]
Wehless Timecelles[4]
Weightrol[4]
X-Trozine[4]
X-Trozine LA[4]
Zantryl[5]

ASPIRIN
8-Hour Bayer Timed Release
217
217 Strong
Acetylsalicylic Acid
Alka-Seltzer Original
Alka-Seltzer Morning Relief
   Medicine

Alka-Seltzer Plus Flu
  Effervescent
Alka-Seltzer PM
Alpha-Phed
Anacin
APAC Improved
APF Arthritic Pain Formula
Arthrinol
Arthrisin
Arthritis Pain Formula
Artria S.R.
A.S.A.
A.S.A. Enseals
Ascriptin
Ascriptin A/D
Aspergum
Astrin
Axotal
Bayer
Bayer Extra Strength Aspirin
Bayer Timed-Release Arthritic
  Pain Formula
Bayer Women's Caplets
  Aspirin Plus Calcium
Buffaprin
Bufferin
Buffets II
Buffinol
Butalgen
Cama Arthritis Reliever
Coryphen
Dristan Formula P
Duradyne
Easprin
Ecotrin
Empirin
Entrophen
Epromate-M
Equagesic
Equazine-M
Excedrin Back & Body
Excedrin Extra Strength Caplets
Excedrin Extra Strength Tablets
Excedrin Migraine
Extra Strength Bayer, Back &
  Body Pain
Extra Strength Bayer PM
Fasprin
Fiorgen PF
Fiorinal
Fiormor
Fortabs
Gelpirin
Gemnisyn
Goody's Extra Strength Tablets
Goody's Headache Powders
Halfprin
Headstart
Heptogesic
Isobutal
Isolin
Isollyl Improved
Laniroif

Lanorinal
Magnaprin
Magnaprin Arthritis Strength
Maprin
Marnal
Measurin
Meprogesic
Meprogesic Q
Micrainin
Nervine
Night-Time Effervescent Cold
Norwich Aspirin
Novasen
P-A-C Revised Formula
Pravigard PAC
Presalin
Riphen
Robaxisal
Sal-Adult
Salatin
Saleto
Sal-Infant
Salocol
Soma Compound
St. Joseph Adult Chewable
  Aspirin
St. Joseph Companion Aspirin
Supac
Supasa
Synalgos-DC
Tecnal
Tenol Plus
Therapy Bayer
Triaphen
Tri-Pain
Trigesic
Ursinus Inlay
Vanquis
Vibutal
Viro-Med
Zorprin

BARBITURATES
GENERIC NAMES
1. AMOBARBITAL
2. APROBARBITAL
3. BUTABARBITAL
4. BUTALBITAL
5. MEPHOBARBITAL
6. METHARBITAL
7. PENTOBARBITAL
8. PHENOBARBITAL
9. SECOBARBITAL
10. SECOBARBITAL &
  AMOBARBITAL
11. TALBUTAL

BRAND NAMES
Alurate[2]
Amaphen[4]
Amytal[1]
Ancalixir[8]
Anolor-300[4]

Anoquan[4]
Arcet[4]
Axotal[4]
Bancap[4]
Barbita[8]
Bucet[4]
Busodium[3]
Butace[4]
Butalan[3]
Butalgen[4]
Butisol[3]
Cafergot PB[7]
Dolmar[4]
Endolor[4]
Esgic[4]
Esgic-Plus4[1]
Ezol[4]
Femcet[4]
Fiorgen PF[4]
Fioricet[4]
Fiorinal[4]
Fiormor[4]
Fortabs[4]
G-1[4]
Gemonil[6]
Isobutal[4]
Isocet[4]
Isolin[4]
Isollyl Improved[4]
Isopap[4]
Laniroif[4]
Lanorinal[4]
Luminal[8]
Marnal[4]
Mebaral[5]
Medigesic[4]
Nembutal[7]
Nova Rectal[7]
Novopentobarb[7]
Novosecobarb[9]
Pacaps[4]
Phrenilin[4]
Phrenilin Forte[4]
Repan[4]
Sarisol No. 2[3]
Seconal[9]
Sedapap[4]
Solfoton[8]
Tecnal[4]
Tencet[4]
Theodrine[8]
Theodrine Pediatric[8]
Theofed[8]
Triad[4]
Triaprin[4]
Tuinal[10]
Two-Dyne[4]
Vibutal[4]

BARBITURATES, ASPIRIN & CODEINE
(Also contains caffeine)

GENERIC NAMES
1. BUTALBITAL, ASPIRIN & CODEINE
2. PHENOBARBITAL, ASPIRIN & CODEINE

BRAND NAMES
Ascomp with Codeine No. 3[1]
B-A-C with Codeine[1]
Butalbital Compound with Codeine[1]
Butinal with Codeine No. 3[1]
Fiorgen with Codeine[1]
Fiorinal with Codeine[1]
Fiorinal with Codeine No. 3[1]
Fiorinal-C1/4[1]
Fiorinal-C1/2[1]
Fiormor with Codeine[1]
Idenal with Codeine[1]
Isollyl with Codeine[1]
Phenaphen with Codeine No. 2[2]
Phenaphen with Codeine No. 3[2]
Phenaphen with Codeine No. 4[2]

BELLADONNA ALKALOIDS & BARBITURATES

GENERIC NAMES
1. ATROPINE & PHENOBARBITAL
2. ATROPINE, HYOSCYAMINE, SCOPOLAMINE & BUTABARBITAL
3. ATROPINE, HYOSCYAMINE, SCOPOLAMINE & PHENOBARBITAL
4. BELLADONNA & AMOBARBITAL
5. BELLADONNA & BUTABARBITAL
6. BELLADONNA & PHENOBARBITAL
7. HYOSCYAMINE & PHENOBARBITAL

BRAND NAMES
Antrocol[1]
Barbidonna[3]
Barbidonna 2[3]
Barophen[3]
Belladenal[7]
Belladenal Spacetabs[6]
Belladenal-S[7]
Bellalphen[3]
Butibel[5]
Chardonna-2[6]
Donnamor[3]
Donnapine[3]
Donna-Sed[6]
Donnatal[3]

Donnatal Elixir[3]
Donnatal Extentabs[3]
Donnatal No. 2[3]
Donphen[3]
Hyosophen[3]
Kinesed[3]
Levsin with Phenobarbital[6]
Levsinex with Phenobarbital Timecaps[7]
Levsin-PB[7]
Malatal[3]
Pheno-Bella[6]
Relaxadon[3]
Spaslin[3]
Spasmolin[3]
Spasmophen[3]
Spasquid[3]
Susano[3]

BENZODIAZEPINES

GENERIC NAMES
1. ALPRAZOLAM
2. BROMAZEPAM
3. CHLORDIAZEPOXIDE
4. CLONAZEPAM
5. CLORAZEPATE
6. DIAZEPAM
7. ESTAZOLAM
8. FLURAZEPAM
9. HALAZEPAM
10. KETAZOLAM
11. LORAZEPAM
12. MIDAZOLAM
13. NITRAZEPAM
14. OXAZEPAM
15. PRAZEPAM
16. QUAZEPAM
17. TEMAZEPAM

BRAND NAMES
Alprazolam Intensol[1]
Apo-Alpraz[1]
Apo-Chlordiazepoxide[3]
Apo-Clorazepate[5]
Apo-Diazepam[6]
Apo-Flurazepam[8]
Apo-Lorazepam[11]
Apo-Oxazepam[14]
Ativan[17]
Centrax[15]
Clindex[3]
Clinoxide[3]
Dalmane[8]
Diastat[6]
Diazemuls[6]
Diazepam Intensol[6]
Doral[16]
Klonopin[4]
Lectopam[2]
Librax[3]
Libritabs[3]
Librium[3]
Lidoxide[3]

Limbitrol[3]
Limbitrol DS[3]
Lipoxide[3]
Loftran[16]
Lorazepam Intensol[11]
Medilium[3]
Meval[6]
Mogadon[15]
Niravam[1]
Niravam Orally Disintegrating Tablets[1]
Novo-Alprazol[1]
Novoclopate[5]
Novodipam[6]
Novoflupam[8]
Novolorazem[11]
Novopoxide[3]
Novoxapam[14]
Nu-Alpraz[1]
Nu-Loraz[11]
Paxipam[9]
PMS Diazepam[6]
Restoril[17]
Rivotril[4]
Serax[14]
Solium[3]
Somnol[8]
T-Quil[6]
Tranxene[5]
Tranxene T-Tab[5]
Tranxene-SD[5]
Valium[6]
Valrelease[6]
Vivol[6]
Xanax[1]
Xanax XR[1]
Zapex[14]
Zebrax[3]
Zetran[6]

BENZOYL PEROXIDE

Acanya
Acetoxyl 2.5 Gel
Acetoxyl 5 Gel
Acetoxyl 10 Gel
Acetoxyl 20 Gel
Acne-5 Lotion
Acne-10 Lotion
Acne-Aid 10 Cream
Acne-Mask
Acnomel B.P. 5 Lotion
Ben-Aqua 2 1/2 Gel
Ben-Aqua 2 1/2 Lotion
Ben-Aqua 5 Gel
Ben-Aqua 5 Lotion
Ben-Aqua 10 Gel
Ben-Aqua 10 Lotion
Ben-Aqua Masque 5
Benoxyl 5 Lotion
Benoxyl 5 Wash
Benoxyl 10 Lotion
Benoxyl 10 Wash

Benoxyl 20 Lotion
Benzac Ac 2½ Gel
Benzac Ac 5 Gel
Benzac Ac 10 Gel
Benzac W 2½ Gel
Benzac W 5 Gel
Benzac W 10 Gel
Benzaclin
Benzagel 5 Acne Lotion
Benzagel 5 Acne Wash
Benzagel 5 Gel
Benzagel 10 Gel
Benzamycin
BenzaShave 5 Cream
BenzaShave 10 Cream
Brevoxyl 4 Gel
Buf-Oxal 10
Cleanse and Treat
Clear By Design 2.5 Gel
Clearasil BP Plus 5 Cream
Clearasil BP Plus 5 Lotion
Clearasil Maximum Strength
  Medicated Anti-Acne 10
  Tinted Cream
Clearasil Maximum Strength
  Medicated Anti-Acne 10
  Vanishing Cream
Clearasil Medicated Anti-Acne
  10 Vanishing Lotion
Cuticura Acne 5 Cream
Del-Aqua-5 Gel
Del-Aqua-10 Gel
Del-Ray
Dermoxyl 2.5 Gel
Dermoxyl 5 Gel
Dermoxyl 10 Gel
Dermoxyl 20 Gel
Dermoxyl Aqua
Desquam-E 2.5 Gel
Desquam-E 5 Gel
Desquam-E 10 Gel
Desquam-X 2.5 Gel
Desquam-X 5 Gel
Desquam-X 5 Wash
Desquam-X 10 Gel
Desquam-X 10 Wash
Dry and Clear 5 Lotion
Dry and Clear Double Strength
  10 Cream
Dryox 5 Gel
Dryox 10 Gel
Dryox 20 Gel
Dryox Wash 5
Dryox Wash 10
Duac Topical Gel
Epiduo
Fostex 5 Gel
Fostex 10 Bar
Fostex 10 Cream
Fostex 10 Gel
Fostex 10 Wash
H₂Oxyl 2.5 Gel
H₂Oxyl 5 Gel

H₂Oxyl 10 Gel
H₂Oxyl 20 Gel
Inova 8/2 ACT
Loroxide 5 Lotion with Flesh
  Tinted Base
Loroxide 5.5 Lotion
NeoBenz Micro
Neutrogena Acne Mask 5
Noxzema Clear-Ups Maximum
  Strength 10
Noxzema Clear-Ups On-the-
  Spot 10 Lotion
Oxy 5 Tinted Lotion
Oxy 5 Vanishing Formula
  Lotion
Oxy 5 Vanishing Lotion
Oxy 10
Oxy 10 Daily Face Wash
Oxy 10 Tinted Lotion
Oxy 10 Vanishing Lotion
Oxyderm 5 Lotion
Oxyderm 10 Lotion
Oxyderm 20 Lotion
PanOxyl 5 Bar
PanOxyl 5 Gel
PanOxyl 10 Bar
PanOxyl 10 Gel
PanOxyl 15 Gel
PanOxyl 20 Gel
PanOxyl AQ 2½ Gel
PanOxyl AQ 5 Gel
Persa-Gel 5
Persa-Gel 10
Persa-Gel W 5
Persa-Gel W 10
pHisoAc BP 10
Propa P.H. 10 Acne Cover Stick
Propa P.H. 10 Liquid Acne Soap
Stri-Dex Maximum Strength
  Treatment 10 Cream
Theroxide 5 Lotion
Theroxide 10 Lotion
Theroxide 10 Wash
Topex 5 Lotion
Topex 10 Lotion
Vanoxide 5 Lotion
Xerac BP 5 Gel
Xerac BP 10 Gel
Zeroxin-5 Gel
Zeroxin-10 Gel
Zoderrm
Zoderm Ready Pads

BETA-ADRENERGIC BLOCKING AGENTS

GENERIC NAMES
1. ACEBUTOLOL
2. ATENOLOL
3. BETAXOLOL
4. BISOPROLOL
5. CARTEOLOL
6. CARVEDILOL
7. LABETALOL
8. LEVOBETAXOLOL
9. METOPROLOL
10. NADOLOL
11. NEBIVOLOL
12. OXPRENOLOL
13. PENBUTOLOL
14. PINDOLOL
15. PROPRANOLOL
16. SOTALOL
17. TIMOLOL

BRAND NAMES
Apo-Atenolol[2]
Apo-Metoprolol[9]
Apo-Propranolol[15]
Apo-Timol[17]
Betaloc[9]
Betaxon[8]
Betapace[16]
Bystolic[11]
Blocadren[17]
Cartrol[5]
Coreg[6]
Coreg CR[6]
Corgard[10]
Detensol[15]
Inderal[15]
Inderal LA[15]
Kerlone[3]
Levatol[13]
Lopressor[9]
Lopressor SR[9]
Monitan[1]
Normodyne[7]
Novo-Atenol[2]
Novometoprol[9]
Novo-Pindol[14]
Novopranol[15]
Novo-Timol[17]
NuMetop[9]
Sectral[1]
Slow-Trasicor[12]
Sotacor[16]
Syn-Nadolol[10]
Syn-Pindolol[14]
Tenormin[2]
Toprol[9]
Toprol XL[9]
Toprol XL-XR[9]
Trandate[7]
Trasicor[12]
Visken[14]
Zebeta[4]

BETA-ADRENERGIC BLOCKING AGENTS & THIAZIDE DIURETICS

GENERIC NAMES
1. ATENOLOL &
   CHLORTHALIDONE
2. BETAXOLOL &
   CHLORTHALIDONE

3. BISOPROLOL &
   HYDROCHLOROTHIAZIDE
4. LABETALOL &
   HYDROCHLOROTHIAZIDE
5. METOPROLOL &
   HYDROCHLOROTHIAZIDE
6. NADOLOL &
   BENDROFLUMETHIAZIDE
7. PINDOLOL &
   HYDROCHLOROTHIAZIDE
8. PROPRANOLOL &
   HYDROCHLOROTHIAZIDE
9. TIMOLOL &
   HYDROCHLOROTHIAZIDE

BRAND NAMES
Co-Betaloc[5]
Corzide[6]
Inderide[8]
Inderide LA[8]
Kerledex[2]
Lopressor HCT[5]
Normozide[4]
Tenoretic[1]
Timolide[9]
Trandate HCT[4]
Viskazide[7]
Ziac[3]

BRONCHODILATORS, ADRENERGIC

GENERIC NAMES
1. ALBUTEROL
2. ARFORMOTEROL
3. BITOLTEROL
4. EPHEDRINE SULFATE
5. EPINEPHRINE
6. ETHYLNOREPINEPHRINE
7. FENOTEROL
8. FORMOTEROL
9. ISOPROTERENOL
10. LEVALBUTEROL
11. METAPROTERENOL
12. PIRBUTEROL
13. PROCATEROL
14. RACEPINEPHRINE
15. SALMETEROL
16. TERBUTALINE

BRAND NAMES
Accuneb[1]
Adrenalin[5]
Advair Diskus[15]
Advair HFA[15]
Alupent[11]
Ana-Guard[5]
Arm-a-Med Metaproterenol[11]
AsthmaHaler[5]
AsthmaNefrin[5]
Berotec[7]
Brethaire[16]
Brethine[16]
Bricanyl[16]

Bronkaid Mist[5]
Bronkaid Mist Suspension[5]
Bronkaid Mistometer[5]
Brovana[3]
Combivent[1]
Dey-Dose Isoproterenol[9]
Dey-Dose Metaproterenol[11]
Dey-Dose Racepinephrine[14]
Dey-Lute Metaproterenol[11]
Dispos-a-Med Isoproterenol[9]
Duoneb[1]
Ephed II[4]
EpiPen Auto-Injector[5]
EpiPen Jr. Auto-Injector[5]
Foradil Aerolizer[8]
Foradil Certihaler[8]
Isuprel[9]
Isuprel Glossets[9]
Isuprel Mistometer[9]
Maxair[12]
Medihaler-Epi[5]
Medihaler-Iso[9]
microNEFRIN[14]
Nephron[5]
Novosalmol[1]
Perforomist Inhalation
   Solution[8]
Primatene Mist[5]
Primatene Mist Suspension[5]
Pro-Air[13]
Proventil[1]
Proventil HFA[1]
Proventil Repetabs[1]
Serevent[15]
Serevent Diskus[15]
Symbicort[8]
Tornalate[3]
Vapo-Iso[9]
Ventolin HFA[1]
Ventolin Rotocaps[1]
Volmax[1]
Xopenex[10]
Xopenex HFA[10]

BRONCHODILATORS, XANTHINE

GENERIC NAMES
1. AMINOPHYLLINE
2. DYPHILLINE
3. OXTRIPHYLLINE
4. THEOPHYLLINE

BRAND NAMES
Accurbron[4]
Aerolate III[4]
Aerolate Jr.[4]
Aerolate Sr.[4]
Aerophyllin[1]
Aminophyllin[1]
Ami Rax[4]
Apo-Oxtriphylline[3]
Aquaphyllin[4]
Asbron G[4]

Asbron G Inlay Tablets[4]
Asmalix[4]
Bronchial[4]
Broncomar GG[4]
Bronkodyl[4]
Choledyl[3]
Choledyl Delayed-Release[3]
Choledyl SA[3]
Constant-T[4]
Corophyllin[1]
Dilor[2]
Dilor-400[2]
Duraphyl[4]
Dyflex 200[2]
Dyflex 400[2]
Ed-Bron G[4]
Elixicon[4]
Elixomin[1]
Elixophyllin[4]
Elixophyllin GG[4]
Elixophyllin SR[4]
Equibron G[4]
Glyceryl T[4]
Lanophyllin[4]
Lixolin[4]
Lufyllin[4]
Lufyllin-400[2]
Marax[4]
Marax D.F.[4]
Mudrane GG2[4]
Neothylline[2]
Novotriphyl[3]
Palaron[1]
Phyllocontin[1]
Phyllocontin-350[1]
PMS Theophylline[4]
Protophylline[2]
Pulmophylline[4]
Quibron[4]
Quibron 300[4]
Quibron-T[4]
Quibron-T Dividose[4]
Quibron-T/SR[4]
Quibron-T/SR Dividose[4]
Respbid[4]
Slo-Bid[4]
Slo-bid Gyrocaps[4]
Slo-phyllin[4]
Slo-Phyllin GG[4]
Slo-Phyllin Gyrocaps[4]
Solu-Phyllin[4]
Somophyllin[1]
Somophyllin-12[1]
Somophyllin-CRT[1]
Somophyllin-DF[1]
Somophyllin-T[1]
Sustaire[4]
Synophylate[4]
Theo-24[4]
Theobid Duracaps[4]
Theobid Jr. Duracaps[4]
Theochron[4]
Theoclear L.A. 130 Cenules[4]

Theoclear L.A. 260 Cenules[4]
Theoclear-80[4]
Theocot[4]
Theo-Dur[4]
Theo-Dur Sprinkle[4]
Theolair[4]
Theolair-SR[4]
Theolate[4]
Theomar[4]
Theon[4]
Theophylline SR[4]
Theo-Sav[4]
Theospan SR[4]
Theo-SR[4]
Theostat[4]
Theostat 80[4]
Theo-Time[4]
Theovent Long-acting[4]
Theox[4]
Thylline[2]
T-Phyl[4]
Truphylline[1]
Truxophyllin[4]
Unidur[4]
Uniphyl[4]

CAFFEINE

222
282
292
692
Actamin Super
Alka-Seltzer Morning Relief
Amaphen
Anacin
Anacin with Codeine
Anolor-300
Anoquan
A.P.C.
Aspirin Free Bayer Select
   Maximum Strength Headache
   Pain Relief Caplets
Aspirin-Free Excedrin Caplets
Cafergot
Cafergot PB
Cafertine
Cafetrate
Caffedrine
Caffefrine Caplets
Citrated Caffeine
Cotanal 65
Darvon-N Compound
Dexitac
Dristan AF
Dristan AF Plus
Dristan Formula P
Enerjets
Ercaf
Ergo-Caff
Esgic
Esgic-Plus
Excedrin Caplets

Excedrin Extra Strength
   Caplets
Excedrin Extra Strength
   Tablets
Excedrin Migraine
Excedrin Tension Headache
Extra Strength Bayer Back &
   Body Pain
Fendol
Fiorinal
Gotamine
Keep Alert
Kolephrin
Lucidex
Migergot
Novo-AC and C
Omnicol
P-A-C Revised Formula
Pacaps
PC-Cap
Pep-Back
Propoxyphene Compound-65
Quick Pep
Repan
S-A-C
Salatin
Saleto
Saleto-D
Salocol
Scot-tussin Original 5-Action
   Cold Medicine
Sinapils
Snap Back
Supac
Synalgos-DC
Tirend
Trigesic
Two-Dyne
Vanquish
Vivarin
Wake-Up
Wigraine

CALCIUM CHANNEL BLOCKERS

GENERIC NAMES
1. AMLODIPINE
2. BEPRIDIL
3. DILTIAZEM
4. FELODIPINE
5. FLUNARIZINE
6. ISRADIPINE
7. NICARDIPINE
8. NIFEDIPINE
9. NISOLDIPINE
10. VERAPAMIL

BRAND NAMES
Adalat[8]
Adalat CC[8]
Adalat FT[8]
Adalat P.A.[8]
Apo-Diltiaz[3]

Apo-Nifed[8]
Apo-Verap[10]
Azor[1]
Bepadin[2]
Caduet[1]
Calan[10]
Calan SR[10]
Cardene[7]
Cardene SR[7]
Cardizem[3]
Cardizem CD[3]
Cardizem LA[3]
Cardizem SR[3]
Cartia XT[3]
Chronovera[10]
Dilacor-XR[3]
Dyna Circ[6]
Exforge[1]
Isoptin[10]
Isoptin SR[10]
Ketorolac[3]
Lotrel[1]
Nifedical[3]
Norvasc[1]
Novo-Diltiazem[3]
Novo-Nifedin[8]
Novo-Veramil[10]
Nu-Diltiaz[3]
Nu-Nifed[8]
Nu-Verap[10]
Plendil[4]
Procardia[8]
Procardia XL[8]
Renedil[4]
Sibelium[5]
Sular[9]
Syn-Diltiazem[3]
Tarka[10]
Teczem[3]
Tiazac[3]
Vascor[2]
Verelan[10]
Verelan PM[10]

CALCIUM SUPPLEMENTS

GENERIC NAMES
1. CALCIUM CARBONATE
2. CALCIUM CITRATE
3. CALCIUM GLUBIONATE
4. CALCIUM GLUCONATE
5. CALCIUM
   GLYCEROPHOSPHATE &
   CALCIUM LACTATE
6. CALCIUM LACTATE
7. DIBASIC CALCIUM
   PHOSPHATE
8. TRIBASIC CALCIUM
   PHOSPHATE

BRAND NAMES
Actonel with Calcium[1]
Apo-Cal[1]

Bayer Women's Caplets Plus
  Calcium[1]
BioCal[1]
Calcarb 600[1]
Calci-Chew[1]
Calciday 667[1]
Calcilac[1]
Calcite 500[1]
Calcium Carbonate/600[1]
Calcium Stanley[4]
Calcium-600[1]
Calcium-Sandoz[3]
Calcium-Sandoz Forte[1,6]
Calglycine[1]
Calphosan[5]
Calsan[1]
Cal-sap[3]
Caltrate[1]
Caltrate-300[1]
Caltrate-600[1]
Caltrate Chewable[1]
Children's Pepto[1]
Chooz[1]
Citracal[2]
Citracal Liquitabs[2]
Gencalc 600[1]
Gramcal[1,6]
Mallamint[1]
Neo-Calglucon[3]
Nephro-Calci[1]
NutraCal[3]
Os-Cal[1]
Os-Cal 500[1]
Os-Cal Chewable[1]
Oysco[1]
Oysco 500 Chewable[1]
Oyst-Cal[1]
Oyst-Cal 500 Chewable[1]
Oystercal 500[1]
Posture[8]
Rolaids-Calcium Rich[1]
Titralac[1]
Tums[1]
Tums E-X[1]

COAL TAR (Topical)

Alphosyl
Aquatar
Balnetar
Balnetar Therapeutic Tar Bath
Cutar Water Dispersible
  Emollient Tar
Denorex
Denorex Extra Strength
  Medicated Shampoo
Denorex Extra Strength
  Medicated Shampoo with
  Conditioners
Denorex Medicated Shampoo
Denorex Medicated Shampoo
  and Conditioner

Denorex Mountain Fresh Herbal
  Scent Medicated Shampoo
DHS Tar Gel Shampoo
DHS Tar Shampoo
Doak Oil
Doak Oil Forte
Doak Oil Forte Therapeutic
  Bath Treatment
Doak Oil Therapeutic Bath
  Treatment For All-Over Body
  Care
Doak Tar Lotion
Doak Tar Shampoo
Doctar
Doctar Hair & Scalp Shampoo
  & Conditioner
Estar
Fototar
Ionil-T Plus
Lavatar
Liquor Carbonis Detergens
Medotar
Pentrax Extra-Strength
  Therapeutic Tar Shampoo
Pentrax Tar Shampoo
Psorent
psoriGel
PsoriNail
Scytera Foam
Tar Doak
Taraphilic
Tarbonis
Tarpaste
Tarpaste Doak
T/Derm Tar Emollient
Tegrin Lotion for Psoriasis
Tegrin Medicated Cream
  Shampoo
Tegrin Medicated Shampoo
  Concentrated Gel
Tegrin Medicated Shampoo
  Extra Conditioning Formula
Tegrin Medicated Shampoo
  Herbal Formula
Tegrin Medicated Shampoo
  Original Formula
Tegrin Medicated Soap for
  Psoriasis
Tegrin Skin Cream for Psoriasis
Tersa-Tar Mild Therapeutic
  Shampoo with Protein and
  Conditioner
Tersa-Tar Soapless Tar
  Shampoo
Tersa-Tar Therapeutic Shampoo
T-Gel
T/Gel Therapeutic Conditioner
T/Gel Therapeutic Shampoo
Theraplex T Shampoo
Zetar
Zetar Emulsion
Zetar Medicated
  Antiseborrheic Shampoo

CONTRACEPTIVES, ORAL & SKIN

GENERIC NAMES
1. DESOGESTREL & ETHINYL
   ESTRADIOL
2. DROSPERINONE &
   ETHINYL ESTRADIOL
3. ETHYNODIOL DIACETATE &
   ETHINYL ESTRADIOL
4. LEVONORGESTREL &
   ETHINYL ESTRADIOL
5. NORELGESTROMIN &
   ETHINYL ESTRADIOL
6. NORETHINDRONE &
   ETHINYL ESTRADIOL
7. NORETHINDRONE &
   MESTRANOL
8. NORETHINDRONE ACETATE
   & ETHINYL ESTRADIOL
9. NORGESTIMATE & ETHINYL
   ESTRADIOL
10. NORGESTREL & ETHINYL
    ESTRADIOL

BRAND NAMES
Alesse[4]
Apri[1]
Aviane[4]
Brevicon[6]
Brevicon 0.5/35[6]
Brevicon 1/35[6]
Cyclen[9]
Cyclessa[1]
Demulen 1/35[3]
Demulen 1/50[3]
Demulen 30[3]
Demulen 50[3]
Desogen 28[1]
Desogen Ortho-Cept[1]
Estrostep[8]
Estrostep Fe[8]
Femcon Fe[6]
GenCept 0.5/35[6]
GenCept 1/35[6]
GenCept 10/11[6]
Genora 0.5/35[6]
Genora 1/35[6]
Genora 1/50[7]
Jenest-28[6]
Levlen[4]
Levlite[4]
Levora[4]
Loestrin 1/20[8]
Loestrin 1.5/30[8]
Loestrin 24 Fe[8]
Lo/Ovral[10]
LoSeasonique[4]
Lybrel[4]
Marvelon[1]
Microgestin Fe[6]
Minestrin 1/20[8]
Min-Ovral[4]
Mircette[1]

ModiCon[6]
Necon 0.5/35-21[6]
Necon 0.5/35-28[6]
Necon 1/35-21[6]
Necon 1/35-28[6]
Necon 1/50-21[7]
Necon 1/50-28[7]
Necon 10/11-21[6]
Necon 10/11-28[6]
N.E.E. 1/35[6]
N.E.E. 1/50[6]
Nelova 0.5/35E[6]
Nelova 1/35E[6]
Nelova 1/50M[7]
Nelova 10/11[6]
Nelulen 1/35E[3]
Nelulen 1/50E[3]
Norcept-E 1/35[8]
Nordette[4]
Norethin 1/35E[6]
Norethin 1/50M[7]
Norinyl 1+35[6]
Norinyl 1+50[7]
Norinyl 1/50[7]
Norlestrin 1/50[8]
Norlestrin 2.5/50[8]
Ortho 0.5/35[6]
Ortho 1/35[6]
Ortho 7/7/7[6]
Ortho 10/11[6]
Ortho-Cept[1]
Ortho-Cyclen[9]
Orthro Evra[5]
Ortho-Novum 0.5[6]
Ortho-Novum 1/35[6]
Ortho-Novum 1/50[7]
Ortho-Novum 1/80[7]
Ortho-Novum 2[6]
Ortho-Novum 7/7/7[6]
Ortho-Novum 10/11[6]
Ortho-Tri-Cyclen 21[7]
Ortho-Tri-Cyclen 28[7]
Orthr-Tri-Cyclen Lo[9]
Ovcon-35[6]
Ovcon-50[6]
Ovral[10]
Previfem[9]
Seasonale[4]
Seasonique[4]
Symphasic[6]
Tri-Cyclen[9]
Tri-Levlen[4]
Tri-Norinyl[6]
Tri-Previfem[9]
Tri-Sprintec[9]
Triphasil[4]
Triquilar[4]
Trivora[4]
Yasmin[2]
Yaz[2]
Zovia 1/35E[3]
Zovia 1/50E[3]

CONTRACEPTIVES, VAGINAL

GENERIC NAMES
1. BENZALKONIUM CHLORIDE
2. ETONOGESTREL & ETHINYL ESTRADIOL
3. NONOXYNOL 9
4. OCTOXYNOL 9

BRAND NAMES
Advantage 24[3]
Because[3]
Conceptrol Gel[3]
Conceptrol-Contraceptive Inserts[3]
Delfen[3]
Emko[3]
Encare[3]
Gynol II Extra Strength[3]
Gynol II Original Formula[3]
Koromex Cream[3]
Koromex Crystal Gel[3]
Koromex Foam[3]
Koromex Jelly[3]
K-Y Plus[3]
NuvaRing[2]
Ortho-Creme[3]
Ortho-Gynol[4]
Pharmatex[1]
Pre-Fil[3]
Ramses Contraceptive Foam[3]
Ramses Contraceptive Vaginal Jelly[3]
Ramses Crystal Clear Gel[3]
Semicid[3]
Shur-Seal[3]
VCF[3]

DEXTROMETHORPHAN
2/G-DM Cough
Alka-Seltzer Plus Cold & Cough Effervescent
Alka-Seltzer Plus Cold & Cough Liquid
Alka-Seltzer Plus Cold & Cough Liquid-Gels
Alka-Seltzer Plus Day & Night Effervescent
Alka-Seltzer Plus Day & Night Liquid Gels
Alka-Seltzer Plus Day Cold Liquid
Alka-Seltzer Plus Flu Effervescent
Alka-Seltzer Plus Nighttime Cold Liquid
Alka-Seltzer Plus Night-Time Effervescent
Alka-Seltzer Plus Night-Time Liquid-Gels
All-Nite Cold Formula

Ambenyl-D Decongestant Cough Formula
Anatuss DM
Anti-Tuss DM Expectorant
Balminil DM
Baytussin DM
Benylin All-In-One Cold & Flu Caplets
Benylin All-In-One Cold & Flu Nightime Syrup
Benylin All-In-One Cold & Flu Syrup
Benylin All-In-One Day & Night Caplets
Benylin DM 12 Hour Nightime Cough Syrup
Benylin DM-D
Benylin DM-D for Children Cough & Cold Syrup
Benylin DM-D-E
Benylin DM-E Chest Cough Syrup
Benylin DM-D-E Extra Strength
Benylin DM-E
Benylin DM-E Chest Cough Syrup
Bromfed-DM
Broncho-Grippol-DM
Carbodec DM Drops
Cerose-DM
Cheracol D Cough
Children's Benylin DM-D
Children's Formula Cough
Children's Hold
Children's Pediacare Chewables
Children's Tylenol Plus Cold & Cough
Children's Tylenol Plus Cough & Runny Nose
Children's Tylenol Plus Cough & Sore Throat
Children's Tylenol Plus Flu
Children's Tylenol Plus Multi-Symptom Plus Cold
Codimal DM
Codistan No. 1
Colrex Cough
Conar
Conar Expectorant
Conar-A
Concentrin
Congespirin
Contac Night Caplets
Contac Severe Cold Formula
Contac Severe Cold Formula Night Strength
Coricidin HBP
Coricidin HBP Chest Congestion & Cough
Cough X
Creo-Terpin
Delsym
Delsym Grape for Adults

Delsym Grape for Children
Diabetic Tussin Cold & Flu
Diabetic Tussin DM
Diabetic Tussin Night Time
 Formula
Dimetapp Children's Elixir
 Cold & Allergy PE
Dimetapp Children's Long
 Acting Cough Plus Cold
DM Cough
DM Syrup
Donatussin
Dondril
Dristan Cold and Flu
Dristan Juice Mix-in Cold, Flu,
 & Cough
Drixoral Cough
Efficol Cough Whip (Cough
 Suppressant/Decongestant)
Efficol Cough Whip (Cough
 Suppressant/Expectorant)
Extra Action Cough
Father John's Medicine Plus
Genatuss DM
Glycotuss-dM
Guiamid D.M. Liquid
Guiatuss-DM
Halotussin-DM Expectorant
Histalet-DM
Hold
Humibid DM Sprinkle
Improved Sino-Tuss
Koffex
Kolephrin GG/DM
Kolephrin/DM Caplets
Kophane Cough and Cold
 Formula
Maximum Strength Mucinex
 DM
Meda Syrup Forte
Medatussin
Mediquell
Mucinex Children's Cough,
 Expectorant & Suppressant
Mucinex Cough Mini-Melts
Mytussin DM
Naldecon Senior DX
Naldecon-DX
NeoCitran DM Coughs & Colds
Neo-DM
Nytcold Medicine
Omnicol
Ornex DM 15
Ornex DM 30
Ornex Severe Cold No
 Drowsiness Caplets
Par Glycerol-DM
PediaCare Long-Acting
 Cough Liquid
Pertussin All Night CS
Pertussin All Night PM
Pertussin Cough Suppressant
Pertussin CS

Pertussin ES
Phanatuss
Phenameth DM
Phenergan with
 Dextromethorphan
Pherazine DM
Prometh with
 Dextromethorphan
Promethazine DM
Queltuss
Remcol-C
Rhinosyn-DM
Rhinosyn-DMX Expectorant
Rhinosyn-X
Robafen DM
Robidex
Robitussin Children's Cough
 Long-Acting
Robitussin Children's Cough
 & Cold Long-Acting
Robitussin Cough & Cold CF
Robitussin Cough & Cold D
Robitussin Cough & Cold
 Long-Acting
Robitussin Cough & Chest
 Congestion
Robitussin Cough & Chest
 Congestion DM
Robitussin Cough & Chest
 Congestion DM Max
Robitussin Cough & Chest
 Congestion Sugar Free DM
Robitussin Cough Cold &
 Flu Nighttime
Robitussin Cough Gels
 Long Acting
Robitussin Cough
 Long Acting
Rondec-DM
Rondec-DM Drops
Ru-Tuss Expectorant
SafeTussin 30
Scot-Tussin DM
Sedatuss
Silexin Cough
Simply Cough
Snaplets-DM
Snaplets-Multi
St. Joseph Cough
 Suppressant for Children
Sucrets Cough Control
Sudafed Multi-Symptom Cold
 & Cough
Sudafed PE Cold & Cough
 Caplets
Suppress Cough with
 Dextromethorphan
Terphan
Theracof Plus Multi-Symptom
 Cough and Cold Reliever
Theraflu Cold & Cough
 Hot Liquid

Theraflu Daytime Severe Cold
 Caplets
Theraflu Daytime Severe Cold
 Caplets
Theraflu Nighttime Severe
 Cold Caplets
Theraflu Thin Strips Daytime
 Cold & Cough
Theraflu Warming Relief
 Daytime
Tolu-Sed DM Cough
Touro DM
Triaminic Cough & Sore
 Throat
Triaminic-D Multi-Symptom
 Cold
Triaminic Day Time Cold &
 Cough
Triaminic Flu, Cough & Fever
Triaminic Long Acting Cough
Triaminic Softchews Cough
 & Runny Nose
Triaminic Softchews Cough
 & Sore Throat
Triaminic Thin Strips
 Daytime Cold & Cough
Triaminic Thin Strips Long
 Acting Cough
Tricodene Sugar Free
Trimedine Liquid
Trocal
Tussar DM
Tuss-DM
Tussi-Bid
Tylenol Cold Head Congestion
 Nighttime
Tylenol Cold Head Congestion
 Severe
Tylenol Cold Multi Symptom
 Daytime
Tylenol Cold Multi Symptom
 Nighttime
Tylenol Cold Multi Symptom
 Severe
Tylenol Cough & Severe
 Congestion Daytime
Tylenol Cough & Sore Throat
 Daytime
Tylenol Cough & Sore Throat
 Nighttime
Tylenol Sinus Severe
 Congestion Daytime
Uni-Tussin DM
Unproco
Vicks Children's NyQuil
Vicks DayQuil Cold/Flu Relief
Vicks DayQuil Cold & Flu
 Symptom Relief Plus
 Vitamin C
Vicks DayQuil Cough
Vicks Formula 44 Custom
 Care Chesty Cough

Vicks Formula 44 Custom
  Care Congestion
Vicks Formula 44 Custom
  Care Cough & Cold PM
Vicks Formula 44 Custom
  Care Dry Cough Suppressant
Vicks NyQuil Cold & Flu Relief
Vicks NyQuil Cold & Flu
  Symptom Relief Plus
  Vitamin C
Vicks NyQuil Cough
Vicks NyQuil D
Vicks Pediatric Formula 44e
  Cough & Chest Congestion
  Relief
Vicks Pediatric Formula 44m
  Cough & Cold Relief
Viravan DM

DICYCLOMINE

Antispas
A-Spas
Bentyl
Bentylol
Byclomine
Dibent
Di-Cyclonex
Dilomine
Di-Spaz
Forulex
Lomine
Neoquess
Or-Tyl
Protylol
Spasmoban
Spasmoject
Viscerol

DIURETICS, THIAZIDE

GENERIC NAMES
1. BENDROFLUMETHIAZIDE
2. BENZTHIAZIDE
3. CHLOROTHIAZIDE
4. CHLORTHALIDONE
5. CYCLOTHIAZIDE
6. HYDROCHLOROTHIAZIDE
7. HYDROFLUMETHIAZIDE
8. METHYCLOTHIAZIDE
9. METOLAZONE
10. POLYTHIAZIDE
11. QUINETHAZONE
12. TRICHLORMETHIAZIDE

BRAND NAMES
Aldoclor[3]
Aldoril[6]
Anhydron[5]
Apo-Chlorthalidone[4]
Apo-Hydro[6]
Aquatensen[8]
Avalide[6]
Benicar HCT[6]

Demi-Regroton[4]
Diovan HCT[6]
Diucardin[7]
Diuchlor H[6]
Diulo[9]
Diupres[5]
Diurese R[12]
Diurigen with Reserpine[3]
Diuril[3]
Diutensen-R[8]
Duretic[8]
Dureticyl[8]
Enduron[8]
Enduronyl[8]
Enduronyl Forte[8]
Esidrix[6]
Exna[2]
Hydrex[2]
Hydro-D[6]
Hydrochlor[6]
HydroDIURIL[6]
Hydromox[11]
Hydropine[7]
Hydropine H.P.[7]
Hydropres[6]
Hygroton[4]
Hyzaar[6]
Metahydrin[12]
Micardis HCT[6]
Micardis Plus[6]
Microzide[6]
Minizide[10]
Mykrox[9]
Naqua[12]
Naturetin[1]
Neo-Codema[6]
Novodoparil[6]
Novo-Hydrazide[6]
Novo-Thalidone[4]
Oretic[6]
Oreticyl[6]
Oreticyl Forte[6]
PMS Dopazide[6]
Rauzide[1]
Regroton[4]
Renese[10]
Renese-R[10]
Saluron[7]
Salutensin[7]
Salutensin-Demi[7]
Supres[3]
Tekturna HCT[6]
Teveten HCT[6]
Thalitone[4]
trichlorex[12]
Uniretic[6]
Uridon[4]
Urozide[6]
Zaroxolyn[9]

ERYTHROMYCINS

GENERIC NAMES
1. ERYTHROMYCIN ESTOLATE
2. ERYTHROMYCIN
   ETHYLSUCCINATE
3. ERYTHROMYCIN
   GLUCEPTATE
4. ERYTHROMYCIN
   LACTOBIONATE
5. ERYTHROMYCIN STEARATE
6. ERYTHROMYCIN-BASE

BRAND NAMES
Apo-Erythro[6]
Apo-Erythro E-C[6]
Apo-Erythro ES[2]
Apo-Erythro-S[5]
E-Base[6]
E.E.S.[2]
E/Gel[6]
Emgel[6]
E-Mycin[6]
Erybid[6]
ERYC[6]
EryPed[2]
Ery-Tab[6]
Erythraderm[6]
Erythro[2]
Erythrocin[5]
Erythrocot[5]
Erythromid[6]
Eryzole[6]
Ilosone[1]
Ilotycin[3]
My-E[5]
Novorythro[5]
PCE Dispersatabs[5]
Pediazole[6]
Sulfimycin[6]
Wintrocin[5]

ESTROGENS

GENERIC NAMES

1. CONJUGATED ESTROGENS
2. DIETHYLSTILBESTROL
3. ESTERIFIED ESTROGENS
4. ESTRADIOL
5. ESTROGEN
6. ESTRONE
7. ESTROPIPATE
8. ETHINYL ESTRADIOL
9. QUINESTROL

BRAND NAMES
Activella[4]
Alora[4]
Angeliq[4]
Cenestin[1]
C.E.S.[1]
Climara[4]
Climara Pro[4]
Clinagen LA 40[4]
CombiPatch[4]

Congest[1]
Deladiol-40[4]
Delestrogen[4]
depGynogen[4]
Depo Estradiol[4]
Depogen[4]
DES[2]
Divigel[4]
Dura-Estrin[4]
Duragen[4]
Duragen-20[4]
Duragen-40[4]
E-Cypionate[4]
Elestrin[4]
Enjuvia[1]
Esclim[4]
Estinyl[8]
Estrace[4]
Estraderm[4]
Estragyn 5[6]
Estragyn LA 5[6]
Estra-L[4]
Estrasorb[4]
Estratab[3]
Estring[4]
Estro-A[6]
Estro-Cyp[4]
Estrofem[4]
Estrogel[4]
Estroject-L.A.[4]
Estro-L.A.[4]
Estro-Span[4]
EvaMist[4]
Femhrt[4]
Femogex[4]
Femring[4]
Femtrace[4]
Gynogen L.A. 20[4]
Gynogen L.A. 40[4]
Honvol [2]
Kestrone-5[6]
Mannest[2]
Menaval-20[4]
Menest[3]
Menostar[4]
Neo-Estrone[3]
Ogen[7]
Ogen 1.25[7]
Ogen 2.5[7]
Ogen 6.25[7]
Ortho-Est[7]
Orthro-Prefest[4]
Premarin[1]
Premarin Vaginal Cream[1]
Premphase[1]
Prempro[1]
SCE-A Vaginal Cream[1]
Stilbestrol[2]
Stilphostrol[2]
Valergen-10[4]
Valergen-20[4]
Valergen-40[4]
Vivelle[4]

Vivelle Dot[4]
Wehgen[6]

GUAIFENESIN
2/G-DM Cough
Adatuss D.C. Expectorant
Ambenyl-D Decongestant
  Cough Formula
Amonidrin
Anatuss DM
Anatuss LA
Anti-Tuss
Anti-Tuss DM Expectorant
Asbron G
Asbron G Inlay Tablets
Balminil Expectorant
Baytussin AC
Baytussin DM
Benylin All-In-One Cold & Flu
  Caplets
Benylin All-In-One Cold & Flu
  Nightime Syrup
Benylin All-In-One Cold & Flu
  Syrup
Benylin All-In-One Day & Night
  Caplets
Benylin Cold And Flu With
  Codeine Narcotic
Benylin DM-D-E
Benylin DM-D-E Extra Strength
Benylin DM-E Chest Cough
  Syrup
Breonesin
Bronchial
Broncholate
Broncomar GG
Brontex
Calmylin with Codeine
Cheracol D Cough
Children's Mucinex Cough
CoActifed Expectorant
Codiclear DH
Codimal Expectorant
Codistan No. 1
Colrex Expectorant
Comtrex Deep Chest Cold
Conar Expectorant
Conar-A
Concentrin
Congess JR
Congess SR
Congestac Caplets
Coricidin HBP Chest
  Congestion and Cough
Deconsal II
Detussin Expectorant
Diabetic Tussin DM
Diabetic Tussin EX
Diabetic Tussin Mucus Relief
Dihistine Expectorant
Dilaudid Cough
Donatussin

Donatussin DC
Donatussin Drops
Duratuss
Duratuss HD
Ed-Bron G
Efficol Cough Whip (Cough
  Suppressant/Decongestant)
Elixophyllin-GG
Entex PSE
Entuss Expectorant
Entuss Pediatric Expectorant
Entuss-D
Equibron G
Extra Action Cough
Father John's Medicine Plus
Fedahist Expectorant
Fedahist Expectorant Pediatric
  Drops
Fendol
Fenesin
Gee-Gee
Genatuss
Genatuss DM
GG-CEN
Glyate
Glyceryl T
Glycotuss
Glycotuss-dM
Glydeine Cough
Glytuss
Guaifed
Guaifed-PD
GuaiMAX-D
Guiamid D.M. Liquid
Guiatuss A.C.
Guiatuss PE
Guiatuss-DM
Halotussin
Halotussin-DM Expectorant
Histalet X
Humibid L.A.
Humibid Sprinkle
Humibid-DM Sprinkle
Hycotuss Expectorant
Hytuss
Hytuss-2X
Kids-EEZE Chest Relief
Kolephrin GG/DM
Kwelcof Liquid
LiquiBid D
LiquiBid PD
Malotuss
Maximum Strength Mucinex
Maximum Strength Mucinex D
Maximum Strength Mucinex
  DM
Meda Syrup Forte
Medatussin
Medatussin Plus
Mucinex
Mucinex Children's Cough,
  Expectorant & Suppressant

Mucinex Children's
  Expectorant
Mucinex Cold Liquid
Mucinex Cough Mini-Melts
Mucinex D
Mucinex DM
Mucinex Junior Strength
  Expectorant
Mucinex Mini-Melts
Mudrane GG2
Mytussin AC
Mytussin DAC
Mytussin DM
Naldecon Senior DX
Naldecon Senior EX
Nasatab LA
NeoCitrin DM Coughs & Colds
Nortussin
Nortussin with Codeine
Novahistine Expectorant
Organidin
Pertussin All Night CS
Phanatuss
Pneumomist
Poly-Histine Expectorant Plain
P-V-Tussin Tablets
Queltuss
Quibron
Quibron 300
Refenesen
Refenesen Chest Congestion
  & Pain Relief PE
Refenesen PE
Respaire-60 SR
Respaire-120 SR
Resyl
Rhinosyn-DMX Expectorant
Rhinosyn-X
Robafen AC Cough
Robafen DAC
Robafen DM
Robafen Syrup
Robitussin Chest
  Congestion
Robitussin Cough & Cold CF
Robitussin Cough & Cold D
Robitussin Cough & Chest
  Congestion
Robitussin Cough & Chest
  Congestion DM
Robitussin Cough & Chest
  Congestion DM Max
Robitussin Cough & Chest
  Congestion Sugar Free DM
Robitussin with Codeine
Ru-Tuss DE
Ru-Tuss Expectorant
Ryna-CX Liquid
SafeTussin 30
Scot-Tussin
Silexin Cough
Sinumist-SR
Sinupan

Sinutab Non-Drying Liquid
  Caps
SINUvent PE
Slo-Phyllin GG
Stamoist E
Sudafed Multi-Symptom Cold
  & Cough
Sudafed Non-Drying Sinus
  Liquid Caps
Sudafed PE Cold & Cough
  Caplets
Theolate
Theracof Plus Multi-Symptom
  Cough and Cold Reliever
Theraflu Flu & Chest
  Congestion Hot Liquid
Tolu-Sed Cough
Tolu-Sed DM Cough
Touro DM
Touro Ex
Touro LA Caplets
Triaminic Chest & Nasal
  Congestion
Tussafed HCG Syrup
Tussafin Expectorant
Tussar SF
Tussar-2
Tuss-DM
Tussi-Bid
Tussi-organidin
Tylenol Chest Congestion
Tylenol Cold Head Congestion
  Severe
Tylenol Cold Multi Symptom
  Severe
Tylenol Cough & Severe
  Congestion Daytime
Tylenol Sinus Congestion &
  Pain Severe
Uni-Tussin
Uni-Tussin DM
Unproco
Versacaps
Vicks Formula 44 Custom
  Care Chesty Cough
Vicks Pediatric Formula 44e
  Cough & Chest Congestion
  Relief
Vicodin-Tuss

INSULIN

Humulin N
Humulin R
Innolet
Insulatard NPH
Insulatard NPH Human
Lente
Lente Iletin I
Lente Iletin II
Mixtard
Mixtard Human
Novolin 70/30

Novolin 70/30 PenFill
Novolin 70/30 Prefilled
Novolin ge NPH PenFill
Novolin ge Toronto PenFill
Novolin N
Novolin N PenFill
Novolin N Prefilled
Novolin R
Novolin R PenFill
Novolin R Prefilled
Protamine Zinc & Iletin
Protamine Zinc & Iletin I
Protamine Zinc & Iletin II
PZI
Regular (Concentrated) Iletin
Regular (Concentrated) Iletin II,
  U-500
Regular Iletin I
Regular Insulin
Semilente
Semilente Iletin
Semilente Iletin I
Ultralente
Ultralente Iletin I

IRON SUPPLEMENTS

GENERIC NAMES
1. CARBONYL IRON
2. FERROUS FUMARATE
3. FERROUS GLUCONATE
4. FERROUS SULFATE
5. IRON DEXTRAN
6. IRON POLYSACCHARIDE
7. IRON SORBITOL

BRAND NAMES
Apo-Ferrous Gluconate[3]
Apo-Ferrous Sulfate[4]
Estrostep Fe[2]
Femiron[2]
Feosol[4]
Feosol Caplet[1]
Feostat[2]
Feostat Drops[2]
Fergon[3]
Fer-In-Sol[4]
Fer-In-Sol Drops[4]
Fer-In-Sol Syrup[4]
Fer-Iron[4]
Fero-folic 500[4]
Fero-Grad[4]
Fero-Gradumet[4]
FerraCap[1]
Ferralet[3]
Ferralet 90[1]
Ferralyn[4]
Ferra-TD[4]
Fertinic[4]
Hemocyte[2]
Hytinic[6]
Icar[1]
Ircon[2]
Jectofer[7]

Loestrin 24 Fe[2]
Neo-Fer[2]
Niferex[6]
Niferex-150[6]
Novoferrogluc[6]
Novoferrosulfa[3]
Novofumar[4]
Nu-Iron[6]
Nu-Iron 150[6]
Palafer[2]
Palmiron[2]
PMS Ferrous Sulfate[4]
Simiron[3]
Slow Fe[4]
Span-FF[2]

KERATOLYTICS

GENERIC NAMES
1. RESORCINOL
2. RESORCINOL & SULFUR
3. SALICYLIC ACID
4. SALICYLIC ACID & SULFUR
5. SULFUR (Topical)

BRAND NAMES
Acne-Aid Gel[2]
AcnoAcnomel Cake[2]
Acnomel Cream[2]
Acnomel Vanishing Cream[2]
Acnomel-Acne Cream[2]
Acnotex[4]
Adult Acne Clearing Gel[3]
Antinea[3]
Aveeno Acne Bar[4]
Aveeno Cleansing Bar[4]
Bensulfoid Cream[2]
Buf-Puf Acne Cleansing Bar
  with Vitamin E[3]
Buf-Puf Medicated Maximum
  Strength Pads[3]
Buf-Puf Medicated Regular
  Strength Pads[3]
Calicylic[3]
Cleanse and Treat[4]
Clear Away[3]
Clear by Design Medicated
  Cleansing Pads[3]
Clearasil Adult Care Medicated
  Blemish Cream[2]
Clearasil Adult Care Medicated
  Blemish Stick[2]
Clearasil Clearstick Maximum[3]
  Strength Topical Solution[3]
Clearasil Clearstick Regular
  Strength Topical Solution[3]
Clearasil Double Textured
  Pads Maximum Strength[3]
Clearasil Double Textured
  Pads Regular Strength[3]
Clearasil Medicated Deep
  Cleanser Topical Solution[3]
Compound W Gel[3]
Compound W Liquid[3]

Creamy SS Shampoo[4]
Cuplex Gel[3]
Cuticura Ointment[5]
Diasporal Cream[4]
Duofilm[3]
Duoplant[3]
Duoplant Topical Solution[3]
Finac[5]
Fostex CM[4]
Fostex Medicated Cleansing
  Bar[4]
Fostex Medicated Cleansing
  Cream[4]
Fostex Medicated Cleansing
  Liquid[4]
Fostex Regular Strength
  Medicated Cleansing Bar[4]
Fostex Regular Strength
  Medicated Cleansing Cream[4]
Fostex Regular Strength
  Medicated Cover-Up[4]
Fostril Cream[5]
Fostril Lotion[5]
Freezone[3]
Gordofilm[3]
Hydrisalic[3]
Inova 8/2 ACT[3]
Ionax Astringent Skin
  Cleanser Topical Solution[3]
Ionil Plus Shampoo[3]
Ionil Shampoo[3]
Keralyt[3]
Keratex Gel[3]
Lactisol[3]
Listerex Golden Scrub Lotion[3]
Listerex Herbal Scrub Lotion[3]
Lotio Asulfa[3]
Mediplast[3]
Meted Maximum Strength Anti-
  Dandruff Shampoo with
  Conditioners[4]
Night Cast R[4]
Night Cast Regular Formula
  Mask-Lotion[4]
Night Cast Special Formula
  Mask-Lotion[2]
Noxzema Anti-Acne Gel[3]
Noxzema Anti-Acne Pads
  Maximum Strength[3]
Noxzema Anti-Acne Pads
  Regular Strength[3]
Occlusal Topical Solution[3]
Occlusal-HP Topical Solution[3]
Off-Ezy Topical Solution Corn
  & Callus Removal Kit[3]
Off-Ezy Topical Solution Wart
  Removal Kit[3]
Oxy Clean Medicated Cleanser[3]
Oxy Clean Medicated Pads
  Maximum Strength[3]
Oxy Clean Medicated Pads
  Sensitive Skin[3]
Oxy Clean Regular Strength[3]

Oxy Clean Regular Strength
  Medicated Cleanser Topical
  Solution[3]
Oxy Clean Regular Strength
  Medicated Pads[3]
Oxy Clean Sensitive Skin
  Cleanser Topical Solution[3]
Oxy Clean Sensitive Skin Pads[3]
Oxy Night Watch Maximum
  Strength Lotion[3]
Oxy Night Watch Night Time
  Acne Medication Extra
  Strength Lotion[3]
Oxy Night Watch Night Time
  Acne Medication Regular
  Strength Lotion[3]
Oxy Night Watch Sensitive
  Skin Lotion[3]
Oxy Sensitive Skin Vanishing
  Formula Lotion[3]
P&S[3]
Paplex[3]
Paplex Ultra[3]
Pernox Lemon Medicated
  Scrub Cleanser[4]
Pernox Lotion Lathering
  Abradant Scrub Cleanser[4]
Pernox Lotion Lathering Scrub
  Cleanser[4]
Pernox Regular Medicated
  Scrub Cleanser[4]
Propa pH Medicated Acne
  Cream Maximum Strength[3]
Propa pH Medicated Cleansing
  Pads Maximum Strength[3]
Propa pH Medicated Cleansing
  Pads Sensitive Skin[3]
Propa pH Perfectly Clear Skin
  Cleanser Topical Solution
  Oily Skin[3]
Propa pH Perfectly Clear Skin
  Cleanser Topical Solution
  Sensitive Skin Formula[3]
R.A.[1]
Rezamid Lotion[2]
Salac[3]
Salacid[3]
Sal-Acid Plaster[3]
Salactic Film Topical Solution[3]
Sal-Clens Plus Shampoo[3]
Sal-Clens Shampoo[3]
Salex Shampoo[3]
Saligel[3]
Salonil[3]
Sal-Plant Gel Topical Solution[3]
Sastid (AL) Scrub[4]
Sastid Plain[4]
Sastid Plain Shampoo and
  Acne Wash[4]
Sastid Soap[4]
Sebasorb Liquid[4]
Sebex[4]
Sebucare[3]

Sebulex Antiseborrheic
Treatment and Conditioning
Shampoo[4]
Sebulex Antiseborrheic
Treatment Shampoo[4]
Sebulex Conditioning Shampoo[4]
Sebulex Cream Medicated
Shampoo[4]
Sebulex Medicated Dandruff
Shampoo with Conditioners[4]
Sebulex Medicated Shampoo[4]
Sebulex Regular Medicated
Dandruff Shampoo[4]
Sebulex Shampoo[4]
Stri-Dex[3]
Stri-Dex Dual Textured Pads
Maximum Strength[3]
Stri-Dex Dual Textured Pads
Regular Strength[3]
Stri-Dex Dual Textured Pads
Sensitive Skin[3]
Stri-Dex Maximum Strength
Pads[3]
Stri-Dex Regular Strength Pads[3]
Stri-Dex Super Scrub Pads[3]
Sulforcin[2]
Sulsal Soap[4]
Tersac Cleansing Gel[3]
Therac Lotion[4]
Trans-Plantar[3]
Trans-Ver-Sal[3]
Vanseb Cream Dandruff
Shampoo[4]
Vanseb Lotion Dandruff
Shampoo[4]
Verukan Topical Solution[3]
Verukan-HP Topical Solution[3]
Viranol[3]
Viranol Ultra[3]
Wart-Off Topical Solution[3]
X-Seb[3]

LAXATIVES, BULK-FORMING

GENERIC NAMES
1. CALCIUM POLYCARBOPHIL
2. CARBOXYMETHYLCELLUOSE
SODIUM
3. MALT SOUP EXTRACT
4. METHYLCELLULOSE
5. POLYCARBOPHIL
6. PSYLLIUM

BRAND NAMES
Cillium[6]
Citrucel Orange Flavor[4]
Citrucel Sugar-Free Orange
Flavor[4]
Cologel[4]
Disolan Forte[2]
Disoplex[2]
Effer-syllium[6]
Equalactin[5]

Fiberall[5]
Fibercon[5]
FiberNorm[5]
Fiberpur[6]
Hydrocil Instant[6]
Karacil[6]
Konsyl[5]
Konsyl Easy Mix Formula[6]
Konsyl-D[6]
Konsyl-Orange[6]
Maalox Daily Fiber Therapy[6]
Maalox Daily Fiber Therapy
Citrus Flavor[6]
Maalox Daily Fiber Therapy
Orange Flavor[6]
Maalox Sugar Free Citrus
Flavor[6]
Maalox Sugar Free Orange
Flavor[6]
Maltsupex[3]
Metamucil[6]
Metamucil Apple Crisp Fiber
Wafers[6]
Metamucil Cinnamon Spice
Fiber Wafers[6]
Metamucil Instant Mix, Orange
Flavor[6]
Metamucil Smooth Citrus
Flavor[6]
Metamucil Smooth Orange
Flavor[6]
Metamucil Smooth, Sugar-Free
Citrus Flavor[6]
Metamucil Smooth, Sugar-Free
Orange Flavor[6]
Metamucil Smooth, Sugar-Free
Regular Flavor[6]
Metamucil Sugar Free[6]
Metamucil Sugar Free Citrus
Flavor[6]
Metamucil Sugar Free Lemon-
Lime Flavor[6]
Metamucil Sugar Free Orange
Flavor[6]
Mitrolan[5]
Modane Bulk[6]
Mylanta Natural Fiber
Supplement[6]
Mylanta Sugar Free Natural
Fiber Supplement[6]
Naturacil[6]
Natural Source Fibre Laxative[6]
Perdiem[6]
Perdiem Fiber[6]
Perdiem Plain[6]
Prodiem[6]
Prodiem Plain[6]
Prodiem Plus[6]
Pro-Lax[6]
Prompt[6]
Reguloid Natural[6]
Reguloid Orange[6]
Reguloid Orange Sugar Free[6]

SennaPrompt[6]
Serutan[6]
Serutan Toasted Granules[6]
Siblin[6]
Syllact[6]
Syllamalt[3]
Versabran[6]
Vitalax Super Smooth Sugar
Free Orange Flavor[6]
Vitalax Unflavored[6]
V-Lax[6]

LAXATIVES, OSMOTIC

GENERIC NAMES
1. GLYCERIN
2. LACTULOSE
3. MAGNESIUM CITRATE
4. MAGNESIUM HYDROXIDE
5. MAGNESIUM OXIDE
6. MAGNESIUM SULFATE
7. MILK OF MAGNESIA
8. MINERAL OIL
9. POLYETHYLENE GLYCOL
3350
10. SODIUM PHOSPHATE

BRAND NAMES
Agarol Plain[7]
Agarol Strawberry[8]
Agarol Vanilla[8]
Bilagog[6]
Cholac[2]
Chronula[2]
Citroma[3]
Citro-Mag[3]
Citro-Nesia[3]
Constilac[2]
Constulose[2]
Duphalac[2]
Evalose[2]
Fleet Phospho-Soda[10]
Generlac[2]
Hayley's M-O[7]
Heptalac[2]
Kristalose[2]
Lactulax[2]
Magnolax[7]
Mag-Ox 400[5]
Maox[5]
Miralax[9]
Phillips' Chewable[4]
Phillips' Concentrated[4]
Phillips' Magnesia Tablets[4]
Phillips' Milk of Magnesia[4]
Portalac[2]

LAXATIVES, SOFTENER/LUBRICANT

GENERIC NAMES
1. CASANTHRANOL &
DOCUSATE
2. DOCUSATE

3. DOCUSATE CALCIUM
4. DOCUSATE POTASSIUM
5. DOCUSATE SODIUM
6. MINERAL OIL
7. POLOXAMER 188

BRAND NAMES
Afko-Lube[2]
Afko-Lube Lax[2]
Agarol Plain[6]
Agarol Marshmallow[6]
Agarol Raspberry[6]
Agarol Strawberry[6]
Agarol Vanilla[6]
Alaxin[7]
Bilax[2]
Colace[5]
Colace Microenema[5]
Correctol Extra Gentle[2]
Dialose[2]
Diocto[2]
Diocto-C[1]
Diocto-K[2]
Diocto-K Plus[1]
Dioeze[2]
Diosuccin[2]
Dio-Sul[2]
Diothron[1]
Disanthrol[1]
Disolan[2]
Disolan Forte[1]
Disonate[2]
Disoplex[2]
Di-Sosul[2]
Di-Sosul Forte[1]
Docu-K Plus[1]
DOK[2]
DOK Softgels[2]
Doss[2]
Doss Tablets[2]
Doxinate[2]
DSMC Plus[1]
Dulcodos[2]
Duosol[2]
Fleet Enema Mineral Oil[7]
Gentlax-S[2]
Kasof[2]
Kondremul[7]
Kondremul with Cascara[7]
Kondremul Plain[7]
Lansoyl[7]
Laxinate 100[2]
Liqui-Doss[7]
Milkinol[7]
Modane Plus[2]
Modane Soft[2]
Molatoc[2]
Molatoc-CST[2]
Neo-Cultol[7]
Neolax[2]
Nujol[7]
Peri-Colase[1]
Pertrogalar Plain[7]

PMS-Docusate Calcium[2]
PMS-Docusate Sodium[2]
Pro-Cal-Sof[2]
Pro-Sof[1]
Pro-Sof Liquid Concentrate[1]
Pro-Sof Plus[1]
Regulace[2]
Regulax SS[2]
Regulex[2]
Regulex-D[2]
Regutol[2]
Senokot-S[2]
Stulex[2]
Sulfolax[2]
Surfak[2]
Therevac Plus[2]
Therevac-SB[2]
Trilax[2]
Zymenol[7]

LAXATIVES, STIMULANT
GENERIC NAMES
1. ALOE
2. BISACODYL
3. CASANTHRANOL
4. CASCARA
5. CASTOR OIL
6. DEHYDROCHOLIC ACID
7. SENNA
8. SENNOSIDES

BRAND NAMES
Afko-Lube Lax[3]
Alphamul[5]
Aromatic Cascara
    Fluidextract[4]
Bilax[6]
Bisac-Evac[2]
Bisacolax[2]
Bisco-Lax[2]
Black Draught[3]
Black-Draught Lax-Senna[7]
Caroid Laxative[2]
Carter's Little Pills[4]
Cascara Aromatic
    Fluidextract[4]
Cascara Sagrada[4]
Cholan-HMB[6]
Dacodyl[2]
Decholin[6]
Deficol[2]
Diocto-C[3]
Diocto-K Plus[1]
Diothron[3]
Disanthrol[3]
Disolan Forte[3]
Di-Sosul Forte[3]
Docu-K Plus[3]
Dosaflex[7]
Dr. Caldwell Senna Laxative[7]
DSMC Plus[3]
Dulcodos[2]
Dulcolax[2]

Emulsoil[5]
Ex-Lax Gentle Nature[8]
Fleet Bisacodyl[2]
Fleet Bisacodyl Prep[2]
Fleet Flavored Castor Oil[5]
Fleet Laxative[2]
Fletcher's Castoria[7]
Gentlax S[7]
Gentle Nature[8]
Glysennid[8]
Hepahydrin[6]
Herbal Laxative[8]
Kellogg's Castor Oil[5]
Kondremul with Cascara[4]
Laxit[2]
Molatoc-CST[3]
Mucinum Herbal[8]
Nature's Remedy[4]
Neolax[6]
Neoloid[5]
Nytilax[8]
Perdiem[7]
Peri-Colace[3]
PMS-Bisacodyl[2]
PMS-Sennosides[8]
Prodiem Plus[7]
Prompt[8]
Pro-Sof Plus[3]
Purge[5]
Regulace[3]
Senexon[7]
SennaPrompt[8]
Senokot[7]
Senokot-S[7]
SenokotXTRA[7]
Senolax[7]
Theralax[2]
Trilax[6]
X-Prep Liquid[7]

MEPROBAMATE
Acabamate
Apo-Meprobamate
Epromate-M
Equagesic
Equanil
Equanil Wyseals
Equazine-M
Heptogesic
Medi-Tran
Meprogesic
Meprogesic Q
Meprospan 200
Meprospan 400
Micrainin
Miltown
Neuramate
Novo-Mepro
Pax 400
Probate
Sedabamate
Trancot
Tranmep

NARCOTIC ANALGESICS

GENERIC NAMES
1. BUPRENORPHINE
2. CODEINE
3. CODEINE & TERPIN HYDRATE
4. DIHYDROCODEINE
5. FENTANYL
6. HYDROCODONE
7. HYDROCODONE & HOMATROPINE
8. HYDROMORPHONE
9. LEVORPHANOL
10. MEPERIDINE
11. METHADONE
12. MORPHINE
13. NALBUPHINE
14. OPIUM
15. OXYCODONE
16. OXYMORPHONE
17. PENTAZOCINE
18. PROPOXYPHENE

BRAND NAMES
642[18]
Actagen-C Cough[2]
Actifed with Codeine Cough[2]
Actiq[5]
Adatuss D.C. Expectorant[6]
Allerfrin with Codeine[2]
Ambay Cough[2]
Ambenyl Cough[2]
Ambophen Expectorant[2]
Anamine HD[6]
Anaplex HD[6]
Aprodrine with Codeine[2]
Astramorph[12]
Astramorph-PF[12]
Avinza[12]
Bayhistine DH[2]
Bayhistine Expectorant[2]
Baytussin AC[2]
Benylin Cold & Flu With Codeine Narcotic[2]
Bromanyl[2]
Brontex[2]
Buprenex[1]
Calcidrine[2]
Calmylin with Codeine[2]
Cheracol[2]
Chlorgest-HD[6]
Citra Forte[6]
CoActifed[2]
CoActifed Expectorant[2]
Codan[7]
Codehist DH[2]
Codeine Sulfate[2]
Codeprex[2]
Codiclear DH[6]
Codimal DH[6]
Codimal PH[2]
Colrex Compound[2]
Combunox[15]

Coristex-DH[6]
Coristine-DH[6]
Cotanal-65[18]
Cotridin[2]
C-Tussin Expectorant[2]
Darvon[18]
Darvon-N[18]
Decohistine DH[2]
Demerol[10]
Deproist Expectorant with Codeine[2]
De-Tuss[6]
Detussin Expectorant[6]
Detussin Liquid[6]
Dihistine DH[2]
Dihistine Expectorant[2]
Dihydromorphinone[8]
Dilaudid[8]
Dilaudid Cough[8]
Dilaudid-HP[8]
Dolophine[11]
Donatussin DC[6]
Doxaphene[18]
Duragesic[5]
Duragesic mc/hr[5]
Duramorph[12]
Duratuss HD[6]
Endagen-HD[6]
Endal-HD[6]
Endal-HD Plus[6]
Entuss Expectorant[6]
Entuss-D[6]
Epimorph[12]
Fentora[5]
Fortral[17]
Glydeine Cough[2]
Guiatuss A.C.[2]
Guiatussin DAC[2]
Guiatussin with Codeine Liquid[2]
Histafed C[2]
Histussin HC[6]
Hycodan[6]
Hycomine Compound[6]
Hycomine-S Pediatric[6]
Hycotuss Expectorant[6]
Hydromet[7]
Hydropane[7]
Hydrostat IR[8]
Ibudone[6]
Isoclor Expectorant[2]
Kadian[12]
Kwelcof Liquid[6]
Laudanum[14]
Levo-Dromoran[9]
Levorphan[9]
Mallergan-VC with Codeine[2]
Methadose[11]
Midahist DH[2]
Morphitec[12]
M.O.S.[12]
M.O.S.-SR[12]
MS Contin[12]
MSIR[12]

MST Continus[12]
Mytussin AC[2]
Mytussin DAC[2]
Nortussin with Codeine[2]
Novagest Expectorant with Codeine[2]
Novahistex C[2]
Novahistex DH[6]
Novahistex DH Expectorant[6]
Novahistine DH Expectorant[6]
Novahistine DH Liquid[2]
Novahistine Expectorant[2]
Nubain[13]
Nucochem[2]
Nucochem Expectorant[2]
Nucochem Pediatric Expectorant[2]
Nucofed[2]
Nucofed Expectorant[2]
Nucofed Pediatric Expectorant[2]
Numorphan[16]
Opana[16]
Opana ER[16]
Oramorph[12]
Oramorph-SR[12]
Oxycontin SR[15]
Pantapon[14]
Paveral[2]
Pediacof Cough[2]
Penazine VC with Cough[2]
Phenameth VC with Codeine[2]
Phenergan VC with Codeine[2]
Phenergan with Codeine[2]
Phenhist DH with Codeine[2]
Phenhist Expectorant[2]
Pherazine VC with Codeine[2]
Pherazine with Codeine[2]
Physeptone[11]
Promehist with Codeine[2]
Prometh VC with Codeine[2]
Propoxycon[18]
Prunicodeine[2]
Pseudodine C Cough[2]
P-V-Tussin[6]
Reprexain[6]
RMS Uniserts[12]
Robafen AC Cough[2]
Robafen DAC[2]
Robidone[6]
Robitussin A-C[2]
Robitussin-DAC[2]
Rolatuss Expectorant[2]
Rolatuss with Hydrocodone[6]
Roxanol[12]
Roxanol SR[12]
Roxicodone[15]
Ryna-C Liquid[2]
Ryna-CX Liquid[2]
Soma Compound[2]
SRC Expectorant[6]
Statex[12]
Statuss Expectorant[2]

Supeudol[15]
Talwin[17]
Talwin-NX[17]
Temgesic[1]
Tolu-Sed Cough[2]
Triacin C Cough[2]
Triafed with Codeine[2]
Tricodene #1[2]
Trifed-C Cough[2]
Tussafed HCG Syrup[6]
Tussafin Expectorant[6]
Tussanil DH[6]
Tussar SF[2]
Tussar-2[2]
TussiCaps[6]
Tussigon[7]
Tussionex[6]
Tussirex with Codeine Liquid[2]
Tyrodone[6]
Vanex Expectorant[6]
Vanex-HD[6]
Vicodin-Tuss[6]
Vicoprofen[8]

NARCOTIC ANALGESICS & ACETAMINOPHEN

GENERIC NAMES
1. ACETAMINOPHEN & CODEINE
2. DIHYDROCODEINE & ACETAMINOPHEN
3. HYDROCODONE & ACETAMINOPHEN
4. MEPERIDINE & ACETAMINOPHEN
5. OXYCODONE & ACETAMINOPHEN
6. PENTAZOCINE & ACETAMINOPHEN
7. PROPOXYPHENE & ACETAMINOPHEN

BRAND NAMES
Allay[3]
Anexsia[3]
Anolor-DH5[3]
APAP with Codeine[1]
Atasol-8[1]
Atasol-15[1]
Atasol-30[1]
Balacet 325[7]
Bancap-HC[3]
Capital with Codeine[1]
Co-Gesic[3]
Compal[3]
Darvocet A500[7]
Darvocet-N 50[7]
Darvocet-N 100[7]
Demerol-APAP[4]
DHCplus[2]
Dolacet[3]
Dolagesic[3]
Dolene-AP 65[7]

Duocet[3]
E-Lor[7]
Empracet 30[1]
Empracet 60[1]
Emtec[1]
Endocet[5]
Exdol-8[1]
Exdol-15[1]
Exdol-30[1]
EZ III[1]
Hycomed[3]
Hyco-Pap[3]
Hydrocet[2]
Hydrocodone with APAP[3]
Hydrogesic[3]
HY-PHEN[3]
Lenoltec with Codeine No. 1[1]
Lenoltec with Codeine No. 2[1]
Lenoltec with Codeine No. 3[1]
Lenoltec with Codeine No. 4[1]
Lorcet[3]
Lorcet 10/650[3]
Lorcet Plus[3]
Lorcet-HD[3]
Lortab[3]
Lortab 5[3]
Lortab 7[3]
Magnacet[5]
Margesic #3[1]
Margesic-H[3]
Maxidone[3]
Norco[3]
Novogesic[1]
Onset[3]
Oxycocet[5]
Panacet 5/500[3]
Panlor[3]
Percocet[5]
Percocet-Demi[5]
Phenaphen with Codeine[1]
Polygesic[3]
Pro Pox with APAP[7]
Propacet 100[7]
Pyregesic-C[1]
Roxicet[5]
Roxilox[5]
Stagesic[3]
Talacen[6]
T-gesic[3]
Tylaprin with Codeine[1]
Tylenol No.1[1]
Tylenol No.1 Forte[1]
Tylenol with Codeine[1]
Tylenol with Codeine No. 1[1]
Tylenol with Codeine No. 2[1]
Tylenol with Codeine No. 3[1]
Tylenol with Codeine No. 4[1]
Tylox[5]
Ugesic[3]
Ultragesic[3]
Vanacet[3]
Vapocet[3]
Veganin[1]

Vendone[3]
Vicodin[3]
Vicodin ES[3]
Wygesic[7]
Xodol[3]
Zydone[3]

NARCOTIC ANALGESICS & ASPIRIN

GENERIC NAMES
1. ASPIRIN & CODEINE
2. BUFFERED ASPIRIN & CODEINE
3. DIHYDROCODEINE & ASPIRIN
4. HYDROCODONE & ASPIRIN
5. OXYCODONE & ASPIRIN
6. PENTAZOCINE & ASPIRIN
7. PROPOXYPHENE & ASPIRIN

BRAND NAMES
222[1]
282[1]
292[1]
293[1]
692[7]
A.C.&C.[1]
Anacin with Codeine[1]
Azdone[1]
Cotanal 65[7]
Damason-P[4]
Darvon Compound[6]
Darvon Compound 65[6]
Darvon with A.S.A.[6]
Darvon-N Compound[7]
Darvon-N with A.S.A.[7]
Drocade and Aspirin[3]
Emcodeine No. 2[1]
Emcodeine No. 3[1]
Emcodeine No. 4[1]
Empirin with Codeine[1]
Empirin with Codeine No. 3[1]
Empirin with Codeine No. 4[1]
Endodan[5]
Lortab ASA[4]
Novo-AC and C[1]
Oxycodan[5]
Panasal 5/500[4]
PC-Cap[7]
Percodan[5]
Percodan-Demi[5]
Propoxyphene Compound-65[7]
Roxiprin[5]
Synalgos-DC[3]
Talwin Compound[6]
Talwin Compound-50[6]

NITRATES

GENERIC NAMES
1. ERYTHRITYL TETRANITRATE
2. ISOSORBIDE DINITRATE
3. ISOSORBIDE MONONITRATE

4. NITROGLYCERIN (GLYCERYL TRINITRATE)

5. PENTAERYTHRITOL TETRANITRATE

BRAND NAMES

Apo-ISDN[2]
BiDil[2]
Cardilate[1]
Cedocard-SR[2]
Coradur[2]
Coronex[2]
Deponit[4]
Dilatrate-SR[2]
Duotrate[5]
Glyceryl Trinitrate[4]
IMDUR[3]
ISMO[3]
Iso-Bid[2]
Isonate[2]
Isorbid[2]
Isordil[2]
Isotrate[2]
Klavikordal[4]
Minitran[4]
Monoket[3]
Niong[4]
Nitro-Bid[4]
Nitrocap[4]
Nitrocap T.D.[4]
Nitrocine[4]
Nitrodisc[4]
Nitro-Dur[4]
Nitro-Dur II[4]
Nitrogard-SR[4]
Nitroglyn[4]
Nitrol[4]
Nitrolin[4]
Nitrolingual[4]
NitroMist[4]
Nitronet[4]
Nitrong[4]
Nitrong SR[4]
Nitrospan[4]
Nitrostat[4]
Novosorbide[2]
NTS[4]
Pentritol[5]
Pentylan[5]
Peritrate[5]
Peritrate Forte[5]
Peritrate SA[5]
P.E.T.N.[5]
Sorbitrate[2]
Sorbitrate SA[2]
Transderm-Nitro[4]
Tridil[4]

OXYMETAZOLINE (Nasal)

4-Way Long Acting Nasal Spray
12-Hour Nostrilla Nasal Decongestant
Afrin 12 Hour Nasal Spray
Afrin 12 Hour Nose Drops
Afrin Cherry Scented Nasal Spray
Afrin Children's Strength 12 Hour Nose Drops
Afrin Children's Strength Nose Drops
Afrin Extra Moisturizing Nasal Decongestant Spray
Afrin Menthol Nasal Spray
Afrin Nasal Spray
Afrin No-Drip Extra Moisturizing
Afrin No-Drip Nasal Decongestant, Severe Congestion with Menthol
Afrin No-Drip Nasal Decongestant Sinus with Vapornase
Afrin No-Drip Sinus
Afrin Nose Drops
Afrin Sinus
Afrin Spray Pump
Allerest 12 Hour Nasal Spray
Cheracol Nasal Spray
Cheracol Nasal Spray Pump Cherry Scented
Coricidin Nasal Mist
Dristan 12-Hour Nasal Spray
Dristan Long Lasting Menthol Nasal Spray
Dristan Long Lasting Nasal Pump Spray
Dristan Long Lasting Nasal Spray
Dristan Long Lasting Nasal Spray 12 Hour Metered Dose Pump
Dristan Mentholated
Drixoral
Duramist Plus Up To 12 Hours Decongestant Nasal Spray
Duration 12 Hour Nasal Spray Pump
Mucinex Full Force Nasal Spray
Mucinex Moisture Smart Nasal Spray
Nasal Decongestant Spray
Nasal Relief
Nasal Spray 12-Hour
Nasal Spray Long Acting
Nasal-12 Hour
Neo-Synephrine 12 Hour Nasal Spray
Neo-Synephrine 12 Hour Nasal Spray Pump
Neo-Synephrine 12 Hour Nose Drops
Neo-Synephrine 12 Hour Vapor Nasal Spray
Nostril Nasal Decongestant Mild
Nostril Nasal Decongestant Regular
NTZ Long Acting Decongestant Nasal Spray
NTZ Long Acting Decongestant Nose Drops
Sinarest 12 Hour Nasal Spray
Vicks Sinex 12-Hour Nasal Spray
Vicks Sinex 12-Hour Ultra Fine Mist
Vicks Sinex Long-Acting 12 Hour Nasal Spray

PENICILLINS

GENERIC NAMES

1. AMOXICILLIN
2. AMPICILLIN
3. BACAMPICILLIN
4. CARBENICILLIN
5. CLOXACILLIN
6. DICLOXACILLIN
7. FLUCLOXACILLIN
8. NAFCILLIN
9. OXACILLIN
10. PENICILLIN G
11. PENICILLIN V
12. PIVAMPICILLIN
13. PIVMECILLINAM

BRAND NAMES

Amoxil[1]
Apo-Amoxi[1]
Apo-Ampi[2]
Apo-Cloxi[5]
Apo-Pen VK[11]
Bactocill[9]
Beepen-VK[11]
Betapen-VK[11]
Cloxapen[5]
DisperMax[1]
Dycill[6]
Dynapen[6]
Fluclox[7]
Geopen Oral[4]
Ledercillin-VK[11]
Megacillin[10]
Moxatag[1]
Nadopen-V[11]
Nadopen-V 200[11]
Nadopen-V 400[11]
Novamoxin[1]
Novo-Ampicillin[2]
Novo-Cloxin[5]
Novo-Pen VK[11]
Nu-Amoxi[11]
Nu-Ampi[2]
Nu-Cloxi[5]
Nu-Pen-VK[11]
Omnipen[2]
Orbenin[5]
Pathocil[6]
Pen Vee[11]
Pen Vee K[11]
Penbritin[2]

Penglobe[3]
Pentids[10]
Polycillin[2]
Pondocillin[12]
Principen[2]
Prostaphlin[9]
PVF[11]
PVF K[11]
Selexld[13]
Spectrobid[3]
Tegopen[5]
Totacillin[2]
Trimox[1]
Unipen[8]
V-Cillin K[11]
Veetids[11]
Wymox[1]

PHENOTHIAZINES

GENERIC NAMES
1. ACETOPHENAZINE
2. CHLORPROMAZINE
3. FLUPHENAZINE
4. MESORIDAZINE
5. METHOTRIMEPRAZINE
6. PERICYAZINE
7. PERPHENAZINE
8. PIPOTIAZINE
9. PROCHLORPERAZINE
10. PROMAZINE
11. THIOPROPAZATE
12. THIOPROPERAZINE
13. THIORIDAZINE
14. TRIFLUOPERAZINE
15. TRIFLUPROMAZINE

BRAND NAMES
Apo-Fluphenazine[3]
Apo-Perphenazine[7]
Apo-Thioridazine[13]
Apo-Trifluoperazine[14]
Chlorpromanyl-5[2]
Chlorpromanyl-20[2]
Chlorpromanyl-40[2]
Compazine[9]
Compazine Spansule[9]
Dartal[11]
Duo-Medihaler
Etrafon[7]
Etrafon-A[7]
Etrafon-D[7]
Etrafon-F[7]
Etrafon-Forte[7]
Largactil[2]
Largactil Liquid[2]
Largactil Oral Drops[2]
Levoprome[5]
Majeptil[12]
Mellaril[13]
Mellaril Concentrate[13]
Mellaril-S[13]
Modecate[3]
Modecate Concentrate[3]

Moditen Enanthate[3]
Moditen HCl[3]
Moditen HCl-H.P.[3]
Neuleptil[6]
Novo-Chlorpromazine[2]
Novo-Flurazine[14]
Novo-Ridazine[13]
Nozinan[5]
Nozinan Liquid[5]
Nozinan Oral Drops[5]
Permitil[3]
Permitil Concentrate[3]
Piportil L[8]
PMS Levazine[7]
PMS Thioridazine[13]
Prolixin[3]
Prolixin Concentrate[3]
Prolixin Decanoate[3]
Prolixin Enanthate[3]
Prorazin[9]
Prozine [10]
Serentil[4]
Serentil Concentrate[4]
Stemetil Liquid[9]
Suprazine[14]
Terfluzine[14]
Terfluzine Concentrate[14]
Thorazine[2]
Thorazine Concentrate[2]
Thorazine Spansule[2]
Thor-Prom[2]
Tindal[2]
Triavil[7]
Trilafon[7]
Trilafon Concentrate[7]
Ultrazine-10[9]
Vesprin[5]

PHENYLEPHRINE

Aclophen
Advanced Formula Dristan
  Caplets
AH-Chew
Alersule
Alka-Seltzer Plus Cold & Sinus
  Effervescent
Alka-Seltzer Plus Night-Time
  Effervescent
Alka-Seltzer Plus Original
  Effervescent
AlleRx Dose Pack PE
AlleRx Suspension
Anamine HD
Atrohist Pediatric
Atrohist Pediatric Suspension
  Dye Free
Atrohist Sprinkle
Benylin All-In-One Cold & Flu
  Night Caplets
Benylin Cold & Sinus
Benylin Cold & Sinus Plus
Cerose-DM
Chlorgest-HD

Citra Forte
Codimal DH
Codimal DM
Codimal PH
Colrex Compound
Colrex Cough
Coltab Children's
Comhist
Comhist LA
Conar
Conar Expectorant
Conar-A
Congespirin for Children Cold
  Tablets
Coristex-DH
Coristine-DH
D.A. Chewable
Dallergy
Dihistine
Doktors
Donatussin
Donatussin DC
Donatussin Drops
Dondril
Dristan Cold Multi-Symptom
  Formula
Dristan Formula P
Dristan-AF
Dristan-AF Plus
Dura-Vent/DA
Ed A-Hist
Endagen-HD
Endal-HD
Endal-HD Plus
Extendryl
Extendryl JR
Extendryl SR
Father John's Medicine Plus
Fendol
Gendecon
Histagesic Modified
Histatab Plus
Histatan
Histor-D
Histor-D Timecelles
Hycomine Compound
Improved Sino-Tuss
Kolephrin
LiquiBid D
LiquiBid PD
Mallergan-VC with Codeine
Meda Syrup Forte
Mucinex Cold Liquid
ND-Gesic
Neocitran A
Neocitran Colds & Flu Calorie
  Reduced
NeoCitran DM Coughs & Colds
NeoCitran Extra Strength
  Colds & Flu
NeoCitran Extra Strength Sinus
Neo-Synephrine Nasal Drops
Neo-Synephrine Pediatric
  Nasal Drops

Nostril Spray Pump
Omnicol
OMNIhist L.A.
Pediacof Cough
Phenameth VC
Phenameth VC with Codeine
Pherazine VC
Pherazine VC with Codeine
Prehist
Prehist D
Prometh VC Plain
Prometh VC with Codeine
Promethazine VC
Refenesen Chest Congestion
  & Pain Relief PE
Refenesen PE
Rhinall
Rhinall Children's Flavored
  Nose Drops
Rhinatate
Rhinogesic
Robitussin Cough & Cold CF
Robitussin Cough & Cold
  Nighttime
Robitussin Cough Cold
  & Flu Nighttime
Rolatuss Expectorant
Rolatuss Plain
R-Tannamine
R-Tannamine Pediatric
R-Tannate
R-Tannate Pediatric
Rynatan
Rynatan Pediatric
Rynatan-S Pediatric
Rynatuss
Rynatuss Pediatric
Salphenyl
Scot-Tussin
Scot-Tussin Original 5-Action
  Cold Medicine
Sinupan
SINUvent PE
Statuss Expectorant
Sudafed PE Cold & Cough
  Caplets
Tanoral
Theracof Plus Multi-Symptom
  Cough and Cold Reliever
TheraFlu Cold & Cough Hot
  Liquid
Theraflu Daytime Severe Cold
  Caplets
Theraflu Daytime Severe
  Cold Hot Liquid
Theraflu Flu & Sore Throat
  Hot Liquid
Theraflu Nighttime Severe
  Cold Caplets
Theraflu Nighttime Severe
  Cold Hot Liquid
Theraflu Thin Strips Daytime
  Cold & Cough

Theraflu Thin Strips Nighttime
  Severe Cold & Cough
Theraflu Warming Relief
  Daytime
Theraflu Warming Relief
  Nighttime
Triaminic Chest & Nasal
  Congestion
Triaminic Cold & Allergy
Triaminic Day Time Cold &
  Cough
Triaminic Night Time Cough
  & Cold
Triaminic Thin Strips Cold
Triaminic Thin Strips Daytime
  Cold & Cough
Triaminic Thin Strips Night
  Time Cold & Cough
Trimedine Liquid
Triotann
Triotann Pediatric
Tritann Pediatric
Tri-Tannate
Tri-Tannate Plus Pediatric
Tussafed HCG Syrup
Tussanil Plain
Tussi-12
Tussirex with Codeine Liquid
Tylenol Allergy Multi-Symptom
Tylenol Allergy Multi-Symptom
  Nighttime
Tylenol Cold Head Congestion
  Daytime
Tylenol Cold Head Congestion
  Nighttime
Tylenol Cold Head Congestion
  Severe
Tylenol Cold Multi Symptom
  Daytime
Tylenol Cold Multi Symptom
  Nighttime
Tylenol Cold Multi Symptom
  Severe
Tylenol Cough & Severe
  Congestion Daytime
Tylenol Sinus Congestion &
  Pain Daytime
Tylenol Sinus Congestion &
  Pain Nighttime
Tylenol Sinus Congestion &
  Pain Severe
Vanex-HD
Vicks DayQuil Cold & Flu
  Symptom Relief Plus
  Vitamin C
Vicks DayQuil Sinus
  LiquiCaps
Vicks Formula 44 Custom
  Care Congestion
Vicks NyQuil Sinus LiquiCaps
Vicks Sinex Nasal Spray
Viravan DM

POTASSIUM SUPPLEMENTS

GENERIC NAMES
1. POTASSIUM ACETATE
2. POTASSIUM BICARBONATE
3. POTASSIUM BICARBONATE
   & POTASSIUM CHLORIDE
4. POTASSIUM BICARBONATE
   & POTASSIUM CITRATE
5. POTASSIUM CHLORIDE
6. POTASSIUM GLUCONATE
7. POTASSIUM GLUCONATE &
   POTASSIUM CHLORIDE
8. POTASSIUM GLUCONATE &
   POTASSIUM CITRATE
9. POTASSIUM TRIPLEX

BRAND NAMES
Apo-K[5]
Cena-K[5]
Effer-K[4]
Gen-K[5]
Glu-K[6]
K+10[5]
K-10[5]
K-8[5]
K+Care[5]
K+Care ET[2]
Kalium Durules[5]
Kaochlor[5]
Kaochlor S-F[5]
Kaochlor-10[5]
Kaochlor-20[5]
Kaochlor-Eff[5]
Kaon[6]
Kaon-Cl[5]
Kaon-Cl 10[5]
Kaon-Cl 20[5]
Kato[5]
Kay Ciel[5]
Kay Ciel Elixir[5]
Kaylixir[6]
KCL[5]
K-Dur[5]
K-Electrolyte[2]
K-G Elixir[6]
K-Lease[5]
K-Long[5]
K-Lor[5]
Klor-Con 8[5]
Klor-Con 10[5]
Klor-Con Powder[5]
Klor-Con/25[5]
Klor-Con/EF[2]
Klorvess[3]
Klorvess 10% Liquid[5]
Klorvess Effervescent Granules[5]
Klotrix[5]
K-Lyte[2]
K-Lyte DS[4]
K-Lyte/Cl[3]
K-Lyte/Cl 50[3]
K-Lyte/CL Powder[5]

K-Med 900[5]
K-Norm[5]
Kolyum[7]
K-Sol[5]
K-Tab[5]
K-Vescent[2]
Micro-K[5]
Micro-K 10[5]
Micro-K LS[5]
Neo-K[3]
Potasalan[5]
Potassium-Rougier[6]
Potassium-Sandoz[3]
Roychlor 10%[5]
Roychlor 20%[5]
Royonate[6]
Rum-K[5]
Slow-K[5]
Ten K[5]
Tri-K[9]
Twin-K[8]

PROGESTINS

GENERIC NAMES
1. DROSPIRENONE
2. ETONOGESTREL
3. HYDROXYPROGESTERONE
4. LEVONORGESTREL
5. MEDROXYPROGESTERONE
6. MEGESTROL
7. NORETHINDRONE
8. NORGESTIMATE
9. NORGESTREL
10. PROGESTERONE

BRAND NAMES
Activella[8]
Amen[5]
Angeliq[1]
Aygestin[7]
CombiPatch[7]
Crinone[10]
Curretab[5]
Cycrin[5]
Depo-Provera[5]
Duralutin[3]
Endometrin[10]
Femhrt[7]
Gesterol 50[10]
Gesterol L.A.[3]
Hy/Gestrone[3]
Hylutin[3]
Hyprogest[3]
Implanon[3]
Megace[6]
Megace ES[6]
Megace Oral Suspension[6]
Micronor[7]
Norlutate[7]
Nor-Q.D.[7]
Ortho-Prefest[8]
Ovrette[9]
Plan B OTC/Rx[4]

Premphase[5]
Prempro[5]
Prodrox[3]
Prometrium[10]
Provera[5]
ProveraPak[5]

PSEUDOEPHEDRINE

Actacin
Actagen
Actagen-C Cough
Advil Cold and Sinus Caplets
Advil Cold and Sinus LiquiGels
Advil Flu & Body Ache
Advil Multi-Symptom Cold
Alavert D-12
Aleve-D Sinus & Cold
Allegra-D
Allegra-D 24 Hour
Allent
Allercon
Allerest Maximum Strength
Allerest No-Drowsiness
Allerphed
AlleRx D
All-Nite Cold Formula
Ambenyl-D Decongestant
  Cough Formula
Amdry-D
Anamine
Anamine T.D.
Anatuss DM
Anatuss LA
Balminil Decongestant
Benylin All-In-One Cold & Flu
  Caplets
Benylin All-In-One Cold & Flu
  Nightime Syrup
Benylin All-In-One Cold & Flu
  Syrup
Benylin All-In-One Day & Night
  Caplets
Benylin Cold And Flu With
  Codeine Narcotic
Benylin DM-D
Benylin DM-D-E
Benylin DM-D-E Extra Strength
Brexin-L.A.
Brofed
Bromatane DX Cough
Bromfed
Bromfed-DM
Bromfed-PD
Carbodec
Carbodec DM Drops
Carbodec TR
Cenafed
Cenafed Plus
Children's Advil Cold
Children's Benadryl Allergy &
  Cold Fastmelt
Children's Motrin Cold
Chlorphedrine SR

Chlor-Trimeton 4 Hour Relief
Chlor-Trimeton 12 Hour Relief
Clarinex D 24 Hour
Claritin-D
Claritin-D 12 Hour
Claritin-D 24 Hour
CoActifed Expectorant
Codehist DH
Codimal-L.A.
Codimal-L.A. Half
Coldrine
Colfed-A
Concentrin
Congess JR
Congess SR
Congestac Caplets
Contac Allergy/Sinus Day
  Caplets
Contac Allergy/Sinus Night
  Caplets
Contac Maximum Strength
  Sinus Caplets
Contac Night Caplets
Contac Non-Drowsy Formula
  Sinus Caplets
Contac Severe Cold Formula
Contac Severe Cold Formula
  Night Strength
Cophene-XP
Cotridin
CoTylenol Cold Medication
Dallergy Jr.
Decohistine DH
Deconamine
Deconamine SR
Deconsal II
Detussin Expectorant
Detussin Liquid
Dexaphen SA
Dexophed
Dihistine DH
Dihistine Expectorant
Disophrol
Disophrol Chronotabs
Dristan Cold and Flu
Dristan Cold Caplets
Dristan Cold Maximum
  Strength Caplets
Dristan Juice Mix-in Cold, Flu,
  & Cough
Dristan Sinus Caplets
Drixoral
Drixoral Cold & Allergy
Drixoral Cold & Flu
Drixoral Nasal Decongestant
Drixoral Non-Drowsy Formula
Drixoral Plus
Drixoral Sinus
Drixtab
Durahist
Duratuss
Duratuss HD
Eltor-120

Entex PSE
Entuss Pediatric Expectorant
Entuss-D
Fedahist
Fedahist Decongestant
Fedahist Expectorant
Fedahist Expectorant Pediatric
  Drops
Fedahist Gyrocaps
Fedahist Timecaps
Genaphed
Guaifed
Guaifed-PD
GuaiMAX-D
Guiatuss PE
Hayfebrol
Histalet
Histalet X
Histalet-DM
Hista-Vent PSE
Isoclor Timesules
Klerist-D
Kolephrin/DM Caplets
Kronofed-A
Kronofed-A Jr.
Lodrane LD
Maxenal
Maximum Strength Mucinex D
Maximum Strength Tylenol
  Allergy Sinus Caplets
Motrin-IB Cold & Sinus
Mucinex D
Mucinex DM
Myfedrine
Mytussin DAC
Nasatab LA
ND Clear T.D.
Novahistine DH Liquid
Novahistine DMX Liquid
Novahistine Expectorant
Nucofed
Nytcold Medicine
Ornex Maximum Strength
  Caplets
Ornex No Drowsiness Caplets
Ornex Severe Cold No
  Drowsiness Caplets
Pertussin All Night PM
Phenapap Sinus Headache &
  Congestion
Phenergan-D
P-V-Tussin
Rescon-JR
Respaire-60 SR
Respaire-120 SR
Rhinosyn
Rhinosyn-DM
Rhinosyn-PD
Rhinosyn-X
Robafen DAC
Robafen DM
Robitussin Cough & Cold D
Rondec

Rondec Drops
Rondec-DM
Rondec-DM Drops
Rondec-TR
Ru-Tuss DE
Ru-Tuss Expectorant
Ryna
Ryna-C Liquid
Ryna-CX Liquid
Semprex-D
Simply Stuffy
Sinus Relief
Sinutab Non-Drying Liquid
  Caps
Stamoist E
Sudafed 12 Hour
Sudafed Multi-Symptom Cold
  & Cough
Sudafed Non-Drying Sinus
  Liquid Caps
Sufedrin
Tavist Allergy/Sinus/Headache
Touro A&H
Touro LA Caplets
Triafed
Triafed with Codeine
Triaminic-D Multi-Symptom
  Cold
Tussafin Expectorant
Tussar DM
Tussar-2
Tussend
Tussend Expectorant
Tussend Liquid
Tyrodone
Versacaps
Vicks NyQuil D
Zyrtec-D

RAUWOLFIA ALKALOIDS

GENERIC NAMES
1. DESERPIDINE
2. RAUWOLFIA SERPENTINA
3. RESERPINE

BRAND NAMES
Demi-Regroton[3]
Diupres[3]
Diurigen with Reserpine[3]
Diutensen-R[3]
Dureticyl[3]
Enduronyl[2]
Enduronyl Forte[2]
Harmonyl[1]
Hydropres[3]
Novoreserpine[3]
Oreticyl[1]
Oreticyl Forte[1]
Raudixin[2]
Rauval[2]
Rauverid[2]
Rauzide[2]
Regroton[3]

Reserfia[3]
Serpalan[3]
Serpasil[3]
Wolfina[2]

SALICYLATES

GENERIC NAMES
1. CHOLINE MAGNESIUM
   SALICYLATES
2. CHOLINE SALICYLATE
3. MAGNESIUM SALICYLATE
4. SALICYLAMIDE
5. SALSALATE
6. SODIUM SALICYLATE

BRAND NAMES
Amigesic[5]
Arthropan[2]
Choline Magnesium
  Trisalicylate[1]
Citra Forte[4]
Diagen[5]
Disalcid[5]
Doan's Pills[3]
Dodd's Pills[6]
Duoprin[4]
Fendol[4]
Improved Sino-Tuss[4]
Kolephrin[4]
Kolephrin NN Liquid[4]
Magan[3]
Mobidin[3]
Mono-Gesic[5]
Omnicol[4]
Presalin[4]
Rhinogesic[4]
Rid-A-Pain Compound[4]
S-A-C[4]
Salcylic Acid[4]
Saleto[4]
Saleto-D[4]
Salflex[5]
Salgesic[4]
Salphenyl[4]
Salsitab[5]
Scot-tussin Original 5-Action
  Cold Medicine[6]
Tricosal[1]
Trilisate[1]
Tri-Pain[4]
Tussanil DH Tablets[4]
Tussirex with Codeine Liquid[6]
Uracel[6]

SCOPOLAMINE
   (Hyoscine)

Barbidonna
Barbidonna 2
Buscopan
Kinesed
Transderm-Scop
Transderm-V

SULFONAMIDES

GENERIC NAMES
1. SULFACYTINE
2. SULFADIAZINE
3. SULFAMETHIZOLE
4. SULFAMETHOXAZOLE
5. SULFISOXAZOLE

BRAND NAMES
Apo-Sulfamethoxazole[4]
Apo-Sulfatrim[4]
Apo-Sulfatrim DS[4]
Apo-Sulfisoxazole[5]
Bactrim[4]
Bactrim DS[4]
Cotrim[4]
Cotrim DS[4]
Co-trimoxazole[4]
Eryzole[5]
Gantanol[4]
Gantrisin[5]
Novo-Soxazole[5]
Novotrimel[4]
Novotrimel DS[4]
Nu-Cotrimox[4]
Nu-Cotrimox DS[4]
Pediazole[5]
Protrin[4]
Renoquid[1]
Roubac[4]
Septra[4]
Septra DS[4]
SMZ-TMP[4]
Sulfamethoprim[4]
Sulfamethoprim DS[4]
Sulfaprim[4]
Sulfaprim DS[4]
Sulfatrim[4]
Sulfatrim DS[4]
Sulfimycin[5]
Sulfizole[5]
Sulfoxaprim[4]
Sulfoxaprim DS[4]
Sulmeprim[4]
Thiosulfil Forte[3]
Triazole[4]
Triazole DS[4]
Trimeth-Sulfa[4]
Trisulfam[4]
Urobak[4]
Uroplus DS[4]
Uroplus SS[4]

SULFONYLUREAS

GENERIC NAMES
1. ACETOHEXAMIDE
2. CHLORPROPAMIDE
3. GLIMEPIRIDE
4. GLIPIZIDE
5. GLYBURIDE
6. TOLAZAMIDE
7. TOLBUTAMIDE

BRAND NAMES
Albert Glyburide[5]
Amaryl[3]
Apo-Chlorpropamide[2]
Apo-Glyburide[5]
Apo-Tolbutamide[7]
Avandaryl[3]
DiaBeta[5]
Diabinese[2]
Dimelor[1]
Duetact[3]
Dymelor[1]
Euglucon[5]
Gen-Glybe[5]
Glucamide[2]
Glucotrol[4]
Glucotrol XL[4]
Glucovance[5]
Glynase PresTab[6]
Metaglip[4]
Micronase[5]
Novo-Butamide[7]
Novo-Glyburide[4]
Novo-Propamide[2]
Orinase[7]
Tolamide[6]
Tolinase[6]

TETRACYCLINES

GENERIC NAMES
1. DEMECLOCYCLINE
2. DOXYCYCLINE
3. MINOCYCLINE
4. OXYTETRACYCLINE
5. TETRACYCLINE

BRAND NAMES
Achromycin[5]
Achromycin V[5]
Apo-Doxy[2]
Apo-Tetra[5]
Arestin[3]
Declomycin[1]
Doryx[2]
Doxy-Caps[2]
Doxycin[2]
Doxy-Tabs[2]
E.P. Mycin[4]
Helidac[5]
Minocin[3]
Monodox[2]
Novodoxlin[2]
Novotetra[5]
Nu-Tetra[5]
Oracea[2]
Panmycin[5]
Periostat[5]
Pylera[5]
Robitet[5]
Solodyn[3]
Sumycin[5]
Terramycin[4]
Tetracyn[5]

Tija[4]
Vibramycin[2]

Additional Drug Interactions

The following lists of drugs and their interactions with other drugs are continuations of lists found in the alphabetized drug charts beginning on page 2. These lists are alphabetized by generic name or drug class name, shown in large capital letters. Only those lists too long for the drug charts are included in this section. For complete information about any generic drug, see the alphabetized charts.

GENERIC NAME OR DRUG CLASS	COMBINED EFFECT	GENERIC NAME OR DRUG CLASS	COMBINED EFFECT

ADRENOCORTICOIDS (Systemic)

GENERIC NAME OR DRUG CLASS	COMBINED EFFECT	GENERIC NAME OR DRUG CLASS	COMBINED EFFECT
Attenuated virus vaccines*	Possible viral infection.	Estrogens*	Increased adreno-corticoid effect.
Azoles	Decreased azole effect.	Foscarnet	Potassium depletion.
Barbiturates*	Decreased prednisone effect. Oversedation.	Glutethimide	Decreased adreno-corticoid effect.
Carbamazepine	Decreased adreno-corticoid effect.	Insulin	Decreased insulin effect.
Carbonic anhydrase inhibitors	Increased loss of calcium.	Insulin lispro	May require increased dosage of insulin.
Chloral hydrate	Decreased adreno-corticoid effect.	Isoniazid	Decreased isoniazid effect.
Chlorthalidone	Potassium depletion.	Mifepristone	Decreased effect of mifepristone.
Cholestyramine	Decreased adreno-corticoid effect.	Mitotane	Decreased adreno-corticoid effect.
Cholinergics*	Decreased cholinergic effect.	Phenobarbital	Decreased adreno-corticoid effect.
Colestipol	Decreased adreno-corticoid effect.	Phenytoin	Decreased adreno-corticoid effect.
Contraceptives, oral*	Increased adreno-corticoid effect.	Potassium supplements*	Decreased potassium effect.
Cyclosporine	Decreased adrenocorticoid effect. Increased cyclosporine effect.	Primidone	Decreased adreno-corticoid effect.
		Rifamycins	Decreased adreno-corticoid effect.
Digitalis preparations*	Dangerous potassium depletion. Possible digitalis toxicity.	Salicylates*	Decreased salicylate effect.
Diuretics	Potassium depletion.	Sympathomimetics*	Possible glaucoma.
Ephedrine	Decreased adreno-corticoid effect.	Thyroid hormones*	May require thyroid hormone dosage change.

AMPHETAMINES

GENERIC NAME OR DRUG CLASS	COMBINED EFFECT	GENERIC NAME OR DRUG CLASS	COMBINED EFFECT
Sympathomimetics*	Seizure risk.	Thyroid hormones*	Irregular heartbeat.

*See Glossary

899

ANGIOTENSIN-CONVERTING ENZYME (ACE) INHIBITORS

GENERIC NAME OR DRUG CLASS	COMBINED EFFECT	GENERIC NAME OR DRUG CLASS	COMBINED EFFECT
Pentoxifylline	Increased anti-hypertensive effect.	Spironolactone	Possible excessive potassium in blood.
Potassium	May raise potassium levels in blood to toxic levels.	Terazosin	Decreased effectiveness of terazosin.
Potassium supplements*	Possible increased potassium in blood.	Tiopronin	Increased risk of toxicity to kidneys.
Sotalol	Increased anti-hypertensive effects of both drugs. Dosages may require adjustment.	Triamterene	Possible excessive potassium in blood.

ANGIOTENSIN-CONVERTING ENZYME (ACE) INHIBITORS & HYDROCHLOROTHIAZIDE

GENERIC NAME OR DRUG CLASS	COMBINED EFFECT	GENERIC NAME OR DRUG CLASS	COMBINED EFFECT
Diuretics*	Decreased blood pressure.	Nitrates*	Excessive blood pressure drop.
Lisinopril	Increased anti-hypertensive effect. Dosage of each may require adjustment.	Potassium supplements*	Excessive potassium in blood.
Lithium	Increased lithium effect.	Probenecid	Decreased probenecid effect.
Monoamine oxidase (MAO) inhibitors*	Increased hydro-chlorothiazide effect.	Sotalol	Increased antihypertensive effects of both drugs. Dosages may require adjustment.
Nicardipine	Blood pressure drop. Dosages may require adjustment.	Spironolactone	Possible excessive potassium in blood.
Nimodipine	Possible irregular heartbeat. May worsen congestive heart failure.	Triamterene	Possible excessive potassium in blood.

ANTICOAGULANTS (Oral)

GENERIC NAME OR DRUG CLASS	COMBINED EFFECT	GENERIC NAME OR DRUG CLASS	COMBINED EFFECT
Cholestyramine	Decreased effect of anticoagulant.	Dextrothyroxine	Increased effect of anticoagulant.
Citalopram	May lessen the effect of warfarin.	Diclofenac	Increased risk of bleeding.
Clofibrate	Increased effect of anticoagulant.	Diflunisal	Increased effect of anticoagulant.
Colestipol	Decreased effect of anticoagulant.	Dipyridamole	Increased risk of hemorrhage.
Contraceptives, oral*	Decreased effect of anticoagulant.	Disulfiram	Increased effect of anticoagulant.
Danazol	Increased effect of anticoagulant.	Erythromycins*	Increased effect of anticoagulant.

*See Glossary

ANTICOAGULANTS (Oral) continued

GENERIC NAME OR DRUG CLASS	COMBINED EFFECT	GENERIC NAME OR DRUG CLASS	COMBINED EFFECT
Estrogens*	Decreased effect of anticoagulant.	Phenylbutazone	Increased effect of anticoagulant.
Fenoprofen	Increased effect of anticoagulant.	Phenytoin	Decreased levels of phenytoin.
Fluoxetine	May cause confusion, agitation, convulsions and high blood pressure. Avoid combining.	Plicamycin	Increased effect of anticoagulant.
		Primidone	Decreased effect of anticoagulant.
Fluvoxamine	Increased effect of warfarin.	Propafenone	May require adjustment of anti-coagulant dosage.
Gemfibrozil	Increased effect of anticoagulant.	Proton pump inhibitors	May cause abnormal bleeding.
Glutethimide	Decreased effect of anticoagulant.	Quinidine	Increased effect of anticoagulant.
Griseofulvin	Decreased effect of anticoagulant.	Raloxifene	May lessen effect of warfarin.
Indomethacin	Increased effect of anticoagulant.	Rifamycins	Decreased effect of anticoagulant.
Leukotriene modifiers	Increased effect of warfarin.	Salicylates*	Increased effect of anticoagulant.
Levamisole	Increased risk of bleeding.	Sulfadoxine and pyrimethamine	Increased risk of toxicity.
Meloxicam	Increased risk of bleeding.	Sulindac	Increased effect of anticoagulant.
Methimazole	Increased effect of anticoagulant.	Suprofen	Increased risk of bleeding.
Metronidazole	Increased effect of anticoagulant.	Testolactone	Increased effect of anticoagulant.
Mifepristone	Increased risk of excessive bleeding.	Thyroid hormones*	Increased effect of anticoagulant.
Mineral oil	Decreased absorption of anticoagulant.	Tolcapone	May require adjustment in dosage of warfarin.
Nalidixic acid	Increased effect of anticoagulant.	Toremifene	May increase time it takes blood to clot.
Nicardipine	Possible increased effect of anticoagulant.	Vitamin E	Increased risk of bleeding.
Nimodipine	Possible increased effect of anticoagulant.	Vitamin K	Decreased effect of anticoagulant.
Nizatidine	Increased effect of anticoagulant.	Zafirlukast	May increase effect of warfarin.
Omeprazole	Increased effect of anticoagulant.	Zileuton	Increased warfarin effect.
Orlistat	Increased anticoagulant effect.	Note: Any medicine	Unpredictable absorption.
Paroxetine	Increased effect of anticoagulant.		

ADDITIONAL DRUG INTERACTIONS

ANTICONVULSANTS, HYDANTOIN

GENERIC NAME OR DRUG CLASS	COMBINED EFFECT	GENERIC NAME OR DRUG CLASS	COMBINED EFFECT
Central nervous system (CNS) depressants*	Oversedation.	Methadone	Decreased methadone effect.
Chloramphenicol	Increased anti-convulsant effect.	Methotrexate	Increased methotrexate effect.
Cimetidine	Increased anti-convulsant toxicity.	Methylphenidate	Increased anti-convulsant effect.
Contraceptives, oral*	Increased seizures.	Mifepristone	Decreased effect of mifepristone.
Cyclosporine	May decrease cyclosporine effect.	Modafinil	Anticonvulsant dose may need adjustment.
Digitalis preparations*	Decreased digitalis effect.	Molindone	Increased phenytoin effect.
Disopyramide	Decreased disopyramide effect.	Monoamine oxidase (MAO) inhibitors*	Increased polythiazide effect.
Disulfiram	Increased anti-convulsant effect.	Nicardipine	Increased anticonvulsant effect.
Estrogens*	Increased estrogen effect.	Nimodipine	Increased anticonvulsant effect.
Felbamate	Increased side effects and adverse reactions.	Nitrates*	Excessive blood pressure drop.
Furosemide	Decreased furosemide effect.	Nitroimidazoles	Decreased effect of phenytoin.
Gold compounds*	Increased anticon-vulsant blood levels. Hydantoin dose may require adjustment.	Nizatidine	Increased effect and toxicity of phenytoin.
Glutethimide	Decreased anti-convulsant effect.	Omeprazole	Delayed excretion of phenytoin causing increased amount of phenytoin in blood.
Griseofulvin	Increased griseofulvin effect.	Oxyphenbutazone	Increased anti-convulsant effect.
Hypoglycemics, oral*	Possible decreased hypoglycemic effect.	Para-aminosalicylic acid (PAS)	Increased anti-convulsant effect.
Hypoglycemics, other*	Possible decreased hypoglycemic effect.	Paroxetine	Decreased anti-convulsant effect.
Isoniazid	Increased anti-convulsant effect.	Phenacemide	Increased risk of paranoid symptoms.
Lamotrigine	Decreased lamotrigine effect with phenytoin.	Phenothiazines*	Increased anti-convulsant effect.
Leucovorin	May counteract the effect of phenytoin or any hydantoin anticonvulsant.	Phenylbutazone	Increased anti-convulsant effect.
		Potassium supplements*	Decreased potassium effect.
Leukotriene modifiers	Increased phenytoin effect.	Probenecid	Decreased probenecid effect.
Loxapine	Decreased anticonvulsant effect.	Methyldopa	Possible decreased methyldopa effect.

*See Glossary

GENERIC NAME OR DRUG CLASS	COMBINED EFFECT	GENERIC NAME OR DRUG CLASS	COMBINED EFFECT

ANTICONVULSANTS, HYDANTOIN continued

GENERIC NAME OR DRUG CLASS	COMBINED EFFECT	GENERIC NAME OR DRUG CLASS	COMBINED EFFECT
Propafenone	Increased effect of both drugs and increased risk of toxicity.	Sucralfate	Decreased anticonvulsant effect.
Propranolol	Increased propranolol effect.	Sulfa drugs*	Increased anticonvulsant effect.
Quetiapine	Decreased quetiapine effect with phenytoin.	Theophylline	Reduced anticonvulsant effect.
Quinidine	Increased quinidine effect.	Trimethoprim	Increased phenytoin effect.
Rifamycins	Decreased anticonvulsant effect.	Valproic acid*	Each drug may need dosage adjusted.
Sedatives*	Increased sedative effect.	Xanthines*	Decreased effects of both drugs.
Sotalol	Decreased sotalol effect.	Zafirlukast	May increase effect of phenytoin.
		Zaleplon	Decreased zaleplon effect.

ANTIDEPRESSANTS, TRICYCLIC

GENERIC NAME OR DRUG CLASS	COMBINED EFFECT	GENERIC NAME OR DRUG CLASS	COMBINED EFFECT
Benzodiazepines*	Increased sedation.	Disulfiram	Delirium.
Bupropion	Increased risk of seizures.	Dofetilide	Increased risk of heart problems.
Central nervous system (CNS) depressants*	Excessive sedation.	Ethchlorvynol	Delirium.
		Fluoxetine	Increased effect of tricyclic antidepressant. Possible toxicity.
Cimetidine	Possible increased tricyclic antidepressant effect and toxicity.	Fluvoxamine	Increased antidepressant effect.
Citalopram	Increased tricyclic antidepressant effect and toxicity.	Furazolidone	Sudden, severe increase in blood pressure.
Clonidine	Blood pressure increase. Avoid combination.	Guanabenz	Decreased guanabenz effect.
Clozapine	Toxic effect on the central nervous system.	Guanadrel	Decreased guanadrel effect.
		Guanethidine	Decreased guanethidine effect.
Contraceptives, oral*	Increased depression.	Leucovorin	High alcohol content of leucovorin may cause adverse effects.
Desmopressin	Increased risk of thirstiness which may lead to drinking excess fluids.	Levodopa	May increase blood pressure. May decrease levodopa effect.
Dextrothyroxine	Increased antidepressant effect. Irregular heartbeat.	Lithium	Possible decreased seizure threshold.

ADDITIONAL DRUG INTERACTIONS

GENERIC NAME OR DRUG CLASS	COMBINED EFFECT	GENERIC NAME OR DRUG CLASS	COMBINED EFFECT

ANTIDEPRESSANTS, TRICYCLIC continued

GENERIC NAME OR DRUG CLASS	COMBINED EFFECT	GENERIC NAME OR DRUG CLASS	COMBINED EFFECT
Methyldopa	Possible decreased methyldopa effect.	Phenytoin	Decreased phenytoin effect.
Methylphenidate	Possible increased tricyclic anti-depressant effect and toxicity.	Procainamide	Possible irregular heartbeat.
		Quinidine	Possible irregular heartbeat.
Modafinil	Increased anti-depressant effect.	Serotonergics*	Increased risk of serotonin syndrome*.
Molindone	Increased molindone effect.	Sertraline	Increased depressive effects of both drugs.
Monoamine oxidase (MAO) inhibitors*	Fever, delirium, convulsions.	Sympathomimetics*	Increased sympatho-mimetic effect.
Narcotics*	Oversedation.	Thyroid hormones*	Irregular heartbeat.
Nicotine	Increased effect of antidepressant (with imipramine).	Tolcapone	May increase incidence of adverse effects of tolcapone.
Phenothiazines*	Possible increased tricyclic anti-depressant effect and toxicity.	Zaleplon	Increased effect of either drug. Avoid.
		Zolpidem	Increased sedative effect. Avoid.

ANTIDYSKINETICS

GENERIC NAME OR DRUG CLASS	COMBINED EFFECT	GENERIC NAME OR DRUG CLASS	COMBINED EFFECT
Imatinib	Increased effect of pimozide.	Monoamine oxidase (MAO) inhibitors*	Increased antidyskinetic effect.
Levodopa	Possible increased levodopa effect.	Telithromycin	Heart problem risk with pimozide. Avoid.

ANTIFUNGALS, AZOLES

GENERIC NAME OR DRUG CLASS	COMBINED EFFECT	GENERIC NAME OR DRUG CLASS	COMBINED EFFECT
Losartan	Decreased losartan effect.	Proton pump inhibitors	Decreased antifungal effect.
Methscopolamine	Decreased azole effect.	Quetiapine	Increased risk of quetiapine toxicity.
Methylprednisolone	Increased effect of methylprednisolone.	Ranitidine	Decreased azole effect.
Mifepristone	Decreased effect of mifepristone.	Rifamycins	Decreased azole effect.
Nizatidine	Decreased azole effect.	Ritonavir	Increased ritonavir effect.
Omeprazole	Decreased azole effect.	Scopolamine	Decreased azole effect.
Phenytoin	May alter effect of both drugs.	Sibutramine	Increased effect of sibutramine.
Propantheline	Decreased azole effect.	Sildenafil	Effects unknown. Consult doctor.

*See Glossary

GENERIC NAME OR DRUG CLASS	COMBINED EFFECT	GENERIC NAME OR DRUG CLASS	COMBINED EFFECT
ANTIFUNGALS, AZOLES continued			
Sodium bicarbonate	Decreased azole effect.	Warfarin	Increased warfarin effect.

ANTIHISTAMINES, PHENOTHIAZINE-DERIVATIVE

Clozapine	Toxic effect on the central nervous system.	Methyprylon	May increase sedative effect to dangerous level. Avoid.
Dronabinol	Increased effects of both drugs. Avoid.	Metyrosine	Increased likelihood of toxic symptoms of each.
Epinephrine	Decreased epinephrine effect.	Mind-altering drugs*	Increased effect of mind-altering drugs.
Ethinamate	Dangerous increased effects of ethinamate. Avoid combining.	Molindone	Increased sedative and antihistamine effect.
Extrapyramidal reaction*-causing medicines	Increased frequency and severity of extra-pyramidal reactions.	Monoamine oxidase (MAO) inhibitors*	Increased anti-histamine effect.
Fluoxetine	Increased depressant effects of both drugs.	Nabilone	Greater depression of central nervous system.
Guanethidine	Decreased guanethidine effect.	Narcotics*	Increased narcotic effect.
Guanfacine	May increase depressant effects of either medicine.	Sedatives*	Increased sedative effect.
Leucovorin	High alcohol content of leucovorin may cause adverse effects.	Sertraline	Increased depressive effects of both drugs.
		Sotalol	Increased antihistamine effect.
Levodopa	Decreased levodopa effect.	Tranquilizers*	Increased tranquilizer effect. Avoid.

ANTI-INFLAMMATORY DRUGS, NONSTEROIDAL (NSAIDs)

Diuretics*	May decrease diuretic effect.	Meloxicam	Increased risk of side effects of meloxicam.
Gold compounds*	Increased risk of kidney toxicity.	Methotrexate	Increased risk of side effects of methotrexate.
Lithium	Increased lithium effect.	Minoxidil	Decreased minoxidil effect.
Losartan	Decreased anti-hypertensive effect.	Probenecid	Increased pain relief.
Meglitinides	Unknown effect. Avoid.		

*See Glossary

905

GENERIC NAME OR DRUG CLASS	COMBINED EFFECT	GENERIC NAME OR DRUG CLASS	COMBINED EFFECT

ANTI-INFLAMMATORY DRUGS, NONSTEROIDAL (NSAIDs) continued

GENERIC NAME OR DRUG CLASS	COMBINED EFFECT	GENERIC NAME OR DRUG CLASS	COMBINED EFFECT
Terazosin	Decreased effectiveness of terazosin. Causes sodium and fluid retention.	Tiopronin	Increased risk of toxicity to kidneys.
Thyroid hormones*	Rapid heartbeat, blood pressure rise.	Triamterene	Reduced triamterene effect.

ASPIRIN

GENERIC NAME OR DRUG CLASS	COMBINED EFFECT	GENERIC NAME OR DRUG CLASS	COMBINED EFFECT
Dextrothyroxine (large doses, continuous use)	Increased dextrothyroxine effect.	Penicillins*	Increased effect of both drugs.
Diclofenac	Increased risk of stomach ulcer.	Phenobarbital	Decreased aspirin effect.
Ethacrynic acid	Possible aspirin toxicity.	Phenytoin	Increased phenytoin effect.
Furosemide	Possible aspirin toxicity. May decrease furosemide effect.	Probenecid	Decreased probenecid effect.
		Propranolol	Decreased aspirin effect.
Gold compounds*	Increased likelihood of kidney damage.	Rauwolfia alkaloids*	Decreased aspirin effect.
Indomethacin	Risk of stomach bleeding and ulcers.	Salicylates*	Likely aspirin toxicity.
Ketoprofen	Increased risk of stomach ulcer.	Sotalol	Decreased anti-hypertensive effect of sotalol.
Levamisole	Increased risk of bleeding.	Spironolactone	Decreased spirono-lactone effect.
Meloxicam	Increased risk of stomach ulcer.	Sulfinpyrazone	Decreased sulfin-pyrazone effect.
Methotrexate	Increased methotrexate effect.	Terazosin	Decreased effectiveness of terazosin. Causes sodium and fluid retention.
Minoxidil	Decreased minoxidil effect.		
Oxprenolol	Decreased anti-hypertensive effect of oxprenolol.	Ticlopidine	Increased effect of both drugs.
		Vitamin C (large doses)	Possible aspirin toxicity.
Para-aminosalicylic acid	Possible aspirin toxicity.	Valproic acid*	May increase valproic acid effect.

ATROPINE, HYOSCYAMINE, METHENAMINE, METHYLENE BLUE, PHENYLSALICYLATE & BENZOIC ACID

GENERIC NAME OR DRUG CLASS	COMBINED EFFECT	GENERIC NAME OR DRUG CLASS	COMBINED EFFECT
Diuretics, thiazide*	Decreased urine acidity.	Gold compounds*	Increased likelihood of kidney damage.
Furosemide	Possible salicylate toxicity.	Haloperidol	Increased internal eye pressure.

ATROPINE, HYOSCYAMINE, METHENAMINE, METHYLENE BLUE, PHENYLSALICYLATE & BENZOIC ACID continued

Generic Name or Drug Class	Combined Effect	Generic Name or Drug Class	Combined Effect
Indomethacin	Risk of stomach bleeding and ulcers.	Pilocarpine	Loss of pilocarpine effect in glaucoma treatment.
Ketoconazole	Reduced ketoconazole effect.	Potassium supplements*	Possible intestinal ulcers with oral potassium tablets.
Meperidine	Increased atropine and hyoscyamine effect.	Probenecid	Decreased probenecid effect.
Methylphenidate	Increased atropine and hyoscyamine effect.	Propranolol	Decreased salicylate effect.
Minoxidil	Decreased minoxidil effect.	Rauwolfia alkaloids*	Decreased salicylate effect.
Monoamine oxidase (MAO) inhibitors*	Increased belladonna and atropine effect.	Salicylates*	Likely salicylate toxicity.
Orphenadrine	Increased atropine and hyoscyamine effect.	Sedatives* or central nervous system (CNS) depressants*	Increased sedative effect of both drugs.
Oxprenolol	Decreased anti-hypertensive effect of oxprenolol.	Sodium bicarbonate	Decreased methenamine effect.
Para-aminosalicylic acid (PAS)	Possible salicylate toxicity.	Spironolactone	Decreased spirono-lactone effect.
Penicillins*	Increased effect of both drugs.	Sulfa drugs*	Possible kidney damage.
Phenobarbital	Decreased salicylate effect.	Sulfinpyrazone	Decreased sulfin-pyrazone effect.
Phenothiazines*	Increased atropine and hyoscyamine effect.	Vitamin C (1 to 4 grams per day)	Increased effect of methenamine, contributing to urine acidity; decreased atropine effect; possible salicylate toxicity.
Phenytoin	Increased phenytoin effect.		

BARBITURATES

Generic Name or Drug Class	Combined Effect	Generic Name or Drug Class	Combined Effect
Meglitinides	Increased blood level of meglitinides.	Nitroimidazoles	Decreased nitroimidazoles effect.
Mifepristone	Decreased effect of mifepristone.	Sertraline	Increased depressive effects of both drugs.
Mind-altering drugs*	Dangerous sedation. Avoid.	Sotalol	Increased barbiturate effect. Dangerous sedation.
Modafinil	Increased modafinil effect.	Valproic acid*	Increased barbiturate effect.
Monoamine oxidase (MAO) inhibitors*	Increased barbiturate effect.	Zaleplon	Decreased zaleplon effect.
Narcotics*	Dangerous sedation. Avoid.		

*See Glossary

ADDITIONAL DRUG INTERACTIONS

BARBITURATES, ASPIRIN & CODEINE (Also contains caffeine)

GENERIC NAME OR DRUG CLASS	COMBINED EFFECT	GENERIC NAME OR DRUG CLASS	COMBINED EFFECT
Anticoagulants, oral*	Increased anti-coagulant effect. Abnormal bleeding.	Mind-altering drugs*	Dangerous sedation. Avoid.
Anticonvulsants*	Changed seizure patterns.	Minoxidil	Decreased minoxidil effect.
Antidepressants*	Decreased anti-depressant effect. Possible dangerous oversedation.	Monoamine oxidase (MAO) inhibitors*	Increased butalbital effect.
Antidiabetics, oral*	Increased butalbital effect. Low blood sugar.	Naltrexone	Decreased analgesic effect.
Antihistamines*	Dangerous sedation. Avoid.	Narcotics*	Dangerous sedation. Avoid.
Anti-inflammatory drugs, nonsteroidal (NSAIDs)*	Risk of stomach bleeding and ulcers.	Nitrates*	Excessive blood pressure drop.
Aspirin, other	Likely aspirin toxicity.	Nitroimidazoles	Decreased nitroimidazole effect.
Beta-adrenergic blocking agents*	Decreased effect of beta-adrenergic blocker.	Pain relievers*	Dangerous sedation. Avoid.
Carteolol	Increased narcotic effect. Dangerous sedation.	Para-aminosalicylic acid	Possible aspirin toxicity.
		Penicillins*	Increased effect of drugs.
Contraceptives, oral*	Decreased contraceptive effect.	Phenobarbital	Decreased aspirin effect.
Digitoxin	Decreased digitoxin effect.	Phenothiazines*	Increased phenothiazine effect.
Doxycycline	Decreased doxycycline effect.	Phenytoin	Increased phenytoin effect.
Dronabinol	Increased effect of drugs.	Probenecid	Decreased probenecid effect.
Furosemide	Possible aspirin toxicity.	Propranolol	Decreased aspirin effect.
Gold compounds*	Increased likelihood of kidney damage.	Rauwolfia alkaloids*	Decreased aspirin effect.
Griseofulvin	Decreased griseofulvin effect.	Salicylates*	Likely aspirin toxicity.
Indapamide	Increased indapamide effect.	Sedatives*	Dangerous sedation. Avoid.
Indomethacin	Risk of stomach bleeding and ulcers.	Sleep inducers*	Dangerous sedation. Avoid.
Lamotrigine	Decreased lamotrigine effect.	Sotalol	Increased narcotic effect. Dangerous sedation.
Methotrexate	Increased methotrexate effect.	Spironolactone	Decreased spirono-lactone effect.
		Sulfinpyrazone	Decreased sulfin-pyrazone effect.

*See Glossary

BARBITURATES, ASPIRIN & CODEINE (Also contains caffeine) continued

GENERIC NAME OR DRUG CLASS	COMBINED EFFECT	GENERIC NAME OR DRUG CLASS	COMBINED EFFECT
Tranquilizers*	Dangerous sedation. Avoid.	Vitamin C (large doses)	Possible aspirin toxicity.
Valproic acid	Increased phenobarbital effect.	Zidovudine	Increased toxicity of both.

BELLADONNA ALKALOIDS & BARBITURATES

GENERIC NAME OR DRUG CLASS	COMBINED EFFECT	GENERIC NAME OR DRUG CLASS	COMBINED EFFECT
Attapulgite	Decreased belladonna effect.	Monoamine oxidase (MAO) inhibitors*	Increased belladonna na and barbiturate effect.
Beta-adrenergic blocking agents*	Decreased effects of beta-adrenergic blocker.	Narcotics*	Dangerous sedation. Avoid.
Carteolol	Increased barbiturate effect. Dangerous sedation.	Nitrates*	Increased internal eye pressure.
Central nervous system (CNS) depressants*	Dangerous sedation. Avoid.	Nizatidine	Increased nizatidine effect.
		Orphenadrine	Increased belladonna effect.
Contraceptives, oral*	Decreased contraceptive effect.	Pain relievers*	Dangerous sedation. Avoid.
Digitoxin	Decreased digitoxin effect.	Phenothiazines*	Increased belladonna effect. Danger of oversedation.
Doxycycline	Decreased doxycycline effect.		
Dronabinol	Increased effects of both drugs. Avoid.	Pilocarpine	Loss of pilocarpine effect in glaucoma treatment.
Furosemide	Possible orthostatic hypotension.	Potassium supplements*	Possible intestinal ulcers with oral potassium tablets.
Griseofulvin	Decreased griseofulvin effect.		
Haloperidol	Increased internal eye pressure.	Quinidine	Increased belladonna effect.
Indapamide	Increased indapamide effect.	Sedatives*	Dangerous sedation. Avoid.
Ketoconazole	Decreased ketoconazole effect.	Sleep inducers*	Dangerous sedation. Avoid.
Meperidine	Increased belladonna effect.	Sotalol	Increased barbiturate effect. Dangerous sedation.
Methylphenidate	Increased belladonna effect.	Tranquilizers*	Dangerous sedation. Avoid.
Metronidazole	Decreased metronidazole effect.	Valproic acid*	Increased barbiturate effect.
Mind-altering drugs*	Dangerous sedation. Avoid.	Vitamin C	Decreased belladonna effect. Avoid large doses of vitamin C.

ADDITIONAL DRUG INTERACTIONS

GENERIC NAME OR DRUG CLASS	COMBINED EFFECT	GENERIC NAME OR DRUG CLASS	COMBINED EFFECT

BENZODIAZEPINES

GENERIC NAME OR DRUG CLASS	COMBINED EFFECT	GENERIC NAME OR DRUG CLASS	COMBINED EFFECT
Levodopa	Decreased levodopa effect.	Proton pump inhibitors	Increased effect of diazepam.
Narcotics*	Increased sedative effect of both drugs.	Telithromycin	Increased effect of benzodiazepine.
Nefazodone	Increased effect of benzodiazepine.	Rifamycins	Decreased effect of benzodiazepine.
Nicotine	Increased effect of benzodiazepine.	Valproic acid*	Increased effect of benzodiazepines.
Omeprazole	Increased effect of benzodiazepine.	Zidovudine	Increased effect of zidovudine.
Probenecid	Increased effect of probenecid and risk of sedation.		

BETA-ADRENERGIC BLOCKING AGENTS

GENERIC NAME OR DRUG CLASS	COMBINED EFFECT	GENERIC NAME OR DRUG CLASS	COMBINED EFFECT
Diazoxide	Additional blood pressure drop.	Nicotine	Increased effect of propranolol.
Estrogens*	May cause blood pressure problems.	Nitrates*	Possible excessive blood pressure drop.
Flecainide	Increased effect of toxicity on heart muscle.	Phenothiazines	Increased effect of both drugs.
Fluvoxamine	Increased beta blocker effect.	Phenytoin	Decreased beta blocker effect.
Guanabenz	May cause blood pressure problems.	Propafenone	Increased beta blocker effect.
Insulin	Hypoglycemic effects may be prolonged.	Quinidine	May cause heart problems.
Leukotriene modifiers	Increased beta blocker effect.	Reserpine	Increased reserpine effect. Excessive sedation and depression. Additional blood pressure drop.
Meglitinides	Increased risk of low blood sugar.		
Miglitol	Decreased effect of propranolol.	Sympathomimetics*	Decreased effects of both drugs.
Molindone	Increased tranquilizer effect.	Telithromycin	Various effects. Use with caution.
Monoamine oxidase (MAO) inhibitors*	High blood pressure following MAO discontinuation.	Warfarin	Increased warfarin effect.
Nefazodone	Dosages of both drugs may require adjustment.	Xanthines (aminophylline, theophylline)	Decreased effects of both drugs.

*See Glossary

BETA-ADRENERGIC BLOCKING AGENTS & THIAZIDE DIURETICS

GENERIC NAME OR DRUG CLASS	COMBINED EFFECT	GENERIC NAME OR DRUG CLASS	COMBINED EFFECT
Antidiabetics*	Increased antidiabetic effect.	Lisinopril	Increased anti-hypertensive effect. Dosage of each may require adjustment.
Antihistamines*	Decreased antihistamine effect.	Metolazone	Increased diuretic effect.
Antihypertensives*	Increased anti-hypertensive effect.	Miglitol	Decreased effect of propranolol.
Anti-inflammatory drugs, nonsteroidal (NSAIDs)*	Decreased antiinflammatory effect.	Monoamine oxidase (MAO) inhibitors*	Increased hydro chlorothiazide effect.
Barbiturates*	Increased barbiturate effect. Dangerous sedation.	Narcotics*	Increased narcotic effect. Dangerous sedation.
Bumetanide	Increased diuretic effect.	Nicardipine	Possible irregular heartbeat and con-gestive heart failure.
Calcium channel blockers*	Increased anti-hypertensive effect. Dosages of both drugs may require adjustments.	Nicotine	Increased beta blocker effect.
Cholestyramine	Decreased hydro-chlorothiazide effect.	Nitrates*	Excessive blood pressure drop.
Diclofenac	Decreased anti-hypertensive effect.	Phenytoin	Increased beta adrenergic effect.
Digitalis preparations*	Excessive potassium loss that causes dangerous heart rhythms. Can either increase or decrease heart rate. Improves irregular heartbeat.	Potassium supplements*	Decreased potassium effect.
		Probenecid	Decreased probenecid effect.
Diuretics, thiazide*	Increased effect of other thiazide diuretics.	Propafenone	Increased beta blocker effect.
Ethacrynic acid	Increased diuretic effect.	Quinidine	Slows heart excessively.
Furosemide	Increased diuretic effect.	Reserpine	Increased reserpine effect. Excessive sedation and depression.
Guanfacine	Increased effect of both drugs.	Sympathomimetics*	Decreased effectiveness of both.
Hypoglycemics, oral*	Decreased ability to lower blood glucose.	Theophylline	Decreased effectiveness of both.
Indapamide	Increased diuretic effect.	Tocainide	May worsen congestive heart failure.
Insulin	Decreased ability to lower blood glucose.	Zinc supplements	Increased need for zinc.

ADDITIONAL DRUG INTERACTIONS

*See Glossary

GENERIC NAME OR DRUG CLASS	COMBINED EFFECT	GENERIC NAME OR DRUG CLASS	COMBINED EFFECT

BRONCHODILATORS, ADRENERGIC

GENERIC NAME OR DRUG CLASS	COMBINED EFFECT	GENERIC NAME OR DRUG CLASS	COMBINED EFFECT
Rauwolfia	Decreased rauwolfia effect.	Theophylline	Increased gastro-intestinal intolerance.
Sympathomimetics*, other	Increased bronchodilator effect.	Thyroid hormones*	Increased bronchodilator effect.
Terazosin	Decreased effectiveness of terazosin.	Tolcapone	May require adjustment in dosage.

BRONCHODILATORS, XANTHINE

GENERIC NAME OR DRUG CLASS	COMBINED EFFECT	GENERIC NAME OR DRUG CLASS	COMBINED EFFECT
Telithromycin	Increased effect of telithromycin.	Zafirlukast	May increase effect of zafirlukast.
Ticlopidine	Increased theophylline effect.	Zileuton	Increased theophylline effect.
Troleandomycin	Increased bronchodilator effect.		

CALCIUM CHANNEL BLOCKERS

GENERIC NAME OR DRUG CLASS	COMBINED EFFECT	GENERIC NAME OR DRUG CLASS	COMBINED EFFECT
Lithium	Possible decreased lithium effect.	Nimodipine	Dangerous blood pressure drop.
Metformin	Increased metformin effect.	Nitrates*	Reduced angina attacks.
Nicardipine	Possible increased effect and toxicity of each drug.		

CALCIUM SUPPLEMENTS

GENERIC NAME OR DRUG CLASS	COMBINED EFFECT	GENERIC NAME OR DRUG CLASS	COMBINED EFFECT
Quinidine	Increased quinidine effect.	Theophylline	May increase effect and toxicity of theophylline.
Rifamycins	Decreased effect of calcium channel blocker.	Vitamin A	Decreased vitamin effect.
Salicylates*	Increased salicylate effect.	Vitamin D	Increased vitamin absorption, sometimes excessively; decreased effect of calcium channel blocker.
Sulfa drugs*	Decreased sulfa effect.		
Tetracyclines*	Decreased tetracycline effect.	Zafirlukast	May increase calcium channel blocker effect.

*See Glossary

CARBAMAZEPINE

GENERIC NAME OR DRUG CLASS	COMBINED EFFECT	GENERIC NAME OR DRUG CLASS	COMBINED EFFECT
Antifungals, azole	Increased effect of carbamazepine. Decreased effect of antifungal.	**Fluoxetine**	Increased carbamazepine effect.
Barbiturates*	Possible increased barbiturate metabolism.	**Fluvoxamine**	Possible toxicity of carbamazepine.
Benzodiazepines	Decreased effect of benzodiazepine.	**Guanfacine**	May increase depressant effects of either drug.
Bupropion	Decreased effect of bupropion.	**Haloperidol**	Decreased effect of haloperidol.
Carbonic anhydrase inhibitors (oral)	Increased risk of bone loss.	**Isoniazid**	Increased effect of carbamazepine.
Central nervous system (CNS) depressants*	Increased sedative effect.	**Lamotrigine**	Decreased lamotrigine effect. Increased risk of side effects.
Cimetidine	Increased carbamazepine effect.	**Leucovorin**	High alcohol content of leucovorin may cause adverse effects.
Citalopram	May lessen effect of citalopram.	**Leukotriene modifiers**	Increased effect of carbamazepine.
Clozapine	Toxic effect on bone marrow and central nervous system.	**Lithium**	Increased risk of side effects.
Contraceptives, oral*	Reduced contraceptive protection. Breakthrough bleeding.	**Mebendazole**	Decreased effect of mebendazole.
Cyclosporine	Decreased effect of cyclosporine.	**Meglitinides**	Blood sugar problems.
Danazol	Increased effect of carbamazepine.	**Methylphenidate**	Decreased effect of methylphenidate.
Desmopressin	May increase desmopressin effect.	**Mifepristone**	Decreased effect of mifepristone.
Digitalis preparations*	Decreased digitalis effect.	**Monoamine oxidase (MAO) Inhibitors***	Dangerous overstimulation. Avoid.
Diltiazem	Increased effect of carbamazepine.	**Phenytoin**	Decreased effect of both drugs.
Doxycycline	Decreased doxycycline effect.	**Phenobarbital**	Decreased carbamazepine effect.
Estrogens*	Decreased estrogen effect.	**Primidone**	Decreased carbamazepine effect.
Erythromycins*	Increased carbamazepine effect.	**Propoxyphene**	Increased toxicity of both. Avoid.
Felbamate	Increased side effects and adverse reactions.	**Rifampin**	Decreased carbamazepine effect.
Felodipine	Decreased effect of felodipine.	**Risperidone**	Decreased risperidone effect.
		Theophylline	Decreases effect of theophylline.

*See Glossary

GENERIC NAME OR DRUG CLASS	COMBINED EFFECT	GENERIC NAME OR DRUG CLASS	COMBINED EFFECT

CARBAMAZEPINE continued

GENERIC NAME OR DRUG CLASS	COMBINED EFFECT	GENERIC NAME OR DRUG CLASS	COMBINED EFFECT
Ticlopidine	Decreased effect of carbamazepine.	Vasopressin	Increased effect of vasopressin.
Tiopronin	Increased risk of toxicity to bone marrow.	Verapamil	Increased effect of carbamazepine.
		Zafirlukast	Increased effect of carbamazepine.
Valproic acid*	Decreased effect of valproic acid.	Zaleplon	Decreased zaleplon effect.

CENTRAL ALPHA AGONISTS

Central nervous system (CNS) depressants*	Increased depressive effects of both drugs.	Monoamine oxidase (MAO) inhibitors*	Dangerous changes in blood pressure. Take at least 14 days apart.

CLONIDINE & CHLORTHALIDONE

Diuretics*	Excessive blood pressure drop.	Nicardipine	Blood pressure drop. Dosage may require adjustment.
Fenfluramine	Possible increased clonidine effect.	Nitrates*	Possible excessive blood pressure drop.
Guanfacine	Impaired blood pressure control.	Potassium supplements*	Decreased potassium effect.
Indapamide	Increased diuretic effect.	Probenecid	Decreased probenecid effect.
Lithium	Increased lithium effect.	Sedatives* or central nervous system (CNS) depressants*	Increased sedative effect of both drugs.
Monoamine oxidase (MAO) inhibitors*	Increased chlorthalidone effect.		
Nabilone	Greater depression of central nervous system.	Sotalol	Decreased antihypertensive effect.
		Terazosin	Decreased terazosin effect.

CONTRACEPTIVES, ORAL & SKIN

Dextrothyroxine	Decreased dextrothyroxine effect.	Meperidine	Increased meperidine effect.
		Meprobamate	Decreased contraceptive effect.
Guanethidine	Decreased guanethidine effect.	Mineral oil	Decreased contraceptive effect.
Hypoglycemics, oral*	Decreased effect of hypoglycemics.	Non-nucleoside reverse transcriptase inhibitors	Decreased contraceptive effect. Use alternative birth control method.
Insulin	Possibly decreased insulin effect.		
Insulin lispro	May need increased dosage of insulin.		

*See Glossary

GENERIC NAME OR DRUG CLASS	COMBINED EFFECT	GENERIC NAME OR DRUG CLASS	COMBINED EFFECT

CONTRACEPTIVES, ORAL & SKIN continued

GENERIC NAME OR DRUG CLASS	COMBINED EFFECT	GENERIC NAME OR DRUG CLASS	COMBINED EFFECT
Phenothiazines*	Increased phenothiazine effect.	Tetracyclines*	Decreased contraceptive effect.
Rifamycins	Decreased contraceptive effect.	Thiazolidinediones	Decreased contraceptive effect.
Sulfadoxine and pyrimethamine	Reduced reliability of the pill.	Ursodiol	Decreased ursodiol effect.
Terazosin	Decreases terazosin effect.	Vitamin A	Vitamin A excess.
		Vitamin C	Possible increased contraceptive effect.

CYCLOSPORINE

GENERIC NAME OR DRUG CLASS	COMBINED EFFECT	GENERIC NAME OR DRUG CLASS	COMBINED EFFECT
Nimodipine	Increased cyclosporine toxicity.	Thiazolidinediones	Decreased effect of cyclosporine.
Nitroimidazoles	Increased cyclosporine effect	Tiopronin	Increased risk of toxicity to kidneys.
Orlistat	Unknown effect. Monitor closely.	Vancomycin	Increased chance of hearing loss or kidney damage.
Rifamycins	Decreased effect of cyclosporine.	Virus vaccines	Increased adverse reactions to vaccine.
Terbinafine (oral)	Decreased effect of cyclosporine.	Zafirlukast	May increase effect of cyclosporine.

DIFENOXIN & ATROPINE

GENERIC NAME OR DRUG CLASS	COMBINED EFFECT	GENERIC NAME OR DRUG CLASS	COMBINED EFFECT
Nitrates*	Increased internal eye pressure.	Potassium supplements*	Possible intestinal ulcers with oral potassium tablets.
Orphenadrine	Increased atropine effect.	Procainamide	Increased atropine effect.
Phenothiazines*	Increased atropine effect.	Sertraline	Increased depressive effects of both drugs.
Pilocarpine	Loss of pilocarpine effect in glaucoma treatment.	Vitamin C	Decreased atropine effect. Avoid large doses of vitamin C.

DIGITALIS PREPARATIONS (Digitalis Glycosides)

GENERIC NAME OR DRUG CLASS	COMBINED EFFECT	GENERIC NAME OR DRUG CLASS	COMBINED EFFECT
Metoclopramide	Decreased digitalis absorption.	Nicardipine	Increased digitalis effect. May need to reduce dose.
Mineral Oil	Decreased digitalis effect.	Nizatidine	Increased digitalis effect.
Nefazodone	Increased effect of digoxin.	Oxyphenbutazone	Decreased digitalis effect.

*See Glossary

GENERIC NAME OR DRUG CLASS	COMBINED EFFECT	GENERIC NAME OR DRUG CLASS	COMBINED EFFECT

DIGITALIS PREPARATIONS (Digitalis Glycosides) continued

GENERIC NAME OR DRUG CLASS	COMBINED EFFECT	GENERIC NAME OR DRUG CLASS	COMBINED EFFECT
Paroxetine	Increased levels of paroxetine in blood.	Spironolactone	Increased digitalis effect. May require digitalis dosage reduction.
Phenobarbital	Decreased digitalis effect.		
Phenylbutazone	Decreased digitalis effect.	Sulfasalazine	Decreased digitalis absorption.
Potassium supplements*	Overdose of either drug may cause severe heartbeat irregularity.	Sympathomimetics*	Increased risk of heartbeat irregularities.
Propafenone	Increased digitalis absorption.	Telithromycin	May increase digoxin effect.
Proton pump inhibitors	Increased effect of digoxin.	Tetracycline	May increase digitalis absorption.
Quinidine	Increased digitalis effect.	Thyroid hormones*	Digitalis toxicity.
Ranolazine	Increased effect of digoxin.	Ticlopidine	Slightly decreased digitalis effect (digoxin only).
Rauwolfia alkaloids*	Increased digitalis effect.	Trazodone	Possible increased digitalis toxicity.
Rifamycins	Possible decreased digitalis effect.	Triamterene	Possible decreased digitalis effect.
Sotalol	Can either increase or decrease heart rate. Improves irregular heartbeat.	Verapamil	Increased digitalis effect.

DIURETICS, LOOP

GENERIC NAME OR DRUG CLASS	COMBINED EFFECT	GENERIC NAME OR DRUG CLASS	COMBINED EFFECT
Meloxicam	Decreased effect of diuretic.	Potassium supplements*	Decreased potassium effect.
Nephrotoxics*	Increased risk of toxicity.	Probenecid	Decreased probenecid effect.
Nimodipine	Dangerous blood pressure drop.	Salicylates* (including aspirin)	Dangerous salicylate retention.
Nitrates*	Excessive blood pressure drop.	Sedatives*	Increased diuretic effect.
Phenytoin	Decreased diuretic effect.		

DIURETICS, POTASSIUM-SPARING & HYDROCHLOROTHIAZIDE

GENERIC NAME OR DRUG CLASS	COMBINED EFFECT	GENERIC NAME OR DRUG CLASS	COMBINED EFFECT
Cholestyramine	Decreased diuretic effect. Take 1 hour before diuretic.	Colestipol	Decreased diuretic effect. Take 1 hour before diuretic.
		Cyclosporine	Increased potassium levels.

*See Glossary

GENERIC NAME OR DRUG CLASS	COMBINED EFFECT	GENERIC NAME OR DRUG CLASS	COMBINED EFFECT

DIURETICS, POTASSIUM-SPARING & HYDROCHLOROTHIAZIDE continued

GENERIC NAME OR DRUG CLASS	COMBINED EFFECT	GENERIC NAME OR DRUG CLASS	COMBINED EFFECT
Digitalis preparations*	Increased digitalis effect.	Lithium	Possible lithium toxicity.
Diuretics*, other	Increased effect of both drugs.	Metformin	Increased metformin effect.
Folic acid	Decreased effect of folic acid.	Potassium-containing medications	Increased potassium levels.

DIURETICS, THIAZIDE

GENERIC NAME OR DRUG CLASS	COMBINED EFFECT	GENERIC NAME OR DRUG CLASS	COMBINED EFFECT
Indapamide	Increased diuretic effect.	Opiates*	Dizziness or weakness when standing up after sitting or lying down.
Indomethacin	Decreased anti-hypertensive effect.	Pentoxifylline	Increased anti-hypertensive effect.
Lithium	Increased effect of lithium.	Potassium supplements*	Decreased potassium effect.
Meglitinides	Increased blood sugar levels.	Probenecid	Decreased probenecid effect.
Memantine	Increased effect of memantine and hydrochlorothiazide.	Sotalol	Increased anti-hypertensive effect.
Monoamine oxidase (MAO) inhibitors*	Increased anti-hypertensive effect.	Terazosin	Decreased terazosin effect.
Nicardipine	Blood pressure drop. Dosages may require adjustment.	Toremifene	Possible increased calcium.
Nimodipine	Dangerous blood pressure drop.	Zinc supplements	Increased need for zinc.
Nitrates*	Excessive blood pressure drop.		

FLUOROQUINOLONES

GENERIC NAME OR DRUG CLASS	COMBINED EFFECT	GENERIC NAME OR DRUG CLASS	COMBINED EFFECT
Cyclosporine	Increased cyclosporine effect.	QT interval prolongation causing drugs*	Heart rhythm problems.
Didanosine	Decreased fluoro-quinolone effect.	Sucralfate	Decreased fluoro-quinolone effect.
Digoxin	Increased digoxin effect.	Theophylline	Increased risk of theophylline toxicity.
Iron supplements	Decreased fluoro-quinolone effect.	Tizanidine	Dangerous increased tizanidine effect with ciprofloxacin
Oxtriphylline	Increased risk of oxtriphylline toxicity.		
Phenytoin	Decreased effect of phenytoin with ciprofloxacin.	Warfarin	Increased warfarin effect.
Probenecid	Increased effect of fluoroquinolone.	Zinc	Decreased fluoro-quinolone effect.

*See Glossary

GENERIC NAME OR DRUG CLASS	COMBINED EFFECT	GENERIC NAME OR DRUG CLASS	COMBINED EFFECT

HALOPERIDOL

GENERIC NAME OR DRUG CLASS	COMBINED EFFECT	GENERIC NAME OR DRUG CLASS	COMBINED EFFECT
Fluoxetine	Increased depressant effects of both drugs.	Loxapine	May increase toxic effects of both drugs.
Guanethidine	Decreased guanethidine effect.	Methyldopa	Possible psychosis.
		Narcotics*	Excessive sedation.
Guanfacine	May increase depressant effects of either drug.	Nefazodone	Unknown effect. May require dosage adjustment.
Leucovorin	High alcohol content of leucovorin may cause adverse effects.	Pergolide	Decreased pergolide effect.
		Procarbazine	Increased sedation.
Levodopa	Decreased levodopa effect.	QT interval prolongation-causing drugs*	Serious heart rhythm problems.
Lithium	Increased toxicity.	Sertraline	Increased depressive effects of both drugs.

HISTAMINE H$_2$ RECEPTOR ANTAGONISTS

GENERIC NAME OR DRUG CLASS	COMBINED EFFECT	GENERIC NAME OR DRUG CLASS	COMBINED EFFECT
Diazepam	Increased effect and toxicity of diazepam.	Metoclopramide	Decreased absorption of histamine H$_2$ receptor antagonist.
Digitalis preparations*	Increased digitalis effect.	Metoprolol	Increased effect and toxicity of metoprolol.
Dofetilide	Increased risk of heart problems.	Miglitol	Decreased effect of ranitidine.
Encainide	Increased effect of histamine H$_2$ receptor antagonist.	Moricizine	Increased concentration of H$_2$ receptor antagonist in the blood.
Flurazepam	Increased effect and toxicity of flurazepam.	Morphine	Increased effect and toxicity of morphine.
Glipizide	Increased effect and toxicity of glipizide.	Nicardipine	Possible increased effect and toxicity of nicardipine.
Itraconazole	Decreased absorption of itraconazole.	Nimodipine	Possible increased effect and toxicity of nimodipine.
Ketoconazole	Decreased ketoconazole absorption.	Nitroimidazoles	Increased nitroimidazole effect
Labetalol	Increased anti-hypertensive effects.	Paroxetine	Increased levels of paroxetine in blood.
Memantine	Increased effect of either drug.	Phenytoin	Increased effect and toxicity of phenytoin
Metformin	Increased metformin effect.	Propafenone	Increased effect of both drugs and increased risk of toxicity.
Methadone	Increased effect and toxicity of methadone.		

*See Glossary

GENERIC NAME OR DRUG CLASS	COMBINED EFFECT	GENERIC NAME OR DRUG CLASS	COMBINED EFFECT

HISTAMINE H₂ RECEPTOR ANTAGONISTS continued

GENERIC NAME OR DRUG CLASS	COMBINED EFFECT	GENERIC NAME OR DRUG CLASS	COMBINED EFFECT
Propranolol	Possible increased propranolol effect.	Triazolam	Increased effect and toxicity of triazolam.
Quinidine	Increased quinidine effect.	Varenicline	May increase effect of varenicline (with cimetidine).
Tacrine	Increased tacrine effect.	Venlafaxine	With cimetidine— Increased risk of adverse reactions.
Tamoxifen	Decreased tamoxifen effect.		
Terbinafine (oral)	Increased effect of terbinafine with cimetidine.	Verapamil	Increased effect and toxicity of verapamil.
Theophylline	Increases theophylline effect.	Zaleplon	Increases zaleplon effect.

HYDRALAZINE

GENERIC NAME OR DRUG CLASS	COMBINED EFFECT	GENERIC NAME OR DRUG CLASS	COMBINED EFFECT
Lisinopril	Increased anti-hypertensive effect. Dosage of each may require adjustment.	Nimodipine	Dangerous blood pressure drop.
		Sotalol	Increased anti-hypertensive effect.
Monoamine oxidase (MAO) inhibitors*	Increased hydralazine effect.	Terazosin	Decreased effectiveness of terazosin.
Nicardipine	Blood pressure drop. Dosages may require adjustment.		

HYDRALAZINE & HYDROCHLOROTHIAZIDE

GENERIC NAME OR DRUG CLASS	COMBINED EFFECT	GENERIC NAME OR DRUG CLASS	COMBINED EFFECT
Barbiturates*	Increased hydrochlorothiazide effect.	Diuretics*, oral	Increased effect of both drugs. When monitored carefully, combination may be beneficial in controlling hypertension.
Carteolol	Decreased antihypertensive effect.		
Cholestyramine	Decreased hydrochlorothiazide effect.	Indapamide	Increased diuretic effect.
Cortisone drugs*	Excessive potassium loss that causes dangerous heart rhythms.	Lisinopril	Increased anti-hypertensive effect. Dosage of each may require adjustment.
Diazoxide	Increased antihypertensive effect.	Lithium	Increased lithium effect.
Digitalis preparations*	Excessive potassium loss that causes dangerous heart rhythms.	Monoamine oxidase (MAO) inhibitors*	Increased effect of drugs.
		Nimodipine	Dangerous blood pressure drop.
		Nitrates*	Excessive blood pressure drop.

ADDITIONAL DRUG INTERACTIONS

GENERIC NAME OR DRUG CLASS	COMBINED EFFECT	GENERIC NAME OR DRUG CLASS	COMBINED EFFECT
HYDRALAZINE & HYDROCHLOROTHIAZIDE continued			
Potassium supplements*	Decreased potassium effect.	Probenecid	Decreased probenecid effect.

IMMUNOSUPPRESSIVE AGENTS

Probenecid	Increased effect of mycophenolate.	Troglitazone	Decreased effect of tacrolimus.
Proton pump inhibitors	Increased effect of tacrolimus.	Vaccinations	Avoid unless doctor approves.
Telithromycin	Increased effect of tacrolimus.		

INDAPAMIDE

Opiates*	Weakness and faintness when arising from bed or chair.	Sotalol	Increased antihypertensive effect.
Probenecid	Decreased probenecid effect.	Terazosin	Decreased effectiveness of terazosin.

KAOLIN, PECTIN, BELLADONNA & OPIUM

Ketoconazole	Decreased ketoconazole effect.	Pilocarpine	Loss of pilocarpine effect in glaucoma treatment.
Lincomycins*	Decreased absorption of lincomycin. Separate doses by at least 2 hours.	Potassium supplements*	Possible intestinal ulcers with oral potassium tablets.
MAO inhibitors*	Increased belladonna effect.	Sedatives*	Excessive sedation.
Meperidine	Increased belladonna effect.	Sleep inducers*	Increased effect of sleep inducers.
Methylphenidate	Increased belladonna effect.	Sotalol	Increased narcotic effect. Dangerous sedation.
Mind-altering drugs*	Increased sedative effect.	Tranquilizers*	Increased tranquilizer effect.
Narcotics, other*	Increased narcotic effect.	Vitamin C	Decreased belladonna effect. Avoid large doses of vitamin C.
Nitrates*	Increased internal eye pressure.	All other oral medicines	Decreased absorption of other medicines. Separate doses by at least 2 hours.
Orphenadrine	Increased belladonna effect.		
Phenothiazines*	Increased sedative effect of paregoric.		

*See Glossary

GENERIC NAME OR DRUG CLASS	COMBINED EFFECT	GENERIC NAME OR DRUG CLASS	COMBINED EFFECT

LITHIUM

GENERIC NAME OR DRUG CLASS	COMBINED EFFECT	GENERIC NAME OR DRUG CLASS	COMBINED EFFECT
Diuretics*	Increased lithium effect or toxicity.	Oxyphenbutazone	Increased lithium effect.
Fluvoxamine	Increased risk of seizure.	Phenothiazines*	Decreased lithium effect.
Haloperidol	Increased toxicity of both drugs.	Phenylbutazone	Increased lithium effect.
Indomethacin	Increased lithium effect.	Phenytoin	Increased lithium effect.
Iodide salts	Increased lithium effects on thyroid function.	Potassium iodide	Increased potassium iodide effect.
Ketoprofen	May increase lithium in blood.	Sodium bicarbonate	Decreased lithium effect.
Meloxicam	Increased lithium effect.	Sumatriptan	Adverse effects unknown. Avoid.
Methyldopa	Increased lithium effect.	Theophylline	Decreased lithium effect.
Molindone	Brain changes.	Tiopronin	Increased risk of toxicity to kidneys.
Nitroimidazoles	Increased lithium effect		

LOXAPINE

GENERIC NAME OR DRUG CLASS	COMBINED EFFECT	GENERIC NAME OR DRUG CLASS	COMBINED EFFECT
Rauwolfia	May increase toxic effects of both drugs.	Thioxanthenes*	May increase toxic effects of both drugs.
Sertraline	Increased depressive effects of both drugs.		

MAPROTILINE

GENERIC NAME OR DRUG CLASS	COMBINED EFFECT	GENERIC NAME OR DRUG CLASS	COMBINED EFFECT
Clonidine	Decreased clonidine effect.	Guanfacine	May increase depressant effects of either drug.
Clozapine	Toxic effect on the central nervous system.	Leucovorin	High alcohol content of leucovorin may cause adverse effects.
Disulfiram	Delirium.		
Diuretics, thiazide*	Increased maprotiline effect.	Levodopa	Decreased levodopa effect.
Ethchlorvynol	Delirium.	Lithium	Possible decreased seizure threshold.
Fluoxetine	Increased depressant effects of both drugs.	Methyldopa	Decreased methyldopa effect.
Guanethidine	Decreased guanethidine effect.	Methylphenidate	Possible increased antidepressant effect and toxicity.

*See Glossary

MAPROTILINE continued

GENERIC NAME OR DRUG CLASS	COMBINED EFFECT	GENERIC NAME OR DRUG CLASS	COMBINED EFFECT
Molindone	Increased tranquilizer effect.	Quinidine	Irregular heartbeat.
Monoamine oxidase (MAO) inhibitors*	Fever, delirium, convulsions.	Selegiline	Fever, delirium, convulsions.
Narcotics*	Dangerous oversedation.	Sertraline	Increased depressive effects of both drugs.
Phenothiazines*	Possible increased antidepressant effect and toxicity.	Sympathomimetics*	Increased sympathomimetic effect.
Phenytoin	Decreased phenytoin effect.	Thyroid hormones*	Irregular heartbeat.

METFORMIN

Penicillins*	Increased risk of methotrexate toxicity.	Trimethoprim	Increased metformin effect.
Quinine	Increased metformin effect.	Vancomycin	Increased metformin effect.
Ranitidine	Increased metformin effect.		

METHOTREXATE

Sulfa drugs*	Possible methotrexate toxicity.	Tiopronin	Increased risk of toxicity to bone marrow and kidneys.
Sulfadoxine and pyrimethamine	Increased risk of toxicity.	Vaccines, live or killed	Increased risk of toxicity or reduced effectiveness of vaccine.
Tetracyclines*	Possible methotrexate toxicity.		

METOCLOPRAMIDE

Phenothiazines*	Increased chance of muscle spasm and trembling.	Tetracyclines*	Slow stomach emptying.
Sertraline	Increased depressive effects of both drugs.	Thiothixenes*	Increased chance of muscle spasm and trembling.

MOLINDONE

Tetracyclines*	Slow stomach emptying.	Thiothixenes*	Increased chance of muscle spasm and trembling.

*See Glossary

MONOAMINE OXIDASE (MAO) INHIBITORS

GENERIC NAME OR DRUG CLASS	COMBINED EFFECT	GENERIC NAME OR DRUG CLASS	COMBINED EFFECT
Central nervous system (CNS) depressants*	Excessive depressant action.	Meglitinides	Increased risk of low blood sugar.
Citalopram	Can cause a life-threatening reaction. Avoid.	Methyldopa	Sudden, severe blood pressure rise.
Clozapine	Toxic effect on the central nervous system.	Methylphenidate	Increased blood pressure.
Doxepin (topical)	Potentially life-threatening. Allow 14 days between use of the 2 drugs.	Mirtazapine	Potentially life-threatening. Allow 14 days between use of 2 drugs.
Dexfenfluramine	Potentially life-threatening. Allow 14 days between use of 2 drugs.	Monoamine oxidase (MAO) inhibitors (others, when taken together)	High fever, convulsions, death.
Dextromethorphan	Very high blood pressure.	Narcotics*	Severe high blood pressure.
Diuretics*	Excessively low blood pressure.	Nefazodone	Potentially life-threatening. Allow 14 days between use of the 2 drugs.
Ephedrine	Increased blood pressure.	Paroxetine	Potentially life-threatening. Avoid.
Fluoxetine	Potentially life-threatening. Avoid.	Phenothiazines*	Possible increased phenothiazine toxicity.
Fluvoxamine	Potentially life-threatening. Avoid.	Pseudoephedrine	Increased blood pressure.
Furazolidone	Sudden, severe increase in blood pressure.	Serotonergics*	Increased risk of serotonin syndrome.
Guanadrel	High blood pressure.	Sertraline	Potentially life-threatening. Avoid.
Guanethidine	Blood pressure rise.	Sympathomimetics*	Blood pressure rise to life-threatening level.
Guanfacine	May increase depressant effects of either drug.	Tolcapone	May reduce effectiveness of MAO inhibitor.
Indapamide	Increased indapamide effect.	Tramadol	Increased risk of seizures.
Insulin	Increased hypoglycemic effect.	Trazodone	Increased risk of mental status changes.
Leucovorin	High alcohol content of leucovorin may cause adverse effects.	Venlafaxine	Increased risk and severity of side effects. Allow 4 weeks between use of the 2 drugs.
Levodopa	Sudden, severe blood pressure rise.		
Maprotiline	Dangerous blood pressure rise.		

ADDITIONAL DRUG INTERACTIONS

*See Glossary

NARCOTIC ANALGESICS

GENERIC NAME OR DRUG CLASS	COMBINED EFFECT	GENERIC NAME OR DRUG CLASS	COMBINED EFFECT
Cimetidine	Possible increased narcotic effect and toxicity.	Naltrexone	Precipitates withdrawal symptoms. May lead to respiratory arrest, coma and death.
Clozapine	Toxic effect on the central nervous system.	Narcotics*, other	Increased narcotic effect.
Ethinamate	Dangerous increased effects of ethinamate. Avoid combining.	Nicotine	Increased effect of pentazocine and propoxyphene.
Fluoxetine	Increased depressant effects of both drugs.	Nitrates*	Excessive blood pressure drop.
Guanfacine	May increase depressant effects of either drug.	Pentazocine	Possibly precipitates withdrawal with chronic narcotic use.
Leucovorin	High alcohol content of leucovorin may cause adverse effects.	Phenothiazines*	Increased sedative effect.
		Phenytoin	Possible decreased narcotic effect.
Methyprylon	Increased sedative effect, perhaps to dangerous level. Avoid.	Rifamycins	Possible decreased narcotic effect.
		Sedatives*	Increased sedative effect.
Metformin	Increased effect of metformin with morphine.	Selegiline	Severe toxicity characterized by breathing difficulties, seizures, coma.
Mind-altering drugs*	Increased sedative effect.	Sertraline	Increased depressive effects of both drugs.
Molindone	Increased narcotic effect.		
Monoamine oxidase (MAO) inhibitors*	Serious toxicity (including death).	Sleep inducers*	Increased sedative effect.
Nabilone	Greater depression of central nervous system.	Sotalol	Increased narcotic effect. Dangerous sedation.
Nalbuphine	Possibly precipitates withdrawal with chronic narcotic use.	Tramadol	Increased sedation.
		Tranquilizers*	Increased sedative effect.

NARCOTIC ANALGESICS & ACETAMINOPHEN

GENERIC NAME OR DRUG CLASS	COMBINED EFFECT	GENERIC NAME OR DRUG CLASS	COMBINED EFFECT
Phenothiazines*	Increased phenothiazine effect.	Sertraline	Increased depressive effects of both drugs.
Sedatives*	Increased sedative effect.	Sleep inducers*	Increased sedative effect.
Selegiline	Severe toxicity characterized by breathing difficulty, seizures, coma.	Sotalol	Increased narcotic effect. Dangerous sedation.

*See Glossary

GENERIC NAME OR DRUG CLASS	COMBINED EFFECT	GENERIC NAME OR DRUG CLASS	COMBINED EFFECT

NARCOTIC ANALGESICS & ACETAMINOPHEN continued

GENERIC NAME OR DRUG CLASS	COMBINED EFFECT	GENERIC NAME OR DRUG CLASS	COMBINED EFFECT
Tetracyclines*	May slow tetracycline absorption. Space doses 2 hours apart.	Tranquilizers*	Increased sedative effect.
Tramadol	Increased sedation.	Zidovudine	Increased toxicity of zidovudine.

NARCOTIC ANALGESICS & ASPIRIN

GENERIC NAME OR DRUG CLASS	COMBINED EFFECT	GENERIC NAME OR DRUG CLASS	COMBINED EFFECT
Antidiabetics*, oral	Low blood sugar.	Rauwolfia alkaloids*	Decreased aspirin effect.
Anti-inflammatory drugs, nonsteroidal (NSAIDs)*	Risk of stomach bleeding and ulcers.	Salicylates, other*	Likely aspirin toxicity.
Aspirin, other	Likely aspirin toxicity.	Sedatives*	Increased sedative effect.
Bumetanide	Possible aspirin toxicity.	Selegiline	Severe toxicity characterized by breathing difficulties, seizures, coma.
Carteolol	Increased narcotic effect. Dangerous sedation.		
Ethacrynic acid	Possible aspirin toxicity.	Sleep inducers*	Increased sedative effect.
Furosemide	Possible aspirin toxicity. May decrease furosemide effect.	Sotalol	Increased narcotic effect. Dangerous sedation.
Gold compounds*	Increased likelihood of kidney damage.	Spironolactone	Decreased spironolactone effect.
Indomethacin	Risk of stomach bleeding and ulcers.	Sulfinpyrazone	Decreased sulfinpyrazone effect.
Methotrexate	Increased methotrexate effect.	Ticlopidine	Decreased effects of both drugs.
Minoxidil	Decreased minoxidil effect.	Tramadol	Increased sedation.
Narcotics*, other	Increased narcotic effect.	Tranquilizers*	Increased sedative effect.
Nitrates*	Excessive blood pressure drop.	Valproic acid*	May increase valproic acid effect.
Propranolol	Decreased aspirin effect.	Vitamin C (large doses)	Possible aspirin toxicity.

NEFAZODONE

GENERIC NAME OR DRUG CLASS	COMBINED EFFECT	GENERIC NAME OR DRUG CLASS	COMBINED EFFECT
Haloperidol	Unknown. May need haloperidol dosage adjusted.	Propranolol	Unknown effect. May need dosage adjustment of both drugs.
Monoamine oxidase (MAO) inhibitors*	Potentially life-threatening. Allow 14 days between use of 2 drugs.	Terfenadine	Increased effect of terfenadine. Avoid.
Pimozide	Increased effect of pimozide. Avoid.	Triazolam	Increased effect of triazolam.

*See Glossary

ADDITIONAL DRUG INTERACTIONS

GENERIC NAME OR DRUG CLASS	COMBINED EFFECT	GENERIC NAME OR DRUG CLASS	COMBINED EFFECT

NICOTINE

Pentazocine	Increased effect of pentazocine.	**Propoxyphene**	Increased effect of propoxyphene.
Phenylephrine	Decreased effect of phenylephrine.	**Theophylline**	Increased effect of theophylline.

NIMODIPINE

Timolol eye drops	May cause increased effect of nimodipine on heart function.	**Tocainide**	Increased likelihood of adverse reaction from either drug.
		Vitamin D (large doses)	Decreased nimodipine effect.

NUCLEOSIDE REVERSE TRANSCRIPTASE INHIBITORS

Peripheral neuropathy-associated drugs*	Increased risk of peripheral neuropathy.	**Tenofovir**	Increased effect of didanosine. Take tenofovir 2 hours before or 1 hour after didanosine.
Probenecid	Increased effect of zalcitabine and zidovudine.	**Tetracyclines**	Decreased antibiotic effect.
Rifamycins	Decreased zidovudine effect.	**Valproic acid***	Increased effect of zidovudine.

OLANZAPINE

Eszopiclone	Decreased alertness.	**Levodopa**	May decrease levodopa effect.
Hepatotoxics*	Risk of liver problems.		

ORPHENADRINE, ASPIRIN & CAFFEINE

Adrenocorticoids, systemic	Increased risk of ulcers. Increased adrenocorticoid effect.	**Antidepressants, tricyclic***	Increased sedation.
		Antidiabetics, oral*	Low blood sugar.
Allopurinol	Decreased allopurinol effect.	**Anti-inflammatory drugs, nonsteroidal (NSAIDs)***	Risk of stomach bleeding and ulcers.
Antacids*	Decreased aspirin effect.	**Aspirin, other**	Likely aspirin toxicity.
Anticholinergics*	Increased anticholinergic effect.	**Chlorpromazine**	Hypoglycemia (low blood sugar).
Anticoagulants*	Increased anticoagulant effect. Abnormal bleeding.	**Contraceptives, oral***	Increased caffeine effect.

*See Glossary

GENERIC NAME OR DRUG CLASS	COMBINED EFFECT	GENERIC NAME OR DRUG CLASS	COMBINED EFFECT

ORPHENADRINE, ASPIRIN & CAFFEINE continued

GENERIC NAME OR DRUG CLASS	COMBINED EFFECT	GENERIC NAME OR DRUG CLASS	COMBINED EFFECT
Furosemide	Possible aspirin toxicity.	Potassium supplements*	Increased possibility of intestinal ulcers with oral potassium tablets.
Gold compounds*	Increased likelihood of kidney damage.		
Griseofulvin	Decreased griseofulvin effect.	Probenecid	Decreased probenecid effect.
Indomethacin	Risk of stomach bleeding and ulcers.	Propoxyphene	Possible confusion, nervousness, tremors.
Isoniazid	Increased caffeine effect.	Propranolol	Decreased aspirin effect.
Levodopa	Increased levodopa effect. (Improves effectiveness in treating Parkinson's disease.)	Rauwolfia alkaloids*	Decreased aspirin effect.
		Salicylates, other*	Likely aspirin toxicity.
		Sedatives*	Decreased sedative effect.
Methotrexate	Increased methotrexate effect.	Sleep inducers*	Decreased sedative effect.
Minoxidil	Decreased minoxidil effect.	Spironolactone	Decreased spirono-lactone effect.
Monoamine oxidase (MAO) inhibitors*	Dangerous blood pressure rise.	Sulfinpyrazone	Decreased sulfin-pyrazone effect.
Nitrates*	Increased internal eye pressure.	Sympathomimetics*	Overstimulation.
Para-aminosalicylic acid (PAS)	Possible aspirin toxicity.	Thyroid hormones*	Increased thyroid effect.
Penicillins*	Increased effect of drugs.	Tranquilizers*	Decreased tranquilizer effect.
Phenobarbital	Decreased aspirin effect.	Valproic acid*	May increase valproic acid effect.
		Vitamin C (large doses)	Possible aspirin toxicity.

PHENOTHIAZINES

GENERIC NAME OR DRUG CLASS	COMBINED EFFECT	GENERIC NAME OR DRUG CLASS	COMBINED EFFECT
Doxepin (topical)	Increased risk of toxicity of both drugs.	Mind-altering drugs*	Increased effect of mind-altering drug.
Duloxetine	Increased effect of duloxetine.	Molindone	Increased tranquilizer effect.
Guanethidine	Increased guanethidine effect.	Narcotics*	Increased narcotic effect.
Isoniazid	Increased risk of liver damage.	Procarbazine	Increased sedation.
Levodopa	Decreased levodopa effect.	Quetiapine	Decreased quetiapine effect.
Lithium	Decreased lithium effect.	Tramadol	Increased sedation.
		Zolpidem	Increased sedation. Avoid.

*See Glossary

GENERIC NAME OR DRUG CLASS	COMBINED EFFECT	GENERIC NAME OR DRUG CLASS	COMBINED EFFECT

POTASSIUM SUPPLEMENTS

GENERIC NAME OR DRUG CLASS	COMBINED EFFECT	GENERIC NAME OR DRUG CLASS	COMBINED EFFECT
Potassium-containing drugs*	Increased potassium levels.	Vitamin B-12	Extended-release tablets may decrease vitamin B-12 absorption and increase vitamin B-12 requirements.
Spironolactone	Dangerous rise in blood potassium.		
Triamterene	Dangerous rise in blood potassium.		

PRIMIDONE

GENERIC NAME OR DRUG CLASS	COMBINED EFFECT	GENERIC NAME OR DRUG CLASS	COMBINED EFFECT
Narcotics*	Increased narcotic effect.	Sedatives*	Increased sedative effect.
Oxyphenbutazone	Decreased oxyphenbutazone effect.	Sertraline	Increased depressive effects of both drugs.
Phenylbutazone	Decreased phenylbutazone effect.	Sleep inducers*	Increased effect of sleep inducer.
Phenytoin	Possible increased primidone toxicity.	Tranquilizers*	Increased tranquilizer effect.
Rifamycins	Possible decreased primidone effect.	Valproic acid*	Increased effect of primidone.

PROBENECID & COLCHICINE

GENERIC NAME OR DRUG CLASS	COMBINED EFFECT	GENERIC NAME OR DRUG CLASS	COMBINED EFFECT
Methotrexate	Increased methotrexate effect.	Salicylates*	Decreased probenecid effect.
Mind-altering drugs*	Oversedation.	Sedatives*	Oversedation.
Narcotics*	Oversedation.	Sleep inducers*	Oversedation.
Nitrofurantoin	Increased nitrofurantoin effect.	Sulfa drugs*	Slows elimination. May cause harmful accumulation of sulfa.
Para-aminosalicylic acid (PAS)	Increased effect of para-aminosalicylic acid.	Thioguanine	More likelihood of toxicity of both drugs.
Penicillins*	Enhanced penicillin effect.	Tranquilizers*	Oversedation.
Phenylbutazone	Decreased antigout effect of colchicine.	Valacyclovir	Increased valacyclovir effect.
Pyrazinamide	Decreased probenecid effect.	Vitamin B-12	Decreased absorption of vitamin B-12.
		Zidovudine	Increased risk of zidovudine toxicity.

*See Glossary

PROCARBAZINE

GENERIC NAME OR DRUG CLASS	COMBINED EFFECT	GENERIC NAME OR DRUG CLASS	COMBINED EFFECT
Diuretics*	Excessively low blood pressure.	Methylphenidate	Excessive high blood pressure.
Doxapram	Increased blood pressure.	Methyprylon	May increase sedative effect to dangerous level. Avoid.
Ethinamate	Dangerous increased effects of ethinamate. Avoid combining.	Monoamine oxidase (MAO) inhibitors, other*	High fever, convulsions, death.
Fluoxetine	Increased depressant effects of both drugs.	Nabilone	Greater depression of central nervous system.
Guanethidine	Blood pressure rise to life-threatening level.	Narcotics*	Increased sedation.
		Phenothiazines*	Increased sedation.
Guanfacine	May increase depressant effects of either medicine.	Rauwolfia alkaloids*	Very high blood pressure.
Leucovorin	High alcohol content of leucovorin may cause adverse effects.	Reserpine	Increased blood pressure, excitation.
		Sertraline	Increased depressive effects of both drugs.
Levamisole	Increased risk of bone marrow depression.	Sumatriptan	Adverse effects unknown. Avoid.
Levodopa	Sudden, severe blood pressure rise.	Sympathomimetics*	Heartbeat abnormalities, severe high blood pressure.
Methyldopa	Severe high blood pressure.	Tiopronin	Increased risk of toxicity to bone marrow.

QUETIAPINE

GENERIC NAME OR DRUG CLASS	COMBINED EFFECT	GENERIC NAME OR DRUG CLASS	COMBINED EFFECT
Levodopa or dopamine agonists*	Decreased effect of levodopa or dopamine agonist.	Phenytoin	Decreased quetiapine effect.
		Thioridazine	Decreased quetiapine effect.

RAUWOLFIA ALKALOIDS

GENERIC NAME OR DRUG CLASS	COMBINED EFFECT	GENERIC NAME OR DRUG CLASS	COMBINED EFFECT
Lisinopril	Increased antihypertensive effect. Dosage of each may require adjustment.	Monoamine oxidase (MAO) inhibitors*	Severe depression.
		Nabilone	Greater depression of central nervous system.
Loxapine	May increase toxic effects of both drugs.	Nicardipine	Blood pressure drop. Dosages may require adjustment.
Methyprylon	May increase sedative effect to dangerous level. Avoid.		
Mind-altering drugs*	Excessive sedation.	Nimodipine	Dangerous blood pressure drop.

ADDITIONAL DRUG INTERACTIONS

*See Glossary

GENERIC NAME OR DRUG CLASS	COMBINED EFFECT	GENERIC NAME OR DRUG CLASS	COMBINED EFFECT
RAUWOLFIA ALKALOIDS continued			
Pergolide	Decreased pergolide effect.	Sotalol	Decreased antihypertensive effect.
Pseudoephedrine	Increased effect of either drug.	Terazosin	Decreased effectiveness of terazosin.
Sertraline	Increased depressive effects of both drugs.		

RESERPINE, HYDRALAZINE & HYDROCHLOROTHIAZIDE

GENERIC NAME OR DRUG CLASS	COMBINED EFFECT	GENERIC NAME OR DRUG CLASS	COMBINED EFFECT
Amphetamines*	Decreased hydralazine effect.	Digitalis preparations*	Excessive potassium loss that causes dangerous heart rhythms.
Anticoagulants*, oral	Unpredictable increased or decreased effect of anticoagulant.	Diuretics, oral*	Increased effects of drugs. When monitored carefully, combination may be beneficial in controlling hypertension.
Anticonvulsants*	Serious change in seizure pattern.		
Antidepressants, tricyclic*	Dangerous drop in blood pressure. Avoid combination unless under medical supervision.	Dronabinol	Increased effects of drugs.
		Indapamide	Increased diuretic effect.
Antihistamines*	Increased antihistamine effect.	Levodopa	Decreased levodopa effect.
Antihypertensives, other*	Increased antihypertensive effect.	Lisinopril	Increased antihypertensive effect. Dosage of each may require adjustment.
Anti-inflammatory drugs, nonsteroidal (NSAIDs)*	Decreased hydralazine effect.		
Aspirin	Decreased aspirin effect.	Lithium	Increased lithium effect.
Barbiturates*	Increased hydrochlorothiazide effect.	Mind-altering drugs*	Excessive sedation.
		Monoamine oxidase (MAO) inhibitors*	Increased effects of both drugs. Severe depression.
Beta-adrenergic blocking agents*	Increased effect of reserpine. Excessive sedation.	Nicardipine	Blood pressure drop. Dosages may require adjustment.
Carteolol	Increased antihypertensive effect.	Nimodipine	Dangerous blood pressure drop.
Cholestyramine	Decreased hydrochlorothiazide effect.	Nitrates*	Excessive blood pressure drop.
Cortisone drugs*	Excessive potassium loss that causes dangerous heart rhythms.	Oxprenolol	Increased antihypertensive effect. Dosages of drugs may require adjustments.
Diazoxide	Increased antihypertensive effect.		

*See Glossary

GENERIC NAME OR DRUG CLASS	COMBINED EFFECT	GENERIC NAME OR DRUG CLASS	COMBINED EFFECT

RESERPINE, HYDRALAZINE & HYDROCHLOROTHIAZIDE continued

GENERIC NAME OR DRUG CLASS	COMBINED EFFECT	GENERIC NAME OR DRUG CLASS	COMBINED EFFECT
Pergolide	Decreased pergolide effect.	Sotalol	Decreased antihypertensive effect.
Potassium supplements*	Decreased potassium effect.	Terazosin	Decreased effectiveness of terazosin.
Probenecid	Decreased probenecid effect.		

RIFAMYCINS

GENERIC NAME OR DRUG CLASS	COMBINED EFFECT	GENERIC NAME OR DRUG CLASS	COMBINED EFFECT
Phenytoin	Decreased phenytoin effect.	Theophyllines*	Decreased theophylline effect.
Probenecid	Possible toxicity to liver.	Tocainide	Possible decreased blood cell production in bone marrow.
Protease inhibitors	Decreased protease inhibitor effect.	Trimethoprim	Decreased trimethoprim effect.
Quinidine	Decreased effect of both drugs.	Valproic acid*	Decreased effect of valproic acid with rifampin.
Quinine	Decreased quinine effect.		
Sildenafil	Decreased sildenafil effect.	Zaleplon	Decreased zaleplon effect.
Tacrolimus	Decreased tacrolimus effect.	Zidovudine	Decreased zidovudine effect.
Telithromycin	Decreased effect of rifampin.		

SALICYLATES

GENERIC NAME OR DRUG CLASS	COMBINED EFFECT	GENERIC NAME OR DRUG CLASS	COMBINED EFFECT
Insulin lispro	May need decreased dosage of insulin.	Rauwolfia alkaloids*	Decreased salicylate effect.
Ketoconazole	Decreased ketoconazole effect with buffered salicylates.	Salicylates*, other	Likely salicylate toxicity.
Methotrexate	Increased methotrexate effect and toxicity.	Sotalol	Decreased antihypertensive effect of sotalol.
Para-aminosalicylic acid	Possible salicylate toxicity.	Spironolactone	Decreased spironolactone effect.
Penicillins*	Increased effect of both drugs.	Sulfinpyrazone	Decreased sulfinpyrazone effect.
Phenobarbital	Decreased salicylate effect.	Terazosin	Decreased effectiveness of terazosin. Causes sodium and fluid retention.
Phenytoin	Increased phenytoin effect.		
Probenecid	Decreased probenecid effect.	Urinary acidifiers*	Decreased excretion. Increased salicylate effect.

ADDITIONAL DRUG INTERACTIONS

GENERIC NAME OR DRUG CLASS	COMBINED EFFECT	GENERIC NAME OR DRUG CLASS	COMBINED EFFECT

SALICYLATES continued

GENERIC NAME OR DRUG CLASS	COMBINED EFFECT	GENERIC NAME OR DRUG CLASS	COMBINED EFFECT
Urinary alkalizers*	Increased excretion. Decreased salicylate effect.	Vitamin C (large doses)	Possible salicylate toxicity.
		Zidovudine	increased zidovudine effect.

SCOPOLAMINE (Hyoscine)

GENERIC NAME OR DRUG CLASS	COMBINED EFFECT	GENERIC NAME OR DRUG CLASS	COMBINED EFFECT
Nabilone	Greater depression of central nervous system.	Potassium supplements*	Possible intestinal ulcers with oral potassium tablets.
Nitrates*	Increased internal eye pressure.	Quinidine	Increased scopolamine effect.
Nizatidine	Increased nizatidine effect.	Sedatives* or central nervous system (CNS) depressants*	Increased sedative effect of both drugs.
Orphenadrine	Increased scopolamine effect.	Sertraline	Increased depressive effects of both drugs.
Phenothiazines*	Increased scopolamine effect.		
Pilocarpine	Loss of pilocarpine effect in glaucoma treatment.	Vitamin C	Decreased scopolamine effect. Avoid large doses of vitamin C.

SELECTIVE SEROTONIN REUPTAKE INHIBITORS (SSRIs)

GENERIC NAME OR DRUG CLASS	COMBINED EFFECT	GENERIC NAME OR DRUG CLASS	COMBINED EFFECT
Buspirone	Increased risk of serotonin syndrome*.	Monoamine oxidase (MAO) inhibitors*	Increased risk of adverse effects. May lead to convulsions and hypertensive crisis. Let 14 days elapse between taking the 2 drugs.
Desmopressin	Increased risk of thirstiness which may lead to drinking excess fluids.		
Dextromethorphan	Increased risk of serotonin syndrome*.	Nefazodone	Increased risk of serotonin syndrome*.
Digoxin	Increased risk of side effects of both drugs.	Pentazocine	Increased risk of serotonin syndrome*.
Levodopa	Increased risk of serotonin syndrome*.	Phenytoin	Increased effect of phenytoin.
Lithium	Increased risk of serotonin syndrome*.	Propranolol	Increased effect of propranolol.
Meperidine	Increased risk of serotonin syndrome*.	Ramelteon	Increased effect of ramelteon. Avoid.
Moclobemide	Increased risk of side effects and serotonin syndrome*.	Serotonergics*	Increased risk of serotonin syndrome*.
		Sumatriptan	Increased risk of serotonin syndrome*.

*See Glossary

SELECTIVE SEROTONIN REUPTAKE INHIBITORS (SSRIs) continued

GENERIC NAME OR DRUG CLASS	COMBINED EFFECT	GENERIC NAME OR DRUG CLASS	COMBINED EFFECT
Theophylline	Increased effect of theophylline.	Tizanidine	Dangerous increased tizanidine effect with fluvoxamine.

SEROTONIN & NOREPINEPHRINE REUPTAKE INHIBITORS (SNRIs)

Serotonergics*	Increased risk of serotonin syndrome*.	Tryptophan	Increased risk of serotonin syndrome*.
Tramadol	Increased risk of serotonin syndrome*.	Venlafaxine	Increased risk of serotonin syndrome*.
Trazodone	Increased risk of serotonin syndrome*.		

SULFONYLUREAS

Insulin	Increased blood sugar lowering.	Phenytoin	Decreased blood sugar lowering.
Insulin lispro	Increased anti-diabetic effect.	Probenecid	Increased blood sugar lowering.
Isoniazid	Decreased blood sugar lowering.	Pyrazinamide	Decreased blood sugar lowering.
Labetalol	Increased blood sugar lowering, may mask hypoglycemia.	Ranitidine	Increased blood sugar lowering.
Leukotriene modifiers	Increased effect of tolbutamide.	Rifamycins	Decreased blood sugar lowering.
MAO inhibitors*	Increased blood sugar lowering.	Sulfa drugs*	Increased blood sugar lowering.
Nicotinic acid	Decreased blood sugar lowering.	Sulfadoxine and pyrimethamine	Increased risk of toxicity.
Oxyphenbutazone	Increased blood sugar lowering.	Sulfaphenazole	Increased blood sugar lowering.
Phenothiazines*	Decreased blood sugar lowering.	Thiazolidinediones*	May decrease plasma glucose concentrations.
Phenylbutazone	Increased blood sugar lowering.	Thyroid hormones*	Decreased blood sugar lowering.
Phenyramidol	Increased blood sugar lowering.	Zafirlukast	May increase effect of tolbutamide.

ADDITIONAL DRUG INTERACTIONS

*See Glossary

GENERIC NAME OR DRUG CLASS	COMBINED EFFECT	GENERIC NAME OR DRUG CLASS	COMBINED EFFECT

TETRACYCLINES

Tiopronin	Increased risk of toxicity to kidneys (except with doxycycline and minocycline).	Zinc supplements	Decreased tetracycline absorption if taken within 2 hours of each other.
Vitamin A	Increased risk of intracranial hypertension.		

THIOTHIXENE

Pergolide	Decreased pergolide effect.	Sertraline	Increased depressive effects of both drugs.
Quinidine	Increased risk of heartbeat irregularities.	Tranquilizers*	Increased thiothixene effect. Excessive sedation.

VALPROIC ACID

Salicylates*	Increased effect of valproic acid.	Zidovudine	Increased effect of zidovudine.

Glossary

Many of the following medical terms are found in the drug charts. Where drug names are listed, they indicate the generic or drug class and not the brand names.

A

ACE Inhibitors—See Angiotensin-Converting Enzyme (ACE) Inhibitors.

Acne Preparations—Creams, lotions and liquids applied to the skin to treat acne. These include adapalene; alcohol and acetone; alcohol and sulfur; azelaic acid; benzoyl peroxide; clindamycin; erythromycin; erythromycin and benzoyl peroxide; isotretinoin; meclocycline; resorcinol; resorcinol and sulfur; salicylic acid gel USP; salicylic acid lotion; salicylic acid ointment; salicylic acid pads; salicylic acid soap; salicylic acid and sulfur bar soap; salicylic acid and sulfur cleansing lotion; salicylic acid and sulfur cleansing suspension; salicylic acid and sulfur lotion; sulfurated lime; sulfur bar soap; sulfur cream; sulfur lotion; tetracycline, oral; tetracycline hydrochloride for topical solution; tretinoin.

Acridine Derivatives—Dyes or stains (usually yellow or orange) used for some medical tests and as antiseptic agents.

Acute—Having a short and relatively severe course.

Addiction—Psychological or physiological dependence upon a drug.

Addictive Drugs—Any drug that can lead to physiological dependence on the drug. These include alcohol, cocaine, marijuana, nicotine, opium, morphine, codeine, heroin (and other narcotics) and others.

Addison's Disease—Changes in the body caused by a deficiency of hormones manufactured by the adrenal gland. Usually fatal if untreated.

Adrenal Cortex—Center of the adrenal gland.

Adrenal Gland—Gland next to the kidney that produces cortisone and epinephrine (adrenalin).

Agranulocytosis—A symptom complex characterized by (1) a sharply decreased number of granulocytes (one of the types of white blood cells), (2) lesions of the throat and other mucous membranes, (3) lesions of the gastrointestinal tract and (4) lesions of the skin. Sometimes also called granulocytopenia.

Alkalizers—These drugs neutralize acidic properties of the blood and urine by making them more alkaline (or basic). Systemic alkalizers include potassium citrate and citric acid, sodium bicarbonate, sodium citrate and citric acid, and tricitrates. Urinary alkalizers include potassium citrate, potassium citrate and citric acid, potassium citrate and sodium citrate, sodium citrate and citric acid.

Alkylating Agent—Chemical used to treat malignant diseases.

Allergy—Excessive sensitivity to a substance that is ordinarily harmless. Reactions include sneezing, stuffy nose, hives, itching.

Alpha-Adrenergic Blocking Agents—A group of drugs used to treat hypertension. These drugs include alfuzosin, prazosin, terazosin, doxazosin and labetalol (an alpha-adrenergic and beta-adrenergic combination drug). Also included are other drugs that produce an alpha-adrenergic blocking action such as haloperidol, loxapine, phenothiazines, thioxanthenes.

Amebiasis—Infection with amoebas, one-celled organisms. Causes diarrhea, fever and abdominal cramps.

Amenorrhea—Abnormal absence of menstrual periods.

Aminoglycosides—A family of antibiotics used for serious infections. Their usefulness is limited because of their relative toxicity compared to some other antibiotics. These drugs include amikacin, gentamicin, kanamycin, neomycin, netilmicin, streptomycin, tobramycin.

Amphetamines—A family of drugs that stimulates the central nervous system, prescribed to treat attention-deficit disorders in children and also for narcolepsy. They are habit-forming, are controlled under U.S. law and are no longer prescribed as appetite suppressants. These drugs include amphetamine, dextroamphetamine, lisdexamfetamine, methamphetamine. They may be ingredients of several combination drugs.

ANA Titers—A test to evaluate the immune system and to detect antinuclear antibodies (ANAs), substances that appear in the blood of some patients with autoimmune disease.

Analgesics—Agents that reduce pain without reducing consciousness.

Anaphylaxis—Severe allergic response to a substance. Symptoms are wheezing, itching, hives, nasal congestion, intense burning of hands and feet, collapse, loss of consciousness and cardiac arrest. Symptoms appear within a few seconds or minutes after exposure. Anaphylaxis is a severe medical emergency. Without appropriate treatment, it can cause death. Instructions for home treatment for anaphylaxis are at the end of the book.

Androgens—Male hormones, including fluoxymesterone, methyltestosterone, testosterone, DHEA.

Anemia—Not enough healthy red blood cells in the bloodstream or too little hemoglobin in the red blood cells. Anemia is caused by an imbalance between blood loss and blood production.

Anemia, Aplastic—A form of anemia in which the bone marrow is unable to manufacture adequate numbers of blood cells of all types—red cells, white cells, and platelets.

Anemia, Hemolytic—Anemia caused by a shortened lifespan of red blood cells. The body can't manufacture new cells fast enough to replace old cells.

Anemia, Iron-Deficiency—Anemia caused when iron necessary to manufacture red blood cells is not available.

Anemia, Pernicious—Anemia caused by a vitamin B-12 deficiency. Symptoms include weakness, fatigue, numbness and tingling of the hands or feet and degeneration of the central nervous system.

Anemia, Sickle-Cell—Anemia caused by defective hemoglobin that deprives red blood cells of oxygen, making them sickle-shaped.

Anesthesias, General—Gases that are used in surgery to render patients unconscious and able to withstand the pain of surgical cutting and manipulation. They include alfentanil, amobarbital, butabarbital, butorphanol, chloral hydrate, enflurane, etomidate, fentanyl, halothane, hydroxyzine, isoflurane, ketamine, levorphanol, meperidine, methohexital, methoxyflurane, midazolam, morphine parenteral, nalbuphine, nitrous oxide, oxymorphone, pentazocine, pentobarbital, phenobarbital, promethazine, propiomazine, propofol, scopolamine, secobarbital, sufentanil, thiamylal, thiopental.

Anesthetics—Drugs that eliminate the sensation of pain.

Angina (Angina Pectoris)—Chest pain with a sensation of suffocation and impending death. Caused by a temporary reduction in the amount of oxygen to the heart muscle through diseased coronary arteries. The pain may also occur in the left shoulder, jaw or arm.

Angiotensin-Converting Enzyme (ACE) Inhibitors—A family of drugs used to treat hypertension and congestive heart failure. Inhibitors decrease the rate of conversion of angiotensin I into angiotensin II, which is the normal process for the angiotensin-converting enzyme. These drugs include benazepril, captopril, enalapril, fosinopril, lisinopril, moexipril, perindopril, quinapril, ramipril, trandolapril.

Antacids—A large family of drugs prescribed to treat hyperacidity, peptic ulcer, esophageal reflux and other conditions. These drugs include alumina and magnesia; alumina, magnesia and calcium carbonate; alumina, magnesia and simethicone; alumina and magnesium carbonate; alumina and magnesium trisilicate; alumina, magnesium trisilicate and sodium bicarbonate; aluminum carbonate; aluminum hydroxide; bismuth subsalicylate; calcium carbonate; calcium carbonate and magnesia; calcium carbonate, magnesia and simethicone; calcium and magnesium carbonates; calcium and magnesium carbonates and magnesium oxide; calcium carbonate and simethicone; dihydroxyaluminum aminoacetate; dihydroxyaluminum sodium carbonate; magaldrate; magaldrate and simethicone; magnesium carbonate and sodium bicarbonate; magnesium hydroxide; magnesium oxide; magnesium trisilicate, alumina and magnesia; simethicone, alumina, calcium carbonate and magnesia; simethicone, alumina, magnesium carbonate and magnesia; sodium bicarbonate.

Antacids, Calcium Carbonate—These antacids include calcium carbonate and magnesium, calcium carbonate and simethicone, calcium carbonate and magnesium carbonates.

Antacids, Magnesium-Containing—These antacids include magnesium carbonate, magnesium hydroxide, magnesium oxide and magnesium trisilicate. All these medicines are designed to treat excess stomach acidity. In addition to being an effective antacid, magnesium can sometimes cause unpleasant side effects and drug interactions. Look for the presence of magnesium in nonprescription drugs.

Anthelmintics—A family of drugs used to treat intestinal parasites. Names of these drugs include niclosamide, piperazine, pyrantel, pyrvinium, quinacrine, mebendazole, metronidazole, oxamniquine, praziquantel, thiabendazole.

Antiacne Topical Preparations—See Acne Preparations.

Antiadrenals—Medicines or drugs that prevent the effects of the hormones produced by the adrenal glands.

Antianginals—A group of drugs used to treat angina pectoris (chest pain that comes and goes, caused by coronary artery disease). These drugs include acebutolol, amlodipine, amyl nitrite, atenolol, bepridil, carteolol, diltiazem, felodipine, isosorbide dinitrate, labetalol, metoprolol, nadolol, nicardipine, nifedipine, nitroglycerin, oxprenolol, penbutolol, pindolol, propranolol, sotalol, timolol, verapamil.

Antianxiety Drugs—A group of drugs prescribed to treat anxiety. These drugs include alprazolam, bromazepam, buspirone, chlordiazepoxide, chlorpromazine, clomipramine, clorazepate, diazepam, halazepam, hydroxyzine, imipramine, ketazolam, lorazepam, meprobamate, oxazepam, prazepam, prochlorperazine, thioridazine, trifluoperazine, venlafaxine.

Antiarrhythmics—A group of drugs used to treat heartbeat irregularities (arrhythmias). These drugs include acebutolol, adenosine, amiodarone, atenolol, atropine, bretylium, deslanoside, digitalis, digitoxin, diltiazem, disopyramide, dofetilide, edrophonium, encainide, esmolol, flecainide, glycopyrrolate, hyoscyamine, lidocaine, methoxamine, metoprolol, mexiletine, nadolol, oxprenolol, phenytoin, propafenone, propranolol, quinidine, scopolamine, sotalol, timolol, verapamil.

Antiasthmatics—Medicines used to treat asthma, which may be tablets, liquids or aerosols (to be inhaled to get directly to the bronchial tubes rather than through the bloodstream). These medicines include adrenocorticoids, glucocorticoid; albuterol; aminophylline; astemizole; beclomethasone; bitolterol; budesonide; cetirizine; corticotropin; cromolyn; dexamethasone; dyphylline; ephedrine;

epinephrine; ethylnorepinephrine; fenoterol; flunisolide; fluticasone; ipratropium, isoetharine; isoproterenol; isoproterenol and phenylephrine; loratadine; metaproterenol; oxtriphylline; oxtriphylline and guaifenesin; pirbuterol; racepinephrine; terbutaline; theophylline; theophylline and guaifenesin; triamcinolone.

Antibacterials (Antibiotics)—A group of drugs prescribed to treat infections. These drugs include, amikacin, amoxicillin, amoxicillin and clavulanate, ampicillin, azlocillin, aztreonam, bacampicillin, carbenicillin, cefaclor, cefadroxil, cefamandole, cefazolin, cefonicid, cefoperazone, ceforanide, cefotaxime, cefotetan, cefoxitin, ceftazidime, ceftibuten, ceftizoxime, ceftriaxone, cefuroxime, cephalexin, cephalothin, cephapirin, cephradine, chloramphenicol, cinoxacin, clindamycin, cloxacillin, cyclacillin, cycloserine, demeclocycline, dicloxacillin, doxycycline, erythromycin, erythromycin and sulfisoxazole, flucloxacillin, fusidic acid, gentamicin, imipenem and cilastatin, kanamycin, lincomycin, methacycline, methenamine, methicillin, metronidazole, mezlocillin, minocycline, moxalactam, nafcillin, nalidixic acid, netilmicin, nitrofurantoin, norfloxacin, oxacillin, oxytetracycline, penicillin G, penicillin V, piperacillin, pivampicillin, rifabutin, rifampin, rifaximin, spectinomycin, streptomycin, sulfacytine, sulfadiazine and trimethoprim, sulfamethoxazole, sulfamethoxazole and trimethoprim, sulfisoxazole, telithromycin, tetracycline, ticarcillin, ticarcillin and clavulanate, tinidazole, tobramycin, trimethoprim, vancomycin.

Antibiotics—Chemicals that inhibit the growth of or kill germs. See Antibacterials.

Anticholinergics—Drugs that work against acetylcholine, a chemical found in many locations in the body, including connections between nerve cells and connections between muscle and nerve cells. Anticholinergic drugs include amantadine, anisotropine, atropine, belladonna, benztropine, biperiden, clidinium, darifenacin, dicyclomine, glycopyrrolate, homatropine, hyoscyamine, ipratropium, isopropamide, mepenzolate, methantheline, methscopolamine, oxybutynin, pirenzepine, propantheline, scopolamine, solifenacin, tolterodine, trihexyphenidyl, trospium.

Anticoagulants—A family of drugs prescribed to slow the rate of blood clotting. These drugs include acenocoumarol, anisindione, dicumarol, dihydroergotamine and heparin, heparin, warfarin.

Anticonvulsants—A group of drugs prescribed to treat or prevent seizures (convulsions). These drugs include these families: barbiturates, carbonic anhydrase inhibitors, diones, hydantoins and succinimides. These are the names of the generic drugs in these families: acetazolamide, amobarbital, carbamazepine, carbonic anhydrase inhibitors, clobazam, clonazepam, clorazepate, diazepam, dichlorphenamide, divalproex, ethosuximide, ethotoin, felbamate, fosphenytoin, gabapentin, lacosamide, lamotrigine, levetiracetam lorazepam, mephenytoin, mephobarbital, metharbital, methsuximide, nitrazepam, oxcarbazepine, paraldehyde, phenacemide, paramethadione, pentobarbital, phenobarbital, phenytoin, primidone, secobarbital, tiagabine, topiramate, trimethadione, valproic acid, zonisamide.

Antidepressants—A group of medicines prescribed to treat mental depression. These drugs include amitriptyline, amoxapine, bupropion, citalopram, clomipramine, desipramine, doxepin, duloxetine, escitalopram, fluoxetine, fluvoxamine, imipramine, isocarboxazid, lithium, maprotiline, mirtazapine, moclobemide, nefazodone, nortriptyline, paroxetine, phenelzine, protriptyline, sertraline, tranylcypromine, trazodone, trimipramine, venlafaxine.

Antidepressants, MAO (Monoamine Oxidase) Inhibitors—A special group of drugs prescribed for mental depression. These are not as popular as in years past because of a relatively high incidence of adverse effects. These drugs include isocarboxazid (Marplan), phenelzine (Nardil), tranylcypromine (Parnate).

Antidepressants, Tricyclic (TCAs)—A group of medicines with similar chemical structure and pharmacologic activity used to treat mental depression. These drugs include amitriptyline, amoxapine, clomipramine, desipramine, doxepin, imipramine, nortriptyline, protriptyline, trimipramine.

Antidiabetic Agents—A group of drugs used in the treatment of diabetes. These medicines all reduce blood sugar. These drugs include acarbose, acetohexamide, chlorpropamide, gliclazide, glimepiride, glipizide, glyburide, insulin, metformin, nateglinide, pioglitazone, repaglinide, rosiglitazone, sitagliptin, tolazamide, tolbutamide, troglitazone.

Antidiarrheal Preparations—Medicines that treat diarrhea symptoms. Most do not cure the cause. Oral medicines include aluminum hydroxide; charcoal, activated; kaolin and pectin; loperamide; polycarbophil; psyllium hydrophilic mucilloid. Systemic medicines include carbohydrates; codeine; difenoxin and atropine; diphenoxylate and atropine; glucose and electrolytes; glycopyrrolate; kaolin, pectin, belladonna alkaloids and opium; kaolin, pectin and paregoric; nitazoxanide, opium tincture; paregoric, rifaximin.

Antidyskinetics—A group of drugs used for treatment of Parkinsonism (paralysis agitans) and drug-induced extrapyramidal reactions (see elsewhere in Glossary). These drugs include amantadine, benztropine, biperiden, bromocriptine, carbidopa and levodopa, diphenhydramine, entacapone, ethopropazine, levodopa, levodopa and benserazide, procyclidine, rasagiline, selegiline, trihexyphenidyl.

Antiemetics—A group of drugs used to treat nausea and vomiting. These drugs include buclizine, cyclizine, chlorpromazine, dimenhydrinate, diphenhydramine, diphenidol, domperidone, dronabinol, haloperidol, hydroxyzine, meclizine, metoclopramide, nabilone, ondansetron, perphenazine, prochlorperazine, promethazine, scopolamine, thiethylperazine, triflupromazine, trimethobenzamide.

Antifibrinolytic Drugs—Drugs that are used to treat serious bleeding. These drugs include aminocaproic acid and tranexamic acid.

Antifungals—A group of drugs used to treat fungus infections. Those listed as systemic are taken orally or given by injection. Those listed as topical are applied directly to the skin and include liquids, powders, creams, ointments and liniments. Those listed as vaginal are used topically inside the vagina and sometimes on the vaginal lips. These drugs include: Systemic—amphotericin B, miconazole, fluconazole, flucytosine, griseofulvin, itraconazole, ketoconazole, potassium iodide, posaconazole, terbinafine. Topical— amphotericin B, carbol-fuchsin, ciclopirox; clioquinol, clotrimazole, econazole, haloprogin, ketoconazole, mafenide, miconazole, naftifine, nystatin, oxiconazole, salicylic acid, silver sulfadiazine, sulconazole, sulfur and coal, terbinafine, tioconazole, tolnaftate, undecylenic acid. Vaginal—butoconazole, clotrimazole, econazole, gentian violet, miconazole, nystatin, terconazole, tioconazole.

Antifungals, Azole—Drugs used to treat certain types of fungal infections. These drugs include fluconazole, itraconazole, ketoconazole, miconazole, posaconazole, sertaconazole, voriconazole.

Antiglaucoma Drugs—Medicines used to treat glaucoma. Those listed as systemic are taken orally or given by injection. Those listed as ophthalmic are for external use. These drugs include: Systemic—acetazolamide, dichlorphenamide, glycerin, mannitol, methazolamide, timolol, urea. Ophthalmic—apraclonidine, betaxolol, brimonidine, brinzolamide, carbachol ophthalmic solution, carteolol, demecarium, dipivefrin, dorzolamide, echothiophate, epinephrine, epinephrine bitartrate, epinephryl borate, isoflurophate, latanoprost, levobetaxolol, levobunolol, metipranolol, physostigmine, pilocarpine, timolol, unoprostone.

Antigout Drugs—Drugs to treat the metabolic disease called gout. Gout causes recurrent attacks of joint pain caused by deposits of uric acid in the joints. Antigout drugs include allopurinol, carprofen, colchicine, febuxostat, fenoprofen, ibuprofen, indomethacin, ketoprofen, naproxen, phenylbutazone, piroxicam, probenecid, probenecid and colchicine, sulfinpyrazone, sulindac.

Antihistamines—A family of drugs used to treat allergic conditions, such as hay fever, allergic conjunctivitis, itching, sneezing, runny nose, motion sickness, dizziness, sedation, insomnia and others. These drugs include astemizole, azatadine, brompheniramine, carbinoxamine, cetirizine, chlorpheniramine, clemastine, cyproheptadine, desloratadine, dexchlorpheniramine, dimenhydrinate, diphenhydramine, diphenylpyraline, doxylamine, fexofenadine, hydroxyzine, loratadine, phenindamine, promethazine, pyrilamine, trimeprazine, tripelennamine, triprolidine.

Antihyperammonemias—Medications that decrease the amount of ammonia in the blood. The ones with this pharmacological property that are available in the United States are lactulose, sodium benzoate and sodium phenylacetate.

Antihyperlipidemics—A group of drugs used to treat hyperlipidemia (high levels of lipids in the blood). These include atorvastatin, cerivastatin, cholestyramine, clofibrate, colesevelam, colestipol, ezetimibe, fenofibrate, fluvastatin, gemfibrozil, lovastatin, niacin, pravastatin, probucol, simvastatin, sodium dichloroacetate.

Antihypertensives—Drugs used to help lower high blood pressure. These medicines can be used singly or in combination with other drugs. They work best if accompanied by a low-salt, low-fat diet plus an active exercise program. These drugs include acebutolol, amiloride, amiloride and hydrochlorothiazide, amlodipine, atenolol, atenolol and chlorthalidone, benazepril, bendroflumethiazide, benzthiazide, betaxolol, bisoprolol, bumetanide, candesartan, captopril, captopril and hydrochlorothiazide, carteolol, carvedilol, chlorothiazide, chlorthalidone, cilazapril, clonidine, clonidine and chlorthalidone, cyclothiazide, debrisoquine, deserpidine, deserpidine and hydrochlorothiazide, deserpidine and methyclothiazide, diazoxide, diltiazem, doxazosin, enalapril, enalapril and hydrochlorothiazide, eplerenone, eprosartan ethacrynic acid, felodipine, fosinopril, furosemide, guanabenz, guanadrel, guanethidine, guanethidine and hydrochlorothiazide, guanfacine, hydralazine, hydralazine and hydrochlorothiazide, hydrochlorothiazide, hydroflumethiazide, indapamide, irbesartan isradipine, labetalol, labetalol and hydrochlorothiazide, lisinopril, lisinopril and hydrochlorothiazide, losartan, losartan and hydrochlorothiazide, mecamylamine, methyclothiazide, methyldopa, methyldopa and chlorothiazide, methyldopa and hydrochlorothiazide, metolazone, metoprolol, metoprolol and hydrochlorothiazide, minoxidil, moexipril, nadolol, nadolol and bendroflumethiazide, nicardipine, nifedipine, nisoldipine, nitroglycerin, nitroprusside, olmesartan, oxprenolol, penbutolol, perindopril, pindolol, pindolol and hydrochlorothiazide, polythiazide, prazosin, prazosin and polythiazide, propranolol, propranolol and hydrochlorothiazide, quinapril, quinethazone, ramipril, rauwolfia serpentina, rauwolfia serpentina and bendroflumethiazide, reserpine, reserpine and chlorothiazide, reserpine and chlorthalidone, reserpine and hydralazine, reserpine, hydralazine and hydrochlorothiazide, reserpine and hydrochlorothiazide, reserpine and hydroflumethiazide, reserpine and methyclothiazide, reserpine and polythiazide, reserpine and quinethazone, reserpine and trichlormethiazide, sotalol, spironolactone, spironolactone and hydrochlorothiazide, telmisartan, terazosin, timolol, timolol and hydrochlorothiazide, torsemide, trandolapril, triamterene, triamterene and hydrochlorothiazide, trichlormethiazide, trimethaphan, valsartan, verapamil.

Anti-Inflammatory Drugs, Nonsteroidal (NSAIDs)—A family of drugs not related to cortisone or other steroids that decrease inflammation wherever it occurs in the body. Used for treatment of pain, fever, arthritis, gout, menstrual cramps and vascular headaches. These drugs include aspirin; aspirin, alumina and magnesia tablets; buffered aspirin; bufexamac; celecoxib; choline salicylate; choline and magnesium salicylates; diclofenac, diflunisal; fenoprofen; flurbiprofen, ibuprofen; indomethacin; ketoprofen; magnesium salicylate; meclofenamate; meloxicam; naproxen; piroxicam; rofecoxib; salsalate; sodium salicylate; sulindac; tolmetin.

Anti-Inflammatory Drugs, Steroidal—A family of drugs with pharmacologic characteristics similar to those of cortisone and cortisone-like drugs. They are used for many purposes to help the body deal with inflammation no matter what the cause. Steroidal drugs may be taken orally or by injection (systemic) or applied locally (topical) for the skin, eyes, ears, bronchial tubes and others. These drugs include: Nasal—beclomethasone, budesonide, dexamethasone, flunisolide, fluticasone, triamcinolone. Ophthalmic (eyes)—betamethasone, dexamethasone, fluorometholone, hydrocortisone, medrysone, prednisolone, rimexolone. Otic (ears)—betamethasone, desonide and acetic acid, dexamethasone, hydrocortisone, hydrocortisone and acetic acid, prednisolone. Systemic—betamethasone, corticotropin, cortisone, dexamethasone, hydrocortisone, methylprednisolone, paramethasone, prednisolone, prednisone, triamcinolone. Topical—alclometasone; amcinonide; beclomethasone; betamethasone; clobetasol; clobetasone; clocortolone; desonide; desoximetasone; dexamethasone; diflorasone; diflucortolone; flumethasone; fluocinolone; fluocinonide; fluocinonide; flurandrenolide; fluticasone; halcinonide; halobetasol; mometasone; procinonide and ciprocinonide; flurandrenolide; halcinonide; hydrocortisone; methylprednisolone; mometasone; triamcinolone.

Antimalarials (also called Antiprotozoals)—A group of drugs used to treat malaria. The choice depends on the precise type of malaria organism and its developmental state. These drugs include amphotericin B, atovaquone and proguanil, clindamycin, chloroquine, dapsone, demeclocycline, doxycycline, halofantrine; hydroxychloroquine, iodoquinol, methacycline, mefloquine, metronidazole, minocycline, oxytetracycline, pentamidine, primaquine, proguanil, pyrimethamine, quinacrine, quinidine, quinine, sulfadoxine and pyrimethamine, sulfamethoxazole, sulfamethoxazole and trimethoprim, sulfisoxazole, tetracycline.

Antimuscarines—Drugs that block the muscarinic action of acetylcholine and therefore decrease spasms of the smooth muscles. They are prescribed for peptic ulcers, dysmenorrhea, dizziness, seasickness, bedwetting, slow heart rate, toxicity from pesticides made from organophosphates and other medical problems. These drugs include anisotropine, atropine, belladonna, clidinium dicyclomine, glycopyrrolate, homatropine, hyoscyamine, hyoscyamine and scopolamine, isopropamide, mepenzolate, methantheline, methscopolamine, oxyphencyclimine, pirenzepine, propantheline, scopolamine, tridihexethyl.

Antimyasthenics—Medicines to treat myasthenia gravis, a muscle disorder (especially of the face and head) with increasing fatigue and weakness as muscles tire from use. These medicines include ambenonium, neostigmine, pyridostigmine.

Antineoplastics—Potent drugs used for malignant disease. Some of these are not described in this book, but they are listed here for completeness. These drugs include: Systemic—amifostine, altretamine, aminoglutethimide, amsacrine, anastrazole, antithyroid agents, asparaginase, azathioprine, bicalutamide, bleomycin, busulfan, capecitabine, carboplatin, carmustine, chlorambucil, chloramphenicol, chlorotrianisene, chromic phosphate, cisplatin, colchicine, cyclophosphamide, cyclosporine, cyproterone, cytarabine, dacarbazine, dactinomycin, daunorubicin, deferoxamine, diethylstilbestrol, docetaxel, doxorubicin, dromostanolone, epirubicin, estradiol, estradiol valerate, estramustine, estrogens (conjugated and esterified), estrone, ethinyl estradiol, etoposide, exemestane, floxuridine, flucytosine, fluorouracil, flutamide, fluoxymesterone, gemcitabine, gold compounds, goserelin, hexamethylmelamine, hydroxyprogesterone, hydroxyurea, ifosfamide, interferon alfa-2a and alfa-2b (recombinant), ketoconazole, letrozole, leucovorin, leuprolide, levamisole, levothyroxine, liothyronine, liotrix, lithium, lomustine, masoprocol, mechlorethamine, medroxyprogesterone, megestrol, melphalan, methyltestosterone, mercaptopurine, methotrexate, mitomycin, mitotane, mitoxantrone, nandrolone, paclitaxel, phenpropionate, penicillamine, plicamycin, porfimer, procarbazine, raltitrexed, sodium iodide I 131, sodium phosphate P 32, streptozocin, tamoxifen, temoporfin, teniposide, testolactone, testosterone, thioguanine, thiotepa, thyroglobulin, thyroid, thyrotropin, topotecan, toremifene, trastuzumab, trimetrexate, triptorelin, uracil mustard, valrubicin, vinblastine, vincristine, vindesine, vinorelbine, zidovudine. Topical—fluorouracil, mechlorethamine.

Antiparkinsonism Drugs—Drugs used to treat Parkinson's disease. A disease of the central nervous system in older adults, it is characterized by gradual progressive muscle rigidity, tremors and clumsiness. These drugs include amantadine, benztropine, biperiden, bromocriptine, carbidopa and levodopa, diphenhydramine, entacapone, ethopropazine, levodopa, levodopa and benserazide, orphenadrine, procyclidine, rasagiline, rotigotine, selegiline, trihexyphenidyl.

Antipsychotic Drugs—A group of drugs used to treat the mental disease of psychosis, including such variants as schizophrenia, manic-depressive illness, anxiety states, severe behavior problems and others. These drugs include acetophenazine, aripiprazole, carbamazepine, chlorpromazine, chlorprothixene, fluphenazine, flupenthixol, fluspirilene, haloperidol, loxapine, mesoridazine, methotrimeprazine, molindone, paliperidone, pericyazine, perphenazine, pimozide, pipotiazine, prochlorperazine, promazine, risperidone, thioproperazine, thioridazine, thiothixene, trifluoperazine, triflupromazine.

Antithyroid Drugs—Drugs that decrease the amount of thyroid hormone produced by the thyroid gland.

Antitussives—A group of drugs used to suppress coughs. These drugs include benzonatate, chlophedianol, codeine (oral), dextromethorphan, diphenhydramine syrup, hydrocodone, hydromorphone, methadone, morphine.

Antiulcer Drugs—A group of medicines used to treat peptic ulcer in the stomach, duodenum or the lower end of the esophagus. These drugs include amitriptyline, antacids, anticholinergics, antispasmodics, bismuth subsalicylate, cimetidine, doxepin, famotidine, lansoprazole,

misoprostol, nizatidine, omeprazole, ranitidine, sucralfate, trimipramine.

Antiurolithics—Medicines that prevent the formation of kidney stones.

Antiviral Drugs—A group of drugs used to treat viral infections. These drugs include: Ophthalmic (eye)—idoxuridine, trifluridine, vidarabine. Systemic—acyclovir, amantadine, didanosine, famciclovir, foscarnet, ganciclovir, oseltamivir, ribavirin, rimantadine, stavudine, zalcitabine, zanamivir, zidovudine. Topical drugs—acyclovir, docosanol.

Antivirals, HIV/AIDS—A group of drugs used to treat human immunodeficiency virus (HIV) and acquired immune deficiency syndrome (AIDS). They work by suppressing the replication of HIV. These drugs include abacavir, darunavir, delavirdine, didanosine, efavirenz, indinavir, lamivudine, maraviroc, nelfinavir, nevirapine, raltegravir, ritonavir, saquinavir, stavudine, tipranavir, zalcitabine, zidovudine.

Appendicitis—Inflammation or infection of the appendix. Symptoms include loss of appetite, nausea, low-grade fever and tenderness in the lower right of the abdomen.

Appetite Suppressants—A group of drugs used to decrease the appetite as part of an overall treatment for obesity. These drugs include amphetamine and dextroamphetamine, benzphetamine, diethylpropion, fenfluramine, mazindol, phendimetrazine, phentermine, phenylpropanolamine, sibutramine.

Artery—Blood vessel carrying blood away from the heart.

Asthma—Recurrent attacks of breathing difficulty due to spasms and contractions of the bronchial tubes.

Attenuated Virus Vaccines—Liquid products of killed germs used for injections to prevent certain diseases.

B

Bacteria—Microscopic organisms. Some bacteria contribute to health; others (germs) cause disease and infection.

Barbiturates—Powerful drugs used for sedation, to help induce sleep and sometimes to prevent seizures. Except for use in seizures (phenobarbital), barbiturates are being used less and less because there are better, less hazardous drugs that produce the same or better effects.

These drugs include amobarbital, aprobarbital, butabarbital, mephobarbital, metharbital, pentobarbital, phenobarbital, secobarbital, secobarbital and amobarbital, talbutal.

Basal Area of Brain—Part of the brain that regulates muscle control and tone.

Benzethonium Chloride—A compound used as a preservative in some drug preparations. It is also used in various concentrations for cleaning cooking and eating utensils and as a disinfectant.

Benzodiazepines—A family of drugs prescribed to treat anxiety and alcohol withdrawal and sometimes prescribed for sedation. These drugs include alprazolam, bromazepam, chlordiazepoxide, clonazepam, clorazepate, diazepam, estazolam, flurazepam, halazepam, ketazolam, lorazepam, nitrazepam, oxazepam, prazepam, quazepam, triazolam.

Beta Agonists—A group of drugs that act directly on cells in the body (beta-adrenergic receptors) to relieve spasms of the bronchial tubes and other organs consisting of smooth muscles. These drugs include albuterol, bitolterol, isoetharine, isoproterenol, metaproterenol, terbutaline.

Beta-Adrenergic Blocking Agents—A family of drugs with similar pharmacological actions with some variations. These drugs are prescribed for angina, heartbeat irregularities (arrhythmias), high blood pressure, hypertrophic subaortic stenosis, vascular headaches (as a preventative, not to treat once the pain begins) and others. Timolol is prescribed for treatment of open-angle glaucoma. These drugs include acebutolol, atenolol, betaxolol, bisoprolol, carteolol, labetalol, levobetaxolol, metoprolol, nadolol, oxprenolol, penbutolol, pindolol, propranolol, sotalol, timolol.

Bile Acids—Components of bile that are derived from cholesterol and formed in the liver. Bile acids aid the digestion of fat.

Blood Count—Laboratory studies to count white blood cells, red blood cells, platelets and other elements of the blood.

Blood Dyscrasia-Causing Medicines—Drugs which cause unpredictable damaging effects to human bone marrow. These effects occur in a small minority of patients and are not dependent upon dosage. These medicines include the following (some of which are not described in this book): ACE inhibitors, acetazolamide, aminopyrine, amodiaquine, anticonvulsants (dione, hydantoin, succinimide), antidepressants (tricyclic), antidiabetic agents (sulfonylurea), anti-inflammatory analgesics, antithyroid agents, bexarotene, captopril, carbamazepine, cephalosporins, chloramphenicol, cisplatin, clopidogrel, clozapine, dapsone, divalproex, felbamate, flecainide acetate, foscarnet, gold compounds, levamisole, loxapine, maprotiline, methicillin, methimazole, methsuximide, metronidazole, mirtazapine, pantoprazole, penicillins (some), penicillamine, pentamidine, phenacemide, phenothiazines, phensuximide, phenytoin, pimozide, primaquine, primidone, propafenone, propylthiouracil, pyrimethamine (large doses), rabeprazole, rifampin, rifapentine, rituximab, sulfamethoxazole and trimethoprim, sulfasalazine, sulfonamides, thioxanthenes, ticlopidine, tiopronin, topiramate, trastuzumab, trimethobenzamide, trimethoprim, valproic acid.

Blood Pressure, Diastolic—Pressure (usually recorded in millimeters of mercury) in the large arteries of the body when the heart muscle is relaxed and filling for the next contraction.

Blood Pressure, Systolic—Pressure (usually recorded in millimeters of mercury) in the large arteries of the body at the instant the heart muscle contracts.

Blood Sugar (Blood Glucose)—Necessary element in the blood to sustain life.

Bone Marrow Depressants—Medicines that affect the bone marrow to depress its normal function of forming blood cells. These medicines include the following (some of which are not described in this book): abacavir, alcohol, aldesleukin, altretamine, amphotericin B (systemic), anticancer drugs, antithyroid drugs, azathioprine, bexarotene, busulfan, capecitabine, carboplatin, carmustine, chlorambucil, chloramphenicol, chromic phosphate, cisplatin, cladribine, clozapine, colchicine, cyclophosphamide, cyproterone, cytarabine, dacarbazine, dactinomycin, daunorubicin, didanosine, docetaxel, doxorubicin, eflornithine, epirubicin, etoposide, floxuridine, flucytosine, fludarabine, fluorouracil, ganciclovir, gemcitabine, hydroxyurea, idarubicin, ifosfamide, imatinib, interferon, irinotecan, lomustine, mechlorethamine, melphalan, mercaptopurine, methotrexate, mitomycin, mitoxantrone, paclitaxel, pentostatin, plicamycin, procarbazine, sirolimus, streptozocin, sulfa drugs, temozolomide, teniposide, thioguanine, thiotepa, topotecan, trimetrexate, uracil mustard, valrubicin, vidarabine (large doses), vinblastine, vincristine, vindesine, vinorelbine, zidovudine, zoledronic acid.

Bone Marrow Depression—Reduction of the blood-producing capacity of human bone marrow. Can be caused by many drugs taken for long periods of time in high doses.

Brain Depressants—Any drug that depresses brain function, such as tranquilizers, narcotics, alcohol and barbiturates.

Bronchodilators—A group of drugs used to dilate the bronchial tubes to treat such problems as asthma, emphysema, bronchitis, bronchiectasis, allergies and others. These drugs include albuterol, aminophylline, arformoterol, bitolterol, cromolyn, dyphylline, ephedrine, epinephrine, ethylnorepinephrine, fenoterol, formoterol, ipratropium, isoetharine, isoproterenol, levalbuterol metaproterenol, nedocromil, oxtriphylline, oxtriphylline and guaifenesin, pirbuterol, procaterol, salmeterol, terbutaline, theophylline and guaifenesin.

Bronchodilators, Xanthine-Derivative—Drugs of similar chemical structure and pharmacological activity that are prescribed to dilate bronchial tubes in disorders such as asthma, bronchitis, emphysema and other chronic lung diseases. These drugs include aminophylline, dyphylline, oxtriphylline, theophylline.

BUN—Abbreviation for blood urea nitrogen. A test often used as a measurement of kidney function.

C

Calcium Channel Blockers—A group of drugs used to treat angina and heartbeat irregularities. These drugs include bepridil, diltiazem, felodipine, flunarizine, isradipine, nicardipine, nifedipine, nimodipine, verapamil.

Calcium Supplements—Supplements used to increase the calcium concentration in the blood in an attempt to make bones denser (as in osteoporosis). These supplements include calcium citrate, calcium glubionate, calcium gluconate, calcium glycerophosphate and calcium lactate, calcium lactate, dibasic calcium phosphate, tribasic calcium phosphate.

Carbamates—A group of drugs derived from carbamic acid and used for anxiety or as sedatives. They include meprobamate and ethinamate.

Carbetapentane—An antitussive (cough suppressing) drug similar to dextromethorphan in action. It is an ingredient in some cough and cold remedies.

Carbonic Anhydrase Inhibitors—Drugs used to treat glaucoma and seizures and to prevent high altitude sickness. They include acetazolamide, brinzolamide, dichlorphenamide, dorzolamide, methazolamide.

Cataract—Loss of transparency in the lens of the eye.

Catecholamines—A group of drugs, also found naturally in the body, used to treat low blood pressure or shock. These drugs include dopamine, norepinephrine and epinephrine.

Cationic Drugs—Drugs removed from the body by the kidneys (called renal tubular secretion). If two of these drugs are taken together, one of them may stay in the body longer and increase its effect. These drugs include digoxin, metformin, morphine, pancuronium, tenofovir, trospium, vancomycin.

Cell—Unit of protoplasm, the essential living matter of all plants and animals.

Central Nervous System (CNS) Depressants—These drugs cause sedation or otherwise diminish brain activity and other parts of the nervous system. These drugs include alcohol, aminoglutethimide, anesthetics (general and injection-local), anticonvulsants, antidepressants (MAO inhibitors, tricyclic), antidyskinetics (except amantadine), antihistamines, apomorphine, azelastine, baclofen, barbiturates, benzodiazepines, beta-adrenergic blocking agents, brimonidine, buclizine, carbamazepine, cetirizine, chlophedianol, chloral hydrate, chlorzoxazone, clonidine, clozapine, cyclizine, cytarabine, difenoxin and atropine, diphenoxylate and atropine, disulfiram, donepezil, dronabinol, droperidol, ethchlorvynol, ethinamate, etomidate, fenfluramine, fluoxetine, glutethimide, guanabenz, guanfacine, haloperidol, hydroxyzine, ifosfamide, interferon, loxapine, magnesium sulfate (injection), maprotiline, meclizine, meprobamate, methyldopa, methyprylon, metoclopramide, metyrosine, mirtazapine, mitotane, molindone, nabilone, nefazodone, olanzapine, opioid (narcotic) analgesics, oxcarbazepine, oxybutynin, paliperidone, paraldehyde, paregoric, pargyline, paroxetine, phenothiazines, pimozide, procarbazine, promethazine, propiomazine, propofol, quetiapine, rauwolfia alkaloids, risperidone, scopolamine, sertraline, skeletal muscle relaxants (centrally acting), thalidomide, thioxanthenes, tramadol, trazodone, trimeprazine, trimethobenzamide, zaleplon, zolpidem, zonisamide, zopiclone.

Central Nervous System (CNS) Stimulants— Drugs that cause excitation, anxiety and nervousness or otherwise stimulate the brain and other parts of the central nervous system. These drugs include amantadine, amphetamines, anesthetics (local), appetite suppressants (except fenfluramine), bronchodilators (xanthine-derivative), bupropion, caffeine, chlophedianol, cocaine, dextroamphetamine, diclofenac, doxapram, dronabinol, dyphylline, entacapone, ephedrine (oral), fluoroquinolones, fluoxetine, meropenem, methamphetamine, methylphenidate, moclobemide, modafinil, nabilone, pemoline, rasagiline, selegiline, sertraline, sympathomimetics, topiramate, tranylcypromine, zonisamide.

Cephalosporins—Antibiotics that kill many bacterial germs that penicillin and sulfa drugs can't destroy.

Cholinergics (Parasympathomimetics)— Chemicals that facilitate passage of nerve impulses through the parasympathetic nervous system.

Cholinesterase Inhibitors—Drugs that prevent the action of cholinesterase (an enzyme that breaks down acetylcholine in the body).

Chronic—Long-term, continuing. Chronic illnesses may not be curable, but they can often be prevented from becoming worse. Symptoms usually can be alleviated or controlled.

Cirrhosis—Disease that scars and destroys liver tissue resulting in abnormal function.

Citrates—Medicines taken orally to make urine more acid. Citrates include potassium citrate, potassium citrate and citric acid, potassium citrate and sodium citrate, sodium citrate and acid, tricitrates.

Coal Tar Preparations—Creams, ointments and lotions used on the skin for various skin ailments.

Cold Urticaria—Hives that appear in areas of the body exposed to the cold.

Colitis, Ulcerative—Chronic, recurring ulcers of the colon for unknown reasons.

Collagen—Support tissue of skin, tendon, bone, cartilage and connective tissue.

Colostomy—Surgical opening from the colon, the large intestine, to the outside of the body.

Coma—A sleeplike state from which a person cannot be aroused.

Compliance—The extent to which a person follows medical advice.

Congestive—Characterized by excess accumulation of fluid. In congestive heart failure, congestion occurs in the lungs, liver, kidneys and other parts of the body to cause shortness of breath, swelling of the ankles and feet, rapid heartbeat and other symptoms.

Constriction—Tightness or pressure.

Contraceptives, Hormonal—Any form of contraception (birth control) that contains hormones (such as ethinyl estradiol and others). These forms include oral, injectable, transdermal and implantable.

Contraceptives, Oral (Birth Control Pills)—A group of hormones used to prevent ovulation, therefore preventing pregnancy. These hormones include drospirenone and ethinyl estradiol, ethynodiol diacetate and ethinyl estradiol, ethynodiol diacetate and mestranol, etonogestrel, levonorgestrel and ethinyl estradiol, medroxyprogesterone, norethindrone tablets, norethindrone acetate and ethinyl estradiol, norethindrone and ethinyl estradiol, norethindrone and mestranol, norethynodrel and mestranol, norgestrel, norgestrel and ethinyl estradiol.

Contraceptives, Vaginal—Topical medications or devices applied inside the vagina to prevent pregnancy.

Convulsions—Violent, uncontrollable contractions of the voluntary muscles.

COPD (Chronic Obstructive Pulmonary Disease)—Lung conditions including emphysema and chronic bronchitis.

Corticosteroids (Adrenocorticosteroids)— Steroid hormones produced by the body's adrenal cortex or their synthetic equivalents.

Cortisone (Adrenocorticoids, Glucocorticoids) and Other Adrenal Steroids—Medicines that mimic the action of the steroid hormone cortisone, manufactured in the cortex of the adrenal gland. These drugs decrease the effects of inflammation within the body. They are available for injection, oral use, topical use for the skin, eyes and nose and inhalation for the bronchial tubes. These drugs include alclometasone; amcinonide; beclomethasone; benzyl benzoate; betamethasone; bismuth; ciclesonide; clobetasol; clobetasone 17-butyrate; clocortolone; cortisone; desonide; desoximetasone; desoxycorticosterone;

dexamethasone; diflorasone; diflucortolone; fludrocortisone; flumethasone; flunisolide; fluocinonide; fluocinonide, procinonide and ciprocinonide; fluorometholone; fluprednisolone, flurandrenolide; halcinonide; hydrocortisone; medrysone; methylprednisolone; mometasone; paramethasone; Peruvian balsam; prednisolone; prednisone; triamcinolone; zinc oxide.

Cycloplegics—Eye drops that prevent the pupils from accommodating to varying degrees of light.

Cystitis—Inflammation of the urinary bladder.

D

Decongestants—Drugs used to relieve congestion by shrinking swollen membranes. These drugs include: Cough-suppressing—phenylephrine and dextromethorphan, phenylpropanolamine (phenylpropanolamine products are being discontinued) and caramiphen, phenylpropanolamine and dextromethorphan, phenylpropanolamine and hydrocodone, pseudoephedrine and codeine, pseudoephedrine and dextromethorphan, pseudoephedrine and hydrocodone. Cough-suppressing and pain-relieving—phenylpropanolamine, dextromethorphan and acetaminophen. Cough-suppressing and sputum-thinning—phenylephrine, dextromethorphan and guaifenesin; phenylephrine, hydrocodone and guaifenesin; phenylpropanolamine, codeine and guaifenesin; phenylpropanolamine, dextromethorphan and guaifenesin; pseudoephedrine, codeine and guaifenesin; pseudoephedrine, dextromethorphan and guaifenesin; pseudoephedrine, hydrocodone and guaifenesin; phenylephrine, dextromethorphan, guaifenesin and acetaminophen; pseudoephedrine, dextromethorphan, guaifenesin and acetaminophen. Sputum-thinning—ephedrine and guaifenesin; ephedrine and potassium iodide; phenylephrine, phenylpropanolamine and guaifenesin; phenylpropanolamine and guaifenesin; pseudoephedrine and guaifenesin. Nasal—ephedrine (oral), phenylpropanolamine, pseudoephedrine. Ophthalmic (eye)—naphazoline, oxymetazoline, phenylephrine. Topical—oxymetazoline, phenylephrine, xylometazoline.

Delirium—Temporary mental disturbance characterized by hallucinations, agitation and incoherence.

Diabetes—Metabolic disorder in which the body can't use carbohydrates efficiently. This leads to a dangerously high level of glucose (a carbohydrate) in the blood.

Dialysis—Procedure to filter waste products from the bloodstream of patients with kidney failure.

Digitalis Preparations (Digitalis Glycosides)—Important drugs to treat heart disease, such as congestive heart failure, heartbeat irregularities and cardiogenic shock. These drugs include digitoxin, digoxin.

Digoxin—One of the digitalis drugs used to treat heart disease. All digitalis products were originally derived from the foxglove plant.

Dilation—Enlargement.

Disulfiram Reaction—Disulfiram (Antabuse) is a drug to treat alcoholism. When alcohol in the bloodstream interacts with disulfiram, it causes a flushed face, severe headache, chest pains, shortness of breath, nausea, vomiting, sweating and weakness. Severe reactions may cause death. A disulfiram reaction is the interaction of any drug with alcohol or another drug to produce these symptoms.

Diuretics—Drugs that act on the kidneys to prevent reabsorption of electrolytes, especially chlorides. They are used to treat edema, high blood pressure, congestive heart failure, kidney and liver failure and others. These drugs include amiloride, amiloride and hydrochlorothiazide, bendroflumethiazide, benzthiazide, bumetanide, chlorothiazide, chlorthalidone, cyclothiazide, ethacrynic acid, furosemide, glycerin, hydrochlorothiazide, hydroflumethiazide, indapamide, mannitol, methyclothiazide, metolazone, polythiazide, quinethazone, spironolactone, spironolactone and hydrochlorothiazide, triamterene, triamterene and hydrochlorothiazide, trichlormethiazide, urea.

Diuretics, Loop—Drugs that act on the kidneys to prevent reabsorption of electrolytes, especially sodium. They are used to treat edema, high blood pressure, congestive heart failure, kidney and liver failure and others. These drugs include bumetanide, ethacrynic acid, furosemide.

Diuretics, Potassium-Sparing—Drugs that act on the kidneys to prevent reabsorption of electrolytes, especially sodium. They are used to treat edema, high blood pressure, congestive heart failure, kidney and liver failure and others.

This particular group of diuretics does not allow the unwanted side effect of low potassium in the blood to occur. These drugs include amiloride, spironolactone, triamterene.

Diuretics, Thiazide—Drugs that act on the kidneys to prevent reabsorption of electrolytes, especially chlorides. They are used to treat edema, high blood pressure, congestive heart failure, kidney and liver failure and others. These drugs include bendroflumethiazide, benzthiazide, chlorothiazide, chlorthalidone, cyclothiazide, hydrochlorothiazide, hydroflumethiazide, methyclothiazide, metolazone, polythiazide, quinethazone, trichlormethiazide.

Dopamine Agonists—Drugs that stimulate activity of dopamine (a brain chemical that helps control movement). These include bromocriptine, cabergoline, ropinirole.

Dopamine Antagonists—Drugs that interfere with dopamine production (brain chemical that helps control movement). These drugs include haloperidol, metoclopramide, phenothiazines, thioxanthenes.

Duodenum—The first 12 inches of the small intestine.

E

ECG (or EKG)—Abbreviation for electrocardiogram or electrocardiograph. An ECG is a graphic tracing representing the electrical current produced by impulses passing through the heart muscle. This is a useful test in the diagnosis of heart disease, but used alone it usually can't make a complete diagnosis. An ECG is most useful in two areas: (1) demonstrating heart rhythm disturbances and (2) demonstrating changes when there is a myocardial infarction (heart attack). It will detect enlargement of either heart chamber, but will not establish a diagnosis of heart failure or disease of the heart valves.

Eczema—Disorder of the skin with redness, itching, blisters, weeping and abnormal pigmentation.

EEG—Electroencephalogram or electro-encephalograph. An EEG is a graphic recording of electrical activity generated spontaneously from nerve cells in the brain. This test is useful in the diagnosis of brain dysfunction, particularly in studying seizure disorders.

Electrolytes—Substances that can transmit electrical impulses when dissolved in body fluids. These include sodium, potassium, chloride, bicarbonate, and carbon dioxide.

Embolism—Sudden blockage of an artery by a clot or foreign material in the blood.

Emphysema—An irreversible disease in which the lung's air sacs lose elasticity and air accumulates in the lungs.

Endometriosis—Condition in which uterus tissue is found outside the uterus. Can cause pain, abnormal menstruation and infertility.

Enzyme Inducers—Drugs that increase the metabolism of another drug in the liver, resulting in a decrease of that drug's effect. Ask your doctor or pharmacist about this possible interaction. Listed here are the more common used drugs in this category. These drugs include: alcohol (chronic use), barbiturates (especially phenobarbital), carbamazepine, darunavir, dexamethasone, efavirenz, glucocorticoids, glutethimide, griseofulvin, insulin, isoniazid, modafinil, nafcillin, nevirapine, norethindrone, omeprazole, oxcarbazepine, phenylbutazone, phenytoin, pioglitazone, prednisone, primidone, rifabutin, rifampin, rifapentine, saquinavir, secobarbital, St. John's wort, tipranavir, troglitazone. Also included are charbroiled meats, cruciferous vegetables (such as broccoli and cabbage) and smoking. There may be other drugs in this category. Consult doctor or pharmacist.

Enzyme Inducing Antiepileptic Drugs—Drugs used for seizure disorders that increase the metabolism of another drug in the liver, resulting in a decrease of that drug's effect. These drugs include carbamazepine, phenytoin, primidone and phenobarbital.

Enzyme Inhibitors—Drugs that decrease the metabolism of another drug in the liver, resulting in an increase of that drug's effect. Ask your doctor or pharmacist about this possible interaction. Listed here are the more common used drugs in this category. These drugs include: amiodarone, antipsychotics, aprepitant, azithromycin, azole antifungals, bupropion, celecoxib, chloramphenicol, chlorpromazine, chlorpheniramine, cimetidine, ciprofloxacin, citalopram, clarithromycin, clemastine, clomipramine, cyclosporine, darunavir, delavirdine, diphenhydramine, diltiazem, disulfiram, doxepin, doxorubicin, duloxetine, enoxacin, erythromycins, escitalopram, fenofibrate, felbamate, fluoroquinolones, gemfibrozil, glitazones, halofantrine, histamine H2 receptor antagonists, HIV antivirals (some), hydroxyzine, imatinib, indomethacin, isoniazid, itraconazole, ketoconazole, lansoprazole, levomepromazine, lovastatin, methadone, methoxsalen, metoclopramide, metronidazole, mibefradil, midodrine, mifepristone, modafinil, montelukast, nefazodone, nelfinavir, norfloxacin, norfluoxetine, omeprazole, oxcarbazepine, pantoprazole, paroxetine, perphenazine, phenothiazines, phenylbutazone, probenecid, protease inhibitors, quinidine, rabeprazole, ranitidine, ranolazine, ritonavir, saquinavir, selective serotonin reuptake inhibitors (SSRIs), sertraline, sulfamethoxazole, telithromycin, teniposide, terbinafine, thiotepa, ticlopidine, topiramate, trimethoprim, tripelennamine, valproic acid, venlafaxine, verapamil, voriconazole, zafirlukast; and grapefruit juice. There may be other drugs in this category. Consult doctor or pharmacist.

Enzymes—Protein chemicals that can accelerate chemical reactions in the body.

Epilepsy—Episodes of brain disturbance that cause convulsions and loss of consciousness.

Erectile Dysfunction Agents—Medicines used to treat male impotence (the inability to develop and sustain an erection). These drugs include: Alprostadil, papaverine, sildenafil citrate, tadalafil, vardenafil, yohimbine.

Ergot Preparations (Alkaloids)—Medicines used to treat migraine and other types of throbbing headaches. Also used after delivery of babies to make the uterus clamp down and reduce excessive bleeding. These drugs include dihydroergotamine, ergoloid mesylates, ergotamine.

Erythromycins—A group of drugs with similar structure used to treat infections. These drugs include erythromycin, erythromycin estolate, erythromycin ethylsuccinate, erythromycin gluceptate, erythromycin lactobionate, erythromycin stearate.

Esophagitis—Inflammation of the lower part of the esophagus, the tube connecting the throat and the stomach.

Estrogens—Female hormones used to replenish the body's stores after the ovaries have been removed or become nonfunctional after menopause. Also used with progesterone in some birth control pills and for other purposes. These drugs include:

Systemic— chlorotrianisene, diethylstilbestrol, estradiol, estrogens (conjugated and esterified), estrone, estropipate, ethinyl estradiol, quinestrol. Vaginal—dienestrol, estradiol, estrogens (conjugated), estrone, estropipate.

Eustachian Tube—Small passage from the middle ear to the sinuses and nasal passages.

Extrapyramidal Reactions—Abnormal reactions in the power and coordination of posture and muscular movements. Movements are not under voluntary control. Some drugs associated with producing extrapyramidal reactions include amoxapine, antidepressants (tricyclic), droperidol, haloperidol, loxapine, metoclopramide, metyrosine, moclobemide, molindone, olanzapine, paliperidone, paroxetine, phenothiazines, pimozide, rauwolfia alkaloids, risperidone, tacrine, thioxanthenes.

Extremity—Arm, leg, hand or foot.

F

Fecal Impaction—Condition in which feces become firmly wedged in the rectum.

Fibrocystic Breast Disease—Overgrowth of fibrous tissue in the breast, producing non- malignant cysts.

Fibroid Tumors—Non-malignant tumors of the muscular layer of the uterus.

Flu (Influenza)—A virus infection of the respiratory tract that lasts three to ten days. Symptoms include headache, fever, runny nose, cough, tiredness and muscle aches.

Fluoroquinolones—A class of drugs used to treat bacterial infections, such as urinary tract infections and some types of bronchitis. These drugs include ciprofloxacin, enoxacin, gatifloxacin, gemifloxacin, levofloxacin, lomefloxacin, moxifloxacin, norfloxacin, ofloxacin, sparfloxacin.

Folate Antagonists—Drugs that impair the body's utilization of folic acid, which is necessary for cell growth. These drugs include dione anticonvulsants, hydantoin anticonvulsants, succinimide anticonvulsants, divalproex, methotrexate, oral contraceptives, phenobarbital (long-term use), pyrimethamine, sulfonamides, triamterene, trimethoprim, trimetrexate, valproic acid.

Folliculitis—Inflammation of a follicle.

Functional Dependence—The development of dependence on a drug for a normal body function. The primary example is the use of laxatives for a prolonged period so that there is a dependence on the laxative for normal bowel action.

G

G6PD—Deficiency of glucose 6-phosphate, which is necessary for glucose metabolism.

Ganglionic Blockers—Medicines that block the passage of nerve impulses through a part of the nerve cell called a ganglion. Ganglionic blockers are used to treat urinary retention and other medical problems. Bethanechol is one of the best ganglionic blockers.

Gastritis—Inflammation of the stomach.

Gastrointestinal—Of the stomach and intestinal tract.

Gland—Organ or group of cells that manufactures and excretes materials not required for its own metabolic needs.

Glaucoma—Eye disease in which increased pressure inside the eye damages the optic nerve, causes pain and changes vision.

Glucagon—Injectable drug that immediately elevates blood sugar by mobilizing glycogen from the liver.

Gold Compounds—Medicines which use gold as their base and are usually used to treat joint or arthritic disorders. These medicines include auranofin, aurothioglucose, gold sodium thiomalate.

H

H₂ Antagonists—Antihistamines that work against H_2 histamine. H_2 histamine may be liberated at any point in the body, but most often in the gastrointestinal tract.

Hangover Effect—The same feelings as a "hangover" after too much alcohol consumption. Symptoms include headache, irritability and nausea.

Hemochromatosis—Disorder of iron metabolism in which excessive iron is deposited in and damages body tissues, particularly of the liver and pancreas.

Hemoglobin—Pigment that carries oxygen in red blood cells.

Hemolytics—Drugs that can destroy red blood cells and separate hemoglobin from the blood cells. These include acetohydroxamic acid, antidiabetic agents (sulfonylurea), doxapram, furazolidone, mefenamic acid, menadiol, methyldopa, nitrofurans, primaquine, quinidine, quinine, sulfonamides (systemic), sulfones, vitamin K.

Hemorrhage—Heavy bleeding.

Hemorheologic Agents—Medicines to help control bleeding.

Hemosiderosis—Increase of iron deposits in body tissues without tissue damage.

Hepatitis—Inflammation of liver cells, usually accompanied by jaundice.

Hepatotoxics—Medications that can possibly cause toxicity or decreased normal function of the liver. These drugs include the following (some of which are not described in this book): acetaminophen (with long-term use); abacavir, acitretin, alcohol; amiodarone; anabolic steroids; androgens; angiotensin-converting enzyme (ACE) inhibitors; acitretin, anti-inflammatory drugs, nonsteroidal (NSAIDs), antithyroid agents, asparaginase, azlocillin, bexarotene, carbamazepine, carmustine; clindamycin; clofibrate; colestipol; cox 2 inhibitors; cyproterone; cytarabine; danazol; dantrolene; dapsone; daunorubicin; disulfiram; divalproex, dofetilide; epirubicin, erythromycins; estrogens; ethionamide; etretinate; felbamate; fenofibrate; fluconazole; flutamide; gold compounds; halothane; HMG-CoA reductase inhibitors; imatinib, iron (overdose) isoniazid; itraconazole; ketoconazole (oral); labetalol; mercaptopurine; methimazole, methotrexate; methyldopa; metronidazole, naltrexone; nevirapine, niacin (high doses); nilutamide, nitrofurans; pemoline; phenothiazines; phenytoin; piperacillin; plicamycin; posaconazole; pravastatin; probucol, rifampin; rosiglitazone, sulfamethoxazole and trimethoprim; sulfonamides; tacrine; tenofovir, testosterone; tizanidine; tolcapone; toremifene; tretinoin; troglitazone; valproic acid; zidovudine, zidovudine and lamivudine.

Hiatal Hernia—Section of the stomach that protrudes into the chest cavity.

Histamine—Chemical in body tissues that dilates the smallest blood vessels, constricts the smooth muscle surrounding the bronchial tubes and stimulates stomach secretions.

History—Past medical events in a patient's life.

Hives—Elevated patches on the skin that are redder or paler than surrounding skin and often itch severely.

HMG-CoA Reductase Inhibitors—A group of prescription drugs used to lower cholesterol. These include Atorvastatin, fluvastatin, lovastatin, pravastatin, pravastatin & aspirin, and simvastatin.

Hoarseness—Husky, gruff, weak voice.

Hormone Replacement Therapy—A medication (estrogen) or combination of medications (estrogen and progestin or estrogen and androgen) used for treatment of premenopausal and menopausal symptoms and for prevention of diseases that affect women in their later years

Hormones—Chemical substances produced in the body to regulate other body functions.

Hypercalcemia—Too much calcium in the blood. This happens with some malignancies and in calcium overdose.

Hyperglycemia-Causing Medications—A group of drugs that may contribute to hyperglycemia (high blood sugar). These include oral estrogen-containing contraceptives, corticosteroids, estrogens, isoniazid, nicotinic acid, phenothiazines, phenytoin, sympathomimetics, thyroid hormones, thiazide diuretics.

Hyperkalemia-Causing Medications—Medicines that cause too much potassium in the bloodstream. These include ACE inhibitors; amiloride, anti-inflammatory drugs, nonsteroidal (NSAIDs); cyclosporine; digitalis glycosides; diuretics (potassium-sparing); pentamidine; spironolactone; succinylcholine chloride; tacrolimus; triamterene; trimethoprim; possibly any medicine that is combined with potassium.

Hypersensitivity—Serious reactions to many medications. The effects of hypersensitivity may be characterized by wheezing, shortness of breath, rapid heart rate, severe itching, faintness, unconsciousness and severe drop in blood pressure.

Hypertension—High blood pressure.

Hypervitaminosis—A condition due to an excess of one or more vitamins. Symptoms may include weakness, fatigue, loss of hair and changes in the skin.

Hypnotics—Drugs used to induce a sleeping state. See Barbiturates.

Hypocalcemia—Abnormally low level of calcium in the blood.

Hypoglycemia—Low blood sugar (blood glucose). A critically low blood sugar level will interfere with normal brain function and can damage the brain permanently.

Hypoglycemia-Causing Medications—A group of drugs that may contribute to hypoglycemia (low blood sugar). These include clofibrate, monoamine oxidase (MAO) inhibitors, probenecid, propranolol, rifabutin, rifampicin, salicylates, sulfonamides (long-acting), sulfonylureas.

Hypoglycemics—Drugs that reduce blood sugar. These include acetohexamide, chlorpropamide, gliclazide, glipizide, glyburide, insulin, metformin, tolazamide, tolbutamide.

Hypokalemia-Causing Medications—Medicines that cause a depletion of potassium in the bloodstream. These include adrenocorticoids (systemic), alcohol, amphotericin B (systemic), bronchodilators (adrenergic), capreomycin, carbonic anhydrase inhibitors, cisplatin, diuretics (loop and thiazide), edetate (long-term use), foscarnet, ifosfamide, indapamide, insulin, insulin lispro, laxatives (if dependent on), penicillins (some), salicylates, sirolimus, sodium bicarbonate, urea, vitamin D (overdose of).

Hypotension—Blood pressure decrease below normal. Symptoms may include weakness, lightheadedness and dizziness.

Hypotension-Causing Drugs—Medications that might cause hypotension (low blood pressure). These include alcohol, alpha adrenergic blocking agents, alprostadil, amantadine, anesthetics (general), angiotensin-converting enzyme inhibitors (ACE inhibitors), angiotensin II receptor antagonists, antidepressants (MAO inhibitors, tricyclic), antihypertensives, benzodiazepines used as preanesthetics, beta-adrenergic blocking agents, brimonidine, bromocriptine, cabergoline, calcium channel-blocking agents, carbidopa and levodopa, clonidine, clozapine, dipyridamole and aspirin, diuretics, docetaxel, droperidol, edetate calcium disodium, edetate disodium, haloperidol, hydralazine, levodopa, lidocaine (systemic), loxapine, magnesium sulfate, maprotiline, mirtazapine, molindone, nabilone (high doses), nefazodone, nitrates, olanzapine, opioid analgesics (including fentanyl, fentanyl and sufentanil), oxcarbazepine, paclitaxel, paliperidone, pentamidine, pentoxifylline, phenothiazines, pimozide, pramipexole, propofol, quetiapine, quinidine, radiopaques (materials used in x-ray studies), ranitidine risperidone, rituximab, ropinirole, sildenafil, thioxanthenes, tizanidine, tolcapone, trazodone, vancomycin, venlafaxine. If you take any of these medications, be sure to tell a dentist, anesthesiologist or anyone else who intends to give you an anesthetic to put you to sleep.

Hypothermia-Causing Medications—Medicines that can cause a significant lowering of body temperature. These drugs include alcohol, alpha-adrenergic blocking agents (dihydroergotamine, ergotamine, labetalol, phenoxybenzamine, phentolamine, prazosin, tolazoline), barbiturates (large amounts), beta-adrenergic blocking agents, clonidine, insulin, minoxidil, narcotic analgesics (with overdose), phenothiazines, vasodilators.

I

Ichthyosis—Skin disorder with dryness, scaling and roughness.

Ileitis—Inflammation of the ileum, the last section of the small intestine.

Ileostomy—Surgical opening from the ileum, the end of the small intestine, to the outside of the body.

Immunosuppressants—Powerful drugs that suppress the immune system. Immuno-suppressants are used in patients who have had organ transplants or severe disease associated with the immune system. These drugs include the following (some of which are not described in this book): azathioprine, basiliximab, betamethasone, chlorambucil, corticotropin, cortisone, cyclophosphamide, cyclosporine, dacliximab, dexamethasone, hydrocortisone, mercaptopurine, methylprednisolone, muromonab, muromonab-CD3, mycophenolate, prednisolone, prednisone, sirolimus, tacrolimus, thalidomide, triamcinolone, ursodiol.

Impotence—Male's inability to achieve or sustain erection of the penis for sexual intercourse.

Insomnia—Sleeplessness.

Interaction—Change in the body's response to one drug when another is taken. Interaction may decrease the effect of one or both drugs, increase the effect of one or both drugs or cause toxicity.

Iron Supplements—Products that contain iron in a form that can be absorbed from the intestinal tract. Supplements include ferrous fumarate,

ferrous gluconate, ferrous sulfate, iron dextran, iron-polysaccharide.

J

Jaundice—Symptoms of liver damage, bile obstruction or destruction of red blood cells. Symptoms include yellowed whites of the eyes, yellow skin, dark urine and light stool.

K

Keratosis—Growth that is an accumulation of cells from the outer skin layers.

Kidney Stones—Small, solid stones made from calcium, cholesterol, cysteine and other body chemicals.

L

Laxatives—Medicines prescribed to treat constipation. These medicines include bisacodyl; bisacodyl and docusate; casanthranol; casanthranol and docusate; cascara sagrada; cascara sagrada and aloe; cascara sagrada and phenolphthalein; castor oil; danthron; danthron and docusate; danthron and poloxamer 188; dehydrocholic acid; dehydrocholic acid and docusate; docusate; docusate and phenolphthalein; docusate and mineral oil; docusate and phenolphthalein; docusate, carboxymethylcellulose and casanthranol; glycerin; lactulose; magnesium citrate; magnesium hydroxide; magnesium hydroxide and mineral oil; magnesium oxide; magnesium sulfate; malt soup extract; malt soup extract and psyllium; methylcellulose; mineral oil; mineral oil and cascara sagrada; mineral oil and phenolphthalein; mineral oil, glycerin and phenolphthalein; phenolphthalein; poloxamer; polycarbophil; potassium bitartrate and sodium bicarbonate; psyllium; psyllium and senna; psyllium hydrophilic mucilloid; psyllium hydrophilic mucilloid and carboxymethyl-cellulose; psyllium hydrophilic mucilloid and sennosides; psyllium hydrophilic mucilloid and senna; senna; senna and docusate; sennosides; sodium phosphate.

LDH—Abbreviation for lactate dehydrogenase. It is a measurement of cardiac enzymes used to confirm some heart conditions.

Lincomycins—A family of antibiotics used to treat certain infections.

Low-Purine Diet—A diet that avoids high-purine foods, such as liver, sweetbreads, kidneys, sardines, oysters and others. If you need a low-purine diet, request instructions from your doctor.

Lupus—Serious disorder of connective tissue that primarily affects women. Varies in severity with skin eruptions, joint inflammation, low white blood cell count and damage to internal organs, especially the kidneys.

Lymph Glands—Glands in the lymph vessels throughout the body that trap foreign and infectious matter and protect the bloodstream from infection.

M

Macrolides—A class of antibiotic (antibacterial) drugs. They include dirithromycin, erythromycin, lincomycin and vancomycin.

Male Hormones—Chemical substances secreted by the testicles, ovaries and adrenal glands in humans. Some male hormones used by humans are derived synthetically. Male hormones include testosterone cypionate and estradiol cypionate, testosterone enanthate and estradiol valerate.

Mania—A mood disturbance characterized by euphoria, agitation, elation, irritability, rapid and confused speech and excessive activity. Mania usually occurs as part of bipolar (manic-depressive) disorder.

Manic-Depressive Illness—Psychosis with alternating cycles of excessive enthusiasm and depression.

MAO Inhibitors—See Monoamine Oxidase (MAO) Inhibitors.

Mast Cell—Connective tissue cell.

Meglitinides—Drugs that stimulate the pancreas to produce insulin. Used to treat Type II (non-insulin dependent) diabetes. These drugs include repaglinide and nateglinide.

Menopause—The end of menstruation in the female, often accompanied by irritability, hot flashes, changes in the skin and bones and vaginal dryness.

Metabolism—Process of using nutrients and energy to build and break down wastes.

Migraine Headaches—Periodic headaches caused by constriction of arteries to the skull. Symptoms include severe pain, vision disturbances, nausea, vomiting and sensitivity to light.

Mind-Altering Drugs—Any drugs that decrease alertness, perception, concentration, contact with reality or muscular coordination.

Mineral Supplements—Mineral substances added to the diet to treat or prevent mineral deficiencies. They include iron, copper, magnesium, calcium, etc.

Monoamine Oxidase (MAO) Inhibitors—Drugs that prevent the activity of the enzyme monoamine oxidase (MAO) in brain tissue. MAO inhibitors include drugs that treat depression, Parkinson's and other conditions. MAOs can cause dangerous interactions with certain foods, beverages and other drugs. Drugs in this class include furazolidone, isocarboxazid, linezolid, methylene blue, phenelzine, procarbazine, rasagiline, selegiline, St. John's wort (acts similar to MAO inhibitors), tranylcypromine.

Muscle Blockers—Same as muscle relaxants or skeletal muscle relaxants.

Muscle Relaxants—Medicines used to lessen painful contractions and spasms of muscles. These include atracurium, carisoprodol, chlorphenesin, chlorzoxazone, cyclobenzaprine, metaxalone, methocarbamol, metocurine, orphenadrine citrate, orphenadrine hydrochloride, pancuronium, phenytoin, succinylcholine, tubocurarine, vecuronium.

Myasthenia Gravis—Disease of the muscles characterized by fatigue and progressive paralysis. It is usually confined to muscles of the face, lips, tongue and neck.

Mydriatics—Eye drops that cause the pupils to dilate (become larger) to a marked degree.

N

Narcotics—A group of habit-forming, addicting drugs used for treatment of pain, diarrhea, cough, acute pulmonary edema and others. They are all derived from opium, a milky exudate in capsules of papaver somniferum. Law requires licensed physicians to dispense by prescription. These drugs include alfentanil, buprenorphine, butorphanol, codeine, fentanyl, hydrocodone, hydromorphone, levorphanol, meperidine, methadone, morphine, nalbuphine, opium, oxycodone, oxymorphone, paregoric, pentazocine, propoxyphene, sufentanil.

Nephrotoxic (Kidney-Poisoning) Medications—Under some circumstances, these medicines can be toxic to the kidneys. These medicines include acetaminophen (in high doses); acyclovir (injection of); aminoglycosides; amphotericin B (given internally); analgesic combinations containing acetaminophen and aspirin or other salicylates (with chronic high-dose use); anti-inflammatory analgesics (nonsteroidal); bacitracin (injection of); capreomycin; carmustine; chlorpropamide; cidofovir; ciprofloxacin; cisplatin; cox 2 inhibitors; cyclosporine; deferoxamine (long-term use); edetate calcium disodium (with high doses); edetate disodium (with high dose); foscarnet; gold compounds; ifosfamide; imipenem; lithium; methicillin, methotrexate (with high dose therapy); methoxyflurane; nafcillin; neomycin (oral); pamidronate; penicillamine; pentamidine; pentostatin, phenacetin; plicamycin; polymyxins (injection of); radiopaques (materials used for special x-ray examinations); rifampin; streptozocin; sulfonamides; tacrolimus; tetracyclines (except doxycycline and minocycline); tiopronin; tretinoin; vancomycin (injection of).

Neuroleptic Malignant Syndrome—Ceaseless involuntary, jerky movements of the tongue, facial muscles and hands.

Neuromuscular Blocking Agents—A group of drugs prescribed to relax skeletal muscles. They are all given by injection, and descriptions are not included in this book. These drugs include atracurium, edrophonium, gallamine, neostigmine, metocurine, pancuronium, pyridostigmine, succinylcholine, tubocurarine, vecuronium.

Neurotoxic Medications—Medicines that cause toxicity to the nerve tissues in the body. These drugs include alcohol (chronic use), allopurinol; altretamine, amantadine; amiodarone; anticonvulsants (hydantoin), capreomycin, carbamazepine, carboplatin, chloramphenicol (oral), chloroquine, cilastatin, ciprofloxacin, cisplatin, cycloserine, cyclosporine, cytarabine, didanosine, disulfiram, docetaxel, ethambutol, ethionamide, fludarabine, hydroxychloroquine, imipenem, interferon, isoniazid, lincomycins, lindane (topical), lithium, meperidine, methotrexate, metronidazole, mexiletine, nitrofurantoin, oxcarbazepine, paclitaxel, pemoline, pentostatin, pyridoxine (large amounts), quinacrine, quinidine, quinine, stavudine, tacrolimus, tetracyclines, thalidomide, vinblastine, vincristine, vindesine, zalcitabine.

Nitrates—Medicines made from a chemical with a nitrogen base. Nitrates include erythrityl tetranitrate, isosorbide dinitrate, nitroglycerin, pentaerythritol tetranitrate.

Nonsteroidal Anti-Inflammatory Drugs (NSAIDs)—See Anti-Inflammatory Drugs, Nonsteroidal.

Nutritional Supplements—Substances used to treat and prevent deficiencies when the body is unable to absorb them by eating a well-balanced, nutritional diet. These supplements include: Vitamins—ascorbic acid, ascorbic acid and sodium ascorbate, calcifediol, calcitriol, calcium pantothenate, cyanocobalamin, dihydrotachysterol, ergocalciferol, folate sodium, folic acid, hydroxocobalamin, niacin, niacinamide, pantothenic, pyridoxine, riboflavin, sodium ascorbate, thiamine, vitamin A, vitamin E. Minerals—calcium carbonate, calcium citrate, calcium glubionate, calcium gluconate, calcium lactate, calcium phosphate (dibasic and tribasic), sodium fluoride. Other—levocarnitine, omega-3 polyunsaturated fatty acids.

O

Opiates—See Narcotics.

Orthostatic Hypotension—Excess drop in blood pressure when arising from a sitting or lying position.

Osteoporosis—Softening of bones caused by a loss of calcium usually found in bone. Bones become brittle and fracture easily.

Ototoxic Medications—These medicines may possibly cause hearing damage. They include aminoglycosides, 4-aminoquinolines, anti-inflammatory analgesics (nonsteroidal), bumetanide (injected), capreomycin, carboplatin, chloroquine, cisplatin, deferoxamine, erythromycins, ethacrynic acid, furosemide, hydroxychloroquine, quinidine, quinine, salicylates, vancomycin (injected).

Ovary—Female sexual gland where eggs mature and ripen for fertilization.

P

Pain Relievers—Non-narcotic medicines used to treat pain.

Palpitations—Rapid, forceful or throbbing heartbeat noticeable to the patient.

Pancreatitis—Serious inflammation or infection of the pancreas that causes upper abdominal pain.

Pancreatitis-associated Drugs—Medications associated with the development of pancreatitis. These include alcohol, asparaginase, azathioprine, didanosine, estrogens, furosemide, methyldopa, nitrofurantoin, sulfonamides, tetracyclines, thiazide diuretics, valproic acid.

Parkinson's Disease or Parkinson's Syndrome—Disease of the central nervous system. Characteristics are a fixed, emotionless expression of the face, tremor, slower muscle movements, weakness, changed gait and a peculiar posture.

Pellagra—Disease caused by a deficiency of the water-soluble vitamin thiamine (vitamin B-1). Symptoms include brain disturbance, diarrhea and skin inflammation.

Penicillin—Chemical substance (antibiotic) originally discovered as a product of mold, that can kill some bacterial germs.

Peripheral Neuropathy (Peripheral Neuritis)—Inflammation and degeneration of the nerve endings or of the terminal nerves. It most often occurs in the nerve tissue of the muscles of the extremities (arms and legs). Symptoms include pain of varying intensity and sensations of numbness, tingling and burning in the hands and feet. It can be caused by certain medications or chemicals, infections, chronic inflammation or nutritive disease.

Peripheral-neuropathy Associated Drugs—Medications that are associated with the development of peripheral neuropathy. These include chloramphenicol, cisplatin, dapsone, didanosine, ethambutol, ethionamide, hydralazine, isoniazid, lithium, metronidazole, nitrofurantoin, nitrous oxide, phenytoin, stavudine, vincristine, zalcitabine.

Phenothiazines—Drugs used to treat mental, nervous and emotional conditions. These drugs include acetophenazine, chlorpromazine, fluphenazine, mesoridazine, methotrimeprazine, pericyazine, perphenazine, prochlorperazine, promazine, thiopropazate, thioproperazine, thioridazine, trifluoperazine, triflupromazine.

Pheochromocytoma—A tumor of the adrenal gland that produces chemicals that cause high blood pressure, headache, nervousness and other symptoms.

Phlegm—Thick mucus secreted by glands in the respiratory tract.

Photophobia—Increased sensitivity to light as perceived by the human eye. Drugs that can cause photophobia include antidiabetic drugs, atropine, belladonna, bromides, chloroquine, ciprofloxacin, chlordiazepoxide, clidinium, clomiphene, dicyclomine, digitalis drugs, doxepin, ethambutol, ethionamide, ethosuximide, etretinate, glycopyrrolate, hydroxychloroquine, hydroxyzine, hyoscyamine, isopropamide, mephenytoin, methenamine, methsuximide, monoamine oxidase (MAO) inhibitors, nalidixic acid, norfloxacin, oral contraceptives, orphenadrine, paramethadione, phenothiazines, propantheline, quinidine, quinine, scopolamine, tetracyclines, tridihexethyl, trimethadione.

Photosensitizing Medications—Medicines that can cause abnormally heightened skin reactions to the effects of sunlight and ultraviolet light. These medicines include acetazolamide, acetohexamide, alprazolam, amantadine, amiloride, amiodarone, amitriptyline, amoxapine, antidiabetic agents (oral), barbiturates, bendroflumethiazide, benzocaine, benzoyl peroxide, benzthiazide, captopril, carbamazepine, chlordiazepoxide, chloroquine, chlorothiazide, chlorpromazine, chlorpropamide, chlortetracycline, chlorthalidone, ciprofloxacin, clindamycin, clofazimine, clofibrate, clomipramine, coal tar, contraceptives (estrogen-containing), cyproheptadine, dacarbazine, dapsone, demeclocycline, desipramine, desoximetasone, diethylstilbestrol, diflunisal, diltiazem, diphenhydramine, disopyramide, doxepin, doxycycline, enoxacin, estrogens, etretinate, flucytosine, fluorescein, fluorouracil, fluphenazine, flutamide, furosemide, glipizide, glyburide, gold preparations, griseofulvin, haloperidol, hexachlorophene, hydrochlorothiazide, hydroflumethiazide, ibuprofen, imipramine, indomethacin, isotretinoin, ketoprofen, lincomycin, lomefloxacin, maprotiline, mesoridazine, methacycline, methotrexate, methoxsalen, methyclothiazide, methyldopa, metolazone, minocycline, minoxidil, nabumetone, nalidixic acid, naproxen, nifedipine, norfloxacin, nortriptyline, ofloxacin, oral contraceptives, oxyphenbutazone, oxytetracycline, perphenazine, phenelzine, phenobarbital, phenylbutazone, phenytoin, piroxicam, polythiazide, prochlorperazine, promazine, promethazine, protriptyline, pyrazinamide, quinidine, quinine, sulfonamides, sulindac, tetracycline, thiabendazole, thioridazine, thiothixene, tolazamide, tolbutamide, tranylcypromine, trazodone, tretinoin, triamterene, trichlormethiazide, trifluoperazine, triflupromazine, trimeprazine, trimethoprim, trimipramine, triprolidine, vinblastine.

Pinworms—Common intestinal parasites that cause rectal itching and irritation.

Pituitary Gland—Gland at the base of the brain that secretes hormones to stimulate growth and other glands to produce hormones.

Platelet—Disc-shaped element of the blood, smaller than a red or white blood cell, necessary for blood clotting.

Polymyxins—A family of antibiotics that kill bacteria.

Polyp—Growth on a mucous membrane.

Porphyria—Inherited metabolic disorder characterized by changes in the nervous system and kidneys.

Post-Partum—Following delivery of a baby.

Potassium—Important chemical found in body cells.

Potassium Foods—Foods high in potassium content, including dried apricots and peaches, lentils, raisins, citrus and whole-grain cereals.

Potassium Supplements—Medicines needed by people who don't have enough potassium in their diets or by those who develop a deficiency due to illness or taking diuretics and other medicines. These supplements include chloride; potassium acetate; potassium bicarbonate; potassium bicarbonate and potassium chloride; potassium bicarbonate and potassium citrate; potassium chloride; potassium chloride, potassium bicarbonate and potassium citrate; potassium gluconate; potassium gluconate and potassium chloride; potassium gluconate and potassium citrate; potassium gluconate, potassium citrate and ammonium; trikates.

Premenstrual Dysphoric Disorder (PMDD)—A severe form of premenstrual syndrome which is characterized by severe monthly mood swings as well as physical symptoms that interfere with everyday life, especially a woman's relationships with her family and friends.

Progesterone—A female steroid sex hormone that is responsible for preparing the uterus for pregnancy.

Progestin—A synthetic hormone that is designed to mimic the actions of progesterone. These include etonogestrel, hydroxy-progesterone, medroxyprogesterone, megestrol, norethindrone, norgestrel and progesterone.

Prostaglandins—A group of drugs used for a variety of therapeutic purposes. These drugs include alprostadil (treats newborns with congenital heart disease), carboprost and dinoprost (both used to induce labor) and dinoprostone (used to induce labor or to induce a late abortion).

Prostate—Gland in the male that surrounds the neck of the bladder and the urethra.

Protease Inhibitors—A class of anti-HIV drugs which inhibit the protease enzyme and stop virus replication. These drugs include: abacavir, atazanavir, darunavir, fosamprenavir, indinavir, lopinavir and ritonavir; nelfinavir, ritonavir, saquinavir and tipranavir.

Protein Bound Drugs—This protein is not to be confused with the protein in your food. If two highly protein bound drugs are given together, they will compete for protein carriers in the body and may possibly cause one or both of the drugs to be less effective and dosages may need to be adjusted. Some of these drugs are clofibrate, diazepam, diazoxide, fluoxetine, ibuprofen, indomethacin, naproxen, raloxifene, tiagabine.

Prothrombin—Blood substance essential in clotting.

Prothrombin Time (Pro Time)—Laboratory study used to follow prothrombin activity and keep coagulation safe.

Psoriasis—Chronic inherited skin disease. Symptoms are lesions with silvery scales on the edges.

Psychosis—Mental disorder characterized by deranged personality, loss of contact with reality and possible delusions, hallucinations or illusions.

Purine Foods—Foods that are metabolized into uric acid. Foods high in purines include anchovies, liver, brains, sweetbreads, sardines, kidneys, oysters, gravy and meat extracts.

Q

QT Interval Prolongation-Causing Drugs—A group of drugs that can cause serious heart rhythm problems. These drugs include amiodarone, calcium channel blockers (especially bepridil), chlorpromazine, clarithromycin, disopyramide, dofetilide, droperidol, erythromycins, fluoroquinolones, halofantrine, haloperidol, maprotiline, mesoridazine, methadone, pentamidine, phenothiazines, pimozide, quinidine, ranolazine, sotalol, sparfloxacin, thioridazine, tricyclic antidepressants and others.

R

Rauwolfia Alkaloids—Drugs that belong to the family of antihypertensives (drugs that lower blood pressure). Rauwolfia alkaloids are not used as extensively as in years past. They include alseroxylon, deserpidine, rauwolfia serpentina, reserpine.

RDA—Recommended daily allowance of a vitamin or mineral.

Rebound Effect—The worsening or return of symptoms when a drug (such as a decongestant) is discontinued or a patient no longer responds to it.

Renal—Pertaining to the kidney.

Retina—Innermost covering of the eyeball on which the image is formed.

Retinoids—A group of drugs that are synthetic vitamin A-like compounds used to treat skin conditions. These drugs include etretinate, isotretinoin and retinoic acid.

Retroperitoneal Imaging—Special x-rays or CT scans of the organs attached to the abdominal wall behind the peritoneum (the covering of the intestinal tract and lining of the walls of the abdominal and pelvic cavities).

Reye's Syndrome—Rare, sometimes fatal, disease of children that causes brain and liver damage.

Rickets—Bone disease caused by vitamin D deficiency. Bones become bent and distorted during infancy or childhood.

S

Salicylates—Medicines to relieve pain and reduce fever. These include aspirin, aspirin and caffeine, buffered aspirin, choline salicylate, choline and magnesium salicylates, magnesium salicylate, salicylamide, salsalate, sodium salicylate.

Sedatives—Drugs that reduce excitement or anxiety. They are used to produce sedation (calmness). These include alprazolam, amobarbital, aprobarbital, bromazepam, butalbital, chloral hydrate, clonazepam, clorazepate, chlordiazepoxide, diazepam, diphenhydramine, doxylamine, estazolam, ethchlorvynol, ethinamate, eszopiclone, flurazepam, glutethimide, halazepam, hydroxyzine, ketazolam, lorazepam, methotrimeprazine, midazolam, nitrazepam, oxazepam, pentobarbital, phenobarbital, prazepam, promethazine, propiomazine, propofol, quazepam, secobarbital, temazepam, triazolam, trimeprazine, zaleplon, zolpidem, zopiclone.

Seizure—A sudden attack as of epilepsy or some other disease can cause changes of consciousness or convulsions.

Seizure threshold lowering drugs—Seizure threshold refers to the minimal conditions required to trigger a seizure. A number of drugs can lower the seizure threshold in susceptible patients and increase the risk for a seizure. These drugs include certain antibiotics, antiasthmatics, antidepressants, antipsychotics, phenothiazines, psychostimulants, hormones, local anesthetics, immunosuppressants, narcotics and others. Herbal remedies may also lower seizure threshold. Consult your doctor about your risks.

Selective Serotonin Reuptake Inhibitors (SSRIs)—Medications used for treatment of depression that work by increasing the serotonin levels in the brain. Serotonin is a neuro-transmitter (brain chemical) having to do with mood and behavior. These drugs include fluoxetine, fluvoxamine, paroxetine, sertraline. More information can be found on the individual drug chart for each drug.

Serotonergics—Drugs that increase the levels of serotonin (a brain chemical). Excess serotonin can lead to serotonin syndrome (a possibly life-threatening condition). These drugs include almotriptan, amitriptyline, amphetamines, bromocriptine, buspirone, citalopram, clomipramine, desvenlafaxine, dextromethorphan, duloxetine, eletriptan, escitalopram, fenfluramine, fluoxetine, fluvoxamine, frovatriptan, imipramine, levodopa, linezolid, lithium, meperidine, moclobemide, monoamine oxidase (MAO) inhibitors, naratriptan, nefazodone, paroxetine, pentazocine, rizatriptan, sertraline, sibutramine, St. John's Wort, sumatriptan, tramadol, trazodone, tricyclic antidepressants, tryptophan, valproic acid, venlafaxine, zolmitriptan and some drugs of abuse (e.g., cocaine, LSD, ecstasy, marijuana and others). Other drugs or herbal supplements may be risk factors also. Ask your doctor or pharmacist about the safety of any drugs you are prescribed and advised them of any herbal supplements you take.

Serotonin Syndrome—A potentially very serious and life-threatening condition caused by drugs that increase serotonin levels in the brain. The syndrome can be caused by an overdose, interaction with other drugs, or rarely, with doses used in treatment. It is more likely to occur when starting a drug or increasing the dosage of a drug. Symptoms often come on quickly and progress rapidly. Symptoms may include confusion, agitation, headache, diarrhea, irritability, muscle rigidity, high body temperature, fast heart beat, rapid change in blood pressure, nausea or vomiting, poor coordination, dilated pupils, restlessness, hallucinations, overactive reflexes, sweating, shivering, tremor, and muscle twitching. More severe symptoms can include seizures, delirium, shock loss of consciousness and other major medical problems.

SGOT—Abbreviation for serum glutamic-oxaloacetic transaminase. Measuring the level in the blood helps demonstrate liver disorders and diagnose recent heart damage.

SGPT—Abbreviation for a laboratory study measuring the blood level of serum glutamic-pyruvic transaminase. Deviations from a normal level may indicate liver disease.

Sick Sinus Syndrome—A complicated, serious heartbeat rhythm disturbance characterized by a slow heart rate alternating with a fast or slow heart rate with heart block.

Sinusitis—Inflammation or infection of the sinus cavities in the skull.

Skeletal Muscle Relaxants (same as Skeletal Muscle Blockers)—A group of drugs prescribed to treat spasms of the skeletal muscles. These drugs include carisoprodol, chlorphenesin, chlorzoxazone, cyclobenzaprine, diazepam, lorazepam, metaxalone, methocarbamol, orphenadrine, phenytoin.

Sleep Inducers—Night-time sedatives to aid in falling asleep.

Sleep-Related Behaviors—Certain behaviors that can occur with the use of sedative-hypnotic drugs. The behaviors include: cooking and eating, using the telephone, having sex and sleep-driving (driving while not fully awake). Typically, the person has no memory of these actions.

Statins—See HMG-CoA Reductase Inhibitors.

Streptococci—A bacteria that can cause infections in the throat, respiratory system and skin. Improperly treated, can lead to disease in the heart, joints and kidneys.

Stroke—Sudden, severe attack, usually sudden paralysis, from injury to the brain or spinal cord caused by a blood clot or hemorrhage in the brain.

Stupor—Near unconsciousness.

Sublingual—Under the tongue. Some drugs are absorbed almost as quickly this way as by injection.

Sulfa Drugs—Shorthand for sulfonamide drugs, which are used to treat infections.

Sulfonamides—Sulfa drugs prescribed to treat infections. They include sulfacytine, sulfamethoxazole, sulfamethoxazole and trimethoprim, sulfasalazine, sulfisoxazole.

Sulfonylureas—A family of drugs that lower blood sugar (hypoglycemic agents). Used in the treatment of some forms of diabetes.

Sympatholytics—A group of drugs that block the action of the sympathetic nervous system. These drugs include beta-blockers, guanethidine, hydralazine and prazosin.

Sympathomimetics—A large group of drugs that mimic the effects of stimulation of the sympathetic part of the autonomic nervous system. These drugs include albuterol, amphetamine, benzphetamine, bitolterol, cocaine, dextroamphetamine, diethylpropion, dobutamine, ephedrine, epinephrine, ethylnorepinephrine, fenfluramine, ipratropium, isoproterenol, isoetharine, mazindol, mephentermine, metaproterenol, metaraminol, methoxamine, norepinephrine, phendimetrazine, phentermine, phenylephrine, pirbuterol, pseudoephedrine, ritodrine, terbutaline.

T

Tardive Dyskinesia—Slow, involuntary movements of the jaw, lips and tongue caused by an unpredictable drug reaction. Drugs that can cause this include haloperidol, phenothiazines, thiothixene.

Tartrazine Dye—A dye used in foods and medicine preparations that may cause an allergic reaction in some people.

Tetracyclines—A group of medicines with similar chemical structure used to treat infections. These drugs include demeclocycline, doxycycline, methacycline, minocycline, oxytetracycline, tetracycline.

Thiazides—A group of chemicals that cause diuresis (loss of water through the kidneys). Frequently used to treat high blood pressure and congestive heart failure. Thiazides include bendroflumethiazide, benzthiazide, chlorothiazide, chlorthalidone, cyclothiazide, hydrochlorothiazide, hydroflumethiazide, methyclothiazide, metolazone, polythiazide, quinethazone, trichlormethiazide.

Thiothixines—See Thioxanthenes.

Thioxanthenes—Drugs used to treat emotional, mental and nervous conditions. These drugs include chlorprothixene, flupenthixol, thiothixene.

Thrombocytopenias—Diseases characterized by inadequate numbers of blood platelets circulating in the bloodstream.

Thrombolytic Agents—Drugs that help to dissolve blood clots. They include alteplase, anistreplase, streptokinase, urokinase.

Thrombophlebitis—Inflammation of a vein caused by a blood clot in the vein.

Thyroid—Gland in the neck that manufactures and secretes several hormones.

Thyroid Hormones—Medications that mimic the action of the thyroid hormone made in the thyroid gland. They include dextrothyroxine, levothyroxine, liothyronine, liotrix, thyroglobulin, thyroid.

Tic Douloureux—Painful condition caused by inflammation of a nerve in the face.

Tolerance—A decreasing response to repeated constant doses of a drug or a need to increase doses to produce the same physical or mental response.

Toxicity—Poisonous reaction to a drug that impairs body functions or damages cells.

Tranquilizers—Drugs that calm a person without clouding consciousness.

Transdermal Patches—Medicated patches that stick to the skin. There are more and more medications in this form. This method produces a prolonged systemic effect. If you are using this form, follow these instructions: Choose an area of skin without cuts, scars or hair, such as the upper arm, chest or behind the ear. Thoroughly clean area where patch is to be applied. If patch gets wet and loose, cover with an additional piece of plastic. Apply a fresh patch if the first one falls off. Apply each dose to a different area of skin if possible.

Tremor—Involuntary trembling.

Trichomoniasis—Infestation of the vagina by trichomonas, an infectious organism. The infection causes itching, vaginal discharge and irritation.

Triglyceride—Fatty chemical manufactured from carbohydrates for storage in fat cells.

Tyramine—Normal chemical component of the body that helps sustain blood pressure. Can rise to fatal levels in combination with some drugs. Tyramine is found in many foods:

Beverages—Alcohol beverages, especially Chianti or robust red wines, vermouth, ale, beer.

Breads—Homemade bread with a lot of yeast and breads or crackers containing cheese.

Fats—Sour cream.

Fruits—Bananas, red plums, avocados, figs, raisins, raspberries.

Meats and meat substitutes—Aged game, liver (if not fresh), canned meats, salami, sausage, aged cheese, salted dried fish, pickled herring, meat tenderizers.

Vegetables—Italian broad beans, green bean pods, eggplant.

Miscellaneous—Yeast concentrates or extracts, marmite, soup cubes, commercial gravy, soy sauce, any protein food that has been stored improperly or is spoiled.

U

Ulcer, Peptic—Open sore on the mucous membrane of the esophagus, stomach or duodenum caused by stomach acid.

Urethra—Hollow tube through which urine (and semen in men) is discharged.

Urethritis—Inflammation or infection of the urethra.

Uricosurics—A group of drugs that promotes excretion of uric acid in the urine. These drugs include probenecid and sulfinpyrazone.

Urinary Acidifiers—Medications that cause urine to become acid. These include ascorbic acid, potassium phosphate, potassium and sodium phosphates, racemethionine.

Urinary Alkalizers—Medications that cause urine to become alkaline. These include potassium citrate, potassium citrate and citric acid, potassium citrate and sodium citrate, sodium bicarbonate, sodium citrate and citric acid, tricitrate.

Uterus—Also called the womb. A hollow muscular organ in the female in which the embryo develops into a fetus.

V

Valproic Acid Drugs—Anticonvulsant drugs that are used to prevent seizures in epilepsy, and as treatment for migraine and bipolar disorder. They include oral drugs divalproex and valproic acid and the injectable drug valproate.

Vascular—Pertaining to blood vessels.

Vascular Headache Preventatives—Medicines prescribed to prevent the occurrence of or reduce the frequency and severity of vascular headaches such as migraines. These drugs include atenolol; clonidine; ergotamine, belladonna alkaloids and phenobarbital; fenoprofen; flunarizine; ibuprofen; indomethacin; isocarboxazid, lithium; mefenamic acid; methysergide; metoprolol; nadolol; naproxen; phenelzine; pizotyline; propranolol; timolol, tranylcypromine, verapamil.

Vascular Headache Treatment—Medicine prescribed to treat vascular headaches such as migraines. These drugs include butalbital (combined with acetaminophen, aspirin, caffeine or codeine); cyproheptadine; diclofenac; diflunisal; dihydroergotamine; ergotamine; ergotamine and caffeine; ergotamine, caffeine, belladonna alkaloids and pentobarbital; etodolac; fenoprofen; ibuprofen; indomethacin (capsules, oral suspension, rectal); isomethcptene, dichloralphenazone and acetaminophen; ketoprofen; meclofenamate; mefenamic acid; metoclopramide; naproxen; phenobarbital; triptans.

Vasoconstrictor—Any agent that causes a narrowing of the blood vessels.

Vasodilator—Any agent that causes a widening of the blood vessels.

Vertigo—A sensation of motion, usually dizziness or whirling either of oneself or one's surroundings.

Virus—Infectious organism that reproduces in the cells of the infected host. Viruses cause many diseases in humans including the common cold.

X

Xanthines—Substances that stimulate muscle tissue, especially that of the heart. Types of xanthines include aminophylline, caffeine, dyphylline, oxtriphylline, theophylline.

Y

Yeast—A single-cell organism that can cause infections of the mouth, vagina, skin and parts of the gastrointestinal system.

GUIDE TO INDEX

To find a drug name in the index, look it up by the brand name, such as Tylenol, or the generic name, such as acetaminophen (the generic name for Tylenol).

The alphabetical entries in the index appear in three different formats:

1. **Drug generic names or drug family names** (a group of similar generic drugs such as antihistamines). These names appear in all capital letters and are followed by their chart page number. An <u>underlined name</u> in the index indicates that it is the title of a drug chart in the book.

Example: <u>HMG-CoA REDUCTASE INHIBITORS</u> 418

Example: ATORVASTATIN - See HMG-CoA REDUCTASE INHIBITORS 418

2. **Drug brand (or trade) names.** These names appear in ***bold italic***, and are followed by the drug chart name and a page number. (The drug chart name may be a single generic drug name or a drug family name.)

Example: ***Bayer*** - See ASPIRIN 150

Many brand name drugs contain two or more generic ingredients. These brand names will be followed by two or more drug chart names. Refer to all the drug charts listed for complete information on that particular brand name.

Example: ***Allent*** - See
ANTIHISTAMINES 106
PSEUDOEPHEDRINE 700

3. **Therapeutic class names.** These names appear in regular type with capital and lower-case letters. The therapeutic class name is followed by drug chart names that are in that class:

Example: Antifungal - See
ANTIFUNGALS, AZOLES 86
CLOTRIMAZOLE (Oral-Local) 264
GRISEOFULVIN 408
NYSTATIN 618

2/G-DM Cough - See
DEXTROMETHORPHAN 310
GUAIFENESIN 410

4-Way Long Acting Nasal Spray - See
OXYMETAZOLINE (Nasal) 634

<u>5-ALPHA REDUCTASE INHIBITORS</u> 2

5-ASA - See MESALAMINE 536

5-FU - See FLUOROURACIL (Topical) 390

6-MP - See MERCAPTOPURINE 534

8-Hour Bayer Timed Release - See ASPIRIN 150

12 Hour Nostrilla Nasal Decongestant - See
OXYMETAZOLINE (Nasal) 634

217 - See ASPIRIN 150

217 Strong - See ASPIRIN 150

222 - See
CAFFEINE 212
NARCOTIC ANALGESICS & ASPIRIN 588

282 - See
CAFFEINE 212
NARCOTIC ANALGESICS & ASPIRIN 588

292 - See
CAFFEINE 212
NARCOTIC ANALGESICS & ASPIRIN 588

293 - See NARCOTIC ANALGESICS & ASPIRIN 588

642 - See NARCOTIC ANALGESICS 584

692 - See
CAFFEINE 212
NARCOTIC ANALGESICS & ASPIRIN 588

9-1-1 - See ADRENOCORTICOIDS (Topical) 18

A

A-200 Gel - See PEDICULICIDES (Topical) 646

A-200 Shampoo - See PEDICULICIDES (Topical) 646

A/B Otic - See ANTIPYRINE & BENZOCAINE (Otic) 130

ABACAVIR - See NUCLEOSIDE REVERSE TRANSCRIPTASE INHIBITORS 614

Abenol - See ACETAMINOPHEN 8

Abilify - See ARIPIPRAZOLE 148

Abilify DiscMelt - See ARIPIPRAZOLE 148

Abilify Oral Solution - See ARIPIPRAZOLE 148

Abitrate - See FIBRATES 382

Abortifacient - See MIFEPRISTONE 554

Abraxane - See PACLITAXEL 636

Abreva - See ANTIVIRALS (Topical) 144

A.C.&C. - See NARCOTIC ANALGESICS & ASPIRIN 588

Acabamate - See MEPROBAMATE 532

ALFACALCIDOL - See VITAMIN D 842

ALFUZOSIN - See ALPHA ADRENERGIC
RECEPTOR BLOCKERS 20

Algenic Alka - See ANTACIDS 50

Algenic Alka Improved - See ANTACIDS 50

Algicon - See ANTACIDS 50

Alinia - See NITAZOXANIDE 604

ALISKIREN - See RENIN INHIBITORS 722

Alka-Butazolidin - See ANTI-INFLAMMATORY
DRUGS, NONSTEROIDAL (NSAIDs) 116

Alkabutazone - See ANTI-INFLAMMATORY
DRUGS, NONSTEROIDAL (NSAIDs) 116

Alkalizer - See SODIUM BICARBONATE 756

Alka-Mints - See ANTACIDS 50

Alka-Phenylbutazone - See ANTI-
INFLAMMATORY DRUGS,
NONSTEROIDAL (NSAIDs) 116

Alka-Seltzer Gas Relief - See SIMETHICONE
754

Alka-Seltzer Morning Relief - See
ASPIRIN 150
CAFFEINE 212

Alka-Seltzer Original - See
ASPIRIN 150
SODIUM BICARBONATE 756

Alka-Seltzer Plus Cold & Cough Effervescent
- See
ACETAMINOPHEN 8
ANTIHISTAMINES 106
DEXTROMETHORPHAN 310
PHENYLEPHRINE 662

Alka-Seltzer Plus Cold & Cough Liquid - See
ACETAMINOPHEN 8
ANTIHISTAMINES 106
DEXTROMETHORPHAN 310
PHENYLEPHRINE 662

Alka-Seltzer Plus Cold & Cough Liquid-Gels -
See
ACETAMINOPHEN 8
ANTIHISTAMINES 106
DEXTROMETHORPHAN 310
PHENYLEPHRINE 662

Alka-Seltzer Plus Day & Night Effervescent -
See
ACETAMINOPHEN 8
DEXTROMETHORPHAN 310
PHENYLEPHRINE 662

Alka-Seltzer Plus Day & Night Liquid Gels -
See
ACETAMINOPHEN 8
DEXTROMETHORPHAN 310
PHENYLEPHRINE 662

Alka-Seltzer Plus Day Cold Liquid - See
ACETAMINOPHEN 8
DEXTROMETHORPHAN 310

PHENYLEPHRINE 662

Alka-Seltzer Plus Flu Effervescent - See
ANTIHISTAMINES 106
ASPIRIN 150
DEXTROMETHORPHAN 310

Alka-Seltzer Plus Night Cold Liquid - See
ACETAMINOPHEN 8
ANTIHISTAMINES 106
DEXTROMETHORPHAN 310
PHENYLEPHRINE 662

Alka-Seltzer Plus Night-Time Effervescent -
See
ACETAMINOPHEN 8
ANTIHISTAMINES 106
DEXTROMETHORPHAN 310
PHENYLEPHRINE 662

Alka-Seltzer Plus Night-Time Liquid-Gels - See
ACETAMINOPHEN 8
ANTIHISTAMINES 106
DEXTROMETHORPHAN 310

Alka-Seltzer Plus Original Effervescent - See
ACETAMINOPHEN 8
ANTIHISTAMINES 106
PHENYLEPHRINE 662

Alka-Seltzer PM - See
ANTIHISTAMINES 106
ASPIRIN 150

Alkeran - See MELPHALAN 528

Alkets - See ANTACIDS 50

Alkets Extra Strength - See ANTACIDS 50

Allay - See NARCOTIC ANALGESICS &
ACETAMINOPHEN 586

Allegra - See ANTIHISTAMINES,
NONSEDATING 110

Allegra-D - See
ANTIHISTAMINES, NONSEDATING 110
PSEUDOEPHEDRINE 700

Allegra-D 24 Hour - See
ANTIHISTAMINES, NONSEDATING 110
PSEUDOEPHEDRINE 700

Allegra ODT - See ANTIHISTAMINES, NON-
SEDATING 110

Allegra Oral Suspension - See
ANTIHISTAMINES, NONSEDATING 110

Allent - See
ANTIHISTAMINES 106
PSEUDOEPHEDRINE 700

Alleract - See ANTIHISTAMINES 106

Aller-Chlor - See ANTIHISTAMINES 106

Allercon - See
ANTIHISTAMINES 106
PSEUDOEPHEDRINE 700

Allercort - See ADRENOCORTICOIDS
(Topical) 18

Allerdryl - See ANTIHISTAMINES 106

Alupent - See BRONCHODILATORS,
   ADRENERGIC 198
Alurate - See BARBITURATES 166
Alu-Tab - See ANTACIDS 50
Alvesco Inhalation - See
   ADRENOCORTICOIDS (Oral Inhalation) 14
AMANTADINE - See ANTIVIRALS FOR
   INFLUENZA 138
Amandron - See ANTIANDROGENS,
   NONSTEROIDAL 60
Amaphen - See
   ACETAMINOPHEN 8
   BARBITURATES 166
   CAFFEINE 212
Amaryl - See SULFONYLUREAS 776
Ambay Cough - See
   ANTIHISTAMINES 106
   NARCOTIC ANALGESICS 584
AMBENONIUM - See ANTIMYASTHENICS 128
Ambenyl Cough - See
   ANTIHISTAMINES 106
   NARCOTIC ANALGESICS 584
Ambenyl-D Decongestant Cough Formula -
   See
   DEXTROMETHORPHAN 310
   GUAIFENESIN 410
   PSEUDOEPHEDRINE 700
Ambien - See ZOLPIDEM 860
Ambien CR - See ZOLPIDEM 860
Ambophen Expectorant - See
   ANTIHISTAMINES 106
   NARCOTIC ANALGESICS 584
AMBRISENTAN - See ENDOTHELIN
   RECEPTOR ANTAGONISTS 350
AMCINONIDE (Topical) - See
   ADRENOCORTICOIDS (Topical) 18
Amdry-D - See
   ANTICHOLINERGICS 72
   PSEUDOEPHEDRINE 700
Amen - See PROGESTINS 686
Amerge - See TRIPTANS 824
Americaine - See ANESTHETICS (Topical) 42
Americaine Hemorrhoidal - See
   ANESTHETICS (Rectal) 40
**Americaine Topical Anesthetic First Aid
   Ointment** - See ANESTHETICS (Topical) 42
Americaine Topical Anesthetic Spray - See
   ANESTHETICS (Topical) 42
Amersol - See ANTI-INFLAMMATORY DRUGS,
   NONSTEROIDAL (NSAIDs) 116
Amethopterin - See METHOTREXATE 542
Amevive - See BIOLOGICS FOR PSORIASIS 186
Amicar - See ANTIFIBRINOLYTIC AGENTS 84
Amidrine - See ISOMETHEPTENE,
   DICHLORALPHENAZONE &

ACETAMINOPHEN 454
Amigesic - See SALICYLATES 742
AMILORIDE - See DIURETICS, POTASSIUM-
   SPARING 332
AMILORIDE & HYDROCHLOROTHIAZIDE - See
   DIURETICS, POTASSIUM-SPARING &
   HYDROCHLOROTHIAZIDE 334
AMINOCAPROIC ACID - See
   ANTIFIBRINOLYTIC AGENTS 84
Aminofen - See ACETAMINOPHEN 8
Aminofen Max - See ACETAMINOPHEN 8
AMINOGLUTETHIMIDE 24
Aminophyllin - See BRONCHODILATORS,
   XANTHINE 200
AMINOPHYLLINE - See BRONCHODILATORS,
   XANTHINE 200
AMIODARONE 26
Ami Rax - See
   BRONCHODILATORS, XANTHINE 200
   EPHEDRINE 352
   HYDROXYZINE 430
Amitiza - See LUBIPROSTONE 508
Amitone - See ANTACIDS 50
AMITRIPTYLINE - See ANTIDEPRESSANTS,
   TRICYCLIC 80
AMLEXANOX 28
AMLODIPINE - See CALCIUM CHANNEL
   BLOCKERS 216
Amnesteem - See ISOTRETINOIN 458
AMOBARBITAL - See BARBITURATES 166
Amogel PG - See KAOLIN, PECTIN,
   BELLADONNA & OPIUM 466
Amonidrin - See GUAIFENESIN 410
AMOXAPINE - See ANTIDEPRESSANTS,
   TRICYCLIC 80
AMOXICILLIN - See PENICILLINS 650
AMOXICILLIN & CLAVULANATE - See
   PENICILLINS & BETA-LACTAMASE
   INHIBITORS 652
Amoxil - See PENICILLINS 650
AMPHETAMINE & DEXTROAMPHETAMINE -
   See AMPHETAMINES 30
AMPHETAMINES 30
Amphojel - See ANTACIDS 50
Amphojel 500 - See ANTACIDS 50
Amphojel Plus - See ANTACIDS 50
AMPHOTERICIN B - See ANTIFUNGALS
   (Topical) 88
AMPICILLIN - See PENICILLINS 650
Amrix - See CYCLOBENZAPRINE 286
Amyotrophic lateral sclerosis therapy agent -
   See RILUZOLE 738
Amylinomimetic - See PRAMLINTIDE 672
Amytal - See BARBITURATES 166
Anabolin - See ANDROGENS 36

INDEX

INDEX

969

INDEX

INDEX

973

ARFORMOTEROL - See BRONCHODILATORS, ADRENERGIC 198

Aricept - See CHOLINESTERASE INHIBITORS 250

Aricept ODT - See CHOLINESTERASE INHIBITORS 250

ARIPIPRAZOLE 148

Aristocort - See ADRENOCORTICOIDS (Systemic) 16 ADRENOCORTICOIDS (Topical) 18

Aristocort A - See ADRENOCORTICOIDS (Topical) 18

Aristocort C - See ADRENOCORTICOIDS (Topical) 18

Aristocort D - See ADRENOCORTICOIDS (Topical) 18

Aristocort R - See ADRENOCORTICOIDS (Topical) 18

Arm & Hammer Pure Baking Soda - See SODIUM BICARBONATE 756

Arm-a-Med Metaproterenol - See BRONCHODILATORS, ADRENERGIC 198

ARMODAFINIL - See STIMULANTS, AMPHETAMINE-RELATED 762

Armour Thyroid - See THYROID HORMONES 796

Aromatic Cascara Fluidextract - See LAXATIVES, STIMULANT 480

Artane - See ANTIDYSKINETICS 82

Artane Sequels - See ANTIDYSKINETICS 82

ArthriCare - See CAPSAICIN 222

Arthrinol - See ASPIRIN 150

Arthrisin - See ASPIRIN 150

Arthritis Pain Formula - See ASPIRIN 150

Arthropan - See SALICYLATES 742

Arthrotec - See ANTI-INFLAMMATORY DRUGS, NONSTEROIDAL (NSAIDs) 116 MISOPROSTOL 564

ARTH-RX - See CAPSAICIN 222

Artificial tears - See PROTECTANT (Ophthalmic) 696

Artificial Tears - See PROTECTANT (Ophthalmic) 696

Artria S.R. - See ASPIRIN 150

A.S.A. - See ASPIRIN 150

A.S.A. Enseals - See ASPIRIN 150

Asacol - See MESALAMINE 536

Asbron G - See BRONCHODILATORS, XANTHINE 200 GUAIFENESIN 410

Asbron G Inlay Tablets - See BRONCHODILATORS, XANTHINE 200 GUAIFENESIN 410

Ascomp with Codeine No. 3 - See BARBITURATES, ASPIRIN & CODEINE (Also contains caffeine) 168

Ascorbicap - See VITAMIN C (Ascorbic Acid) 840

Ascriptin - See ASPIRIN 150

Ascriptin A/D - See ASPIRIN 150

Asendin - See ANTIDEPRESSANTS, TRICYCLIC 80

Asmalix - See BRONCHODILATORS, XANTHINE 200

Asmanex - See ADRENOCORTICOIDS (Nasal Inhalation) 12

A-Spas - See DICYCLOMINE 314

Aspergum - See ASPIRIN 150

ASPIRIN 150

ASPIRIN & CODEINE - See NARCOTIC ANALGESICS & ASPIRIN 588

Aspirin Free Anacin Maximum Strength Caplets - See ACETAMINOPHEN 8

Aspirin Free Anacin Maximum Strength Tablets - See ACETAMINOPHEN 8

Aspirin Free Bayer Select Maximum Strength Headache Pain Relief Caplets - See CAFFEINE 212

Aspirin Free Bayer Select Maximum Strength Headache Plus Caplets - See ACETAMINOPHEN 8

Aspirin-Free Excedrin Caplets - See ACETAMINOPHEN 8 CAFFEINE 212

Astelin - See ANTIHISTAMINES (Nasal) 108

Astepro - See ANTIHISTAMINES (Nasal) 108

AsthmaHaler - See BRONCHODILATORS, ADRENERGIC 198

AsthmaNefrin - See BRONCHODILATORS, ADRENERGIC 198

Astramorph - See NARCOTIC ANALGESICS 584

Astramorph-PF - See NARCOTIC ANALGESICS 584

Astrin - See ASPIRIN 150

Atabrine - See QUINACRINE 708

Atacand - See ANGIOTENSIN II RECEPTOR ANTAGONISTS 44

Atapryl - See MONOAMINE OXIDASE TYPE B (MAO-B) INHIBITORS 572

Atarax - See HYDROXYZINE 430

Atasol Caplets - See ACETAMINOPHEN 8

Atasol Drops - See ACETAMINOPHEN 8

Atasol Forte - See ACETAMINOPHEN 8

Atasol Forte Caplets - See ACETAMINOPHEN 8

Atasol Forte Tablets - See ACETAMINOPHEN 8

Atasol Oral Solution - See ACETAMINOPHEN 8

Atasol Tablets - See ACETAMINOPHEN 8

INDEX

Avirax - See ANTIVIRALS FOR HERPES VIRUS 136

Avita - See RETINOIDS (Topical) 728

Avlosulfon - See DAPSONE 302

Avodart - See 5-ALPHA REDUCTASE INHIBITORS 2

Axert - See TRIPTANS 824

Axid - See HISTAMINE H$_2$ RECEPTOR ANTAGONISTS 416

Axotal - See
ASPIRIN 150
BARBITURATES 166

Axsain - See CAPSAICIN 222

Aygestin - See PROGESTINS 686

Azaline - See SULFASALAZINE 768

Azasan - See AZATHIOPRINE 160

AzaSite - See ANTIBACTERIALS (Ophthalmic) 66

AZATADINE - See ANTIHISTAMINES 106

AZATHIOPRINE 160

Azdone - See NARCOTIC ANALGESICS & ASPIRIN 588

AZELAIC ACID 162

AZELASTINE - See ANTIHISTAMINES (Nasal) 108

AZELASTINE (Ophthalmic) - See ANTI-ALLERGIC AGENTS (Ophthalmic) 58

Azelex - See AZELAIC ACID 162

Azilect - See MONOAMINE OXIDASE TYPE B (MAO-B) INHIBITORS 572

AZITHROMYCIN - See MACROLIDE ANTIBIOTICS 510

AZITHROMYCIN (Ophthalmic) - See ANTIBACTERIALS (Ophthalmic) 66

Azmacort - See ADRENOCORTICOIDS (Oral Inhalation) 14

Azo Gantanol - See SULFONAMIDES & PHENAZOPYRIDINE 774

Azo-Cheragan - See PHENAZOPYRIDINE 658

Azo-Gantrisin - See
PHENAZOPYRIDINE 658
SULFONAMIDES & PHENAZOPYRIDINE 774

Azopt - See ANTIGLAUCOMA, CARBONIC ANHYDRASE INHIBITORS 98

Azor - See
ANGIOTENSIN II RECEPTOR ANTAGONISTS 44
CALCIUM CHANNEL BLOCKERS 216

Azo-Standard - See PHENAZOPYRIDINE 658

Azo-Sulfamethoxazole - See SULFONAMIDES & PHENAZOPYRIDINE 774

Azo-Sulfisoxazol - See SULFONAMIDES & PHENAZOPYRIDINE 774

Azo-Truxazole - See SULFONAMIDES & PHENAZOPYRIDINE 774

AZT - See NUCLEOSIDE REVERSE TRANSCRIPTASE INHIBITORS 614

Azulfidine - See SULFASALAZINE 768

Azulfidine En-Tabs - See SULFASALAZINE 768

B

Baby Anbesol - See ANESTHETICS (Mucosal-Local) 38

Baby Orabase - See ANESTHETICS (Mucosal-Local) 38

Baby Oragel - See ANESTHETICS (Mucosal-Local) 38

Baby Oragel Nighttime Formula - See ANESTHETICS (Mucosal-Local) 38

B-A-C with Codeine - See BARBITURATES, ASPIRIN & CODEINE (Also contains caffeine) 168

BACAMPICILLIN - See PENICILLINS 650

BACLOFEN 164

Bactine - See ADRENOCORTICOIDS (Topical) 18

Bactine First Aid - See ANTIBACTERIALS (Topical) 70

Bactocill - See PENICILLINS 650

Bactrim - See
SULFONAMIDES 772
TRIMETHOPRIM 822

Bactrim DS - See
SULFONAMIDES 772
TRIMETHOPRIM 822

Bactroban - See ANTIBACTERIALS (Topical) 70

Bactroban Nasal - See ANTIBACTERIALS (Topical) 70

Balacet 325 - See NARCOTIC ANALGESICS & ACETAMINOPHEN 586

Baldex - See ANTI-INFLAMMATORY DRUGS, STEROIDAL (Ophthalmic) 122

Balminil Decongestant - See PSEUDOEPHEDRINE 700

Balminil DM - See DEXTROMETHORPHAN 310

Balminil Expectorant - See GUAIFENESIN 410

Balnetar - See COAL TAR (Topical) 268

Balnetar Therapeutic Tar Bath - See COAL TAR (Topical) 268

Bancap - See
ACETAMINOPHEN 8
BARBITURATES 166

Bancap-HC - See NARCOTIC ANALGESICS & ACETAMINOPHEN 586

Banesin - See ACETAMINOPHEN 8

Banflex - See ORPHENADRINE 628

Banophen - See ANTIHISTAMINES 106

Banophen Caplets - See ANTIHISTAMINES 106

Banthine - See ANTICHOLINERGICS 72

Barbidonna - See
  BELLADONNA ALKALOIDS &
    BARBITURATES 172
  HYOSCYAMINE 432
  SCOPOLAMINE (Hyoscine) 744
Barbidonna 2 - See
  BELLADONNA ALKALOIDS &
    BARBITURATES 172
  HYOSCYAMINE 432
  SCOPOLAMINE (Hyoscine) 744
Barbita - See BARBITURATES 166
Barbiturate - See
  BARBITURATES 166
  BARBITURATES, ASPIRIN & CODEINE (Also
    contains caffeine) 168
BARBITURATES 166
BARBITURATES, ASPIRIN & CODEINE (Also
  contains caffeine) 168
Barc - See PEDICULICIDES (Topical) 646
Baridium - See PHENAZOPYRIDINE 658
Barophen - See BELLADONNA ALKALOIDS &
  BARBITURATES 172
Barr - See NALTREXONE 582
Barriere-HC - See ADRENOCORTICOIDS
  (Topical) 18
Basaljel - See ANTACIDS 50
Bayer - See ASPIRIN 150
Bayer Extra Strength Aspirin - See ASPIRIN 150
*Bayer Select Maximum Strength Pain Relief
  Formula* - See ACETAMINOPHEN 8
Bayer Timed-Release Arthritic Pain Formula -
  See ASPIRIN 150
Bayer Women's Caplets, Aspirin Plus Calcium
  See
  ASPIRIN 150
  CALCIUM SUPPLEMENTS 218
Baytussin AC - See
  GUAIFENESIN 410
  NARCOTIC ANALGESICS 584
Baytussin DM - See
  DEXTROMETHORPHAN 310
  GUAIFENESIN 410
Beben - See ADRENOCORTICOIDS (Topical) 18
BECAPLERMIN 170
Because - See CONTRACEPTIVES,
  VAGINAL 280
Beclodisk - See ADRENOCORTICOIDS (Oral
  Inhalation) 14
Becloforte - See ADRENOCORTICOIDS (Oral
  Inhalation) 14
BECLOMETHASONE (Nasal) - See
  ADRENOCORTICOIDS (Nasal Inhalation) 12
BECLOMETHASONE (Oral Inhalation) - See
  ADRENOCORTICOIDS (Oral Inhalation) 14

BECLOMETHASONE (Topical) - See
  ADRENOCORTICOIDS (Topical) 18
Beconase - See ADRENOCORTICOIDS (Nasal
  Inhalation) 12
Beconase AQ - See ADRENOCORTICOIDS
  (Nasal Inhalation) 12
Bedoz - See VITAMIN B-12 (Cyanocobalamin)
  838
Beepen-VK - See PENICILLINS 650
Beesix - See PYRIDOXINE (Vitamin B-6) 704
Beldin - See ANTIHISTAMINES 106
Belix - See ANTIHISTAMINES 106
Belladenal - See
  BELLADONNA ALKALOIDS &
    BARBITURATES 172
  HYOSCYAMINE 432
Belladenal Spacetabs - See BELLADONNA
  ALKALOIDS & BARBITURATES 172
Belladenal-S - See BELLADONNA ALKALOIDS
  & BARBITURATES 172
BELLADONNA & AMOBARBITAL - See
  BELLADONNA ALKALOIDS &
    BARBITURATES 172
BELLADONNA & BUTABARBITAL - See
  BELLADONNA ALKALOIDS &
    BARBITURATES 172
BELLADONNA & PHENOBARBITAL - See
  BELLADONNA ALKALOIDS &
    BARBITURATES 172
BELLADONNA ALKALOIDS & BARBITURATES
  172
Bellalphen - See BELLADONNA ALKALOIDS &
  BARBITURATES 172
Bell/ans - See SODIUM BICARBONATE 756
Bena-D 10 - See ANTIHISTAMINES 106
Bena-D 50 - See ANTIHISTAMINES 106
Benadryl Allergy & Cold Caplet - See
  ACETAMINOPHEN 8
  ANTIHISTAMINES 106
  PHENYLEPHRINE 662
Benadryl Allergy & Sinus Headache Gelcap -
  See
  ACETAMINOPHEN 8
  ANTIHISTAMINES 106
  PSEUDOEPHEDRINE 700
Benadryl Allergy Dye-Free Liqui-gel - See
  ANTIHISTAMINES 106
Benadryl Allergy Kapseals - See
  ANTIHISTAMINES 106
Benadryl Allergy Quick Dissolve Strips - See
  ANTIHISTAMINES 106
Benadryl Allergy Ultratab Tablets - See
  ANTIHISTAMINES 106

INDEX

INDEX

BETAMETHASONE (Ophthalmic) - See
    ANTI-INFLAMMATORY DRUGS,
    STEROIDAL (Ophthalmic) 122
BETAMETHASONE (Otic) - See ANTI-
    INFLAMMATORY DRUGS, STEROIDAL
    (Otic) 124
BETAMETHASONE (Topical) - See
    ADRENOCORTICOIDS (Topical) 18
Betapace - See BETA-ADRENERGIC
    BLOCKING AGENTS 180
Betapen-VK - See PENICILLINS 650
Beta-Tim - See ANTIGLAUCOMA,
    BETA BLOCKERS 96
Betatrex - See ADRENOCORTICOIDS (Topical)
    18
Beta-Val - See ADRENOCORTICOIDS (Topical)
    18
Betaxin - See THIAMINE (Vitamin B-1) 788
BETAXOLOL - See BETA-ADRENERGIC
    BLOCKING AGENTS 180
BETAXOLOL & CHLORTHALIDONE - See
    BETA-ADRENERGIC BLOCKING AGENTS
    & THIAZIDE DIURETICS 182
BETAXOLOL (Ophthalmic) - See
    ANTIGLAUCOMA, BETA BLOCKERS 96
Betaxon - See BETA-ADRENERGIC
    BLOCKING AGENTS 180
BETHANECHOL 184
Bethaprim - See TRIMETHOPRIM 822
Betimol - See ANTIGLAUCOMA, BETA
    BLOCKERS 96
Betnelan - See ADRENOCORTICOIDS
    (Systemic) 16
Betnesol - See
    ADRENOCORTICOIDS (Systemic) 16
    ANTI-INFLAMMATORY DRUGS, STEROIDAL
    (Ophthalmic) 122
    ANTI-INFLAMMATORY DRUGS, STEROIDAL
    (Otic) 124
Betnovate - See ADRENOCORTICOIDS
    (Topical) 18
Betnovate 1/2 - See ADRENOCORTICOIDS
    (Topical) 18
Betoptic - See ANTIGLAUCOMA, BETA
    BLOCKERS 96
Betoptic S - See ANTIGLAUCOMA,
    BETA BLOCKERS 96
Bewon - See THIAMINE (Vitamin B-1) 788
BEXAROTENE - See RETINOIDS (Topical) 728
Biamine - See THIAMINE (Vitamin B-1) 788
Biaxin - See MACROLIDE ANTIBIOTICS 510
BICALUTAMIDE - See ANTIANDROGENS,
    NONSTEROIDAL 60
Bicitra - See CITRATES 254

BiDil - See
    HYDRALAZINE 420
    NITRATES 606
Bilagog - See LAXATIVES, OSMOTIC 476
Bilax - See
    LAXATIVES, SOFTENER/LUBRICANT 478
    LAXATIVES, STIMULANT 480
BIMATOPROST - See ANTIGLAUCOMA,
    PROSTAGLANDINS 102
BioCal - See CALCIUM SUPPLEMENTS 218
Biologic response modifier- See
    ANAKINRA 34
    TUMOR NECROSIS FACTOR BLOCKERS
    826
BIOLOGICS FOR PSORIASIS 186
Bion Tears - See PROTECTANT (Ophthalmic)
    696
Bio-Syn - See ADRENOCORTICOIDS (Topical)
    18
BIPERIDEN - See ANTIDYSKINETICS 82
Bisac-Evac - See LAXATIVES, STIMULANT
    480
BISACODYL - See LAXATIVES, STIMULANT
    480
Bisacolax - See LAXATIVES, STIMULANT 480
Bisco-Lax - See LAXATIVES, STIMULANT 480
BISKALCITRATE - See BISMUTH SALTS 188
Bismatrol - See BISMUTH SALTS 188
BISMUTH SALTS 188
BISMUTH SUBSALICYLATE - See BISMUTH
    SALTS 188
BISOPROLOL - See BETA-ADRENERGIC
    BLOCKING AGENTS 180
BISOPROLOL & HYDROCHLOROTHIAZIDE -
    See BETA-ADRENERGIC BLOCKING
    AGENTS & THIAZIDE DIURETICS 182
BISPHOSPHONATES 190
BITOLTEROL - See BRONCHODILATORS,
    ADRENERGIC 198
Black Draught - See LAXATIVES, STIMULANT
    480
Black-Draught Lax-Senna - See LAXATIVES,
    STIMULANT 480
Blanex - See ORPHENADRINE 628
Bleph-10 - See ANTIBACTERIALS (Ophthalmic)
    66
Blocadren - See BETA-ADRENERGIC
    BLOCKING AGENTS 180
Blue - See PEDICULICIDES (Topical) 646
Bonamine - See ANTIHISTAMINES,
    PIPERAZINE (Antinausea) 114
BONE FORMATION AGENTS 192
Bonine - See ANTIHISTAMINES,
    PIPERAZINE (Antinausea) 114
Boniva - See BISPHOSPHONATES 190

INDEX

CAPTOPRIL & HYDROCHLOROTHIAZIDE -
See ANGIOTENSIN-CONVERTING
ENZYME (ACE) INHIBITORS &
HYDROCHLOROTHIAZIDE 48

Carafate - See SUCRALFATE 764

CARBACHOL - See ANTIGLAUCOMA,
CHOLINERGIC AGONISTS 100

Carbacot - See MUSCLE RELAXANTS,
SKELETAL 576

CARBAMAZEPINE 224

Carbastat - See ANTIGLAUCOMA,
CHOLINERGIC AGONISTS 100

Carbatrol - See CARBAMAZEPINE 224

CARBENICILLIN - See PENICILLINS 650

Carbex - See MONOAMINE OXIDASE
TYPE B (MAO-B) INHIBITORS 572

CARBIDOPA & LEVODOPA 226

CARBINOXAMINE - See ANTIHISTAMINES 106

Carbodec - See
ANTIHISTAMINES 106
PSEUDOEPHEDRINE 700

Carbodec DM Drops - See
ANTIHISTAMINES 106
DEXTROMETHORPHAN 310
PSEUDOEPHEDRINE 700

Carbodec TR - See
ANTIHISTAMINES 106
PSEUDOEPHEDRINE 700

Carbolith - See LITHIUM 500

Carbonic anhydrase inhibitor - See CARBONIC
ANHYDRASE INHIBITORS 228

CARBONIC ANHYDRASE INHIBITORS 228

CARBONYL IRON - See IRON SUPPLEMENTS
452

Carboptic - See ANTIGLAUCOMA,
CHOLINERGIC AGONISTS 100

CARBOXYMETHYLCELLULOSE SODIUM - See
LAXATIVES, BULK-FORMING 474

Cardene - See CALCIUM CHANNEL
BLOCKERS 216

Cardene SR - See CALCIUM CHANNEL
BLOCKERS 216

Cardilate1 - See NITRATES 606

Cardioquin - See QUINIDINE 710

Cardizem - See CALCIUM CHANNEL
BLOCKERS 216

Cardizem CD - See CALCIUM CHANNEL
BLOCKERS 216

Cardizem LA - See CALCIUM CHANNEL
BLOCKERS 216

Cardizem SR - See CALCIUM CHANNEL
BLOCKERS 216

Cardura - See ALPHA ADRENERGIC
RECEPTOR BLOCKERS 20

Cardura XL- See ALPHA ADRENERGIC
RECEPTOR BLOCKERS 20

CARISOPRODOL - See MUSCLE RELAXANTS,
SKELETAL 576

Cari-Tab - See VITAMINS & FLUORIDE 850

Carmol-HC - See ADRENOCORTICOIDS
(Topical) 18

Carnitor - See LEVOCARNITINE 492

Carnitor Sugar-free Oral Solution - See
LEVOCARNITINE 492

Caroid Laxative - See LAXATIVES,
STIMULANT 480

CARTEOLOL - See BETA-ADRENERGIC
BLOCKING AGENTS 180

CARTEOLOL (Ophthalmic) - See
ANTIGLAUCOMA, BETA BLOCKERS 96

Carter's Little Pills - See LAXATIVES,
STIMULANT 480

Cartia XT - See CALCIUM CHANNEL
BLOCKERS 216

Cartrol - See BETA-ADRENERGIC BLOCKING
AGENTS 180

CARVEDILOL - See BETA-ADRENERGIC
BLOCKING AGENTS 180

CASANTHRANOL - See LAXATIVES,
STIMULANT 480

CASANTHRANOL & DOCUSATE - See
LAXATIVES, SOFTENER/LUBRICANT 478

CASCARA - See LAXATIVES, STIMULANT 480

Cascara Aromatic Fluidextract - See
LAXATIVES, STIMULANT 480

Cascara Sagrada - See LAXATIVES,
STIMULANT 480

Casodex - See ANTIANDROGENS,
NONSTEROIDAL 60

CASTOR OIL - See LAXATIVES, STIMULANT
480

Cataflam - See ANTI-INFLAMMATORY DRUGS,
NONSTEROIDAL (NSAIDs) 116

Catapres - See CENTRAL ALPHA AGONISTS
232

Catapres-TTS - See CENTRAL ALPHA
AGONISTS 232

Caverject - See ALPROSTADIL 22

CCNU - See LOMUSTINE 502

Ceclor - See CEPHALOSPORINS 234

Ceclor CD - See CEPHALOSPORINS 234

Cecon - See VITAMIN C (Ascorbic Acid) 840

Cedax - See CEPHALOSPORINS 234

Cedocard-SR - See NITRATES 606

CeeNU - See LOMUSTINE 502

CEFACLOR - See CEPHALOSPORINS 234

CEFADROXIL - See CEPHALOSPORINS 234

Cefanex - See CEPHALOSPORINS 234

CEFDINIR - See CEPHALOSPORINS 234

INDEX

CIPROFLOXACIN & DEXAMETHASONE - See
  ANTIBACTERIALS (Otic) 68
CIPROFLOXACIN & HYDROCORTISONE
  (Otic) - See ANTIBACTERIALS (Otic) 68
CITALOPRAM - See SELECTIVE SEROTONIN
  REUPTAKE INHIBITORS (SSRIs) 746
Citra Forte - See
  ANTIHISTAMINES 106
  CITRATES 254
  NARCOTIC ANALGESICS 584
  PHENYLEPHRINE 662
  SALICYLATES 742
Citracal - See CALCIUM SUPPLEMENTS 218
Citracal Liquitabs - See CALCIUM
  SUPPLEMENTS 218
Citrated Caffeine - See CAFFEINE 212
CITRATES 254
Citrocarbonate - See SODIUM BICARBONATE
  756
Citrocovorin Calcium - See LEUCOVORIN 484
Citrolith - See CITRATES 254
Citroma - See LAXATIVES, OSMOTIC 476
Citro-Mag - See LAXATIVES, OSMOTIC 476
Citro-Nesia - See LAXATIVES, OSMOTIC 476
Citrovorum Factor - See LEUCOVORIN 484
Citrucel Orange Flavor - See LAXATIVES,
  BULK-FORMING 474
Citrucel Sugar-Free Orange Flavor - See
  LAXATIVES, BULK-FORMING 474
Claravis - See ISOTRETINOIN 458
Clarinex - See ANTIHISTAMINES,
  NONSEDATING 110
Clarinex-D 12 Hour - See
  ANTIHISTAMINES, NONSEDATING 110
  PSEUDOEPHEDRINE 700
Clarinex-D 24 Hour - See
  ANTIHISTAMINES, NONSEDATING 110
  PSEUDOEPHEDRINE 700
Clarinex RediTabs - See ANTIHISTAMINES,
  NONSEDATING 110
Clarinex Syrup - See ANTIHISTAMINES,
  NONSEDATING 110
Claripex - See FIBRATES 382
CLARITHROMYCIN - See MACROLIDE
  ANTIBIOTICS 510
Claritin - See ANTIHISTAMINES,
  NONSEDATING 110
Claritin-D - See
  ANTIHISTAMINES, NONSEDATING 110
  PSEUDOEPHEDRINE 700
Claritin-D 12 Hour - See
  ANTIHISTAMINES, NONSEDATING 110
  PSEUDOEPHEDRINE 700
Claritin-D 24 Hour - See
  ANTIHISTAMINES, NONSEDATING 110

PSEUDOEPHEDRINE 700
Claritin Extra- See ANTIHISTAMINES,
  NONSEDATING 110
Claritin Hives Relief - See ANTIHISTAMINES,
  NONSEDATING 110
Claritin Liqui-Gels - See ANTIHISTAMINES,
  NONSEDATING 110
Claritin RediTabs - See ANTIHISTAMINES,
  NONSEDATING 110
Claritin Syrup - See ANTIHISTAMINES,
  NONSEDATING 110
Clavulin - See PENICILLINS & BETA-
  LACTAMASE INHIBITORS 652
Cleanse and Treat - See
  BENZOYL PEROXIDE 176
  KERATOLYTICS 468
Clear Away - See KERATOLYTICS 468
Clear by Design 2.5 Gel - See BENZOYL
  PEROXIDE 176
Clear by Design Medicated Cleansing Pads -
  See KERATOLYTICS 468
Clear Eyes - See DECONGESTANTS
  (Ophthalmic) 304
*Clearasil Adult Care Medicated Blemish
  Cream* - See KERATOLYTICS 468
Clearasil Adult Care Medicated Blemish Stick
  - See KERATOLYTICS 468
Clearasil BP Plus 5 Cream - See BENZOYL
  PEROXIDE 176
Clearasil BP Plus 5 Lotion - See BENZOYL
  PEROXIDE 176
*Clearasil Clearstick Maximum Strength
  Topical Solution* - See KERATOLYTICS 468
*Clearasil Clearstick Regular Strength Topical
  Solution* - See KERATOLYTICS 468
*Clearasil Double Textured Pads Maximum
  Strength* - See KERATOLYTICS 468
*Clearasil Double Textured Pads Regular
  Strength* - See KERATOLYTICS 468
*Clearasil Maximum Strength Medicated Anti-
  Acne 10 Tinted Cream* - See BENZOYL
  PEROXIDE 176
*Clearasil Maximum Strength Medicated Anti-
  Acne 10 Vanishing Cream* - See
  BENZOYL PEROXIDE 176
*Clearasil Medicated Anti-Acne 10 Vanishing
  Lotion* - See BENZOYL PEROXIDE 176
*Clearasil Medicated Deep Cleanser Topical
  Solution* - See KERATOLYTICS 468
CLEMASTINE FUMARATE - See
  ANTIHISTAMINES 106
Cleocin - See CLINDAMYCIN 258
Cleocin Pediatric - See CLINDAMYCIN 258
Cleocin T Gel - See ANTIBACTERIALS FOR
  ACNE (Topical) 64

INDEX

Dermtex HC - See ADRENOCORTICOIDS
(Topical) 18

Deronil - See ADRENOCORTICOIDS
(Systemic) 16

DES - See ESTROGENS 368

Desenex Aerosol Powder - See
ANTIFUNGALS (Topical) 88

Desenex Antifungal Cream - See
ANTIFUNGALS (Topical) 88

Desenex Antifungal Liquid - See
ANTIFUNGALS (Topical) 88

Desenex Antifungal Ointment - See
ANTIFUNGALS (Topical) 88

Desenex Antifungal Penetrating Foam - See
ANTIFUNGALS (Topical) 88

Desenex Antifungal Powder - See
ANTIFUNGALS (Topical) 88

Desenex Antifungal Spray Powder - See
ANTIFUNGALS (Topical) 88

Desenex Ointment - See ANTIFUNGALS
(Topical) 88

Desenex Powder - See ANTIFUNGALS
(Topical) 88

Desenex Solution - See ANTIFUNGALS
(Topical) 88

DESERPIDINE - See RAUWOLFIA ALKALOIDS
720

DESIPRAMINE - See ANTIDEPRESSANTS,
TRICYCLIC 80

DESLORATADINE - See ANTIHISTAMINES,
NONSEDATING 110

DESMOPRESSIN 308

Desogen 28 - See CONTRACEPTIVES, ORAL
& SKIN 278

Desogen Ortho-Cept - See
CONTRACEPTIVES, ORAL & SKIN 278

DESOGESTREL & ETHINYL ESTRADIOL - See
CONTRACEPTIVES, ORAL & SKIN 278

Desonate - See ADRENOCORTICOIDS
(Topical) 18

DESONIDE (Topical) - See
ADRENOCORTICOIDS (Topical) 18

DesOwen - See ADRENOCORTICOIDS
(Topical) 18

DESOXIMETASONE (Topical) - See
ADRENOCORTICOIDS (Topical) 18

Desoxyn - See AMPHETAMINES 30

Desoxyn Gradumet - See AMPHETAMINES 30

Desquam-E 2.5 Gel - See BENZOYL
PEROXIDE 176

Desquam-E 5 Gel - See BENZOYL PEROXIDE
176

Desquam-E 10 Gel - See BENZOYL
PEROXIDE 176

Desquam-X 2.5 Gel - See BENZOYL
PEROXIDE 176

Desquam-X 5 Gel - See BENZOYL PEROXIDE
176

Desquam-X 5 Wash - See BENZOYL
PEROXIDE 176

Desquam-X 10 Gel - See BENZOYL
PEROXIDE 176

Desquam-X 10 Wash - See BENZOYL
PEROXIDE 176

DESVENLAFAXINE- See SEROTONIN &
NOREPINEPHRINE REUPTAKE
INHIBITORS (SNRIs) 750

DETEMIR - See INSULIN ANALOGS 442

Detensol - See BETA-ADRENERGIC
BLOCKING AGENTS 180

Detrol - See - See MUSCARINIC RECEPTOR
ANTAGONISTS 574

Detrol LA - See MUSCARINIC RECEPTOR
ANTAGONISTS 574

Detussin Expectorant - See
GUAIFENESIN 410
NARCOTIC ANALGESICS 584
PSEUDOEPHEDRINE 700

Detussin Liquid - See
NARCOTIC ANALGESICS 584
PSEUDOEPHEDRINE 700

Dexacort Turbinaire - See
ADRENOCORTICOIDS (Nasal Inhalation) 12

Dexair - See ANTI-INFLAMMATORY DRUGS,
STEROIDAL (Ophthalmic) 122

DEXAMETHASONE - See
ADRENOCORTICOIDS (Systemic) 16

DEXAMETHASONE (Nasal) - See
ADRENOCORTICOIDS (Nasal Inhalation) 12

DEXAMETHASONE (Ophthalmic) - See
ANTI-INFLAMMATORY DRUGS,
STEROIDAL (Ophthalmic) 122

DEXAMETHASONE (Oral Inhalation) - See
ADRENOCORTICOIDS (Oral Inhalation) 14

DEXAMETHASONE (Otic) - See ANTI-
INFLAMMATORY DRUGS, STEROIDAL
(Otic) 124

DEXAMETHASONE (Topical) - See
ADRENOCORTICOIDS (Topical) 18

Dexaphen SA - See
ANTIHISTAMINES 106
PSEUDOEPHEDRINE 700

Dexasone - See ADRENOCORTICOIDS
(Systemic) 16

DEXBROMPHENIRAMINE - See
ANTIHISTAMINES 106

Dexchlor - See ANTIHISTAMINES 106

DEXCHLORPHENIRAMINE - See
ANTIHISTAMINES 106

DEXTROMETHORPHAN 310
Dimetapp Cold & Allergy - See
ANTIHISTAMINES 106
PHENYLEPHRINE 662
Dimetapp Cold & Cough DM Elixir - See
ANTIHISTAMINES 106
DEXTROMETHORPHAN 310
PHENYLEPHRINE 662
Dimetapp Long Acting Cough Plus Cold - See
ANTIHISTAMINES 106
DEXTROMETHORPHAN 310
Dimetapp Nighttime Flu Syrup - See
ACETAMINOPHEN 8
ANTIHISTAMINES 106
DEXTROMETHORPHAN 310
PHENYLEPHRINE 662
Dinate - See ANTIHISTAMINES 106
Diocto - See LAXATIVES, SOFTENER/
LUBRICANT 478
Diocto-C - See
LAXATIVES, SOFTENER/LUBRICANT 478
LAXATIVES, STIMULANT 480
Diocto-K - See LAXATIVES, SOFTENER/
LUBRICANT 478
Diocto-K Plus - See
LAXATIVES, SOFTENER/LUBRICANT 478
LAXATIVES, STIMULANT 480
Diodex - See ANTI-INFLAMMATORY DRUGS,
STEROIDAL (Ophthalmic) 122
Diodoquin - See IODOQUINOL 448
Dioeze - See LAXATIVES, SOFTENER/
LUBRICANT 478
Dionephrine - See PHENYLEPHRINE
(Ophthalmic) 664
Diosuccin - See LAXATIVES, SOFTENER/
LUBRICANT 478
Dio-Sul - See LAXATIVES, SOFTENER/
LUBRICANT 478
Diothron - See
LAXATIVES, SOFTENER/LUBRICANT 478
LAXATIVES, STIMULANT 480
Diovan - See ANGIOTENSIN II RECEPTOR
ANTAGONISTS 44
Diovan HCT - See
ANGIOTENSIN II RECEPTOR
ANTAGONISTS 44
DIURETICS. THIAZIDE 336
Diovan Oral - See ANGIOTENSIN II
RECEPTOR ANTAGONISTS 44
Diovol Ex - See ANTACIDS 50
Diovol Plus - See ANTACIDS 50
Dipentum - See OLSALAZINE 622
Diphen Cough - See ANTIHISTAMINES 106
Diphenacen-10 - See ANTIHISTAMINES 106
Diphenacen-50 - See ANTIHISTAMINES 106

Diphenadryl - See ANTIHISTAMINES 106
Diphenatol - See DIPHENOXYLATE &
ATROPINE 322
DIPHENHYDRAMINE - See ANTIHISTAMINES
106
DIPHENIDOL 320
DIPHENOXYLATE & ATROPINE 322
Diphenylan - See ANTICONVULSANTS,
HYDANTOIN 76
DIPHENYLPYRALINE - See ANTIHISTAMINES
106
Dipimol - See DIPYRIDAMOLE 324
DIPIVEFRIN - See ANTIGLAUCOMA,
ADRENERGIC AGONISTS 92
Dipridacot - See DIPYRIDAMOLE 324
Diprolene - See ADRENOCORTICOIDS
(Topical) 18
Diprolene AF - See ADRENOCORTICOIDS
(Topical) 18
Diprosone - See ADRENOCORTICOIDS
(Topical) 18
DIPYRIDAMOLE 324
Diquinol - See IODOQUINOL 448
DIRITHROMYCIN - See MACROLIDE
ANTIBIOTICS 510
Disalcid - See SALICYLATES 742
Disanthrol - See
LAXATIVES, SOFTENER/LUBRICANT 478
LAXATIVES, STIMULANT 480
Disipal - See ORPHENADRINE 628
Disolan - See LAXATIVES, SOFTENER/
LUBRICANT 478
Disolan Forte - See
LAXATIVES, BULK-FORMING 474
LAXATIVES, SOFTENER/LUBRICANT 478
LAXATIVES, STIMULANT 480
Disonate - See LAXATIVES, SOFTENER/
LUBRICANT 478
Disophrol - See
ANTIHISTAMINES 106
PSEUDOEPHEDRINE 700
Disophrol Chronotabs - See
ANTIHISTAMINES 106
PSEUDOEPHEDRINE 700
Disoplex - See
LAXATIVES, BULK-FORMING 474
LAXATIVES, SOFTENER/LUBRICANT 478
DISOPYRAMIDE 326
Di-Sosul - See LAXATIVES, SOFTENER/
LUBRICANT 478
Di-Sosul Forte - See
LAXATIVES, SOFTENER/LUBRICANT 478
LAXATIVES, STIMULANT 480
Dispatabs - See VITAMIN A 836
Di-Spaz - See DICYCLOMINE 314

DisperMox - See PENICILLINS 650
Dispos-a-Med Isoproterenol - See
   BRONCHODILATORS, ADRENERGIC 198
DISULFIRAM 328
Dital - See APPETITE SUPPRESSANTS 146
Dithranol - See ANTHRALIN (Topical) 54
Ditropan - See - See MUSCARINIC
   RECEPTOR ANTAGONISTS 574
Ditropan XL - See - See MUSCARINIC
   RECEPTOR ANTAGONISTS 574
Diucardin - See DIURETICS, THIAZIDE 336
Diuchlor H - See DIURETICS, THIAZIDE 336
Diulo - See DIURETICS, THIAZIDE 336
Diupres - See
   DIURETICS, THIAZIDE 336
   RAUWOLFIA ALKALOIDS 720
Diuretic - See
   CLONIDINE & CHLORTHALIDONE 262
   DIURETICS, POTASSIUM-SPARING 332
   DIURETICS, POTASSIUM-SPARING &
      HYDROCHLOROTHIAZIDE 334
   HYDRALAZINE & HYDROCHLOROTHIAZIDE
      422
   INDAPAMIDE 438
Diuretic (Loop) - See DIURETICS, LOOP 330
DIURETICS, LOOP 330
DIURETICS, POTASSIUM-SPARING 332
DIURETICS, POTASSIUM-SPARING &
   HYDROCHLOROTHIAZIDE 334
Diuretic (Thiazide) - See
   BETA-ADRENERGIC BLOCKING AGENTS &
      THIAZIDE DIURETICS 182
   DIURETICS, THIAZIDE 336
DIURETICS, THIAZIDE 336
Diurigen with Reserpine - See
   DIURETICS, THIAZIDE 336
   RAUWOLFIA ALKALOIDS 720
Diuril - See DIURETICS, THIAZIDE 336
Diutensen-R - See
   DIURETICS, THIAZIDE 336
   RAUWOLFIA ALKALOIDS 720
DIVALPROEX 338
Divigel - See ESTROGENS 368
Dixarit - See CENTRAL ALPHA AGONISTS
   232
DM Cough - See DEXTROMETHORPHAN 310
DM Syrup - See DEXTROMETHORPHAN 310
Doak Oil - See COAL TAR (Topical) 268
Doak Oil Forte - See COAL TAR (Topical) 268
Doak Oil Forte Therapeutic Bath Treatment -
   See COAL TAR (Topical) 268
**Doak Oil Therapeutic Bath Treatment For All-
   Over Body Care** - See COAL TAR (Topical)
   268
Doak Tar Lotion - See COAL TAR (Topical) 268

Doak Tar Shampoo - See COAL TAR (Topical)
   268
Doan's Pills - See SALICYLATES 742
DOCOSANOL (Topical) - See ANTIVIRALS
   (Topical) 144
Doctar - See COAL TAR (Topical) 268
Doctar Hair & Scalp Shampoo & Conditioner -
   See COAL TAR (Topical) 268
Docucal-P - See
   LAXATIVES, SOFTENER/LUBRICANT 478
   LAXATIVES, STIMULANT 480
Docu-K Plus - See
   LAXATIVES, SOFTENER/LUBRICANT 478
   LAXATIVES, STIMULANT 480
DOCUSATE - See LAXATIVES, SOFTENER/
   LUBRICANT 478
DOCUSATE CALCIUM - See LAXATIVES,
   SOFTENER/LUBRICANT 478
DOCUSATE POTASSIUM - See LAXATIVES,
   SOFTENER/LUBRICANT 478
DOCUSATE SODIUM - See LAXATIVES,
   SOFTENER/LUBRICANT 478
Dodd's Pills - See SALICYLATES 742
DOFETILIDE 340
DOK - See LAXATIVES, SOFTENER/
   LUBRICANT 478
DOK Softgels - See LAXATIVES, SOFTENER/
   LUBRICANT 478
Doktors - See PHENYLEPHRINE 662
Dolacet - See NARCOTIC ANALGESICS &
   ACETAMINOPHEN 586
Dolagesic - See NARCOTIC ANALGESICS &
   ACETAMINOPHEN 586
Dolanex - See ACETAMINOPHEN 8
Dolene-AP 65 - See NARCOTIC ANALGESICS
   & ACETAMINOPHEN 586
Dolgesic - See ANTI-INFLAMMATORY DRUGS,
   NONSTEROIDAL (NSAIDs) 116
Dolmar - See
   ACETAMINOPHEN 8
   BARBITURATES 166
Dolobid - See ANTI-INFLAMMATORY DRUGS,
   NONSTEROIDAL (NSAIDs) 116
Dolophine - See NARCOTIC ANALGESICS 584
Dolotic - See ANTIPYRINE & BENZOCAINE
   (Otic) 130
Dolsed - See ATROPINE, HYOSCYAMINE,
   METHENAMINE, METHYLENE BLUE,
   PHENYLSALICYLATE & BENZOIC ACID 156
Domeboro - See ANTIBACTERIALS (Otic) 68
Dommanate - See ANTIHISTAMINES 106
Donatussin - See
   ANTIHISTAMINES 106
   DEXTROMETHORPHAN 310
   GUAIFENESIN 410

INDEX

Dristan Cold Multi-Symptom Formula - See
ACETAMINOPHEN 8
ANTIHISTAMINES 106
PHENYLEPHRINE 662
Dristan Formula P - See
ANTIHISTAMINES 106
ASPIRIN 150
CAFFEINE 212
PHENYLEPHRINE 662
Dristan Juice Mix-in Cold, Flu, & Cough - See
ACETAMINOPHEN 8
DEXTROMETHORPHAN 310
PSEUDOEPHEDRINE 700
Dristan Long Lasting Menthol Nasal Spray -
See OXYMETAZOLINE (Nasal) 634
Dristan Long Lasting Nasal Pump Spray - See
OXYMETAZOLINE (Nasal) 634
Dristan Long Lasting Nasal Spray - See
OXYMETAZOLINE (Nasal) 634
Dristan Long Lasting Nasal Spray 12 Hour
Metered Dose Pump - See
OXYMETAZOLINE (Nasal) 634
Dristan Mentholated - See OXYMETAZOLINE
(Nasal) 634
Dristan Sinus Caplets - See
ANTI-INFLAMMATORY DRUGS,
NONSTEROIDAL (NSAIDs) 116
PSEUDOEPHEDRINE 700
Dristan-AF - See
ACETAMINOPHEN 8
ANTIHISTAMINES 106
CAFFEINE 212
PHENYLEPHRINE 662
Dristan-AF Plus - See
ACETAMINOPHEN 8
CAFFEINE 212
PHENYLEPHRINE 662
Drithocreme - See ANTHRALIN (Topical) 54
Drithocreme HP - See ANTHRALIN (Topical) 54
Dritho-Scalp - See ANTHRALIN (Topical) 54
Drixoral - See
ANTIHISTAMINES 106
OXYMETAZOLINE (Nasal) 634
PSEUDOEPHEDRINE 700
Drixoral Cold and Allergy - See
ANTIHISTAMINES 106
PSEUDOEPHEDRINE 700
Drixoral Cold and Flu - See
ACETAMINOPHEN 8
ANTIHISTAMINES 106
PSEUDOEPHEDRINE 700
Drixoral Cough - See DEXTROMETHORPHAN
310
Drixoral Nasal Decongestant - See
PSEUDOEPHEDRINE 700

Drixoral Non-Drowsy Formula - See
PSEUDOEPHEDRINE 700
Drixoral Plus - See
ACETAMINOPHEN 8
ANTIHISTAMINES 106
PSEUDOEPHEDRINE 700
Drixoral Sinus - See
ACETAMINOPHEN 8
ANTIHISTAMINES 106
PSEUDOEPHEDRINE 700
Drixtab - See
ANTIHISTAMINES 106
PSEUDOEPHEDRINE 700
Drocade and Aspirin - See NARCOTIC
ANALGESICS & ASPIRIN 588
DRONABINOL (THC, Marijuana) 346
DROSPIRENONE - See PROGESTINS 686
DROSPIRENONE & ETHINYL ESTRADIOL - See
CONTRACEPTIVES, ORAL & SKIN 278
Drotic - See ANTIBACTERIALS (Otic) 68
Droxia - See HYDROXYUREA 428
Droxomin - See VITAMIN B-12
(Cyanocobalamin) 838
Dry and Clear 5 Lotion - See BENZOYL
PEROXIDE 176
Dry and Clear Double Strength 10 Cream -
See BENZOYL PEROXIDE 176
Dryox 5 Gel - See BENZOYL PEROXIDE 176
Dryox 10 Gel - See BENZOYL PEROXIDE 176
Dryox 20 Gel - See BENZOYL PEROXIDE 176
Dryox Wash 5 - See BENZOYL PEROXIDE 176
Dryox Wash 10 - See BENZOYL PEROXIDE 176
Dryphen - See
ACETAMINOPHEN 8
ANTIHISTAMINES 106
PHENYLEPHRINE 662
DSMC Plus - See
LAXATIVES, SOFTENER/LUBRICANT 478
LAXATIVES, STIMULANT 480
DUAC Topical Gel - See
ANTIBACTERIALS FOR ACNE (Topical) 64
BENZOYL PEROXIDE 176
Duagen - See 5-ALPHA REDUCTASE
INHIBITORS 2
Duetact - See
SULFONYLUREAS 776
THIAZOLIDINEDIONES 790
Dulcodos - See
LAXATIVES, SOFTENER/LUBRICANT 478
LAXATIVES, STIMULANT 480
Dulcolax - See LAXATIVES, STIMULANT 480
DULOXETINE - See SEROTONIN &
NOREPINEPHRINE REUPTAKE
INHIBITORS (SNRIs) 750

INDEX

INDEX

INDEX

INDEX

FOSINOPRIL - See ANGIOTENSIN-
CONVERTING ENZYME (ACE)
INHIBITORS 46
Fostex 5 Gel - See BENZOYL PEROXIDE 176
Fostex 10 Bar - See BENZOYL PEROXIDE 176
Fostex 10 Cream - See BENZOYL PEROXIDE
176
Fostex 10 Gel - See BENZOYL PEROXIDE 176
Fostex 10 Wash - See BENZOYL PEROXIDE
176
Fostex CM - See KERATOLYTICS 468
Fostex Medicated Cleansing Bar - See
KERATOLYTICS 468
Fostex Medicated Cleansing Cream - See
KERATOLYTICS 468
Fostex Medicated Cleansing Liquid - See
KERATOLYTICS 468
*Fostex Regular Strength Medicated
Cleansing Bar* - See KERATOLYTICS 468
*Fostex Regular Strength Medicated Cleansing
Cream* - See KERATOLYTICS 468
Fostex Regular Strength Medicated Cover-Up
- See KERATOLYTICS 468
Fostril Cream - See KERATOLYTICS 468
Fostril Lotion - See KERATOLYTICS 468
Fototar - See COAL TAR (Topical) 268
Fowlers Diarrhea Tablets - See ATTAPULGITE
158
Freezone - See KERATOLYTICS 468
Froben - See ANTI-INFLAMMATORY DRUGS,
NONSTEROIDAL (NSAIDs) 116
Froben SR - See ANTI-INFLAMMATORY
DRUGS, NONSTEROIDAL (NSAIDs) 116
Frova - See TRIPTANS 824
FROVATRIPTAN - See TRIPTANS 824
Fulvicin P/G - See GRISEOFULVIN 408
Fulvicin U/F - See GRISEOFULVIN 408
Fungizone - See ANTIFUNGALS (Topical) 88
Furadantin - See NITROFURANTOIN 608
Furalan - See NITROFURANTOIN 608
Furaloid - See NITROFURANTOIN 608
Furan - See NITROFURANTOIN 608
Furanite - See NITROFURANTOIN 608
Furantoin - See NITROFURANTOIN 608
Furatine - See NITROFURANTOIN 608
Furaton - See NITROFURANTOIN 608
FURAZOLIDONE 394
FUROSEMIDE - See DIURETICS, LOOP 330
Furoside - See DIURETICS, LOOP 330
Furoxone - See FURAZOLIDONE 394
Furoxone Liquid - See FURAZOLIDONE 394
FUSION INHIBITOR 396
Fusion inhibitor - See FUSION INHIBITOR 396
Fuzeon - See FUSION INHIBITOR 396
Fynex - See ANTIHISTAMINES 106

G

G-1 - See BARBITURATES 166
GABAPENTIN 398
Gabitril - See TIAGABINE 798
GALANTAMINE - See CHOLINESTERASE
INHIBITORS 250
Galzin - See ZINC SUPPLEMENTS 856
GANCICLOVIR - See ANTIVIRALS FOR
HERPES VIRUS 136
Gantanol - See SULFONAMIDES 772
Gantrisin - See
ANTIBACTERIALS (Ophthalmic) 66
SULFONAMIDES 772
Garamycin - See
ANTIBACTERIALS (Ophthalmic) 66
ANTIBACTERIALS (Topical) 70
Gas Aid - See SIMETHICONE 754
Gas Relief - See SIMETHICONE 754
Gastrocrom - See CROMOLYN 282
Gastrointestinal selective receptor agonist - See
TEGASEROD 780
Gastrosed - See HYOSCYAMINE 432
Gastrozepin - See ANTICHOLINERGICS 72
Gas-X - See SIMETHICONE 754
Gas-X Extra Strength - See SIMETHICONE
754
Gas-X Thin Strips - See SIMETHICONE 754
Gas-X with Maalox - See
ANTACIDS 50
SIMETHICONE 754
GATIFLOXACIN (Ophthalmic) - See
ANTIBACTERIALS (Ophthalmic) 66
Gaviscon - See ANTACIDS 50
Gaviscon Extra Strength Relief Formula - See
ANTACIDS 50
Gaviscon-2 - See ANTACIDS 50
GBH - See PEDICULICIDES (Topical) 646
Gee-Gee - See GUAIFENESIN 410
Gelnique - See MUSCARINIC RECEPTOR
ANTAGONISTS 574
Gelpirin - See
ACETAMINOPHEN 8
ASPIRIN 150
Gelusil - See
ANTACIDS 50
SIMETHICONE 754
Gelusil Extra-Strength - See ANTACIDS 50
GEMFIBROZIL 400
GEMIFLOXACIN - See FLUOROQUINOLONES
388
Gemnisyn - See
ACETAMINOPHEN 8
ASPIRIN 150
Gemonil - See BARBITURATES 166
Genabid - See PAPAVERINE 642

GLYBURIDE - See SULFONYLUREAS 776
Glycate - See ANTACIDS 50
GLYCERIN - See LAXATIVES, OSMOTIC 476
Glyceryl T - See
  BRONCHODILATORS, XANTHINE 200
  GUAIFENESIN 410
Glyceryl Trinitrate - See NITRATES 606
GLYCOPYRROLATE 404
Gly-Cort - See ADRENOCORTICOIDS (Topical)
  18
Glycotuss - See GUAIFENESIN 410
Glycotuss-dM - See
  DEXTROMETHORPHAN 310
  GUAIFENESIN 410
Glydeine Cough - See
  GUAIFENESIN 410
  NARCOTIC ANALGESICS 584
Glynase PresTab - See SULFONYLUREAS 776
Glysennid - See LAXATIVES, STIMULANT 480
Glyset - See MIGLITOL 556
Glytuss - See GUAIFENESIN 410
G-Myticin Antibiotic - See ANTIBACTERIALS
  (Topical) 70
Gold compounds - See GOLD COMPOUNDS
  406
GOLD COMPOUNDS 406
GOLD SODIUM THIOMALATE - See GOLD
  COMPOUNDS 406
Gonad stimulant - See CLOMIPHENE 260
Gonadotropin inhibitor - See
  DANAZOL 298
  NAFARELIN 580
Gonak - See PROTECTANT (Ophthalmic) 696
Goniosoft - See PROTECTANT (Ophthalmic)
  696
Goniosol - See PROTECTANT (Ophthalmic) 696
Goody's Extra Strength Tablet - See
  ACETAMINOPHEN 8
  ASPIRIN 150
Goody's Headache Powders - See
  ACETAMINOPHEN 8
  ASPIRIN 150
Gordochom Solution - See ANTIFUNGALS
  (Topical) 88
Gordofilm - See KERATOLYTICS 468
Gotamine - See
  CAFFEINE 212
  ERGOTAMINE 362
Gramcal - See CALCIUM SUPPLEMENTS 218
Gravol - See ANTIHISTAMINES 106
Gravol L/A - See ANTIHISTAMINES 106
Grifulvin V - See GRISEOFULVIN 408
Grisactin - See GRISEOFULVIN 408
Grisactin Ultra - See GRISEOFULVIN 408
GRISEOFULVIN 408

Grisovin-FP - See GRISEOFULVIN 408
Gris-PEG - See GRISEOFULVIN 408
Guaifed - See
  GUAIFENESIN 410
  PSEUDOEPHEDRINE 700
Guaifed-PD - See
  GUAIFENESIN 410
  PSEUDOEPHEDRINE 700
GUAIFENESIN 410
GuaiMAX-D - See
  GUAIFENESIN 410
  PSEUDOEPHEDRINE 700
GUANABENZ - See CENTRAL ALPHA
  AGONISTS 232
GUANADREL 412
GUANFACINE - See CENTRAL ALPHA
  AGONISTS 232
Guiamid D.M. Liquid - See
  DEXTROMETHORPHAN 310
  GUAIFENESIN 410
Guiatuss A.C. - See
  GUAIFENESIN 410
  NARCOTIC ANALGESICS 584
Guiatuss PE - See
  GUAIFENESIN 410
  PSEUDOEPHEDRINE 700
Guiatuss-DM - See
  DEXTROMETHORPHAN 310
  GUAIFENESIN 410
G-Well - See PEDICULICIDES (Topical) 646
Gynecort - See ADRENOCORTICOIDS
  (Topical) 18
Gynecort 10 - See ADRENOCORTICOIDS
  (Topical) 18
Gyne-Lotrimin - See ANTIFUNGALS (Vaginal)
  90
Gyne-Lotrimin 3 - See ANTIFUNGALS
  (Vaginal) 90
Gynergen - See ERGOTAMINE 362
Gyno-Trosyd - See ANTIFUNGALS (Vaginal) 90
Gynogen L.A. 20 - See ESTROGENS 368
Gynogen L.A. 40 - See ESTROGENS 368
Gynol II Extra Strength - See
  CONTRACEPTIVES, VAGINAL 280
Gynol II Original Formula - See
  CONTRACEPTIVES, VAGINAL 280

H

H_2Oxyl 2.5 Gel - See BENZOYL PEROXIDE
  176
H_2Oxyl 5 Gel - See BENZOYL PEROXIDE 176
H_2Oxyl 10 Gel - See BENZOYL PEROXIDE 176
Habitrol - See NICOTINE 600
Hair growth stimulant - See
  ANTHRALIN (Topical) 54

INDEX

ISONIAZID 456

Isopap - See
  ACETAMINOPHEN 8
  BARBITURATES 166

ISOPROPAMIDE - See ANTICHOLINERGICS
  72

ISOPROPYL UNOPROSTONE - See
  ANTIGLAUCOMA, PROSTAGLANDINS 102

ISOPROTERENOL - See
  BRONCHODILATORS, ADRENERGIC 198

Isoptin - See CALCIUM CHANNEL BLOCKERS
  216

Isoptin SR - See CALCIUM CHANNEL
  BLOCKERS 216

Isopto Alkaline - See PROTECTANT
  (Ophthalmic) 696

Isopto Atropine - See CYCLOPLEGIC,
  MYDRIATIC (Ophthalmic) 292

Isopto Carbachol - See ANTIGLAUCOMA,
  CHOLINERGIC AGONISTS 100

Isopto Carpine - See ANTIGLAUCOMA,
  CHOLINERGIC AGONISTS 100

Isopto Frin - See PHENYLEPHRINE
  (Ophthalmic) 664

Isopto Homatropine - See CYCLOPLEGIC,
  MYDRIATIC (Ophthalmic) 292

Isopto Hyoscine - See CYCLOPLEGIC,
  MYDRIATIC (Ophthalmic) 292

Isopto Plain - See PROTECTANT (Ophthalmic)
  696

Isopto Tears - See PROTECTANT (Ophthalmic)
  696

Isorbid - See NITRATES 606

Isordil - See NITRATES 606

ISOSORBIDE DINITRATE - See NITRATES 606

ISOSORBIDE MONONITRATE - See
  NITRATES 606

Isotamine - See ISONIAZID 456

Isotrate - See NITRATES 606

ISOTRETINOIN 458

ISOXSUPRINE 460

ISRADIPINE - See CALCIUM CHANNEL
  BLOCKERS 216

Istalol - See ANTIGLAUCOMA, BETA
  BLOCKERS 96

I-Sulfacet - See ANTIBACTERIALS
  (Ophthalmic) 66

Isuprel - See BRONCHODILATORS,
  ADRENERGIC 198

Isuprel Glossets - See BRONCHODILATORS,
  ADRENERGIC 198

Isuprel Mistometer - See
  BRONCHODILATORS, ADRENERGIC 198

ITRACONAZOLE - See ANTIFUNGALS,
  AZOLES 86

I-Tropine - See CYCLOPLEGIC, MYDRIATIC
  (Ophthalmic) 292

IVERMECTIN - See ANTHELMINTICS 52

J

Janumet - See
  DPP-4 INHIBITORS 344
  METFORMIN 538

Januvia - See DPP-4 INHIBITORS 344

Jectofer - See IRON SUPPLEMENTS 452

Jenest-28 - See CONTRACEPTIVES, ORAL &
  SKIN 278

Junior Strength Advil - See ANTI-
  INFLAMMATORY DRUGS,
  NONSTEROIDAL (NSAIDs) 116

Junior Tylenol - See ACETAMINOPHEN 8

Just Tears - See PROTECTANT (Ophthalmic)
  696

K

K-10 - See POTASSIUM SUPPLEMENTS 670

K+10 - See POTASSIUM SUPPLEMENTS 670

K+Care - See POTASSIUM SUPPLEMENTS
  670

K+Care ET - See POTASSIUM SUPPLEMENTS
  670

Kabolin - See ANDROGENS 36

Kadian - See NARCOTIC ANALGESICS 584

Kaletra - See PROTEASE INHIBITORS 694

Kalium Durules - See POTASSIUM
  SUPPLEMENTS 670

KANAMYCIN 462

Kantrex - See KANAMYCIN 462

Kaochlor - See POTASSIUM SUPPLEMENTS
  670

Kaochlor S-F - See POTASSIUM
  SUPPLEMENTS 670

Kaochlor-10 - See POTASSIUM
  SUPPLEMENTS 670

Kaochlor-20 - See POTASSIUM
  SUPPLEMENTS 670

Kaochlor-Eff - See POTASSIUM
  SUPPLEMENTS 670

Kao-Con - See KAOLIN & PECTIN 464

KAOLIN & PECTIN 464

KAOLIN, PECTIN, BELLADONNA & OPIUM 466

Kaon - See POTASSIUM SUPPLEMENTS 670

Kaon-Cl - See POTASSIUM SUPPLEMENTS
  670

Kaon-Cl 10 - See POTASSIUM
  SUPPLEMENTS 670

Kaon-Cl 20 - See POTASSIUM
  SUPPLEMENTS 670

Kaopectate - See ATTAPULGITE 158

INDEX

Maximum Strength Mucinex DM - See
DEXTROMETHORPHAN 310
GUAIFENESIN 410
Maximum Strength Mucinex D - See
GUAIFENESIN 410
PSEUDOEPHEDRINE 700
Maximum Strength Mylanta Gas Relief - See
SIMETHICONE 754
Maximum Strength Phazyme - See
SIMETHICONE 754
Maximum Strength Tylenol Allergy Sinus
Caplets - See
ACETAMINOPHEN 8
ANTIHISTAMINES 106
PSEUDOEPHEDRINE 700
Maxivate - See ADRENOCORTICOIDS
(Topical) 18
Maxzide - See DIURETICS, POTASSIUM-
SPARING & HYDROCHLOROTHIAZIDE 334
Mazanor - See APPETITE SUPPRESSANTS
146
Mazepine - See CARBAMAZEPINE 224
MAZINDOL - See APPETITE SUPPRESSANTS
146
Measurin - See ASPIRIN 150
Mebaral - See BARBITURATES 166
Mebendacin - See ANTHELMINTICS 52
MEBENDAZOLE - See ANTHELMINTICS 52
Mebutar - See ANTHELMINTICS 52
MECAMYLAMINE 518
MECHLORETHAMINE (Topical) 520
Meclan - See ANTIBACTERIALS FOR
ACNE (Topical) 64
MECLIZINE - See ANTIHISTAMINES,
PIPERAZINE (Antinausea) 114
MECLOCYCLINE (Topical)- See ANTI-
BACTERIALS FOR ACNE (Topical) 64
Meclofen - See ANTI-INFLAMMATORY
DRUGS, NONSTEROIDAL (NSAIDs) 116
MECLOFENAMATE - See ANTI-
INFLAMMATORY DRUGS,
NONSTEROIDAL (NSAIDs) 116
Meclomen - See ANTI-INFLAMMATORY
DRUGS, NONSTEROIDAL (NSAIDs) 116
Med Tamoxifen - See TAMOXIFEN 778
Meda Cap - See ACETAMINOPHEN 8
Meda Syrup Forte - See
ANTIHISTAMINES 106
DEXTROMETHORPHAN 310
GUAIFENESIN 410
PHENYLEPHRINE 662
Meda Tab - See ACETAMINOPHEN 8
Medatussin - See
DEXTROMETHORPHAN 310
GUAIFENESIN 410

Medatussin Plus - See GUAIFENESIN 410
Meclicot - See ANTIHISTAMINES,
PIPERAZINE (Antinausea) 114
Medigesic - See
ACETAMINOPHEN 8
BARBITURATES 166
Medihaler Ergotamine - See ERGOTAMINE 362
Medihaler-Epi - See BRONCHODILATORS,
ADRENERGIC 198
Medihaler-Iso - See BRONCHODILATORS,
ADRENERGIC 198
Medilium - See BENZODIAZEPINES 174
Mediplast - See KERATOLYTICS 468
Medipren - See ANTI-INFLAMMATORY
DRUGS, NONSTEROIDAL (NSAIDs) 116
Medipren Caplets - See ANTI-INFLAMMATORY
DRUGS, NONSTEROIDAL (NSAIDs) 116
Mediquell - See DEXTROMETHORPHAN 310
Medi-Tran - See MEPROBAMATE 532
Medivert - See ANTIHISTAMINES,
PIPERAZINE (Antinausea) 114
Medotar - See COAL TAR (Topical) 268
Medrol - See ADRENOCORTICOIDS
(Systemic) 16
MEDROXYPROGESTERONE - See
PROGESTINS 686
MEDRYSONE - See ANTI-INFLAMMATORY
DRUGS, STEROIDAL (Ophthalmic) 122
Med-Timolol - See ANTIGLAUCOMA, BETA
BLOCKERS 96
MEFENAMIC ACID - See ANTI-INFLAMMATORY
DRUGS, NONSTEROIDAL (NSAIDs) 116
MEFLOQUINE - See ANTIMALARIAL 126
Megace - See PROGESTINS 686
Megace ES - See PROGESTINS 686
Megace Oral Suspension - See PROGESTINS
686
Megacillin - See PENICILLINS 650
MEGESTROL - See PROGESTINS 686
MEGLITINIDES 522
MELATONIN 524
Melatonin receptor agonist - See RAMELTEON
716
Melfiat-105 Unicelles - See APPETITE
SUPPRESSANTS 146
Mellaril - See PHENOTHIAZINES 660
Mellaril Concentrate - See PHENOTHIAZINES
660
Mellaril-S - See PHENOTHIAZINES 660
MELOXICAM 526
MELPHALAN 528
MEMANTINE 530
MENADIOL - See VITAMIN K 848
Menaval-20 - See ESTROGENS 368
Menest - See ESTROGENS 368

METHYLCELLULOSE - See LAXATIVES,
BULK-FORMING 474
METHYLDOPA - See CENTRAL ALPHA
AGONISTS 232
Methylergometrine - See
METHYLERGONOVINE 544
METHYLERGONOVINE 544
Methylin Chewable - See STIMULANT
MEDICATIONS 760
Methylin ER - See STIMULANT MEDICATIONS
760
Methylin Oral Suspension - See STIMULANT
MEDICATIONS 760
METHYLPHENIDATE - See STIMULANT
MEDICATIONS 760
METHYLPREDNISOLONE - See
ADRENOCORTICOIDS (Systemic) 16
ADRENOCORTICOIDS (Topical) 18
METHYLTESTOSTERONE - See ANDROGENS
36
METHYSERGIDE 546
Meticorten - See ADRENOCORTICOIDS
(Systemic) 16
METIPRANOLOL (Ophthalmic) - See
ANTIGLAUCOMA, BETA BLOCKERS 96
Metizol - See NITROIMIDAZOLES 610
METOCLOPRAMIDE 548
METOLAZONE - See DIURETICS, THIAZIDE
336
Metopirone - See METYRAPONE 550
METOPROLOL - See BETA-ADRENERGIC
BLOCKING AGENTS 180
METOPROLOL & HYDROCHLOROTHIAZIDE -
See BETA-ADRENERGIC BLOCKING
AGENTS & THIAZIDE DIURETICS 182
Metosyn - See ADRENOCORTICOIDS (Topical)
18
Metosyn FAPG - See ADRENOCORTICOIDS
(Topical) 18
Metra - See APPETITE SUPPRESSANTS 146
Metric 21 - See NITROIMIDAZOLES 610
Metro Cream - See NITROIMIDAZOLES 610
MetroGel - See NITROIMIDAZOLES 610
MetroGel-Vaginal - See NITROIMIDAZOLES
610
METRONIDAZOLE - See NITROIMIDAZOLES
610
METYRAPONE 550
Mevacor - See HMG-CoA REDUCTASE
INHIBITORS 418
Meval - See BENZODIAZEPINES 174
Mevinolin - See HMG-CoA REDUCTASE
INHIBITORS 418
Mexate - See METHOTREXATE 542
Mexate AQ - See METHOTREXATE 542

MEXILETINE 552
Mexitil - See MEXILETINE 552
Miacalcin - See CALCITONIN 214
Mi-Acid - See ANTACIDS 50
Mi-Acid Double Strength - See ANTACIDS 50
Micanol - See ANTHRALIN (Topical) 54
Micardis - See ANGIOTENSIN II RECEPTOR
ANTAGONISTS 44
Micardis HCT - See
ANGIOTENSIN II RECEPTOR
ANTAGONISTS 44
DIURETICS, THIAZIDE 336
Micardis Plus- See
ANGIOTENSIN II RECEPTOR
ANTAGONISTS 44
DIURETICS, THIAZIDE 336
Micatin - See ANTIFUNGALS (Topical) 88
MICONAZOLE - See
ANTIFUNGALS (Topical) 88
ANTIFUNGALS (Vaginal) 90
Micrainin - See
ASPIRIN 150
MEPROBAMATE 532
Microgestin Fe - See CONTRACEPTIVES,
ORAL & SKIN 278
Micro-K - See POTASSIUM SUPPLEMENTS
670
Micro-K 10 - See POTASSIUM SUPPLEMENTS
670
Micro-K LS - See POTASSIUM
SUPPLEMENTS 670
Micronase - See SULFONYLUREAS 776
microNEFRIN - See BRONCHODILATORS,
ADRENERGIC 198
Micronor - See PROGESTINS 686
Midamor - See DIURETICS, POTASSIUM-
SPARING 332
MIDAZOLAM - See BENZODIAZEPINES 174
Midchlor - See ISOMETHEPTENE,
DICHLORALPHENAZONE &
ACETAMINOPHEN 454
Midol 200 - See ANTI-INFLAMMATORY
DRUGS, NONSTEROIDAL (NSAIDs) 116
Midol-IB - See ANTI-INFLAMMATORY DRUGS,
NONSTEROIDAL (NSAIDs) 116
Midquin - See ISOMETHEPTENE,
DICHLORALPHENAZONE &
ACETAMINOPHEN 454
Midrin - See ISOMETHEPTENE,
DICHLORALPHENAZONE &
ACETAMINOPHEN 454
Mifeprex - See MIFEPRISTONE 554
MIFEPRISTONE 554
Migergot - See
CAFFEINE 212

ERGOTAMINE 362
MIGLITOL 556
Migquin - See ISOMETHEPTENE,
    DICHLORALPHENAZONE &
    ACETAMINOPHEN 454
Migrapap - See ISOMETHEPTENE,
    DICHLORALPHENAZONE &
    ACETAMINOPHEN 454
Migratine - See ISOMETHEPTENE,
    DICHLORALPHENAZONE &
    ACETAMINOPHEN 454
Migrazone - See ISOMETHEPTENE,
    DICHLORALPHENAZONE &
    ACETAMINOPHEN 454
Migrend - See ISOMETHEPTENE,
    DICHLORALPHENAZONE &
    ACETAMINOPHEN 454
Migrex - See ISOMETHEPTENE,
    DICHLORALPHENAZONE &
    ACETAMINOPHEN 454
MILK OF MAGNESIA - See LAXATIVES,
    OSMOTIC 476
Milkinol - See LAXATIVES, SOFTENER/
    LUBRICANT 478
MILNACIPRAN - See SEROTONIN &
    NOREPINEPHRINE REUPTAKE
    INHIBITORS (SNRIs) 750
Milophene - See CLOMIPHENE 260
Miltown - See MEPROBAMATE 532
MINERAL OIL - See
    LAXATIVES, OSMOTIC 476
    LAXATIVES, SOFTENER/LUBRICANT 478
Mineral supplement (Iron) - See IRON
    SUPPLEMENTS 452
Mineral supplement (Potassium) - See
    POTASSIUM SUPPLEMENTS 670
Minestrin 1/20 - See CONTRACEPTIVES,
    ORAL & SKIN 278
Minims Atropine - See CYCLOPLEGIC,
    MYDRIATIC (Ophthalmic) 292
Minims Cyclopentolate - See
    CYCLOPENTOLATE (Ophthalmic) 288
Minims Homatropine - See CYCLOPLEGIC,
    MYDRIATIC (Ophthalmic) 292
Minims Phenylephrine - See
    PHENYLEPHRINE (Ophthalmic) 664
Minims - See ANTIGLAUCOMA,
    CHOLINERGIC AGONISTS 100
Minipress - See ALPHA ADRENERGIC
    RECEPTOR BLOCKERS 20
Minitran - See NITRATES 606
Minizide - See
    ALPHA ADRENERGIC RECEPTOR
    BLOCKERS 20
    DIURETICS, THIAZIDE 336

Minocin - See TETRACYCLINES 786
MINOCYCLINE - See TETRACYCLINES 786
Min-Ovral - See CONTRACEPTIVES, ORAL &
    SKIN 278
MINOXIDIL 558
MINOXIDIL (Topical) 560
Mintezol - See ANTHELMINTICS 52
Mintezol Topical - See ANTHELMINTICS 52
Mintox - See ANTACIDS 50
Mintox Extra Strength - See ANTACIDS 50
Minzolum - See ANTHELMINTICS 52
Miocarpine - See ANTIGLAUCOMA,
    CHOLINERGIC AGONISTS 100
Miostat - See ANTIGLAUCOMA,
    CHOLINERGIC AGONISTS 100
Miradon - See ANTICOAGULANTS (Oral) 74
Miralax - See LAXATIVES, OSMOTIC 476
Mirapex - See ANTIDYSKINETICS 82
Mircette- See CONTRACEPTIVES, ORAL &
    SKIN 278
MIRTAZAPINE 562
MISOPROSTOL 564
MITOTANE 566
Mitride - See ISOMETHEPTENE,
    DICHLORALPHENAZONE &
    ACETAMINOPHEN 454
Mitrolan - See LAXATIVES, BULK-FORMING
    474
Mixtard - See INSULIN 440
Mixtard Human - See INSULIN 440
Moban - See MOLINDONE 568
Moban Concentrate - See MOLINDONE 568
Mobic - See MELOXICAM 526
Mobidin - See SALICYLATES 742
Mobiflex - See ANTI-INFLAMMATORY DRUGS,
    NONSTEROIDAL (NSAIDs) 116
MODAFINIL- See STIMULANTS,
AMPHETAMINE-RELATED 762
Modane Bulk - See LAXATIVES, BULK-
    FORMING 474
Modane Plus - See LAXATIVES, SOFTENER/
    LUBRICANT 478
Modane Soft - See LAXATIVES, SOFTENER/
    LUBRICANT 478
Modecate - See PHENOTHIAZINES 660
Modecate Concentrate - See
    PHENOTHIAZINES 660
ModiCon - See CONTRACEPTIVES, ORAL &
    SKIN 278
Modified Shohl's Solution - See CITRATES
    254
Moditen Enanthate - See PHENOTHIAZINES
    660
Moditen HCl - See PHENOTHIAZINES 660
Moditen HCl-H.P - See PHENOTHIAZINES 660

INDEX

Modrastane - See TRILOSTANE 818

Moduret - See DIURETICS, POTASSIUM-SPARING & HYDROCHLOROTHIAZIDE 334

Moduretic - See DIURETICS, POTASSIUM-SPARING & HYDROCHLOROTHIAZIDE 334

MOEXIPRIL - See ANGIOTENSIN-CONVERTING ENZYME (ACE) INHIBITORS 46

Mogadon - See BENZODIAZEPINES 174

Moisture Drops - See PROTECTANT (Ophthalmic) 696

Molatoc - See LAXATIVES, SOFTENER/LUBRICANT 478

Molatoc-CST - See
LAXATIVES, SOFTENER/LUBRICANT 478
LAXATIVES, STIMULANT 480

MOLINDONE 568

MOMETASONE - See ADRENOCORTICOIDS (Nasal Inhalation) 12

MOMETASONE (Topical) - See ADRENOCORTICOIDS (Topical) 18

Monistat - See ANTIFUNGALS (Vaginal) 90

Monistat 1 - See ANTIFUNGALS (Vaginal) 90

Monistat 3 - See ANTIFUNGALS (Vaginal) 90

Monistat 5 - See ANTIFUNGALS (Vaginal) 90

Monistat 7 - See ANTIFUNGALS (Vaginal) 90

Monistat-Derm - See ANTIFUNGALS (Topical) 88

Monitan - See BETA-ADRENERGIC BLOCKING AGENTS 180

MONOAMINE OXIDASE (MAO) INHIBITORS 570

MONOAMINE OXIDASE TYPE B (MAO-B) INHIBITORS 572

Monodox - See TETRACYCLINES 786

Mono-Gesic - See SALICYLATES 742

Monoket - See NITRATES 606

Monopril - See ANGIOTENSIN-CONVERTING ENZYME (ACE) INHIBITORS 46

MONTELUKAST - See LEUKOTRIENE MODIFIERS 486

Mood stabilizer - See LITHIUM 500

M-Orexic - See APPETITE SUPPRESSANTS 146

MORPHINE - See NARCOTIC ANALGESICS 584

Morphitec - See NARCOTIC ANALGESICS 584

M.O.S. - See NARCOTIC ANALGESICS 584

M.O.S.-SR - See NARCOTIC ANALGESICS 584

Motion-Aid - See ANTIHISTAMINES 106

Motofen - See DIFENOXIN & ATROPINE 316

Motrin-IB - See ANTI-INFLAMMATORY DRUGS, NONSTEROIDAL (NSAIDs) 116

Motrin-IB Cold & Sinus - See
ANTI-INFLAMMATORY DRUGS, NONSTEROIDAL (NSAIDs) 116
PSEUDOEPHEDRINE 700

Movergan - See MONOAMINE OXIDASE TYPE B (MAO-B) INHIBITORS 572

Moxatag - See PENICILLINS 650

MOXIFLOXACIN - See FLUOROQUINOLONES 388

MS Contin - See NARCOTIC ANALGESICS 584

MSIR - See NARCOTIC ANALGESICS 584

MST Continus - See NARCOTIC ANALGESICS 584

Mucinex - See GUAIFENESIN 410

Mucinex Children's Cough, Expectorant and Suppressant - See
DEXTROMETHORPHAN 310
GUAIFENESIN 410

Mucinex Children's Expectorant - See
GUAIFENESIN 410

Mucinex Cold Liquid - See
GUAIFENESIN 410
PHENYLEPHRINE 662

Mucinex Cough Mini-Melts - See
DEXTROMETHORPHAN 310
GUAIFENESIN 410

Mucinex D - See
GUAIFENESIN 410
PSEUDOEPHEDRINE 700

Mucinex DM
DEXTROMETHORPHAN 310
GUAIFENESIN 410

Mucinex Full Force Nasal Spray - See
OXYMETAZOLINE (Nasal) 634

Mucinex Junior Strength Expectorant - See
GUAIFENESIN 410

Mucinex Mini-Melts - See GUAIFENESIN 410

Mucinex Moisture Smart Nasal Spray - See
OXYMETAZOLINE (Nasal 634

Mucinum - See LAXATIVES, STIMULANT 480

Mucinum Herbal - See LAXATIVES, STIMULANT 480

Mucolysin - See TIOPRONIN 800

Mudrane GG2 - See
BRONCHODILATORS, XANTHINE 200
GUAIFENESIN 410

Multipax - See HYDROXYZINE 430

Mulvidren-F - See VITAMINS & FLUORIDE 850

MUPIROCIN - See ANTIBACTERIALS (Topical) 70

Murine Plus - See DECONGESTANTS (Ophthalmic) 304

Muro's Opcon - See DECONGESTANTS (Ophthalmic) 304

MUSCARINIC RECEPTOR ANTAGONISTS 574

INDEX

INDEX

Nix Cream Rinse - See PEDICULICIDES
(Topical) 646

NIZATIDINE - See HISTAMINE H$_2$ RECEPTOR
ANTAGONISTS 416

Nizoral - See ANTIFUNGALS, AZOLES 86

Nizoral A-D - See ANTIFUNGALS (Topical) 88

Nizoral Shampoo - See ANTIFUNGALS
(Topical) 88

N-methyl-D-aspartate (NMDA) receptor
antagonist - See MEMANTINE 530

Noctec - See CHLORAL HYDRATE 238

Nolahist - See ANTIHISTAMINES 106

Nonbenzodiazepine hypnotic - See
RAMELTEON 716

NON-NUCLEOSIDE REVERSE
TRANSCRIPTASE INHIBITORS 612

NONOXYNOL 9 - See CONTRACEPTIVES,
VAGINAL 280

Nonsteroidal anti-inflammatory drug (NSAID),
topical - See DICLOFENAC (Topical) 312

Noradex - See ORPHENADRINE 628

Noradryl - See ANTIHISTAMINES 106

Norafed - See ANTIHISTAMINES 106

Norcept-E 1/35 - See CONTRACEPTIVES,
ORAL & SKIN 278

Norco - See NARCOTIC ANALGESICS &
ACETAMINOPHEN 586

Nordette - See CONTRACEPTIVES, ORAL &
SKIN 278

Nordryl - See ANTIHISTAMINES 106

Nordryl Cough - See ANTIHISTAMINES 106

NORELGESTROMIN & ETHINYL ESTRADIOL -
See CONTRACEPTIVES, ORAL & SKIN
278

Norethin 1/35E - See CONTRACEPTIVES,
ORAL & SKIN 278

Norethin 1/50M - See CONTRACEPTIVES,
ORAL & SKIN 278

NORETHINDRONE - See PROGESTINS 686

NORETHINDRONE & ETHINYL ESTRADIOL -
See CONTRACEPTIVES, ORAL & SKIN
278

NORETHINDRONE & MESTRANOL - See
CONTRACEPTIVES, ORAL & SKIN 278

NORETHINDRONE ACETATE & ETHINYL
ESTRADIOL - See CONTRACEPTIVES,
ORAL & SKIN 278

Norflex - See ORPHENADRINE 628

NORFLOXACIN - See FLUOROQUINOLONES
388

NORFLOXACIN (Ophthalmic) - See
ANTIBACTERIALS (Ophthalmic) 66

Norfranil - See ANTIDEPRESSANTS,
TRICYCLIC 80

Norgesic - See ORPHENADRINE, ASPIRIN &
CAFFEINE 630

Norgesic Forte - See ORPHENADRINE,
ASPIRIN & CAFFEINE 630

NORGESTIMATE - See PROGESTINS 686

NORGESTIMATE & ETHINYL ESTRADIOL - See
CONTRACEPTIVES, ORAL & SKIN 278

NORGESTREL - See PROGESTINS 686

NORGESTREL & ETHINYL ESTRADIOL - See
CONTRACEPTIVES, ORAL & SKIN 278

Norinyl 1+35 - See CONTRACEPTIVES, ORAL
& SKIN 278

Norinyl 1+50 - See CONTRACEPTIVES, ORAL
& SKIN 278

Norinyl 1/50 - See CONTRACEPTIVES, ORAL
& SKIN 278

Noritate - See NITROIMIDAZOLES 610

Norlestrin 1/50 - See CONTRACEPTIVES,
ORAL & SKIN 278

Norlestrin 2.5/50 - See CONTRACEPTIVES,
ORAL & SKIN 278

Norlutate - See PROGESTINS 686

Nor-Mil - See DIPHENOXYLATE & ATROPINE
322

Normodyne - See BETA-ADRENERGIC
BLOCKING AGENTS 180

Normozide - See BETA-ADRENERGIC
BLOCKING AGENTS & THIAZIDE
DIURETICS 182

Noroxin - See FLUOROQUINOLONES 388

Norpace - See DISOPYRAMIDE 326

Norpace CR - See DISOPYRAMIDE 326

Norphadrine - See ORPHENADRINE, ASPIRIN
& CAFFEINE 630

Norphadrine Forte - See ORPHENADRINE,
ASPIRIN & CAFFEINE 630

Norpramin - See ANTIDEPRESSANTS,
TRICYCLIC 80

Nor-Pred-TBA - See ADRENOCORTICOIDS
(Systemic) 16

Nor-Q.D. - See PROGESTINS 686

NORTRIPTYLINE - See ANTIDEPRESSANTS,
TRICYCLIC 80

Nortussin - See GUAIFENESIN 410

Nortussin with Codeine - See
GUAIFENESIN 410
NARCOTIC ANALGESICS 584

Norvasc - See CALCIUM CHANNEL
BLOCKERS 216

Norvir - See PROTEASE INHIBITORS 694

Norwich Aspirin - See ASPIRIN 150

Nostril Nasal Decongestant Mild - See
OXYMETAZOLINE (Nasal) 634

Nostril Nasal Decongestant Regular - See
OXYMETAZOLINE (Nasal) 634

INDEX

Ortho Evra - See CONTRACEPTIVES, ORAL & SKIN 278

Ortho-Gynol - See CONTRACEPTIVES, VAGINAL 280

Ortho-Novum 0.5 - See CONTRACEPTIVES, ORAL & SKIN 278

Ortho-Novum 1/35 - See CONTRACEPTIVES, ORAL & SKIN 278

Ortho-Novum 1/50 - See CONTRACEPTIVES, ORAL & SKIN 278

Ortho-Novum 1/80 - See CONTRACEPTIVES, ORAL & SKIN 278

Ortho-Novum 2 - See CONTRACEPTIVES, ORAL & SKIN 278

Ortho-Novum 7/7/7 - See CONTRACEPTIVES, ORAL & SKIN 278

Ortho-Novum 10/11 - See CONTRACEPTIVES, ORAL & SKIN 278

Ortho-Prefest - See
ESTROGENS 368
PROGESTINS 686

Ortho-Tri-Cyclen 21 - See CONTRACEPTIVES, ORAL & SKIN 278

Ortho-Tri-Cyclen 28 - See CONTRACEPTIVES, ORAL & SKIN 278

Ortho Tri-Cyclen Lo - See CONTRACEPTIVES, ORAL & SKIN 278

Or-Tyl - See DICYCLOMINE 314

Orudis - See ANTI-INFLAMMATORY DRUGS, NONSTEROIDAL (NSAIDs) 116

Orudis-E - See ANTI-INFLAMMATORY DRUGS, NONSTEROIDAL (NSAIDs) 116

Orudis-KT - See ANTI-INFLAMMATORY DRUGS, NONSTEROIDAL (NSAIDs) 116

Orudis-SR - See ANTI-INFLAMMATORY DRUGS, NONSTEROIDAL (NSAIDs) 116

Oruvail - See ANTI-INFLAMMATORY DRUGS, NONSTEROIDAL (NSAIDs) 116

Os-Cal - See CALCIUM SUPPLEMENTS 218

Os-Cal 500 - See CALCIUM SUPPLEMENTS 218

Os-Cal Chewable - See CALCIUM SUPPLEMENTS 218

OSELTAMIVIR - See ANTIVIRALS FOR INFLUENZA, NEURAMINIDASE INHIBITORS 140

Osteopenia therapy - See BISPHOSPHONATES 190

Osteoporosis therapy - See
BONE FORMATION AGENTS 192
CALCITONIN 214
RALOXIFENE 714

Osteoporosis therapy, bisphosphonate - See BISPHOSPHONATES 190

Osto Forte - See VITAMIN D 842

Oticair - See ANTIBACTERIALS (Otic) 68

Otimar - See ANTIBACTERIALS (Otic) 68

Otiprin - See ANTIPYRINE & BENZOCAINE (Otic) 130

Otobione - See ANTIBACTERIALS (Otic) 68

Otocalm - See ANTIPYRINE & BENZOCAINE (Otic) 130

Otocidin - See ANTIBACTERIALS (Otic) 68

Otocort - See ANTIBACTERIALS (Otic) 68

Otrivin Decongestant Nose Drops - See XYLOMETAZOLINE 852

Otrivin Nasal Drops - See XYLOMETAZOLINE 852

Otrivin Nasal Spray - See XYLOMETAZOLINE 852

Otrivin Pediatric Decongestant Nose Drops - See XYLOMETAZOLINE 852

Otrivin Pediatric Nasal Drops - See XYLOMETAZOLINE 852

Otrivin Pediatric Nasal Spray - See XYLOMETAZOLINE 852

Otrivin with M-D Pump - See XYLOMETAZOLINE 852

Ovcon-35 - See CONTRACEPTIVES, ORAL & SKIN 278

Ovcon-50 - See CONTRACEPTIVES, ORAL & SKIN 278

Ovide - See PEDICULICIDES (Topical) 646

Ovol - See SIMETHICONE 754

Ovol-40 - See SIMETHICONE 754

Ovol-80 - See SIMETHICONE 754

Ovral - See CONTRACEPTIVES, ORAL & SKIN 278

Ovrette - See PROGESTINS 686

OXACILLIN - See PENICILLINS 650

OXANDROLONE - See ANDROGENS 36

OXAPROZIN - See ANTI-INFLAMMATORY DRUGS, NONSTEROIDAL (NSAIDs) 116

OXAZEPAM - See BENZODIAZEPINES 174

OXCARBAZEPINE 632

OXICONAZOLE (Topical) - See ANTIFUNGALS (Topical) 88

Oxistat - See ANTIFUNGALS (Topical) 88

OXPRENOLOL - See BETA-ADRENERGIC BLOCKING AGENTS 180

Oxsoralen - See PSORALENS 702

Oxsoralen Topical - See PSORALENS 702

Oxsoralen Ultra - See PSORALENS 702

OXTRIPHYLLINE - See BRONCHODILATORS, XANTHINE 200

Oxy 5 Tinted Lotion - See BENZOYL PEROXIDE 176

Oxy 5 Vanishing Formula Lotion - See BENZOYL PEROXIDE 176

INDEX

Panadol - See ACETAMINOPHEN 8
Panadol Extra Strength - See
ACETAMINOPHEN 8
Panadol Junior Strength Caplets - See
ACETAMINOPHEN 8
Panadol Maximum Strength Caplets - See
ACETAMINOPHEN 8
Panadol Maximum Strength Tablets - See
ACETAMINOPHEN 8
Panasal 5/500 - See NARCOTIC ANALGESICS
& ASPIRIN 588
Pancoate - See PANCRELIPASE 638
Pancrease MT4 - See PANCRELIPASE 638
Pancrease MT10 - See PANCRELIPASE 638
Pancrease MT16 - See PANCRELIPASE 638
PANCRELIPASE 638
Pandel - See ADRENOCORTICOIDS (Topical)
18
Panectyl - See ANTIHISTAMINES,
PHENOTHIAZINE-DERIVATIVE 112
Panex - See ACETAMINOPHEN 8
Panex 500 - See ACETAMINOPHEN 8
Panlor - See NARCOTIC ANALGESICS &
ACETAMINOPHEN 586
Panmycin - See TETRACYCLINES 786
PanOxyl 5 Bar - See BENZOYL PEROXIDE
176
PanOxyl 10 Bar - See BENZOYL PEROXIDE
176
PanOxyl 5 Gel - See BENZOYL PEROXIDE 176
PanOxyl 10 Gel - See BENZOYL PEROXIDE
176
PanOxyl 15 Gel - See BENZOYL PEROXIDE
176
PanOxyl 20 Gel - See BENZOYL PEROXIDE
176
PanOxyl AQ 21/2 Gel - See BENZOYL
PEROXIDE 176
PanOxyl AQ 5 Gel - See BENZOYL PEROXIDE
176
Panrexin M - See APPETITE SUPPRESSANTS
146
Panrexin MTP - See APPETITE
SUPPRESSANTS 146
Panshape - See APPETITE SUPPRESSANTS
146
Pantapon - See NARCOTIC ANALGESICS 584
Pantoloc - See PROTON PUMP INHIBITORS
698
PANTOPRAZOLE - See PROTON PUMP
INHIBITORS 698
PANTOTHENIC ACID (Vitamin B-5) 640
Panwarfarin - See ANTICOAGULANTS (Oral)
74
PAPAVERINE 642

Paplex - See KERATOLYTICS 468
Paplex Ultra - See KERATOLYTICS 468
Papulex - See NIACIN (Vitamin B-3, Nicotinic
Acid, Nicotinamide) 598
Par Glycerol-DM - See
DEXTROMETHORPHAN 310
Paracetamol - See ACETAMINOPHEN 8
Paraflex - See MUSCLE RELAXANTS,
SKELETAL 576
Parafon Forte - See
ACETAMINOPHEN 8
MUSCLE RELAXANTS, SKELETAL 576
Parepectolin - See
KAOLIN & PECTIN 464
PAREGORIC 644
Parcopa - See CARBIDOPA & LEVODOPA 226
PAREGORIC 644
Parlodel - See BROMOCRIPTINE 196
Parlodel Snaptabs - See BROMOCRIPTINE 196
Parnate - See MONOAMINE OXIDASE (MAO)
INHIBITORS 570
PAROXETINE - See SELECTIVE SEROTONIN
REUPTAKE INHIBITORS (SSRIs) 746
Parsidol - See ANTIDYSKINETICS 82
Parsitan - See ANTIDYSKINETICS 82
Parzine - See APPETITE SUPPRESSANTS 146
Pataday - See ANTIALLERGIC AGENTS
(Ophthalmic) 58
Patanase - See ANTIHISTAMINES (Nasal) 108
Patanol - See ANTIALLERGIC AGENTS
(Ophthalmic) 58
Pathilon - See ANTICHOLINERGICS 72
Pathocil - See PENICILLINS 650
Pavabid - See PAPAVERINE 642
Pavabid Plateau Caps - See PAPAVERINE 642
Pavacot - See PAPAVERINE 642
Pavagen - See PAPAVERINE 642
Pavarine - See PAPAVERINE 642
Pavased - See PAPAVERINE 642
Pavatine - See PAPAVERINE 642
Pavatym - See PAPAVERINE 642
Paveral - See NARCOTIC ANALGESICS 584
Paverolan - See PAPAVERINE 642
Pax 400 - See MEPROBAMATE 532
Paxil - See SELECTIVE SEROTONIN
REUPTAKE INHIBITORS (SSRIs) 746
Paxil CR - See SELECTIVE SEROTONIN
REUPTAKE INHIBITORS (SSRIs) 746
Paxipam - See BENZODIAZEPINES 174
Paxofen - See ANTI-INFLAMMATORY DRUGS,
NONSTEROIDAL (NSAIDs) 116
PBZ - See ANTIHISTAMINES 106
PBZ-SR - See ANTIHISTAMINES 106
PC-Cap - See
CAFFEINE 212

Percocet-Demi - See NARCOTIC ANALGESICS & ACETAMINOPHEN 586

Percodan - See NARCOTIC ANALGESICS & ASPIRIN 588

Percodan-Demi - See NARCOTIC ANALGESICS & ASPIRIN 588

Perdiem - See
LAXATIVES, BULK-FORMING 474
LAXATIVES, STIMULANT 480

Perdiem Fiber - See LAXATIVES, BULK-FORMING 474

Perdiem Plain - See LAXATIVES, BULK-FORMING 474

Perforomist Inhalation Solution - See BRONCHODILATORS, ADRENERGIC 198

Periactin - See ANTIHISTAMINES 106

Peri-Colace - See LAXATIVES, STIMULANT 480

Peri-Colase - See LAXATIVES, SOFTENER/ LUBRICANT 478

PERICYAZINE - See PHENOTHIAZINES 660

Peridex - See CHLORHEXIDINE 244

Peridol - See HALOPERIDOL 414

PERINDOPRIL - See ANGIOTENSIN-CONVERTING ENZYME (ACE) INHIBITORS 46

Periochip - See CHLORHEXIDINE 244

Periogard - See CHLORHEXIDINE 244

Periostat - See TETRACYCLINES 786

Peritrate - See NITRATES 606

Peritrate Forte - See NITRATES 606

Peritrate SA - See NITRATES 606

PERMETHRIN - See PEDICULICIDES (Topical) 646

Permitil - See PHENOTHIAZINES 660

Permitil Concentrate - See PHENOTHIAZINES 660

Pernox Lemon Medicated Scrub Cleanser - See KERATOLYTICS 468

Pernox Lotion Lathering Abradant Scrub Cleanser - See KERATOLYTICS 468

Pernox Lotion Lathering Scrub Cleanser - See KERATOLYTICS 468

Pernox Regular Medicated Scrub Cleanser - See KERATOLYTICS 468

PERPHENAZINE - See PHENOTHIAZINES 660

Persa-Gel 5 - See BENZOYL PEROXIDE 176

Persa-Gel 10 - See BENZOYL PEROXIDE 176

Persa-Gel W 5 - See BENZOYL PEROXIDE 176

Persa-Gel W 10 - See BENZOYL PEROXIDE 176

Persantine - See DIPYRIDAMOLE 324

Pertofrane - See ANTIDEPRESSANTS, TRICYCLIC 80

Pertrogalar Plain - See LAXATIVES, SOFTENER/LUBRICANT 478

Pertussin All Night CS - See
DEXTROMETHORPHAN 310
GUAIFENESIN 410

Pertussin All Night PM - See
ACETAMINOPHEN 8
ANTIHISTAMINES 106
DEXTROMETHORPHAN 310
PSEUDOEPHEDRINE 700

Pertussin Cough Suppressant - See DEXTROMETHORPHAN 310

Pertussin CS - See DEXTROMETHORPHAN 310

Pertussin ES - See DEXTROMETHORPHAN 310

P.E.T.N. - See NITRATES 606

Pfeiffer's Allergy - See ANTIHISTAMINES 106

Phanatuss - See
DEXTROMETHORPHAN 310
GUAIFENESIN 410

Pharma-Cort - See ADRENOCORTICOIDS (Topical) 18

Pharmatex - See CONTRACEPTIVES, VAGINAL 280

Phazyme - See SIMETHICONE 754

Phazyme 55 - See SIMETHICONE 754

Phazyme 95 - See SIMETHICONE 754

Phenameth DM - See
ANTIHISTAMINES, PHENOTHIAZINE-DERIVATIVE 112
DEXTROMETHORPHAN 310

Phenameth VC - See PHENYLEPHRINE 662

Phenameth VC with Codeine - See
ANTIHISTAMINES, PHENOTHIAZINE-DERIVATIVE 112
NARCOTIC ANALGESICS 584
PHENYLEPHRINE 662

Phenapap Sinus Headache & Congestion - See
ACETAMINOPHEN 8
ANTIHISTAMINES 106
PSEUDOEPHEDRINE 700

Phenaphen - See ACETAMINOPHEN 8

Phenaphen with Codeine - See NARCOTIC ANALGESICS & ACETAMINOPHEN 586

Phenaphen with Codeine No. 2 - See BARBITURATES, ASPIRIN & CODEINE (Also contains caffeine) 168

Phenaphen with Codeine No. 3 - See BARBITURATES, ASPIRIN & CODEINE (Also contains caffeine) 168

Phenaphen with Codeine No. 4 - See BARBITURATES, ASPIRIN & CODEINE (Also contains caffeine) 168

Phenazine 25 - See ANTIHISTAMINES, PHENOTHIAZINE-DERIVATIVE 112

INDEX

RASAGILINE - See MONOAMINE OXIDASE TYPE B (MAO-B) INHIBITORS 572
Raudixin - See RAUWOLFIA ALKALOIDS 720
Rauval - See RAUWOLFIA ALKALOIDS 720
Rauverid - See RAUWOLFIA ALKALOIDS 720
RAUWOLFIA ALKALOIDS 720
RAUWOLFIA SERPENTINA - See RAUWOLFIA ALKALOIDS 720
Rauzide - See
  DIURETICS, THIAZIDE 336
  RAUWOLFIA ALKALOIDS 720
Razadyne ER - See CHOLINESTERASE INHIBITORS 250
Reactine - See ANTIHISTAMINES, NONSEDATING 110
Reclast - See BISPHOSPHONATES 190
Reclomide - See METOCLOPRAMIDE 548
Rectocort - See HYDROCORTISONE (Rectal) 424
Rederm - See ADRENOCORTICOIDS (Topical) 18
Redisol - See VITAMIN B-12 (Cyanocobalamin) 838
Redoxon - See VITAMIN C (Ascorbic Acid) 840
Redutemp - See ACETAMINOPHEN 8
Reese's Pinworm Medicine - See ANTHELMINTICS 52
Refenesen - See GUAIFENESIN 410
Refenesen Chest Congestion & Pain Relief PE - See
  ACETAMINOPHEN 8
  GUAIFENESIN 410
  PHENYLEPHRINE 662
Refenesen PE - See
  GUAIFENESIN 410
  PHENYLEPHRINE 662
Refresh Eye Itch - See ANTIALLERGIC AGENTS (Ophthalmic) 58
Reglan - See METOCLOPRAMIDE 548
Regonol - See ANTIMYASTHENICS 128
Regranex - See BECAPLERMIN 170
Regroton - See RAUWOLFIA ALKALOIDS 720
Regulace - See
  LAXATIVES, SOFTENER/LUBRICANT 478
  LAXATIVES, STIMULANT 480
Regular - See INSULIN 440
Regular (Concentrated) Iletin - See INSULIN 440
Regular (Concentrated) Iletin II, U-500 - See INSULIN 440
Regular Iletin I - See INSULIN 440
Regular Iletin II - See INSULIN 440
Regular Insulin - See INSULIN 440
Regulax SS - See LAXATIVES, SOFTENER/LUBRICANT 478

Regulex - See LAXATIVES, SOFTENER/LUBRICANT 478
Regulex-D - See LAXATIVES, SOFTENER/LUBRICANT 478
Reguloid Natural - See LAXATIVES, BULK-FORMING 474
Reguloid Orange - See LAXATIVES, BULK-FORMING 474
Reguloid Orange Sugar Free - See LAXATIVES, BULK-FORMING 474
Regutol - See LAXATIVES, SOFTENER/LUBRICANT 478
Rela - See MUSCLE RELAXANTS, SKELETAL 576
Relaxadon - See BELLADONNA ALKALOIDS & BARBITURATES 172
Relenza - See ANTIVIRALS FOR INFLUENZA, NEURAMINIDASE INHIBITORS 140
Relief Eye Drops for Red Eyes - See PHENYLEPHRINE (Ophthalmic) 664
Relpax - See TRIPTANS 824
Remcol-C - See
  ACETAMINOPHEN 8
  ANTIHISTAMINES 106
  DEXTROMETHORPHAN 310
Remeron - See MIRTAZAPINE 562
Remeron SolTab - See MIRTAZAPINE 562
Remicade - See TUMOR NECROSIS FACTOR BLOCKERS 826
Reminyl - See CHOLINESTERASE INHIBITORS 250
Renedil - See CALCIUM CHANNEL BLOCKERS 216
Renese - See DIURETICS, THIAZIDE 336
Renese-R - See RAUWOLFIA ALKALOIDS 720
Renin Inhibitor - See RENIN INHIBITORS 722
RENIN INHIBITORS 722
Renoquid - See SULFONAMIDES 772
Renova - See RETINOIDS (Topical) 728
REPAGLINIDE - See MEGLITINIDES 522
Repan - See
  ACETAMINOPHEN 8
  BARBITURATES 166
  CAFFEINE 212
Repigmenting agent (Psoralen) - See PSORALENS 702
Reprexain CIII - See
  ANTI-INFLAMMATORY DRUGS, NONSTEROIDAL (NSAIDs) 116
  NARCOTIC ANALGESICS 584
Requip - See ANTIDYSKINETICS 82
Requip XL - See ANTIDYSKINETICS 82
Rescon-JR - See
  ANTIHISTAMINES 106
  PSEUDOEPHEDRINE 700

Ridaura-Oral - See GOLD COMPOUNDS 406
Rifadin - See RIFAMYCINS 734
Rifamate - See
  ISONIAZID 456
  RIFAMYCINS 734
Rifampicin - See RIFAMYCINS 734
RIFAMPIN - See RIFAMYCINS 734
<u>RIFAMYCINS</u> 734
RIFAPENTINE - See RIFAMYCINS 734
<u>RIFAXIMIN</u> 736
Rilutek - See RILUZOLE 738
<u>RILUZOLE</u> 738
Rimactane - See RIFAMYCINS 734
RIMANTADINE - See ANTIVIRALS FOR
  INFLUENZA 138
RIMEXOLONE - See ANTI-INFLAMMATORY
  DRUGS, STEROIDAL (Ophthalmic) 122
Riomet - See METFORMIN 538
Riopan - See ANTACIDS 50
Riopan Extra Strength - See ANTACIDS 50
Riopan Plus - See
  ANTACIDS 50
  SIMETHICONE 754
Riopan Plus Double Strength - See
  ANTACIDS 50
Riopan Plus Extra Strength - See ANTACIDS
  50
Riphen - See ASPIRIN 150
RISEDRONATE - See BISPHOSPHONATES 190
Risperdal - See SEROTONIN-DOPAMINE
  ANTAGONISTS 748
Risperdal Consta - See SEROTONIN-
  DOPAMINE ANTAGONISTS 748
Risperdal M-TAB - See SEROTONIN-
  DOPAMINE ANTAGONISTS 748
RISPERIDONE - See SEROTONIN-DOPAMINE
  ANTAGONISTS 748
Ritalin - See STIMULANT MEDICATIONS 760
Ritalin LA - See STIMULANT MEDICATIONS
  760
Ritalin SR - See STIMULANT MEDICATIONS
  760
<u>RITODRINE</u> 740
RITONAVIR - See PROTEASE INHIBITORS
  694
RIVASTIGMINE - See CHOLINESTERASE
  INHIBITORS 250
Rivotril - See BENZODIAZEPINES 174
RIZATRIPTAN - See TRIPTANS 824
RMS Uniserts - See NARCOTIC ANALGESICS
  584
Ro-Antoin - See NITROFURANTOIN 608
Robafen AC Cough - See
  GUAIFENESIN 410
  NARCOTIC ANALGESICS 584

Robafen DAC - See
  GUAIFENESIN 410
  NARCOTIC ANALGESICS 584
  PSEUDOEPHEDRINE 700
Robafen DM - See
  DEXTROMETHORPHAN 310
  GUAIFENESIN 410
  PSEUDOEPHEDRINE 700
Robafen Syrup - See
  GUAIFENESIN 410
Robamol - See MUSCLE RELAXANTS,
  SKELETAL 576
Robaxin - See MUSCLE RELAXANTS,
  SKELETAL 576
Robaxisal - See
  ASPIRIN 150
  MUSCLE RELAXANTS, SKELETAL 576
Robidex - See DEXTROMETHORPHAN 310
Robidone - See NARCOTIC ANALGESICS 584
Robigesic - See ACETAMINOPHEN 8
Robinul - See GLYCOPYRROLATE 404
Robinul Forte - See GLYCOPYRROLATE 404
Robitet - See TETRACYCLINES 786
Robitussin Chest Congestion - See
  GUAIFENESIN 410
Robitussin Children's Cough Long-Acting
  See DEXTROMETHORPHAN 310
Robitussin Children's Cough & Cold
  Long-Acting - See
  ANTIHISTAMINES 106
  DEXTROMETHORPHAN 310
Robitussin Cough & Chest Congestion DM
  See
  DEXTROMETHORPHAN 310
  GUAIFENESIN 410
Robitussin Cough & Chest Congestion
  DM Max - See
  DEXTROMETHORPHAN 310
  GUAIFENESIN 410
Robitussin Cough & Chest Congestion
  Sugar Free DM - See
  DEXTROMETHORPHAN 310
  GUAIFENESIN 410
Robitussin Cough & Cold CF - See
  DEXTROMETHORPHAN 310
  GUAIFENESIN 410
  PHENYLEPHRINE 662
Robitussin Cough & Cold D - See
  DEXTROMETHORPHAN 310
  GUAIFENESIN 410
  PSEUDOEPHEDRINE 700
Robitussin Cough & Cold Long-Acting - See
  ANTIHISTAMINES 106
  DEXTROMETHORPHAN 310

Rubramin-PC - See VITAMIN B-12
  (Cyanocobalamin) 838
Rufen - See ANTI-INFLAMMATORY DRUGS,
  NONSTEROIDAL (NSAIDs) 116
Rulox - See ANTACIDS 50
Rulox No. 1 - See ANTACIDS 50
Rulox No. 2 - See ANTACIDS 50
Rulox Plus - See ANTACIDS 50
Rum-K - See POTASSIUM SUPPLEMENTS 670
Ru-Tuss DE - See
  GUAIFENESIN 410
  PSEUDOEPHEDRINE 700
Ru-Tuss Expectorant - See
  DEXTROMETHORPHAN 310
  GUAIFENESIN 410
  PSEUDOEPHEDRINE 700
Rycotin - See NIACIN (Vitamin B-3, Nicotinic
  Acid, Nicotinamide) 598
Ryna - See
  ANTIHISTAMINES 106
  PSEUDOEPHEDRINE 700
Ryna-C Liquid - See
  ANTIHISTAMINES 106
  NARCOTIC ANALGESICS 584
  PSEUDOEPHEDRINE 700
Ryna-CX Liquid - See
  GUAIFENESIN 410
  NARCOTIC ANALGESICS 584
  PSEUDOEPHEDRINE 700
Rynacrom - See CROMOLYN 282
Rynatan - See
  ANTIHISTAMINES 106
  PHENYLEPHRINE 662
Rynatan Pediatric - See
  ANTIHISTAMINES 106
  PHENYLEPHRINE 662
Rynatan-S Pediatric - See
  ANTIHISTAMINES 106
  PHENYLEPHRINE 662
Rynatuss - See
  ANTIHISTAMINES 106
  EPHEDRINE 352
  PHENYLEPHRINE 662
Rynatuss Pediatric - See
  ANTIHISTAMINES 106
  EPHEDRINE 352
  PHENYLEPHRINE 662
Rythmodan - See DISOPYRAMIDE 326
Rythmodan-LA - See DISOPYRAMIDE 326
Ryzolt - See TRAMADOL 812

S

S-A-C - See
  ACETAMINOPHEN 8
  CAFFEINE 212

SALICYLATES 742
SafeTussin 30 - See
  DEXTROMETHORPHAN 310
  GUAIFENESIN 410
Salac - See KERATOLYTICS 468
Salacid - See KERATOLYTICS 468
Sal-Acid Plaster - See KERATOLYTICS 468
Salactic Film Topical Solution - See
  KERATOLYTICS 468
Sal-Adult - See ASPIRIN 150
Salagen - See PILOCARPINE (Oral) 666
Salatin - See
  ASPIRIN 150
  CAFFEINE 212
Salazopyrin - See SULFASALAZINE 768
Salazosulfapyridine - See SULFASALAZINE
  768
Sal-Clens Plus Shampoo - See
  KERATOLYTICS 468
Sal-Clens Shampoo - See KERATOLYTICS 468
Salcylic Acid - See SALICYLATES 742
Saleto - See
  ACETAMINOPHEN 8
  ASPIRIN 150
  CAFFEINE 212
Saleto-200 - See ANTI-INFLAMMATORY
  DRUGS, NONSTEROIDAL (NSAIDs) 116
Saleto-400 - See ANTI-INFLAMMATORY
  DRUGS, NONSTEROIDAL (NSAIDs) 116
Saleto-600 - See ANTI-INFLAMMATORY
  DRUGS, NONSTEROIDAL (NSAIDs) 116
Saleto-800 - See ANTI-INFLAMMATORY
  DRUGS, NONSTEROIDAL (NSAIDs) 116
Salflex - See SALICYLATES 742
Salgesic - See SALICYLATES 742
SALICYLAMIDE - See SALICYLATES 742
SALICYLATES 742
Salicylazosulfapyridine - See
  SULFASALAZINE 768
SALICYLIC ACID - See KERATOLYTICS 468
SALICYLIC ACID & SULFUR - See
  KERATOLYTICS 468
SALICYLIC ACID, SULFUR & COAL TAR - See
  ANTISEBORRHEICS (Topical) 132
Saligel - See KERATOLYTICS 468
Sal-Infant - See ASPIRIN 150
SALMETEROL - See BRONCHODILATORS,
  ADRENERGIC 198
Salocol - See
  ASPIRIN 150
  CAFFEINE 212
Salofalk - See MESALAMINE 536
Salonil - See KERATOLYTICS 468
Salphenyl - See
  ACETAMINOPHEN 8

INDEX

Sedative-hypnotic agent - See
  BARBITURATES 166
  CHLORAL HYDRATE 238
  ESZOPICLONE 370
  TRIAZOLAM 816
  ZOLPIDEM 860
Sedatuss - See DEXTROMETHORPHAN 310
Selective aldosterone blocker - See
  EPLERENONE 354
Selective norepinephrine reuptake inhibitor - See
  ATOMOXETINE 152
SELECTIVE SEROTONIN REUPTAKE
  INHIBITORS (SSRIs) 746
SELEGILINE - See MONOAMINE OXIDASE
  TYPE B (MAO-B) INHIBITORS 572
SELENIUM SULFIDE - See
  ANTISEBORRHEICS (Topical) 132
Selexid - See PENICILLINS 650
Selpak - See MONOAMINE OXIDASE TYPE B
  (MAO-B) INHIBITORS 572
Selsun - See ANTISEBORRHEICS (Topical)
  132
Selsun Blue - See ANTISEBORRHEICS
  (Topical) 132
Selsun Blue Dry Formula - See
  ANTISEBORRHEICS (Topical) 132
Selsun Blue Extra Conditioning Formula -
  See ANTISEBORRHEICS (Topical) 132
Selsun Blue Extra Medicated Formula - See
  ANTISEBORRHEICS (Topical) 132
Selsun Blue Oily Formula - See
  ANTISEBORRHEICS (Topical) 132
Selsun Blue Regular Formula - See
  ANTISEBORRHEICS (Topical) 132
Selzentry - See MARAVIROC 514
Semcet - See ACETAMINOPHEN 8
Semicid - See CONTRACEPTIVES, VAGINAL
  280
Semilente - See INSULIN 440
Semilente Iletin - See INSULIN 440
Semilente Iletin I - See INSULIN 440
Semprex-D - See
  ANTIHISTAMINES 106
  PSEUDOEPHEDRINE 700
Senexon - See LAXATIVES, STIMULANT 480
SENNA - See LAXATIVES, STIMULANT 480
SennaPrompt - See
  LAXATIVES, BULK-FORMING 474
  LAXATIVES, STIMULANT 480
SENNOSIDES - See LAXATIVES, STIMULANT
  480
Senokot - See LAXATIVES, STIMULANT 480
Senokot-S - See
  LAXATIVES, SOFTENER/LUBRICANT 478
  LAXATIVES, STIMULANT 480

SenokotXTRA - See LAXATIVES, STIMULANT
  480
Senolax - See LAXATIVES, STIMULANT 480
SensoGARD Canker Sore Relief - See
  ANESTHETICS (Mucosal-Local) 38
Sential - See ADRENOCORTICOIDS (Topical)
  18
Septra - See
  SULFONAMIDES 772
  TRIMETHOPRIM 822
Septra DS - See
  SULFONAMIDES 772
  TRIMETHOPRIM 822
Ser-A-Gen - See RESERPINE, HYDRALAZINE
  & HYDROCHLOROTHIAZIDE 724
Seralazide - See RESERPINE, HYDRALAZINE
  & HYDROCHLOROTHIAZIDE 724
Serax - See BENZODIAZEPINES 174
Serentil - See PHENOTHIAZINES 660
Serentil Concentrate - See PHENOTHIAZINES
  660
Serevent - See BRONCHODILATORS,
  ADRENERGIC 198
Serevent Diskus - See BRONCHODILATORS,
  ADRENERGIC 198
Seromycin - See CYCLOSERINE 294
Serophene - See CLOMIPHENE 260
Seroquel - See QUETIAPINE 706
Seroquel XR - See QUETIAPINE 706
SEROTONIN-DOPAMINE ANTAGONISTS 748
SEROTONIN & NOREPINEPHRINE
  REUPTAKE INHIBITORS (SNRIs) 750
Serpalan - See RAUWOLFIA ALKALOIDS 720
Serpasil - See RAUWOLFIA ALKALOIDS 720
Serpazide - See RESERPINE, HYDRALAZINE
  & HYDROCHLOROTHIAZIDE 724
SERTACONAZOLE - See ANTIFUNGALS
  (Topical) 88
Sertan - See PRIMIDONE 678
SERTRALINE - See SELECTIVE SEROTONIN
  REUPTAKE INHIBITORS (SSRIs) 746
Serutan - See LAXATIVES, BULK-FORMING
  474
Serutan Toasted Granules - See LAXATIVES,
  BULK-FORMING 474
Serzone - See NEFAZODONE 592
Shogan - See ANTIHISTAMINES,
  PHENOTHIAZINE-DERIVATIVE 112
Shur-Seal - See CONTRACEPTIVES, VAGINAL
  280
Sibelium - See CALCIUM CHANNEL
  BLOCKERS 216
Siblin - See LAXATIVES, BULK-FORMING 474
SIBUTRAMINE 752
Siladryl - See ANTIHISTAMINES 106

Solium - See BENZODIAZEPINES 174

Solodyn - See TETRACYCLINES 786

Soltamox - See TAMOXIFEN 778

Solu-Phyllin - See BRONCHODILATORS, XANTHINE 200

Solurex - See ADRENOCORTICOIDS (Systemic) 16

Solurex LA - See ADRENOCORTICOIDS (Systemic) 16

Soma - See MUSCLE RELAXANTS, SKELETAL 576

Soma Compound - See
ASPIRIN 150
NARCOTIC ANALGESICS 584

Soma Compound with Codeine - See MUSCLE RELAXANTS, SKELETAL 576

Sominex Formula 2 - See ANTIHISTAMINES 106

Somnol - See BENZODIAZEPINES 174

Somophyllin - See BRONCHODILATORS, XANTHINE 200

Somophyllin-12 - See BRONCHODILATORS, XANTHINE 200

Somophyllin-CRT - See BRONCHODILATORS, XANTHINE 200

Somophyllin-DF - See BRONCHODILATORS, XANTHINE 200

Somophyllin-T - See BRONCHODILATORS, XANTHINE 200

Sonata - See ZALEPLON 854

Sopamycetin Ophthalmic Ointment - See ANTIBACTERIALS (Ophthalmic) 66

Sopamycetin Ophthalmic Solution - See ANTIBACTERIALS (Ophthalmic) 66

Sopridol - See MUSCLE RELAXANTS, SKELETAL 576

Sorbitrate - See NITRATES 606

Sorbitrate SA - See NITRATES 606

Soriatane - See RETINOIDS (Oral) 726

Soridol - See MUSCLE RELAXANTS, SKELETAL 576

Sotacor - See BETA-ADRENERGIC BLOCKING AGENTS 180

SOTALOL - See BETA-ADRENERGIC BLOCKING AGENTS 180

Sotret - See ISOTRETINOIN 458

Spancap - See AMPHETAMINES 30

Span-FF - See IRON SUPPLEMENTS 452

Span-Niacin - See NIACIN (Vitamin B-3, Nicotinic Acid, Nicotinamide) 598

SPARFLOXACIN - See FLUOROQUINOLONES 388

Sparlon - See STIMULANTS, AMPHETAMINE RELATED 762

Spaslin - See BELLADONNA ALKALOIDS & BARBITURATES 172

Spasmoban - See DICYCLOMINE 314

Spasmoject - See DICYCLOMINE 314

Spasmolin - See BELLADONNA ALKALOIDS & BARBITURATES 172

Spasmophen - See BELLADONNA ALKALOIDS & BARBITURATES 172

Spasquid - See BELLADONNA ALKALOIDS & BARBITURATES 172

Spec-T Sore Throat Anesthetic - See ANESTHETICS (Mucosal-Local) 38

Spectazole - See ANTIFUNGALS (Topical) 88

Spectracef - See CEPHALOSPORINS 234

Spectrobid - See PENICILLINS 650

Spectro-Chlor Ophthalmic Ointment - See ANTIBACTERIALS (Ophthalmic) 66

Spectro-Chlor Ophthalmic Solution - See ANTIBACTERIALS (Ophthalmic) 66

Spectro-Genta - See ANTIBACTERIALS (Ophthalmic) 66

Spectro-Homatropine - See CYCLOPLEGIC, MYDRIATIC (Ophthalmic) 292

Spectro-Pentolate - See CYCLOPENTOLATE (Ophthalmic) 288

Spectro-Sporin - See ANTIBACTERIALS (Ophthalmic) 66

Spectro-Sulf - See ANTIBACTERIALS (Ophthalmic) 66

Spersadex - See ANTI-INFLAMMATORY DRUGS, STEROIDAL (Ophthalmic) 122

Spersaphrine - See PHENYLEPHRINE (Ophthalmic) 664

Spiriva - See TIOTROPIUM 802

SPIRONOLACTONE - See DIURETICS, POTASSIUM-SPARING 332

SPIRONOLACTONE & HYDROCHLOROTHIAZIDE - See DIURETICS, POTASSIUM-SPARING & HYDROCHLOROTHIAZIDE 334

Spirozide - See DIURETICS, POTASSIUM-SPARING & HYDROCHLOROTHIAZIDE 334

Sporanox - See ANTIFUNGALS, AZOLES 86

SSD - See ANTIBACTERIALS, ANTIFUNGALS (Topical) 62

SSD AF - See ANTIBACTERIALS, ANTIFUNGALS (Topical) 62

SSKI - See POTASSIUM SUPPLEMENTS 670

S-T Cort - See ADRENOCORTICOIDS (Topical) 18

St. Joseph Adult Chewable Aspirin - See ASPIRIN 150

St. Joseph Antidiarrheal - See ATTAPULGITE 158

Sudafed PE Nighttime Cold Caplets - See
ACETAMINOPHEN 8
ANTIHISTAMINES 106
PHENYLEPHRINE 662
**Sudafed PE Nighttime Nasal Decongestant
Tablets** - See
ANTIHISTAMINES 106
PHENYLEPHRINE 662
**Sudafed PE Quick Dissolve Strips Cherry
Menthol** - See PHENYLEPHRINE 662
Sudafed PE Severe Cold Caplets - See
ACETAMINOPHEN 8
ANTIHISTAMINES 106
PHENYLEPHRINE 662
Sudafed PE Sinus & Allergy Tablets - See
ANTIHISTAMINES 106
PHENYLEPHRINE 662
Sudafed PE Sinus Headache Caplets - See
ACETAMINOPHEN 8
PHENYLEPHRINE 662
Sufedrin - See PSEUDOEPHEDRINE 700
Sular - See CALCIUM CHANNEL BLOCKERS
216
Sul-Azo - See SULFONAMIDES &
PHENAZOPYRIDINE 774
SULCONAZOLE - See ANTIFUNGALS (Topical)
88
Sulcrate - See SUCRALFATE 764
Sulcrate Suspension Plus - See
SUCRALFATE 764
Sulf-10 - See ANTIBACTERIALS (Ophthalmic)
66
SULFACETAMIDE (Ophthalmic) - See
ANTIBACTERIALS (Ophthalmic) 66
Sulfa (Sulfonamide) - See
SULFASALAZINE 768
SULFONAMIDES 772
SULFACYTINE - See SULFONAMIDES 772
SULFADIAZINE - See
ANTIBACTERIALS, ANTIFUNGALS (Topical)
62
SULFONAMIDES 772
SULFADOXINE & PYRIMETHAMINE 766
Sulfair - See ANTIBACTERIALS (Ophthalmic)
66
Sulfair 10 - See ANTIBACTERIALS
(Ophthalmic) 66
Sulfair 15 - See ANTIBACTERIALS
(Ophthalmic) 66
Sulfair Forte - See ANTIBACTERIALS
(Ophthalmic) 66
SULFAMETHIZOLE - See SULFONAMIDES 772
Sulfamethoprim - See
SULFONAMIDES 772
TRIMETHOPRIM 822

Sulfamethoprim DS - See
SULFONAMIDES 772
TRIMETHOPRIM 822
SULFAMETHOXAZOLE - See SULFONAMIDES
772
SULFAMETHOXAZOLE & PHENAZOPYRIDINE
- See SULFONAMIDES &
PHENAZOPYRIDINE 774
Sulfamide - See ANTIBACTERIALS
(Ophthalmic) 66
Sulfaprim - See
SULFONAMIDES 772
TRIMETHOPRIM 822
Sulfaprim DS - See
SULFONAMIDES 772
TRIMETHOPRIM 822
SULFASALAZINE 768
Sulfatrim - See
SULFONAMIDES 772
TRIMETHOPRIM 822
Sulfatrim DS - See
SULFONAMIDES 772
TRIMETHOPRIM 822
Sulfex - See ANTIBACTERIALS (Ophthalmic) 66
Sulfimycin - See
ERYTHROMYCINS 364
SULFONAMIDES 772
SULFINPYRAZONE 770
SULFISOXAZOLE - See SULFONAMIDES 772
SULFISOXAZOLE & PHENAZOPYRIDINE - See
SULFONAMIDES & PHENAZOPYRIDINE
774
SULFISOXAZOLE (Ophthalmic) - See
ANTIBACTERIALS (Ophthalmic) 66
Sulfizole - See SULFONAMIDES 772
Sulfolax - See LAXATIVES, SOFTENER/
LUBRICANT 478
Sulfonamide - See SULFONAMIDES &
PHENAZOPYRIDINE 774
SULFONAMIDES 772
SULFONAMIDES & PHENAZOPYRIDINE 774
Sulfone - See DAPSONE 302
SULFONYLUREAS 776
Sulforcin - See KERATOLYTICS 468
Sulfoxaprim - See
SULFONAMIDES 772
TRIMETHOPRIM 822
Sulfoxaprim DS - See
SULFONAMIDES 772
TRIMETHOPRIM 822
SULFUR (Topical) - See KERATOLYTICS 468
SULFURATED LIME - See ANTIACNE,
CLEANSING (Topical) 56
SULINDAC - See ANTI-INFLAMMATORY
DRUGS, NONSTEROIDAL (NSAIDs) 116

INDEX

T

Taclonex - See
 ADRENOCORTICOIDS (Topical) 18
 VITAMIN D (Topical) 844
TACRINE - See CHOLINESTERASE
 INHIBITORS 250
TACROLIMUS - See IMMUNOSUPPRESSIVE
 AGENTS 436
TADALAFIL - See ERECTILE DYSFUNCTION
 AGENTS 356
Tagamet - See HISTAMINE H$_2$ RECEPTOR
 ANTAGONISTS 416
Tagamet HB - See HISTAMINE H$_2$ RECEPTOR
 ANTAGONISTS 416
Talacen - See NARCOTIC ANALGESICS &
 ACETAMINOPHEN 586
TALBUTAL - See BARBITURATES 166
Talwin - See NARCOTIC ANALGESICS 584
Talwin Compound - See NARCOTIC
 ANALGESICS & ASPIRIN 588
Talwin Compound-50 - See NARCOTIC
 ANALGESICS & ASPIRIN 588
Talwin-NX - See NARCOTIC ANALGESICS 584
Tambocor - See FLECAINIDE ACETATE 386
Tamiflu - See ANTIVIRALS FOR INFLUENZA,
 NEURAMINIDASE INHIBITORS 140
Tamofen - See TAMOXIFEN 778
Tamone - See TAMOXIFEN 778
Tamoplex - See TAMOXIFEN 778
TAMOXIFEN 778
TAMSULOSIN - See ALPHA ADRENERGIC
 RECEPTOR BLOCKERS 20
Tanoral - See
 ANTIHISTAMINES 106
 PHENYLEPHRINE 662
Tapanol - See ACETAMINOPHEN 8
Tapanol Extra Strength - See
 ACETAMINOPHEN 8
Tapar - See ACETAMINOPHEN 8
Tapazole - See ANTITHYROID DRUGS 134
Tar Doak - See COAL TAR (Topical) 268
Taraphilic - See COAL TAR (Topical) 268
Tarbonis - See COAL TAR (Topical) 268
Targretin - See RETINOIDS (Topical) 728
Tarka - See
 ANGIOTENSIN-CONVERTING ENZYME
 (ACE) INHIBITORS 46
 CALCIUM CHANNEL BLOCKERS 216
Taro-Carbamazepine - See CARBAMAZEPINE
 224
Tarpaste - See COAL TAR (Topical) 268
Tarpaste Doak - See COAL TAR (Topical) 268
Tasmar - See TOLCAPONE 806
Tavist - See ANTIHISTAMINES 106

Tavist Allergy/Sinus/Headache - See
 ACETAMINOPHEN 8
 ANTIHISTAMINES 106
 PSEUDOEPHEDRINE 700
Tavist-1 - See ANTIHISTAMINES 106
Taxol - See PACLITAXEL 636
TAZAROTENE - See RETINOIDS (Topical) 728
Tazorac - See RETINOIDS (Topical) 728
T-Cypionate - See ANDROGENS 36
T/Derm Tar Emollient - See COAL TAR
 (Topical) 268
T-Diet - See APPETITE SUPPRESSANTS 146
Tearisol - See PROTECTANT (Ophthalmic) 696
Tears Naturale - See PROTECTANT
 (Ophthalmic) 696
Tears Naturale Free - See PROTECTANT
 (Ophthalmic) 696
Tears Naturale II - See PROTECTANT
 (Ophthalmic) 696
Tears Renewed - See PROTECTANT
 (Ophthalmic) 696
Tecnal - See
 ASPIRIN 150
 BARBITURATES 166
Teczem - See
 ANGIOTENSIN-CONVERTING ENZYME
 (ACE) INHIBITORS 46
 CALCIUM CHANNEL BLOCKERS 216
Tega-Flex - See ORPHENADRINE 628
Tega-Nil - See APPETITE SUPPRESSANTS 146
TEGASEROD 780
Tega-Span - See NIACIN (Vitamin B-3, Nicotinic
 Acid, Nicotinamide) 598
Tega-Vert - See ANTIHISTAMINES 106
Tegopen - See PENICILLINS 650
Tegretol - See CARBAMAZEPINE 224
Tegretol Chewtabs - See CARBAMAZEPINE
 224
Tegretol CR - See CARBAMAZEPINE 224
Tegretol XR - See CARBAMAZEPINE 224
Tegrin Lotion for Psoriasis - See COAL TAR
 (Topical) 268
Tegrin Medicated Cream Shampoo - See
 COAL TAR (Topical) 268
**Tegrin Medicated Shampoo Concentrated
 Gel** - See COAL TAR (Topical) 268
**Tegrin Medicated Shampoo Extra
 Conditioning Formula** - See COAL TAR
 (Topical) 268
Tegrin Medicated Shampoo Herbal Formula -
 See COAL TAR (Topical) 268
Tegrin Medicated Shampoo Original Formula
 - See COAL TAR (Topical) 268
Tegrin Medicated Soap for Psoriasis - See
 COAL TAR (Topical) 268

INDEX

1071

Triafed with Codeine - See
  ANTIHISTAMINES 106
  NARCOTIC ANALGESICS 584
  PSEUDOEPHEDRINE 700
Trialodine - See TRAZODONE 814
TRIAMCINOLONE - See
  ADRENOCORTICOIDS (Systemic) 16
TRIAMCINOLONE (Dental) - See
  ADRENOCORTICOIDS (Topical) 18
TRIAMCINOLONE (Nasal) - See
  ADRENOCORTICOIDS (Nasal Inhalation) 12
TRIAMCINOLONE (Oral Inhalation) - See
  ADRENOCORTICOIDS (Oral Inhalation) 14
TRIAMCINOLONE (Topical) - See
  ADRENOCORTICOIDS (Topical) 18
Triaminic Chest & Nasal Congestion - See
  GUAIFENESIN 410
  PHENYLEPHRINE 662
Triaminic Cold & Allergy - See
  ANTIHISTAMINES 106
  PHENYLEPHRINE 662
Triaminic Cough & Sore Throat - See
  ACETAMINOPHEN 8
  DEXTROMETHORPHAN 310
Triaminic-D Multi-Symptom Cold - See
  ANTIHISTAMINES 106
  DEXTROMETHORPHAN 310
  PSEUDOEPHEDRINE 700
Triaminic Day Time Cold & Cough - See
  DEXTROMETHORPHAN 310
  PHENYLEPHRINE 662
*Triaminic Decongestant Spray Nasal & Sinus
  Congestion* - See XYLOMETAZOLINE 852
Triaminic Flu, Cough & Fever - See
  ACETAMINOPHEN 8
  ANTIHISTAMINES 106
  DEXTROMETHORPHAN 310
Triaminic Long Acting Cough - See
  DEXTROMETHORPHAN 310
Triaminic Night Time Cough & Cold - See
  ANTIHISTAMINES 106
  PHENYLEPHRINE 662
Triaminic Softchews Cough & Runny Nose -
  See
  ANTIHISTAMINES 106
  DEXTROMETHORPHAN 310
Triaminic Softchews Cough & Sore Throat -
  See
  ACETAMINOPHEN 8
  DEXTROMETHORPHAN 310
Triaminic Thin Strips Cold - See
  PHENYLEPHRINE 662
Triaminic Thin Strips Daytime Cold & Cough
  See
  DEXTROMETHORPHAN 310

PHENYLEPHRINE 662
*Triaminic Thin Strips Cough & Runny
  Nose* - See ANTIHISTAMINES 106
Triaminic Thin Strips Long Acting Cough -
  See DEXTROMETHORPHAN 310
*Triaminic Thin Strips Night Time Cold &
  Cough* - See
  ANTIHISTAMINES 106
  PHENYLEPHRINE 662
TRIAMTERENE - See DIURETICS,
  POTASSIUM-SPARING 332
TRIAMTERENE & HYDROCHLOROTHIAZIDE -
  See DIURETICS, POTASSIUM-SPARING &
  HYDROCHLOROTHIAZIDE 334
Trianide Mild - See ADRENOCORTICOIDS
  (Topical) 18
Trianide Regular - See ADRENOCORTICOIDS
  (Topical) 18
Triaphen - See ASPIRIN 150
Triaprin - See
  ACETAMINOPHEN 8
  BARBITURATES 166
Triasox - See ANTHELMINTICS 52
Triavil - See
  ANTIDEPRESSANTS, TRICYCLIC 80
  PHENOTHIAZINES 660
TRIAZOLAM 816
Triazole - See
  SULFONAMIDES 772
  TRIMETHOPRIM 822
Triazole DS - See
  SULFONAMIDES 772
  TRIMETHOPRIM 822
Tri-B3 - See NIACIN (Vitamin B-3, Nicotinic
  Acid, Nicotinamide) 598
TRIBASIC CALCIUM PHOSPHATE - See
  CALCIUM SUPPLEMENTS 218
Tribavirin - See RIBAVIRIN 730
Tribiotic - See ANTIBACTERIALS (Ophthalmic)
  66
TRICHLORMETHIAZIDE - See DIURETICS,
  THIAZIDE 336
TRICITRATES - See CITRATES 254
Tricodene #1 - See NARCOTIC ANALGESICS
  584
Tricodene Sugar Free - See
  ANTIHISTAMINES 106
  DEXTROMETHORPHAN 310
Tricom Caplets - See PSEUDOEPHEDRINE
  700
Tricom Tablets - See
  ACETAMINOPHEN 8
  ANTIHISTAMINES 106
Triconsil - See ANTACIDS 50
Tricor - See FIBRATES 382

INDEX

Vusion - See ANTIFUNGALS (Topical) 88
Vytorin - See
 EZETIMIBE 378
 HMG-CoA REDUCTASE INHIBITORS 418
Vyvanse - See AMPHETAMINES 30

W

Wake-Up - See CAFFEINE 212
WARFARIN SODIUM - See
 ANTICOAGULANTS (Oral) 74
Warfilone - See ANTICOAGULANTS (Oral) 74
Wart-Off Topical Solution - See
 KERATOLYTICS 468
Wehamine - See ANTIHISTAMINES 106
Wehdryl - See ANTIHISTAMINES 106
Wehdryl-10 - See ANTIHISTAMINES 106
Wehdryl-50 - See ANTIHISTAMINES 106
Wehgen - See ESTROGENS 368
Wehless - See APPETITE SUPPRESSANTS
 146
Wehless Timecelles - See APPETITE
 SUPPRESSANTS 146
Weightrol - See APPETITE SUPPRESSANTS
 146
Welchol - See COLESEVELAM 272
Wellbutrin - See BUPROPION 204
Wellbutrin SR - See BUPROPION 204
Wellbutrin XL - See BUPROPION 204
Wellcovorin - See LEUCOVORIN 484
Westcort - See ADRENOCORTICOIDS
 (Topical) 18
Westhroid - See THYROID HORMONES 796
Wigraine - See
 CAFFEINE 212
 ERGOTAMINE 362
Winpred - See ADRENOCORTICOIDS
 (Systemic) 16
Winstrol - See ANDROGENS 36
Wintrocin - See ERYTHROMYCINS 364
Wolfina - See RAUWOLFIA ALKALOIDS 720
Women's Tylenol Menstrual Relief Caplets -
 See ACETAMINOPHEN 8
Wygesic - See NARCOTIC ANALGESICS &
 ACETAMINOPHEN 586
Wymox - See PENICILLINS 650
Wytensin - CENTRAL ALPHA AGONISTS 232

X

Xalatan - See ANTIGLAUCOMA,
 PROSTAGLANDINS 102
Xalcom - See
 ANTIGLAUCOMA, BETA BLOCKERS 96
 ANTIGLAUCOMA, PROSTAGLANDINS 102
Xanax - See BENZODIAZEPINES 174
Xanax XR - See BENZODIAZEPINES 174

Xeloda - See CAPECITABINE 220
Xenical - See ORLISTAT 626
Xerac BP 5 Gel - See BENZOYL PEROXIDE
 176
Xerac BP 10 Gel - See BENZOYL PEROXIDE
 176
Xibrom - See ANTI-INFLAMMATORY DRUGS,
 NONSTEROIDAL (NSAIDs) (Ophthalmic)
 120
Xifaxan - See RIFAXIMIN 736
Xodol - See NARCOTIC ANALGESICS &
 ACETAMINOPHEN 586
Xolegel Gel - See ANTIFUNGALS (Topical) 88
Xopenex - See BRONCHODILATORS,
 ADRENERGIC 198
Xopenex HFA - See BRONCHODILATORS,
 ADRENERGIC 198
X-Prep Liquid - See LAXATIVES, STIMULANT
 480
X-Seb - See KERATOLYTICS 468
X-Trozine - See APPETITE SUPPRESSANTS
 146
X-Trozine LA - See APPETITE
 SUPPRESSANTS 146
Xylocaine - See
 ANESTHETICS (Mucosal-Local) 38
 ANESTHETICS (Topical) 42
Xylocaine Viscous - See ANESTHETICS
 (Mucosal-Local) 38
XYLOMETAZOLINE 852
Xyralid Cream - See
 ADRENOCORTICOIDS (Topical) 18
 ANESTHETICS (Topical) 42
Xyralid LP Lotion - See
 ADRENOCORTICOIDS (Topical) 18
 ANESTHETICS (Topical) 42
Xyralid RC - See
 ANESTHETICS (Rectal) 40
 HYDROCORTISONE (Rectal) 424
Xyzal - See ANTIHISTAMINES, NON-
 SEDATING 110

Y

Yasmin - See CONTRACEPTIVES, ORAL &
 SKIN 278
Yaz - See CONTRACEPTIVES, ORAL & SKIN
 278
Yodoquinol - See IODOQUINOL 448
Yodoxin - See IODOQUINOL 448
Yutopar - See RITODRINE 740

Z

Zaditor - See ANTIALLERGIC AGENTS
 (Ophthalmic) 58
Zagam - See FLUOROQUINOLONES 388

Emergency Guide for Overdose Victims

These are basic steps in recognizing and treating immediate effects of drug overdose.

Take just 5 to 10 seconds to check for a response from the victim. In an adult, check for *normal* breathing. In a child, check for the *presence* or *absence* of breathing (a child may be breathing in a pattern that is not normal, but is adequate).

IF VICTIM IS NOT BREATHING:
Adults and children over age 1:
1. Call 911. The emergency dispatcher can help coach you through CPR (cardiopulmonary resuscitation) until experienced help arrives. If there are other persons available, have one call 911 and one or more persons perform CPR .
2. Begin CPR. Open the victim's airway—tilt the head back and lift chin. Pinch the victim's nose and prepare to give two rescue breaths. Give the first rescue breath (last one second) into his or her mouth. The chest should rise. If it does, give the second breath. If the chest does not rise after the first breath, reopen the airway.
3. Then place your hands on the breastbone in the middle of the chest. Use the heel of both hands (stacked) and push down on the chest 1½ to 2 inches 30 times right between the nipples. Pump hard and fast at the rate of 100/minute (faster than once per second). Let the chest rebound between pumps. For a child ages 1 to 8, use 1 hand or 2 hands as needed to compress the chest one third to one half its depth.
4. Continue with 2 breaths and 30 pumps until victim is breathing or medical help arrives. This ratio is the same for one-person and two-person CPR. In two-person CPR the person pumping the chest stops while the other gives mouth-to-mouth breathing.

Infants under age 1 (excluding newborns):
1. If there are other persons present, have one call 911 and one or more persons begin CPR. If you are alone, perform about 5 cycles or 2 minutes of CPR and then call 911.
2. Begin CPR. Place infant on his or her back. Open the airway—tilt head back and lift chin. Do not tilt the head too far back. Cover the infant's mouth and nose with your mouth. Give 2 small gentle breaths. Each breath should be 1 second long. The infant's chest should rise with each breath.
3. Then place two fingers in the center of the chest just below the nipples. Give 30 gentle chest compressions at the rate of 100 per minute. Press down about one-third the depth of the chest.
4. Continue with 2 breaths and 30 pumps until victim is breathing or medical help arrives. This ratio is the same for one-person and two-person CPR. In two-person CPR the person pumping the chest stops while the other gives mouth-to-mouth breathing.

Note: For all victims, don't try to make the victim vomit. If vomiting does occur, turn the victim's head to the side and try to sweep out or wipe off the vomit. Continue with CPR. Save vomit to take to emergency room for analysis. Take medicine or empty pill bottles with you to emergency room.

IF VICTIM IS UNCONSCIOUS AND BREATHING:

1. Call 911 for medical help.
2. If you are in a location where you can't get emergency help immediately, take victim to the nearest emergency room. Monitor the victim's breathing.
3. Don't try to make victim vomit. If vomiting occurs, save vomit to take to emergency room for analysis.
4. Take medicine or empty pill bottles with you to emergency room.

IF VICTIM IS DROWSY:

1. Call 911 for medical help.
2. If you are in a location where you can't get emergency help immediately, take victim to the nearest emergency room. Monitor the victim's breathing.
3. Don't try to make victim vomit. If vomiting occurs, save vomit to take to emergency room for analysis.
4. Take medicine or empty pill bottles with you to emergency room.

IF VICTIM IS ALERT:

1. Call 911 for medical help or call Poison Control Center–1-800-222-1222 (in the United States) for instructions.
2. If you can't get medical help quickly, take victim to nearest emergency room.
3. Take medicine or empty pill bottles with you to emergency room.

IF VICTIM HAS NO SYMPTOMS, BUT YOU SUSPECT AN OVERDOSE:

1. Call Poison Control Center 1-800-222-1222 (in the United States).
2. Describe the suspect drug with as much information as you can quickly gather. The center will give emergency instructions.
3. Consider calling the victim's doctor or your doctor for instructions.
4. If you have no telephone, take victim to the nearest emergency room.
5. Take medicine or empty pill bottles with you to emergency room.

A note about CPR training: Just about everyone can benefit by taking a certified course in first aid and learn to perform cardiopulmonary resuscitation (CPR). Courses taught by certified instructors are the best way to learn CPR. To find a course in your area, contact:

American Heart Association: 800-242-8721 or check website at www.americanheart.org.

American Red Cross: call the local office or check website at www.redcross.org.

Also, classes are offered in almost every city and town, at YMCAs, civic centers, schools, doctors' offices, and elsewhere.

Emergency Guide for Anaphylaxis Victims

The following are basic steps in recognizing and treating immediate effects of a severe allergic reaction, which is called *anaphylaxis*.

Some people may be highly sensitive to drugs. An anaphylactic reaction to a drug can be life-threatening! Persons suffering these allergic symptoms need immediate emergency treatment!

Symptoms of anaphylaxis:

- **Itching**
- **Rash**
- **Hives**
- **Runny nose**
- **Wheezing**
- **Paleness**
- **Cold sweats**
- **Low blood pressure**
- **Coma**
- **Cardiac arrest**

IF VICTIM IS UNCONSCIOUS AND NOT BREATHING:

1. Call 911. The emergency dispatcher may be able to coach you through CPR until experienced help arrives. If there are other persons available, have one call 911 and one or more persons perform CPR (cardiopulmonary resuscitation).
2. Check to see if the person is carrying special medication (e.g., Epi-Pen or allergy kit) to inject to counter the effects of the allergic attack. If so, inject it if you know how to do so. Avoid oral medication if the person is not breathing.
3. Begin CPR. See instructions 2 through 4 under Emergency Guide for Overdose Victims on page 1088 (2nd previous page).

IF VICTIM IS UNCONSCIOUS AND BREATHING:

1. Call 911 for medical help.
2. Check to see if the person is carrying special medication to inject to counter the effects of the allergic attack. If so, inject it if you know how to do so.
3. Take medicine or empty bottles with you to emergency room for analysis.

IF VICTIM IS CONSCIOUS:

1. Ask the person if he or she is carrying special medication to inhale, swallow or inject to counter the effects of the allergic attack. Help the person use the medication.
2. Give the person an antihistamine pill, if it is available.
3. Encourage the person to breathe slowly and deeply. Stay calm and be reassuring.

DISCLAIMER: The information provided in Emergency Guide for Overdose Victims and Emergency Guide for Anaphylaxis Victims is of a general nature and should not be used as a substitute for professional medical advice, emergency treatment instructions, or formal first aid training. If you think you or a family member may suffer from an allergic or other disease that requires attention, you should discuss it with your health care provider.